HEALTH CARE STATE RANKINGS
2001

Health Care in the 50 United States

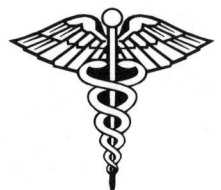

Kathleen O'Leary Morgan and Scott Morgan, Editors

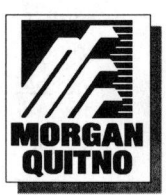

Morgan Quitno Press
© Copyright 2001, All Rights Reserved

512 East 9th Street, P.O. Box 1656
Lawrence, KS 66044-8656
USA
800-457-0742 or 785-841-3534
www.statestats.com
Ninth Edition

ISBN: 0-7401-0030-0
ISSN: 1065-1403

Health Care State Rankings 2001 sells for $52.95 ($5.00 shipping) and is only available in paper binding. For those who prefer ranking information tailored to a particular state, we also offer *Health Care State Perspectives*, state-specific reports for each of the 50 states. These individual guides provide information on a state's data and rank for each of the categories featured in the national *Health Care State Rankings* volume. Perspectives sell for $19.00 or $9.50 if ordered with *Health Care State Rankings*. If crime statistics are your interest, please ask about our annual *Crime State Rankings* ($52.95 paper). If you are interested in city and metropolitan crime data, we offer *City Crime Rankings* ($39.95 paper). For a general view of the states, please ask about our annual *State Rankings* reference book ($52.95 paper). All of our data sets are also available in machine readable format. Shipping and handling is $5.00 per order.

Ninth Edition
Printed in the United States of America
April 2001

PREFACE

Health Care State Rankings 2001 features a huge collection of state health care statistics covering hundreds of health care-related issues. Births and reproductive health, deaths, disease, insurance and finance, health care providers, facilities and physical fitness are compared state-by-state in this newly-revised, ninth edition. In all, more than 500 tables of state comparisons give you all the information you need for virtually every aspect of health care in the 50 United States.

Important Notes About *Health Care State Rankings 2001*

Health Care State Rankings 2001 presents information from government and private sector sources in one user-friendly volume. Most tables have been updated, some are brand new, while others were deleted. Regular subscribers will note (and rejoice) that the finance chapter in this updated *Health Care State Rankings* book at last has new state health care expenditure data. In August of 2000, HCFA released its 1998 estimates. A number of tables incorporating this newly released information are included.

Our goal in publishing *Health Care State Rankings* is to make complicated and often convoluted health care data easier to use and understand. The book is designed with that goal in mind. Source information and other pertinent footnotes are clearly shown at the bottom of each page and national totals, rates and percentages are prominently displayed at the top of each table. Every other line is shaded in gray for easier reading. In addition, numerous information-finding tools are provided: a thorough table of contents, table listings at the beginning of each chapter, a roster of sources with addresses and phone numbers, a detailed index and a chapter thumb index.

As in all of our reference books, the numbers shown in *Health Care State Rankings* require no additional calculations to convert them from millions, thousands, etc. All states are ranked on a high to low basis, with any ties among the states listed alphabetically for a given ranking. Negative numbers are shown in parentheses "( )." For tables with national totals (as opposed to rates, per capitas, etc.) a separate column is included showing what percent of the national total each individual state's total represents. This column is headed by "% of USA." This percentage figure is particularly interesting when compared with a state's share of the nation's population for a particular year (provided in an appendix).

For those who need information for just one state, check out our *Health Care State Perspective* series of publications. These 21-page comb bound reports feature data and ranking information for an individual state, as reported in *Health Care State Rankings 2001*. (For example *California Health Care in Perspective* features information about the state of California only.) They serve as handy, quick reference guides for those who do not want to page through the entire *Health Care State Rankings* volume searching for information for their particular state. When purchased by themselves, *Health Care State Perspectives* sell for $19. When purchased with a copy of *Health Care State Rankings*, these handy quick reference guides are just $9.50. For additional information, please call us toll-free at 1-800-457-0742.

Other Books From Morgan Quitno Press

In addition to *Health Care State Rankings*, our company offers three other rankings reference books. The first of these, *State Rankings*, provides a general view of the states. Statistics for a wide variety of categories are featured, including agriculture, transportation, government finance, health, population, crime, education, social welfare, energy and environment. Our annual compilation of state crime data is presented in *Crime State Rankings*. This reference volume offers a huge collection of user-friendly statistics on law enforcement personnel and expenditures, corrections, juvenile crime and delinquency, arrests and offenses. If city and metro area crime are your interest, *City Crime Rankings* compares crime in all metropolitan areas and cities of 75,000 or more population (approx. 300 cities). Numbers of crimes, crime rates, changes in crime rates over one and five years are presented for all major crime categories reported by the FBI. Final 1999 crime data are featured in the most recent 7th edition.

City Crime Rankings sells for $39.95. The *State Rankings* and *Crime State Rankings* books each are available for $52.95. (paper; S/H $5 per order). For true data aficionados, the information in our books also is available CD-ROM. These electronic editions provide a searchable PDF version of each book as well as the raw data in .dbf, Excel and ASCII formats. CD-ROM and book sets are $152.95 for each of the state books and $139.95 for the *City Crime Rankings* volume.

State Statistical Trends is our popular monthly journal that examines changes in life and government for the 50 United States. Each 100-page monthly issue focuses on a different subject and provides a collection of tables, graphics and commentary showing state multi-year trends. For further information about *Trends* or any of our other publications, please call us toll-free at 1-800-457-0742 or check out our web site at www.statestats.com.

Finally, we would like to extend a big "thank you" to the librarians, government and health care industry officials who help us each year with the development, design and production of this book. Your guidance is invaluable. Thanks also to you, our readers. We always welcome your thoughts and suggestions, so please give us a call, send us an e-mail or drop us a note with your ideas.

- THE EDITORS

WHICH STATE IS HEALTHIEST?

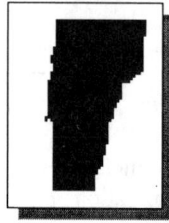

For eight of the nine years we have issued the Healthiest State Award, Vermont has ranked among the top six states. This year Vermont finally beats out its sister states and comes in as our 2001 Healthiest State. Last year's winner, New Hampshire, dropped to third, while Minnesota placed second. Mississippi brings up the less healthy end of the rankings for the second year in a row. It is preceded by South Carolina in 49th and Louisiana 48th.

Each year we take a step back from our objective reporting of health statistics, feed some basic figures into our computer and determine which is the Healthiest State. While we never claim our findings are indisputable, we do believe they provide an interesting statistical match-up of how the states are doing with regard to health care.

Methodology

The Healthiest State designation is awarded based on 21 factors chosen from the year 2001 edition of our annual reference book, *Health Care State Rankings*. These factors reflect access to health care providers,

2001 HEALTHIEST STATE AWARD

RANK	STATE	SUM	'00	RANK	STATE	SUM	'00
1	Vermont	16.62	2	26	Idaho	1.30	20
2	Minnesota	15.39	3	27	Michigan	0.63	31
3	New Hampshire	15.02	1	28	Arizona	0.25	27
4	Hawaii	14.92	4	29	Indiana	0.20	25
5	Iowa	14.27	15	30	West Virginia	(0.17)	35
6	Nebraska	13.53	10	31	Kentucky	(0.67)	33
7	Kansas	12.65	11	32	Illinois	(1.54)	26
8	Maine	11.31	6	33	Maryland	(1.56)	28
9	North Dakota	10.17	23	34	New York	(1.80)	42
10	Massachusetts	8.84	8	35	North Carolina	(2.35)	34
11	Washington	8.46	7	36	Oklahoma	(2.53)	29
12	Utah	8.15	5	37	Alaska	(3.32)	18
13	Montana	7.98	32	38	Missouri	(3.81)	36
14	Connecticut	7.96	9	39	Tennessee	(5.15)	40
15	Rhode Island	7.91	13	40	Arkansas	(5.92)	44
16	New Jersey	6.62	17	41	Georgia	(6.61)	45
17	California	6.53	19	42	Texas	(6.82)	41
18	Oregon	6.25	14	43	Delaware	(8.68)	37
18	Virginia	6.25	16	44	Florida	(10.04)	43
20	Pennsylvania	4.49	30	45	New Mexico	(12.66)	39
21	Colorado	3.57	12	46	Nevada	(14.89)	46
22	Ohio	3.02	21	47	Alabama	(15.67)	48
23	South Dakota	2.95	38	48	Louisiana	(17.51)	49
24	Wisconsin	2.79	22	49	South Carolina	(18.30)	47
25	Wyoming	1.91	23	50	Mississippi	(22.44)	50

factors reflect access to health care providers, affordability of health care and a generally healthy population (see box below.) Nineteen of the 21 factors are the same as last year. Two of the factors changed slightly. For the second factor, we switched from "Births to Teenage Mothers as a Percent of Live Births" to "Teenage Birth Rate." We also switched from "Percent of Adults Overweight" to "Percent of Adults Overweight or Obese." The 21 factors were divided into two groups: those that are "negative" for which a high ranking would be considered bad for a state, and those that are "positive" for which a high ranking would be considered good for a state. Rates for each of the 21 factors were processed through a formula that measures how a state compares to the national average for a given category. The positive and negative nature of each factor was taken into account as part of the formula. Once these computations were made, the factors then were weighted (factors were weighted equally.) These weighted scores were then added together to get a state's final score ("SUM" on the table above.) This way, states are assessed based on how they stack up against the national average. The end result is that the farther below the national average a state's health ranking is, the lower (and less healthy) it ranks. The farther above the national average, the higher (and healthier) a state ranks. This same methodology was used for our Dangerous State and Safest/Dangerous City Awards.

The table above shows how each state fared in the 2001 Healthiest State Award as well as its placement in 2000. We wish the citizens of the Green Mountain State continued good health!

THE EDITORS

POSITIVE (+) AND NEGATIVE (-) FACTORS CONSIDERED:

1. Births of Low Birthweight as a Percent of All Births (Table 13) -
2. Teenage Birth Rate (Table 27) -
3. Percent of Mothers Receiving Late or No Prenatal Care (Table 55) -
4. Age-Adjusted Death Rate (Table 81) -
5. Infant Mortality Rate (Table 85) -
6. Age-Adjusted Death Rate by Malignant Neoplasms (Table 153) -
7. Age-Adjusted Death Rate by Suicide (Table 177) -
8. Health Care Expenditures as a Percent of Gross State Product (Table 240) -
9. Per Capita Personal Health Expenditures (Table 243) -
10. Percent of Population Not Covered by Health Insurance (Table 303) -
11. Estimated Rate of New Cancer Cases (Table 356) -

12. AIDS Rate (Table 378) -
13. Sexually Transmitted Disease Rate (Table 413) -
14. Percent of Population Lacking Access to Primary Care (Table 442) -
15. Percent of Adults Who Are Binge Drinkers (Table 502) -
16. Percent of Adults Who Smoke (Table 504) -
17. Percent of Adults Overweight or Obese (Table 507) -
18. Number of Days in Past Month When Physical Health was "Not Good" (Table 510) -
19. Beds in Community Hospitals per 100,000 Population (Table 205) +
20. Percent of Children Aged 19-35 Months Fully Immunized (Table 411) +
21. Safety Belt Usage Rate (Table 512) +

TABLE OF CONTENTS

I. Births and Reproductive Health

TABLE OF CONTENTS (continued)

Abortions

II. Deaths

TABLE OF CONTENTS (continued)

TABLE OF CONTENTS (continued)

III. Facilities

TABLE OF CONTENTS (continued)

IV. Finance

TABLE OF CONTENTS (continued)

TABLE OF CONTENTS (continued)

V. Incidence of Disease

TABLE OF CONTENTS (continued)

TABLE OF CONTENTS (continued)

VII. Physical Fitness

VIII. Appendix

IX. Sources

X. Index

I. BIRTHS AND REPRODUCTIVE HEALTH

I. BIRTHS AND REPRODUCTIVE HEALTH
(CONTINUED)

Abortions

Births in 1999

National Total = 3,957,829 Live Births*

<u>ALPHA ORDER</u>

RANK	STATE	BIRTHS	% of USA
24	Alabama	62,123	1.6%
47	Alaska	9,953	0.3%
14	Arizona	81,225	2.1%
34	Arkansas	36,832	0.9%
1	California	518,229	13.1%
23	Colorado	62,161	1.6%
30	Connecticut	43,471	1.1%
45	Delaware	10,675	0.3%
4	Florida	197,014	5.0%
9	Georgia	126,744	3.2%
40	Hawaii	17,047	0.4%
39	Idaho	19,871	0.5%
5	Illinois	182,174	4.6%
13	Indiana	86,040	2.2%
33	Iowa	37,541	0.9%
32	Kansas	38,788	1.0%
26	Kentucky	54,344	1.4%
21	Louisiana	66,913	1.7%
42	Maine	13,615	0.3%
19	Maryland	72,207	1.8%
15	Massachusetts	80,998	2.0%
8	Michigan	133,562	3.4%
22	Minnesota	65,966	1.7%
31	Mississippi	42,694	1.1%
18	Missouri	75,352	1.9%
44	Montana	10,789	0.3%
37	Nebraska	23,907	0.6%
35	Nevada	29,357	0.7%
41	New Hampshire	14,071	0.4%
10	New Jersey	114,097	2.9%
36	New Mexico	27,065	0.7%
3	New York	258,412	6.5%
11	North Carolina	113,800	2.9%
48	North Dakota	7,637	0.2%
6	Ohio	150,292	3.8%
27	Oklahoma	49,054	1.2%
29	Oregon	45,205	1.1%
7	Pennsylvania	145,497	3.7%
43	Rhode Island	12,356	0.3%
25	South Carolina	54,984	1.4%
46	South Dakota	10,523	0.3%
17	Tennessee	77,839	2.0%
2	Texas	346,774	8.8%
28	Utah	46,289	1.2%
49	Vermont	6,565	0.2%
12	Virginia	95,538	2.4%
16	Washington	79,603	2.0%
38	West Virginia	20,764	0.5%
20	Wisconsin	68,216	1.7%
50	Wyoming	6,135	0.2%

<u>RANK ORDER</u>

RANK	STATE	BIRTHS	% of USA
1	California	518,229	13.1%
2	Texas	346,774	8.8%
3	New York	258,412	6.5%
4	Florida	197,014	5.0%
5	Illinois	182,174	4.6%
6	Ohio	150,292	3.8%
7	Pennsylvania	145,497	3.7%
8	Michigan	133,562	3.4%
9	Georgia	126,744	3.2%
10	New Jersey	114,097	2.9%
11	North Carolina	113,800	2.9%
12	Virginia	95,538	2.4%
13	Indiana	86,040	2.2%
14	Arizona	81,225	2.1%
15	Massachusetts	80,998	2.0%
16	Washington	79,603	2.0%
17	Tennessee	77,839	2.0%
18	Missouri	75,352	1.9%
19	Maryland	72,207	1.8%
20	Wisconsin	68,216	1.7%
21	Louisiana	66,913	1.7%
22	Minnesota	65,966	1.7%
23	Colorado	62,161	1.6%
24	Alabama	62,123	1.6%
25	South Carolina	54,984	1.4%
26	Kentucky	54,344	1.4%
27	Oklahoma	49,054	1.2%
28	Utah	46,289	1.2%
29	Oregon	45,205	1.1%
30	Connecticut	43,471	1.1%
31	Mississippi	42,694	1.1%
32	Kansas	38,788	1.0%
33	Iowa	37,541	0.9%
34	Arkansas	36,832	0.9%
35	Nevada	29,357	0.7%
36	New Mexico	27,065	0.7%
37	Nebraska	23,907	0.6%
38	West Virginia	20,764	0.5%
39	Idaho	19,871	0.5%
40	Hawaii	17,047	0.4%
41	New Hampshire	14,071	0.4%
42	Maine	13,615	0.3%
43	Rhode Island	12,356	0.3%
44	Montana	10,789	0.3%
45	Delaware	10,675	0.3%
46	South Dakota	10,523	0.3%
47	Alaska	9,953	0.3%
48	North Dakota	7,637	0.2%
49	Vermont	6,565	0.2%
50	Wyoming	6,135	0.2%
	District of Columbia	7,523	0.2%

Source: U.S. Department of Health and Human Services, National Center for Health Statistics
"National Vital Statistics Reports" (Vol. 48, No. 14, August 8, 2000)
Data are preliminary estimates by state of residence.

Birth Rate in 1999

National Rate = 14.5 Live Births per 1,000 Population*

ALPHA ORDER				RANK ORDER		
RANK	STATE	RATE		RANK	STATE	RATE
22	Alabama	14.2		1	Utah	21.7
6	Alaska	16.1		2	Texas	17.3
3	Arizona	17.0		3	Arizona	17.0
18	Arkansas	14.4		4	Georgia	16.3
8	California	15.6		5	Nevada	16.2
11	Colorado	15.3		6	Alaska	16.1
37	Connecticut	13.2		7	Idaho	15.9
22	Delaware	14.2		8	California	15.6
40	Florida	13.0		8	New Mexico	15.6
4	Georgia	16.3		10	Mississippi	15.4
18	Hawaii	14.4		11	Colorado	15.3
7	Idaho	15.9		11	Louisiana	15.3
13	Illinois	15.0		13	Illinois	15.0
17	Indiana	14.5		14	North Carolina	14.9
38	Iowa	13.1		15	Kansas	14.6
15	Kansas	14.6		15	Oklahoma	14.6
33	Kentucky	13.7		17	Indiana	14.5
11	Louisiana	15.3		18	Arkansas	14.4
50	Maine	10.9		18	Hawaii	14.4
27	Maryland	14.0		18	South Dakota	14.4
38	Massachusetts	13.1		21	Nebraska	14.3
35	Michigan	13.5		22	Alabama	14.2
30	Minnesota	13.8		22	Delaware	14.2
10	Mississippi	15.4		22	New York	14.2
30	Missouri	13.8		22	South Carolina	14.2
44	Montana	12.2		22	Tennessee	14.2
21	Nebraska	14.3		27	Maryland	14.0
5	Nevada	16.2		27	New Jersey	14.0
47	New Hampshire	11.7		29	Virginia	13.9
27	New Jersey	14.0		30	Minnesota	13.8
8	New Mexico	15.6		30	Missouri	13.8
22	New York	14.2		30	Washington	13.8
14	North Carolina	14.9		33	Kentucky	13.7
45	North Dakota	12.1		34	Oregon	13.6
36	Ohio	13.4		35	Michigan	13.5
15	Oklahoma	14.6		36	Ohio	13.4
34	Oregon	13.6		37	Connecticut	13.2
45	Pennsylvania	12.1		38	Iowa	13.1
43	Rhode Island	12.5		38	Massachusetts	13.1
22	South Carolina	14.2		40	Florida	13.0
18	South Dakota	14.4		40	Wisconsin	13.0
22	Tennessee	14.2		42	Wyoming	12.8
2	Texas	17.3		43	Rhode Island	12.5
1	Utah	21.7		44	Montana	12.2
49	Vermont	11.1		45	North Dakota	12.1
29	Virginia	13.9		45	Pennsylvania	12.1
30	Washington	13.8		47	New Hampshire	11.7
48	West Virginia	11.5		48	West Virginia	11.5
40	Wisconsin	13.0		49	Vermont	11.1
42	Wyoming	12.8		50	Maine	10.9
					District of Columbia	14.5

Source: U.S. Department of Health and Human Services, National Center for Health Statistics
"National Vital Statistics Reports" (Vol. 48, No. 14, August 8, 2000)
*Data are preliminary estimates by state of residence.

Births in 1998

National Total = 3,941,553 Live Births*

ALPHA ORDER

RANK	STATE	BIRTHS	% of USA
23	Alabama	62,074	1.6%
47	Alaska	9,926	0.3%
16	Arizona	78,243	2.0%
34	Arkansas	36,865	0.9%
1	California	521,661	13.2%
24	Colorado	59,577	1.5%
30	Connecticut	43,820	1.1%
45	Delaware	10,578	0.3%
4	Florida	195,637	5.0%
9	Georgia	122,368	3.1%
40	Hawaii	17,583	0.4%
39	Idaho	19,391	0.5%
5	Illinois	182,588	4.6%
13	Indiana	85,122	2.2%
33	Iowa	37,282	0.9%
32	Kansas	38,422	1.0%
25	Kentucky	54,329	1.4%
21	Louisiana	66,888	1.7%
42	Maine	13,733	0.3%
19	Maryland	71,972	1.8%
14	Massachusetts	81,411	2.1%
8	Michigan	133,666	3.4%
22	Minnesota	65,202	1.7%
31	Mississippi	42,939	1.1%
18	Missouri	75,358	1.9%
44	Montana	10,795	0.3%
37	Nebraska	23,534	0.6%
35	Nevada	28,699	0.7%
41	New Hampshire	14,429	0.4%
10	New Jersey	114,550	2.9%
36	New Mexico	27,318	0.7%
3	New York	258,207	6.6%
11	North Carolina	111,688	2.8%
48	North Dakota	7,932	0.2%
6	Ohio	152,794	3.9%
27	Oklahoma	49,461	1.3%
28	Oregon	45,273	1.1%
7	Pennsylvania	145,899	3.7%
43	Rhode Island	12,599	0.3%
26	South Carolina	53,877	1.4%
46	South Dakota	10,288	0.3%
17	Tennessee	77,396	2.0%
2	Texas	342,283	8.7%
29	Utah	45,165	1.1%
49	Vermont	6,582	0.2%
12	Virginia	94,351	2.4%
15	Washington	79,663	2.0%
38	West Virginia	20,747	0.5%
20	Wisconsin	67,450	1.7%
50	Wyoming	6,252	0.2%

RANK ORDER

RANK	STATE	BIRTHS	% of USA
1	California	521,661	13.2%
2	Texas	342,283	8.7%
3	New York	258,207	6.6%
4	Florida	195,637	5.0%
5	Illinois	182,588	4.6%
6	Ohio	152,794	3.9%
7	Pennsylvania	145,899	3.7%
8	Michigan	133,666	3.4%
9	Georgia	122,368	3.1%
10	New Jersey	114,550	2.9%
11	North Carolina	111,688	2.8%
12	Virginia	94,351	2.4%
13	Indiana	85,122	2.2%
14	Massachusetts	81,411	2.1%
15	Washington	79,663	2.0%
16	Arizona	78,243	2.0%
17	Tennessee	77,396	2.0%
18	Missouri	75,358	1.9%
19	Maryland	71,972	1.8%
20	Wisconsin	67,450	1.7%
21	Louisiana	66,888	1.7%
22	Minnesota	65,202	1.7%
23	Alabama	62,074	1.6%
24	Colorado	59,577	1.5%
25	Kentucky	54,329	1.4%
26	South Carolina	53,877	1.4%
27	Oklahoma	49,461	1.3%
28	Oregon	45,273	1.1%
29	Utah	45,165	1.1%
30	Connecticut	43,820	1.1%
31	Mississippi	42,939	1.1%
32	Kansas	38,422	1.0%
33	Iowa	37,282	0.9%
34	Arkansas	36,865	0.9%
35	Nevada	28,699	0.7%
36	New Mexico	27,318	0.7%
37	Nebraska	23,534	0.6%
38	West Virginia	20,747	0.5%
39	Idaho	19,391	0.5%
40	Hawaii	17,583	0.4%
41	New Hampshire	14,429	0.4%
42	Maine	13,733	0.3%
43	Rhode Island	12,599	0.3%
44	Montana	10,795	0.3%
45	Delaware	10,578	0.3%
46	South Dakota	10,288	0.3%
47	Alaska	9,926	0.3%
48	North Dakota	7,932	0.2%
49	Vermont	6,582	0.2%
50	Wyoming	6,252	0.2%
	District of Columbia	7,686	0.2%

Source: U.S. Department of Health and Human Services, National Center for Health Statistics
"National Vital Statistics Reports" (Vol. 48, No. 3, March 28, 2000)
Final data by state of residence.

Birth Rate in 1998

National Rate = 14.6 Live Births per 1,000 Population*

ALPHA ORDER

RANK	STATE	RATE
20	Alabama	14.3
5	Alaska	16.2
3	Arizona	16.8
18	Arkansas	14.5
6	California	16.0
13	Colorado	15.0
37	Connecticut	13.4
22	Delaware	14.2
39	Florida	13.1
6	Georgia	16.0
16	Hawaii	14.7
8	Idaho	15.8
12	Illinois	15.2
19	Indiana	14.4
40	Iowa	13.0
17	Kansas	14.6
32	Kentucky	13.8
11	Louisiana	15.3
50	Maine	11.0
26	Maryland	14.0
38	Massachusetts	13.2
35	Michigan	13.6
32	Minnesota	13.8
10	Mississippi	15.6
29	Missouri	13.9
45	Montana	12.3
22	Nebraska	14.2
4	Nevada	16.4
46	New Hampshire	12.2
25	New Jersey	14.1
9	New Mexico	15.7
22	New York	14.2
14	North Carolina	14.8
44	North Dakota	12.4
35	Ohio	13.6
14	Oklahoma	14.8
32	Oregon	13.8
46	Pennsylvania	12.2
43	Rhode Island	12.7
26	South Carolina	14.0
29	South Dakota	13.9
20	Tennessee	14.3
2	Texas	17.3
1	Utah	21.5
49	Vermont	11.1
29	Virginia	13.9
26	Washington	14.0
48	West Virginia	11.5
42	Wisconsin	12.9
40	Wyoming	13.0

RANK ORDER

RANK	STATE	RATE
1	Utah	21.5
2	Texas	17.3
3	Arizona	16.8
4	Nevada	16.4
5	Alaska	16.2
6	California	16.0
6	Georgia	16.0
8	Idaho	15.8
9	New Mexico	15.7
10	Mississippi	15.6
11	Louisiana	15.3
12	Illinois	15.2
13	Colorado	15.0
14	North Carolina	14.8
14	Oklahoma	14.8
16	Hawaii	14.7
17	Kansas	14.6
18	Arkansas	14.5
19	Indiana	14.4
20	Alabama	14.3
20	Tennessee	14.3
22	Delaware	14.2
22	Nebraska	14.2
22	New York	14.2
25	New Jersey	14.1
26	Maryland	14.0
26	South Carolina	14.0
26	Washington	14.0
29	Missouri	13.9
29	South Dakota	13.9
29	Virginia	13.9
32	Kentucky	13.8
32	Minnesota	13.8
32	Oregon	13.8
35	Michigan	13.6
35	Ohio	13.6
37	Connecticut	13.4
38	Massachusetts	13.2
39	Florida	13.1
40	Iowa	13.0
40	Wyoming	13.0
42	Wisconsin	12.9
43	Rhode Island	12.7
44	North Dakota	12.4
45	Montana	12.3
46	New Hampshire	12.2
46	Pennsylvania	12.2
48	West Virginia	11.5
49	Vermont	11.1
50	Maine	11.0
	District of Columbia	14.7

Source: U.S. Department of Health and Human Services, National Center for Health Statistics
"National Vital Statistics Reports" (Vol. 48, No. 3, March 28, 2000)
*Final data by state of residence.

Birth Rate in 1990

National Rate = 16.7 Births per 1,000 Population*

ALPHA ORDER			RANK ORDER		
RANK	**STATE**	**RATE**	**RANK**	**STATE**	**RATE**
26	Alabama	15.7	1	Alaska	21.6
1	Alaska	21.6	2	Utah	21.1
4	Arizona	18.8	3	California	20.6
29	Arkansas	15.5	4	Arizona	18.8
3	California	20.6	5	Texas	18.6
20	Colorado	16.2	6	Hawaii	18.5
38	Connecticut	15.2	7	New Mexico	18.1
15	Delaware	16.7	8	Nevada	18.0
32	Florida	15.4	9	Georgia	17.4
9	Georgia	17.4	10	Illinois	17.1
6	Hawaii	18.5	10	Louisiana	17.1
18	Idaho	16.3	12	Mississippi	16.9
10	Illinois	17.1	13	Maryland	16.8
28	Indiana	15.6	13	South Carolina	16.8
48	Iowa	14.2	15	Delaware	16.7
26	Kansas	15.7	16	Michigan	16.5
43	Kentucky	14.8	16	New York	16.5
10	Louisiana	17.1	18	Idaho	16.3
49	Maine	14.1	18	Washington	16.3
13	Maryland	16.8	20	Colorado	16.2
32	Massachusetts	15.4	21	Virginia	16.1
16	Michigan	16.5	22	New Hampshire	15.8
29	Minnesota	15.5	22	New Jersey	15.8
12	Mississippi	16.9	22	North Carolina	15.8
29	Missouri	15.5	22	South Dakota	15.8
45	Montana	14.5	26	Alabama	15.7
32	Nebraska	15.4	26	Kansas	15.7
8	Nevada	18.0	28	Indiana	15.6
22	New Hampshire	15.8	29	Arkansas	15.5
22	New Jersey	15.8	29	Minnesota	15.5
7	New Mexico	18.1	29	Missouri	15.5
16	New York	16.5	32	Florida	15.4
22	North Carolina	15.8	32	Massachusetts	15.4
45	North Dakota	14.5	32	Nebraska	15.4
32	Ohio	15.4	32	Ohio	15.4
39	Oklahoma	15.1	32	Tennessee	15.4
39	Oregon	15.1	32	Wyoming	15.4
45	Pennsylvania	14.5	38	Connecticut	15.2
39	Rhode Island	15.1	39	Oklahoma	15.1
13	South Carolina	16.8	39	Oregon	15.1
22	South Dakota	15.8	39	Rhode Island	15.1
32	Tennessee	15.4	42	Wisconsin	14.9
5	Texas	18.6	43	Kentucky	14.8
2	Utah	21.1	44	Vermont	14.7
44	Vermont	14.7	45	Montana	14.5
21	Virginia	16.1	45	North Dakota	14.5
18	Washington	16.3	45	Pennsylvania	14.5
50	West Virginia	12.6	48	Iowa	14.2
42	Wisconsin	14.9	49	Maine	14.1
32	Wyoming	15.4	50	West Virginia	12.6
				District of Columbia	19.5

Source: U.S. Department of Health and Human Services, National Center for Health Statistics
"Monthly Vital Statistics Report" (Vol. 41, No. 9, Supplement, February 25, 1993)
*Final data by state of residence.

Birth Rate in 1980

National Rate = 15.9 Births per 1,000 Population*

ALPHA ORDER

RANK	STATE	RATE
27	Alabama	16.3
2	Alaska	23.7
11	Arizona	18.4
27	Arkansas	16.3
18	California	17.0
15	Colorado	17.2
50	Connecticut	12.5
33	Delaware	15.8
45	Florida	13.5
19	Georgia	16.9
10	Hawaii	18.8
4	Idaho	21.4
20	Illinois	16.6
30	Indiana	16.1
24	Iowa	16.4
15	Kansas	17.2
27	Kentucky	16.3
6	Louisiana	19.5
41	Maine	14.6
43	Maryland	14.2
49	Massachusetts	12.7
34	Michigan	15.7
20	Minnesota	16.6
9	Mississippi	19.0
30	Missouri	16.1
13	Montana	18.1
14	Nebraska	17.4
20	Nevada	16.6
39	New Hampshire	14.9
47	New Jersey	13.2
5	New Mexico	20.0
44	New York	13.6
42	North Carolina	14.4
11	North Dakota	18.4
34	Ohio	15.7
15	Oklahoma	17.2
24	Oregon	16.4
46	Pennsylvania	13.4
48	Rhode Island	12.9
20	South Carolina	16.6
7	South Dakota	19.2
37	Tennessee	15.1
7	Texas	19.2
1	Utah	28.6
36	Vermont	15.4
40	Virginia	14.7
24	Washington	16.4
37	West Virginia	15.1
32	Wisconsin	15.9
3	Wyoming	22.5

RANK ORDER

RANK	STATE	RATE
1	Utah	28.6
2	Alaska	23.7
3	Wyoming	22.5
4	Idaho	21.4
5	New Mexico	20.0
6	Louisiana	19.5
7	South Dakota	19.2
7	Texas	19.2
9	Mississippi	19.0
10	Hawaii	18.8
11	Arizona	18.4
11	North Dakota	18.4
13	Montana	18.1
14	Nebraska	17.4
15	Colorado	17.2
15	Kansas	17.2
15	Oklahoma	17.2
18	California	17.0
19	Georgia	16.9
20	Illinois	16.6
20	Minnesota	16.6
20	Nevada	16.6
20	South Carolina	16.6
24	Iowa	16.4
24	Oregon	16.4
24	Washington	16.4
27	Alabama	16.3
27	Arkansas	16.3
27	Kentucky	16.3
30	Indiana	16.1
30	Missouri	16.1
32	Wisconsin	15.9
33	Delaware	15.8
34	Michigan	15.7
34	Ohio	15.7
36	Vermont	15.4
37	Tennessee	15.1
37	West Virginia	15.1
39	New Hampshire	14.9
40	Virginia	14.7
41	Maine	14.6
42	North Carolina	14.4
43	Maryland	14.2
44	New York	13.6
45	Florida	13.5
46	Pennsylvania	13.4
47	New Jersey	13.2
48	Rhode Island	12.9
49	Massachusetts	12.7
50	Connecticut	12.5
	District of Columbia	14.7

Source: U.S. Department of Health and Human Services, National Center for Health Statistics
   "Vital Statistics of the United States, 1980" and "Monthly Vital Statistics Report"
*Live births by state of residence.

Fertility Rate in 1999

National Rate = 65.8 Live Births per 1,000 Women 15 to 44 Years Old*

ALPHA ORDER

RANK	STATE	RATE
27	Alabama	63.3
5	Alaska	74.3
2	Arizona	81.1
15	Arkansas	67.8
9	California	69.4
8	Colorado	69.7
32	Connecticut	62.1
34	Delaware	61.7
22	Florida	65.1
11	Georgia	68.8
11	Hawaii	68.8
6	Idaho	73.2
13	Illinois	68.1
21	Indiana	65.2
30	Iowa	62.2
18	Kansas	67.5
35	Kentucky	61.4
18	Louisiana	67.5
49	Maine	49.4
38	Maryland	60.6
43	Massachusetts	58.5
37	Michigan	60.7
29	Minnesota	62.6
14	Mississippi	67.9
28	Missouri	62.9
40	Montana	59.8
20	Nebraska	66.6
3	Nevada	78.3
48	New Hampshire	51.0
24	New Jersey	64.5
7	New Mexico	71.9
25	New York	64.3
17	North Carolina	67.6
45	North Dakota	57.3
39	Ohio	60.5
10	Oklahoma	69.0
23	Oregon	64.8
44	Pennsylvania	57.4
46	Rhode Island	57.1
30	South Carolina	62.2
16	South Dakota	67.7
26	Tennessee	63.5
4	Texas	77.1
1	Utah	93.1
50	Vermont	49.2
41	Virginia	59.7
32	Washington	62.1
47	West Virginia	54.8
42	Wisconsin	59.4
36	Wyoming	60.8

RANK ORDER

RANK	STATE	RATE
1	Utah	93.1
2	Arizona	81.1
3	Nevada	78.3
4	Texas	77.1
5	Alaska	74.3
6	Idaho	73.2
7	New Mexico	71.9
8	Colorado	69.7
9	California	69.4
10	Oklahoma	69.0
11	Georgia	68.8
11	Hawaii	68.8
13	Illinois	68.1
14	Mississippi	67.9
15	Arkansas	67.8
16	South Dakota	67.7
17	North Carolina	67.6
18	Kansas	67.5
18	Louisiana	67.5
20	Nebraska	66.6
21	Indiana	65.2
22	Florida	65.1
23	Oregon	64.8
24	New Jersey	64.5
25	New York	64.3
26	Tennessee	63.5
27	Alabama	63.3
28	Missouri	62.9
29	Minnesota	62.6
30	Iowa	62.2
30	South Carolina	62.2
32	Connecticut	62.1
32	Washington	62.1
34	Delaware	61.7
35	Kentucky	61.4
36	Wyoming	60.8
37	Michigan	60.7
38	Maryland	60.6
39	Ohio	60.5
40	Montana	59.8
41	Virginia	59.7
42	Wisconsin	59.4
43	Massachusetts	58.5
44	Pennsylvania	57.4
45	North Dakota	57.3
46	Rhode Island	57.1
47	West Virginia	54.8
48	New Hampshire	51.0
49	Maine	49.4
50	Vermont	49.2
	District of Columbia	60.0

Source: U.S. Department of Health and Human Services, National Center for Health Statistics
"National Vital Statistics Reports" (Vol. 48, No. 14, August 8, 2000)
*Data are preliminary estimates by state of residence.

Births to White Women in 1999

National Total = 3,130,100 Live Births to White Women*

ALPHA ORDER

RANK	STATE	BIRTHS	% of USA
25	Alabama	41,729	1.3%
47	Alaska	6,529	0.2%
13	Arizona	71,125	2.3%
33	Arkansas	28,476	0.9%
1	California	420,188	13.4%
21	Colorado	56,706	1.8%
29	Connecticut	36,502	1.2%
45	Delaware	7,678	0.2%
4	Florida	146,663	4.7%
11	Georgia	81,140	2.6%
50	Hawaii	4,001	0.1%
39	Idaho	19,211	0.6%
5	Illinois	140,805	4.5%
12	Indiana	75,448	2.4%
30	Iowa	35,348	1.1%
32	Kansas	34,611	1.1%
22	Kentucky	48,747	1.6%
28	Louisiana	38,408	1.2%
41	Maine	13,241	0.4%
23	Maryland	44,296	1.4%
15	Massachusetts	68,218	2.2%
8	Michigan	105,293	3.4%
20	Minnesota	57,491	1.8%
36	Mississippi	22,668	0.7%
17	Missouri	62,531	2.0%
43	Montana	9,387	0.3%
37	Nebraska	21,727	0.7%
34	Nevada	24,975	0.8%
40	New Hampshire	13,657	0.4%
9	New Jersey	84,103	2.7%
35	New Mexico	22,791	0.7%
3	New York	186,128	5.9%
10	North Carolina	81,232	2.6%
46	North Dakota	6,742	0.2%
6	Ohio	126,636	4.0%
27	Oklahoma	38,628	1.2%
26	Oregon	41,410	1.3%
7	Pennsylvania	121,063	3.9%
42	Rhode Island	10,796	0.3%
31	South Carolina	34,987	1.1%
44	South Dakota	8,669	0.3%
18	Tennessee	59,998	1.9%
2	Texas	297,150	9.5%
24	Utah	44,033	1.4%
48	Vermont	6,469	0.2%
16	Virginia	68,199	2.2%
14	Washington	68,227	2.2%
38	West Virginia	19,828	0.6%
19	Wisconsin	58,777	1.9%
49	Wyoming	5,745	0.2%

RANK ORDER

RANK	STATE	BIRTHS	% of USA
1	California	420,188	13.4%
2	Texas	297,150	9.5%
3	New York	186,128	5.9%
4	Florida	146,663	4.7%
5	Illinois	140,805	4.5%
6	Ohio	126,636	4.0%
7	Pennsylvania	121,063	3.9%
8	Michigan	105,293	3.4%
9	New Jersey	84,103	2.7%
10	North Carolina	81,232	2.6%
11	Georgia	81,140	2.6%
12	Indiana	75,448	2.4%
13	Arizona	71,125	2.3%
14	Washington	68,227	2.2%
15	Massachusetts	68,218	2.2%
16	Virginia	68,199	2.2%
17	Missouri	62,531	2.0%
18	Tennessee	59,998	1.9%
19	Wisconsin	58,777	1.9%
20	Minnesota	57,491	1.8%
21	Colorado	56,706	1.8%
22	Kentucky	48,747	1.6%
23	Maryland	44,296	1.4%
24	Utah	44,033	1.4%
25	Alabama	41,729	1.3%
26	Oregon	41,410	1.3%
27	Oklahoma	38,628	1.2%
28	Louisiana	38,408	1.2%
29	Connecticut	36,502	1.2%
30	Iowa	35,348	1.1%
31	South Carolina	34,987	1.1%
32	Kansas	34,611	1.1%
33	Arkansas	28,476	0.9%
34	Nevada	24,975	0.8%
35	New Mexico	22,791	0.7%
36	Mississippi	22,668	0.7%
37	Nebraska	21,727	0.7%
38	West Virginia	19,828	0.6%
39	Idaho	19,211	0.6%
40	New Hampshire	13,657	0.4%
41	Maine	13,241	0.4%
42	Rhode Island	10,796	0.3%
43	Montana	9,387	0.3%
44	South Dakota	8,669	0.3%
45	Delaware	7,678	0.2%
46	North Dakota	6,742	0.2%
47	Alaska	6,529	0.2%
48	Vermont	6,469	0.2%
49	Wyoming	5,745	0.2%
50	Hawaii	4,001	0.1%
	District of Columbia	1,687	0.1%

Source: U.S. Department of Health and Human Services, National Center for Health Statistics
   "National Vital Statistics Reports" (Vol. 48, No. 14, August 8, 2000)
*Preliminary data by state of residence. By race of mother.

White Births as a Percent of All Births in 1999

National Percent = 79.1% of Live Births*

ALPHA ORDER

RANK	STATE	PERCENT
43	Alabama	67.2
44	Alaska	65.6
16	Arizona	87.6
34	Arkansas	77.3
31	California	81.1
10	Colorado	91.2
27	Connecticut	84.0
40	Delaware	71.9
37	Florida	74.4
45	Georgia	64.0
50	Hawaii	23.5
4	Idaho	96.7
34	Illinois	77.3
15	Indiana	87.7
7	Iowa	94.2
13	Kansas	89.2
12	Kentucky	89.7
48	Louisiana	57.4
2	Maine	97.3
47	Maryland	61.3
25	Massachusetts	84.2
32	Michigan	78.8
18	Minnesota	87.2
49	Mississippi	53.1
29	Missouri	83.0
19	Montana	87.0
11	Nebraska	90.9
23	Nevada	85.1
3	New Hampshire	97.1
38	New Jersey	73.7
25	New Mexico	84.2
39	New York	72.0
41	North Carolina	71.4
14	North Dakota	88.3
24	Ohio	84.3
33	Oklahoma	78.7
9	Oregon	91.6
28	Pennsylvania	83.2
17	Rhode Island	87.4
46	South Carolina	63.6
30	South Dakota	82.4
36	Tennessee	77.1
21	Texas	85.7
6	Utah	95.1
1	Vermont	98.5
41	Virginia	71.4
21	Washington	85.7
5	West Virginia	95.5
20	Wisconsin	86.2
8	Wyoming	93.6

RANK ORDER

RANK	STATE	PERCENT
1	Vermont	98.5
2	Maine	97.3
3	New Hampshire	97.1
4	Idaho	96.7
5	West Virginia	95.5
6	Utah	95.1
7	Iowa	94.2
8	Wyoming	93.6
9	Oregon	91.6
10	Colorado	91.2
11	Nebraska	90.9
12	Kentucky	89.7
13	Kansas	89.2
14	North Dakota	88.3
15	Indiana	87.7
16	Arizona	87.6
17	Rhode Island	87.4
18	Minnesota	87.2
19	Montana	87.0
20	Wisconsin	86.2
21	Texas	85.7
21	Washington	85.7
23	Nevada	85.1
24	Ohio	84.3
25	Massachusetts	84.2
25	New Mexico	84.2
27	Connecticut	84.0
28	Pennsylvania	83.2
29	Missouri	83.0
30	South Dakota	82.4
31	California	81.1
32	Michigan	78.8
33	Oklahoma	78.7
34	Arkansas	77.3
34	Illinois	77.3
36	Tennessee	77.1
37	Florida	74.4
38	New Jersey	73.7
39	New York	72.0
40	Delaware	71.9
41	North Carolina	71.4
41	Virginia	71.4
43	Alabama	67.2
44	Alaska	65.6
45	Georgia	64.0
46	South Carolina	63.6
47	Maryland	61.3
48	Louisiana	57.4
49	Mississippi	53.1
50	Hawaii	23.5
	District of Columbia	22.4

Source: Morgan Quitno Press using data from U.S. Dept. of Health and Human Services, Nat'l Center for Health Statistics
"National Vital Statistics Reports" (Vol. 48, No. 14, August 8, 2000)
*Preliminary data by state of residence. By race of mother.

Births to Black Women in 1999

National Total = 606,720 Live Births to Black Women*

ALPHA ORDER

RANK	STATE	BIRTHS	% of USA
15	Alabama	19,771	3.3%
40	Alaska	460	0.1%
31	Arizona	2,803	0.5%
22	Arkansas	7,717	1.3%
5	California	35,991	5.9%
29	Colorado	2,900	0.5%
24	Connecticut	5,314	0.9%
32	Delaware	2,688	0.4%
2	Florida	45,095	7.4%
3	Georgia	42,113	6.9%
40	Hawaii	460	0.1%
47	Idaho	77	0.0%
6	Illinois	34,254	5.6%
20	Indiana	9,323	1.5%
35	Iowa	1,165	0.2%
30	Kansas	2,858	0.5%
25	Kentucky	4,959	0.8%
8	Louisiana	27,225	4.5%
44	Maine	106	0.0%
9	Maryland	24,568	4.0%
21	Massachusetts	8,292	1.4%
10	Michigan	24,057	4.0%
27	Minnesota	4,034	0.7%
16	Mississippi	19,417	3.2%
19	Missouri	11,253	1.9%
50	Montana	35	0.0%
34	Nebraska	1,281	0.2%
33	Nevada	2,223	0.4%
43	New Hampshire	139	0.0%
12	New Jersey	21,385	3.5%
39	New Mexico	497	0.1%
1	New York	53,798	8.9%
7	North Carolina	28,446	4.7%
46	North Dakota	86	0.0%
13	Ohio	21,020	3.5%
26	Oklahoma	4,649	0.8%
37	Oregon	905	0.1%
14	Pennsylvania	20,608	3.4%
36	Rhode Island	967	0.2%
17	South Carolina	19,103	3.1%
45	South Dakota	89	0.0%
18	Tennessee	16,537	2.7%
4	Texas	38,883	6.4%
42	Utah	270	0.0%
49	Vermont	40	0.0%
11	Virginia	22,498	3.7%
28	Washington	3,363	0.6%
38	West Virginia	752	0.1%
23	Wisconsin	6,509	1.1%
48	Wyoming	73	0.0%

RANK ORDER

RANK	STATE	BIRTHS	% of USA
1	New York	53,798	8.9%
2	Florida	45,095	7.4%
3	Georgia	42,113	6.9%
4	Texas	38,883	6.4%
5	California	35,991	5.9%
6	Illinois	34,254	5.6%
7	North Carolina	28,446	4.7%
8	Louisiana	27,225	4.5%
9	Maryland	24,568	4.0%
10	Michigan	24,057	4.0%
11	Virginia	22,498	3.7%
12	New Jersey	21,385	3.5%
13	Ohio	21,020	3.5%
14	Pennsylvania	20,608	3.4%
15	Alabama	19,771	3.3%
16	Mississippi	19,417	3.2%
17	South Carolina	19,103	3.1%
18	Tennessee	16,537	2.7%
19	Missouri	11,253	1.9%
20	Indiana	9,323	1.5%
21	Massachusetts	8,292	1.4%
22	Arkansas	7,717	1.3%
23	Wisconsin	6,509	1.1%
24	Connecticut	5,314	0.9%
25	Kentucky	4,959	0.8%
26	Oklahoma	4,649	0.8%
27	Minnesota	4,034	0.7%
28	Washington	3,363	0.6%
29	Colorado	2,900	0.5%
30	Kansas	2,858	0.5%
31	Arizona	2,803	0.5%
32	Delaware	2,688	0.4%
33	Nevada	2,223	0.4%
34	Nebraska	1,281	0.2%
35	Iowa	1,165	0.2%
36	Rhode Island	967	0.2%
37	Oregon	905	0.1%
38	West Virginia	752	0.1%
39	New Mexico	497	0.1%
40	Alaska	460	0.1%
40	Hawaii	460	0.1%
42	Utah	270	0.0%
43	New Hampshire	139	0.0%
44	Maine	106	0.0%
45	South Dakota	89	0.0%
46	North Dakota	86	0.0%
47	Idaho	77	0.0%
48	Wyoming	73	0.0%
49	Vermont	40	0.0%
50	Montana	35	0.0%
	District of Columbia	5,662	0.9%

Source: U.S. Department of Health and Human Services, National Center for Health Statistics
   "National Vital Statistics Reports" (Vol. 48, No. 14, August 8, 2000)
*Preliminary data by state of residence. By race of mother.

Black Births as a Percent of All Births in 1999

National Percent = 15.3% of Live Births*

ALPHA ORDER

RANK	STATE	PERCENT
6	Alabama	31.8
34	Alaska	4.6
37	Arizona	3.5
12	Arkansas	.21.0
30	California	6.9
33	Colorado	4.7
20	Connecticut	12.2
7	Delaware	25.2
10	Florida	22.9
5	Georgia	33.2
39	Hawaii	2.7
49	Idaho	0.4
14	Illinois	18.8
22	Indiana	10.8
38	Iowa	3.1
29	Kansas	7.4
26	Kentucky	9.1
2	Louisiana	40.7
45	Maine	0.8
4	Maryland	34.0
23	Massachusetts	10.2
16	Michigan	18.0
31	Minnesota	6.1
1	Mississippi	45.5
17	Missouri	14.9
50	Montana	0.3
32	Nebraska	5.4
28	Nevada	7.6
44	New Hampshire	1.0
15	New Jersey	18.7
41	New Mexico	1.8
13	New York	20.8
8	North Carolina	25.0
43	North Dakota	1.1
19	Ohio	14.0
24	Oklahoma	9.5
40	Oregon	2.0
18	Pennsylvania	14.2
27	Rhode Island	7.8
3	South Carolina	34.7
45	South Dakota	0.8
11	Tennessee	21.2
21	Texas	11.2
47	Utah	0.6
47	Vermont	0.6
9	Virginia	23.5
35	Washington	4.2
36	West Virginia	3.6
24	Wisconsin	9.5
42	Wyoming	1.2

RANK ORDER

RANK	STATE	PERCENT
1	Mississippi	45.5
2	Louisiana	40.7
3	South Carolina	34.7
4	Maryland	34.0
5	Georgia	33.2
6	Alabama	31.8
7	Delaware	25.2
8	North Carolina	25.0
9	Virginia	23.5
10	Florida	22.9
11	Tennessee	21.2
12	Arkansas	21.0
13	New York	20.8
14	Illinois	18.8
15	New Jersey	18.7
16	Michigan	18.0
17	Missouri	14.9
18	Pennsylvania	14.2
19	Ohio	14.0
20	Connecticut	12.2
21	Texas	11.2
22	Indiana	10.8
23	Massachusetts	10.2
24	Oklahoma	9.5
24	Wisconsin	9.5
26	Kentucky	9.1
27	Rhode Island	7.8
28	Nevada	7.6
29	Kansas	7.4
30	California	6.9
31	Minnesota	6.1
32	Nebraska	5.4
33	Colorado	4.7
34	Alaska	4.6
35	Washington	4.2
36	West Virginia	3.6
37	Arizona	3.5
38	Iowa	3.1
39	Hawaii	2.7
40	Oregon	2.0
41	New Mexico	1.8
42	Wyoming	1.2
43	North Dakota	1.1
44	New Hampshire	1.0
45	Maine	0.8
45	South Dakota	0.8
47	Utah	0.6
47	Vermont	0.6
49	Idaho	0.4
50	Montana	0.3

District of Columbia   75.3

Source: Morgan Quitno Press using data from U.S. Dept. of Health and Human Services, Nat'l Center for Health Statistics
"National Vital Statistics Reports" (Vol. 48, No. 14, August 8, 2000)
*Preliminary data by state of residence. By race of mother.

Births of Low Birthweight in 1999

National Total = 300,795 Live Births*

ALPHA ORDER					RANK ORDER			
RANK	STATE		BIRTHS	% of USA	RANK	STATE	BIRTHS	% of USA
18	Alabama		5,777	1.9%	1	California	31,612	10.5%
47	Alaska		577	0.2%	2	Texas	25,315	8.4%
20	Arizona		5,686	1.9%	3	New York	20,156	6.7%
30	Arkansas		3,168	1.1%	4	Florida	16,155	5.4%
1	California		31,612	10.5%	5	Illinois	14,574	4.8%
22	Colorado		5,159	1.7%	6	Ohio	11,572	3.8%
29	Connecticut		3,304	1.1%	7	Pennsylvania	11,349	3.8%
41	Delaware		918	0.3%	8	Georgia	11,027	3.7%
4	Florida		16,155	5.4%	9	Michigan	10,819	3.6%
8	Georgia		11,027	3.7%	10	North Carolina	10,128	3.4%
39	Hawaii		1,279	0.4%	11	New Jersey	9,242	3.1%
40	Idaho		1,232	0.4%	12	Virginia	7,452	2.5%
5	Illinois		14,574	4.8%	13	Tennessee	7,161	2.4%
14	Indiana		6,797	2.3%	14	Indiana	6,797	2.3%
34	Iowa		2,328	0.8%	15	Louisiana	6,691	2.2%
32	Kansas		2,754	0.9%	16	Maryland	6,499	2.2%
25	Kentucky		4,456	1.5%	17	Missouri	5,802	1.9%
15	Louisiana		6,691	2.2%	18	Alabama	5,777	1.9%
44	Maine		817	0.3%	19	Massachusetts	5,751	1.9%
16	Maryland		6,499	2.2%	20	Arizona	5,686	1.9%
19	Massachusetts		5,751	1.9%	21	South Carolina	5,388	1.8%
9	Michigan		10,819	3.6%	22	Colorado	5,159	1.7%
27	Minnesota		4,024	1.3%	23	Washington	4,617	1.5%
26	Mississippi		4,397	1.5%	24	Wisconsin	4,570	1.5%
17	Missouri		5,802	1.9%	25	Kentucky	4,456	1.5%
45	Montana		734	0.2%	26	Mississippi	4,397	1.5%
38	Nebraska		1,602	0.5%	27	Minnesota	4,024	1.3%
35	Nevada		2,231	0.7%	28	Oklahoma	3,630	1.2%
43	New Hampshire		872	0.3%	29	Connecticut	3,304	1.1%
11	New Jersey		9,242	3.1%	30	Arkansas	3,168	1.1%
36	New Mexico		2,084	0.7%	31	Utah	3,148	1.0%
3	New York		20,156	6.7%	32	Kansas	2,754	0.9%
10	North Carolina		10,128	3.4%	33	Oregon	2,441	0.8%
49	North Dakota		473	0.2%	34	Iowa	2,328	0.8%
6	Ohio		11,572	3.8%	35	Nevada	2,231	0.7%
28	Oklahoma		3,630	1.2%	36	New Mexico	2,084	0.7%
33	Oregon		2,441	0.8%	37	West Virginia	1,661	0.6%
7	Pennsylvania		11,349	3.8%	38	Nebraska	1,602	0.5%
42	Rhode Island		902	0.3%	39	Hawaii	1,279	0.4%
21	South Carolina		5,388	1.8%	40	Idaho	1,232	0.4%
46	South Dakota		621	0.2%	41	Delaware	918	0.3%
13	Tennessee		7,161	2.4%	42	Rhode Island	902	0.3%
2	Texas		25,315	8.4%	43	New Hampshire	872	0.3%
31	Utah		3,148	1.0%	44	Maine	817	0.3%
50	Vermont		374	0.1%	45	Montana	734	0.2%
12	Virginia		7,452	2.5%	46	South Dakota	621	0.2%
23	Washington		4,617	1.5%	47	Alaska	577	0.2%
37	West Virginia		1,661	0.6%	48	Wyoming	515	0.2%
24	Wisconsin		4,570	1.5%	49	North Dakota	473	0.2%
48	Wyoming		515	0.2%	50	Vermont	374	0.1%
						District of Columbia	986	0.3%

Source: Morgan Quitno Press using data from U.S. Dept. of Health and Human Services, Nat'l Center for Health Statistics "National Vital Statistics Reports" (Vol. 48, No. 14, August 8, 2000)
Births of less than 2,500 grams (5 pounds 8 ounces). Preliminary data by state of residence. Calculated by the editors by multiplying total number of births by percent of such births reported as being low birthweight.

Births of Low Birthweight as a Percent of All Births in 1999

National Percent = 7.6% of Live Births*

ALPHA ORDER			RANK ORDER		
RANK	STATE	PERCENT	RANK	STATE	PERCENT
4	Alabama	9.3	1	Mississippi	10.3
47	Alaska	5.8	2	Louisiana	10.0
34	Arizona	7.0	3	South Carolina	9.8
9	Arkansas	8.6	4	Alabama	9.3
43	California	6.1	5	Tennessee	9.2
12	Colorado	8.3	6	Maryland	9.0
26	Connecticut	7.6	7	North Carolina	8.9
9	Delaware	8.6	8	Georgia	8.7
13	Florida	8.2	9	Arkansas	8.6
8	Georgia	8.7	9	Delaware	8.6
28	Hawaii	7.5	11	Wyoming	8.4
39	Idaho	6.2	12	Colorado	8.3
17	Illinois	8.0	13	Florida	8.2
19	Indiana	7.9	13	Kentucky	8.2
39	Iowa	6.2	15	Michigan	8.1
32	Kansas	7.1	15	New Jersey	8.1
13	Kentucky	8.2	17	Illinois	8.0
2	Louisiana	10.0	17	West Virginia	8.0
45	Maine	6.0	19	Indiana	7.9
6	Maryland	9.0	20	New York	7.8
32	Massachusetts	7.1	20	Pennsylvania	7.8
15	Michigan	8.1	20	Virginia	7.8
43	Minnesota	6.1	23	Missouri	7.7
1	Mississippi	10.3	23	New Mexico	7.7
23	Missouri	7.7	23	Ohio	7.7
35	Montana	6.8	26	Connecticut	7.6
37	Nebraska	6.7	26	Nevada	7.6
26	Nevada	7.6	28	Hawaii	7.5
39	New Hampshire	6.2	29	Oklahoma	7.4
15	New Jersey	8.1	30	Rhode Island	7.3
23	New Mexico	7.7	30	Texas	7.3
20	New York	7.8	32	Kansas	7.1
7	North Carolina	8.9	32	Massachusetts	7.1
39	North Dakota	6.2	34	Arizona	7.0
23	Ohio	7.7	35	Montana	6.8
29	Oklahoma	7.4	35	Utah	6.8
50	Oregon	5.4	37	Nebraska	6.7
20	Pennsylvania	7.8	37	Wisconsin	6.7
30	Rhode Island	7.3	39	Idaho	6.2
3	South Carolina	9.8	39	Iowa	6.2
46	South Dakota	5.9	39	New Hampshire	6.2
5	Tennessee	9.2	39	North Dakota	6.2
30	Texas	7.3	43	California	6.1
35	Utah	6.8	43	Minnesota	6.1
49	Vermont	5.7	45	Maine	6.0
20	Virginia	7.8	46	South Dakota	5.9
47	Washington	5.8	47	Alaska	5.8
17	West Virginia	8.0	47	Washington	5.8
37	Wisconsin	6.7	49	Vermont	5.7
11	Wyoming	8.4	50	Oregon	5.4
				District of Columbia	13.1

Source: U.S. Department of Health and Human Services, National Center for Health Statistics
   "National Vital Statistics Reports" (Vol. 48, No. 14, August 8, 2000)
*Estimates based on preliminary data by state of residence. Births of less than 2,500 grams (5 pounds 8 ounces).

Births of Low Birthweight to White Women in 1999

National Total = 206,587 Live Births*

ALPHA ORDER

RANK ORDER

RANK	STATE	BIRTHS	% of USA		RANK	STATE	BIRTHS	% of USA
23	Alabama	3,046	1.5%		1	California	23,110	11.2%
49	Alaska	346	0.2%		2	Texas	19,612	9.5%
13	Arizona	4,765	2.3%		3	New York	12,471	6.0%
32	Arkansas	2,107	1.0%		4	Florida	10,120	4.9%
1	California	23,110	11.2%		5	Illinois	9,152	4.4%
15	Colorado	4,536	2.2%		6	Ohio	8,611	4.2%
29	Connecticut	2,482	1.2%		7	Pennsylvania	8,111	3.9%
44	Delaware	530	0.3%		8	Michigan	6,949	3.4%
4	Florida	10,120	4.9%		9	North Carolina	5,849	2.8%
11	Georgia	5,436	2.6%		10	New Jersey	5,719	2.8%
50	Hawaii	220	0.1%		11	Georgia	5,436	2.6%
39	Idaho	1,172	0.6%		12	Indiana	5,432	2.6%
5	Illinois	9,152	4.4%		13	Arizona	4,765	2.3%
12	Indiana	5,432	2.6%		14	Tennessee	4,740	2.3%
33	Iowa	2,086	1.0%		15	Colorado	4,536	2.2%
30	Kansas	2,319	1.1%		16	Massachusetts	4,502	2.2%
20	Kentucky	3,705	1.8%		17	Virginia	4,365	2.1%
27	Louisiana	2,650	1.3%		18	Missouri	4,190	2.0%
41	Maine	794	0.4%		19	Washington	3,752	1.8%
24	Maryland	2,968	1.4%		20	Kentucky	3,705	1.8%
16	Massachusetts	4,502	2.2%		21	Wisconsin	3,468	1.7%
8	Michigan	6,949	3.4%		22	Minnesota	3,219	1.6%
22	Minnesota	3,219	1.6%		23	Alabama	3,046	1.5%
36	Mississippi	1,677	0.8%		24	Maryland	2,968	1.4%
18	Missouri	4,190	2.0%		25	Utah	2,950	1.4%
43	Montana	638	0.3%		26	Oklahoma	2,743	1.3%
38	Nebraska	1,391	0.7%		27	Louisiana	2,650	1.3%
34	Nevada	1,773	0.9%		28	South Carolina	2,519	1.2%
40	New Hampshire	847	0.4%		29	Connecticut	2,482	1.2%
10	New Jersey	5,719	2.8%		30	Kansas	2,319	1.1%
35	New Mexico	1,755	0.8%		31	Oregon	2,195	1.1%
3	New York	12,471	6.0%		32	Arkansas	2,107	1.0%
9	North Carolina	5,849	2.8%		33	Iowa	2,086	1.0%
47	North Dakota	418	0.2%		34	Nevada	1,773	0.9%
6	Ohio	8,611	4.2%		35	New Mexico	1,755	0.8%
26	Oklahoma	2,743	1.3%		36	Mississippi	1,677	0.8%
31	Oregon	2,195	1.1%		37	West Virginia	1,566	0.8%
7	Pennsylvania	8,111	3.9%		38	Nebraska	1,391	0.7%
42	Rhode Island	734	0.4%		39	Idaho	1,172	0.6%
28	South Carolina	2,519	1.2%		40	New Hampshire	847	0.4%
45	South Dakota	511	0.2%		41	Maine	794	0.4%
14	Tennessee	4,740	2.3%		42	Rhode Island	734	0.4%
2	Texas	19,612	9.5%		43	Montana	638	0.3%
25	Utah	2,950	1.4%		44	Delaware	530	0.3%
48	Vermont	369	0.2%		45	South Dakota	511	0.2%
17	Virginia	4,365	2.1%		46	Wyoming	465	0.2%
19	Washington	3,752	1.8%		47	North Dakota	418	0.2%
37	West Virginia	1,566	0.8%		48	Vermont	369	0.2%
21	Wisconsin	3,468	1.7%		49	Alaska	346	0.2%
46	Wyoming	465	0.2%		50	Hawaii	220	0.1%
						District of Columbia	105	0.1%

Source: Morgan Quitno Press using data from U.S. Dept. of Health and Human Services, Nat'l Center for Health Statistics "National Vital Statistics Reports" (Vol. 48, No. 14, August 8, 2000)

*Births of less than 2,500 grams (5 pounds 8 ounces). Preliminary data by state of residence. Calculated by the editors by multiplying total number of births to white women by percent of births to white women reported as being low birthweight.

Births of Low Birthweight to White Women
As a Percent of All Births to White Women in 1999
National Percent = 6.6% of Live Births to White Women*

<table>
<tr><td colspan="3">ALPHA ORDER</td><td colspan="3">RANK ORDER</td></tr>
<tr><td>RANK</td><td>STATE</td><td>PERCENT</td><td>RANK</td><td>STATE</td><td>PERCENT</td></tr>
<tr><td>9</td><td>Alabama</td><td>7.3</td><td>1</td><td>Wyoming</td><td>8.1</td></tr>
<tr><td>49</td><td>Alaska</td><td>5.3</td><td>2</td><td>Colorado</td><td>8.0</td></tr>
<tr><td>23</td><td>Arizona</td><td>6.7</td><td>3</td><td>Tennessee</td><td>7.9</td></tr>
<tr><td>7</td><td>Arkansas</td><td>7.4</td><td>3</td><td>West Virginia</td><td>7.9</td></tr>
<tr><td>46</td><td>California</td><td>5.5</td><td>5</td><td>New Mexico</td><td>7.7</td></tr>
<tr><td>2</td><td>Colorado</td><td>8.0</td><td>6</td><td>Kentucky</td><td>7.6</td></tr>
<tr><td>18</td><td>Connecticut</td><td>6.8</td><td>7</td><td>Arkansas</td><td>7.4</td></tr>
<tr><td>15</td><td>Delaware</td><td>6.9</td><td>7</td><td>Mississippi</td><td>7.4</td></tr>
<tr><td>15</td><td>Florida</td><td>6.9</td><td>9</td><td>Alabama</td><td>7.3</td></tr>
<tr><td>23</td><td>Georgia</td><td>6.7</td><td>10</td><td>Indiana</td><td>7.2</td></tr>
<tr><td>46</td><td>Hawaii</td><td>5.5</td><td>10</td><td>North Carolina</td><td>7.2</td></tr>
<tr><td>39</td><td>Idaho</td><td>6.1</td><td>10</td><td>South Carolina</td><td>7.2</td></tr>
<tr><td>34</td><td>Illinois</td><td>6.5</td><td>13</td><td>Nevada</td><td>7.1</td></tr>
<tr><td>10</td><td>Indiana</td><td>7.2</td><td>13</td><td>Oklahoma</td><td>7.1</td></tr>
<tr><td>41</td><td>Iowa</td><td>5.9</td><td>15</td><td>Delaware</td><td>6.9</td></tr>
<tr><td>23</td><td>Kansas</td><td>6.7</td><td>15</td><td>Florida</td><td>6.9</td></tr>
<tr><td>6</td><td>Kentucky</td><td>7.6</td><td>15</td><td>Louisiana</td><td>6.9</td></tr>
<tr><td>15</td><td>Louisiana</td><td>6.9</td><td>18</td><td>Connecticut</td><td>6.8</td></tr>
<tr><td>40</td><td>Maine</td><td>6.0</td><td>18</td><td>Montana</td><td>6.8</td></tr>
<tr><td>23</td><td>Maryland</td><td>6.7</td><td>18</td><td>New Jersey</td><td>6.8</td></tr>
<tr><td>31</td><td>Massachusetts</td><td>6.6</td><td>18</td><td>Ohio</td><td>6.8</td></tr>
<tr><td>31</td><td>Michigan</td><td>6.6</td><td>18</td><td>Rhode Island</td><td>6.8</td></tr>
<tr><td>45</td><td>Minnesota</td><td>5.6</td><td>23</td><td>Arizona</td><td>6.7</td></tr>
<tr><td>7</td><td>Mississippi</td><td>7.4</td><td>23</td><td>Georgia</td><td>6.7</td></tr>
<tr><td>23</td><td>Missouri</td><td>6.7</td><td>23</td><td>Kansas</td><td>6.7</td></tr>
<tr><td>18</td><td>Montana</td><td>6.8</td><td>23</td><td>Maryland</td><td>6.7</td></tr>
<tr><td>35</td><td>Nebraska</td><td>6.4</td><td>23</td><td>Missouri</td><td>6.7</td></tr>
<tr><td>13</td><td>Nevada</td><td>7.1</td><td>23</td><td>New York</td><td>6.7</td></tr>
<tr><td>37</td><td>New Hampshire</td><td>6.2</td><td>23</td><td>Pennsylvania</td><td>6.7</td></tr>
<tr><td>18</td><td>New Jersey</td><td>6.8</td><td>23</td><td>Utah</td><td>6.7</td></tr>
<tr><td>5</td><td>New Mexico</td><td>7.7</td><td>31</td><td>Massachusetts</td><td>6.6</td></tr>
<tr><td>23</td><td>New York</td><td>6.7</td><td>31</td><td>Michigan</td><td>6.6</td></tr>
<tr><td>10</td><td>North Carolina</td><td>7.2</td><td>31</td><td>Texas</td><td>6.6</td></tr>
<tr><td>37</td><td>North Dakota</td><td>6.2</td><td>34</td><td>Illinois</td><td>6.5</td></tr>
<tr><td>18</td><td>Ohio</td><td>6.8</td><td>35</td><td>Nebraska</td><td>6.4</td></tr>
<tr><td>13</td><td>Oklahoma</td><td>7.1</td><td>35</td><td>Virginia</td><td>6.4</td></tr>
<tr><td>49</td><td>Oregon</td><td>5.3</td><td>37</td><td>New Hampshire</td><td>6.2</td></tr>
<tr><td>23</td><td>Pennsylvania</td><td>6.7</td><td>37</td><td>North Dakota</td><td>6.2</td></tr>
<tr><td>18</td><td>Rhode Island</td><td>6.8</td><td>39</td><td>Idaho</td><td>6.1</td></tr>
<tr><td>10</td><td>South Carolina</td><td>7.2</td><td>40</td><td>Maine</td><td>6.0</td></tr>
<tr><td>41</td><td>South Dakota</td><td>5.9</td><td>41</td><td>Iowa</td><td>5.9</td></tr>
<tr><td>3</td><td>Tennessee</td><td>7.9</td><td>41</td><td>South Dakota</td><td>5.9</td></tr>
<tr><td>31</td><td>Texas</td><td>6.6</td><td>41</td><td>Wisconsin</td><td>5.9</td></tr>
<tr><td>23</td><td>Utah</td><td>6.7</td><td>44</td><td>Vermont</td><td>5.7</td></tr>
<tr><td>44</td><td>Vermont</td><td>5.7</td><td>45</td><td>Minnesota</td><td>5.6</td></tr>
<tr><td>35</td><td>Virginia</td><td>6.4</td><td>46</td><td>California</td><td>5.5</td></tr>
<tr><td>46</td><td>Washington</td><td>5.5</td><td>46</td><td>Hawaii</td><td>5.5</td></tr>
<tr><td>3</td><td>West Virginia</td><td>7.9</td><td>46</td><td>Washington</td><td>5.5</td></tr>
<tr><td>41</td><td>Wisconsin</td><td>5.9</td><td>49</td><td>Alaska</td><td>5.3</td></tr>
<tr><td>1</td><td>Wyoming</td><td>8.1</td><td>49</td><td>Oregon</td><td>5.3</td></tr>
<tr><td></td><td></td><td></td><td></td><td>District of Columbia</td><td>6.2</td></tr>
</table>

Source: U.S. Department of Health and Human Services, National Center for Health Statistics
"National Vital Statistics Reports" (Vol. 48, No. 14, August 8, 2000)
Estimates based on preliminary data by state of residence. Births of less than 2,500 grams (5 pounds 8 ounces).

Births of Low Birthweight to Black Women in 1999

National Total = 79,480 Live Births*

ALPHA ORDER

RANK ORDER

RANK	STATE	BIRTHS	% of USA		RANK	STATE	BIRTHS	% of USA
15	Alabama	2,689	3.4%		1	New York	6,294	7.9%
40	Alaska	49	0.1%		2	Florida	5,502	6.9%
32	Arizona	345	0.4%		3	Georgia	5,348	6.7%
21	Arkansas	1,003	1.3%		4	Texas	4,899	6.2%
6	California	4,175	5.3%		5	Illinois	4,864	6.1%
28	Colorado	397	0.5%		6	California	4,175	5.3%
24	Connecticut	701	0.9%		7	Louisiana	3,920	4.9%
29	Delaware	368	0.5%		8	North Carolina	3,897	4.9%
2	Florida	5,502	6.9%		9	Michigan	3,536	4.4%
3	Georgia	5,348	6.7%		10	Maryland	3,317	4.2%
41	Hawaii	44	0.1%		11	Pennsylvania	2,947	3.7%
NA	Idaho**	NA	NA		12	Ohio	2,817	3.5%
5	Illinois	4,864	6.1%		13	South Carolina	2,808	3.5%
20	Indiana	1,203	1.5%		14	New Jersey	2,780	3.5%
35	Iowa	148	0.2%		15	Alabama	2,689	3.4%
30	Kansas	346	0.4%		16	Mississippi	2,680	3.4%
25	Kentucky	689	0.9%		17	Virginia	2,677	3.4%
7	Louisiana	3,920	4.9%		18	Tennessee	2,332	2.9%
NA	Maine**	NA	NA		19	Missouri	1,542	1.9%
10	Maryland	3,317	4.2%		20	Indiana	1,203	1.5%
22	Massachusetts	896	1.1%		21	Arkansas	1,003	1.3%
9	Michigan	3,536	4.4%		22	Massachusetts	896	1.1%
27	Minnesota	444	0.6%		23	Wisconsin	872	1.1%
16	Mississippi	2,680	3.4%		24	Connecticut	701	0.9%
19	Missouri	1,542	1.9%		25	Kentucky	689	0.9%
NA	Montana**	NA	NA		26	Oklahoma	549	0.7%
34	Nebraska	164	0.2%		27	Minnesota	444	0.6%
33	Nevada	271	0.3%		28	Colorado	397	0.5%
NA	New Hampshire**	NA	NA		29	Delaware	368	0.5%
14	New Jersey	2,780	3.5%		30	Kansas	346	0.4%
39	New Mexico	62	0.1%		30	Washington	346	0.4%
1	New York	6,294	7.9%		32	Arizona	345	0.4%
8	North Carolina	3,897	4.9%		33	Nevada	271	0.3%
NA	North Dakota**	NA	NA		34	Nebraska	164	0.2%
12	Ohio	2,817	3.5%		35	Iowa	148	0.2%
26	Oklahoma	549	0.7%		36	Rhode Island	107	0.1%
37	Oregon	97	0.1%		37	Oregon	97	0.1%
11	Pennsylvania	2,947	3.7%		38	West Virginia	92	0.1%
36	Rhode Island	107	0.1%		39	New Mexico	62	0.1%
13	South Carolina	2,808	3.5%		40	Alaska	49	0.1%
NA	South Dakota**	NA	NA		41	Hawaii	44	0.1%
18	Tennessee	2,332	2.9%		42	Utah	36	0.0%
4	Texas	4,899	6.2%		NA	Idaho**	NA	NA
42	Utah	36	0.0%		NA	Maine**	NA	NA
NA	Vermont**	NA	NA		NA	Montana**	NA	NA
17	Virginia	2,677	3.4%		NA	New Hampshire**	NA	NA
30	Washington	346	0.4%		NA	North Dakota**	NA	NA
38	West Virginia	92	0.1%		NA	South Dakota**	NA	NA
23	Wisconsin	872	1.1%		NA	Vermont**	NA	NA
NA	Wyoming**	NA	NA		NA	Wyoming**	NA	NA
						District of Columbia	866	1.1%

Source: Morgan Quitno Press using data from U.S. Dept. of Health and Human Services, Nat'l Center for Health Statistics "National Vital Statistics Reports" (Vol. 48, No. 14, August 8, 2000)
Births of less than 2,500 grams (5 pounds 8 ounces). Preliminary data by state of residence. Calculated by the editors by multiplying total number of births to black women by percent of births to black women reported as being low birthweight.
***Insufficient data.*

Births of Low Birthweight to Black Women
As a Percent of All Births to Black Women in 1999
National Percent = 13.1% of Live Births to Black Women*

ALPHA ORDER

RANK	STATE	PERCENT
13	Alabama	13.6
39	Alaska	10.7
27	Arizona	12.3
19	Arkansas	13.0
35	California	11.6
9	Colorado	13.7
18	Connecticut	13.2
9	Delaware	13.7
29	Florida	12.2
23	Georgia	12.7
42	Hawaii	9.6
NA	Idaho**	NA
5	Illinois	14.2
21	Indiana	12.9
23	Iowa	12.7
31	Kansas	12.1
7	Kentucky	13.9
3	Louisiana	14.4
NA	Maine**	NA
14	Maryland	13.5
38	Massachusetts	10.8
1	Michigan	14.7
37	Minnesota	11.0
8	Mississippi	13.8
9	Missouri	13.7
NA	Montana**	NA
22	Nebraska	12.8
29	Nevada	12.2
NA	New Hampshire**	NA
19	New Jersey	13.0
26	New Mexico	12.4
34	New York	11.7
9	North Carolina	13.7
NA	North Dakota**	NA
15	Ohio	13.4
33	Oklahoma	11.8
39	Oregon	10.7
4	Pennsylvania	14.3
36	Rhode Island	11.1
1	South Carolina	14.7
NA	South Dakota**	NA
6	Tennessee	14.1
25	Texas	12.6
17	Utah	13.3
NA	Vermont**	NA
32	Virginia	11.9
41	Washington	10.3
27	West Virginia	12.3
15	Wisconsin	13.4
NA	Wyoming**	NA

RANK ORDER

RANK	STATE	PERCENT
1	Michigan	14.7
1	South Carolina	14.7
3	Louisiana	14.4
4	Pennsylvania	14.3
5	Illinois	14.2
6	Tennessee	14.1
7	Kentucky	13.9
8	Mississippi	13.8
9	Colorado	13.7
9	Delaware	13.7
9	Missouri	13.7
9	North Carolina	13.7
13	Alabama	13.6
14	Maryland	13.5
15	Ohio	13.4
15	Wisconsin	13.4
17	Utah	13.3
18	Connecticut	13.2
19	Arkansas	13.0
19	New Jersey	13.0
21	Indiana	12.9
22	Nebraska	12.8
23	Georgia	12.7
23	Iowa	12.7
25	Texas	12.6
26	New Mexico	12.4
27	Arizona	12.3
27	West Virginia	12.3
29	Florida	12.2
29	Nevada	12.2
31	Kansas	12.1
32	Virginia	11.9
33	Oklahoma	11.8
34	New York	11.7
35	California	11.6
36	Rhode Island	11.1
37	Minnesota	11.0
38	Massachusetts	10.8
39	Alaska	10.7
39	Oregon	10.7
41	Washington	10.3
42	Hawaii	9.6
NA	Idaho**	NA
NA	Maine**	NA
NA	Montana**	NA
NA	New Hampshire**	NA
NA	North Dakota**	NA
NA	South Dakota**	NA
NA	Vermont**	NA
NA	Wyoming**	NA
	District of Columbia	15.3

Source: U.S. Department of Health and Human Services, National Center for Health Statistics
"National Vital Statistics Reports" (Vol. 48, No. 14, August 8, 2000)
Estimates based on preliminary data by state of residence. Births of less than 2,500 grams (5 pounds 8 ounces).
***Insufficient data.*

Births to Unmarried Women in 1999

National Total = 1,306,084 Live Births*

ALPHA ORDER

ALPHA ORDER

RANK	STATE	BIRTHS	% of USA
22	Alabama	20,687	1.6%
46	Alaska	3,294	0.3%
12	Arizona	31,434	2.4%
30	Arkansas	12,965	1.0%
1	California	170,497	13.1%
28	Colorado	15,789	1.2%
31	Connecticut	12,563	1.0%
42	Delaware	4,153	0.3%
4	Florida	73,880	5.7%
8	Georgia	46,388	3.6%
39	Hawaii	5,574	0.4%
40	Idaho	4,292	0.3%
5	Illinois	62,121	4.8%
14	Indiana	29,684	2.3%
35	Iowa	10,324	0.8%
33	Kansas	11,093	0.8%
26	Kentucky	16,466	1.3%
13	Louisiana	29,977	2.3%
41	Maine	4,261	0.3%
18	Maryland	25,200	1.9%
19	Massachusetts	21,464	1.6%
9	Michigan	44,209	3.4%
25	Minnesota	17,019	1.3%
24	Mississippi	19,639	1.5%
17	Missouri	25,695	2.0%
47	Montana	3,204	0.2%
38	Nebraska	6,192	0.5%
34	Nevada	10,480	0.8%
44	New Hampshire	3,405	0.3%
11	New Jersey	32,175	2.5%
32	New Mexico	12,179	0.9%
3	New York	94,320	7.2%
10	North Carolina	37,782	2.9%
48	North Dakota	2,100	0.2%
6	Ohio	51,099	3.9%
27	Oklahoma	16,139	1.2%
29	Oregon	13,742	1.1%
7	Pennsylvania	47,869	3.7%
43	Rhode Island	4,115	0.3%
20	South Carolina	21,444	1.6%
45	South Dakota	3,346	0.3%
16	Tennessee	26,932	2.1%
2	Texas	107,500	8.2%
36	Utah	7,730	0.6%
49	Vermont	1,904	0.1%
15	Virginia	28,470	2.2%
21	Washington	21,095	1.6%
37	West Virginia	6,582	0.5%
23	Wisconsin	19,919	1.5%
50	Wyoming	1,785	0.1%

RANK ORDER

RANK	STATE	BIRTHS	% of USA
1	California	170,497	13.1%
2	Texas	107,500	8.2%
3	New York	94,320	7.2%
4	Florida	73,880	5.7%
5	Illinois	62,121	4.8%
6	Ohio	51,099	3.9%
7	Pennsylvania	47,869	3.7%
8	Georgia	46,388	3.6%
9	Michigan	44,209	3.4%
10	North Carolina	37,782	2.9%
11	New Jersey	32,175	2.5%
12	Arizona	31,434	2.4%
13	Louisiana	29,977	2.3%
14	Indiana	29,684	2.3%
15	Virginia	28,470	2.2%
16	Tennessee	26,932	2.1%
17	Missouri	25,695	2.0%
18	Maryland	25,200	1.9%
19	Massachusetts	21,464	1.6%
20	South Carolina	21,444	1.6%
21	Washington	21,095	1.6%
22	Alabama	20,687	1.6%
23	Wisconsin	19,919	1.5%
24	Mississippi	19,639	1.5%
25	Minnesota	17,019	1.3%
26	Kentucky	16,466	1.3%
27	Oklahoma	16,139	1.2%
28	Colorado	15,789	1.2%
29	Oregon	13,742	1.1%
30	Arkansas	12,965	1.0%
31	Connecticut	12,563	1.0%
32	New Mexico	12,179	0.9%
33	Kansas	11,093	0.8%
34	Nevada	10,480	0.8%
35	Iowa	10,324	0.8%
36	Utah	7,730	0.6%
37	West Virginia	6,582	0.5%
38	Nebraska	6,192	0.5%
39	Hawaii	5,574	0.4%
40	Idaho	4,292	0.3%
41	Maine	4,261	0.3%
42	Delaware	4,153	0.3%
43	Rhode Island	4,115	0.3%
44	New Hampshire	3,405	0.3%
45	South Dakota	3,346	0.3%
46	Alaska	3,294	0.3%
47	Montana	3,204	0.2%
48	North Dakota	2,100	0.2%
49	Vermont	1,904	0.1%
50	Wyoming	1,785	0.1%
	District of Columbia	4,642	0.4%

Source: Morgan Quitno Press using data from U.S. Dept. of Health and Human Services, Nat'l Center for Health Statistics
"National Vital Statistics Reports" (Vol. 48, No. 14, August 8, 2000)
*Preliminary data by state of residence. Calculated by the editors by multiplying total number of births by reported percent of births to unmarried women.

Births to Unmarried Women as a Percent of All Births in 1999

National Percent = 33.0% of Live Births*

ALPHA ORDER

ALPHA ORDER

RANK ORDER

RANK	STATE	PERCENT		RANK	STATE	PERCENT
18	Alabama	33.3		1	Mississippi	46.0
21	Alaska	33.1		2	New Mexico	45.0
6	Arizona	38.7		3	Louisiana	44.8
11	Arkansas	35.2		4	South Carolina	39.0
23	California	32.9		5	Delaware	38.9
47	Colorado	25.4		6	Arizona	38.7
38	Connecticut	28.9		7	Florida	37.5
5	Delaware	38.9		8	Georgia	36.6
7	Florida	37.5		9	New York	36.5
8	Georgia	36.6		10	Nevada	35.7
26	Hawaii	32.7		11	Arkansas	35.2
49	Idaho	21.6		12	Maryland	34.9
15	Illinois	34.1		13	Tennessee	34.6
14	Indiana	34.5		14	Indiana	34.5
41	Iowa	27.5		15	Illinois	34.1
39	Kansas	28.6		15	Missouri	34.1
32	Kentucky	30.3		17	Ohio	34.0
3	Louisiana	44.8		18	Alabama	33.3
29	Maine	31.3		18	Rhode Island	33.3
12	Maryland	34.9		20	North Carolina	33.2
43	Massachusetts	26.5		21	Alaska	33.1
21	Michigan	33.1		21	Michigan	33.1
46	Minnesota	25.8		23	California	32.9
1	Mississippi	46.0		23	Oklahoma	32.9
15	Missouri	34.1		23	Pennsylvania	32.9
34	Montana	29.7		26	Hawaii	32.7
45	Nebraska	25.9		27	South Dakota	31.8
10	Nevada	35.7		28	West Virginia	31.7
48	New Hampshire	24.2		29	Maine	31.3
40	New Jersey	28.2		30	Texas	31.0
2	New Mexico	45.0		31	Oregon	30.4
9	New York	36.5		32	Kentucky	30.3
20	North Carolina	33.2		33	Virginia	29.8
41	North Dakota	27.5		34	Montana	29.7
17	Ohio	34.0		35	Wisconsin	29.2
23	Oklahoma	32.9		36	Wyoming	29.1
31	Oregon	30.4		37	Vermont	29.0
23	Pennsylvania	32.9		38	Connecticut	28.9
18	Rhode Island	33.3		39	Kansas	28.6
4	South Carolina	39.0		40	New Jersey	28.2
27	South Dakota	31.8		41	Iowa	27.5
13	Tennessee	34.6		41	North Dakota	27.5
30	Texas	31.0		43	Massachusetts	26.5
50	Utah	16.7		43	Washington	26.5
37	Vermont	29.0		45	Nebraska	25.9
33	Virginia	29.8		46	Minnesota	25.8
43	Washington	26.5		47	Colorado	25.4
28	West Virginia	31.7		48	New Hampshire	24.2
35	Wisconsin	29.2		49	Idaho	21.6
36	Wyoming	29.1		50	Utah	16.7
					District of Columbia	61.7

*Source: U.S. Department of Health and Human Services, National Center for Health Statistics
"National Vital Statistics Reports" (Vol. 48, No. 14, August 8, 2000)
Preliminary data by state of residence.

Births to Unmarried White Women in 1999

National Total = 835,737 Live Births*

ALPHA ORDER

RANK	STATE	BIRTHS	% of USA
33	Alabama	7,177	0.9%
49	Alaska	1,502	0.2%
9	Arizona	25,605	3.1%
35	Arkansas	7,034	0.8%
1	California	137,401	16.4%
19	Colorado	13,666	1.6%
29	Connecticut	8,833	1.1%
44	Delaware	2,150	0.3%
4	Florida	42,532	5.1%
11	Georgia	17,770	2.1%
50	Hawaii	704	0.1%
40	Idaho	4,054	0.5%
5	Illinois	35,060	4.2%
10	Indiana	22,257	2.7%
28	Iowa	9,190	1.1%
30	Kansas	8,791	1.1%
22	Kentucky	12,723	1.5%
25	Louisiana	9,640	1.2%
39	Maine	4,118	0.5%
26	Maryland	9,568	1.1%
16	Massachusetts	15,758	1.9%
8	Michigan	25,902	3.1%
21	Minnesota	12,820	1.5%
38	Mississippi	4,760	0.6%
15	Missouri	16,696	2.0%
43	Montana	2,281	0.3%
37	Nebraska	4,932	0.6%
31	Nevada	8,292	1.0%
41	New Hampshire	3,319	0.4%
12	New Jersey	17,746	2.1%
27	New Mexico	9,413	1.1%
3	New York	54,722	6.5%
13	North Carolina	17,709	2.1%
48	North Dakota	1,544	0.2%
6	Ohio	34,698	4.2%
24	Oklahoma	10,430	1.2%
23	Oregon	12,382	1.5%
7	Pennsylvania	31,355	3.8%
42	Rhode Island	3,228	0.4%
32	South Carolina	7,802	0.9%
45	South Dakota	2,046	0.2%
17	Tennessee	14,580	1.7%
2	Texas	82,013	9.8%
34	Utah	7,045	0.8%
46	Vermont	1,870	0.2%
18	Virginia	13,981	1.7%
14	Washington	17,125	2.0%
36	West Virginia	5,988	0.7%
20	Wisconsin	13,636	1.6%
47	Wyoming	1,563	0.2%

RANK ORDER

RANK	STATE	BIRTHS	% of USA
1	California	137,401	16.4%
2	Texas	82,013	9.8%
3	New York	54,722	6.5%
4	Florida	42,532	5.1%
5	Illinois	35,060	4.2%
6	Ohio	34,698	4.2%
7	Pennsylvania	31,355	3.8%
8	Michigan	25,902	3.1%
9	Arizona	25,605	3.1%
10	Indiana	22,257	2.7%
11	Georgia	17,770	2.1%
12	New Jersey	17,746	2.1%
13	North Carolina	17,709	2.1%
14	Washington	17,125	2.0%
15	Missouri	16,696	2.0%
16	Massachusetts	15,758	1.9%
17	Tennessee	14,580	1.7%
18	Virginia	13,981	1.7%
19	Colorado	13,666	1.6%
20	Wisconsin	13,636	1.6%
21	Minnesota	12,820	1.5%
22	Kentucky	12,723	1.5%
23	Oregon	12,382	1.5%
24	Oklahoma	10,430	1.2%
25	Louisiana	9,640	1.2%
26	Maryland	9,568	1.1%
27	New Mexico	9,413	1.1%
28	Iowa	9,190	1.1%
29	Connecticut	8,833	1.1%
30	Kansas	8,791	1.1%
31	Nevada	8,292	1.0%
32	South Carolina	7,802	0.9%
33	Alabama	7,177	0.9%
34	Utah	7,045	0.8%
35	Arkansas	7,034	0.8%
36	West Virginia	5,988	0.7%
37	Nebraska	4,932	0.6%
38	Mississippi	4,760	0.6%
39	Maine	4,118	0.5%
40	Idaho	4,054	0.5%
41	New Hampshire	3,319	0.4%
42	Rhode Island	3,228	0.4%
43	Montana	2,281	0.3%
44	Delaware	2,150	0.3%
45	South Dakota	2,046	0.2%
46	Vermont	1,870	0.2%
47	Wyoming	1,563	0.2%
48	North Dakota	1,544	0.2%
49	Alaska	1,502	0.2%
50	Hawaii	704	0.1%
	District of Columbia	240	0.0%

Source: Morgan Quitno Press using data from U.S. Dept. of Health and Human Services, Nat'l Center for Health Statistics "National Vital Statistics Reports" (Vol. 48, No. 14, August 8, 2000)
Preliminary data by state of residence. Calculated by the editors by multiplying total number of births to white women by percent of such births reported as being to unmarried white women.

Births to Unmarried White Women
As a Percent of All Births to White Women in 1999
National Percent = 26.7% of Live Births*

ALPHA ORDER

RANK	STATE	PERCENT
49	Alabama	17.2
36	Alaska	23.0
2	Arizona	36.0
26	Arkansas	24.7
4	California	32.7
32	Colorado	24.1
31	Connecticut	24.2
13	Delaware	28.0
11	Florida	29.0
41	Georgia	21.9
48	Hawaii	17.6
44	Idaho	21.1
25	Illinois	24.9
9	Indiana	29.5
20	Iowa	26.0
22	Kansas	25.4
19	Kentucky	26.1
23	Louisiana	25.1
5	Maine	31.1
43	Maryland	21.6
35	Massachusetts	23.1
27	Michigan	24.6
39	Minnesota	22.3
46	Mississippi	21.0
18	Missouri	26.7
28	Montana	24.3
38	Nebraska	22.7
3	Nevada	33.2
28	New Hampshire	24.3
44	New Jersey	21.1
1	New Mexico	41.3
10	New York	29.4
42	North Carolina	21.8
37	North Dakota	22.9
15	Ohio	27.4
17	Oklahoma	27.0
7	Oregon	29.9
21	Pennsylvania	25.9
7	Rhode Island	29.9
39	South Carolina	22.3
33	South Dakota	23.6
28	Tennessee	24.3
14	Texas	27.6
50	Utah	16.0
12	Vermont	28.9
47	Virginia	20.5
23	Washington	25.1
6	West Virginia	30.2
34	Wisconsin	23.2
16	Wyoming	27.2

RANK ORDER

RANK	STATE	PERCENT
1	New Mexico	41.3
2	Arizona	36.0
3	Nevada	33.2
4	California	32.7
5	Maine	31.1
6	West Virginia	30.2
7	Oregon	29.9
7	Rhode Island	29.9
9	Indiana	29.5
10	New York	29.4
11	Florida	29.0
12	Vermont	28.9
13	Delaware	28.0
14	Texas	27.6
15	Ohio	27.4
16	Wyoming	27.2
17	Oklahoma	27.0
18	Missouri	26.7
19	Kentucky	26.1
20	Iowa	26.0
21	Pennsylvania	25.9
22	Kansas	25.4
23	Louisiana	25.1
23	Washington	25.1
25	Illinois	24.9
26	Arkansas	24.7
27	Michigan	24.6
28	Montana	24.3
28	New Hampshire	24.3
28	Tennessee	24.3
31	Connecticut	24.2
32	Colorado	24.1
33	South Dakota	23.6
34	Wisconsin	23.2
35	Massachusetts	23.1
36	Alaska	23.0
37	North Dakota	22.9
38	Nebraska	22.7
39	Minnesota	22.3
39	South Carolina	22.3
41	Georgia	21.9
42	North Carolina	21.8
43	Maryland	21.6
44	Idaho	21.1
44	New Jersey	21.1
46	Mississippi	21.0
47	Virginia	20.5
48	Hawaii	17.6
49	Alabama	17.2
50	Utah	16.0
	District of Columbia	14.2

Source: U.S. Department of Health and Human Services, National Center for Health Statistics
"National Vital Statistics Reports" (Vol. 48, No. 14, August 8, 2000)
*Preliminary data by state of residence.

Births to Unmarried Black Women in 1999

National Total = 417,423 Live Births*

ALPHA ORDER

RANK	STATE	BIRTHS	% of USA	RANK	STATE	BIRTHS	% of USA
17	Alabama	13,405	3.2%	1	New York	36,529	8.8%
40	Alaska	211	0.1%	2	Florida	30,259	7.2%
30	Arizona	1,780	0.4%	3	Georgia	28,089	6.7%
21	Arkansas	5,749	1.4%	4	Illinois	26,410	6.3%
6	California	22,314	5.3%	5	Texas	24,224	5.8%
32	Colorado	1,583	0.4%	6	California	22,314	5.3%
25	Connecticut	3,555	0.9%	7	Louisiana	20,038	4.8%
29	Delaware	1,957	0.5%	8	North Carolina	18,888	4.5%
2	Florida	30,259	7.2%	9	Michigan	17,489	4.2%
3	Georgia	28,089	6.7%	10	Pennsylvania	16,012	3.8%
42	Hawaii	114	0.0%	11	Ohio	15,996	3.8%
46	Idaho	32	0.0%	12	Maryland	15,232	3.6%
4	Illinois	26,410	6.3%	13	Mississippi	14,640	3.5%
20	Indiana	7,179	1.7%	14	Virginia	14,039	3.4%
35	Iowa	829	0.2%	15	New Jersey	13,815	3.3%
28	Kansas	1,975	0.5%	16	South Carolina	13,487	3.2%
24	Kentucky	3,620	0.9%	17	Alabama	13,405	3.2%
7	Louisiana	20,038	4.8%	18	Tennessee	12,122	2.9%
43	Maine	52	0.0%	19	Missouri	8,609	2.1%
12	Maryland	15,232	3.6%	20	Indiana	7,179	1.7%
23	Massachusetts	4,917	1.2%	21	Arkansas	5,749	1.4%
9	Michigan	17,489	4.2%	22	Wisconsin	5,435	1.3%
27	Minnesota	2,493	0.6%	23	Massachusetts	4,917	1.2%
13	Mississippi	14,640	3.5%	24	Kentucky	3,620	0.9%
19	Missouri	8,609	2.1%	25	Connecticut	3,555	0.9%
NA	Montana**	NA	NA	26	Oklahoma	3,278	0.8%
34	Nebraska	894	0.2%	27	Minnesota	2,493	0.6%
33	Nevada	1,512	0.4%	28	Kansas	1,975	0.5%
43	New Hampshire	52	0.0%	29	Delaware	1,957	0.5%
15	New Jersey	13,815	3.3%	30	Arizona	1,780	0.4%
39	New Mexico	315	0.1%	31	Washington	1,698	0.4%
1	New York	36,529	8.8%	32	Colorado	1,583	0.4%
8	North Carolina	18,888	4.5%	33	Nevada	1,512	0.4%
48	North Dakota	23	0.0%	34	Nebraska	894	0.2%
11	Ohio	15,996	3.8%	35	Iowa	829	0.2%
26	Oklahoma	3,278	0.8%	36	Rhode Island	628	0.2%
38	Oregon	570	0.1%	37	West Virginia	584	0.1%
10	Pennsylvania	16,012	3.8%	38	Oregon	570	0.1%
36	Rhode Island	628	0.2%	39	New Mexico	315	0.1%
16	South Carolina	13,487	3.2%	40	Alaska	211	0.1%
46	South Dakota	32	0.0%	41	Utah	138	0.0%
18	Tennessee	12,122	2.9%	42	Hawaii	114	0.0%
5	Texas	24,224	5.8%	43	Maine	52	0.0%
41	Utah	138	0.0%	43	New Hampshire	52	0.0%
49	Vermont	22	0.0%	45	Wyoming	39	0.0%
14	Virginia	14,039	3.4%	46	Idaho	32	0.0%
31	Washington	1,698	0.4%	46	South Dakota	32	0.0%
37	West Virginia	584	0.1%	48	North Dakota	23	0.0%
22	Wisconsin	5,435	1.3%	49	Vermont	22	0.0%
45	Wyoming	39	0.0%	NA	Montana**	NA	NA
					District of Columbia	4,371	1.0%

Source: Morgan Quitno Press using data from U.S. Dept. of Health and Human Services, Nat'l Center for Health Statistics "National Vital Statistics Reports" (Vol. 48, No. 14, August 8, 2000)
Preliminary data by state of residence. Calculated by the editors by multiplying total number of births to black women by percent of such births reported as being to unmarried black women.
**Not available.*

Births to Unmarried Black Women
As a Percent of All Births to Black Women in 1999
National Percent = 68.8% of Live Births*

RANK	STATE	PERCENT
22	Alabama	67.8
44	Alaska	45.9
29	Arizona	63.5
9	Arkansas	74.5
34	California	62.0
39	Colorado	54.6
24	Connecticut	66.9
13	Delaware	72.8
23	Florida	67.1
25	Georgia	66.7
49	Hawaii	24.8
45	Idaho	41.6
4	Illinois	77.1
5	Indiana	77.0
15	Iowa	71.2
19	Kansas	69.1
12	Kentucky	73.0
10	Louisiana	73.6
43	Maine	49.1
34	Maryland	62.0
37	Massachusetts	59.3
14	Michigan	72.7
36	Minnesota	61.8
8	Mississippi	75.4
6	Missouri	76.5
NA	Montana**	NA
18	Nebraska	69.8
20	Nevada	68.0
46	New Hampshire	37.4
28	New Jersey	64.6
30	New Mexico	63.3
21	New York	67.9
26	North Carolina	66.4
48	North Dakota	26.7
7	Ohio	76.1
17	Oklahoma	70.5
31	Oregon	63.0
2	Pennsylvania	77.7
27	Rhode Island	64.9
16	South Carolina	70.6
47	South Dakota	36.0
11	Tennessee	73.3
33	Texas	62.3
41	Utah	51.1
38	Vermont	55.0
32	Virginia	62.4
42	Washington	50.5
2	West Virginia	77.7
1	Wisconsin	83.5
40	Wyoming	54.1

RANK	STATE	PERCENT
1	Wisconsin	83.5
2	Pennsylvania	77.7
2	West Virginia	77.7
4	Illinois	77.1
5	Indiana	77.0
6	Missouri	76.5
7	Ohio	76.1
8	Mississippi	75.4
9	Arkansas	74.5
10	Louisiana	73.6
11	Tennessee	73.3
12	Kentucky	73.0
13	Delaware	72.8
14	Michigan	72.7
15	Iowa	71.2
16	South Carolina	70.6
17	Oklahoma	70.5
18	Nebraska	69.8
19	Kansas	69.1
20	Nevada	68.0
21	New York	67.9
22	Alabama	67.8
23	Florida	67.1
24	Connecticut	66.9
25	Georgia	66.7
26	North Carolina	66.4
27	Rhode Island	64.9
28	New Jersey	64.6
29	Arizona	63.5
30	New Mexico	63.3
31	Oregon	63.0
32	Virginia	62.4
33	Texas	62.3
34	California	62.0
34	Maryland	62.0
36	Minnesota	61.8
37	Massachusetts	59.3
38	Vermont	55.0
39	Colorado	54.6
40	Wyoming	54.1
41	Utah	51.1
42	Washington	50.5
43	Maine	49.1
44	Alaska	45.9
45	Idaho	41.6
46	New Hampshire	37.4
47	South Dakota	36.0
48	North Dakota	26.7
49	Hawaii	24.8
NA	Montana**	NA
	District of Columbia	77.2

Source: U.S. Department of Health and Human Services, National Center for Health Statistics
"National Vital Statistics Reports" (Vol. 48, No. 14, August 8, 2000)
Data are preliminary estimates by state of residence. By race of mother.
**Too few births for a reliable figure.*

Births to Teenage Mothers in 1999

National Total = 482,855 Live Births*

ALPHA ORDER

RANK	STATE	BIRTHS	% of USA
17	Alabama	10,064	2.1%
46	Alaska	1,145	0.2%
11	Arizona	12,021	2.5%
27	Arkansas	6,556	1.4%
1	California	57,523	11.9%
25	Colorado	7,335	1.5%
36	Connecticut	3,478	0.7%
41	Delaware	1,420	0.3%
3	Florida	25,415	5.3%
7	Georgia	18,505	3.8%
40	Hawaii	1,773	0.4%
39	Idaho	2,424	0.5%
5	Illinois	21,861	4.5%
14	Indiana	11,357	2.4%
34	Iowa	3,979	0.8%
31	Kansas	4,965	1.0%
22	Kentucky	8,152	1.7%
13	Louisiana	11,777	2.4%
42	Maine	1,321	0.3%
24	Maryland	7,437	1.5%
29	Massachusetts	5,589	1.2%
10	Michigan	14,825	3.1%
28	Minnesota	5,607	1.2%
20	Mississippi	8,411	1.7%
15	Missouri	10,173	2.1%
43	Montana	1,262	0.3%
38	Nebraska	2,510	0.5%
35	Nevada	3,846	0.8%
47	New Hampshire	999	0.2%
21	New Jersey	8,329	1.7%
32	New Mexico	4,845	1.0%
4	New York	22,223	4.6%
8	North Carolina	15,363	3.2%
49	North Dakota	710	0.1%
6	Ohio	18,937	3.9%
23	Oklahoma	7,947	1.6%
30	Oregon	5,560	1.2%
9	Pennsylvania	14,986	3.1%
44	Rhode Island	1,199	0.2%
18	South Carolina	8,687	1.8%
45	South Dakota	1,189	0.2%
12	Tennessee	11,987	2.5%
2	Texas	55,137	11.4%
33	Utah	4,305	0.9%
50	Vermont	558	0.1%
16	Virginia	10,127	2.1%
19	Washington	8,597	1.8%
37	West Virginia	3,073	0.6%
26	Wisconsin	7,299	1.5%
48	Wyoming	853	0.2%

RANK ORDER

RANK	STATE	BIRTHS	% of USA
1	California	57,523	11.9%
2	Texas	55,137	11.4%
3	Florida	25,415	5.3%
4	New York	22,223	4.6%
5	Illinois	21,861	4.5%
6	Ohio	18,937	3.9%
7	Georgia	18,505	3.8%
8	North Carolina	15,363	3.2%
9	Pennsylvania	14,986	3.1%
10	Michigan	14,825	3.1%
11	Arizona	12,021	2.5%
12	Tennessee	11,987	2.5%
13	Louisiana	11,777	2.4%
14	Indiana	11,357	2.4%
15	Missouri	10,173	2.1%
16	Virginia	10,127	2.1%
17	Alabama	10,064	2.1%
18	South Carolina	8,687	1.8%
19	Washington	8,597	1.8%
20	Mississippi	8,411	1.7%
21	New Jersey	8,329	1.7%
22	Kentucky	8,152	1.7%
23	Oklahoma	7,947	1.6%
24	Maryland	7,437	1.5%
25	Colorado	7,335	1.5%
26	Wisconsin	7,299	1.5%
27	Arkansas	6,556	1.4%
28	Minnesota	5,607	1.2%
29	Massachusetts	5,589	1.2%
30	Oregon	5,560	1.2%
31	Kansas	4,965	1.0%
32	New Mexico	4,845	1.0%
33	Utah	4,305	0.9%
34	Iowa	3,979	0.8%
35	Nevada	3,846	0.8%
36	Connecticut	3,478	0.7%
37	West Virginia	3,073	0.6%
38	Nebraska	2,510	0.5%
39	Idaho	2,424	0.5%
40	Hawaii	1,773	0.4%
41	Delaware	1,420	0.3%
42	Maine	1,321	0.3%
43	Montana	1,262	0.3%
44	Rhode Island	1,199	0.2%
45	South Dakota	1,189	0.2%
46	Alaska	1,145	0.2%
47	New Hampshire	999	0.2%
48	Wyoming	853	0.2%
49	North Dakota	710	0.1%
50	Vermont	558	0.1%
	District of Columbia	1,113	0.2%

Source: Morgan Quitno Press using data from U.S. Dept. of Health and Human Services, Nat'l Center for Health Statistics "National Vital Statistics Reports" (Vol. 48, No. 14, August 8, 2000)

*Preliminary data. Live births to women under the age of 20 years old. These numbers were calculated by the editors by multiplying the percent of live births to teenage women times total births. These are rough estimates and differ from other teenage birth numbers in this book in that they include births to women under the age of 15.

Percent of Births to Teenage Mothers in 1999

National Percent = 12.2% of Live Births*

<table>
<tr><td colspan="3">ALPHA ORDER</td><td colspan="3">RANK ORDER</td></tr>
<tr><td>RANK</td><td>STATE</td><td>PERCENT</td><td>RANK</td><td>STATE</td><td>PERCENT</td></tr>
<tr><td>5</td><td>Alabama</td><td>16.2</td><td>1</td><td>Mississippi</td><td>19.7</td></tr>
<tr><td>28</td><td>Alaska</td><td>11.5</td><td>2</td><td>New Mexico</td><td>17.9</td></tr>
<tr><td>11</td><td>Arizona</td><td>14.8</td><td>3</td><td>Arkansas</td><td>17.8</td></tr>
<tr><td>3</td><td>Arkansas</td><td>17.8</td><td>4</td><td>Louisiana</td><td>17.6</td></tr>
<tr><td>30</td><td>California</td><td>11.1</td><td>5</td><td>Alabama</td><td>16.2</td></tr>
<tr><td>26</td><td>Colorado</td><td>11.8</td><td>5</td><td>Oklahoma</td><td>16.2</td></tr>
<tr><td>47</td><td>Connecticut</td><td>8.0</td><td>7</td><td>Texas</td><td>15.9</td></tr>
<tr><td>17</td><td>Delaware</td><td>13.3</td><td>8</td><td>South Carolina</td><td>15.8</td></tr>
<tr><td>20</td><td>Florida</td><td>12.9</td><td>9</td><td>Tennessee</td><td>15.4</td></tr>
<tr><td>13</td><td>Georgia</td><td>14.6</td><td>10</td><td>Kentucky</td><td>15.0</td></tr>
<tr><td>37</td><td>Hawaii</td><td>10.4</td><td>11</td><td>Arizona</td><td>14.8</td></tr>
<tr><td>24</td><td>Idaho</td><td>12.2</td><td>11</td><td>West Virginia</td><td>14.8</td></tr>
<tr><td>25</td><td>Illinois</td><td>12.0</td><td>13</td><td>Georgia</td><td>14.6</td></tr>
<tr><td>18</td><td>Indiana</td><td>13.2</td><td>14</td><td>Wyoming</td><td>13.9</td></tr>
<tr><td>34</td><td>Iowa</td><td>10.6</td><td>15</td><td>Missouri</td><td>13.5</td></tr>
<tr><td>21</td><td>Kansas</td><td>12.8</td><td>15</td><td>North Carolina</td><td>13.5</td></tr>
<tr><td>10</td><td>Kentucky</td><td>15.0</td><td>17</td><td>Delaware</td><td>13.3</td></tr>
<tr><td>4</td><td>Louisiana</td><td>17.6</td><td>18</td><td>Indiana</td><td>13.2</td></tr>
<tr><td>40</td><td>Maine</td><td>9.7</td><td>19</td><td>Nevada</td><td>13.1</td></tr>
<tr><td>38</td><td>Maryland</td><td>10.3</td><td>20</td><td>Florida</td><td>12.9</td></tr>
<tr><td>50</td><td>Massachusetts</td><td>6.9</td><td>21</td><td>Kansas</td><td>12.8</td></tr>
<tr><td>30</td><td>Michigan</td><td>11.1</td><td>22</td><td>Ohio</td><td>12.6</td></tr>
<tr><td>45</td><td>Minnesota</td><td>8.5</td><td>23</td><td>Oregon</td><td>12.3</td></tr>
<tr><td>1</td><td>Mississippi</td><td>19.7</td><td>24</td><td>Idaho</td><td>12.2</td></tr>
<tr><td>15</td><td>Missouri</td><td>13.5</td><td>25</td><td>Illinois</td><td>12.0</td></tr>
<tr><td>27</td><td>Montana</td><td>11.7</td><td>26</td><td>Colorado</td><td>11.8</td></tr>
<tr><td>36</td><td>Nebraska</td><td>10.5</td><td>27</td><td>Montana</td><td>11.7</td></tr>
<tr><td>19</td><td>Nevada</td><td>13.1</td><td>28</td><td>Alaska</td><td>11.5</td></tr>
<tr><td>49</td><td>New Hampshire</td><td>7.1</td><td>29</td><td>South Dakota</td><td>11.3</td></tr>
<tr><td>48</td><td>New Jersey</td><td>7.3</td><td>30</td><td>California</td><td>11.1</td></tr>
<tr><td>2</td><td>New Mexico</td><td>17.9</td><td>30</td><td>Michigan</td><td>11.1</td></tr>
<tr><td>44</td><td>New York</td><td>8.6</td><td>32</td><td>Washington</td><td>10.8</td></tr>
<tr><td>15</td><td>North Carolina</td><td>13.5</td><td>33</td><td>Wisconsin</td><td>10.7</td></tr>
<tr><td>42</td><td>North Dakota</td><td>9.3</td><td>34</td><td>Iowa</td><td>10.6</td></tr>
<tr><td>22</td><td>Ohio</td><td>12.6</td><td>34</td><td>Virginia</td><td>10.6</td></tr>
<tr><td>5</td><td>Oklahoma</td><td>16.2</td><td>36</td><td>Nebraska</td><td>10.5</td></tr>
<tr><td>23</td><td>Oregon</td><td>12.3</td><td>37</td><td>Hawaii</td><td>10.4</td></tr>
<tr><td>38</td><td>Pennsylvania</td><td>10.3</td><td>38</td><td>Maryland</td><td>10.3</td></tr>
<tr><td>40</td><td>Rhode Island</td><td>9.7</td><td>38</td><td>Pennsylvania</td><td>10.3</td></tr>
<tr><td>8</td><td>South Carolina</td><td>15.8</td><td>40</td><td>Maine</td><td>9.7</td></tr>
<tr><td>29</td><td>South Dakota</td><td>11.3</td><td>40</td><td>Rhode Island</td><td>9.7</td></tr>
<tr><td>9</td><td>Tennessee</td><td>15.4</td><td>42</td><td>North Dakota</td><td>9.3</td></tr>
<tr><td>7</td><td>Texas</td><td>15.9</td><td>42</td><td>Utah</td><td>9.3</td></tr>
<tr><td>42</td><td>Utah</td><td>9.3</td><td>44</td><td>New York</td><td>8.6</td></tr>
<tr><td>45</td><td>Vermont</td><td>8.5</td><td>45</td><td>Minnesota</td><td>8.5</td></tr>
<tr><td>34</td><td>Virginia</td><td>10.6</td><td>45</td><td>Vermont</td><td>8.5</td></tr>
<tr><td>32</td><td>Washington</td><td>10.8</td><td>47</td><td>Connecticut</td><td>8.0</td></tr>
<tr><td>11</td><td>West Virginia</td><td>14.8</td><td>48</td><td>New Jersey</td><td>7.3</td></tr>
<tr><td>33</td><td>Wisconsin</td><td>10.7</td><td>49</td><td>New Hampshire</td><td>7.1</td></tr>
<tr><td>14</td><td>Wyoming</td><td>13.9</td><td>50</td><td>Massachusetts</td><td>6.9</td></tr>
<tr><td></td><td></td><td></td><td></td><td>District of Columbia</td><td>14.8</td></tr>
</table>

Source: U.S. Department of Health and Human Services, National Center for Health Statistics
"National Vital Statistics Reports" (Vol. 48, No. 14, August 8, 2000)
*Births to women 19 years old and younger.

Births to Teenage Mothers in 1998

National Total = 484,895 Live Births*

ALPHA ORDER

RANK	STATE	BIRTHS	% of USA
15	Alabama	10,393	2.1%
46	Alaska	1,101	0.2%
14	Arizona	11,561	2.4%
27	Arkansas	6,691	1.4%
1	California	58,170	12.0%
25	Colorado	7,060	1.5%
36	Connecticut	3,555	0.7%
41	Delaware	1,347	0.3%
3	Florida	25,228	5.2%
7	Georgia	17,867	3.7%
40	Hawaii	1,849	0.4%
38	Idaho	2,457	0.5%
5	Illinois	22,180	4.6%
13	Indiana	11,570	2.4%
34	Iowa	3,900	0.8%
32	Kansas	4,805	1.0%
22	Kentucky	8,250	1.7%
12	Louisiana	12,033	2.5%
42	Maine	1,326	0.3%
24	Maryland	7,139	1.5%
28	Massachusetts	5,823	1.2%
9	Michigan	15,261	3.1%
30	Minnesota	5,522	1.1%
21	Mississippi	8,318	1.7%
16	Missouri	10,281	2.1%
43	Montana	1,316	0.3%
39	Nebraska	2,451	0.5%
35	Nevada	3,700	0.8%
47	New Hampshire	1,094	0.2%
18	New Jersey	8,708	1.8%
31	New Mexico	4,865	1.0%
4	New York	22,344	4.6%
8	North Carolina	15,325	3.2%
49	North Dakota	775	0.2%
6	Ohio	19,564	4.0%
23	Oklahoma	7,954	1.6%
29	Oregon	5,571	1.1%
10	Pennsylvania	14,849	3.1%
44	Rhode Island	1,293	0.3%
20	South Carolina	8,391	1.7%
45	South Dakota	1,214	0.3%
11	Tennessee	12,046	2.5%
2	Texas	54,004	11.1%
33	Utah	4,389	0.9%
50	Vermont	514	0.1%
17	Virginia	9,945	2.1%
19	Washington	8,591	1.8%
37	West Virginia	3,225	0.7%
26	Wisconsin	6,941	1.4%
48	Wyoming	1,006	0.2%

RANK ORDER

RANK	STATE	BIRTHS	% of USA
1	California	58,170	12.0%
2	Texas	54,004	11.1%
3	Florida	25,228	5.2%
4	New York	22,344	4.6%
5	Illinois	22,180	4.6%
6	Ohio	19,564	4.0%
7	Georgia	17,867	3.7%
8	North Carolina	15,325	3.2%
9	Michigan	15,261	3.1%
10	Pennsylvania	14,849	3.1%
11	Tennessee	12,046	2.5%
12	Louisiana	12,033	2.5%
13	Indiana	11,570	2.4%
14	Arizona	11,561	2.4%
15	Alabama	10,393	2.1%
16	Missouri	10,281	2.1%
17	Virginia	9,945	2.1%
18	New Jersey	8,708	1.8%
19	Washington	8,591	1.8%
20	South Carolina	8,391	1.7%
21	Mississippi	8,318	1.7%
22	Kentucky	8,250	1.7%
23	Oklahoma	7,954	1.6%
24	Maryland	7,139	1.5%
25	Colorado	7,060	1.5%
26	Wisconsin	6,941	1.4%
27	Arkansas	6,691	1.4%
28	Massachusetts	5,823	1.2%
29	Oregon	5,571	1.1%
30	Minnesota	5,522	1.1%
31	New Mexico	4,865	1.0%
32	Kansas	4,805	1.0%
33	Utah	4,389	0.9%
34	Iowa	3,900	0.8%
35	Nevada	3,700	0.8%
36	Connecticut	3,555	0.7%
37	West Virginia	3,225	0.7%
38	Idaho	2,457	0.5%
39	Nebraska	2,451	0.5%
40	Hawaii	1,849	0.4%
41	Delaware	1,347	0.3%
42	Maine	1,326	0.3%
43	Montana	1,316	0.3%
44	Rhode Island	1,293	0.3%
45	South Dakota	1,214	0.3%
46	Alaska	1,101	0.2%
47	New Hampshire	1,094	0.2%
48	Wyoming	1,006	0.2%
49	North Dakota	775	0.2%
50	Vermont	514	0.1%
	District of Columbia	1,133	0.2%

Source: U.S. Dept of Health & Human Services, National Center for Health Statistics
    (unpublished data)
*Live births to women age 15 to 19 years old by state of residence.

Teenage Birth Rate in 1998

National Rate = 51.1 Births per 1,000 Teenage Women*

ALPHA ORDER

RANK	STATE	RATE
7	Alabama	65.5
32	Alaska	42.4
4	Arizona	70.5
3	Arkansas	70.8
17	California	53.5
22	Colorado	48.7
41	Connecticut	35.8
16	Delaware	53.9
15	Florida	55.5
8	Georgia	65.4
27	Hawaii	45.7
28	Idaho	44.8
19	Illinois	53.2
18	Indiana	53.3
42	Iowa	35.2
26	Kansas	47.0
14	Kentucky	57.0
8	Louisiana	65.4
47	Maine	30.4
30	Maryland	43.1
45	Massachusetts	30.8
31	Michigan	42.6
46	Minnesota	30.6
1	Mississippi	73.0
20	Missouri	51.2
38	Montana	37.1
39	Nebraska	37.0
6	Nevada	65.7
49	New Hampshire	27.1
44	New Jersey	34.6
5	New Mexico	69.0
36	New York	38.5
12	North Carolina	61.0
47	North Dakota	30.4
23	Ohio	48.1
11	Oklahoma	61.6
25	Oregon	47.4
40	Pennsylvania	36.9
34	Rhode Island	41.0
13	South Carolina	60.4
36	South Dakota	38.5
10	Tennessee	64.3
2	Texas	70.9
35	Utah	40.9
50	Vermont	24.4
29	Virginia	43.5
33	Washington	41.7
21	West Virginia	49.2
43	Wisconsin	34.8
24	Wyoming	47.8

RANK ORDER

RANK	STATE	RATE
1	Mississippi	73.0
2	Texas	70.9
3	Arkansas	70.8
4	Arizona	70.5
5	New Mexico	69.0
6	Nevada	65.7
7	Alabama	65.5
8	Georgia	65.4
8	Louisiana	65.4
10	Tennessee	64.3
11	Oklahoma	61.6
12	North Carolina	61.0
13	South Carolina	60.4
14	Kentucky	57.0
15	Florida	55.5
16	Delaware	53.9
17	California	53.5
18	Indiana	53.3
19	Illinois	53.2
20	Missouri	51.2
21	West Virginia	49.2
22	Colorado	48.7
23	Ohio	48.1
24	Wyoming	47.8
25	Oregon	47.4
26	Kansas	47.0
27	Hawaii	45.7
28	Idaho	44.8
29	Virginia	43.5
30	Maryland	43.1
31	Michigan	42.6
32	Alaska	42.4
33	Washington	41.7
34	Rhode Island	41.0
35	Utah	40.9
36	New York	38.5
36	South Dakota	38.5
38	Montana	37.1
39	Nebraska	37.0
40	Pennsylvania	36.9
41	Connecticut	35.8
42	Iowa	35.2
43	Wisconsin	34.8
44	New Jersey	34.6
45	Massachusetts	30.8
46	Minnesota	30.6
47	Maine	30.4
47	North Dakota	30.4
49	New Hampshire	27.1
50	Vermont	24.4

| | District of Columbia | 86.7 |

Source: U.S. Department of Health and Human Services, National Center for Health Statistics
"National Vital Statistics Reports" (Vol. 48, No. 3, March 28, 2000)
*Women aged 15 to 19 years old.

Births to Teenage Mothers as a Percent of Births in 1998

National Percent = 12.3% of Live Births*

ALPHA ORDER				RANK ORDER		
RANK	STATE	PERCENT		RANK	STATE	PERCENT
5	Alabama	16.7		1	Mississippi	19.4
31	Alaska	11.1		2	Arkansas	18.2
13	Arizona	14.8		3	Louisiana	18.0
2	Arkansas	18.2		4	New Mexico	17.8
30	California	11.2		5	Alabama	16.7
27	Colorado	11.9		6	Oklahoma	16.1
46	Connecticut	8.1		6	Wyoming	16.1
21	Delaware	12.7		8	Texas	15.8
18	Florida	12.9		9	South Carolina	15.6
14	Georgia	14.6		9	Tennessee	15.6
33	Hawaii	10.5		11	West Virginia	15.5
21	Idaho	12.7		12	Kentucky	15.2
26	Illinois	12.1		13	Arizona	14.8
16	Indiana	13.6		14	Georgia	14.6
33	Iowa	10.5		15	North Carolina	13.7
23	Kansas	12.5		16	Indiana	13.6
12	Kentucky	15.2		16	Missouri	13.6
3	Louisiana	18.0		18	Florida	12.9
42	Maine	9.7		18	Nevada	12.9
40	Maryland	9.9		20	Ohio	12.8
50	Massachusetts	7.2		21	Delaware	12.7
29	Michigan	11.4		21	Idaho	12.7
45	Minnesota	8.5		23	Kansas	12.5
1	Mississippi	19.4		24	Oregon	12.3
16	Missouri	13.6		25	Montana	12.2
25	Montana	12.2		26	Illinois	12.1
36	Nebraska	10.4		27	Colorado	11.9
18	Nevada	12.9		28	South Dakota	11.8
48	New Hampshire	7.6		29	Michigan	11.4
48	New Jersey	7.6		30	California	11.2
4	New Mexico	17.8		31	Alaska	11.1
44	New York	8.7		32	Washington	10.8
15	North Carolina	13.7		33	Hawaii	10.5
41	North Dakota	9.8		33	Iowa	10.5
20	Ohio	12.8		33	Virginia	10.5
6	Oklahoma	16.1		36	Nebraska	10.4
24	Oregon	12.3		37	Rhode Island	10.3
39	Pennsylvania	10.2		37	Wisconsin	10.3
37	Rhode Island	10.3		39	Pennsylvania	10.2
9	South Carolina	15.6		40	Maryland	9.9
28	South Dakota	11.8		41	North Dakota	9.8
9	Tennessee	15.6		42	Maine	9.7
8	Texas	15.8		42	Utah	9.7
42	Utah	9.7		44	New York	8.7
47	Vermont	7.8		45	Minnesota	8.5
33	Virginia	10.5		46	Connecticut	8.1
32	Washington	10.8		47	Vermont	7.8
11	West Virginia	15.5		48	New Hampshire	7.6
37	Wisconsin	10.3		48	New Jersey	7.6
6	Wyoming	16.1		50	Massachusetts	7.2
					District of Columbia	14.7

Source: Morgan Quitno Press using data from U.S. Dept of Health & Human Services, National Center for Health Statistics (unpublished data)
*Live births to women age 15 to 19 years old by state of residence.

Births to White Teenage Mothers in 1998

National Total = 340,694 Live Births*

ALPHA ORDER

RANK	STATE	BIRTHS	% of USA
20	Alabama	5,479	1.6%
47	Alaska	586	0.2%
9	Arizona	9,806	2.9%
26	Arkansas	4,446	1.3%
1	California	48,633	14.3%
17	Colorado	6,247	1.8%
37	Connecticut	2,554	0.7%
46	Delaware	714	0.2%
3	Florida	15,693	4.6%
10	Georgia	9,248	2.7%
50	Hawaii	207	0.1%
38	Idaho	2,363	0.7%
6	Illinois	13,146	3.9%
11	Indiana	9,210	2.7%
32	Iowa	3,545	1.0%
31	Kansas	3,969	1.2%
16	Kentucky	7,062	2.1%
22	Louisiana	4,857	1.4%
40	Maine	1,283	0.4%
34	Maryland	3,072	0.9%
25	Massachusetts	4,528	1.3%
8	Michigan	10,029	2.9%
30	Minnesota	4,031	1.2%
33	Mississippi	3,210	0.9%
14	Missouri	7,517	2.2%
43	Montana	1,011	0.3%
39	Nebraska	2,062	0.6%
35	Nevada	3,038	0.9%
41	New Hampshire	1,069	0.3%
23	New Jersey	4,792	1.4%
27	New Mexico	4,113	1.2%
4	New York	14,169	4.2%
12	North Carolina	8,704	2.6%
48	North Dakota	579	0.2%
5	Ohio	14,019	4.1%
18	Oklahoma	5,657	1.7%
21	Oregon	5,063	1.5%
7	Pennsylvania	10,172	3.0%
42	Rhode Island	1,038	0.3%
29	South Carolina	4,040	1.2%
45	South Dakota	795	0.2%
13	Tennessee	7,919	2.3%
2	Texas	44,783	13.1%
28	Utah	4,101	1.2%
49	Vermont	507	0.1%
19	Virginia	5,598	1.6%
15	Washington	7,284	2.1%
36	West Virginia	3,027	0.9%
24	Wisconsin	4,684	1.4%
44	Wyoming	922	0.3%

RANK ORDER

RANK	STATE	BIRTHS	% of USA
1	California	48,633	14.3%
2	Texas	44,783	13.1%
3	Florida	15,693	4.6%
4	New York	14,169	4.2%
5	Ohio	14,019	4.1%
6	Illinois	13,146	3.9%
7	Pennsylvania	10,172	3.0%
8	Michigan	10,029	2.9%
9	Arizona	9,806	2.9%
10	Georgia	9,248	2.7%
11	Indiana	9,210	2.7%
12	North Carolina	8,704	2.6%
13	Tennessee	7,919	2.3%
14	Missouri	7,517	2.2%
15	Washington	7,284	2.1%
16	Kentucky	7,062	2.1%
17	Colorado	6,247	1.8%
18	Oklahoma	5,657	1.7%
19	Virginia	5,598	1.6%
20	Alabama	5,479	1.6%
21	Oregon	5,063	1.5%
22	Louisiana	4,857	1.4%
23	New Jersey	4,792	1.4%
24	Wisconsin	4,684	1.4%
25	Massachusetts	4,528	1.3%
26	Arkansas	4,446	1.3%
27	New Mexico	4,113	1.2%
28	Utah	4,101	1.2%
29	South Carolina	4,040	1.2%
30	Minnesota	4,031	1.2%
31	Kansas	3,969	1.2%
32	Iowa	3,545	1.0%
33	Mississippi	3,210	0.9%
34	Maryland	3,072	0.9%
35	Nevada	3,038	0.9%
36	West Virginia	3,027	0.9%
37	Connecticut	2,554	0.7%
38	Idaho	2,363	0.7%
39	Nebraska	2,062	0.6%
40	Maine	1,283	0.4%
41	New Hampshire	1,069	0.3%
42	Rhode Island	1,038	0.3%
43	Montana	1,011	0.3%
44	Wyoming	922	0.3%
45	South Dakota	795	0.2%
46	Delaware	714	0.2%
47	Alaska	586	0.2%
48	North Dakota	579	0.2%
49	Vermont	507	0.1%
50	Hawaii	207	0.1%
	District of Columbia	113	0.0%

Source: U.S. Dept of Health & Human Services, National Center for Health Statistics
    (unpublished data)
*Live births to women age 15 to 19 years old by state of residence.

29

White Teenage Birth Rate in 1998

National Rate = 45.4 Births per 1,000 White Teenage Women*

ALPHA ORDER			RANK ORDER		
RANK	STATE	RATE	RANK	STATE	RATE
11	Alabama	53.8	1	Texas	71.4
36	Alaska	31.9	2	Arizona	70.4
2	Arizona	70.4	3	New Mexico	69.7
5	Arkansas	62.2	4	Nevada	65.1
6	California	58.1	5	Arkansas	62.2
17	Colorado	47.4	6	California	58.1
38	Connecticut	30.5	7	Oklahoma	56.0
29	Delaware	39.0	8	Tennessee	55.0
19	Florida	46.5	9	Georgia	54.7
9	Georgia	54.7	10	Kentucky	54.1
50	Hawaii	17.2	11	Alabama	53.8
22	Idaho	44.6	12	Mississippi	53.7
26	Illinois	40.7	13	North Carolina	50.6
16	Indiana	48.0	14	West Virginia	48.5
35	Iowa	33.5	15	South Carolina	48.2
24	Kansas	43.3	16	Indiana	48.0
10	Kentucky	54.1	17	Colorado	47.4
21	Louisiana	45.4	18	Oregon	46.9
39	Maine	30.0	19	Florida	46.5
40	Maryland	29.6	20	Wyoming	45.9
43	Massachusetts	27.5	21	Louisiana	45.4
31	Michigan	34.6	22	Idaho	44.6
49	Minnesota	24.5	23	Missouri	44.2
12	Mississippi	53.7	24	Kansas	43.3
23	Missouri	44.2	25	Washington	40.9
37	Montana	31.6	26	Illinois	40.7
34	Nebraska	33.7	27	Ohio	40.6
4	Nevada	65.1	28	Utah	40.1
44	New Hampshire	27.2	29	Delaware	39.0
46	New Jersey	25.6	30	Rhode Island	36.9
3	New Mexico	69.7	31	Michigan	34.6
33	New York	33.9	32	Virginia	34.4
13	North Carolina	50.6	33	New York	33.9
47	North Dakota	24.6	34	Nebraska	33.7
27	Ohio	40.6	35	Iowa	33.5
7	Oklahoma	56.0	36	Alaska	31.9
18	Oregon	46.9	37	Montana	31.6
41	Pennsylvania	29.3	38	Connecticut	30.5
30	Rhode Island	36.9	39	Maine	30.0
15	South Carolina	48.2	40	Maryland	29.6
42	South Dakota	28.7	41	Pennsylvania	29.3
8	Tennessee	55.0	42	South Dakota	28.7
1	Texas	71.4	43	Massachusetts	27.5
28	Utah	40.1	44	New Hampshire	27.2
47	Vermont	24.6	45	Wisconsin	26.2
32	Virginia	34.4	46	New Jersey	25.6
25	Washington	40.9	47	North Dakota	24.6
14	West Virginia	48.5	47	Vermont	24.6
45	Wisconsin	26.2	49	Minnesota	24.5
20	Wyoming	45.9	50	Hawaii	17.2
				District of Columbia	20.9

Source: U.S. Department of Health and Human Services, National Center for Health Statistics
    "National Vital Statistics Reports" (Vol. 48, No. 6, April 24, 2000)
*Women aged 15 to 19 years old.

Births to White Teenage Mothers as a Percent of White Births in 1998

National Percent = 10.9% of White Live Births*

ALPHA ORDER			RANK ORDER		
RANK	**STATE**	**PERCENT**	**RANK**	**STATE**	**PERCENT**
11	Alabama	13.2	1	New Mexico	17.9
37	Alaska	8.8	2	Arkansas	15.7
8	Arizona	14.4	2	Wyoming	15.7
2	Arkansas	15.7	4	Texas	15.3
21	California	11.5	5	West Virginia	15.2
21	Colorado	11.5	6	Kentucky	14.5
46	Connecticut	6.9	6	Oklahoma	14.5
36	Delaware	9.3	8	Arizona	14.4
25	Florida	10.7	9	Mississippi	14.0
18	Georgia	11.8	10	Tennessee	13.4
50	Hawaii	5.0	11	Alabama	13.2
13	Idaho	12.6	12	Louisiana	12.7
34	Illinois	9.4	13	Idaho	12.6
15	Indiana	12.3	14	Nevada	12.5
28	Iowa	10.1	15	Indiana	12.3
20	Kansas	11.6	16	Oregon	12.2
6	Kentucky	14.5	17	Missouri	12.0
12	Louisiana	12.7	18	Georgia	11.8
29	Maine	9.6	18	South Carolina	11.8
46	Maryland	6.9	20	Kansas	11.6
48	Massachusetts	6.5	21	California	11.5
32	Michigan	9.5	21	Colorado	11.5
45	Minnesota	7.0	23	North Carolina	11.0
9	Mississippi	14.0	23	Ohio	11.0
17	Missouri	12.0	25	Florida	10.7
25	Montana	10.7	25	Montana	10.7
29	Nebraska	9.6	27	Washington	10.6
14	Nevada	12.5	28	Iowa	10.1
43	New Hampshire	7.6	29	Maine	9.6
49	New Jersey	5.6	29	Nebraska	9.6
1	New Mexico	17.9	29	Utah	9.6
43	New York	7.6	32	Michigan	9.5
23	North Carolina	11.0	32	South Dakota	9.5
40	North Dakota	8.2	34	Illinois	9.4
23	Ohio	11.0	34	Rhode Island	9.4
6	Oklahoma	14.5	36	Delaware	9.3
16	Oregon	12.2	37	Alaska	8.8
38	Pennsylvania	8.4	38	Pennsylvania	8.4
34	Rhode Island	9.4	39	Virginia	8.3
18	South Carolina	11.8	40	North Dakota	8.2
32	South Dakota	9.5	41	Wisconsin	8.1
10	Tennessee	13.4	42	Vermont	7.8
4	Texas	15.3	43	New Hampshire	7.6
29	Utah	9.6	43	New York	7.6
42	Vermont	7.8	45	Minnesota	7.0
39	Virginia	8.3	46	Connecticut	6.9
27	Washington	10.6	46	Maryland	6.9
5	West Virginia	15.2	48	Massachusetts	6.5
41	Wisconsin	8.1	49	New Jersey	5.6
2	Wyoming	15.7	50	Hawaii	5.0
				District of Columbia	5.5

Source: Morgan Quitno Press using data from U.S. Dept of Health & Human Services, National Center for Health Statistics (unpublished data)
*Live births to women age 15 to 19 years old by state of residence.

Births to Black Teenage Mothers in 1998

National Total = 126,937 Live Births*

ALPHA ORDER

RANK	STATE	BIRTHS	% of USA
12	Alabama	4,863	3.8%
41	Alaska	54	0.0%
31	Arizona	575	0.5%
21	Arkansas	2,158	1.7%
7	California	6,078	4.8%
30	Colorado	579	0.5%
26	Connecticut	942	0.7%
29	Delaware	624	0.5%
1	Florida	9,193	7.2%
4	Georgia	8,486	6.7%
42	Hawaii	51	0.0%
46	Idaho	13	0.0%
2	Illinois	8,843	7.0%
20	Indiana	2,294	1.8%
35	Iowa	269	0.2%
28	Kansas	688	0.5%
23	Kentucky	1,153	0.9%
6	Louisiana	7,025	5.5%
46	Maine	13	0.0%
17	Maryland	3,971	3.1%
25	Massachusetts	1,082	0.9%
11	Michigan	4,955	3.9%
27	Minnesota	756	0.6%
10	Mississippi	5,030	4.0%
19	Missouri	2,662	2.1%
48	Montana	12	0.0%
34	Nebraska	271	0.2%
33	Nevada	440	0.3%
44	New Hampshire	14	0.0%
18	New Jersey	3,780	3.0%
39	New Mexico	119	0.1%
5	New York	7,698	6.1%
8	North Carolina	6,014	4.7%
43	North Dakota	17	0.0%
9	Ohio	5,369	4.2%
24	Oklahoma	1,096	0.9%
36	Oregon	204	0.2%
13	Pennsylvania	4,510	3.6%
38	Rhode Island	158	0.1%
14	South Carolina	4,274	3.4%
44	South Dakota	14	0.0%
16	Tennessee	4,028	3.2%
3	Texas	8,759	6.9%
40	Utah	56	0.0%
50	Vermont	3	0.0%
15	Virginia	4,178	3.3%
32	Washington	558	0.4%
37	West Virginia	190	0.1%
22	Wisconsin	1,791	1.4%
48	Wyoming	12	0.0%

RANK ORDER

RANK	STATE	BIRTHS	% of USA
1	Florida	9,193	7.2%
2	Illinois	8,843	7.0%
3	Texas	8,759	6.9%
4	Georgia	8,486	6.7%
5	New York	7,698	6.1%
6	Louisiana	7,025	5.5%
7	California	6,078	4.8%
8	North Carolina	6,014	4.7%
9	Ohio	5,369	4.2%
10	Mississippi	5,030	4.0%
11	Michigan	4,955	3.9%
12	Alabama	4,863	3.8%
13	Pennsylvania	4,510	3.6%
14	South Carolina	4,274	3.4%
15	Virginia	4,178	3.3%
16	Tennessee	4,028	3.2%
17	Maryland	3,971	3.1%
18	New Jersey	3,780	3.0%
19	Missouri	2,662	2.1%
20	Indiana	2,294	1.8%
21	Arkansas	2,158	1.7%
22	Wisconsin	1,791	1.4%
23	Kentucky	1,153	0.9%
24	Oklahoma	1,096	0.9%
25	Massachusetts	1,082	0.9%
26	Connecticut	942	0.7%
27	Minnesota	756	0.6%
28	Kansas	688	0.5%
29	Delaware	624	0.5%
30	Colorado	579	0.5%
31	Arizona	575	0.5%
32	Washington	558	0.4%
33	Nevada	440	0.3%
34	Nebraska	271	0.2%
35	Iowa	269	0.2%
36	Oregon	204	0.2%
37	West Virginia	190	0.1%
38	Rhode Island	158	0.1%
39	New Mexico	119	0.1%
40	Utah	56	0.0%
41	Alaska	54	0.0%
42	Hawaii	51	0.0%
43	North Dakota	17	0.0%
44	New Hampshire	14	0.0%
44	South Dakota	14	0.0%
46	Idaho	13	0.0%
46	Maine	13	0.0%
48	Montana	12	0.0%
48	Wyoming	12	0.0%
50	Vermont	3	0.0%
	District of Columbia	1,015	0.8%

Source: U.S. Dept of Health & Human Services, National Center for Health Statistics
(unpublished data)
*Live births to women age 15 to 19 years old by state of residence.

Black Teenage Birth Rate in 1998

National Rate = 85.4 Births per 1,000 Black Teenage Women*

<table>
<tr><td colspan="3">ALPHA ORDER</td><td colspan="3">RANK ORDER</td></tr>
<tr><td>RANK</td><td>STATE</td><td>RATE</td><td>RANK</td><td>STATE</td><td>RATE</td></tr>
<tr><td>16</td><td>Alabama</td><td>88.6</td><td>1</td><td>Wisconsin</td><td>126.7</td></tr>
<tr><td>40</td><td>Alaska</td><td>49.3</td><td>2</td><td>Minnesota</td><td>115.4</td></tr>
<tr><td>28</td><td>Arizona</td><td>76.4</td><td>3</td><td>Illinois</td><td>113.7</td></tr>
<tr><td>6</td><td>Arkansas</td><td>99.6</td><td>4</td><td>Delaware</td><td>104.0</td></tr>
<tr><td>36</td><td>California</td><td>64.0</td><td>5</td><td>Indiana</td><td>102.9</td></tr>
<tr><td>29</td><td>Colorado</td><td>76.3</td><td>6</td><td>Arkansas</td><td>99.6</td></tr>
<tr><td>27</td><td>Connecticut</td><td>77.3</td><td>7</td><td>Tennessee</td><td>98.9</td></tr>
<tr><td>4</td><td>Delaware</td><td>104.0</td><td>8</td><td>Pennsylvania</td><td>98.8</td></tr>
<tr><td>17</td><td>Florida</td><td>88.1</td><td>9</td><td>Missouri</td><td>97.6</td></tr>
<tr><td>18</td><td>Georgia</td><td>87.0</td><td>10</td><td>Ohio</td><td>96.8</td></tr>
<tr><td>41</td><td>Hawaii</td><td>34.7</td><td>11</td><td>Kansas</td><td>96.6</td></tr>
<tr><td>NA</td><td>Idaho**</td><td>NA</td><td>12</td><td>Louisiana</td><td>95.8</td></tr>
<tr><td>3</td><td>Illinois</td><td>113.7</td><td>13</td><td>Mississippi</td><td>95.1</td></tr>
<tr><td>5</td><td>Indiana</td><td>102.9</td><td>14</td><td>Iowa</td><td>93.4</td></tr>
<tr><td>14</td><td>Iowa</td><td>93.4</td><td>15</td><td>Kentucky</td><td>89.1</td></tr>
<tr><td>11</td><td>Kansas</td><td>96.6</td><td>16</td><td>Alabama</td><td>88.6</td></tr>
<tr><td>15</td><td>Kentucky</td><td>89.1</td><td>17</td><td>Florida</td><td>88.1</td></tr>
<tr><td>12</td><td>Louisiana</td><td>95.8</td><td>18</td><td>Georgia</td><td>87.0</td></tr>
<tr><td>NA</td><td>Maine**</td><td>NA</td><td>19</td><td>Oklahoma</td><td>85.0</td></tr>
<tr><td>32</td><td>Maryland</td><td>73.5</td><td>20</td><td>North Carolina</td><td>84.7</td></tr>
<tr><td>35</td><td>Massachusetts</td><td>71.3</td><td>21</td><td>Michigan</td><td>84.6</td></tr>
<tr><td>21</td><td>Michigan</td><td>84.6</td><td>22</td><td>Nebraska</td><td>81.9</td></tr>
<tr><td>2</td><td>Minnesota</td><td>115.4</td><td>23</td><td>Nevada</td><td>81.3</td></tr>
<tr><td>13</td><td>Mississippi</td><td>95.1</td><td>24</td><td>Texas</td><td>80.7</td></tr>
<tr><td>9</td><td>Missouri</td><td>97.6</td><td>25</td><td>New Jersey</td><td>80.4</td></tr>
<tr><td>NA</td><td>Montana**</td><td>NA</td><td>26</td><td>South Carolina</td><td>80.3</td></tr>
<tr><td>22</td><td>Nebraska</td><td>81.9</td><td>27</td><td>Connecticut</td><td>77.3</td></tr>
<tr><td>23</td><td>Nevada</td><td>81.3</td><td>28</td><td>Arizona</td><td>76.4</td></tr>
<tr><td>NA</td><td>New Hampshire**</td><td>NA</td><td>29</td><td>Colorado</td><td>76.3</td></tr>
<tr><td>25</td><td>New Jersey</td><td>80.4</td><td>30</td><td>Virginia</td><td>74.6</td></tr>
<tr><td>39</td><td>New Mexico</td><td>57.1</td><td>31</td><td>Rhode Island</td><td>74.2</td></tr>
<tr><td>38</td><td>New York</td><td>61.4</td><td>32</td><td>Maryland</td><td>73.5</td></tr>
<tr><td>20</td><td>North Carolina</td><td>84.7</td><td>33</td><td>West Virginia</td><td>72.4</td></tr>
<tr><td>NA</td><td>North Dakota**</td><td>NA</td><td>34</td><td>Oregon</td><td>72.2</td></tr>
<tr><td>10</td><td>Ohio</td><td>96.8</td><td>35</td><td>Massachusetts</td><td>71.3</td></tr>
<tr><td>19</td><td>Oklahoma</td><td>85.0</td><td>36</td><td>California</td><td>64.0</td></tr>
<tr><td>34</td><td>Oregon</td><td>72.2</td><td>37</td><td>Washington</td><td>62.9</td></tr>
<tr><td>8</td><td>Pennsylvania</td><td>98.8</td><td>38</td><td>New York</td><td>61.4</td></tr>
<tr><td>31</td><td>Rhode Island</td><td>74.2</td><td>39</td><td>New Mexico</td><td>57.1</td></tr>
<tr><td>26</td><td>South Carolina</td><td>80.3</td><td>40</td><td>Alaska</td><td>49.3</td></tr>
<tr><td>NA</td><td>South Dakota**</td><td>NA</td><td>41</td><td>Hawaii</td><td>34.7</td></tr>
<tr><td>7</td><td>Tennessee</td><td>98.9</td><td>NA</td><td>Idaho**</td><td>NA</td></tr>
<tr><td>24</td><td>Texas</td><td>80.7</td><td>NA</td><td>Maine**</td><td>NA</td></tr>
<tr><td>NA</td><td>Utah**</td><td>NA</td><td>NA</td><td>Montana**</td><td>NA</td></tr>
<tr><td>NA</td><td>Vermont**</td><td>NA</td><td>NA</td><td>New Hampshire**</td><td>NA</td></tr>
<tr><td>30</td><td>Virginia</td><td>74.6</td><td>NA</td><td>North Dakota**</td><td>NA</td></tr>
<tr><td>37</td><td>Washington</td><td>62.9</td><td>NA</td><td>South Dakota**</td><td>NA</td></tr>
<tr><td>33</td><td>West Virginia</td><td>72.4</td><td>NA</td><td>Utah**</td><td>NA</td></tr>
<tr><td>1</td><td>Wisconsin</td><td>126.7</td><td>NA</td><td>Vermont**</td><td>NA</td></tr>
<tr><td>NA</td><td>Wyoming**</td><td>NA</td><td>NA</td><td>Wyoming**</td><td>NA</td></tr>
<tr><td></td><td></td><td></td><td></td><td>District of Columbia</td><td>141.7</td></tr>
</table>

Source: U.S. Department of Health and Human Services, National Center for Health Statistics
    "National Vital Statistics Reports" (Vol. 48, No. 6, April 24, 2000)

*Women aged 15 to 19 years old.

**Insufficient data.

Births to Black Teenage Mothers as a Percent of Black Births in 1998

National Percent = 20.8% of Black Live Births*

ALPHA ORDER

RANK	STATE	PERCENT
11	Alabama	24.3
47	Alaska	13.5
23	Arizona	21.7
3	Arkansas	27.0
39	California	16.5
31	Colorado	20.2
38	Connecticut	17.2
13	Delaware	23.8
27	Florida	20.7
28	Georgia	20.6
50	Hawaii	9.1
43	Idaho	15.9
7	Illinois	24.8
7	Indiana	24.8
10	Iowa	24.6
9	Kansas	24.7
14	Kentucky	23.7
5	Louisiana	25.6
44	Maine	14.3
39	Maryland	16.5
46	Massachusetts	13.7
30	Michigan	20.4
28	Minnesota	20.6
4	Mississippi	26.0
16	Missouri	23.4
2	Montana	27.3
21	Nebraska	21.9
33	Nevada	19.6
49	New Hampshire	10.4
37	New Jersey	17.6
16	New Mexico	23.4
45	New York	14.1
25	North Carolina	21.3
34	North Dakota	19.5
15	Ohio	23.6
18	Oklahoma	22.8
26	Oregon	21.1
23	Pennsylvania	21.7
42	Rhode Island	16.3
19	South Carolina	22.7
39	South Dakota	16.5
12	Tennessee	23.9
22	Texas	21.8
32	Utah	19.9
48	Vermont	12.5
35	Virginia	19.0
36	Washington	17.9
6	West Virginia	25.0
1	Wisconsin	27.4
20	Wyoming	22.2

RANK ORDER

RANK	STATE	PERCENT
1	Wisconsin	27.4
2	Montana	27.3
3	Arkansas	27.0
4	Mississippi	26.0
5	Louisiana	25.6
6	West Virginia	25.0
7	Illinois	24.8
7	Indiana	24.8
9	Kansas	24.7
10	Iowa	24.6
11	Alabama	24.3
12	Tennessee	23.9
13	Delaware	23.8
14	Kentucky	23.7
15	Ohio	23.6
16	Missouri	23.4
16	New Mexico	23.4
18	Oklahoma	22.8
19	South Carolina	22.7
20	Wyoming	22.2
21	Nebraska	21.9
22	Texas	21.8
23	Arizona	21.7
23	Pennsylvania	21.7
25	North Carolina	21.3
26	Oregon	21.1
27	Florida	20.7
28	Georgia	20.6
28	Minnesota	20.6
30	Michigan	20.4
31	Colorado	20.2
32	Utah	19.9
33	Nevada	19.6
34	North Dakota	19.5
35	Virginia	19.0
36	Washington	17.9
37	New Jersey	17.6
38	Connecticut	17.2
39	California	16.5
39	Maryland	16.5
39	South Dakota	16.5
42	Rhode Island	16.3
43	Idaho	15.9
44	Maine	14.3
45	New York	14.1
46	Massachusetts	13.7
47	Alaska	13.5
48	Vermont	12.5
49	New Hampshire	10.4
50	Hawaii	9.1
	District of Columbia	18.6

Source: Morgan Quitno Press using data from U.S. Dept of Health & Human Services, National Center for Health Statistics (unpublished data)

*Live births to women age 15 to 19 years old by state of residence.

Pregnancy Rate for 15 to 19 Year Old Women in 1997

National rate = 71.3 Births and Abortions per 1,000 Women 15-19 Years Old*

ALPHA ORDER

RANK	STATE	RATE
9	Alabama	83.1
29	Alaska	57.9
8	Arizona	83.7
5	Arkansas	85.7
NA	California**	NA
25	Colorado	63.3
22	Connecticut	66.1
1	Delaware	107.9
NA	Florida**	NA
2	Georgia	92.0
19	Hawaii	69.7
40	Idaho	47.2
NA	Illinois**	NA
22	Indiana	66.1
NA	Iowa**	NA
17	Kansas	73.8
20	Kentucky	69.4
13	Louisiana	78.3
42	Maine	46.2
33	Maryland	55.0
30	Massachusetts	56.9
27	Michigan	59.8
41	Minnesota	47.1
12	Mississippi	81.1
26	Missouri	60.7
31	Montana	56.7
35	Nebraska	53.3
4	Nevada	90.5
NA	New Hampshire**	NA
32	New Jersey	55.3
7	New Mexico	84.9
11	New York	82.9
6	North Carolina	85.6
44	North Dakota	40.6
21	Ohio	68.7
NA	Oklahoma**	NA
16	Oregon	74.7
34	Pennsylvania	54.4
14	Rhode Island	76.9
15	South Carolina	75.0
39	South Dakota	47.6
9	Tennessee	83.1
3	Texas	91.6
36	Utah	48.8
36	Vermont	48.8
24	Virginia	65.7
18	Washington	70.1
28	West Virginia	58.7
38	Wisconsin	48.6
43	Wyoming	44.5

RANK ORDER

RANK	STATE	RATE
1	Delaware	107.9
2	Georgia	92.0
3	Texas	91.6
4	Nevada	90.5
5	Arkansas	85.7
6	North Carolina	85.6
7	New Mexico	84.9
8	Arizona	83.7
9	Alabama	83.1
9	Tennessee	83.1
11	New York	82.9
12	Mississippi	81.1
13	Louisiana	78.3
14	Rhode Island	76.9
15	South Carolina	75.0
16	Oregon	74.7
17	Kansas	73.8
18	Washington	70.1
19	Hawaii	69.7
20	Kentucky	69.4
21	Ohio	68.7
22	Connecticut	66.1
22	Indiana	66.1
24	Virginia	65.7
25	Colorado	63.3
26	Missouri	60.7
27	Michigan	59.8
28	West Virginia	58.7
29	Alaska	57.9
30	Massachusetts	56.9
31	Montana	56.7
32	New Jersey	55.3
33	Maryland	55.0
34	Pennsylvania	54.4
35	Nebraska	53.3
36	Utah	48.8
36	Vermont	48.8
38	Wisconsin	48.6
39	South Dakota	47.6
40	Idaho	47.2
41	Minnesota	47.1
42	Maine	46.2
43	Wyoming	44.5
44	North Dakota	40.6
NA	California**	NA
NA	Florida**	NA
NA	Illinois**	NA
NA	Iowa**	NA
NA	New Hampshire**	NA
NA	Oklahoma**	NA

District of Columbia   211.9

Source: Morgan Quitno Press using data from US Dept of Health & Human Serv's, Centers for Disease Control-Prevention "Abortion Surveillance-United States, 1997" (Morbidity Mortality Weekly Report, Vol. 49, No. SS-11, 12/08/00)
*The sum of live births and legal induced abortions per 1,000 women aged 15-19 years old. Births by state of residence, abortions by state of occurrence. Miscarriages are not included in these rates. National rate includes only states reporting abortions and births.
**Not available.

Percent Change in Pregnancy Rate for 15 to 19 Year Old Women: 1992 to 1997

National Percent Change = 10.5% Decrease*

ALPHA ORDER

RANK	STATE	PERCENT CHANGE
5	Alabama	(10.8)
NA	Alaska**	NA
27	Arizona	(19.1)
1	Arkansas	(5.5)
NA	California**	NA
33	Colorado	(20.7)
NA	Connecticut**	NA
NA	Delaware**	NA
NA	Florida**	NA
11	Georgia	(13.9)
29	Hawaii	(19.3)
35	Idaho	(20.9)
NA	Illinois**	NA
4	Indiana	(8.4)
NA	Iowa**	NA
17	Kansas	(15.2)
16	Kentucky	(15.1)
18	Louisiana	(15.4)
20	Maine	(16.3)
40	Maryland	(28.5)
25	Massachusetts	(18.1)
38	Michigan	(25.0)
14	Minnesota	(14.7)
30	Mississippi	(19.5)
36	Missouri	(22.2)
28	Montana	(19.2)
19	Nebraska	(15.9)
13	Nevada	(14.6)
NA	New Hampshire**	NA
33	New Jersey	(20.7)
21	New Mexico	(16.6)
12	New York	(14.2)
26	North Carolina	(18.2)
39	North Dakota	(25.1)
3	Ohio	(7.9)
NA	Oklahoma**	NA
2	Oregon	(7.8)
37	Pennsylvania	(24.1)
10	Rhode Island	(12.7)
15	South Carolina	(14.8)
31	South Dakota	(19.9)
7	Tennessee	(11.6)
8	Texas	(11.7)
9	Utah	(12.2)
41	Vermont	(29.0)
22	Virginia	(16.8)
24	Washington	(17.6)
6	West Virginia	(11.2)
32	Wisconsin	(20.1)
23	Wyoming	(17.1)

RANK ORDER

RANK	STATE	PERCENT CHANGE
1	Arkansas	(5.5)
2	Oregon	(7.8)
3	Ohio	(7.9)
4	Indiana	(8.4)
5	Alabama	(10.8)
6	West Virginia	(11.2)
7	Tennessee	(11.6)
8	Texas	(11.7)
9	Utah	(12.2)
10	Rhode Island	(12.7)
11	Georgia	(13.9)
12	New York	(14.2)
13	Nevada	(14.6)
14	Minnesota	(14.7)
15	South Carolina	(14.8)
16	Kentucky	(15.1)
17	Kansas	(15.2)
18	Louisiana	(15.4)
19	Nebraska	(15.9)
20	Maine	(16.3)
21	New Mexico	(16.6)
22	Virginia	(16.8)
23	Wyoming	(17.1)
24	Washington	(17.6)
25	Massachusetts	(18.1)
26	North Carolina	(18.2)
27	Arizona	(19.1)
28	Montana	(19.2)
29	Hawaii	(19.3)
30	Mississippi	(19.5)
31	South Dakota	(19.9)
32	Wisconsin	(20.1)
33	Colorado	(20.7)
33	New Jersey	(20.7)
35	Idaho	(20.9)
36	Missouri	(22.2)
37	Pennsylvania	(24.1)
38	Michigan	(25.0)
39	North Dakota	(25.1)
40	Maryland	(28.5)
41	Vermont	(29.0)
NA	Alaska**	NA
NA	California**	NA
NA	Connecticut**	NA
NA	Delaware**	NA
NA	Florida**	NA
NA	Illinois**	NA
NA	Iowa**	NA
NA	New Hampshire**	NA
NA	Oklahoma**	NA

District of Columbia   1.7

Source: Morgan Quitno Press using data from US Dept of Health & Human Serv's, Centers for Disease Control-Prevention
"Abortion Surveillance-United States, 1997" (Morbidity Mortality Weekly Report, Vol. 49, No. SS-11, 12/08/00)
*The sum of live births and legal induced abortions per 1,000 women aged 15-19 years old. Births by state of
residence, abortions by state of occurrence. Miscarriages are not included in these rates. National rate includes
only states reporting abortions and births.
**Not available.

Births to Teenage Mothers in 1990

National Total = 521,826 Live Births*

<table>
<tr><td colspan="4">ALPHA ORDER</td><td colspan="4">RANK ORDER</td></tr>
<tr><td>RANK</td><td>STATE</td><td>BIRTHS</td><td>% of USA</td><td>RANK</td><td>STATE</td><td>BIRTHS</td><td>% of USA</td></tr>
<tr><td>15</td><td>Alabama</td><td>11,252</td><td>2.2%</td><td>1</td><td>California</td><td>69,712</td><td>13.4%</td></tr>
<tr><td>47</td><td>Alaska</td><td>1,142</td><td>0.2%</td><td>2</td><td>Texas</td><td>48,302</td><td>9.3%</td></tr>
<tr><td>19</td><td>Arizona</td><td>9,612</td><td>1.8%</td><td>3</td><td>Florida</td><td>27,017</td><td>5.2%</td></tr>
<tr><td>27</td><td>Arkansas</td><td>7,011</td><td>1.3%</td><td>4</td><td>New York</td><td>26,608</td><td>5.1%</td></tr>
<tr><td>1</td><td>California</td><td>69,712</td><td>13.4%</td><td>5</td><td>Illinois</td><td>24,967</td><td>4.8%</td></tr>
<tr><td>28</td><td>Colorado</td><td>5,975</td><td>1.1%</td><td>6</td><td>Ohio</td><td>22,690</td><td>4.3%</td></tr>
<tr><td>33</td><td>Connecticut</td><td>4,038</td><td>0.8%</td><td>7</td><td>Michigan</td><td>20,312</td><td>3.9%</td></tr>
<tr><td>44</td><td>Delaware</td><td>1,277</td><td>0.2%</td><td>8</td><td>Georgia</td><td>18,369</td><td>3.5%</td></tr>
<tr><td>3</td><td>Florida</td><td>27,017</td><td>5.2%</td><td>9</td><td>Pennsylvania</td><td>18,216</td><td>3.5%</td></tr>
<tr><td>8</td><td>Georgia</td><td>18,369</td><td>3.5%</td><td>10</td><td>North Carolina</td><td>16,506</td><td>3.2%</td></tr>
<tr><td>39</td><td>Hawaii</td><td>2,122</td><td>0.4%</td><td>11</td><td>Tennessee</td><td>12,928</td><td>2.5%</td></tr>
<tr><td>40</td><td>Idaho</td><td>2,009</td><td>0.4%</td><td>12</td><td>Indiana</td><td>12,335</td><td>2.4%</td></tr>
<tr><td>5</td><td>Illinois</td><td>24,967</td><td>4.8%</td><td>13</td><td>Louisiana</td><td>12,270</td><td>2.4%</td></tr>
<tr><td>12</td><td>Indiana</td><td>12,335</td><td>2.4%</td><td>14</td><td>Virginia</td><td>11,353</td><td>2.2%</td></tr>
<tr><td>34</td><td>Iowa</td><td>3,989</td><td>0.8%</td><td>15</td><td>Alabama</td><td>11,252</td><td>2.2%</td></tr>
<tr><td>31</td><td>Kansas</td><td>4,722</td><td>0.9%</td><td>16</td><td>Missouri</td><td>11,227</td><td>2.2%</td></tr>
<tr><td>20</td><td>Kentucky</td><td>9,349</td><td>1.8%</td><td>17</td><td>New Jersey</td><td>10,068</td><td>1.9%</td></tr>
<tr><td>13</td><td>Louisiana</td><td>12,270</td><td>2.4%</td><td>18</td><td>South Carolina</td><td>9,721</td><td>1.9%</td></tr>
<tr><td>41</td><td>Maine</td><td>1,857</td><td>0.4%</td><td>19</td><td>Arizona</td><td>9,612</td><td>1.8%</td></tr>
<tr><td>23</td><td>Maryland</td><td>8,143</td><td>1.6%</td><td>20</td><td>Kentucky</td><td>9,349</td><td>1.8%</td></tr>
<tr><td>26</td><td>Massachusetts</td><td>7,266</td><td>1.4%</td><td>21</td><td>Mississippi</td><td>8,909</td><td>1.7%</td></tr>
<tr><td>7</td><td>Michigan</td><td>20,312</td><td>3.9%</td><td>22</td><td>Washington</td><td>8,397</td><td>1.6%</td></tr>
<tr><td>29</td><td>Minnesota</td><td>5,342</td><td>1.0%</td><td>23</td><td>Maryland</td><td>8,143</td><td>1.6%</td></tr>
<tr><td>21</td><td>Mississippi</td><td>8,909</td><td>1.7%</td><td>24</td><td>Oklahoma</td><td>7,590</td><td>1.5%</td></tr>
<tr><td>16</td><td>Missouri</td><td>11,227</td><td>2.2%</td><td>25</td><td>Wisconsin</td><td>7,281</td><td>1.4%</td></tr>
<tr><td>43</td><td>Montana</td><td>1,331</td><td>0.3%</td><td>26</td><td>Massachusetts</td><td>7,266</td><td>1.4%</td></tr>
<tr><td>38</td><td>Nebraska</td><td>2,352</td><td>0.5%</td><td>27</td><td>Arkansas</td><td>7,011</td><td>1.3%</td></tr>
<tr><td>37</td><td>Nevada</td><td>2,663</td><td>0.5%</td><td>28</td><td>Colorado</td><td>5,975</td><td>1.1%</td></tr>
<tr><td>45</td><td>New Hampshire</td><td>1,258</td><td>0.2%</td><td>29</td><td>Minnesota</td><td>5,342</td><td>1.0%</td></tr>
<tr><td>17</td><td>New Jersey</td><td>10,068</td><td>1.9%</td><td>30</td><td>Oregon</td><td>5,084</td><td>1.0%</td></tr>
<tr><td>32</td><td>New Mexico</td><td>4,367</td><td>0.8%</td><td>31</td><td>Kansas</td><td>4,722</td><td>0.9%</td></tr>
<tr><td>4</td><td>New York</td><td>26,608</td><td>5.1%</td><td>32</td><td>New Mexico</td><td>4,367</td><td>0.8%</td></tr>
<tr><td>10</td><td>North Carolina</td><td>16,506</td><td>3.2%</td><td>33</td><td>Connecticut</td><td>4,038</td><td>0.8%</td></tr>
<tr><td>49</td><td>North Dakota</td><td>793</td><td>0.2%</td><td>34</td><td>Iowa</td><td>3,989</td><td>0.8%</td></tr>
<tr><td>6</td><td>Ohio</td><td>22,690</td><td>4.3%</td><td>35</td><td>West Virginia</td><td>3,976</td><td>0.8%</td></tr>
<tr><td>24</td><td>Oklahoma</td><td>7,590</td><td>1.5%</td><td>36</td><td>Utah</td><td>3,707</td><td>0.7%</td></tr>
<tr><td>30</td><td>Oregon</td><td>5,084</td><td>1.0%</td><td>37</td><td>Nevada</td><td>2,663</td><td>0.5%</td></tr>
<tr><td>9</td><td>Pennsylvania</td><td>18,216</td><td>3.5%</td><td>38</td><td>Nebraska</td><td>2,352</td><td>0.5%</td></tr>
<tr><td>42</td><td>Rhode Island</td><td>1,564</td><td>0.3%</td><td>39</td><td>Hawaii</td><td>2,122</td><td>0.4%</td></tr>
<tr><td>18</td><td>South Carolina</td><td>9,721</td><td>1.9%</td><td>40</td><td>Idaho</td><td>2,009</td><td>0.4%</td></tr>
<tr><td>46</td><td>South Dakota</td><td>1,172</td><td>0.2%</td><td>41</td><td>Maine</td><td>1,857</td><td>0.4%</td></tr>
<tr><td>11</td><td>Tennessee</td><td>12,928</td><td>2.5%</td><td>42</td><td>Rhode Island</td><td>1,564</td><td>0.3%</td></tr>
<tr><td>2</td><td>Texas</td><td>48,302</td><td>9.3%</td><td>43</td><td>Montana</td><td>1,331</td><td>0.3%</td></tr>
<tr><td>36</td><td>Utah</td><td>3,707</td><td>0.7%</td><td>44</td><td>Delaware</td><td>1,277</td><td>0.2%</td></tr>
<tr><td>50</td><td>Vermont</td><td>702</td><td>0.1%</td><td>45</td><td>New Hampshire</td><td>1,258</td><td>0.2%</td></tr>
<tr><td>14</td><td>Virginia</td><td>11,353</td><td>2.2%</td><td>46</td><td>South Dakota</td><td>1,172</td><td>0.2%</td></tr>
<tr><td>22</td><td>Washington</td><td>8,397</td><td>1.6%</td><td>47</td><td>Alaska</td><td>1,142</td><td>0.2%</td></tr>
<tr><td>35</td><td>West Virginia</td><td>3,976</td><td>0.8%</td><td>48</td><td>Wyoming</td><td>943</td><td>0.2%</td></tr>
<tr><td>25</td><td>Wisconsin</td><td>7,281</td><td>1.4%</td><td>49</td><td>North Dakota</td><td>793</td><td>0.2%</td></tr>
<tr><td>48</td><td>Wyoming</td><td>943</td><td>0.2%</td><td>50</td><td>Vermont</td><td>702</td><td>0.1%</td></tr>
<tr><td></td><td></td><td></td><td></td><td></td><td>District of Columbia</td><td>2,030</td><td>0.4%</td></tr>
</table>

Source: U.S. Department of Health and Human Services, Centers for Disease Control and Prevention
    "Surveillance for Pregnancy and Birth Rates Among Teenagers" (MMWR, Vol. 42, No. SS-6, 12/17/93)
*Women aged 15 to 19 years old.

Teenage Birth Rate in 1990

National Rate = 59.9 Live Births per 1,000 Teenage Women*

ALPHA ORDER				RANK ORDER		
RANK	STATE	RATE		RANK	STATE	RATE
11	Alabama	71.0		1	Mississippi	81.0
17	Alaska	65.3		2	Arkansas	80.1
4	Arizona	75.5		3	New Mexico	78.2
2	Arkansas	80.1		4	Arizona	75.5
12	California	70.6		4	Georgia	75.5
28	Colorado	54.5		6	Texas	75.3
45	Connecticut	38.8		7	Louisiana	74.2
28	Delaware	54.5		8	Nevada	73.3
13	Florida	69.1		9	Tennessee	72.3
4	Georgia	75.5		10	South Carolina	71.3
20	Hawaii	61.2		11	Alabama	71.0
33	Idaho	50.6		12	California	70.6
18	Illinois	62.9		13	Florida	69.1
22	Indiana	58.6		14	Kentucky	67.6
43	Iowa	40.5		14	North Carolina	67.6
26	Kansas	56.1		16	Oklahoma	66.8
14	Kentucky	67.6		17	Alaska	65.3
7	Louisiana	74.2		18	Illinois	62.9
40	Maine	43.0		19	Missouri	62.8
30	Maryland	53.2		20	Hawaii	61.2
48	Massachusetts	35.1		21	Michigan	59.0
21	Michigan	59.0		22	Indiana	58.6
46	Minnesota	36.3		23	Ohio	57.9
1	Mississippi	81.0		24	West Virginia	57.3
19	Missouri	62.8		25	Wyoming	56.3
35	Montana	48.4		26	Kansas	56.1
42	Nebraska	42.3		27	Oregon	54.6
8	Nevada	73.3		28	Colorado	54.5
50	New Hampshire	33.0		28	Delaware	54.5
43	New Jersey	40.5		30	Maryland	53.2
3	New Mexico	78.2		31	Washington	53.1
39	New York	43.6		32	Virginia	52.9
14	North Carolina	67.6		33	Idaho	50.6
47	North Dakota	35.4		34	Utah	48.5
23	Ohio	57.9		35	Montana	48.4
16	Oklahoma	66.8		36	South Dakota	46.8
27	Oregon	54.6		37	Pennsylvania	44.9
37	Pennsylvania	44.9		38	Rhode Island	43.9
38	Rhode Island	43.9		39	New York	43.6
10	South Carolina	71.3		40	Maine	43.0
36	South Dakota	46.8		41	Wisconsin	42.6
9	Tennessee	72.3		42	Nebraska	42.3
6	Texas	75.3		43	Iowa	40.5
34	Utah	48.5		43	New Jersey	40.5
49	Vermont	34.0		45	Connecticut	38.8
32	Virginia	52.9		46	Minnesota	36.3
31	Washington	53.1		47	North Dakota	35.4
24	West Virginia	57.3		48	Massachusetts	35.1
41	Wisconsin	42.6		49	Vermont	34.0
25	Wyoming	56.3		50	New Hampshire	33.0
					District of Columbia	93.1

Source: U.S. Department of Health and Human Services, Centers for Disease Control and Prevention
   "Surveillance for Pregnancy and Birth Rates Among Teenagers" (MMWR, Vol. 42, No. SS-6, 12/17/93)
*Women aged 15 to 19 years old.

Percent Change in Teenage Birth Rate: 1990 to 1998

National Percent Change = 14.7% Decrease*

ALPHA ORDER

RANK ORDER

RANK	STATE	PERCENT CHANGE		RANK	STATE	PERCENT CHANGE
5	Alabama	(7.7)		1	Delaware	(1.1)
50	Alaska	(35.1)		2	Texas	(5.8)
3	Arizona	(6.6)		3	Arizona	(6.6)
15	Arkansas	(11.6)		3	Rhode Island	(6.6)
45	California	(24.2)		5	Alabama	(7.7)
12	Colorado	(10.6)		5	Connecticut	(7.7)
5	Connecticut	(7.7)		7	Oklahoma	(7.8)
1	Delaware	(1.1)		8	Indiana	(9.0)
42	Florida	(19.7)		9	North Carolina	(9.8)
23	Georgia	(13.4)		10	Mississippi	(9.9)
46	Hawaii	(25.3)		11	Nevada	(10.4)
14	Idaho	(11.5)		12	Colorado	(10.6)
29	Illinois	(15.4)		13	Tennessee	(11.1)
8	Indiana	(9.0)		14	Idaho	(11.5)
21	Iowa	(13.1)		15	Arkansas	(11.6)
33	Kansas	(16.2)		16	New York	(11.7)
30	Kentucky	(15.7)		17	New Mexico	(11.8)
18	Louisiana	(11.9)		18	Louisiana	(11.9)
49	Maine	(29.3)		19	Massachusetts	(12.3)
41	Maryland	(19.0)		20	Nebraska	(12.5)
19	Massachusetts	(12.3)		21	Iowa	(13.1)
47	Michigan	(27.8)		22	Oregon	(13.2)
30	Minnesota	(15.7)		23	Georgia	(13.4)
10	Mississippi	(9.9)		24	North Dakota	(14.1)
40	Missouri	(18.5)		24	West Virginia	(14.1)
44	Montana	(23.3)		26	New Jersey	(14.6)
20	Nebraska	(12.5)		27	Wyoming	(15.1)
11	Nevada	(10.4)		28	South Carolina	(15.3)
38	New Hampshire	(17.9)		29	Illinois	(15.4)
26	New Jersey	(14.6)		30	Kentucky	(15.7)
17	New Mexico	(11.8)		30	Minnesota	(15.7)
16	New York	(11.7)		30	Utah	(15.7)
9	North Carolina	(9.8)		33	Kansas	(16.2)
24	North Dakota	(14.1)		34	Ohio	(16.9)
34	Ohio	(16.9)		35	South Dakota	(17.7)
7	Oklahoma	(7.8)		36	Pennsylvania	(17.8)
22	Oregon	(13.2)		36	Virginia	(17.8)
36	Pennsylvania	(17.8)		38	New Hampshire	(17.9)
3	Rhode Island	(6.6)		39	Wisconsin	(18.3)
28	South Carolina	(15.3)		40	Missouri	(18.5)
35	South Dakota	(17.7)		41	Maryland	(19.0)
13	Tennessee	(11.1)		42	Florida	(19.7)
2	Texas	(5.8)		43	Washington	(21.5)
30	Utah	(15.7)		44	Montana	(23.3)
48	Vermont	(28.2)		45	California	(24.2)
36	Virginia	(17.8)		46	Hawaii	(25.3)
43	Washington	(21.5)		47	Michigan	(27.8)
24	West Virginia	(14.1)		48	Vermont	(28.2)
39	Wisconsin	(18.3)		49	Maine	(29.3)
27	Wyoming	(15.1)		50	Alaska	(35.1)

District of Columbia   (6.9)

Source: Morgan Quitno Press using data from U.S. Department of Health and Human Services
   "National Vital Statistics Reports" (Vol. 48, No. 3, March 28, 2000)
   "Surveillance for Pregnancy and Birth Rates Among Teenagers" (MMWR, Vol. 42, No. SS-6, 12/17/93)
*Women aged 15 to 19 years old.

Births to Teenage Mothers in 1980

National Total = 562,330 Live Births*

ALPHA ORDER

RANK	STATE	BIRTHS	% of USA
15	Alabama	13,096	2.3%
49	Alaska	1,123	0.2%
25	Arizona	8,235	1.5%
26	Arkansas	8,060	1.4%
1	California	56,138	10.0%
29	Colorado	6,592	1.2%
36	Connecticut	4,408	0.8%
45	Delaware	1,572	0.3%
6	Florida	24,042	4.3%
9	Georgia	19,137	3.4%
40	Hawaii	2,085	0.4%
38	Idaho	2,645	0.5%
3	Illinois	29,798	5.3%
12	Indiana	15,331	2.7%
31	Iowa	5,962	1.1%
30	Kansas	6,090	1.1%
16	Kentucky	12,559	2.2%
10	Louisiana	16,504	2.9%
39	Maine	2,522	0.4%
23	Maryland	8,885	1.6%
27	Massachusetts	7,765	1.4%
8	Michigan	20,401	3.6%
28	Minnesota	7,048	1.3%
19	Mississippi	11,079	2.0%
14	Missouri	13,312	2.4%
43	Montana	1,761	0.3%
37	Nebraska	3,313	0.6%
41	Nevada	2,048	0.4%
47	New Hampshire	1,475	0.3%
18	New Jersey	11,904	2.1%
34	New Mexico	4,758	0.8%
4	New York	28,206	5.0%
11	North Carolina	16,192	2.9%
48	North Dakota	1,304	0.2%
5	Ohio	26,567	4.7%
21	Oklahoma	10,206	1.8%
33	Oregon	5,731	1.0%
7	Pennsylvania	22,029	3.9%
46	Rhode Island	1,502	0.3%
20	South Carolina	10,282	1.8%
42	South Dakota	1,797	0.3%
13	Tennessee	13,792	2.5%
2	Texas	50,125	8.9%
35	Utah	4,594	0.8%
50	Vermont	1,024	0.2%
17	Virginia	12,138	2.2%
24	Washington	8,495	1.5%
32	West Virginia	5,911	1.1%
22	Wisconsin	9,220	1.6%
44	Wyoming	1,634	0.3%

RANK ORDER

RANK	STATE	BIRTHS	% of USA
1	California	56,138	10.0%
2	Texas	50,125	8.9%
3	Illinois	29,798	5.3%
4	New York	28,206	5.0%
5	Ohio	26,567	4.7%
6	Florida	24,042	4.3%
7	Pennsylvania	22,029	3.9%
8	Michigan	20,401	3.6%
9	Georgia	19,137	3.4%
10	Louisiana	16,504	2.9%
11	North Carolina	16,192	2.9%
12	Indiana	15,331	2.7%
13	Tennessee	13,792	2.5%
14	Missouri	13,312	2.4%
15	Alabama	13,096	2.3%
16	Kentucky	12,559	2.2%
17	Virginia	12,138	2.2%
18	New Jersey	11,904	2.1%
19	Mississippi	11,079	2.0%
20	South Carolina	10,282	1.8%
21	Oklahoma	10,206	1.8%
22	Wisconsin	9,220	1.6%
23	Maryland	8,885	1.6%
24	Washington	8,495	1.5%
25	Arizona	8,235	1.5%
26	Arkansas	8,060	1.4%
27	Massachusetts	7,765	1.4%
28	Minnesota	7,048	1.3%
29	Colorado	6,592	1.2%
30	Kansas	6,090	1.1%
31	Iowa	5,962	1.1%
32	West Virginia	5,911	1.1%
33	Oregon	5,731	1.0%
34	New Mexico	4,758	0.8%
35	Utah	4,594	0.8%
36	Connecticut	4,408	0.8%
37	Nebraska	3,313	0.6%
38	Idaho	2,645	0.5%
39	Maine	2,522	0.4%
40	Hawaii	2,085	0.4%
41	Nevada	2,048	0.4%
42	South Dakota	1,797	0.3%
43	Montana	1,761	0.3%
44	Wyoming	1,634	0.3%
45	Delaware	1,572	0.3%
46	Rhode Island	1,502	0.3%
47	New Hampshire	1,475	0.3%
48	North Dakota	1,304	0.2%
49	Alaska	1,123	0.2%
50	Vermont	1,024	0.2%
	District of Columbia	1,933	0.3%

Source: U.S. Department of Health and Human Services, National Center for Health Statistics
    "Vital Statistics of the United States, 1980" (Vol. I-Natality, issued 1984)
*Births to women age 15 to 19 years old.

Teenage Birth Rate in 1980

National Rate = 53.0 Live Births per 1,000 Teenage Women*

ALPHA ORDER

RANK	STATE	RATE
10	Alabama	68.3
15	Alaska	64.4
12	Arizona	65.5
5	Arkansas	74.5
25	California	53.3
31	Colorado	49.9
49	Connecticut	30.5
28	Delaware	51.2
18	Florida	58.5
8	Georgia	71.9
30	Hawaii	50.7
17	Idaho	59.5
24	Illinois	55.8
21	Indiana	57.5
39	Iowa	43.0
23	Kansas	56.8
7	Kentucky	72.3
3	Louisiana	76.0
34	Maine	47.4
38	Maryland	43.4
50	Massachusetts	28.1
37	Michigan	45.0
44	Minnesota	35.4
1	Mississippi	83.7
20	Missouri	57.8
32	Montana	48.5
36	Nebraska	45.1
18	Nevada	58.5
47	New Hampshire	33.6
45	New Jersey	35.2
9	New Mexico	71.8
46	New York	34.8
21	North Carolina	57.5
40	North Dakota	41.7
27	Ohio	52.5
4	Oklahoma	74.6
29	Oregon	50.9
41	Pennsylvania	40.5
48	Rhode Island	33.0
14	South Carolina	64.8
26	South Dakota	52.6
16	Tennessee	64.1
6	Texas	74.3
13	Utah	65.2
42	Vermont	39.5
33	Virginia	48.3
35	Washington	46.7
11	West Virginia	67.8
42	Wisconsin	39.5
2	Wyoming	78.7

RANK ORDER

RANK	STATE	RATE
1	Mississippi	83.7
2	Wyoming	78.7
3	Louisiana	76.0
4	Oklahoma	74.6
5	Arkansas	74.5
6	Texas	74.3
7	Kentucky	72.3
8	Georgia	71.9
9	New Mexico	71.8
10	Alabama	68.3
11	West Virginia	67.8
12	Arizona	65.5
13	Utah	65.2
14	South Carolina	64.8
15	Alaska	64.4
16	Tennessee	64.1
17	Idaho	59.5
18	Florida	58.5
18	Nevada	58.5
20	Missouri	57.8
21	Indiana	57.5
21	North Carolina	57.5
23	Kansas	56.8
24	Illinois	55.8
25	California	53.3
26	South Dakota	52.6
27	Ohio	52.5
28	Delaware	51.2
29	Oregon	50.9
30	Hawaii	50.7
31	Colorado	49.9
32	Montana	48.5
33	Virginia	48.3
34	Maine	47.4
35	Washington	46.7
36	Nebraska	45.1
37	Michigan	45.0
38	Maryland	43.4
39	Iowa	43.0
40	North Dakota	41.7
41	Pennsylvania	40.5
42	Vermont	39.5
42	Wisconsin	39.5
44	Minnesota	35.4
45	New Jersey	35.2
46	New York	34.8
47	New Hampshire	33.6
48	Rhode Island	33.0
49	Connecticut	30.5
50	Massachusetts	28.1
	District of Columbia	62.4

Source: U.S. Department of Health and Human Services, Centers for Disease Control and Prevention
    "Surveillance for Pregnancy and Birth Rates Among Teenagers" (MMWR, Vol. 42, No. SS-6, 12/17/93)
*Women aged 15 to 19 years old.

Births to Women 35 to 54 Years Old in 1998

National Total = 509,699 Live Births*

RANK	STATE	BIRTHS	% of USA
27	Alabama	5,142	1.0%
44	Alaska	1,329	0.3%
17	Arizona	8,693	1.7%
38	Arkansas	2,708	0.5%
1	California	79,100	15.5%
19	Colorado	8,521	1.7%
20	Connecticut	8,474	1.7%
46	Delaware	1,294	0.3%
4	Florida	26,115	5.1%
12	Georgia	13,247	2.6%
37	Hawaii	2,813	0.6%
41	Idaho	1,807	0.4%
5	Illinois	24,451	4.8%
22	Indiana	8,022	1.6%
32	Iowa	3,888	0.8%
29	Kansas	4,366	0.9%
28	Kentucky	4,471	0.9%
24	Louisiana	5,788	1.1%
42	Maine	1,737	0.3%
13	Maryland	12,097	2.4%
9	Massachusetts	16,328	3.2%
10	Michigan	15,865	3.1%
16	Minnesota	9,587	1.9%
34	Mississippi	3,002	0.6%
21	Missouri	8,176	1.6%
45	Montana	1,302	0.3%
36	Nebraska	2,817	0.6%
33	Nevada	3,205	0.6%
39	New Hampshire	2,355	0.5%
6	New Jersey	22,174	4.4%
35	New Mexico	2,898	0.6%
2	New York	45,078	8.8%
14	North Carolina	11,691	2.3%
49	North Dakota	879	0.2%
8	Ohio	17,175	3.4%
31	Oklahoma	4,067	0.8%
25	Oregon	5,558	1.1%
7	Pennsylvania	20,883	4.1%
40	Rhode Island	1,973	0.4%
26	South Carolina	5,339	1.0%
47	South Dakota	1,082	0.2%
23	Tennessee	7,086	1.4%
3	Texas	34,566	6.8%
30	Utah	4,323	0.8%
48	Vermont	1,007	0.2%
11	Virginia	13,949	2.7%
15	Washington	11,128	2.2%
43	West Virginia	1,625	0.3%
18	Wisconsin	8,651	1.7%
50	Wyoming	557	0.1%

RANK	STATE	BIRTHS	% of USA
1	California	79,100	15.5%
2	New York	45,078	8.8%
3	Texas	34,566	6.8%
4	Florida	26,115	5.1%
5	Illinois	24,451	4.8%
6	New Jersey	22,174	4.4%
7	Pennsylvania	20,883	4.1%
8	Ohio	17,175	3.4%
9	Massachusetts	16,328	3.2%
10	Michigan	15,865	3.1%
11	Virginia	13,949	2.7%
12	Georgia	13,247	2.6%
13	Maryland	12,097	2.4%
14	North Carolina	11,691	2.3%
15	Washington	11,128	2.2%
16	Minnesota	9,587	1.9%
17	Arizona	8,693	1.7%
18	Wisconsin	8,651	1.7%
19	Colorado	8,521	1.7%
20	Connecticut	8,474	1.7%
21	Missouri	8,176	1.6%
22	Indiana	8,022	1.6%
23	Tennessee	7,086	1.4%
24	Louisiana	5,788	1.1%
25	Oregon	5,558	1.1%
26	South Carolina	5,339	1.0%
27	Alabama	5,142	1.0%
28	Kentucky	4,471	0.9%
29	Kansas	4,366	0.9%
30	Utah	4,323	0.8%
31	Oklahoma	4,067	0.8%
32	Iowa	3,888	0.8%
33	Nevada	3,205	0.6%
34	Mississippi	3,002	0.6%
35	New Mexico	2,898	0.6%
36	Nebraska	2,817	0.6%
37	Hawaii	2,813	0.6%
38	Arkansas	2,708	0.5%
39	New Hampshire	2,355	0.5%
40	Rhode Island	1,973	0.4%
41	Idaho	1,807	0.4%
42	Maine	1,737	0.3%
43	West Virginia	1,625	0.3%
44	Alaska	1,329	0.3%
45	Montana	1,302	0.3%
46	Delaware	1,294	0.3%
47	South Dakota	1,082	0.2%
48	Vermont	1,007	0.2%
49	North Dakota	879	0.2%
50	Wyoming	557	0.1%
	District of Columbia	1,310	0.3%

Source: Morgan Quitno Press using data from U.S. Dept of Health & Human Services, National Center for Health Statistics (unpublished data)
*By state of residence.

Births to Women 35 to 54 Years Old as a Percent of All Births in 1998

National Percent = 12.9% of Live Births*

ALPHA ORDER			RANK ORDER		
RANK	STATE	PERCENT	RANK	STATE	PERCENT
45	Alabama	8.3	1	Massachusetts	20.1
16	Alaska	13.4	2	New Jersey	19.4
29	Arizona	11.1	3	Connecticut	19.3
49	Arkansas	7.3	4	New York	17.5
10	California	15.2	5	Maryland	16.8
13	Colorado	14.3	6	New Hampshire	16.3
3	Connecticut	19.3	7	Hawaii	16.0
22	Delaware	12.2	8	Rhode Island	15.7
18	Florida	13.3	9	Vermont	15.3
31	Georgia	10.8	10	California	15.2
7	Hawaii	16.0	11	Virginia	14.8
41	Idaho	9.3	12	Minnesota	14.7
16	Illinois	13.4	13	Colorado	14.3
40	Indiana	9.4	13	Pennsylvania	14.3
36	Iowa	10.4	15	Washington	14.0
26	Kansas	11.4	16	Alaska	13.4
46	Kentucky	8.2	16	Illinois	13.4
44	Louisiana	8.7	18	Florida	13.3
20	Maine	12.6	19	Wisconsin	12.8
5	Maryland	16.8	20	Maine	12.6
1	Massachusetts	20.1	21	Oregon	12.3
25	Michigan	11.9	22	Delaware	12.2
12	Minnesota	14.7	23	Montana	12.1
50	Mississippi	7.0	24	Nebraska	12.0
31	Missouri	10.8	25	Michigan	11.9
23	Montana	12.1	26	Kansas	11.4
24	Nebraska	12.0	27	Nevada	11.2
27	Nevada	11.2	27	Ohio	11.2
6	New Hampshire	16.3	29	Arizona	11.1
2	New Jersey	19.4	29	North Dakota	11.1
33	New Mexico	10.6	31	Georgia	10.8
4	New York	17.5	31	Missouri	10.8
34	North Carolina	10.5	33	New Mexico	10.6
29	North Dakota	11.1	34	North Carolina	10.5
27	Ohio	11.2	34	South Dakota	10.5
46	Oklahoma	8.2	36	Iowa	10.4
21	Oregon	12.3	37	Texas	10.1
13	Pennsylvania	14.3	38	South Carolina	9.9
8	Rhode Island	15.7	39	Utah	9.6
38	South Carolina	9.9	40	Indiana	9.4
34	South Dakota	10.5	41	Idaho	9.3
42	Tennessee	9.2	42	Tennessee	9.2
37	Texas	10.1	43	Wyoming	8.9
39	Utah	9.6	44	Louisiana	8.7
9	Vermont	15.3	45	Alabama	8.3
11	Virginia	14.8	46	Kentucky	8.2
15	Washington	14.0	46	Oklahoma	8.2
48	West Virginia	7.8	48	West Virginia	7.8
19	Wisconsin	12.8	49	Arkansas	7.3
43	Wyoming	8.9	50	Mississippi	7.0
				District of Columbia	17.0

Source: Morgan Quitno Press using data from U.S. Dept of Health & Human Services, National Center for Health Statistics
(unpublished data)
*By state of residence.

43

Multiple Birth Rate in 1997

National Rate = 27.3 Multiple Births per 1,000 Live Births*

ALPHA ORDER

RANK	STATE	RATE
25	Alabama	27.0
35	Alaska	24.8
38	Arizona	24.5
34	Arkansas	25.0
38	California	24.5
8	Colorado	30.6
2	Connecticut	35.0
5	Delaware	31.5
32	Florida	26.2
26	Georgia	26.9
50	Hawaii	19.1
47	Idaho	22.3
9	Illinois	30.2
27	Indiana	26.8
13	Iowa	29.2
20	Kansas	27.4
33	Kentucky	25.6
20	Louisiana	27.4
16	Maine	28.4
6	Maryland	31.0
1	Massachusetts	35.3
12	Michigan	29.4
9	Minnesota	30.2
42	Mississippi	24.2
19	Missouri	27.6
44	Montana	24.0
4	Nebraska	33.5
45	Nevada	23.9
18	New Hampshire	28.0
3	New Jersey	34.3
49	New Mexico	21.4
7	New York	30.7
23	North Carolina	27.2
9	North Dakota	30.2
17	Ohio	28.3
46	Oklahoma	23.1
37	Oregon	24.6
14	Pennsylvania	29.0
15	Rhode Island	28.6
30	South Carolina	26.4
27	South Dakota	26.8
30	Tennessee	26.4
40	Texas	24.4
43	Utah	24.1
48	Vermont	22.1
20	Virginia	27.4
36	Washington	24.7
40	West Virginia	24.4
23	Wisconsin	27.2
29	Wyoming	26.6

RANK ORDER

RANK	STATE	RATE
1	Massachusetts	35.3
2	Connecticut	35.0
3	New Jersey	34.3
4	Nebraska	33.5
5	Delaware	31.5
6	Maryland	31.0
7	New York	30.7
8	Colorado	30.6
9	Illinois	30.2
9	Minnesota	30.2
9	North Dakota	30.2
12	Michigan	29.4
13	Iowa	29.2
14	Pennsylvania	29.0
15	Rhode Island	28.6
16	Maine	28.4
17	Ohio	28.3
18	New Hampshire	28.0
19	Missouri	27.6
20	Kansas	27.4
20	Louisiana	27.4
20	Virginia	27.4
23	North Carolina	27.2
23	Wisconsin	27.2
25	Alabama	27.0
26	Georgia	26.9
27	Indiana	26.8
27	South Dakota	26.8
29	Wyoming	26.6
30	South Carolina	26.4
30	Tennessee	26.4
32	Florida	26.2
33	Kentucky	25.6
34	Arkansas	25.0
35	Alaska	24.8
36	Washington	24.7
37	Oregon	24.6
38	Arizona	24.5
38	California	24.5
40	Texas	24.4
40	West Virginia	24.4
42	Mississippi	24.2
43	Utah	24.1
44	Montana	24.0
45	Nevada	23.9
46	Oklahoma	23.1
47	Idaho	22.3
48	Vermont	22.1
49	New Mexico	21.4
50	Hawaii	19.1

District of Columbia   29.5

Source: Morgan Quitno Press using data from U.S. Dept. of Health and Human Services, Nat'l Center for Health Statistics "National Vital Statistics Reports" (Vol. 47, No. 24, September 14, 1999)
*By state of residence of mother. Multiple births include all births of twins, triplets or more. Rate is based on a three-year average of rates for 1995 through 1997.

Percent Change in Multiple Birth Rate: 1993 to 1997

National Percent Change = 11.4% Increase*

ALPHA ORDER

RANK ORDER

RANK	STATE	PERCENT CHANGE
25	Alabama	10.4
18	Alaska	12.2
22	Arizona	11.4
32	Arkansas	9.0
29	California	9.7
5	Colorado	27.1
7	Connecticut	24.0
9	Delaware	22.3
17	Florida	13.1
27	Georgia	10.1
50	Hawaii	(11.8)
30	Idaho	9.5
19	Illinois	12.1
36	Indiana	8.6
11	Iowa	15.1
15	Kansas	14.0
24	Kentucky	10.7
34	Louisiana	8.9
16	Maine	13.8
10	Maryland	17.1
8	Massachusetts	23.4
25	Michigan	10.4
6	Minnesota	24.1
48	Mississippi	(6.0)
39	Missouri	7.3
41	Montana	7.1
1	Nebraska	32.9
45	Nevada	3.3
34	New Hampshire	8.9
4	New Jersey	28.3
32	New Mexico	9.0
12	New York	14.8
38	North Carolina	7.7
2	North Dakota	29.6
42	Ohio	6.7
47	Oklahoma	(1.0)
46	Oregon	0.0
20	Pennsylvania	12.0
13	Rhode Island	14.4
44	South Carolina	4.6
28	South Dakota	10.0
31	Tennessee	9.2
23	Texas	11.2
43	Utah	6.2
49	Vermont	(11.2)
20	Virginia	12.0
14	Washington	14.2
39	West Virginia	7.3
37	Wisconsin	7.8
3	Wyoming	28.7

RANK	STATE	PERCENT CHANGE
1	Nebraska	32.9
2	North Dakota	29.6
3	Wyoming	28.7
4	New Jersey	28.3
5	Colorado	27.1
6	Minnesota	24.1
7	Connecticut	24.0
8	Massachusetts	23.4
9	Delaware	22.3
10	Maryland	17.1
11	Iowa	15.1
12	New York	14.8
13	Rhode Island	14.4
14	Washington	14.2
15	Kansas	14.0
16	Maine	13.8
17	Florida	13.1
18	Alaska	12.2
19	Illinois	12.1
20	Pennsylvania	12.0
20	Virginia	12.0
22	Arizona	11.4
23	Texas	11.2
24	Kentucky	10.7
25	Alabama	10.4
25	Michigan	10.4
27	Georgia	10.1
28	South Dakota	10.0
29	California	9.7
30	Idaho	9.5
31	Tennessee	9.2
32	Arkansas	9.0
32	New Mexico	9.0
34	Louisiana	8.9
34	New Hampshire	8.9
36	Indiana	8.6
37	Wisconsin	7.8
38	North Carolina	7.7
39	Missouri	7.3
39	West Virginia	7.3
41	Montana	7.1
42	Ohio	6.7
43	Utah	6.2
44	South Carolina	4.6
45	Nevada	3.3
46	Oregon	0.0
47	Oklahoma	(1.0)
48	Mississippi	(6.0)
49	Vermont	(11.2)
50	Hawaii	(11.8)

District of Columbia 15.8

Source: Morgan Quitno Press using data from U.S. Dept. of Health and Human Services, Nat'l Center for Health Statistics
"National Vital Statistics Report" (Vol. 47, No. 24, September 14, 1999) and
"Vital Statistics of the United States: Volume I-Natality" (various years)
*By state of residence of mother. Multiple births include all births of twins, triplets or more. Rate is based on a three-year average of rates for 1991-1993 and 1995-1997.

Births by Vaginal Delivery in 1998

National Total = 3,105,944 Live Births*

ALPHA ORDER

RANK	STATE	BIRTHS	% of USA
24	Alabama	47,176	1.5%
45	Alaska	8,467	0.3%
15	Arizona	64,942	2.1%
34	Arkansas	27,686	0.9%
1	California	408,461	13.2%
22	Colorado	49,806	1.6%
30	Connecticut	35,012	1.1%
46	Delaware	8,124	0.3%
4	Florida	151,814	4.9%
9	Georgia	96,915	3.1%
40	Hawaii	14,840	0.5%
38	Idaho	16,347	0.5%
5	Illinois	147,166	4.7%
13	Indiana	68,098	2.2%
33	Iowa	29,975	1.0%
32	Kansas	31,276	1.0%
25	Kentucky	41,942	1.4%
23	Louisiana	49,497	1.6%
42	Maine	11,028	0.4%
20	Maryland	56,642	1.8%
16	Massachusetts	64,396	2.1%
8	Michigan	106,131	3.4%
21	Minnesota	53,466	1.7%
31	Mississippi	31,345	1.0%
18	Missouri	59,834	1.9%
44	Montana	8,755	0.3%
37	Nebraska	18,686	0.6%
36	Nevada	22,557	0.7%
41	New Hampshire	11,760	0.4%
11	New Jersey	85,454	2.8%
35	New Mexico	22,838	0.7%
3	New York	199,078	6.4%
10	North Carolina	87,675	2.8%
48	North Dakota	6,393	0.2%
6	Ohio	123,916	4.0%
27	Oklahoma	38,184	1.2%
29	Oregon	37,214	1.2%
7	Pennsylvania	117,303	3.8%
43	Rhode Island	10,142	0.3%
26	South Carolina	41,270	1.3%
47	South Dakota	8,076	0.3%
17	Tennessee	59,905	1.9%
2	Texas	261,846	8.4%
28	Utah	37,939	1.2%
49	Vermont	5,496	0.2%
12	Virginia	74,349	2.4%
14	Washington	65,403	2.1%
39	West Virginia	15,747	0.5%
19	Wisconsin	56,658	1.8%
50	Wyoming	5,089	0.2%

RANK ORDER

RANK	STATE	BIRTHS	% of USA
1	California	408,461	13.2%
2	Texas	261,846	8.4%
3	New York	199,078	6.4%
4	Florida	151,814	4.9%
5	Illinois	147,166	4.7%
6	Ohio	123,916	4.0%
7	Pennsylvania	117,303	3.8%
8	Michigan	106,131	3.4%
9	Georgia	96,915	3.1%
10	North Carolina	87,675	2.8%
11	New Jersey	85,454	2.8%
12	Virginia	74,349	2.4%
13	Indiana	68,098	2.2%
14	Washington	65,403	2.1%
15	Arizona	64,942	2.1%
16	Massachusetts	64,396	2.1%
17	Tennessee	59,905	1.9%
18	Missouri	59,834	1.9%
19	Wisconsin	56,658	1.8%
20	Maryland	56,642	1.8%
21	Minnesota	53,466	1.7%
22	Colorado	49,806	1.6%
23	Louisiana	49,497	1.6%
24	Alabama	47,176	1.5%
25	Kentucky	41,942	1.4%
26	South Carolina	41,270	1.3%
27	Oklahoma	38,184	1.2%
28	Utah	37,939	1.2%
29	Oregon	37,214	1.2%
30	Connecticut	35,012	1.1%
31	Mississippi	31,345	1.0%
32	Kansas	31,276	1.0%
33	Iowa	29,975	1.0%
34	Arkansas	27,686	0.9%
35	New Mexico	22,838	0.7%
36	Nevada	22,557	0.7%
37	Nebraska	18,686	0.6%
38	Idaho	16,347	0.5%
39	West Virginia	15,747	0.5%
40	Hawaii	14,840	0.5%
41	New Hampshire	11,760	0.4%
42	Maine	11,028	0.4%
43	Rhode Island	10,142	0.3%
44	Montana	8,755	0.3%
45	Alaska	8,467	0.3%
46	Delaware	8,124	0.3%
47	South Dakota	8,076	0.3%
48	North Dakota	6,393	0.2%
49	Vermont	5,496	0.2%
50	Wyoming	5,089	0.2%
	District of Columbia	6,087	0.2%

Source: Morgan Quitno Press using data from U.S. Dept of Health & Human Services, National Center for Health Statistics unpublished data

*By state of residence. Includes VBACs (vaginal births after cesarean).

Percent of Births by Vaginal Delivery in 1998

National Percent = 78.8% of Live Births*

ALPHA ORDER				RANK ORDER		
RANK	STATE	PERCENT		RANK	STATE	PERCENT
45	Alabama	76.0		1	Alaska	85.3
1	Alaska	85.3		2	Hawaii	84.4
9	Arizona	83.0		3	Idaho	84.3
47	Arkansas	75.1		4	Utah	84.0
36	California	78.3		4	Wisconsin	84.0
6	Colorado	83.6		6	Colorado	83.6
25	Connecticut	79.9		6	New Mexico	83.6
42	Delaware	76.8		8	Vermont	83.5
37	Florida	77.6		9	Arizona	83.0
29	Georgia	79.2		10	Oregon	82.2
2	Hawaii	84.4		11	Washington	82.1
3	Idaho	84.3		12	Minnesota	82.0
18	Illinois	80.6		13	New Hampshire	81.5
24	Indiana	80.0		14	Kansas	81.4
21	Iowa	80.4		14	Wyoming	81.4
14	Kansas	81.4		16	Montana	81.1
39	Kentucky	77.2		16	Ohio	81.1
49	Louisiana	74.0		18	Illinois	80.6
23	Maine	80.3		18	North Dakota	80.6
32	Maryland	78.7		20	Rhode Island	80.5
30	Massachusetts	79.1		21	Iowa	80.4
26	Michigan	79.4		21	Pennsylvania	80.4
12	Minnesota	82.0		23	Maine	80.3
50	Mississippi	73.0		24	Indiana	80.0
26	Missouri	79.4		25	Connecticut	79.9
16	Montana	81.1		26	Michigan	79.4
26	Nebraska	79.4		26	Missouri	79.4
33	Nevada	78.6		26	Nebraska	79.4
13	New Hampshire	81.5		29	Georgia	79.2
48	New Jersey	74.6		30	Massachusetts	79.1
6	New Mexico	83.6		31	Virginia	78.8
41	New York	77.1		32	Maryland	78.7
34	North Carolina	78.5		33	Nevada	78.6
18	North Dakota	80.6		34	North Carolina	78.5
16	Ohio	81.1		34	South Dakota	78.5
39	Oklahoma	77.2		36	California	78.3
10	Oregon	82.2		37	Florida	77.6
21	Pennsylvania	80.4		38	Tennessee	77.4
20	Rhode Island	80.5		39	Kentucky	77.2
43	South Carolina	76.6		39	Oklahoma	77.2
34	South Dakota	78.5		41	New York	77.1
38	Tennessee	77.4		42	Delaware	76.8
44	Texas	76.5		43	South Carolina	76.6
4	Utah	84.0		44	Texas	76.5
8	Vermont	83.5		45	Alabama	76.0
31	Virginia	78.8		46	West Virginia	75.9
11	Washington	82.1		47	Arkansas	75.1
46	West Virginia	75.9		48	New Jersey	74.6
4	Wisconsin	84.0		49	Louisiana	74.0
14	Wyoming	81.4		50	Mississippi	73.0
					District of Columbia	79.2

Source: Morgan Quitno Press using data from U.S. Dept of Health & Human Services, National Center for Health Statistics unpublished data

*By state of residence. Includes VBACs (vaginal births after cesarean).

Births by Cesarean Delivery in 1998

National Total = 835,609 Live Cesarean Births*

ALPHA ORDER					RANK ORDER			

RANK	STATE	BIRTHS	% of USA		RANK	STATE	BIRTHS	% of USA
19	Alabama	14,898	1.8%		1	California	113,200	13.5%
48	Alaska	1,459	0.2%		2	Texas	80,437	9.6%
21	Arizona	13,301	1.6%		3	New York	59,129	7.1%
29	Arkansas	9,179	1.1%		4	Florida	43,823	5.2%
1	California	113,200	13.5%		5	Illinois	35,422	4.2%
28	Colorado	9,771	1.2%		6	New Jersey	29,096	3.5%
30	Connecticut	8,808	1.1%		7	Ohio	28,878	3.5%
44	Delaware	2,454	0.3%		8	Pennsylvania	28,596	3.4%
4	Florida	43,823	5.2%		9	Michigan	27,535	3.3%
10	Georgia	25,453	3.0%		10	Georgia	25,453	3.0%
40	Hawaii	2,743	0.3%		11	North Carolina	24,013	2.9%
39	Idaho	3,044	0.4%		12	Virginia	20,002	2.4%
5	Illinois	35,422	4.2%		13	Tennessee	17,491	2.1%
15	Indiana	17,024	2.0%		14	Louisiana	17,391	2.1%
32	Iowa	7,307	0.9%		15	Indiana	17,024	2.0%
34	Kansas	7,146	0.9%		16	Massachusetts	17,015	2.0%
23	Kentucky	12,387	1.5%		17	Missouri	15,524	1.9%
14	Louisiana	17,391	2.1%		18	Maryland	15,330	1.8%
41	Maine	2,705	0.3%		19	Alabama	14,898	1.8%
18	Maryland	15,330	1.8%		20	Washington	14,260	1.7%
16	Massachusetts	17,015	2.0%		21	Arizona	13,301	1.6%
9	Michigan	27,535	3.3%		22	South Carolina	12,607	1.5%
24	Minnesota	11,736	1.4%		23	Kentucky	12,387	1.5%
25	Mississippi	11,594	1.4%		24	Minnesota	11,736	1.4%
17	Missouri	15,524	1.9%		25	Mississippi	11,594	1.4%
46	Montana	2,040	0.2%		26	Oklahoma	11,277	1.3%
37	Nebraska	4,848	0.6%		27	Wisconsin	10,792	1.3%
35	Nevada	6,142	0.7%		28	Colorado	9,771	1.2%
42	New Hampshire	2,669	0.3%		29	Arkansas	9,179	1.1%
6	New Jersey	29,096	3.5%		30	Connecticut	8,808	1.1%
38	New Mexico	4,480	0.5%		31	Oregon	8,059	1.0%
3	New York	59,129	7.1%		32	Iowa	7,307	0.9%
11	North Carolina	24,013	2.9%		33	Utah	7,226	0.9%
47	North Dakota	1,539	0.2%		34	Kansas	7,146	0.9%
7	Ohio	28,878	3.5%		35	Nevada	6,142	0.7%
26	Oklahoma	11,277	1.3%		36	West Virginia	5,000	0.6%
31	Oregon	8,059	1.0%		37	Nebraska	4,848	0.6%
8	Pennsylvania	28,596	3.4%		38	New Mexico	4,480	0.5%
43	Rhode Island	2,457	0.3%		39	Idaho	3,044	0.4%
22	South Carolina	12,607	1.5%		40	Hawaii	2,743	0.3%
45	South Dakota	2,212	0.3%		41	Maine	2,705	0.3%
13	Tennessee	17,491	2.1%		42	New Hampshire	2,669	0.3%
2	Texas	80,437	9.6%		43	Rhode Island	2,457	0.3%
33	Utah	7,226	0.9%		44	Delaware	2,454	0.3%
50	Vermont	1,086	0.1%		45	South Dakota	2,212	0.3%
12	Virginia	20,002	2.4%		46	Montana	2,040	0.2%
20	Washington	14,260	1.7%		47	North Dakota	1,539	0.2%
36	West Virginia	5,000	0.6%		48	Alaska	1,459	0.2%
27	Wisconsin	10,792	1.3%		49	Wyoming	1,163	0.1%
49	Wyoming	1,163	0.1%		50	Vermont	1,086	0.1%
						District of Columbia	1,599	0.2%

Source: Morgan Quitno Press using data from U.S. Dept of Health & Human Services, National Center for Health Statistics
unpublished data
*By state of residence.

Percent of Births by Cesarean Delivery in 1998

National Percent = 21.2% of Live Births*

RANK	STATE	PERCENT
6	Alabama	24.0
50	Alaska	14.7
42	Arizona	17.0
4	Arkansas	24.9
15	California	21.7
44	Colorado	16.4
26	Connecticut	20.1
9	Delaware	23.2
14	Florida	22.4
22	Georgia	20.8
49	Hawaii	15.6
48	Idaho	15.7
32	Illinois	19.4
27	Indiana	20.0
29	Iowa	19.6
36	Kansas	18.6
11	Kentucky	22.8
2	Louisiana	26.0
28	Maine	19.7
19	Maryland	21.3
21	Massachusetts	20.9
23	Michigan	20.6
39	Minnesota	18.0
1	Mississippi	27.0
23	Missouri	20.6
34	Montana	18.9
23	Nebraska	20.6
18	Nevada	21.4
38	New Hampshire	18.5
3	New Jersey	25.4
44	New Mexico	16.4
10	New York	22.9
16	North Carolina	21.5
32	North Dakota	19.4
34	Ohio	18.9
11	Oklahoma	22.8
41	Oregon	17.8
29	Pennsylvania	19.6
31	Rhode Island	19.5
8	South Carolina	23.4
16	South Dakota	21.5
13	Tennessee	22.6
7	Texas	23.5
46	Utah	16.0
43	Vermont	16.5
20	Virginia	21.2
40	Washington	17.9
5	West Virginia	24.1
46	Wisconsin	16.0
36	Wyoming	18.6

RANK	STATE	PERCENT
1	Mississippi	27.0
2	Louisiana	26.0
3	New Jersey	25.4
4	Arkansas	24.9
5	West Virginia	24.1
6	Alabama	24.0
7	Texas	23.5
8	South Carolina	23.4
9	Delaware	23.2
10	New York	22.9
11	Kentucky	22.8
11	Oklahoma	22.8
13	Tennessee	22.6
14	Florida	22.4
15	California	21.7
16	North Carolina	21.5
16	South Dakota	21.5
18	Nevada	21.4
19	Maryland	21.3
20	Virginia	21.2
21	Massachusetts	20.9
22	Georgia	20.8
23	Michigan	20.6
23	Missouri	20.6
23	Nebraska	20.6
26	Connecticut	20.1
27	Indiana	20.0
28	Maine	19.7
29	Iowa	19.6
29	Pennsylvania	19.6
31	Rhode Island	19.5
32	Illinois	19.4
32	North Dakota	19.4
34	Montana	18.9
34	Ohio	18.9
36	Kansas	18.6
36	Wyoming	18.6
38	New Hampshire	18.5
39	Minnesota	18.0
40	Washington	17.9
41	Oregon	17.8
42	Arizona	17.0
43	Vermont	16.5
44	Colorado	16.4
44	New Mexico	16.4
46	Utah	16.0
46	Wisconsin	16.0
48	Idaho	15.7
49	Hawaii	15.6
50	Alaska	14.7
	District of Columbia	20.8

Source: U.S. Department of Health and Human Services, National Center for Health Statistics
"National Vital Statistics Reports" (Vol. 48, No. 3, March 28, 2000)
*By state of residence.

Percent Change in Rate of Cesarean Births: 1994 to 1998

National Percent Change = 0.0% Change*

ALPHA ORDER			RANK ORDER		
RANK	STATE	PERCENT CHANGE	RANK	STATE	PERCENT CHANGE
13	Alabama	3.4	1	Rhode Island	12.7
48	Alaska	(9.8)	2	Nevada	11.5
21	Arizona	1.2	3	Nebraska	10.2
40	Arkansas	(3.9)	4	Minnesota	9.1
12	California	4.3	5	Colorado	7.2
5	Colorado	7.2	6	Tennessee	7.1
10	Connecticut	5.2	7	New Jersey	6.3
8	Delaware	5.9	8	Delaware	5.9
23	Florida	0.9	8	Washington	5.9
32	Georgia	(2.3)	10	Connecticut	5.2
47	Hawaii	(9.3)	11	Wyoming	4.5
16	Idaho	2.6	12	California	4.3
35	Illinois	(3.5)	13	Alabama	3.4
43	Indiana	(5.7)	14	Iowa	3.2
14	Iowa	3.2	15	Mississippi	3.1
50	Kansas	(10.1)	16	Idaho	2.6
20	Kentucky	1.3	17	Oregon	2.3
46	Louisiana	(8.1)	18	Wisconsin	1.9
42	Maine	(4.8)	19	South Dakota	1.4
45	Maryland	(5.8)	20	Kentucky	1.3
22	Massachusetts	1.0	21	Arizona	1.2
27	Michigan	(0.5)	22	Massachusetts	1.0
4	Minnesota	9.1	23	Florida	0.9
15	Mississippi	3.1	23	South Carolina	0.9
29	Missouri	(1.0)	25	West Virginia	0.8
27	Montana	(0.5)	26	New York	0.0
3	Nebraska	10.2	27	Michigan	(0.5)
2	Nevada	11.5	27	Montana	(0.5)
41	New Hampshire	(4.1)	29	Missouri	(1.0)
7	New Jersey	6.3	30	Utah	(1.2)
43	New Mexico	(5.7)	31	Oklahoma	(1.7)
26	New York	0.0	32	Georgia	(2.3)
33	North Carolina	(2.7)	33	North Carolina	(2.7)
35	North Dakota	(3.5)	34	Pennsylvania	(3.0)
49	Ohio	(10.0)	35	Illinois	(3.5)
31	Oklahoma	(1.7)	35	North Dakota	(3.5)
17	Oregon	2.3	35	Vermont	(3.5)
34	Pennsylvania	(3.0)	38	Virginia	(3.6)
1	Rhode Island	12.7	39	Texas	(3.7)
23	South Carolina	0.9	40	Arkansas	(3.9)
19	South Dakota	1.4	41	New Hampshire	(4.1)
6	Tennessee	7.1	42	Maine	(4.8)
39	Texas	(3.7)	43	Indiana	(5.7)
30	Utah	(1.2)	43	New Mexico	(5.7)
35	Vermont	(3.5)	45	Maryland	(5.8)
38	Virginia	(3.6)	46	Louisiana	(8.1)
8	Washington	5.9	47	Hawaii	(9.3)
25	West Virginia	0.8	48	Alaska	(9.8)
18	Wisconsin	1.9	49	Ohio	(10.0)
11	Wyoming	4.5	50	Kansas	(10.1)
				District of Columbia	(7.1)

Source: Morgan Quitno Press using data from US Dept of Health & Human Services, National Center for Health Statistics
   "National Vital Statistics Reports" (Vol. 48, No. 3, March 28, 2000) and unpublished data
*By state of residence.

Percent of Vaginal Births After a Cesarean (VBAC) in 1998

National Percent = 26.3% of Live Births to Women Who Have Had a Cesarean*

ALPHA ORDER

RANK	STATE	PERCENT
42	Alabama	21.6
6	Alaska	35.2
34	Arizona	23.9
46	Arkansas	19.5
47	California	18.4
8	Colorado	34.9
17	Connecticut	31.8
22	Delaware	30.8
39	Florida	22.8
36	Georgia	23.3
2	Hawaii	39.7
4	Idaho	36.4
19	Illinois	31.6
31	Indiana	27.6
22	Iowa	30.8
35	Kansas	23.8
38	Kentucky	22.9
50	Louisiana	13.1
26	Maine	30.3
26	Maryland	30.3
15	Massachusetts	32.8
33	Michigan	25.8
29	Minnesota	29.4
49	Mississippi	15.0
28	Missouri	29.6
17	Montana	31.8
30	Nebraska	28.0
45	Nevada	19.8
3	New Hampshire	38.5
13	New Jersey	33.4
6	New Mexico	35.2
16	New York	32.0
32	North Carolina	27.2
25	North Dakota	30.6
10	Ohio	34.2
41	Oklahoma	22.0
5	Oregon	36.0
9	Pennsylvania	34.3
21	Rhode Island	30.9
44	South Carolina	21.5
42	South Dakota	21.6
40	Tennessee	22.6
48	Texas	18.2
12	Utah	33.5
1	Vermont	40.6
24	Virginia	30.7
13	Washington	33.4
37	West Virginia	23.1
11	Wisconsin	33.8
20	Wyoming	31.0

RANK ORDER

RANK	STATE	PERCENT
1	Vermont	40.6
2	Hawaii	39.7
3	New Hampshire	38.5
4	Idaho	36.4
5	Oregon	36.0
6	Alaska	35.2
6	New Mexico	35.2
8	Colorado	34.9
9	Pennsylvania	34.3
10	Ohio	34.2
11	Wisconsin	33.8
12	Utah	33.5
13	New Jersey	33.4
13	Washington	33.4
15	Massachusetts	32.8
16	New York	32.0
17	Connecticut	31.8
17	Montana	31.8
19	Illinois	31.6
20	Wyoming	31.0
21	Rhode Island	30.9
22	Delaware	30.8
22	Iowa	30.8
24	Virginia	30.7
25	North Dakota	30.6
26	Maine	30.3
26	Maryland	30.3
28	Missouri	29.6
29	Minnesota	29.4
30	Nebraska	28.0
31	Indiana	27.6
32	North Carolina	27.2
33	Michigan	25.8
34	Arizona	23.9
35	Kansas	23.8
36	Georgia	23.3
37	West Virginia	23.1
38	Kentucky	22.9
39	Florida	22.8
40	Tennessee	22.6
41	Oklahoma	22.0
42	Alabama	21.6
42	South Dakota	21.6
44	South Carolina	21.5
45	Nevada	19.8
46	Arkansas	19.5
47	California	18.4
48	Texas	18.2
49	Mississippi	15.0
50	Louisiana	13.1
	District of Columbia	25.6

Source: U.S. Department of Health and Human Services, National Center for Health Statistics
    "National Vital Statistics Reports" (Vol. 48, No. 3, March 28, 2000)
Vaginal births after a cesarean delivery as a percent of all births to women with a previous cesarean delivery giving birth in 1998.

Percent of Mothers Beginning Prenatal Care in First Trimester in 1999

National Percent = 83.2% of Mothers*

RANK	STATE	PERCENT
30	Alabama	83.2
45	Alaska	79.3
48	Arizona	76.0
47	Arkansas	79.1
28	California	83.6
35	Colorado	81.7
4	Connecticut	89.3
27	Delaware	83.7
25	Florida	83.9
8	Georgia	87.3
15	Hawaii	85.7
42	Idaho	80.5
34	Illinois	82.5
44	Indiana	80.0
7	Iowa	87.7
14	Kansas	85.8
11	Kentucky	86.6
33	Louisiana	82.9
5	Maine	89.2
10	Maryland	87.0
3	Massachusetts	89.4
24	Michigan	84.0
20	Minnesota	84.5
37	Mississippi	81.5
9	Missouri	87.1
25	Montana	83.9
21	Nebraska	84.4
49	Nevada	75.2
2	New Hampshire	90.7
35	New Jersey	81.7
50	New Mexico	66.8
38	New York	81.0
19	North Carolina	85.0
13	North Dakota	86.3
12	Ohio	86.5
40	Oklahoma	80.6
39	Oregon	80.9
17	Pennsylvania	85.1
1	Rhode Island	91.5
40	South Carolina	80.6
29	South Dakota	83.4
22	Tennessee	84.3
45	Texas	79.3
42	Utah	80.5
6	Vermont	88.0
16	Virginia	85.3
31	Washington	83.0
17	West Virginia	85.1
23	Wisconsin	84.1
31	Wyoming	83.0

RANK	STATE	PERCENT
1	Rhode Island	91.5
2	New Hampshire	90.7
3	Massachusetts	89.4
4	Connecticut	89.3
5	Maine	89.2
6	Vermont	88.0
7	Iowa	87.7
8	Georgia	87.3
9	Missouri	87.1
10	Maryland	87.0
11	Kentucky	86.6
12	Ohio	86.5
13	North Dakota	86.3
14	Kansas	85.8
15	Hawaii	85.7
16	Virginia	85.3
17	Pennsylvania	85.1
17	West Virginia	85.1
19	North Carolina	85.0
20	Minnesota	84.5
21	Nebraska	84.4
22	Tennessee	84.3
23	Wisconsin	84.1
24	Michigan	84.0
25	Florida	83.9
25	Montana	83.9
27	Delaware	83.7
28	California	83.6
29	South Dakota	83.4
30	Alabama	83.2
31	Washington	83.0
31	Wyoming	83.0
33	Louisiana	82.9
34	Illinois	82.5
35	Colorado	81.7
35	New Jersey	81.7
37	Mississippi	81.5
38	New York	81.0
39	Oregon	80.9
40	Oklahoma	80.6
40	South Carolina	80.6
42	Idaho	80.5
42	Utah	80.5
44	Indiana	80.0
45	Alaska	79.3
45	Texas	79.3
47	Arkansas	79.1
48	Arizona	76.0
49	Nevada	75.2
50	New Mexico	66.8
	District of Columbia	71.9

Source: U.S. Department of Health and Human Services, National Center for Health Statistics
"National Vital Statistics Reports" (Vol. 48, No. 14, August 8, 2000)
Preliminary data by state of residence.

Percent of White Mothers Beginning Prenatal Care in First Trimester in 1999

National Percent = 85.1% of White Mothers*

ALPHA ORDER

RANK	STATE	PERCENT
12	Alabama	88.9
40	Alaska	82.2
48	Arizona	76.7
42	Arkansas	81.8
37	California	83.6
41	Colorado	82.0
6	Connecticut	90.5
27	Delaware	86.6
21	Florida	87.1
7	Georgia	90.4
3	Hawaii	91.0
46	Idaho	80.7
33	Illinois	85.4
43	Indiana	81.7
15	Iowa	88.3
26	Kansas	86.7
19	Kentucky	87.5
8	Louisiana	89.7
9	Maine	89.5
2	Maryland	91.5
5	Massachusetts	90.9
23	Michigan	87.0
21	Minnesota	87.1
10	Mississippi	89.1
10	Missouri	89.1
30	Montana	85.8
33	Nebraska	85.4
49	Nevada	75.5
3	New Hampshire	91.0
31	New Jersey	85.6
50	New Mexico	68.0
35	New York	84.2
14	North Carolina	88.4
15	North Dakota	88.3
17	Ohio	88.2
39	Oklahoma	82.7
45	Oregon	81.2
19	Pennsylvania	87.5
1	Rhode Island	92.7
29	South Carolina	85.9
23	South Dakota	87.0
23	Tennessee	87.0
47	Texas	79.4
44	Utah	81.5
18	Vermont	88.0
13	Virginia	88.8
36	Washington	83.9
31	West Virginia	85.6
27	Wisconsin	86.6
38	Wyoming	83.4

RANK ORDER

RANK	STATE	PERCENT
1	Rhode Island	92.7
2	Maryland	91.5
3	Hawaii	91.0
3	New Hampshire	91.0
5	Massachusetts	90.9
6	Connecticut	90.5
7	Georgia	90.4
8	Louisiana	89.7
9	Maine	89.5
10	Mississippi	89.1
10	Missouri	89.1
12	Alabama	88.9
13	Virginia	88.8
14	North Carolina	88.4
15	Iowa	88.3
15	North Dakota	88.3
17	Ohio	88.2
18	Vermont	88.0
19	Kentucky	87.5
19	Pennsylvania	87.5
21	Florida	87.1
21	Minnesota	87.1
23	Michigan	87.0
23	South Dakota	87.0
23	Tennessee	87.0
26	Kansas	86.7
27	Delaware	86.6
27	Wisconsin	86.6
29	South Carolina	85.9
30	Montana	85.8
31	New Jersey	85.6
31	West Virginia	85.6
33	Illinois	85.4
33	Nebraska	85.4
35	New York	84.2
36	Washington	83.9
37	California	83.6
38	Wyoming	83.4
39	Oklahoma	82.7
40	Alaska	82.2
41	Colorado	82.0
42	Arkansas	81.8
43	Indiana	81.7
44	Utah	81.5
45	Oregon	81.2
46	Idaho	80.7
47	Texas	79.4
48	Arizona	76.7
49	Nevada	75.5
50	New Mexico	68.0

| | District of Columbia | 87.4 |

Source: U.S. Department of Health and Human Services, National Center for Health Statistics
"National Vital Statistics Reports" (Vol. 48, No. 14, August 8, 2000)
*Preliminary data by state of residence.

Percent of Black Mothers Beginning Prenatal Care in First Trimester in 1999

National Percent = 74.0% of Black Mothers*

<u>ALPHA ORDER</u>

RANK	STATE	PERCENT
36	Alabama	71.4
3	Alaska	83.6
28	Arizona	73.7
44	Arkansas	69.4
7	California	81.2
21	Colorado	75.4
7	Connecticut	81.2
21	Delaware	75.4
30	Florida	73.6
9	Georgia	81.0
1	Hawaii	91.2
24	Idaho	74.7
41	Illinois	70.0
47	Indiana	66.1
23	Iowa	74.8
13	Kansas	77.0
11	Kentucky	78.4
31	Louisiana	73.2
5	Maine	83.0
12	Maryland	78.0
10	Massachusetts	79.8
42	Michigan	69.9
46	Minnesota	66.3
34	Mississippi	72.6
16	Missouri	76.3
2	Montana	85.7
28	Nebraska	73.7
43	Nevada	69.5
33	New Hampshire	72.9
48	New Jersey	65.0
50	New Mexico	62.5
38	New York	71.0
17	North Carolina	76.1
35	North Dakota	72.1
17	Ohio	76.1
31	Oklahoma	73.2
17	Oregon	76.1
37	Pennsylvania	71.1
4	Rhode Island	83.5
39	South Carolina	70.9
27	South Dakota	74.2
25	Tennessee	74.6
15	Texas	76.5
49	Utah	64.3
6	Vermont	81.6
26	Virginia	74.4
20	Washington	75.5
39	West Virginia	70.9
45	Wisconsin	69.1
14	Wyoming	76.6

<u>RANK ORDER</u>

RANK	STATE	PERCENT
1	Hawaii	91.2
2	Montana	85.7
3	Alaska	83.6
4	Rhode Island	83.5
5	Maine	83.0
6	Vermont	81.6
7	California	81.2
7	Connecticut	81.2
9	Georgia	81.0
10	Massachusetts	79.8
11	Kentucky	78.4
12	Maryland	78.0
13	Kansas	77.0
14	Wyoming	76.6
15	Texas	76.5
16	Missouri	76.3
17	North Carolina	76.1
17	Ohio	76.1
17	Oregon	76.1
20	Washington	75.5
21	Colorado	75.4
21	Delaware	75.4
23	Iowa	74.8
24	Idaho	74.7
25	Tennessee	74.6
26	Virginia	74.4
27	South Dakota	74.2
28	Arizona	73.7
28	Nebraska	73.7
30	Florida	73.6
31	Louisiana	73.2
31	Oklahoma	73.2
33	New Hampshire	72.9
34	Mississippi	72.6
35	North Dakota	72.1
36	Alabama	71.4
37	Pennsylvania	71.1
38	New York	71.0
39	South Carolina	70.9
39	West Virginia	70.9
41	Illinois	70.0
42	Michigan	69.9
43	Nevada	69.5
44	Arkansas	69.4
45	Wisconsin	69.1
46	Minnesota	66.3
47	Indiana	66.1
48	New Jersey	65.0
49	Utah	64.3
50	New Mexico	62.5
	District of Columbia	66.9

Source: U.S. Department of Health and Human Services, National Center for Health Statistics
"National Vital Statistics Reports" (Vol. 48, No. 14, August 8, 2000)
*Preliminary data by state of residence.

Percent of Mothers Receiving Late or No Prenatal Care in 1998

National Percent = 3.9% of Mothers*

<table>
<tr><td colspan="3">ALPHA ORDER</td><td colspan="3">RANK ORDER</td></tr>
<tr><td>RANK</td><td>STATE</td><td>PERCENT</td><td>RANK</td><td>STATE</td><td>PERCENT</td></tr>
<tr><td>18</td><td>Alabama</td><td>3.9</td><td>1</td><td>New Mexico</td><td>8.5</td></tr>
<tr><td>9</td><td>Alaska</td><td>4.5</td><td>2</td><td>Arizona</td><td>7.2</td></tr>
<tr><td>2</td><td>Arizona</td><td>7.2</td><td>3</td><td>Nevada</td><td>7.0</td></tr>
<tr><td>5</td><td>Arkansas</td><td>5.1</td><td>4</td><td>Texas</td><td>5.3</td></tr>
<tr><td>22</td><td>California</td><td>3.6</td><td>5</td><td>Arkansas</td><td>5.1</td></tr>
<tr><td>11</td><td>Colorado</td><td>4.3</td><td>5</td><td>Oklahoma</td><td>5.1</td></tr>
<tr><td>35</td><td>Connecticut</td><td>3.0</td><td>7</td><td>New York</td><td>4.8</td></tr>
<tr><td>22</td><td>Delaware</td><td>3.6</td><td>8</td><td>New Jersey</td><td>4.6</td></tr>
<tr><td>25</td><td>Florida</td><td>3.5</td><td>9</td><td>Alaska</td><td>4.5</td></tr>
<tr><td>40</td><td>Georgia</td><td>2.8</td><td>10</td><td>Idaho</td><td>4.4</td></tr>
<tr><td>34</td><td>Hawaii</td><td>3.1</td><td>11</td><td>Colorado</td><td>4.3</td></tr>
<tr><td>10</td><td>Idaho</td><td>4.4</td><td>12</td><td>Ohio</td><td>4.2</td></tr>
<tr><td>18</td><td>Illinois</td><td>3.9</td><td>12</td><td>South Carolina</td><td>4.2</td></tr>
<tr><td>16</td><td>Indiana</td><td>4.0</td><td>14</td><td>Utah</td><td>4.1</td></tr>
<tr><td>45</td><td>Iowa</td><td>2.4</td><td>14</td><td>Wyoming</td><td>4.1</td></tr>
<tr><td>40</td><td>Kansas</td><td>2.8</td><td>16</td><td>Indiana</td><td>4.0</td></tr>
<tr><td>43</td><td>Kentucky</td><td>2.5</td><td>16</td><td>Mississippi</td><td>4.0</td></tr>
<tr><td>18</td><td>Louisiana</td><td>3.9</td><td>18</td><td>Alabama</td><td>3.9</td></tr>
<tr><td>49</td><td>Maine</td><td>1.7</td><td>18</td><td>Illinois</td><td>3.9</td></tr>
<tr><td>35</td><td>Maryland</td><td>3.0</td><td>18</td><td>Louisiana</td><td>3.9</td></tr>
<tr><td>45</td><td>Massachusetts</td><td>2.4</td><td>21</td><td>Oregon</td><td>3.8</td></tr>
<tr><td>27</td><td>Michigan</td><td>3.4</td><td>22</td><td>California</td><td>3.6</td></tr>
<tr><td>37</td><td>Minnesota</td><td>2.9</td><td>22</td><td>Delaware</td><td>3.6</td></tr>
<tr><td>16</td><td>Mississippi</td><td>4.0</td><td>22</td><td>Tennessee</td><td>3.6</td></tr>
<tr><td>37</td><td>Missouri</td><td>2.9</td><td>25</td><td>Florida</td><td>3.5</td></tr>
<tr><td>30</td><td>Montana</td><td>3.2</td><td>25</td><td>Pennsylvania</td><td>3.5</td></tr>
<tr><td>30</td><td>Nebraska</td><td>3.2</td><td>27</td><td>Michigan</td><td>3.4</td></tr>
<tr><td>3</td><td>Nevada</td><td>7.0</td><td>27</td><td>Wisconsin</td><td>3.4</td></tr>
<tr><td>48</td><td>New Hampshire</td><td>1.9</td><td>29</td><td>Virginia</td><td>3.3</td></tr>
<tr><td>8</td><td>New Jersey</td><td>4.6</td><td>30</td><td>Montana</td><td>3.2</td></tr>
<tr><td>1</td><td>New Mexico</td><td>8.5</td><td>30</td><td>Nebraska</td><td>3.2</td></tr>
<tr><td>7</td><td>New York</td><td>4.8</td><td>30</td><td>South Dakota</td><td>3.2</td></tr>
<tr><td>37</td><td>North Carolina</td><td>2.9</td><td>30</td><td>Washington</td><td>3.2</td></tr>
<tr><td>43</td><td>North Dakota</td><td>2.5</td><td>34</td><td>Hawaii</td><td>3.1</td></tr>
<tr><td>12</td><td>Ohio</td><td>4.2</td><td>35</td><td>Connecticut</td><td>3.0</td></tr>
<tr><td>5</td><td>Oklahoma</td><td>5.1</td><td>35</td><td>Maryland</td><td>3.0</td></tr>
<tr><td>21</td><td>Oregon</td><td>3.8</td><td>37</td><td>Minnesota</td><td>2.9</td></tr>
<tr><td>25</td><td>Pennsylvania</td><td>3.5</td><td>37</td><td>Missouri</td><td>2.9</td></tr>
<tr><td>50</td><td>Rhode Island</td><td>1.5</td><td>37</td><td>North Carolina</td><td>2.9</td></tr>
<tr><td>12</td><td>South Carolina</td><td>4.2</td><td>40</td><td>Georgia</td><td>2.8</td></tr>
<tr><td>30</td><td>South Dakota</td><td>3.2</td><td>40</td><td>Kansas</td><td>2.8</td></tr>
<tr><td>22</td><td>Tennessee</td><td>3.6</td><td>42</td><td>West Virginia</td><td>2.6</td></tr>
<tr><td>4</td><td>Texas</td><td>5.3</td><td>43</td><td>Kentucky</td><td>2.5</td></tr>
<tr><td>14</td><td>Utah</td><td>4.1</td><td>43</td><td>North Dakota</td><td>2.5</td></tr>
<tr><td>47</td><td>Vermont</td><td>2.0</td><td>45</td><td>Iowa</td><td>2.4</td></tr>
<tr><td>29</td><td>Virginia</td><td>3.3</td><td>45</td><td>Massachusetts</td><td>2.4</td></tr>
<tr><td>30</td><td>Washington</td><td>3.2</td><td>47</td><td>Vermont</td><td>2.0</td></tr>
<tr><td>42</td><td>West Virginia</td><td>2.6</td><td>48</td><td>New Hampshire</td><td>1.9</td></tr>
<tr><td>27</td><td>Wisconsin</td><td>3.4</td><td>49</td><td>Maine</td><td>1.7</td></tr>
<tr><td>14</td><td>Wyoming</td><td>4.1</td><td>50</td><td>Rhode Island</td><td>1.5</td></tr>
<tr><td></td><td></td><td></td><td></td><td>District of Columbia</td><td>10.2</td></tr>
</table>

Source: U.S. Department of Health and Human Services, National Center for Health Statistics
  "National Vital Statistics Reports" (Vol. 48, No. 3, March 28, 2000)
*Final data by state of residence. "Late" means care begun in third trimester.

Percent of White Mothers Receiving Late or No Prenatal Care in 1998

National Percent = 3.3% of White Mothers*

RANK	STATE	PERCENT
31	Alabama	2.3
10	Alaska	3.7
2	Arizona	6.9
6	Arkansas	4.3
10	California	3.7
8	Colorado	4.1
20	Connecticut	2.8
22	Delaware	2.7
25	Florida	2.6
42	Georgia	1.9
37	Hawaii	2.1
6	Idaho	4.3
20	Illinois	2.8
15	Indiana	3.5
35	Iowa	2.2
26	Kansas	2.5
31	Kentucky	2.3
45	Louisiana	1.8
48	Maine	1.7
45	Maryland	1.8
39	Massachusetts	2.0
29	Michigan	2.4
35	Minnesota	2.2
48	Mississippi	1.7
37	Missouri	2.1
29	Montana	2.4
18	Nebraska	2.9
3	Nevada	6.8
42	New Hampshire	1.9
17	New Jersey	3.0
1	New Mexico	7.9
10	New York	3.7
39	North Carolina	2.0
42	North Dakota	1.9
16	Ohio	3.1
5	Oklahoma	4.5
10	Oregon	3.7
22	Pennsylvania	2.7
50	Rhode Island	1.3
31	South Carolina	2.3
45	South Dakota	1.8
26	Tennessee	2.5
4	Texas	5.2
10	Utah	3.7
39	Vermont	2.0
31	Virginia	2.3
18	Washington	2.9
26	West Virginia	2.5
22	Wisconsin	2.7
9	Wyoming	3.8

RANK	STATE	PERCENT
1	New Mexico	7.9
2	Arizona	6.9
3	Nevada	6.8
4	Texas	5.2
5	Oklahoma	4.5
6	Arkansas	4.3
6	Idaho	4.3
8	Colorado	4.1
9	Wyoming	3.8
10	Alaska	3.7
10	California	3.7
10	New York	3.7
10	Oregon	3.7
10	Utah	3.7
15	Indiana	3.5
16	Ohio	3.1
17	New Jersey	3.0
18	Nebraska	2.9
18	Washington	2.9
20	Connecticut	2.8
20	Illinois	2.8
22	Delaware	2.7
22	Pennsylvania	2.7
22	Wisconsin	2.7
25	Florida	2.6
26	Kansas	2.5
26	Tennessee	2.5
26	West Virginia	2.5
29	Michigan	2.4
29	Montana	2.4
31	Alabama	2.3
31	Kentucky	2.3
31	South Carolina	2.3
31	Virginia	2.3
35	Iowa	2.2
35	Minnesota	2.2
37	Hawaii	2.1
37	Missouri	2.1
39	Massachusetts	2.0
39	North Carolina	2.0
39	Vermont	2.0
42	Georgia	1.9
42	New Hampshire	1.9
42	North Dakota	1.9
45	Louisiana	1.8
45	Maryland	1.8
45	South Dakota	1.8
48	Maine	1.7
48	Mississippi	1.7
50	Rhode Island	1.3

| | District of Columbia | 5.0 |

Source: U.S. Department of Health and Human Services, National Center for Health Statistics
    "National Vital Statistics Reports" (Vol. 48, No. 3, March 28, 2000)
*Final data by state of residence. "Late" means care begun in third trimester.

Percent of Black Mothers Receiving Late or No Prenatal Care in 1998

National Percent = 7.0% of Black Mothers*

ALPHA ORDER

RANK	STATE	PERCENT
18	Alabama	7.1
34	Alaska	5.1
17	Arizona	7.4
10	Arkansas	8.3
37	California	4.5
23	Colorado	6.5
36	Connecticut	4.6
26	Delaware	6.1
23	Florida	6.5
38	Georgia	4.4
NA	Hawaii**	NA
NA	Idaho**	NA
11	Illinois	8.2
8	Indiana	8.4
25	Iowa	6.3
29	Kansas	5.7
39	Kentucky	4.2
19	Louisiana	7.0
NA	Maine**	NA
33	Maryland	5.2
30	Massachusetts	5.6
12	Michigan	7.9
12	Minnesota	7.9
21	Mississippi	6.7
20	Missouri	6.9
NA	Montana**	NA
21	Nebraska	6.7
5	Nevada	9.5
NA	New Hampshire**	NA
1	New Jersey	11.1
1	New Mexico	11.1
7	New York	8.5
32	North Carolina	5.4
NA	North Dakota**	NA
4	Ohio	10.4
15	Oklahoma	7.5
40	Oregon	4.1
8	Pennsylvania	8.4
41	Rhode Island	3.9
15	South Carolina	7.5
NA	South Dakota**	NA
14	Tennessee	7.7
26	Texas	6.1
3	Utah	10.7
NA	Vermont**	NA
26	Virginia	6.1
35	Washington	5.0
31	West Virginia	5.5
6	Wisconsin	8.7
NA	Wyoming**	NA

RANK ORDER

RANK	STATE	PERCENT
1	New Jersey	11.1
1	New Mexico	11.1
3	Utah	10.7
4	Ohio	10.4
5	Nevada	9.5
6	Wisconsin	8.7
7	New York	8.5
8	Indiana	8.4
8	Pennsylvania	8.4
10	Arkansas	8.3
11	Illinois	8.2
12	Michigan	7.9
12	Minnesota	7.9
14	Tennessee	7.7
15	Oklahoma	7.5
15	South Carolina	7.5
17	Arizona	7.4
18	Alabama	7.1
19	Louisiana	7.0
20	Missouri	6.9
21	Mississippi	6.7
21	Nebraska	6.7
23	Colorado	6.5
23	Florida	6.5
25	Iowa	6.3
26	Delaware	6.1
26	Texas	6.1
26	Virginia	6.1
29	Kansas	5.7
30	Massachusetts	5.6
31	West Virginia	5.5
32	North Carolina	5.4
33	Maryland	5.2
34	Alaska	5.1
35	Washington	5.0
36	Connecticut	4.6
37	California	4.5
38	Georgia	4.4
39	Kentucky	4.2
40	Oregon	4.1
41	Rhode Island	3.9
NA	Hawaii**	NA
NA	Idaho**	NA
NA	Maine**	NA
NA	Montana**	NA
NA	New Hampshire**	NA
NA	North Dakota**	NA
NA	South Dakota**	NA
NA	Vermont**	NA
NA	Wyoming**	NA

District of Columbia   12.3

Source: U.S. Department of Health and Human Services, National Center for Health Statistics
     "National Vital Statistics Reports" (Vol. 48, No. 3, March 28, 2000)
*Final data by state of residence. "Late" means care begun in third trimester.
**Insufficient data.

Percent of Births Attended by Midwives in 1999

National Percent = 7.5% of Live Births*

RANK	STATE	PERCENT
45	Alabama	2.7
3	Alaska	17.0
14	Arizona	9.3
46	Arkansas	2.0
16	California	8.9
15	Colorado	9.0
19	Connecticut	8.0
19	Delaware	8.0
9	Florida	12.1
5	Georgia	15.8
36	Hawaii	4.2
35	Idaho	4.3
40	Illinois	3.3
44	Indiana	2.8
41	Iowa	3.0
47	Kansas	1.9
38	Kentucky	4.0
48	Louisiana	1.6
10	Maine	12.0
18	Maryland	8.3
7	Massachusetts	13.7
25	Michigan	6.8
17	Minnesota	8.5
48	Mississippi	1.6
50	Missouri	1.0
12	Montana	10.7
43	Nebraska	2.9
26	Nevada	6.7
4	New Hampshire	16.5
29	New Jersey	5.6
1	New Mexico	22.8
11	New York	11.1
22	North Carolina	7.6
27	North Dakota	6.1
31	Ohio	5.4
37	Oklahoma	4.1
6	Oregon	14.6
22	Pennsylvania	7.6
8	Rhode Island	12.5
30	South Carolina	5.5
38	South Dakota	4.0
34	Tennessee	4.6
33	Texas	5.0
24	Utah	7.1
2	Vermont	17.4
28	Virginia	5.9
13	Washington	9.5
19	West Virginia	8.0
32	Wisconsin	5.3
41	Wyoming	3.0

RANK	STATE	PERCENT
1	New Mexico	22.8
2	Vermont	17.4
3	Alaska	17.0
4	New Hampshire	16.5
5	Georgia	15.8
6	Oregon	14.6
7	Massachusetts	13.7
8	Rhode Island	12.5
9	Florida	12.1
10	Maine	12.0
11	New York	11.1
12	Montana	10.7
13	Washington	9.5
14	Arizona	9.3
15	Colorado	9.0
16	California	8.9
17	Minnesota	8.5
18	Maryland	8.3
19	Connecticut	8.0
19	Delaware	8.0
19	West Virginia	8.0
22	North Carolina	7.6
22	Pennsylvania	7.6
24	Utah	7.1
25	Michigan	6.8
26	Nevada	6.7
27	North Dakota	6.1
28	Virginia	5.9
29	New Jersey	5.6
30	South Carolina	5.5
31	Ohio	5.4
32	Wisconsin	5.3
33	Texas	5.0
34	Tennessee	4.6
35	Idaho	4.3
36	Hawaii	4.2
37	Oklahoma	4.1
38	Kentucky	4.0
38	South Dakota	4.0
40	Illinois	3.3
41	Iowa	3.0
41	Wyoming	3.0
43	Nebraska	2.9
44	Indiana	2.8
45	Alabama	2.7
46	Arkansas	2.0
47	Kansas	1.9
48	Louisiana	1.6
48	Mississippi	1.6
50	Missouri	1.0
	District of Columbia	2.5

Source: U.S. Department of Health and Human Services, National Center for Health Statistics
   unpublished data
*Includes certified nurse midwives and other midwives.

Reported Legal Abortions in 1997

National Total = 1,186,039 Abortions*

ALPHA ORDER

RANK	STATE	ABORTIONS	% of USA
21	Alabama	13,063	1.1%
46	Alaska	1,632	0.1%
23	Arizona	11,266	0.9%
33	Arkansas	5,782	0.5%
1	California	275,739	23.2%
29	Colorado	9,183	0.8%
18	Connecticut	13,802	1.2%
36	Delaware	5,138	0.4%
4	Florida	81,692	6.9%
8	Georgia	35,702	3.0%
38	Hawaii	4,520	0.4%
49	Idaho	878	0.1%
5	Illinois	50,147	4.2%
20	Indiana	13,208	1.1%
26	Iowa	10,022	0.8%
24	Kansas	11,249	0.9%
30	Kentucky	7,033	0.6%
22	Louisiana	11,739	1.0%
43	Maine	2,545	0.2%
27	Maryland	9,869	0.8%
12	Massachusetts	28,477	2.4%
11	Michigan	29,528	2.5%
17	Minnesota	14,229	1.2%
39	Mississippi	4,325	0.4%
25	Missouri	10,202	0.9%
41	Montana	2,809	0.2%
37	Nebraska	5,129	0.4%
31	Nevada	6,887	0.6%
44	New Hampshire	2,069	0.2%
10	New Jersey	30,654	2.6%
35	New Mexico	5,382	0.5%
2	New York	140,834	11.9%
9	North Carolina	31,495	2.7%
47	North Dakota	1,226	0.1%
6	Ohio	38,242	3.2%
32	Oklahoma	6,428	0.5%
16	Oregon	14,834	1.3%
7	Pennsylvania	37,135	3.1%
34	Rhode Island	5,478	0.5%
28	South Carolina	9,212	0.8%
48	South Dakota	919	0.1%
15	Tennessee	18,283	1.5%
3	Texas	84,680	7.1%
40	Utah	3,408	0.3%
45	Vermont	1,955	0.2%
14	Virginia	26,089	2.2%
13	Washington	26,932	2.3%
42	West Virginia	2,808	0.2%
19	Wisconsin	13,218	1.1%
50	Wyoming	192	0.0%

RANK ORDER

RANK	STATE	ABORTIONS	% of USA
1	California	275,739	23.2%
2	New York	140,834	11.9%
3	Texas	84,680	7.1%
4	Florida	81,692	6.9%
5	Illinois	50,147	4.2%
6	Ohio	38,242	3.2%
7	Pennsylvania	37,135	3.1%
8	Georgia	35,702	3.0%
9	North Carolina	31,495	2.7%
10	New Jersey	30,654	2.6%
11	Michigan	29,528	2.5%
12	Massachusetts	28,477	2.4%
13	Washington	26,932	2.3%
14	Virginia	26,089	2.2%
15	Tennessee	18,283	1.5%
16	Oregon	14,834	1.3%
17	Minnesota	14,229	1.2%
18	Connecticut	13,802	1.2%
19	Wisconsin	13,218	1.1%
20	Indiana	13,208	1.1%
21	Alabama	13,063	1.1%
22	Louisiana	11,739	1.0%
23	Arizona	11,266	0.9%
24	Kansas	11,249	0.9%
25	Missouri	10,202	0.9%
26	Iowa	10,022	0.8%
27	Maryland	9,869	0.8%
28	South Carolina	9,212	0.8%
29	Colorado	9,183	0.8%
30	Kentucky	7,033	0.6%
31	Nevada	6,887	0.6%
32	Oklahoma	6,428	0.5%
33	Arkansas	5,782	0.5%
34	Rhode Island	5,478	0.5%
35	New Mexico	5,382	0.5%
36	Delaware	5,138	0.4%
37	Nebraska	5,129	0.4%
38	Hawaii	4,520	0.4%
39	Mississippi	4,325	0.4%
40	Utah	3,408	0.3%
41	Montana	2,809	0.2%
42	West Virginia	2,808	0.2%
43	Maine	2,545	0.2%
44	New Hampshire	2,069	0.2%
45	Vermont	1,955	0.2%
46	Alaska	1,632	0.1%
47	North Dakota	1,226	0.1%
48	South Dakota	919	0.1%
49	Idaho	878	0.1%
50	Wyoming	192	0.0%
	District of Columbia	8,771	0.7%

Source: U.S. Department of Health and Human Services, Centers for Disease Control and Prevention
   "Abortion Surveillance-United States, 1997" (Morbidity Mortality Weekly Report, Vol. 49, No. SS-11, 12/08/00)
By state of occurrence.

Reported Legal Abortions per 1,000 Live Births in 1997

National Rate = 306 Abortions per 1,000 Live Births*

ALPHA ORDER

RANK	STATE	RATE
28	Alabama	214
34	Alaska	164
38	Arizona	149
36	Arkansas	159
2	California	525
35	Colorado	162
9	Connecticut	320
3	Delaware	501
5	Florida	425
10	Georgia	302
18	Hawaii	260
49	Idaho	47
15	Illinois	277
37	Indiana	158
16	Iowa	273
10	Kansas	302
45	Kentucky	132
32	Louisiana	178
31	Maine	186
41	Maryland	141
6	Massachusetts	354
25	Michigan	221
25	Minnesota	221
46	Mississippi	104
42	Missouri	138
19	Montana	259
27	Nebraska	220
21	Nevada	256
40	New Hampshire	145
17	New Jersey	271
29	New Mexico	200
1	New York	547
13	North Carolina	294
39	North Dakota	147
23	Ohio	252
44	Oklahoma	133
8	Oregon	339
20	Pennsylvania	257
4	Rhode Island	440
33	South Carolina	176
47	South Dakota	90
24	Tennessee	245
22	Texas	254
48	Utah	79
12	Vermont	296
14	Virginia	284
7	Washington	344
43	West Virginia	135
30	Wisconsin	199
50	Wyoming	30

RANK ORDER

RANK	STATE	RATE
1	New York	547
2	California	525
3	Delaware	501
4	Rhode Island	440
5	Florida	425
6	Massachusetts	354
7	Washington	344
8	Oregon	339
9	Connecticut	320
10	Georgia	302
10	Kansas	302
12	Vermont	296
13	North Carolina	294
14	Virginia	284
15	Illinois	277
16	Iowa	273
17	New Jersey	271
18	Hawaii	260
19	Montana	259
20	Pennsylvania	257
21	Nevada	256
22	Texas	254
23	Ohio	252
24	Tennessee	245
25	Michigan	221
25	Minnesota	221
27	Nebraska	220
28	Alabama	214
29	New Mexico	200
30	Wisconsin	199
31	Maine	186
32	Louisiana	178
33	South Carolina	176
34	Alaska	164
35	Colorado	162
36	Arkansas	159
37	Indiana	158
38	Arizona	149
39	North Dakota	147
40	New Hampshire	145
41	Maryland	141
42	Missouri	138
43	West Virginia	135
44	Oklahoma	133
45	Kentucky	132
46	Mississippi	104
47	South Dakota	90
48	Utah	79
49	Idaho	47
50	Wyoming	30
	District of Columbia**	NA

Source: U.S. Department of Health and Human Services, Centers for Disease Control and Prevention
  "Abortion Surveillance-United States, 1997" (Morbidity Mortality Weekly Report, Vol. 49, No. SS-11, 12/08/00)
*By state of occurrence.
**The District of Columbia's ratio was not listed but was noted as being greater than 1,000 abortions per 1,000 live births.

Reported Legal Abortions per 1,000 Women Ages 15 to 44 in 1997

National Rate = 20 Abortions per 1,000 Women Ages 15 to 44*

ALPHA ORDER

RANK ORDER

RANK	STATE	RATE
27	Alabama	13
30	Alaska	12
32	Arizona	11
32	Arkansas	11
1	California	38
36	Colorado	10
11	Connecticut	19
3	Delaware	30
4	Florida	27
8	Georgia	20
16	Hawaii	18
49	Idaho	3
11	Illinois	19
36	Indiana	10
18	Iowa	16
8	Kansas	20
42	Kentucky	8
30	Louisiana	12
38	Maine	9
42	Maryland	8
8	Massachusetts	20
27	Michigan	13
27	Minnesota	13
45	Mississippi	7
38	Missouri	9
20	Montana	15
24	Nebraska	14
11	Nevada	19
42	New Hampshire	8
17	New Jersey	17
24	New Mexico	14
2	New York	35
11	North Carolina	19
38	North Dakota	9
20	Ohio	15
38	Oklahoma	9
6	Oregon	21
24	Pennsylvania	14
5	Rhode Island	25
32	South Carolina	11
48	South Dakota	6
20	Tennessee	15
11	Texas	19
45	Utah	7
20	Vermont	15
18	Virginia	16
6	Washington	21
45	West Virginia	7
32	Wisconsin	11
50	Wyoming	2

RANK	STATE	RATE
1	California	38
2	New York	35
3	Delaware	30
4	Florida	27
5	Rhode Island	25
6	Oregon	21
6	Washington	21
8	Georgia	20
8	Kansas	20
8	Massachusetts	20
11	Connecticut	19
11	Illinois	19
11	Nevada	19
11	North Carolina	19
11	Texas	19
16	Hawaii	18
17	New Jersey	17
18	Iowa	16
18	Virginia	16
20	Montana	15
20	Ohio	15
20	Tennessee	15
20	Vermont	15
24	Nebraska	14
24	New Mexico	14
24	Pennsylvania	14
27	Alabama	13
27	Michigan	13
27	Minnesota	13
30	Alaska	12
30	Louisiana	12
32	Arizona	11
32	Arkansas	11
32	South Carolina	11
32	Wisconsin	11
36	Colorado	10
36	Indiana	10
38	Maine	9
38	Missouri	9
38	North Dakota	9
38	Oklahoma	9
42	Kentucky	8
42	Maryland	8
42	New Hampshire	8
45	Mississippi	7
45	Utah	7
45	West Virginia	7
48	South Dakota	6
49	Idaho	3
50	Wyoming	2

| | District of Columbia | 68 |

Source: U.S. Department of Health and Human Services, Centers for Disease Control and Prevention
"Abortion Surveillance-United States, 1997" (Morbidity Mortality Weekly Report, Vol. 49, No. SS-11, 12/08/00)
By state of occurrence.

Percent of Legal Abortions Obtained by Out-Of-State Residents in 1997

National Percent = 8.1% of Abortions*

<u>ALPHA ORDER</u>

RANK	STATE	PERCENT
11	Alabama	15.0
NA	Alaska**	NA
41	Arizona	1.9
16	Arkansas	10.4
NA	California**	NA
20	Colorado	9.3
38	Connecticut	3.4
2	Delaware	34.5
NA	Florida**	NA
18	Georgia	9.9
42	Hawaii	0.4
32	Idaho	4.3
23	Illinois	7.8
33	Indiana	4.1
NA	Iowa**	NA
1	Kansas	44.2
6	Kentucky	21.5
NA	Louisiana**	NA
39	Maine	3.2
35	Maryland	4.0
26	Massachusetts	6.2
36	Michigan	3.9
21	Minnesota	8.6
28	Mississippi	5.2
17	Missouri	10.1
9	Montana	17.3
5	Nebraska	22.0
14	Nevada	11.3
NA	New Hampshire**	NA
40	New Jersey	2.4
29	New Mexico	5.1
NA	New York**	NA
15	North Carolina	11.2
3	North Dakota	32.4
24	Ohio	6.6
NA	Oklahoma**	NA
12	Oregon	12.0
31	Pennsylvania	4.5
7	Rhode Island	18.9
25	South Carolina	6.3
4	South Dakota	23.9
8	Tennessee	18.3
36	Texas	3.9
22	Utah	8.0
10	Vermont	17.1
27	Virginia	5.7
30	Washington	4.6
13	West Virginia	11.7
33	Wisconsin	4.1
19	Wyoming	9.4

<u>RANK ORDER</u>

RANK	STATE	PERCENT
1	Kansas	44.2
2	Delaware	34.5
3	North Dakota	32.4
4	South Dakota	23.9
5	Nebraska	22.0
6	Kentucky	21.5
7	Rhode Island	18.9
8	Tennessee	18.3
9	Montana	17.3
10	Vermont	17.1
11	Alabama	15.0
12	Oregon	12.0
13	West Virginia	11.7
14	Nevada	11.3
15	North Carolina	11.2
16	Arkansas	10.4
17	Missouri	10.1
18	Georgia	9.9
19	Wyoming	9.4
20	Colorado	9.3
21	Minnesota	8.6
22	Utah	8.0
23	Illinois	7.8
24	Ohio	6.6
25	South Carolina	6.3
26	Massachusetts	6.2
27	Virginia	5.7
28	Mississippi	5.2
29	New Mexico	5.1
30	Washington	4.6
31	Pennsylvania	4.5
32	Idaho	4.3
33	Indiana	4.1
33	Wisconsin	4.1
35	Maryland	4.0
36	Michigan	3.9
36	Texas	3.9
38	Connecticut	3.4
39	Maine	3.2
40	New Jersey	2.4
41	Arizona	1.9
42	Hawaii	0.4
NA	Alaska**	NA
NA	California**	NA
NA	Florida**	NA
NA	Iowa**	NA
NA	Louisiana**	NA
NA	New Hampshire**	NA
NA	New York**	NA
NA	Oklahoma**	NA

District of Columbia	42.1

Source: U.S. Department of Health and Human Services, Centers for Disease Control and Prevention
    "Abortion Surveillance-United States, 1997" (Morbidity Mortality Weekly Report, Vol. 49, No. SS-11, 12/08/00)
*By state of occurrence.
**Not reported.

Percent of Reported Legal Abortions Obtained by White Women in 1997

Reporting States' Percent = 56.3% of Abortions*

ALPHA ORDER				RANK ORDER		
RANK	STATE	PERCENT		RANK	STATE	PERCENT
30	Alabama	51.6		1	Vermont	96.7
NA	Alaska**	NA		2	Idaho	93.3
12	Arizona	79.9		3	Maine	92.9
23	Arkansas	62.3		4	West Virginia	88.2
NA	California**	NA		5	North Dakota	88.1
16	Colorado	74.4		6	Wyoming	87.5
NA	Connecticut**	NA		7	Oregon	86.9
22	Delaware	63.0		8	New Mexico	86.3
NA	Florida**	NA		9	Utah	85.7
33	Georgia	42.9		10	South Dakota	85.6
38	Hawaii	27.0		11	Montana	83.1
2	Idaho	93.3		12	Arizona	79.9
NA	Illinois**	NA		13	Nevada	77.9
21	Indiana	64.5		14	Rhode Island	76.9
NA	Iowa**	NA		15	Kansas	75.4
15	Kansas	75.4		16	Colorado	74.4
17	Kentucky	73.9		17	Kentucky	73.9
32	Louisiana	45.3		18	Minnesota	73.3
3	Maine	92.9		19	Wisconsin	71.8
35	Maryland	34.6		20	Texas	71.1
NA	Massachusetts**	NA		21	Indiana	64.5
NA	Michigan**	NA		22	Delaware	63.0
18	Minnesota	73.3		23	Arkansas	62.3
36	Mississippi	32.8		24	Missouri	61.7
24	Missouri	61.7		25	Ohio	59.9
11	Montana	83.1		26	Pennsylvania	56.3
NA	Nebraska**	NA		27	Tennessee	56.0
13	Nevada	77.9		28	South Carolina	53.9
NA	New Hampshire**	NA		29	Virginia	53.2
37	New Jersey	32.5		30	Alabama	51.6
8	New Mexico	86.3		31	North Carolina	50.5
34	New York**	39.7		32	Louisiana	45.3
31	North Carolina	50.5		33	Georgia	42.9
5	North Dakota	88.1		34	New York**	39.7
25	Ohio	59.9		35	Maryland	34.6
NA	Oklahoma**	NA		36	Mississippi	32.8
7	Oregon	86.9		37	New Jersey	32.5
26	Pennsylvania	56.3		38	Hawaii	27.0
14	Rhode Island	76.9		NA	Alaska**	NA
28	South Carolina	53.9		NA	California**	NA
10	South Dakota	85.6		NA	Connecticut**	NA
27	Tennessee	56.0		NA	Florida**	NA
20	Texas	71.1		NA	Illinois**	NA
9	Utah	85.7		NA	Iowa**	NA
1	Vermont	96.7		NA	Massachusetts**	NA
29	Virginia	53.2		NA	Michigan**	NA
NA	Washington**	NA		NA	Nebraska**	NA
4	West Virginia	88.2		NA	New Hampshire**	NA
19	Wisconsin	71.8		NA	Oklahoma**	NA
6	Wyoming	87.5		NA	Washington**	NA
					District of Columbia	7.6

Source: U.S. Department of Health and Human Services, Centers for Disease Control and Prevention
"Abortion Surveillance-United States, 1997" (Morbidity Mortality Weekly Report, Vol. 49, No. SS-11, 12/08/00)
*By state of occurrence. Includes those of Hispanic ethnicity. National percent is for reporting states only.
**Not reported. New York's number is for New York City only.

Percent of Reported Legal Abortions Obtained by Black Women in 1997

Reporting States' Percent = 34.6% of Abortions*

ALPHA ORDER

RANK	STATE	PERCENT
7	Alabama	46.0
NA	Alaska**	NA
28	Arizona	4.8
13	Arkansas	34.9
NA	California**	NA
26	Colorado	6.2
NA	Connecticut**	NA
15	Delaware	33.7
NA	Florida**	NA
3	Georgia	54.4
29	Hawaii	3.2
35	Idaho	1.1
NA	Illinois**	NA
17	Indiana	25.4
NA	Iowa**	NA
21	Kansas	18.7
20	Kentucky	21.5
4	Louisiana	52.5
34	Maine	1.4
2	Maryland	56.5
NA	Massachusetts**	NA
NA	Michigan**	NA
22	Minnesota	13.9
1	Mississippi	65.9
14	Missouri	33.8
37	Montana	0.3
NA	Nebraska**	NA
25	Nevada	8.0
NA	New Hampshire**	NA
6	New Jersey	47.3
31	New Mexico	2.7
5	New York	47.4
11	North Carolina	39.7
33	North Dakota	1.5
16	Ohio	32.4
NA	Oklahoma**	NA
27	Oregon	5.4
10	Pennsylvania	40.4
23	Rhode Island	13.1
8	South Carolina	43.7
29	South Dakota	3.2
9	Tennessee	41.7
19	Texas	21.7
32	Utah	1.7
35	Vermont	1.1
12	Virginia	39.3
NA	Washington**	NA
24	West Virginia	10.5
18	Wisconsin	22.6
38	Wyoming	0.0

RANK ORDER

RANK	STATE	PERCENT
1	Mississippi	65.9
2	Maryland	56.5
3	Georgia	54.4
4	Louisiana	52.5
5	New York	47.4
6	New Jersey	47.3
7	Alabama	46.0
8	South Carolina	43.7
9	Tennessee	41.7
10	Pennsylvania	40.4
11	North Carolina	39.7
12	Virginia	39.3
13	Arkansas	34.9
14	Missouri	33.8
15	Delaware	33.7
16	Ohio	32.4
17	Indiana	25.4
18	Wisconsin	22.6
19	Texas	21.7
20	Kentucky	21.5
21	Kansas	18.7
22	Minnesota	13.9
23	Rhode Island	13.1
24	West Virginia	10.5
25	Nevada	8.0
26	Colorado	6.2
27	Oregon	5.4
28	Arizona	4.8
29	Hawaii	3.2
29	South Dakota	3.2
31	New Mexico	2.7
32	Utah	1.7
33	North Dakota	1.5
34	Maine	1.4
35	Idaho	1.1
35	Vermont	1.1
37	Montana	0.3
38	Wyoming	0.0
NA	Alaska**	NA
NA	California**	NA
NA	Connecticut**	NA
NA	Florida**	NA
NA	Illinois**	NA
NA	Iowa**	NA
NA	Massachusetts**	NA
NA	Michigan**	NA
NA	Nebraska**	NA
NA	New Hampshire**	NA
NA	Oklahoma**	NA
NA	Washington**	NA

District of Columbia	76.4

Source: U.S. Department of Health and Human Services, Centers for Disease Control and Prevention
"Abortion Surveillance-United States, 1997" (Morbidity Mortality Weekly Report, Vol. 49, No. SS-11, 12/08/00)
*By state of occurrence. National percent is for reporting states only.
**Not reported. New York's number is for New York City only.

Percent of Reported Legal Abortions Obtained by Married Women in 1997

Reporting States' Percent = 18.5% of Abortions*

ALPHA ORDER

RANK ORDER

RANK	STATE	PERCENT		RANK	STATE	PERCENT
27	Alabama	17.2		1	Utah	35.0
NA	Alaska**	NA		2	Nevada	23.2
NA	Arizona**	NA		3	Oregon	22.1
19	Arkansas	18.2		4	South Dakota	21.9
NA	California**	NA		5	Vermont	21.7
13	Colorado	19.1		6	Missouri	20.6
NA	Connecticut**	NA		7	North Dakota	20.5
36	Delaware	15.7		8	North Carolina	20.3
NA	Florida**	NA		9	Texas	20.2
19	Georgia	18.2		10	Massachusetts	20.1
26	Hawaii	17.5		11	Kansas	19.8
15	Idaho	19.0		12	Tennessee	19.2
35	Illinois	16.3		13	Colorado	19.1
37	Indiana	14.1		13	New York**	19.1
NA	Iowa**	NA		15	Idaho	19.0
11	Kansas	19.8		15	Minnesota	19.0
28	Kentucky	17.1		17	Wyoming	18.8
NA	Louisiana**	NA		18	Maryland	18.3
22	Maine	17.9		19	Arkansas	18.2
18	Maryland	18.3		19	Georgia	18.2
10	Massachusetts	20.1		21	Rhode Island	18.1
34	Michigan	16.5		22	Maine	17.9
15	Minnesota	19.0		22	South Carolina	17.9
38	Mississippi	13.0		24	Montana	17.7
6	Missouri	20.6		24	Wisconsin	17.7
24	Montana	17.7		26	Hawaii	17.5
NA	Nebraska**	NA		27	Alabama	17.2
2	Nevada	23.2		28	Kentucky	17.1
NA	New Hampshire**	NA		28	New Jersey	17.1
28	New Jersey	17.1		30	New Mexico	16.9
30	New Mexico	16.9		31	Ohio	16.8
13	New York**	19.1		32	West Virginia	16.7
8	North Carolina	20.3		33	Pennsylvania	16.6
7	North Dakota	20.5		34	Michigan	16.5
31	Ohio	16.8		35	Illinois	16.3
NA	Oklahoma**	NA		36	Delaware	15.7
3	Oregon	22.1		37	Indiana	14.1
33	Pennsylvania	16.6		38	Mississippi	13.0
21	Rhode Island	18.1		NA	Alaska**	NA
22	South Carolina	17.9		NA	Arizona**	NA
4	South Dakota	21.9		NA	California**	NA
12	Tennessee	19.2		NA	Connecticut**	NA
9	Texas	20.2		NA	Florida**	NA
1	Utah	35.0		NA	Iowa**	NA
5	Vermont	21.7		NA	Louisiana**	NA
NA	Virginia**	NA		NA	Nebraska**	NA
NA	Washington**	NA		NA	New Hampshire**	NA
32	West Virginia	16.7		NA	Oklahoma**	NA
24	Wisconsin	17.7		NA	Virginia**	NA
17	Wyoming	18.8		NA	Washington**	NA
					District of Columbia**	NA

Source: U.S. Department of Health and Human Services, Centers for Disease Control and Prevention
"Abortion Surveillance-United States, 1997" (Morbidity Mortality Weekly Report, Vol. 49, No. SS-11, 12/08/00)
*By state of occurrence. National percent is for reporting states only.
**Not reported. New York's percentage is for New York City only.

Percent of Reported Legal Abortions Obtained by Unmarried Women in 1997

Reporting States' Percent = 78.8% of Abortions*

ALPHA ORDER

RANK ORDER

RANK	STATE	PERCENT
10	Alabama	82.0
NA	Alaska**	NA
NA	Arizona**	NA
17	Arkansas	80.4
NA	California**	NA
18	Colorado	80.2
NA	Connecticut**	NA
2	Delaware	84.3
NA	Florida**	NA
11	Georgia	81.8
7	Hawaii	82.2
14	Idaho	81.0
13	Illinois	81.1
33	Indiana	73.1
NA	Iowa**	NA
19	Kansas	80.1
12	Kentucky	81.3
NA	Louisiana**	NA
29	Maine	76.2
21	Maryland	79.6
36	Massachusetts	72.1
4	Michigan	83.0
22	Minnesota	79.1
1	Mississippi	86.9
25	Missouri	77.7
30	Montana	75.8
NA	Nebraska**	NA
32	Nevada	74.5
NA	New Hampshire**	NA
6	New Jersey	82.6
8	New Mexico	82.1
24	New York**	78.2
37	North Carolina	70.3
23	North Dakota	79.0
20	Ohio	79.7
NA	Oklahoma**	NA
31	Oregon	74.8
3	Pennsylvania	83.3
33	Rhode Island	73.1
8	South Carolina	82.1
25	South Dakota	77.7
15	Tennessee	80.8
27	Texas	77.5
38	Utah	65.0
35	Vermont	72.3
NA	Virginia**	NA
NA	Washington**	NA
4	West Virginia	83.0
27	Wisconsin	77.5
16	Wyoming	80.7

RANK	STATE	PERCENT
1	Mississippi	86.9
2	Delaware	84.3
3	Pennsylvania	83.3
4	Michigan	83.0
4	West Virginia	83.0
6	New Jersey	82.6
7	Hawaii	82.2
8	New Mexico	82.1
8	South Carolina	82.1
10	Alabama	82.0
11	Georgia	81.8
12	Kentucky	81.3
13	Illinois	81.1
14	Idaho	81.0
15	Tennessee	80.8
16	Wyoming	80.7
17	Arkansas	80.4
18	Colorado	80.2
19	Kansas	80.1
20	Ohio	79.7
21	Maryland	79.6
22	Minnesota	79.1
23	North Dakota	79.0
24	New York**	78.2
25	Missouri	77.7
25	South Dakota	77.7
27	Texas	77.5
27	Wisconsin	77.5
29	Maine	76.2
30	Montana	75.8
31	Oregon	74.8
32	Nevada	74.5
33	Indiana	73.1
33	Rhode Island	73.1
35	Vermont	72.3
36	Massachusetts	72.1
37	North Carolina	70.3
38	Utah	65.0
NA	Alaska**	NA
NA	Arizona**	NA
NA	California**	NA
NA	Connecticut**	NA
NA	Florida**	NA
NA	Iowa**	NA
NA	Louisiana**	NA
NA	Nebraska**	NA
NA	New Hampshire**	NA
NA	Oklahoma**	NA
NA	Virginia**	NA
NA	Washington**	NA
	District of Columbia**	NA

Source: U.S. Department of Health and Human Services, Centers for Disease Control and Prevention
   "Abortion Surveillance-United States, 1997" (Morbidity Mortality Weekly Report, Vol. 49, No. SS-11, 12/08/00)
*By state of occurrence. National percent is for reporting states only.
**Not reported. New York's percentage is for New York City only.

Reported Legal Abortions Obtained by Teenagers in 1997

Reporting States' Total = 150,531 Abortions Obtained by Teenagers*

ALPHA ORDER

RANK	STATE	ABORTIONS	% of USA
15	Alabama	2,832	1.9%
40	Alaska	349	0.2%
21	Arizona	2,248	1.5%
28	Arkansas	1,327	0.9%
NA	California**	NA	NA
22	Colorado	2,189	1.5%
14	Connecticut	3,038	2.0%
27	Delaware	1,334	0.9%
NA	Florida**	NA	NA
5	Georgia	7,043	4.7%
33	Hawaii	1,088	0.7%
43	Idaho	236	0.2%
NA	Illinois**	NA	NA
17	Indiana	2,759	1.8%
NA	Iowa**	NA	NA
18	Kansas	2,672	1.8%
26	Kentucky	1,569	1.0%
20	Louisiana	2,432	1.6%
38	Maine	632	0.4%
25	Maryland	1,912	1.3%
11	Massachusetts	4,849	3.2%
7	Michigan	6,026	4.0%
16	Minnesota	2,763	1.8%
34	Mississippi	957	0.6%
24	Missouri	1,985	1.3%
36	Montana	695	0.5%
31	Nebraska	1,106	0.7%
29	Nevada	1,248	0.8%
NA	New Hampshire**	NA	NA
9	New Jersey	5,207	3.5%
30	New Mexico	1,198	0.8%
1	New York	26,440	17.6%
6	North Carolina	6,332	4.2%
41	North Dakota	280	0.2%
3	Ohio	8,149	5.4%
NA	Oklahoma**	NA	NA
13	Oregon	3,335	2.2%
4	Pennsylvania	7,174	4.8%
32	Rhode Island	1,096	0.7%
23	South Carolina	2,056	1.4%
42	South Dakota	249	0.2%
12	Tennessee	3,732	2.5%
2	Texas	15,020	10.0%
35	Utah	732	0.5%
39	Vermont	461	0.3%
10	Virginia	5,031	3.3%
8	Washington	5,728	3.8%
37	West Virginia	691	0.5%
19	Wisconsin	2,666	1.8%
44	Wyoming	33	0.0%

RANK ORDER

RANK	STATE	ABORTIONS	% of USA
1	New York	26,440	17.6%
2	Texas	15,020	10.0%
3	Ohio	8,149	5.4%
4	Pennsylvania	7,174	4.8%
5	Georgia	7,043	4.7%
6	North Carolina	6,332	4.2%
7	Michigan	6,026	4.0%
8	Washington	5,728	3.8%
9	New Jersey	5,207	3.5%
10	Virginia	5,031	3.3%
11	Massachusetts	4,849	3.2%
12	Tennessee	3,732	2.5%
13	Oregon	3,335	2.2%
14	Connecticut	3,038	2.0%
15	Alabama	2,832	1.9%
16	Minnesota	2,763	1.8%
17	Indiana	2,759	1.8%
18	Kansas	2,672	1.8%
19	Wisconsin	2,666	1.8%
20	Louisiana	2,432	1.6%
21	Arizona	2,248	1.5%
22	Colorado	2,189	1.5%
23	South Carolina	2,056	1.4%
24	Missouri	1,985	1.3%
25	Maryland	1,912	1.3%
26	Kentucky	1,569	1.0%
27	Delaware	1,334	0.9%
28	Arkansas	1,327	0.9%
29	Nevada	1,248	0.8%
30	New Mexico	1,198	0.8%
31	Nebraska	1,106	0.7%
32	Rhode Island	1,096	0.7%
33	Hawaii	1,088	0.7%
34	Mississippi	957	0.6%
35	Utah	732	0.5%
36	Montana	695	0.5%
37	West Virginia	691	0.5%
38	Maine	632	0.4%
39	Vermont	461	0.3%
40	Alaska	349	0.2%
41	North Dakota	280	0.2%
42	South Dakota	249	0.2%
43	Idaho	236	0.2%
44	Wyoming	33	0.0%
NA	California**	NA	NA
NA	Florida**	NA	NA
NA	Illinois**	NA	NA
NA	Iowa**	NA	NA
NA	New Hampshire**	NA	NA
NA	Oklahoma**	NA	NA
	District of Columbia	1,632	1.1%

Source: U.S. Department of Health and Human Services, Centers for Disease Control and Prevention
"Abortion Surveillance-United States, 1997" (Morbidity Mortality Weekly Report, Vol. 49, No. SS-11, 12/08/00)
*Nineteen years old and younger by state of occurrence. National total is for reporting states only.
**Not reported.

Percent of Reported Legal Abortions Obtained by Teenagers in 1997

Reporting States' Percent = 19.8% of Abortions*

ALPHA ORDER				RANK ORDER		
RANK	STATE	PERCENT		RANK	STATE	PERCENT
19	Alabama	21.7		1	South Dakota	27.1
22	Alaska	21.4		2	Idaho	26.9
31	Arizona	20.0		3	Delaware	26.0
11	Arkansas	23.0		4	Maine	24.8
NA	California**	NA		5	Montana	24.7
8	Colorado	23.8		6	West Virginia	24.6
18	Connecticut	22.0		7	Hawaii	24.1
3	Delaware	26.0		8	Colorado	23.8
NA	Florida**	NA		8	Kansas	23.8
33	Georgia	19.7		10	Vermont	23.6
7	Hawaii	24.1		11	Arkansas	23.0
2	Idaho	26.9		12	North Dakota	22.8
NA	Illinois**	NA		13	Oregon	22.5
25	Indiana	20.9		14	Kentucky	22.3
NA	Iowa**	NA		14	New Mexico	22.3
8	Kansas	23.8		14	South Carolina	22.3
14	Kentucky	22.3		17	Mississippi	22.1
26	Louisiana	20.7		18	Connecticut	22.0
4	Maine	24.8		19	Alabama	21.7
35	Maryland	19.4		20	Nebraska	21.6
43	Massachusetts	17.0		21	Utah	21.5
27	Michigan	20.4		22	Alaska	21.4
35	Minnesota	19.4		23	Ohio	21.3
17	Mississippi	22.1		23	Washington	21.3
34	Missouri	19.5		25	Indiana	20.9
5	Montana	24.7		26	Louisiana	20.7
20	Nebraska	21.6		27	Michigan	20.4
40	Nevada	18.1		27	Tennessee	20.4
NA	New Hampshire**	NA		29	Wisconsin	20.2
43	New Jersey	17.0		30	North Carolina	20.1
14	New Mexico	22.3		31	Arizona	20.0
39	New York	18.8		31	Rhode Island	20.0
30	North Carolina	20.1		33	Georgia	19.7
12	North Dakota	22.8		34	Missouri	19.5
23	Ohio	21.3		35	Maryland	19.4
NA	Oklahoma**	NA		35	Minnesota	19.4
13	Oregon	22.5		37	Pennsylvania	19.3
37	Pennsylvania	19.3		37	Virginia	19.3
31	Rhode Island	20.0		39	New York	18.8
14	South Carolina	22.3		40	Nevada	18.1
1	South Dakota	27.1		41	Texas	17.7
27	Tennessee	20.4		42	Wyoming	17.2
41	Texas	17.7		43	Massachusetts	17.0
21	Utah	21.5		43	New Jersey	17.0
10	Vermont	23.6		NA	California**	NA
37	Virginia	19.3		NA	Florida**	NA
23	Washington	21.3		NA	Illinois**	NA
6	West Virginia	24.6		NA	Iowa**	NA
29	Wisconsin	20.2		NA	New Hampshire**	NA
42	Wyoming	17.2		NA	Oklahoma**	NA

District of Columbia	18.6

Source: Morgan Quitno Press using data from US Dept of Health & Human Serv's, Centers for Disease Control-Prevention "Abortion Surveillance-United States, 1997" (Morbidity Mortality Weekly Report, Vol. 49, No. SS-11, 12/08/00)
*Nineteen and younger by state of occurrence. National percent is for reporting states only.
**Not reported.

Reported Legal Abortions Obtained by Teenagers 17 Years and Younger in 1997

Reporting States' Total = 61,341 Abortions*

ALPHA ORDER

RANK	STATE	ABORTIONS	% of USA
16	Alabama	1,135	1.9%
40	Alaska	144	0.2%
22	Arizona	885	1.4%
30	Arkansas	548	0.9%
NA	California**	NA	NA
20	Colorado	1,011	1.6%
14	Connecticut	1,340	2.2%
27	Delaware	609	1.0%
NA	Florida**	NA	NA
4	Georgia	3,032	4.9%
31	Hawaii	476	0.8%
43	Idaho	101	0.2%
NA	Illinois**	NA	NA
19	Indiana	1,024	1.7%
NA	Iowa**	NA	NA
15	Kansas	1,146	1.9%
26	Kentucky	634	1.0%
21	Louisiana	946	1.5%
37	Maine	290	0.5%
24	Maryland	793	1.3%
11	Massachusetts	1,925	3.1%
8	Michigan	2,372	3.9%
17	Minnesota	1,083	1.8%
33	Mississippi	380	0.6%
25	Missouri	782	1.3%
35	Montana	302	0.5%
32	Nebraska	461	0.8%
29	Nevada	552	0.9%
NA	New Hampshire**	NA	NA
9	New Jersey	2,023	3.3%
28	New Mexico	553	0.9%
1	New York	11,388	18.6%
7	North Carolina	2,433	4.0%
41	North Dakota	115	0.2%
3	Ohio	3,444	5.6%
NA	Oklahoma**	NA	NA
13	Oregon	1,412	2.3%
5	Pennsylvania	2,594	4.2%
34	Rhode Island	355	0.6%
23	South Carolina	871	1.4%
42	South Dakota	114	0.2%
12	Tennessee	1,513	2.5%
2	Texas	5,505	9.0%
38	Utah	269	0.4%
39	Vermont	186	0.3%
10	Virginia	1,995	3.3%
6	Washington	2,560	4.2%
36	West Virginia	294	0.5%
18	Wisconsin	1,071	1.7%
44	Wyoming	18	0.0%

RANK ORDER

RANK	STATE	ABORTIONS	% of USA
1	New York	11,388	18.6%
2	Texas	5,505	9.0%
3	Ohio	3,444	5.6%
4	Georgia	3,032	4.9%
5	Pennsylvania	2,594	4.2%
6	Washington	2,560	4.2%
7	North Carolina	2,433	4.0%
8	Michigan	2,372	3.9%
9	New Jersey	2,023	3.3%
10	Virginia	1,995	3.3%
11	Massachusetts	1,925	3.1%
12	Tennessee	1,513	2.5%
13	Oregon	1,412	2.3%
14	Connecticut	1,340	2.2%
15	Kansas	1,146	1.9%
16	Alabama	1,135	1.9%
17	Minnesota	1,083	1.8%
18	Wisconsin	1,071	1.7%
19	Indiana	1,024	1.7%
20	Colorado	1,011	1.6%
21	Louisiana	946	1.5%
22	Arizona	885	1.4%
23	South Carolina	871	1.4%
24	Maryland	793	1.3%
25	Missouri	782	1.3%
26	Kentucky	634	1.0%
27	Delaware	609	1.0%
28	New Mexico	553	0.9%
29	Nevada	552	0.9%
30	Arkansas	548	0.9%
31	Hawaii	476	0.8%
32	Nebraska	461	0.8%
33	Mississippi	380	0.6%
34	Rhode Island	355	0.6%
35	Montana	302	0.5%
36	West Virginia	294	0.5%
37	Maine	290	0.5%
38	Utah	269	0.4%
39	Vermont	186	0.3%
40	Alaska	144	0.2%
41	North Dakota	115	0.2%
42	South Dakota	114	0.2%
43	Idaho	101	0.2%
44	Wyoming	18	0.0%
NA	California**	NA	NA
NA	Florida**	NA	NA
NA	Illinois**	NA	NA
NA	Iowa**	NA	NA
NA	New Hampshire**	NA	NA
NA	Oklahoma**	NA	NA
	District of Columbia	657	1.1%

Source: Morgan Quitno Press using data from US Dept of Health & Human Serv's, Centers for Disease Control-Prevention "Abortion Surveillance-United States, 1997" (Morbidity Mortality Weekly Report, Vol. 49, No. SS-11, 12/08/00)
*By state of occurrence. National total is for reporting states only.
**Not reported.

Percent of Reported Legal Abortions Obtained
By Teenagers 17 Years and Younger in 1997
Reporting States' Percent = 8.1% of Abortions*

ALPHA ORDER

RANK	STATE	PERCENT
24	Alabama	8.7
22	Alaska	8.8
33	Arizona	7.9
12	Arkansas	9.5
NA	California**	NA
5	Colorado	11.0
11	Connecticut	9.7
2	Delaware	11.9
NA	Florida**	NA
25	Georgia	8.5
7	Hawaii	10.5
3	Idaho	11.5
NA	Illinois**	NA
35	Indiana	7.8
NA	Iowa**	NA
10	Kansas	10.2
19	Kentucky	9.0
27	Louisiana	8.1
4	Maine	11.4
30	Maryland	8.0
41	Massachusetts	6.8
30	Michigan	8.0
38	Minnesota	7.6
22	Mississippi	8.8
36	Missouri	7.7
6	Montana	10.8
19	Nebraska	9.0
30	Nevada	8.0
NA	New Hampshire**	NA
42	New Jersey	6.6
9	New Mexico	10.3
27	New York	8.1
36	North Carolina	7.7
17	North Dakota	9.4
19	Ohio	9.0
NA	Oklahoma**	NA
12	Oregon	9.5
40	Pennsylvania	7.0
43	Rhode Island	6.5
12	South Carolina	9.5
1	South Dakota	12.4
26	Tennessee	8.3
43	Texas	6.5
33	Utah	7.9
12	Vermont	9.5
38	Virginia	7.6
12	Washington	9.5
7	West Virginia	10.5
27	Wisconsin	8.1
17	Wyoming	9.4

RANK ORDER

RANK	STATE	PERCENT
1	South Dakota	12.4
2	Delaware	11.9
3	Idaho	11.5
4	Maine	11.4
5	Colorado	11.0
6	Montana	10.8
7	Hawaii	10.5
7	West Virginia	10.5
9	New Mexico	10.3
10	Kansas	10.2
11	Connecticut	9.7
12	Arkansas	9.5
12	Oregon	9.5
12	South Carolina	9.5
12	Vermont	9.5
12	Washington	9.5
17	North Dakota	9.4
17	Wyoming	9.4
19	Kentucky	9.0
19	Nebraska	9.0
19	Ohio	9.0
22	Alaska	8.8
22	Mississippi	8.8
24	Alabama	8.7
25	Georgia	8.5
26	Tennessee	8.3
27	Louisiana	8.1
27	New York	8.1
27	Wisconsin	8.1
30	Maryland	8.0
30	Michigan	8.0
30	Nevada	8.0
33	Arizona	7.9
33	Utah	7.9
35	Indiana	7.8
36	Missouri	7.7
36	North Carolina	7.7
38	Minnesota	7.6
38	Virginia	7.6
40	Pennsylvania	7.0
41	Massachusetts	6.8
42	New Jersey	6.6
43	Rhode Island	6.5
43	Texas	6.5
NA	California**	NA
NA	Florida**	NA
NA	Illinois**	NA
NA	Iowa**	NA
NA	New Hampshire**	NA
NA	Oklahoma**	NA
	District of Columbia	7.5

Source: Morgan Quitno Press using data from US Dept of Health & Human Serv's, Centers for Disease Control-Prevention "Abortion Surveillance-United States, 1997" (Morbidity Mortality Weekly Report, Vol. 49, No. SS-11, 12/08/00)
*By state of occurrence. National percent is for reporting states only.
**Not reported.

Percent of Teenage Abortions Obtained
By Teenagers 17 Years and Younger in 1997
Reporting States' Percent = 40.7% of Teenage Abortions*

ALPHA ORDER

RANK	STATE	PERCENT
29	Alabama	40.1
22	Alaska	41.3
33	Arizona	39.4
22	Arkansas	41.3
NA	California**	NA
2	Colorado	46.2
9	Connecticut	44.1
6	Delaware	45.7
NA	Florida**	NA
13	Georgia	43.0
10	Hawaii	43.8
15	Idaho	42.8
NA	Illinois**	NA
40	Indiana	37.1
NA	Iowa**	NA
14	Kansas	42.9
26	Kentucky	40.4
37	Louisiana	38.9
4	Maine	45.9
21	Maryland	41.5
30	Massachusetts	39.7
33	Michigan	39.4
36	Minnesota	39.2
30	Mississippi	39.7
33	Missouri	39.4
11	Montana	43.5
20	Nebraska	41.7
8	Nevada	44.2
NA	New Hampshire**	NA
37	New Jersey	38.9
2	New Mexico	46.2
12	New York	43.1
39	North Carolina	38.4
24	North Dakota	41.1
18	Ohio	42.3
NA	Oklahoma**	NA
18	Oregon	42.3
43	Pennsylvania	36.2
44	Rhode Island	32.4
17	South Carolina	42.4
5	South Dakota	45.8
25	Tennessee	40.5
41	Texas	36.7
41	Utah	36.7
27	Vermont	40.3
30	Virginia	39.7
7	Washington	44.7
16	West Virginia	42.5
28	Wisconsin	40.2
1	Wyoming	54.5

RANK ORDER

RANK	STATE	PERCENT
1	Wyoming	54.5
2	Colorado	46.2
2	New Mexico	46.2
4	Maine	45.9
5	South Dakota	45.8
6	Delaware	45.7
7	Washington	44.7
8	Nevada	44.2
9	Connecticut	44.1
10	Hawaii	43.8
11	Montana	43.5
12	New York	43.1
13	Georgia	43.0
14	Kansas	42.9
15	Idaho	42.8
16	West Virginia	42.5
17	South Carolina	42.4
18	Ohio	42.3
18	Oregon	42.3
20	Nebraska	41.7
21	Maryland	41.5
22	Alaska	41.3
22	Arkansas	41.3
24	North Dakota	41.1
25	Tennessee	40.5
26	Kentucky	40.4
27	Vermont	40.3
28	Wisconsin	40.2
29	Alabama	40.1
30	Massachusetts	39.7
30	Mississippi	39.7
30	Virginia	39.7
33	Arizona	39.4
33	Michigan	39.4
33	Missouri	39.4
36	Minnesota	39.2
37	Louisiana	38.9
37	New Jersey	38.9
39	North Carolina	38.4
40	Indiana	37.1
41	Texas	36.7
41	Utah	36.7
43	Pennsylvania	36.2
44	Rhode Island	32.4
NA	California**	NA
NA	Florida**	NA
NA	Illinois**	NA
NA	Iowa**	NA
NA	New Hampshire**	NA
NA	Oklahoma**	NA

District of Columbia 40.3

Source: Morgan Quitno Press using data from US Dept of Health & Human Serv's, Centers for Disease Control-Prevention "Abortion Surveillance-United States, 1997" (Morbidity Mortality Weekly Report, Vol. 49, No. SS-11, 12/08/00)
*By state of occurrence. National percent is for reporting states only.
**Not reported.

Reported Legal Abortions Performed at 12 Weeks or Less of Gestation in 1997

Reporting States' Total = 616,419 Abortions*

ALPHA ORDER

RANK	STATE	ABORTIONS	% of USA
16	Alabama	11,460	1.9%
NA	Alaska**	NA	NA
18	Arizona	9,618	1.6%
28	Arkansas	4,704	0.8%
NA	California**	NA	NA
24	Colorado	7,808	1.3%
14	Connecticut	12,482	2.0%
30	Delaware	4,493	0.7%
NA	Florida**	NA	NA
5	Georgia	29,515	4.8%
31	Hawaii	4,015	0.7%
40	Idaho	838	0.1%
NA	Illinois**	NA	NA
13	Indiana	12,518	2.0%
NA	Iowa**	NA	NA
23	Kansas	9,105	1.5%
26	Kentucky	5,741	0.9%
20	Louisiana	9,389	1.5%
34	Maine	2,511	0.4%
19	Maryland	9,412	1.5%
NA	Massachusetts**	NA	NA
6	Michigan	26,076	4.2%
15	Minnesota	12,399	2.0%
32	Mississippi	3,827	0.6%
21	Missouri	9,310	1.5%
35	Montana	2,485	0.4%
NA	Nebraska**	NA	NA
25	Nevada	6,041	1.0%
NA	New Hampshire**	NA	NA
9	New Jersey	23,673	3.8%
29	New Mexico	4,524	0.7%
1	New York	117,345	19.0%
7	North Carolina	25,495	4.1%
38	North Dakota	1,072	0.2%
4	Ohio	32,300	5.2%
NA	Oklahoma**	NA	NA
12	Oregon	13,028	2.1%
3	Pennsylvania	32,726	5.3%
27	Rhode Island	4,925	0.8%
22	South Carolina	9,123	1.5%
39	South Dakota	915	0.1%
11	Tennessee	17,317	2.8%
2	Texas	73,643	11.9%
33	Utah	3,088	0.5%
37	Vermont	1,870	0.3%
8	Virginia	24,974	4.1%
10	Washington	22,973	3.7%
36	West Virginia	2,384	0.4%
17	Wisconsin	11,113	1.8%
41	Wyoming	184	0.0%

RANK ORDER

RANK	STATE	ABORTIONS	% of USA
1	New York	117,345	19.0%
2	Texas	73,643	11.9%
3	Pennsylvania	32,726	5.3%
4	Ohio	32,300	5.2%
5	Georgia	29,515	4.8%
6	Michigan	26,076	4.2%
7	North Carolina	25,495	4.1%
8	Virginia	24,974	4.1%
9	New Jersey	23,673	3.8%
10	Washington	22,973	3.7%
11	Tennessee	17,317	2.8%
12	Oregon	13,028	2.1%
13	Indiana	12,518	2.0%
14	Connecticut	12,482	2.0%
15	Minnesota	12,399	2.0%
16	Alabama	11,460	1.9%
17	Wisconsin	11,113	1.8%
18	Arizona	9,618	1.6%
19	Maryland	9,412	1.5%
20	Louisiana	9,389	1.5%
21	Missouri	9,310	1.5%
22	South Carolina	9,123	1.5%
23	Kansas	9,105	1.5%
24	Colorado	7,808	1.3%
25	Nevada	6,041	1.0%
26	Kentucky	5,741	0.9%
27	Rhode Island	4,925	0.8%
28	Arkansas	4,704	0.8%
29	New Mexico	4,524	0.7%
30	Delaware	4,493	0.7%
31	Hawaii	4,015	0.7%
32	Mississippi	3,827	0.6%
33	Utah	3,088	0.5%
34	Maine	2,511	0.4%
35	Montana	2,485	0.4%
36	West Virginia	2,384	0.4%
37	Vermont	1,870	0.3%
38	North Dakota	1,072	0.2%
39	South Dakota	915	0.1%
40	Idaho	838	0.1%
41	Wyoming	184	0.0%
NA	Alaska**	NA	NA
NA	California**	NA	NA
NA	Florida**	NA	NA
NA	Illinois**	NA	NA
NA	Iowa**	NA	NA
NA	Massachusetts**	NA	NA
NA	Nebraska**	NA	NA
NA	New Hampshire**	NA	NA
NA	Oklahoma**	NA	NA
	District of Columbia**	NA	NA

Source: Morgan Quitno Press using data from US Dept of Health & Human Serv's, Centers for Disease Control-Prevention "Abortion Surveillance-United States, 1997" (Morbidity Mortality Weekly Report, Vol. 49, No. SS-11, 12/08/00)
*By state of occurrence. National total is for reporting states only.
**Not reported.

Percent of Reported Legal Abortions Performed
At 12 Weeks or Less of Gestation in 1997
Reporting States' Percent = 86.2% of Abortions*

ALPHA ORDER				RANK ORDER		
RANK	STATE	PERCENT		RANK	STATE	PERCENT
21	Alabama	87.7		1	South Dakota	99.6
NA	Alaska**	NA		2	South Carolina	99.0
28	Arizona	85.4		3	Maine	98.7
37	Arkansas	81.4		4	Wyoming	95.8
NA	California**	NA		5	Vermont	95.7
30	Colorado	85.0		5	Virginia	95.7
13	Connecticut	90.4		7	Idaho	95.4
24	Delaware	87.4		7	Maryland	95.4
NA	Florida**	NA		9	Indiana	94.8
35	Georgia	82.7		10	Tennessee	94.7
15	Hawaii	88.8		11	Missouri	91.3
7	Idaho	95.4		12	Utah	90.6
NA	Illinois**	NA		13	Connecticut	90.4
9	Indiana	94.8		14	Rhode Island	89.9
NA	Iowa**	NA		15	Hawaii	88.8
38	Kansas	80.9		16	Mississippi	88.5
36	Kentucky	81.6		16	Montana	88.5
40	Louisiana	80.0		18	Michigan	88.3
3	Maine	98.7		19	Pennsylvania	88.1
7	Maryland	95.4		20	Oregon	87.8
NA	Massachusetts**	NA		21	Alabama	87.7
18	Michigan	88.3		21	Nevada	87.7
26	Minnesota	87.1		21	Wisconsin	87.7
16	Mississippi	88.5		24	Delaware	87.4
11	Missouri	91.3		24	North Dakota	87.4
16	Montana	88.5		26	Minnesota	87.1
NA	Nebraska**	NA		27	Texas	87.0
21	Nevada	87.7		28	Arizona	85.4
NA	New Hampshire**	NA		29	Washington	85.3
41	New Jersey	77.2		30	Colorado	85.0
33	New Mexico	84.1		31	West Virginia	84.9
34	New York	83.3		32	Ohio	84.5
38	North Carolina	80.9		33	New Mexico	84.1
24	North Dakota	87.4		34	New York	83.3
32	Ohio	84.5		35	Georgia	82.7
NA	Oklahoma**	NA		36	Kentucky	81.6
20	Oregon	87.8		37	Arkansas	81.4
19	Pennsylvania	88.1		38	Kansas	80.9
14	Rhode Island	89.9		38	North Carolina	80.9
2	South Carolina	99.0		40	Louisiana	80.0
1	South Dakota	99.6		41	New Jersey	77.2
10	Tennessee	94.7		NA	Alaska**	NA
27	Texas	87.0		NA	California**	NA
12	Utah	90.6		NA	Florida**	NA
5	Vermont	95.7		NA	Illinois**	NA
5	Virginia	95.7		NA	Iowa**	NA
29	Washington	85.3		NA	Massachusetts**	NA
31	West Virginia	84.9		NA	Nebraska**	NA
21	Wisconsin	87.7		NA	New Hampshire**	NA
4	Wyoming	95.8		NA	Oklahoma**	NA
				District of Columbia**		NA

Source: Morgan Quitno Press using data from US Dept of Health & Human Serv's, Centers for Disease Control-Prevention
"Abortion Surveillance-United States, 1997" (Morbidity Mortality Weekly Report, Vol. 49, No. SS-11, 12/08/00)
*By state of occurrence. National percent is for reporting states only.
**Not reported.

Reported Legal Abortions Performed At or After 21 Weeks of Gestation in 1997

Reporting States' Total = 9,985 Abortions*

ALPHA ORDER

RANK	STATE	ABORTIONS	% of USA
19	Alabama	53	0.5%
NA	Alaska**	NA	NA
38	Arizona	0	0.0%
29	Arkansas	8	0.1%
NA	California**	NA	NA
13	Colorado	152	1.5%
30	Connecticut	4	0.0%
27	Delaware	10	0.1%
NA	Florida**	NA	NA
2	Georgia	1,376	13.8%
22	Hawaii	28	0.3%
30	Idaho	4	0.0%
NA	Illinois**	NA	NA
38	Indiana	0	0.0%
NA	Iowa**	NA	NA
4	Kansas	807	8.1%
15	Kentucky	129	1.3%
8	Louisiana	339	3.4%
34	Maine	1	0.0%
34	Maryland	1	0.0%
NA	Massachusetts**	NA	NA
11	Michigan	221	2.2%
16	Minnesota	102	1.0%
26	Mississippi	15	0.2%
21	Missouri	45	0.5%
20	Montana	47	0.5%
NA	Nebraska**	NA	NA
18	Nevada	69	0.7%
NA	New Hampshire**	NA	NA
5	New Jersey	660	6.6%
22	New Mexico	28	0.3%
1	New York	2,506	25.1%
12	North Carolina	217	2.2%
38	North Dakota	0	0.0%
6	Ohio	647	6.5%
NA	Oklahoma**	NA	NA
10	Oregon	266	2.7%
9	Pennsylvania	285	2.9%
28	Rhode Island	9	0.1%
22	South Carolina	28	0.3%
38	South Dakota	0	0.0%
25	Tennessee	19	0.2%
3	Texas	1,047	10.5%
32	Utah	3	0.0%
33	Vermont	2	0.0%
17	Virginia	96	1.0%
7	Washington	607	6.1%
34	West Virginia	1	0.0%
13	Wisconsin	152	1.5%
34	Wyoming	1	0.0%

RANK ORDER

RANK	STATE	ABORTIONS	% of USA
1	New York	2,506	25.1%
2	Georgia	1,376	13.8%
3	Texas	1,047	10.5%
4	Kansas	807	8.1%
5	New Jersey	660	6.6%
6	Ohio	647	6.5%
7	Washington	607	6.1%
8	Louisiana	339	3.4%
9	Pennsylvania	285	2.9%
10	Oregon	266	2.7%
11	Michigan	221	2.2%
12	North Carolina	217	2.2%
13	Colorado	152	1.5%
13	Wisconsin	152	1.5%
15	Kentucky	129	1.3%
16	Minnesota	102	1.0%
17	Virginia	96	1.0%
18	Nevada	69	0.7%
19	Alabama	53	0.5%
20	Montana	47	0.5%
21	Missouri	45	0.5%
22	Hawaii	28	0.3%
22	New Mexico	28	0.3%
22	South Carolina	28	0.3%
25	Tennessee	19	0.2%
26	Mississippi	15	0.2%
27	Delaware	10	0.1%
28	Rhode Island	9	0.1%
29	Arkansas	8	0.1%
30	Connecticut	4	0.0%
30	Idaho	4	0.0%
32	Utah	3	0.0%
33	Vermont	2	0.0%
34	Maine	1	0.0%
34	Maryland	1	0.0%
34	West Virginia	1	0.0%
34	Wyoming	1	0.0%
38	Arizona	0	0.0%
38	Indiana	0	0.0%
38	North Dakota	0	0.0%
38	South Dakota	0	0.0%
NA	Alaska**	NA	NA
NA	California**	NA	NA
NA	Florida**	NA	NA
NA	Illinois**	NA	NA
NA	Iowa**	NA	NA
NA	Massachusetts**	NA	NA
NA	Nebraska**	NA	NA
NA	New Hampshire**	NA	NA
NA	Oklahoma**	NA	NA
	District of Columbia**	NA	NA

Source: U.S. Department of Health and Human Services, Centers for Disease Control and Prevention
    "Abortion Surveillance-United States, 1997" (Morbidity Mortality Weekly Report, Vol. 49, No. SS-11, 12/08/00)
*By state of occurrence. National total is for reporting states only.
**Not reported.

Percent of Reported Legal Abortions Performed At or After
21 Weeks of Gestation in 1997
Reporting States' Percent = 1.4% of Abortions*

ALPHA ORDER

RANK	STATE	PERCENT
23	Alabama	0.4
NA	Alaska**	NA
34	Arizona	0.0
30	Arkansas	0.1
NA	California**	NA
9	Colorado	1.7
34	Connecticut	0.0
28	Delaware	0.2
NA	Florida**	NA
2	Georgia	3.9
19	Hawaii	0.6
20	Idaho	0.5
NA	Illinois**	NA
34	Indiana	0.0
NA	Iowa**	NA
1	Kansas	7.2
6	Kentucky	1.8
3	Louisiana	2.9
34	Maine	0.0
34	Maryland	0.0
NA	Massachusetts**	NA
16	Michigan	0.7
16	Minnesota	0.7
26	Mississippi	0.3
23	Missouri	0.4
9	Montana	1.7
NA	Nebraska**	NA
14	Nevada	1.0
NA	New Hampshire**	NA
5	New Jersey	2.2
20	New Mexico	0.5
6	New York	1.8
16	North Carolina	0.7
34	North Dakota	0.0
9	Ohio	1.7
NA	Oklahoma**	NA
6	Oregon	1.8
15	Pennsylvania	0.8
28	Rhode Island	0.2
26	South Carolina	0.3
34	South Dakota	0.0
30	Tennessee	0.1
12	Texas	1.2
30	Utah	0.1
30	Vermont	0.1
23	Virginia	0.4
4	Washington	2.3
34	West Virginia	0.0
12	Wisconsin	1.2
20	Wyoming	0.5

RANK ORDER

RANK	STATE	PERCENT
1	Kansas	7.2
2	Georgia	3.9
3	Louisiana	2.9
4	Washington	2.3
5	New Jersey	2.2
6	Kentucky	1.8
6	New York	1.8
6	Oregon	1.8
9	Colorado	1.7
9	Montana	1.7
9	Ohio	1.7
12	Texas	1.2
12	Wisconsin	1.2
14	Nevada	1.0
15	Pennsylvania	0.8
16	Michigan	0.7
16	Minnesota	0.7
16	North Carolina	0.7
19	Hawaii	0.6
20	Idaho	0.5
20	New Mexico	0.5
20	Wyoming	0.5
23	Alabama	0.4
23	Missouri	0.4
23	Virginia	0.4
26	Mississippi	0.3
26	South Carolina	0.3
28	Delaware	0.2
28	Rhode Island	0.2
30	Arkansas	0.1
30	Tennessee	0.1
30	Utah	0.1
30	Vermont	0.1
34	Arizona	0.0
34	Connecticut	0.0
34	Indiana	0.0
34	Maine	0.0
34	Maryland	0.0
34	North Dakota	0.0
34	South Dakota	0.0
34	West Virginia	0.0
NA	Alaska**	NA
NA	California**	NA
NA	Florida**	NA
NA	Illinois**	NA
NA	Iowa**	NA
NA	Massachusetts**	NA
NA	Nebraska**	NA
NA	New Hampshire**	NA
NA	Oklahoma**	NA
	District of Columbia**	NA

Source: Morgan Quitno Press using data from US Dept of Health & Human Serv's, Centers for Disease Control-Prevention
"Abortion Surveillance-United States, 1997" (Morbidity Mortality Weekly Report, Vol. 49, No. SS-11, 12/08/00)
*By state of occurrence. National percent is for reporting states only.
**Not reported.

II. DEATHS

II. DEATHS (Continued)

Deaths in 1999

National Total = 2,396,096 Deaths*

ALPHA ORDER					RANK ORDER			
RANK	STATE	DEATHS	% of USA		RANK	STATE	DEATHS	% of USA
18	Alabama	44,698	1.9%		1	California	232,146	9.7%
50	Alaska	2,684	0.1%		2	Florida	162,983	6.8%
22	Arizona	40,033	1.7%		3	New York	159,985	6.7%
31	Arkansas	27,828	1.2%		4	Texas	148,994	6.2%
1	California	232,146	9.7%		5	Pennsylvania	130,268	5.4%
32	Colorado	27,082	1.1%		6	Ohio	108,583	4.5%
27	Connecticut	29,410	1.2%		7	Illinois	108,372	4.5%
46	Delaware	6,589	0.3%		8	Michigan	87,300	3.6%
2	Florida	162,983	6.8%		9	New Jersey	74,170	3.1%
11	Georgia	61,977	2.6%		10	North Carolina	69,537	2.9%
43	Hawaii	8,268	0.3%		11	Georgia	61,977	2.6%
41	Idaho	9,636	0.4%		12	Missouri	55,961	2.3%
7	Illinois	108,372	4.5%		13	Massachusetts	55,843	2.3%
15	Indiana	55,377	2.3%		14	Virginia	55,399	2.3%
29	Iowa	28,383	1.2%		15	Indiana	55,377	2.3%
33	Kansas	24,525	1.0%		16	Tennessee	53,766	2.2%
23	Kentucky	39,368	1.6%		17	Wisconsin	46,479	1.9%
21	Louisiana	41,098	1.7%		18	Alabama	44,698	1.9%
38	Maine	12,272	0.5%		19	Washington	43,865	1.8%
20	Maryland	43,241	1.8%		20	Maryland	43,241	1.8%
13	Massachusetts	55,843	2.3%		21	Louisiana	41,098	1.7%
8	Michigan	87,300	3.6%		22	Arizona	40,033	1.7%
24	Minnesota	38,616	1.6%		23	Kentucky	39,368	1.6%
30	Mississippi	28,292	1.2%		24	Minnesota	38,616	1.6%
12	Missouri	55,961	2.3%		25	South Carolina	36,125	1.5%
44	Montana	8,108	0.3%		26	Oklahoma	34,705	1.4%
35	Nebraska	15,545	0.6%		27	Connecticut	29,410	1.2%
36	Nevada	14,934	0.6%		28	Oregon	29,336	1.2%
42	New Hampshire	9,584	0.4%		29	Iowa	28,383	1.2%
9	New Jersey	74,170	3.1%		30	Mississippi	28,292	1.2%
37	New Mexico	13,645	0.6%		31	Arkansas	27,828	1.2%
3	New York	159,985	6.7%		32	Colorado	27,082	1.1%
10	North Carolina	69,537	2.9%		33	Kansas	24,525	1.0%
47	North Dakota	6,098	0.3%		34	West Virginia	21,199	0.9%
6	Ohio	108,583	4.5%		35	Nebraska	15,545	0.6%
26	Oklahoma	34,705	1.4%		36	Nevada	14,934	0.6%
28	Oregon	29,336	1.2%		37	New Mexico	13,645	0.6%
5	Pennsylvania	130,268	5.4%		38	Maine	12,272	0.5%
40	Rhode Island	9,733	0.4%		39	Utah	12,013	0.5%
25	South Carolina	36,125	1.5%		40	Rhode Island	9,733	0.4%
45	South Dakota	7,017	0.3%		41	Idaho	9,636	0.4%
16	Tennessee	53,766	2.2%		42	New Hampshire	9,584	0.4%
4	Texas	148,994	6.2%		43	Hawaii	8,268	0.3%
39	Utah	12,013	0.5%		44	Montana	8,108	0.3%
48	Vermont	4,856	0.2%		45	South Dakota	7,017	0.3%
14	Virginia	55,399	2.3%		46	Delaware	6,589	0.3%
19	Washington	43,865	1.8%		47	North Dakota	6,098	0.3%
34	West Virginia	21,199	0.9%		48	Vermont	4,856	0.2%
17	Wisconsin	46,479	1.9%		49	Wyoming	4,074	0.2%
49	Wyoming	4,074	0.2%		50	Alaska	2,684	0.1%
						District of Columbia	6,096	0.3%

Source: U.S. Department of Health and Human Services, National Center for Health Statistics
"National Vital Statistics Reports" (Vol. 48, No. 19, February 22, 2001)
*Preliminary data by state of residence.

Death Rate in 1999

National Rate = 878.7 Deaths per 100,000 Population*

<u>ALPHA ORDER</u>

RANK	STATE	RATE
7	Alabama	1,022.9
50	Alaska	433.3
34	Arizona	837.8
2	Arkansas	1,090.7
46	California	700.4
48	Colorado	667.7
26	Connecticut	896.1
32	Delaware	874.4
4	Florida	1,078.6
41	Georgia	795.8
47	Hawaii	697.4
43	Idaho	769.8
27	Illinois	893.5
19	Indiana	931.8
10	Iowa	989.2
21	Kansas	924.1
9	Kentucky	993.9
17	Louisiana	940.0
13	Maine	979.4
35	Maryland	836.1
25	Massachusetts	904.3
29	Michigan	885.1
38	Minnesota	808.6
8	Mississippi	1,021.9
6	Missouri	1,023.4
22	Montana	918.5
18	Nebraska	933.1
36	Nevada	825.4
40	New Hampshire	797.9
23	New Jersey	910.8
42	New Mexico	784.3
31	New York	879.2
24	North Carolina	908.9
15	North Dakota	962.3
14	Ohio	964.6
5	Oklahoma	1,033.5
30	Oregon	884.6
3	Pennsylvania	1,086.1
11	Rhode Island	982.3
20	South Carolina	929.7
16	South Dakota	957.1
12	Tennessee	980.5
45	Texas	743.3
49	Utah	564.0
37	Vermont	817.9
39	Virginia	806.0
44	Washington	762.0
1	West Virginia	1,173.2
28	Wisconsin	885.2
33	Wyoming	849.5

<u>RANK ORDER</u>

RANK	STATE	RATE
1	West Virginia	1,173.2
2	Arkansas	1,090.7
3	Pennsylvania	1,086.1
4	Florida	1,078.6
5	Oklahoma	1,033.5
6	Missouri	1,023.4
7	Alabama	1,022.9
8	Mississippi	1,021.9
9	Kentucky	993.9
10	Iowa	989.2
11	Rhode Island	982.3
12	Tennessee	980.5
13	Maine	979.4
14	Ohio	964.6
15	North Dakota	962.3
16	South Dakota	957.1
17	Louisiana	940.0
18	Nebraska	933.1
19	Indiana	931.8
20	South Carolina	929.7
21	Kansas	924.1
22	Montana	918.5
23	New Jersey	910.8
24	North Carolina	908.9
25	Massachusetts	904.3
26	Connecticut	896.1
27	Illinois	893.5
28	Wisconsin	885.2
29	Michigan	885.1
30	Oregon	884.6
31	New York	879.2
32	Delaware	874.4
33	Wyoming	849.5
34	Arizona	837.8
35	Maryland	836.1
36	Nevada	825.4
37	Vermont	817.9
38	Minnesota	808.6
39	Virginia	806.0
40	New Hampshire	797.9
41	Georgia	795.8
42	New Mexico	784.3
43	Idaho	769.8
44	Washington	762.0
45	Texas	743.3
46	California	700.4
47	Hawaii	697.4
48	Colorado	667.7
49	Utah	564.0
50	Alaska	433.3

District of Columbia   1,174.6

Source: Morgan Quitno Press using data from U.S. Dept. of Health & Human Services, National Center for Health Statistics "National Vital Statistics Reports" (Vol. 48, No. 19, February 22, 2001)
Preliminary data by state of residence. Not age-adjusted.

Births to Deaths Ratio in 1999

National Ratio = 1.65 Births for Every Death in 1999

RANK	STATE (ALPHA ORDER)	RATIO		RANK	STATE (RANK ORDER)	RATIO
37	Alabama	1.39		1	Utah	3.85
2	Alaska	3.71		2	Alaska	3.71
9	Arizona	2.03		3	Texas	2.33
43	Arkansas	1.32		4	Colorado	2.30
5	California	2.23		5	California	2.23
4	Colorado	2.30		6	Hawaii	2.06
31	Connecticut	1.48		6	Idaho	2.06
19	Delaware	1.62		8	Georgia	2.05
47	Florida	1.21		9	Arizona	2.03
8	Georgia	2.05		10	New Mexico	1.98
6	Hawaii	2.06		11	Nevada	1.97
6	Idaho	2.06		12	Washington	1.81
15	Illinois	1.68		13	Virginia	1.72
22	Indiana	1.55		14	Minnesota	1.71
43	Iowa	1.32		15	Illinois	1.68
21	Kansas	1.58		16	Maryland	1.67
38	Kentucky	1.38		17	North Carolina	1.64
18	Louisiana	1.63		18	Louisiana	1.63
49	Maine	1.11		19	Delaware	1.62
16	Maryland	1.67		19	New York	1.62
34	Massachusetts	1.45		21	Kansas	1.58
26	Michigan	1.53		22	Indiana	1.55
14	Minnesota	1.71		23	Nebraska	1.54
28	Mississippi	1.51		23	New Jersey	1.54
40	Missouri	1.35		23	Oregon	1.54
42	Montana	1.33		26	Michigan	1.53
23	Nebraska	1.54		27	South Carolina	1.52
11	Nevada	1.97		28	Mississippi	1.51
32	New Hampshire	1.47		28	Wyoming	1.51
23	New Jersey	1.54		30	South Dakota	1.50
10	New Mexico	1.98		31	Connecticut	1.48
19	New York	1.62		32	New Hampshire	1.47
17	North Carolina	1.64		32	Wisconsin	1.47
46	North Dakota	1.25		34	Massachusetts	1.45
38	Ohio	1.38		34	Tennessee	1.45
36	Oklahoma	1.41		36	Oklahoma	1.41
23	Oregon	1.54		37	Alabama	1.39
48	Pennsylvania	1.12		38	Kentucky	1.38
45	Rhode Island	1.27		38	Ohio	1.38
27	South Carolina	1.52		40	Missouri	1.35
30	South Dakota	1.50		40	Vermont	1.35
34	Tennessee	1.45		42	Montana	1.33
3	Texas	2.33		43	Arkansas	1.32
1	Utah	3.85		43	Iowa	1.32
40	Vermont	1.35		45	Rhode Island	1.27
13	Virginia	1.72		46	North Dakota	1.25
12	Washington	1.81		47	Florida	1.21
50	West Virginia	0.98		48	Pennsylvania	1.12
32	Wisconsin	1.47		49	Maine	1.11
28	Wyoming	1.51		50	West Virginia	0.98
					District of Columbia	1.23

Source: Morgan Quitno Press using data from U.S. Dept. of Health & Human Services, National Center for Health Statistics
"National Vital Statistics Reports" (Vol. 48, No. 19, February 22, 2001)
*Preliminary data by state of residence.

Deaths in 1998

National Total = 2,337,256 Deaths*

ALPHA ORDER

ALPHA ORDER

RANK	STATE	DEATHS	% of USA
18	Alabama	43,950	1.9%
50	Alaska	2,571	0.1%
22	Arizona	38,300	1.6%
31	Arkansas	27,510	1.2%
1	California	226,954	9.7%
32	Colorado	26,640	1.1%
27	Connecticut	29,710	1.3%
46	Delaware	6,578	0.3%
2	Florida	158,167	6.8%
11	Georgia	60,428	2.6%
43	Hawaii	8,091	0.3%
42	Idaho	9,155	0.4%
7	Illinois	104,480	4.5%
15	Indiana	53,477	2.3%
29	Iowa	28,362	1.2%
33	Kansas	24,057	1.0%
23	Kentucky	37,832	1.6%
21	Louisiana	40,337	1.7%
38	Maine	12,135	0.5%
20	Maryland	42,059	1.8%
12	Massachusetts	55,237	2.4%
8	Michigan	85,160	3.6%
24	Minnesota	37,195	1.6%
30	Mississippi	27,847	1.2%
13	Missouri	55,070	2.4%
44	Montana	7,981	0.3%
35	Nebraska	15,198	0.7%
36	Nevada	14,464	0.6%
41	New Hampshire	9,495	0.4%
9	New Jersey	71,611	3.1%
37	New Mexico	12,907	0.6%
3	New York	156,619	6.7%
10	North Carolina	67,993	2.9%
47	North Dakota	5,920	0.3%
6	Ohio	105,891	4.5%
26	Oklahoma	33,929	1.5%
28	Oregon	29,383	1.3%
5	Pennsylvania	126,700	5.4%
40	Rhode Island	9,604	0.4%
25	South Carolina	34,827	1.5%
45	South Dakota	6,867	0.3%
16	Tennessee	53,415	2.3%
4	Texas	142,605	6.1%
39	Utah	11,824	0.5%
48	Vermont	4,948	0.2%
14	Virginia	54,446	2.3%
19	Washington	42,706	1.8%
34	West Virginia	20,767	0.9%
17	Wisconsin	45,947	2.0%
49	Wyoming	3,853	0.2%

RANK ORDER

RANK	STATE	DEATHS	% of USA
1	California	226,954	9.7%
2	Florida	158,167	6.8%
3	New York	156,619	6.7%
4	Texas	142,605	6.1%
5	Pennsylvania	126,700	5.4%
6	Ohio	105,891	4.5%
7	Illinois	104,480	4.5%
8	Michigan	85,160	3.6%
9	New Jersey	71,611	3.1%
10	North Carolina	67,993	2.9%
11	Georgia	60,428	2.6%
12	Massachusetts	55,237	2.4%
13	Missouri	55,070	2.4%
14	Virginia	54,446	2.3%
15	Indiana	53,477	2.3%
16	Tennessee	53,415	2.3%
17	Wisconsin	45,947	2.0%
18	Alabama	43,950	1.9%
19	Washington	42,706	1.8%
20	Maryland	42,059	1.8%
21	Louisiana	40,337	1.7%
22	Arizona	38,300	1.6%
23	Kentucky	37,832	1.6%
24	Minnesota	37,195	1.6%
25	South Carolina	34,827	1.5%
26	Oklahoma	33,929	1.5%
27	Connecticut	29,710	1.3%
28	Oregon	29,383	1.3%
29	Iowa	28,362	1.2%
30	Mississippi	27,847	1.2%
31	Arkansas	27,510	1.2%
32	Colorado	26,640	1.1%
33	Kansas	24,057	1.0%
34	West Virginia	20,767	0.9%
35	Nebraska	15,198	0.7%
36	Nevada	14,464	0.6%
37	New Mexico	12,907	0.6%
38	Maine	12,135	0.5%
39	Utah	11,824	0.5%
40	Rhode Island	9,604	0.4%
41	New Hampshire	9,495	0.4%
42	Idaho	9,155	0.4%
43	Hawaii	8,091	0.3%
44	Montana	7,981	0.3%
45	South Dakota	6,867	0.3%
46	Delaware	6,578	0.3%
47	North Dakota	5,920	0.3%
48	Vermont	4,948	0.2%
49	Wyoming	3,853	0.2%
50	Alaska	2,571	0.1%
	District of Columbia	6,054	0.3%

Source: U.S. Department of Health and Human Services, National Center for Health Statistics
"National Vital Statistics Reports" (Vol. 48, No. 11, July 24, 2000)
Final data by state of residence.

Death Rate in 1998

National Rate = 864.7 Deaths per 100,000 Population*

Source: U.S. Department of Health and Human Services, National Center for Health Statistics
     "National Vital Statistics Reports" (Vol. 48, No. 11, July 24, 2000)
*Final data by state of residence. Not age-adjusted.

ALPHA ORDER

RANK	STATE	RATE
8	Alabama	1,009.9
50	Alaska	418.7
35	Arizona	820.4
2	Arkansas	1,083.8
46	California	694.8
48	Colorado	670.9
21	Connecticut	907.4
27	Delaware	884.6
3	Florida	1,060.4
40	Georgia	790.7
47	Hawaii	678.2
43	Idaho	745.1
31	Illinois	867.4
22	Indiana	906.5
9	Iowa	990.8
18	Kansas	915.0
13	Kentucky	961.1
17	Louisiana	923.3
11	Maine	975.3
36	Maryland	819.1
25	Massachusetts	898.6
30	Michigan	867.5
41	Minnesota	787.1
7	Mississippi	1,011.8
6	Missouri	1,012.6
22	Montana	906.5
19	Nebraska	914.0
34	Nevada	828.0
38	New Hampshire	801.2
28	New Jersey	882.5
44	New Mexico	743.1
32	New York	861.7
24	North Carolina	901.0
16	North Dakota	927.5
14	Ohio	944.7
5	Oklahoma	1,013.8
26	Oregon	895.3
4	Pennsylvania	1,055.7
12	Rhode Island	971.6
20	South Carolina	907.9
15	South Dakota	930.3
10	Tennessee	983.6
45	Texas	721.7
49	Utah	563.1
33	Vermont	837.4
37	Virginia	801.7
42	Washington	750.6
1	West Virginia	1,146.6
29	Wisconsin	879.6
38	Wyoming	801.2

RANK ORDER

RANK	STATE	RATE
1	West Virginia	1,146.6
2	Arkansas	1,083.8
3	Florida	1,060.4
4	Pennsylvania	1,055.7
5	Oklahoma	1,013.8
6	Missouri	1,012.6
7	Mississippi	1,011.8
8	Alabama	1,009.9
9	Iowa	990.8
10	Tennessee	983.6
11	Maine	975.3
12	Rhode Island	971.6
13	Kentucky	961.1
14	Ohio	944.7
15	South Dakota	930.3
16	North Dakota	927.5
17	Louisiana	923.3
18	Kansas	915.0
19	Nebraska	914.0
20	South Carolina	907.9
21	Connecticut	907.4
22	Indiana	906.5
22	Montana	906.5
24	North Carolina	901.0
25	Massachusetts	898.6
26	Oregon	895.3
27	Delaware	884.6
28	New Jersey	882.5
29	Wisconsin	879.6
30	Michigan	867.5
31	Illinois	867.4
32	New York	861.7
33	Vermont	837.4
34	Nevada	828.0
35	Arizona	820.4
36	Maryland	819.1
37	Virginia	801.7
38	New Hampshire	801.2
38	Wyoming	801.2
40	Georgia	790.7
41	Minnesota	787.1
42	Washington	750.6
43	Idaho	745.1
44	New Mexico	743.1
45	Texas	721.7
46	California	694.8
47	Hawaii	678.2
48	Colorado	670.9
49	Utah	563.1
50	Alaska	418.7
	District of Columbia	1,157.3

Age-Adjusted Death Rate in 1998

National Rate = 471.7 Deaths per 100,000 Population*

ALPHA ORDER

RANK	STATE	RATE
3	Alabama	565.9
34	Alaska	441.9
25	Arizona	461.7
5	Arkansas	551.0
41	California	425.4
46	Colorado	419.0
40	Connecticut	425.6
14	Delaware	496.9
26	Florida	458.4
8	Georgia	539.8
50	Hawaii	370.1
42	Idaho	424.4
19	Illinois	480.5
15	Indiana	496.5
45	Iowa	421.6
30	Kansas	447.8
10	Kentucky	533.6
2	Louisiana	575.2
24	Maine	462.4
16	Maryland	494.8
44	Massachusetts	421.9
18	Michigan	484.6
49	Minnesota	394.5
1	Mississippi	606.6
13	Missouri	511.1
29	Montana	449.9
39	Nebraska	431.9
9	Nevada	539.1
35	New Hampshire	440.0
31	New Jersey	445.3
27	New Mexico	457.5
32	New York	443.5
12	North Carolina	518.6
47	North Dakota	414.8
17	Ohio	489.8
11	Oklahoma	529.5
28	Oregon	451.4
21	Pennsylvania	475.4
38	Rhode Island	433.5
6	South Carolina	550.8
33	South Dakota	442.6
4	Tennessee	557.0
22	Texas	475.3
48	Utah	404.5
36	Vermont	434.4
20	Virginia	480.0
43	Washington	423.2
7	West Virginia	547.9
37	Wisconsin	433.9
23	Wyoming	464.8

RANK ORDER

RANK	STATE	RATE
1	Mississippi	606.6
2	Louisiana	575.2
3	Alabama	565.9
4	Tennessee	557.0
5	Arkansas	551.0
6	South Carolina	550.8
7	West Virginia	547.9
8	Georgia	539.8
9	Nevada	539.1
10	Kentucky	533.6
11	Oklahoma	529.5
12	North Carolina	518.6
13	Missouri	511.1
14	Delaware	496.9
15	Indiana	496.5
16	Maryland	494.8
17	Ohio	489.8
18	Michigan	484.6
19	Illinois	480.5
20	Virginia	480.0
21	Pennsylvania	475.4
22	Texas	475.3
23	Wyoming	464.8
24	Maine	462.4
25	Arizona	461.7
26	Florida	458.4
27	New Mexico	457.5
28	Oregon	451.4
29	Montana	449.9
30	Kansas	447.8
31	New Jersey	445.3
32	New York	443.5
33	South Dakota	442.6
34	Alaska	441.9
35	New Hampshire	440.0
36	Vermont	434.4
37	Wisconsin	433.9
38	Rhode Island	433.5
39	Nebraska	431.9
40	Connecticut	425.6
41	California	425.4
42	Idaho	424.4
43	Washington	423.2
44	Massachusetts	421.9
45	Iowa	421.6
46	Colorado	419.0
47	North Dakota	414.8
48	Utah	404.5
49	Minnesota	394.5
50	Hawaii	370.1
	District of Columbia	684.8

Source: U.S. Department of Health and Human Services, National Center for Health Statistics
   "National Vital Statistics Reports" (Vol. 48, No. 11, July 24, 2000)
*Final data by state of residence. Age-adjusted rates eliminate the distorting effects of the aging of the population.

Death Rate in 1990

National Rate = 863 Deaths per 100,000 Population*

ALPHA ORDER

RANK ORDER

RANK	STATE	RATE
7	Alabama	974
50	Alaska	398
37	Arizona	784
2	Arkansas	1,048
44	California	719
47	Colorado	655
32	Connecticut	840
27	Delaware	864
3	Florida	1,038
35	Georgia	799
48	Hawaii	611
42	Idaho	740
19	Illinois	900
21	Indiana	894
8	Iowa	968
20	Kansas	899
11	Kentucky	951
22	Louisiana	890
18	Maine	905
34	Maryland	803
24	Massachusetts	884
31	Michigan	847
36	Minnesota	795
6	Mississippi	976
5	Missouri	984
29	Montana	859
14	Nebraska	936
38	Nevada	775
40	New Hampshire	765
16	New Jersey	910
46	New Mexico	701
13	New York	938
27	North Carolina	864
22	North Dakota	890
15	Ohio	911
9	Oklahoma	966
24	Oregon	884
4	Pennsylvania	1,026
10	Rhode Island	954
30	South Carolina	852
17	South Dakota	909
12	Tennessee	949
43	Texas	738
49	Utah	533
33	Vermont	817
38	Virginia	775
41	Washington	762
1	West Virginia	1,080
26	Wisconsin	874
45	Wyoming	706

RANK	STATE	RATE
1	West Virginia	1,080
2	Arkansas	1,048
3	Florida	1,038
4	Pennsylvania	1,026
5	Missouri	984
6	Mississippi	976
7	Alabama	974
8	Iowa	968
9	Oklahoma	966
10	Rhode Island	954
11	Kentucky	951
12	Tennessee	949
13	New York	938
14	Nebraska	936
15	Ohio	911
16	New Jersey	910
17	South Dakota	909
18	Maine	905
19	Illinois	900
20	Kansas	899
21	Indiana	894
22	Louisiana	890
22	North Dakota	890
24	Massachusetts	884
24	Oregon	884
26	Wisconsin	874
27	Delaware	864
27	North Carolina	864
29	Montana	859
30	South Carolina	852
31	Michigan	847
32	Connecticut	840
33	Vermont	817
34	Maryland	803
35	Georgia	799
36	Minnesota	795
37	Arizona	784
38	Nevada	775
38	Virginia	775
40	New Hampshire	765
41	Washington	762
42	Idaho	740
43	Texas	738
44	California	719
45	Wyoming	706
46	New Mexico	701
47	Colorado	655
48	Hawaii	611
49	Utah	533
50	Alaska	398

| District of Columbia | 1,200 |

Source: U.S. Department of Health and Human Services, National Center for Health Statistics
    "Monthly Vital Statistics Report" (Vol. 41, No. 7(S), January 7, 1993)
*Final data by state of residence. Not age adjusted.

Death Rate in 1980

National Rate = 877 Deaths per 100,000 Population*

<u>ALPHA ORDER</u>

RANK	STATE	RATE
18	Alabama	912
50	Alaska	425
40	Arizona	784
4	Arkansas	994
39	California	786
47	Colorado	654
23	Connecticut	877
27	Delaware	847
1	Florida	1,072
35	Georgia	809
49	Hawaii	515
44	Idaho	715
20	Illinois	899
25	Indiana	862
14	Iowa	930
14	Kansas	930
16	Kentucky	922
28	Louisiana	846
8	Maine	960
36	Maryland	806
9	Massachusetts	959
34	Michigan	811
33	Minnesota	817
11	Mississippi	937
3	Missouri	1,008
28	Montana	846
17	Nebraska	920
43	Nevada	735
30	New Hampshire	830
12	New Jersey	936
45	New Mexico	696
6	New York	984
32	North Carolina	823
26	North Dakota	856
19	Ohio	911
13	Oklahoma	932
31	Oregon	827
2	Pennsylvania	1,041
6	Rhode Island	984
37	South Carolina	805
10	South Dakota	947
22	Tennessee	887
42	Texas	758
48	Utah	554
21	Vermont	895
38	Virginia	794
41	Washington	773
5	West Virginia	987
24	Wisconsin	867
46	Wyoming	684

<u>RANK ORDER</u>

RANK	STATE	RATE
1	Florida	1,072
2	Pennsylvania	1,041
3	Missouri	1,008
4	Arkansas	994
5	West Virginia	987
6	New York	984
6	Rhode Island	984
8	Maine	960
9	Massachusetts	959
10	South Dakota	947
11	Mississippi	937
12	New Jersey	936
13	Oklahoma	932
14	Iowa	930
14	Kansas	930
16	Kentucky	922
17	Nebraska	920
18	Alabama	912
19	Ohio	911
20	Illinois	899
21	Vermont	895
22	Tennessee	887
23	Connecticut	877
24	Wisconsin	867
25	Indiana	862
26	North Dakota	856
27	Delaware	847
28	Louisiana	846
28	Montana	846
30	New Hampshire	830
31	Oregon	827
32	North Carolina	823
33	Minnesota	817
34	Michigan	811
35	Georgia	809
36	Maryland	806
37	South Carolina	805
38	Virginia	794
39	California	786
40	Arizona	784
41	Washington	773
42	Texas	758
43	Nevada	735
44	Idaho	715
45	New Mexico	696
46	Wyoming	684
47	Colorado	654
48	Utah	554
49	Hawaii	515
50	Alaska	425

District of Columbia   1,109

Source: U.S. Department of Health and Human Services, National Center for Health Statistics
   "Vital Statistics of the United States 1980" and "Monthly Vital Statistics Report"
*Final data by state of residence. Not age adjusted.

Infant Deaths in 1999

National Total = 28,100 Infant Deaths*

RANK	STATE	DEATHS	% of USA
17	Alabama	596	2.1%
48	Alaska	55	0.2%
20	Arizona	552	2.0%
30	Arkansas	275	1.0%
1	California	2,851	10.1%
25	Colorado	406	1.4%
31	Connecticut	265	0.9%
41	Delaware	109	0.4%
5	Florida	1,457	5.2%
10	Georgia	1,038	3.7%
40	Hawaii	121	0.4%
39	Idaho	133	0.5%
4	Illinois	1,557	5.5%
13	Indiana	676	2.4%
34	Iowa	222	0.8%
29	Kansas	280	1.0%
28	Kentucky	390	1.4%
14	Louisiana	629	2.2%
46	Maine	64	0.2%
16	Maryland	608	2.2%
23	Massachusetts	416	1.5%
7	Michigan	1,084	3.9%
27	Minnesota	394	1.4%
22	Mississippi	446	1.6%
18	Missouri	593	2.1%
44	Montana	75	0.3%
38	Nebraska	148	0.5%
35	Nevada	202	0.7%
45	New Hampshire	73	0.3%
11	New Jersey	782	2.8%
36	New Mexico	190	0.7%
3	New York	1,618	5.8%
8	North Carolina	1,053	3.7%
47	North Dakota	58	0.2%
6	Ohio	1,259	4.5%
24	Oklahoma	413	1.5%
32	Oregon	255	0.9%
9	Pennsylvania	1,041	3.7%
43	Rhode Island	82	0.3%
19	South Carolina	560	2.0%
42	South Dakota	100	0.4%
15	Tennessee	615	2.2%
2	Texas	2,200	7.8%
33	Utah	223	0.8%
50	Vermont	36	0.1%
12	Virginia	686	2.4%
26	Washington	402	1.4%
37	West Virginia	170	0.6%
21	Wisconsin	456	1.6%
49	Wyoming	39	0.1%

RANK	STATE	DEATHS	% of USA
1	California	2,851	10.1%
2	Texas	2,200	7.8%
3	New York	1,618	5.8%
4	Illinois	1,557	5.5%
5	Florida	1,457	5.2%
6	Ohio	1,259	4.5%
7	Michigan	1,084	3.9%
8	North Carolina	1,053	3.7%
9	Pennsylvania	1,041	3.7%
10	Georgia	1,038	3.7%
11	New Jersey	782	2.8%
12	Virginia	686	2.4%
13	Indiana	676	2.4%
14	Louisiana	629	2.2%
15	Tennessee	615	2.2%
16	Maryland	608	2.2%
17	Alabama	596	2.1%
18	Missouri	593	2.1%
19	South Carolina	560	2.0%
20	Arizona	552	2.0%
21	Wisconsin	456	1.6%
22	Mississippi	446	1.6%
23	Massachusetts	416	1.5%
24	Oklahoma	413	1.5%
25	Colorado	406	1.4%
26	Washington	402	1.4%
27	Minnesota	394	1.4%
28	Kentucky	390	1.4%
29	Kansas	280	1.0%
30	Arkansas	275	1.0%
31	Connecticut	265	0.9%
32	Oregon	255	0.9%
33	Utah	223	0.8%
34	Iowa	222	0.8%
35	Nevada	202	0.7%
36	New Mexico	190	0.7%
37	West Virginia	170	0.6%
38	Nebraska	148	0.5%
39	Idaho	133	0.5%
40	Hawaii	121	0.4%
41	Delaware	109	0.4%
42	South Dakota	100	0.4%
43	Rhode Island	82	0.3%
44	Montana	75	0.3%
45	New Hampshire	73	0.3%
46	Maine	64	0.2%
47	North Dakota	58	0.2%
48	Alaska	55	0.2%
49	Wyoming	39	0.1%
50	Vermont	36	0.1%
	District of Columbia	106	0.4%

Source: U.S. Department of Health and Human Services, National Center for Health Statistics
  "National Vital Statistics Reports" (Vol. 48, No. 19, February 22, 2001)
*For 12 months ending December 1999. Provisional data. Deaths under 1 year old by state of residence.

Infant Mortality Rate in 1999

National Rate = 7.1 Infant Deaths per 1,000 Live Births*

ALPHA ORDER

RANK	STATE	RATE
4	Alabama	9.6
43	Alaska	5.5
30	Arizona	6.8
19	Arkansas	7.4
43	California	5.5
34	Colorado	6.5
39	Connecticut	6.1
3	Delaware	10.1
19	Florida	7.4
13	Georgia	8.2
24	Hawaii	7.1
31	Idaho	6.7
8	Illinois	8.5
17	Indiana	7.8
41	Iowa	5.9
25	Kansas	7.0
21	Kentucky	7.2
6	Louisiana	9.4
50	Maine	4.7
8	Maryland	8.5
47	Massachusetts	5.1
14	Michigan	8.1
40	Minnesota	6.0
1	Mississippi	10.5
15	Missouri	8.0
27	Montana	6.9
37	Nebraska	6.2
27	Nevada	6.9
46	New Hampshire	5.2
27	New Jersey	6.9
25	New Mexico	7.0
35	New York	6.3
7	North Carolina	9.2
18	North Dakota	7.5
11	Ohio	8.3
10	Oklahoma	8.4
42	Oregon	5.7
21	Pennsylvania	7.2
31	Rhode Island	6.7
2	South Carolina	10.2
5	South Dakota	9.5
16	Tennessee	7.9
37	Texas	6.2
49	Utah	4.8
43	Vermont	5.5
21	Virginia	7.2
48	Washington	5.0
11	West Virginia	8.3
31	Wisconsin	6.7
35	Wyoming	6.3

RANK ORDER

RANK	STATE	RATE
1	Mississippi	10.5
2	South Carolina	10.2
3	Delaware	10.1
4	Alabama	9.6
5	South Dakota	9.5
6	Louisiana	9.4
7	North Carolina	9.2
8	Illinois	8.5
8	Maryland	8.5
10	Oklahoma	8.4
11	Ohio	8.3
11	West Virginia	8.3
13	Georgia	8.2
14	Michigan	8.1
15	Missouri	8.0
16	Tennessee	7.9
17	Indiana	7.8
18	North Dakota	7.5
19	Arkansas	7.4
19	Florida	7.4
21	Kentucky	7.2
21	Pennsylvania	7.2
21	Virginia	7.2
24	Hawaii	7.1
25	Kansas	7.0
25	New Mexico	7.0
27	Montana	6.9
27	Nevada	6.9
27	New Jersey	6.9
30	Arizona	6.8
31	Idaho	6.7
31	Rhode Island	6.7
31	Wisconsin	6.7
34	Colorado	6.5
35	New York	6.3
35	Wyoming	6.3
37	Nebraska	6.2
37	Texas	6.2
39	Connecticut	6.1
40	Minnesota	6.0
41	Iowa	5.9
42	Oregon	5.7
43	Alaska	5.5
43	California	5.5
43	Vermont	5.5
46	New Hampshire	5.2
47	Massachusetts	5.1
48	Washington	5.0
49	Utah	4.8
50	Maine	4.7

	District of Columbia	13.2

Source: U.S. Department of Health and Human Services, National Center for Health Statistics
  "National Vital Statistics Reports" (Vol. 48, No. 19, February 22, 2001)
*For 12 months ending December 1999. Provisional data. Deaths under 1 year old by state of residence.

Infant Deaths in 1998

National Total = 28,371 Infant Deaths*

ALPHA ORDER

ALPHA ORDER

RANK	STATE	DEATHS	% of USA
15	Alabama	633	2.2%
48	Alaska	59	0.2%
18	Arizona	590	2.1%
29	Arkansas	329	1.2%
1	California	3,007	10.6%
27	Colorado	399	1.4%
30	Connecticut	307	1.1%
41	Delaware	102	0.4%
5	Florida	1,417	5.0%
10	Georgia	1,035	3.6%
40	Hawaii	121	0.4%
39	Idaho	140	0.5%
4	Illinois	1,539	5.4%
13	Indiana	649	2.3%
33	Iowa	246	0.9%
31	Kansas	270	1.0%
26	Kentucky	409	1.4%
17	Louisiana	609	2.1%
44	Maine	87	0.3%
16	Maryland	616	2.2%
25	Massachusetts	416	1.5%
7	Michigan	1,098	3.9%
28	Minnesota	386	1.4%
23	Mississippi	435	1.5%
19	Missouri	577	2.0%
45	Montana	80	0.3%
37	Nebraska	172	0.6%
35	Nevada	200	0.7%
47	New Hampshire	63	0.2%
11	New Jersey	734	2.6%
36	New Mexico	197	0.7%
3	New York	1,623	5.7%
9	North Carolina	1,038	3.7%
46	North Dakota	68	0.2%
6	Ohio	1,221	4.3%
24	Oklahoma	420	1.5%
34	Oregon	245	0.9%
8	Pennsylvania	1,043	3.7%
43	Rhode Island	88	0.3%
20	South Carolina	515	1.8%
42	South Dakota	94	0.3%
14	Tennessee	635	2.2%
2	Texas	2,185	7.7%
32	Utah	255	0.9%
49	Vermont	46	0.2%
12	Virginia	722	2.5%
22	Washington	455	1.6%
38	West Virginia	166	0.6%
21	Wisconsin	489	1.7%
50	Wyoming	45	0.2%

RANK ORDER

RANK	STATE	DEATHS	% of USA
1	California	3,007	10.6%
2	Texas	2,185	7.7%
3	New York	1,623	5.7%
4	Illinois	1,539	5.4%
5	Florida	1,417	5.0%
6	Ohio	1,221	4.3%
7	Michigan	1,098	3.9%
8	Pennsylvania	1,043	3.7%
9	North Carolina	1,038	3.7%
10	Georgia	1,035	3.6%
11	New Jersey	734	2.6%
12	Virginia	722	2.5%
13	Indiana	649	2.3%
14	Tennessee	635	2.2%
15	Alabama	633	2.2%
16	Maryland	616	2.2%
17	Louisiana	609	2.1%
18	Arizona	590	2.1%
19	Missouri	577	2.0%
20	South Carolina	515	1.8%
21	Wisconsin	489	1.7%
22	Washington	455	1.6%
23	Mississippi	435	1.5%
24	Oklahoma	420	1.5%
25	Massachusetts	416	1.5%
26	Kentucky	409	1.4%
27	Colorado	399	1.4%
28	Minnesota	386	1.4%
29	Arkansas	329	1.2%
30	Connecticut	307	1.1%
31	Kansas	270	1.0%
32	Utah	255	0.9%
33	Iowa	246	0.9%
34	Oregon	245	0.9%
35	Nevada	200	0.7%
36	New Mexico	197	0.7%
37	Nebraska	172	0.6%
38	West Virginia	166	0.6%
39	Idaho	140	0.5%
40	Hawaii	121	0.4%
41	Delaware	102	0.4%
42	South Dakota	94	0.3%
43	Rhode Island	88	0.3%
44	Maine	87	0.3%
45	Montana	80	0.3%
46	North Dakota	68	0.2%
47	New Hampshire	63	0.2%
48	Alaska	59	0.2%
49	Vermont	46	0.2%
50	Wyoming	45	0.2%
	District of Columbia	96	0.3%

Source: U.S. Department of Health and Human Services, National Center for Health Statistics
    "National Vital Statistics Reports" (Vol. 48, No. 11, July 24, 2000)
*Final data. Deaths under 1 year old by state of residence.

Infant Mortality Rate in 1998

National Rate = 7.2 Infant Deaths per 1,000 Live Births*

ALPHA ORDER

RANK	STATE	RATE
1	Alabama	10.2
43	Alaska	5.9
21	Arizona	7.5
8	Arkansas	8.9
45	California	5.8
37	Colorado	6.7
31	Connecticut	7.0
3	Delaware	9.6
25	Florida	7.2
11	Georgia	8.5
36	Hawaii	6.9
25	Idaho	7.2
13	Illinois	8.4
20	Indiana	7.6
38	Iowa	6.6
31	Kansas	7.0
21	Kentucky	7.5
6	Louisiana	9.1
41	Maine	6.3
9	Maryland	8.6
49	Massachusetts	5.1
14	Michigan	8.2
43	Minnesota	5.9
2	Mississippi	10.1
18	Missouri	7.7
23	Montana	7.4
24	Nebraska	7.3
31	Nevada	7.0
50	New Hampshire	4.4
39	New Jersey	6.4
25	New Mexico	7.2
41	New York	6.3
5	North Carolina	9.3
9	North Dakota	8.6
16	Ohio	8.0
11	Oklahoma	8.5
48	Oregon	5.4
30	Pennsylvania	7.1
31	Rhode Island	7.0
3	South Carolina	9.6
6	South Dakota	9.1
14	Tennessee	8.2
39	Texas	6.4
47	Utah	5.6
31	Vermont	7.0
18	Virginia	7.7
46	Washington	5.7
16	West Virginia	8.0
25	Wisconsin	7.2
25	Wyoming	7.2

RANK ORDER

RANK	STATE	RATE
1	Alabama	10.2
2	Mississippi	10.1 ·
3	Delaware	9.6
3	South Carolina	9.6
5	North Carolina	9.3
6	Louisiana	9.1
6	South Dakota	9.1
8	Arkansas	8.9
9	Maryland	8.6
9	North Dakota	8.6
11	Georgia	8.5
11	Oklahoma	8.5
13	Illinois	8.4
14	Michigan	8.2
14	Tennessee	8.2
16	Ohio	8.0
16	West Virginia	8.0
18	Missouri	7.7
18	Virginia	7.7
20	Indiana	7.6
21	Arizona	7.5
21	Kentucky	7.5
23	Montana	7.4
24	Nebraska	7.3
25	Florida	7.2
25	Idaho	7.2
25	New Mexico	7.2
25	Wisconsin	7.2
25	Wyoming	7.2
30	Pennsylvania	7.1
31	Connecticut	7.0
31	Kansas	7.0
31	Nevada	7.0
31	Rhode Island	7.0
31	Vermont	7.0
36	Hawaii	6.9
37	Colorado	6.7
38	Iowa	6.6
39	New Jersey	6.4
39	Texas	6.4
41	Maine	6.3
41	New York	6.3
43	Alaska	5.9
43	Minnesota	5.9
45	California	5.8
46	Washington	5.7
47	Utah	5.6
48	Oregon	5.4
49	Massachusetts	5.1
50	New Hampshire	4.4

District of Columbia 12.5

Source: U.S. Department of Health and Human Services, National Center for Health Statistics
   "National Vital Statistics Reports" (Vol. 48, No. 11, July 24, 2000)
*Final data. Deaths under 1 year old by state of residence.

Infant Mortality Rate in 1990

National Rate = 9.2 Infant Deaths per 1,000 Live Births*

ALPHA ORDER

RANK	STATE	RATE	RANK	STATE	RATE
5	Alabama	10.8	1	Georgia	12.4
9	Alaska	10.5	2	Mississippi	12.1
27	Arizona	8.8	3	South Carolina	11.7
22	Arkansas	9.2	4	Louisiana	11.1
41	California	7.9	5	Alabama	10.8
27	Colorado	8.8	5	Illinois	10.8
41	Connecticut	7.9	7	Michigan	10.7
12	Delaware	10.1	8	North Carolina	10.6
16	Florida	9.6	9	Alaska	10.5
1	Georgia	12.4	10	Tennessee	10.3
48	Hawaii	6.7	11	Virginia	10.2
29	Idaho	8.7	12	Delaware	10.1
5	Illinois	10.8	12	South Dakota	10.1
16	Indiana	9.6	14	West Virginia	9.9
37	Iowa	8.1	15	Ohio	9.8
32	Kansas	8.4	16	Florida	9.6
31	Kentucky	8.5	16	Indiana	9.6
4	Louisiana	11.1	16	Maryland	9.6
50	Maine	6.2	16	New York	9.6
16	Maryland	9.6	16	Pennsylvania	9.6
47	Massachusetts	7.0	21	Missouri	9.4
7	Michigan	10.7	22	Arkansas	9.2
45	Minnesota	7.3	22	Oklahoma	9.2
2	Mississippi	12.1	24	Montana	9.0
21	Missouri	9.4	24	New Jersey	9.0
24	Montana	9.0	24	New Mexico	9.0
34	Nebraska	8.3	27	Arizona	8.8
32	Nevada	8.4	27	Colorado	8.8
46	New Hampshire	7.1	29	Idaho	8.7
24	New Jersey	9.0	30	Wyoming	8.6
24	New Mexico	9.0	31	Kentucky	8.5
16	New York	9.6	32	Kansas	8.4
8	North Carolina	10.6	32	Nevada	8.4
40	North Dakota	8.0	34	Nebraska	8.3
15	Ohio	9.8	34	Oregon	8.3
22	Oklahoma	9.2	36	Wisconsin	8.2
34	Oregon	8.3	37	Iowa	8.1
16	Pennsylvania	9.6	37	Rhode Island	8.1
37	Rhode Island	8.1	37	Texas	8.1
3	South Carolina	11.7	40	North Dakota	8.0
12	South Dakota	10.1	41	California	7.9
10	Tennessee	10.3	41	Connecticut	7.9
37	Texas	8.1	43	Washington	7.8
44	Utah	7.5	44	Utah	7.5
49	Vermont	6.4	45	Minnesota	7.3
11	Virginia	10.2	46	New Hampshire	7.1
43	Washington	7.8	47	Massachusetts	7.0
14	West Virginia	9.9	48	Hawaii	6.7
36	Wisconsin	8.2	49	Vermont	6.4
30	Wyoming	8.6	50	Maine	6.2
				District of Columbia	20.7

RANK ORDER

Source: U.S. Department of Health and Human Services, National Center for Health Statistics
   "Monthly Vital Statistics Report" (Vol. 41, No. 7(S), January 7, 1993)
*Final data by state of residence. Infant deaths are those under 1 year old.

Infant Mortality Rate in 1980

National Rate = 12.6 Infant Deaths per 1,000 Live Births*

ALPHA ORDER

RANK	STATE	RATE
3	Alabama	15.2
24	Alaska	12.3
21	Arizona	12.4
17	Arkansas	12.7
35	California	11.1
46	Colorado	10.1
34	Connecticut	11.2
10	Delaware	13.9
5	Florida	14.6
6	Georgia	14.5
44	Hawaii	10.3
38	Idaho	10.7
4	Illinois	14.8
28	Indiana	11.9
29	Iowa	11.8
42	Kansas	10.4
14	Kentucky	12.9
8	Louisiana	14.3
50	Maine	9.2
9	Maryland	14.1
41	Massachusetts	10.5
15	Michigan	12.8
47	Minnesota	10.0
1	Mississippi	17.0
21	Missouri	12.4
21	Montana	12.4
32	Nebraska	11.5
38	Nevada	10.7
48	New Hampshire	9.9
19	New Jersey	12.5
32	New Mexico	11.5
19	New York	12.5
6	North Carolina	14.5
27	North Dakota	12.1
15	Ohio	12.8
17	Oklahoma	12.7
25	Oregon	12.2
13	Pennsylvania	13.2
36	Rhode Island	11.0
2	South Carolina	15.6
37	South Dakota	10.9
12	Tennessee	13.5
25	Texas	12.2
42	Utah	10.4
38	Vermont	10.7
11	Virginia	13.6
29	Washington	11.8
29	West Virginia	11.8
44	Wisconsin	10.3
49	Wyoming	9.8

RANK ORDER

RANK	STATE	RATE
1	Mississippi	17.0
2	South Carolina	15.6
3	Alabama	15.2
4	Illinois	14.8
5	Florida	14.6
6	Georgia	14.5
6	North Carolina	14.5
8	Louisiana	14.3
9	Maryland	14.1
10	Delaware	13.9
11	Virginia	13.6
12	Tennessee	13.5
13	Pennsylvania	13.2
14	Kentucky	12.9
15	Michigan	12.8
15	Ohio	12.8
17	Arkansas	12.7
17	Oklahoma	12.7
19	New Jersey	12.5
19	New York	12.5
21	Arizona	12.4
21	Missouri	12.4
21	Montana	12.4
24	Alaska	12.3
25	Oregon	12.2
25	Texas	12.2
27	North Dakota	12.1
28	Indiana	11.9
29	Iowa	11.8
29	Washington	11.8
29	West Virginia	11.8
32	Nebraska	11.5
32	New Mexico	11.5
34	Connecticut	11.2
35	California	11.1
36	Rhode Island	11.0
37	South Dakota	10.9
38	Idaho	10.7
38	Nevada	10.7
38	Vermont	10.7
41	Massachusetts	10.5
42	Kansas	10.4
42	Utah	10.4
44	Hawaii	10.3
44	Wisconsin	10.3
46	Colorado	10.1
47	Minnesota	10.0
48	New Hampshire	9.9
49	Wyoming	9.8
50	Maine	9.2

District of Columbia	25.0

Source: U.S. Department of Health and Human Services, National Center for Health Statistics
"Monthly Vital Statistics Report"
*Final data by state of residence. Deaths under 1 year old, exclusive of fetal deaths.

Percent Change in Infant Mortality Rate: 1990 to 1998

National Percent Change = 21.7% Decrease*

ALPHA ORDER

RANK	STATE	PERCENT CHANGE
7	Alabama	(5.6)
50	Alaska	(43.8)
17	Arizona	(14.8)
5	Arkansas	(3.3)
42	California	(26.6)
37	Colorado	(23.9)
11	Connecticut	(11.4)
6	Delaware	(5.0)
39	Florida	(25.0)
46	Georgia	(31.5)
3	Hawaii	3.0
22	Idaho	(17.2)
35	Illinois	(22.2)
33	Indiana	(20.8)
28	Iowa	(18.5)
20	Kansas	(16.7)
12	Kentucky	(11.8)
25	Louisiana	(18.0)
4	Maine	1.6
10	Maryland	(10.4)
44	Massachusetts	(27.1)
36	Michigan	(23.4)
29	Minnesota	(19.2)
19	Mississippi	(16.5)
26	Missouri	(18.1)
23	Montana	(17.8)
13	Nebraska	(12.0)
20	Nevada	(16.7)
49	New Hampshire	(38.0)
45	New Jersey	(28.9)
31	New Mexico	(20.0)
47	New York	(34.4)
15	North Carolina	(12.3)
2	North Dakota	7.5
27	Ohio	(18.4)
8	Oklahoma	(7.6)
48	Oregon	(34.9)
41	Pennsylvania	(26.0)
16	Rhode Island	(13.6)
24	South Carolina	(17.9)
9	South Dakota	(9.9)
32	Tennessee	(20.4)
34	Texas	(21.0)
40	Utah	(25.3)
1	Vermont	9.4
38	Virginia	(24.5)
43	Washington	(26.9)
29	West Virginia	(19.2)
14	Wisconsin	(12.2)
18	Wyoming	(16.3)

RANK ORDER

RANK	STATE	PERCENT CHANGE
1	Vermont	9.4
2	North Dakota	7.5
3	Hawaii	3.0
4	Maine	1.6
5	Arkansas	(3.3)
6	Delaware	(5.0)
7	Alabama	(5.6)
8	Oklahoma	(7.6)
9	South Dakota	(9.9)
10	Maryland	(10.4)
11	Connecticut	(11.4)
12	Kentucky	(11.8)
13	Nebraska	(12.0)
14	Wisconsin	(12.2)
15	North Carolina	(12.3)
16	Rhode Island	(13.6)
17	Arizona	(14.8)
18	Wyoming	(16.3)
19	Mississippi	(16.5)
20	Kansas	(16.7)
20	Nevada	(16.7)
22	Idaho	(17.2)
23	Montana	(17.8)
24	South Carolina	(17.9)
25	Louisiana	(18.0)
26	Missouri	(18.1)
27	Ohio	(18.4)
28	Iowa	(18.5)
29	Minnesota	(19.2)
29	West Virginia	(19.2)
31	New Mexico	(20.0)
32	Tennessee	(20.4)
33	Indiana	(20.8)
34	Texas	(21.0)
35	Illinois	(22.2)
36	Michigan	(23.4)
37	Colorado	(23.9)
38	Virginia	(24.5)
39	Florida	(25.0)
40	Utah	(25.3)
41	Pennsylvania	(26.0)
42	California	(26.6)
43	Washington	(26.9)
44	Massachusetts	(27.1)
45	New Jersey	(28.9)
46	Georgia	(31.5)
47	New York	(34.4)
48	Oregon	(34.9)
49	New Hampshire	(38.0)
50	Alaska	(43.8)

District of Columbia (39.6)

Source: Morgan Quitno Press using data from US Dept of Health & Human Services, National Center for Health Statistics "Monthly Vital Statistics Report" (Vol. 41, No. 7(S), January 7, 1993) and "National Vital Statistics Reports" (Vol. 48, No. 11, July 24, 2000)

*By state of residence. Infant deaths are those under 1 year old.

Percent Change in Infant Mortality Rate: 1980 to 1998

National Percent Change = 42.9% Decrease*

ALPHA ORDER

RANK	STATE	PERCENT CHANGE
11	Alabama	(32.9)
48	Alaska	(52.0)
30	Arizona	(39.5)
4	Arkansas	(29.9)
42	California	(47.7)
14	Colorado	(33.7)
24	Connecticut	(37.5)
6	Delaware	(30.9)
45	Florida	(50.7)
34	Georgia	(41.4)
12	Hawaii	(33.0)
9	Idaho	(32.7)
36	Illinois	(43.2)
19	Indiana	(36.1)
38	Iowa	(44.1)
9	Kansas	(32.7)
35	Kentucky	(41.9)
20	Louisiana	(36.4)
7	Maine	(31.5)
28	Maryland	(39.0)
46	Massachusetts	(51.4)
17	Michigan	(35.9)
33	Minnesota	(41.0)
32	Mississippi	(40.6)
26	Missouri	(37.9)
31	Montana	(40.3)
22	Nebraska	(36.5)
15	Nevada	(34.6)
49	New Hampshire	(55.6)
43	New Jersey	(48.8)
23	New Mexico	(37.4)
44	New York	(49.6)
17	North Carolina	(35.9)
3	North Dakota	(28.9)
24	Ohio	(37.5)
13	Oklahoma	(33.1)
50	Oregon	(55.7)
39	Pennsylvania	(46.2)
20	Rhode Island	(36.4)
27	South Carolina	(38.5)
1	South Dakota	(16.5)
29	Tennessee	(39.3)
41	Texas	(47.5)
39	Utah	(46.2)
15	Vermont	(34.6)
37	Virginia	(43.4)
47	Washington	(51.7)
8	West Virginia	(32.2)
5	Wisconsin	(30.1)
2	Wyoming	(26.5)

RANK ORDER

RANK	STATE	PERCENT CHANGE
1	South Dakota	(16.5)
2	Wyoming	(26.5)
3	North Dakota	(28.9)
4	Arkansas	(29.9)
5	Wisconsin	(30.1)
6	Delaware	(30.9)
7	Maine	(31.5)
8	West Virginia	(32.2)
9	Idaho	(32.7)
9	Kansas	(32.7)
11	Alabama	(32.9)
12	Hawaii	(33.0)
13	Oklahoma	(33.1)
14	Colorado	(33.7)
15	Nevada	(34.6)
15	Vermont	(34.6)
17	Michigan	(35.9)
17	North Carolina	(35.9)
19	Indiana	(36.1)
20	Louisiana	(36.4)
20	Rhode Island	(36.4)
22	Nebraska	(36.5)
23	New Mexico	(37.4)
24	Connecticut	(37.5)
24	Ohio	(37.5)
26	Missouri	(37.9)
27	South Carolina	(38.5)
28	Maryland	(39.0)
29	Tennessee	(39.3)
30	Arizona	(39.5)
31	Montana	(40.3)
32	Mississippi	(40.6)
33	Minnesota	(41.0)
34	Georgia	(41.4)
35	Kentucky	(41.9)
36	Illinois	(43.2)
37	Virginia	(43.4)
38	Iowa	(44.1)
39	Pennsylvania	(46.2)
39	Utah	(46.2)
41	Texas	(47.5)
42	California	(47.7)
43	New Jersey	(48.8)
44	New York	(49.6)
45	Florida	(50.7)
46	Massachusetts	(51.4)
47	Washington	(51.7)
48	Alaska	(52.0)
49	New Hampshire	(55.6)
50	Oregon	(55.7)

District of Columbia (50.0)

Source: Morgan Quitno Press using data from US Dept of Health & Human Services, National Center for Health Statistics
"National Vital Statistics Reports" (Vol. 48, No. 11, July 24, 2000)
"Vital Statistics of the United States, 1980" (Vol. I-Natality, issued 1984) and unpublished data
*Final data by state of residence. Infant deaths are those occurring under 1 year, exclusive of fetal deaths.

White Infant Deaths in 1998

National Total = 18,561 Deaths*

ALPHA ORDER

RANK ORDER

RANK	STATE	DEATHS	% of USA
22	Alabama	318	1.7%
49	Alaska	31	0.2%
12	Arizona	469	2.5%
31	Arkansas	215	1.2%
1	California	2,239	12.1%
19	Colorado	346	1.9%
32	Connecticut	208	1.1%
46	Delaware	53	0.3%
6	Florida	857	4.6%
11	Georgia	470	2.5%
50	Hawaii	22	0.1%
39	Idaho	134	0.7%
4	Illinois	901	4.9%
10	Indiana	482	2.6%
30	Iowa	218	1.2%
26	Kansas	240	1.3%
21	Kentucky	332	1.8%
29	Louisiana	219	1.2%
40	Maine	85	0.5%
27	Maryland	233	1.3%
20	Massachusetts	341	1.8%
8	Michigan	668	3.6%
24	Minnesota	294	1.6%
37	Mississippi	145	0.8%
15	Missouri	382	2.1%
41	Montana	68	0.4%
38	Nebraska	143	0.8%
36	Nevada	146	0.8%
44	New Hampshire	60	0.3%
13	New Jersey	428	2.3%
34	New Mexico	159	0.9%
3	New York	980	5.3%
9	North Carolina	514	2.8%
45	North Dakota	58	0.3%
5	Ohio	888	4.8%
23	Oklahoma	316	1.7%
28	Oregon	221	1.2%
7	Pennsylvania	710	3.8%
41	Rhode Island	68	0.4%
33	South Carolina	206	1.1%
43	South Dakota	63	0.3%
16	Tennessee	375	2.0%
2	Texas	1,678	9.0%
25	Utah	243	1.3%
47	Vermont	44	0.2%
14	Virginia	386	2.1%
17	Washington	358	1.9%
35	West Virginia	158	0.9%
18	Wisconsin	347	1.9%
48	Wyoming	34	0.2%

RANK	STATE	DEATHS	% of USA
1	California	2,239	12.1%
2	Texas	1,678	9.0%
3	New York	980	5.3%
4	Illinois	901	4.9%
5	Ohio	888	4.8%
6	Florida	857	4.6%
7	Pennsylvania	710	3.8%
8	Michigan	668	3.6%
9	North Carolina	514	2.8%
10	Indiana	482	2.6%
11	Georgia	470	2.5%
12	Arizona	469	2.5%
13	New Jersey	428	2.3%
14	Virginia	386	2.1%
15	Missouri	382	2.1%
16	Tennessee	375	2.0%
17	Washington	358	1.9%
18	Wisconsin	347	1.9%
19	Colorado	346	1.9%
20	Massachusetts	341	1.8%
21	Kentucky	332	1.8%
22	Alabama	318	1.7%
23	Oklahoma	316	1.7%
24	Minnesota	294	1.6%
25	Utah	243	1.3%
26	Kansas	240	1.3%
27	Maryland	233	1.3%
28	Oregon	221	1.2%
29	Louisiana	219	1.2%
30	Iowa	218	1.2%
31	Arkansas	215	1.2%
32	Connecticut	208	1.1%
33	South Carolina	206	1.1%
34	New Mexico	159	0.9%
35	West Virginia	158	0.9%
36	Nevada	146	0.8%
37	Mississippi	145	0.8%
38	Nebraska	143	0.8%
39	Idaho	134	0.7%
40	Maine	85	0.5%
41	Montana	68	0.4%
41	Rhode Island	68	0.4%
43	South Dakota	63	0.3%
44	New Hampshire	60	0.3%
45	North Dakota	58	0.3%
46	Delaware	53	0.3%
47	Vermont	44	0.2%
48	Wyoming	34	0.2%
49	Alaska	31	0.2%
50	Hawaii	22	0.1%
	District of Columbia	8	0.0%

Source: U.S. Department of Health and Human Services, National Center for Health Statistics
   "National Vital Statistics Reports" (Vol. 48, No. 11, July 24, 2000)
*Final data. Deaths of infants under 1 year old, exclusive of fetal deaths. Based on race of the mother.

White Infant Mortality Rate in 1998

National Rate = 6.0 White Infant Deaths per 1,000 White Live Births*

ALPHA ORDER

RANK	STATE	RATE
4	Alabama	7.7
49	Alaska	4.7
11	Arizona	6.9
5	Arkansas	7.6
40	California	5.3
19	Colorado	6.4
39	Connecticut	5.6
11	Delaware	6.9
32	Florida	5.9
28	Georgia	6.0
40	Hawaii	5.3
8	Idaho	7.1
19	Illinois	6.4
17	Indiana	6.5
25	Iowa	6.2
9	Kansas	7.0
14	Kentucky	6.8
36	Louisiana	5.7
19	Maine	6.4
44	Maryland	5.2
48	Massachusetts	4.9
22	Michigan	6.3
46	Minnesota	5.1
22	Mississippi	6.3
27	Missouri	6.1
7	Montana	7.2
16	Nebraska	6.7
28	Nevada	6.0
50	New Hampshire	4.3
47	New Jersey	5.0
11	New Mexico	6.9
40	New York	5.3
17	North Carolina	6.5
1	North Dakota	8.2
9	Ohio	7.0
2	Oklahoma	8.1
40	Oregon	5.3
33	Pennsylvania	5.8
25	Rhode Island	6.2
28	South Carolina	6.0
6	South Dakota	7.5
22	Tennessee	6.3
33	Texas	5.8
36	Utah	5.7
14	Vermont	6.8
36	Virginia	5.7
44	Washington	5.2
3	West Virginia	8.0
28	Wisconsin	6.0
33	Wyoming	5.8

RANK ORDER

RANK	STATE	RATE
1	North Dakota	8.2
2	Oklahoma	8.1
3	West Virginia	8.0
4	Alabama	7.7
5	Arkansas	7.6
6	South Dakota	7.5
7	Montana	7.2
8	Idaho	7.1
9	Kansas	7.0
9	Ohio	7.0
11	Arizona	6.9
11	Delaware	6.9
11	New Mexico	6.9
14	Kentucky	6.8
14	Vermont	6.8
16	Nebraska	6.7
17	Indiana	6.5
17	North Carolina	6.5
19	Colorado	6.4
19	Illinois	6.4
19	Maine	6.4
22	Michigan	6.3
22	Mississippi	6.3
22	Tennessee	6.3
25	Iowa	6.2
25	Rhode Island	6.2
27	Missouri	6.1
28	Georgia	6.0
28	Nevada	6.0
28	South Carolina	6.0
28	Wisconsin	6.0
32	Florida	5.9
33	Pennsylvania	5.8
33	Texas	5.8
33	Wyoming	5.8
36	Louisiana	5.7
36	Utah	5.7
36	Virginia	5.7
39	Connecticut	5.6
40	California	5.3
40	Hawaii	5.3
40	New York	5.3
40	Oregon	5.3
44	Maryland	5.2
44	Washington	5.2
46	Minnesota	5.1
47	New Jersey	5.0
48	Massachusetts	4.9
49	Alaska	4.7
50	New Hampshire	4.3
	District of Columbia**	NA

Source: U.S. Department of Health and Human Services, National Center for Health Statistics
       "National Vital Statistics Reports" (Vol. 48, No. 11, July 24, 2000)
*Final data. Deaths of infants under 1 year old, exclusive of fetal deaths. Based on race of the mother.
**Not available, fewer than 20 white infant deaths.

Black Infant Deaths in 1998

National Total = 8,726 Deaths*

ALPHA ORDER

RANK	STATE	DEATHS	% of USA
14	Alabama	311	3.6%
40	Alaska	6	0.1%
27	Arizona	53	0.6%
22	Arkansas	112	1.3%
5	California	505	5.8%
30	Colorado	46	0.5%
23	Connecticut	95	1.1%
28	Delaware	49	0.6%
4	Florida	548	6.3%
3	Georgia	553	6.3%
41	Hawaii	5	0.1%
42	Idaho	2	0.0%
1	Illinois	614	7.0%
20	Indiana	160	1.8%
35	Iowa	20	0.2%
33	Kansas	28	0.3%
24	Kentucky	75	0.9%
9	Louisiana	385	4.4%
42	Maine	2	0.0%
10	Maryland	367	4.2%
25	Massachusetts	65	0.7%
8	Michigan	407	4.7%
28	Minnesota	49	0.6%
16	Mississippi	286	3.3%
19	Missouri	191	2.2%
48	Montana	1	0.0%
34	Nebraska	24	0.3%
32	Nevada	39	0.4%
42	New Hampshire	2	0.0%
17	New Jersey	274	3.1%
38	New Mexico	9	0.1%
2	New York	591	6.8%
6	North Carolina	497	5.7%
50	North Dakota	0	0.0%
12	Ohio	323	3.7%
25	Oklahoma	65	0.7%
37	Oregon	13	0.1%
13	Pennsylvania	320	3.7%
36	Rhode Island	17	0.2%
15	South Carolina	306	3.5%
42	South Dakota	2	0.0%
18	Tennessee	253	2.9%
7	Texas	466	5.3%
42	Utah	2	0.0%
48	Vermont	1	0.0%
11	Virginia	328	3.8%
31	Washington	42	0.5%
39	West Virginia	8	0.1%
21	Wisconsin	122	1.4%
42	Wyoming	2	0.0%

RANK ORDER

RANK	STATE	DEATHS	% of USA
1	Illinois	614	7.0%
2	New York	591	6.8%
3	Georgia	553	6.3%
4	Florida	548	6.3%
5	California	505	5.8%
6	North Carolina	497	5.7%
7	Texas	466	5.3%
8	Michigan	407	4.7%
9	Louisiana	385	4.4%
10	Maryland	367	4.2%
11	Virginia	328	3.8%
12	Ohio	323	3.7%
13	Pennsylvania	320	3.7%
14	Alabama	311	3.6%
15	South Carolina	306	3.5%
16	Mississippi	286	3.3%
17	New Jersey	274	3.1%
18	Tennessee	253	2.9%
19	Missouri	191	2.2%
20	Indiana	160	1.8%
21	Wisconsin	122	1.4%
22	Arkansas	112	1.3%
23	Connecticut	95	1.1%
24	Kentucky	75	0.9%
25	Massachusetts	65	0.7%
25	Oklahoma	65	0.7%
27	Arizona	53	0.6%
28	Delaware	49	0.6%
28	Minnesota	49	0.6%
30	Colorado	46	0.5%
31	Washington	42	0.5%
32	Nevada	39	0.4%
33	Kansas	28	0.3%
34	Nebraska	24	0.3%
35	Iowa	20	0.2%
36	Rhode Island	17	0.2%
37	Oregon	13	0.1%
38	New Mexico	9	0.1%
39	West Virginia	8	0.1%
40	Alaska	6	0.1%
41	Hawaii	5	0.1%
42	Idaho	2	0.0%
42	Maine	2	0.0%
42	New Hampshire	2	0.0%
42	South Dakota	2	0.0%
42	Utah	2	0.0%
42	Wyoming	2	0.0%
48	Montana	1	0.0%
48	Vermont	1	0.0%
50	North Dakota	0	0.0%
	District of Columbia	85	1.0%

Source: U.S. Department of Health and Human Services, National Center for Health Statistics
   "National Vital Statistics Reports" (Vol. 48, No. 11, July 24, 2000)
*Final data. Deaths of infants under 1 year old, exclusive of fetal deaths. Based on race of the mother.

Black Infant Mortality Rate in 1998

National Rate = 14.3 Black Infant Deaths per 1,000 Black Live Births*

ALPHA ORDER			RANK ORDER		
RANK	STATE	RATE	RANK	STATE	RATE
15	Alabama	15.5	1	Arizona	20.0
NA	Alaska**	NA	2	Nebraska	19.4
1	Arizona	20.0	3	Delaware	18.7
23	Arkansas	14.0	3	Wisconsin	18.7
25	California	13.7	5	Iowa	18.3
14	Colorado	16.0	6	North Carolina	17.6
7	Connecticut	17.4	7	Connecticut	17.4
3	Delaware	18.7	8	Indiana	17.3
31	Florida	12.3	8	Nevada	17.3
28	Georgia	13.4	10	Illinois	17.2
NA	Hawaii**	NA	11	Michigan	16.8
NA	Idaho**	NA	11	Missouri	16.8
10	Illinois	17.2	13	South Carolina	16.2
8	Indiana	17.3	14	Colorado	16.0
5	Iowa	18.3	15	Alabama	15.5
34	Kansas	10.0	16	Kentucky	15.4
16	Kentucky	15.4	16	Pennsylvania	15.4
23	Louisiana	14.0	18	Maryland	15.3
NA	Maine**	NA	19	Tennessee	15.0
18	Maryland	15.3	20	Virginia	14.9
35	Massachusetts	8.3	21	Mississippi	14.8
11	Michigan	16.8	22	Ohio	14.2
28	Minnesota	13.4	23	Arkansas	14.0
21	Mississippi	14.8	23	Louisiana	14.0
11	Missouri	16.8	25	California	13.7
NA	Montana**	NA	26	Oklahoma	13.5
2	Nebraska	19.4	26	Washington	13.5
8	Nevada	17.3	28	Georgia	13.4
NA	New Hampshire**	NA	28	Minnesota	13.4
30	New Jersey	12.8	30	New Jersey	12.8
NA	New Mexico**	NA	31	Florida	12.3
33	New York	10.9	32	Texas	11.6
6	North Carolina	17.6	33	New York	10.9
NA	North Dakota**	NA	34	Kansas	10.0
22	Ohio	14.2	35	Massachusetts	8.3
26	Oklahoma	13.5	NA	Alaska**	NA
NA	Oregon**	NA	NA	Hawaii**	NA
16	Pennsylvania	15.4	NA	Idaho**	NA
NA	Rhode Island**	NA	NA	Maine**	NA
13	South Carolina	16.2	NA	Montana**	NA
NA	South Dakota**	NA	NA	New Hampshire**	NA
19	Tennessee	15.0	NA	New Mexico**	NA
32	Texas	11.6	NA	North Dakota**	NA
NA	Utah**	NA	NA	Oregon**	NA
NA	Vermont**	NA	NA	Rhode Island**	NA
20	Virginia	14.9	NA	South Dakota**	NA
26	Washington	13.5	NA	Utah**	NA
NA	West Virginia**	NA	NA	Vermont**	NA
3	Wisconsin	18.7	NA	West Virginia**	NA
NA	Wyoming**	NA	NA	Wyoming**	NA
				District of Columbia	15.5

Source: U.S. Department of Health and Human Services, National Center for Health Statistics
"National Vital Statistics Reports" (Vol. 48, No. 11, July 24, 2000)
*Final data. Deaths of infants under 1 year old, exclusive of fetal deaths. Based on race of the mother.
**Not available, fewer than 20 black infant deaths.

Percent Change in White Infant Mortality Rate: 1990 to 1998

National Percent Change = 22.1% Decrease*

ALPHA ORDER				RANK ORDER		
RANK	STATE	PERCENT CHANGE		RANK	STATE	PERCENT CHANGE
8	Alabama	(7.2)		1	Vermont	4.6
50	Alaska	(44.7)		2	Hawaii	3.9
15	Arizona	(15.9)		3	North Dakota	3.8
5	Arkansas	(5.0)		4	Maine	3.2
43	California	(30.3)		5	Arkansas	(5.0)
31	Colorado	(23.8)		6	Delaware	(5.5)
14	Connecticut	(15.2)		7	Nebraska	(6.9)
6	Delaware	(5.5)		8	Alabama	(7.2)
29	Florida	(22.4)		9	Kansas	(9.1)
46	Georgia	(34.1)		10	South Dakota	(12.8)
2	Hawaii	3.9		11	Oklahoma	(13.8)
21	Idaho	(18.4)		12	Ohio	(14.6)
19	Illinois	(16.9)		13	Kentucky	(15.0)
41	Indiana	(27.0)		14	Connecticut	(15.2)
24	Iowa	(20.5)		15	Arizona	(15.9)
9	Kansas	(9.1)		16	Montana	(16.3)
13	Kentucky	(15.0)		17	West Virginia	(16.7)
28	Louisiana	(21.9)		17	Wisconsin	(16.7)
4	Maine	3.2		19	Illinois	(16.9)
22	Maryland	(20.0)		20	Texas	(18.3)
40	Massachusetts	(26.9)		21	Idaho	(18.4)
23	Michigan	(20.3)		22	Maryland	(20.0)
32	Minnesota	(23.9)		23	Michigan	(20.3)
37	Mississippi	(25.9)		24	Iowa	(20.5)
27	Missouri	(21.8)		25	Tennessee	(21.3)
16	Montana	(16.3)		26	North Carolina	(21.7)
7	Nebraska	(6.9)		27	Missouri	(21.8)
37	Nevada	(25.9)		28	Louisiana	(21.9)
49	New Hampshire	(40.3)		29	Florida	(22.4)
39	New Jersey	(26.5)		30	Utah	(23.0)
36	New Mexico	(25.8)		31	Colorado	(23.8)
44	New York	(31.2)		32	Minnesota	(23.9)
26	North Carolina	(21.7)		33	Virginia	(24.0)
3	North Dakota	3.8		34	Rhode Island	(25.3)
12	Ohio	(14.6)		35	Pennsylvania	(25.6)
11	Oklahoma	(13.8)		36	New Mexico	(25.8)
48	Oregon	(34.6)		37	Mississippi	(25.9)
35	Pennsylvania	(25.6)		37	Nevada	(25.9)
34	Rhode Island	(25.3)		39	New Jersey	(26.5)
42	South Carolina	(27.7)		40	Massachusetts	(26.9)
10	South Dakota	(12.8)		41	Indiana	(27.0)
25	Tennessee	(21.3)		42	South Carolina	(27.7)
20	Texas	(18.3)		43	California	(30.3)
30	Utah	(23.0)		44	New York	(31.2)
1	Vermont	4.6		45	Washington	(31.6)
33	Virginia	(24.0)		46	Georgia	(34.1)
45	Washington	(31.6)		46	Wyoming	(34.1)
17	West Virginia	(16.7)		48	Oregon	(34.6)
17	Wisconsin	(16.7)		49	New Hampshire	(40.3)
46	Wyoming	(34.1)		50	Alaska	(44.7)
					District of Columbia**	NA

Source: Morgan Quitno Press using data from US Dept of Health & Human Services, National Center for Health Statistics
   "National Vital Statistics Reports" (Vol. 48, No. 11, July 24, 2000) and "Vital Statistics of the United States"
*Final data. Deaths of infants under 1 year old, exclusive of fetal deaths. Based on race of the mother.
**Not available, fewer than 20 white infant deaths.

Percent Change in Black Infant Mortality Rate: 1990 to 1998

National Percent Change = 16.5% Decrease*

ALPHA ORDER				RANK ORDER		
RANK	STATE	PERCENT CHANGE		RANK	STATE	PERCENT CHANGE
12	Alabama	(2.5)		1	Nevada	38.4
NA	Alaska**	NA		2	Arizona	19.8
2	Arizona	19.8		3	Nebraska	15.5
9	Arkansas	2.9		4	Kentucky	13.2
14	California	(3.5)		5	North Carolina	10.0
13	Colorado	(3.0)		6	Connecticut	8.8
6	Connecticut	8.8		7	Indiana	8.1
15	Delaware	(3.6)		8	Wisconsin	3.3
30	Florida	(24.1)		9	Arkansas	2.9
31	Georgia	(25.6)		10	Oklahoma	2.3
NA	Hawaii**	NA		11	Iowa	1.7
NA	Idaho**	NA		12	Alabama	(2.5)
25	Illinois	(20.0)		13	Colorado	(3.0)
7	Indiana	8.1		14	California	(3.5)
11	Iowa	1.7		15	Delaware	(3.6)
34	Kansas	(35.1)		16	Missouri	(4.0)
4	Kentucky	13.2		17	South Carolina	(5.3)
22	Louisiana	(15.2)		18	Maryland	(6.1)
NA	Maine**	NA		19	Washington	(6.9)
18	Maryland	(6.1)		20	Mississippi	(8.1)
27	Massachusetts	(20.2)		21	Tennessee	(14.3)
25	Michigan	(20.0)		22	Louisiana	(15.2)
33	Minnesota	(32.0)		23	Texas	(16.5)
20	Mississippi	(8.1)		24	Pennsylvania	(18.1)
16	Missouri	(4.0)		25	Illinois	(20.0)
NA	Montana**	NA		25	Michigan	(20.0)
3	Nebraska	15.5		27	Massachusetts	(20.2)
1	Nevada	38.4		28	Virginia	(20.7)
NA	New Hampshire**	NA		29	Ohio	(22.4)
32	New Jersey	(26.0)		30	Florida	(24.1)
NA	New Mexico**	NA		31	Georgia	(25.6)
35	New York	(37.0)		32	New Jersey	(26.0)
5	North Carolina	10.0		33	Minnesota	(32.0)
NA	North Dakota**	NA		34	Kansas	(35.1)
29	Ohio	(22.4)		35	New York	(37.0)
10	Oklahoma	2.3		NA	Alaska**	NA
NA	Oregon**	NA		NA	Hawaii**	NA
24	Pennsylvania	(18.1)		NA	Idaho**	NA
NA	Rhode Island**	NA		NA	Maine**	NA
17	South Carolina	(5.3)		NA	Montana**	NA
NA	South Dakota**	NA		NA	New Hampshire**	NA
21	Tennessee	(14.3)		NA	New Mexico**	NA
23	Texas	(16.5)		NA	North Dakota**	NA
NA	Utah**	NA		NA	Oregon**	NA
NA	Vermont**	NA		NA	Rhode Island**	NA
28	Virginia	(20.7)		NA	South Dakota**	NA
19	Washington	(6.9)		NA	Utah**	NA
NA	West Virginia**	NA		NA	Vermont**	NA
8	Wisconsin	3.3		NA	West Virginia**	NA
NA	Wyoming**	NA		NA	Wyoming**	NA
					District of Columbia	(36.5)

Source: Morgan Quitno Press using data from US Dept of Health & Human Services, National Center for Health Statistics "National Vital Statistics Reports" (Vol. 48, No. 11, July 24, 2000) and "Vital Statistics of the United States"
*Final data. Deaths of infants under 1 year old, exclusive of fetal deaths. Based on race of the mother.
**Not available, fewer than 20 black infant deaths.

Neonatal Deaths in 1998

National Total = 18,918 Deaths*

<table>
<tr><td colspan="4"><u>ALPHA ORDER</u></td><td colspan="4"><u>RANK ORDER</u></td></tr>
<tr><td>RANK</td><td>STATE</td><td>DEATHS</td><td>% of USA</td><td>RANK</td><td>STATE</td><td>DEATHS</td><td>% of USA</td></tr>
<tr><td>16</td><td>Alabama</td><td>414</td><td>2.2%</td><td>1</td><td>California</td><td>2,003</td><td>10.6%</td></tr>
<tr><td>49</td><td>Alaska</td><td>29</td><td>0.2%</td><td>2</td><td>Texas</td><td>1,363</td><td>7.2%</td></tr>
<tr><td>18</td><td>Arizona</td><td>376</td><td>2.0%</td><td>3</td><td>New York</td><td>1,151</td><td>6.1%</td></tr>
<tr><td>30</td><td>Arkansas</td><td>202</td><td>1.1%</td><td>4</td><td>Illinois</td><td>1,020</td><td>5.4%</td></tr>
<tr><td>1</td><td>California</td><td>2,003</td><td>10.6%</td><td>5</td><td>Florida</td><td>935</td><td>4.9%</td></tr>
<tr><td>27</td><td>Colorado</td><td>264</td><td>1.4%</td><td>6</td><td>Ohio</td><td>820</td><td>4.3%</td></tr>
<tr><td>29</td><td>Connecticut</td><td>224</td><td>1.2%</td><td>7</td><td>Pennsylvania</td><td>731</td><td>3.9%</td></tr>
<tr><td>41</td><td>Delaware</td><td>73</td><td>0.4%</td><td>8</td><td>North Carolina</td><td>720</td><td>3.8%</td></tr>
<tr><td>5</td><td>Florida</td><td>935</td><td>4.9%</td><td>9</td><td>Michigan</td><td>713</td><td>3.8%</td></tr>
<tr><td>10</td><td>Georgia</td><td>706</td><td>3.7%</td><td>10</td><td>Georgia</td><td>706</td><td>3.7%</td></tr>
<tr><td>39</td><td>Hawaii</td><td>89</td><td>0.5%</td><td>11</td><td>New Jersey</td><td>518</td><td>2.7%</td></tr>
<tr><td>39</td><td>Idaho</td><td>89</td><td>0.5%</td><td>12</td><td>Virginia</td><td>509</td><td>2.7%</td></tr>
<tr><td>4</td><td>Illinois</td><td>1,020</td><td>5.4%</td><td>13</td><td>Maryland</td><td>449</td><td>2.4%</td></tr>
<tr><td>14</td><td>Indiana</td><td>439</td><td>2.3%</td><td>14</td><td>Indiana</td><td>439</td><td>2.3%</td></tr>
<tr><td>32</td><td>Iowa</td><td>170</td><td>0.9%</td><td>15</td><td>Tennessee</td><td>434</td><td>2.3%</td></tr>
<tr><td>31</td><td>Kansas</td><td>178</td><td>0.9%</td><td>16</td><td>Alabama</td><td>414</td><td>2.2%</td></tr>
<tr><td>25</td><td>Kentucky</td><td>265</td><td>1.4%</td><td>17</td><td>Louisiana</td><td>396</td><td>2.1%</td></tr>
<tr><td>17</td><td>Louisiana</td><td>396</td><td>2.1%</td><td>18</td><td>Arizona</td><td>376</td><td>2.0%</td></tr>
<tr><td>43</td><td>Maine</td><td>58</td><td>0.3%</td><td>19</td><td>Missouri</td><td>373</td><td>2.0%</td></tr>
<tr><td>13</td><td>Maryland</td><td>449</td><td>2.4%</td><td>20</td><td>South Carolina</td><td>362</td><td>1.9%</td></tr>
<tr><td>22</td><td>Massachusetts</td><td>316</td><td>1.7%</td><td>21</td><td>Wisconsin</td><td>344</td><td>1.8%</td></tr>
<tr><td>9</td><td>Michigan</td><td>713</td><td>3.8%</td><td>22</td><td>Massachusetts</td><td>316</td><td>1.7%</td></tr>
<tr><td>28</td><td>Minnesota</td><td>263</td><td>1.4%</td><td>23</td><td>Washington</td><td>287</td><td>1.5%</td></tr>
<tr><td>25</td><td>Mississippi</td><td>265</td><td>1.4%</td><td>24</td><td>Oklahoma</td><td>267</td><td>1.4%</td></tr>
<tr><td>19</td><td>Missouri</td><td>373</td><td>2.0%</td><td>25</td><td>Kentucky</td><td>265</td><td>1.4%</td></tr>
<tr><td>46</td><td>Montana</td><td>45</td><td>0.2%</td><td>25</td><td>Mississippi</td><td>265</td><td>1.4%</td></tr>
<tr><td>36</td><td>Nebraska</td><td>114</td><td>0.6%</td><td>27</td><td>Colorado</td><td>264</td><td>1.4%</td></tr>
<tr><td>37</td><td>Nevada</td><td>100</td><td>0.5%</td><td>28</td><td>Minnesota</td><td>263</td><td>1.4%</td></tr>
<tr><td>44</td><td>New Hampshire</td><td>49</td><td>0.3%</td><td>29</td><td>Connecticut</td><td>224</td><td>1.2%</td></tr>
<tr><td>11</td><td>New Jersey</td><td>518</td><td>2.7%</td><td>30</td><td>Arkansas</td><td>202</td><td>1.1%</td></tr>
<tr><td>35</td><td>New Mexico</td><td>120</td><td>0.6%</td><td>31</td><td>Kansas</td><td>178</td><td>0.9%</td></tr>
<tr><td>3</td><td>New York</td><td>1,151</td><td>6.1%</td><td>32</td><td>Iowa</td><td>170</td><td>0.9%</td></tr>
<tr><td>8</td><td>North Carolina</td><td>720</td><td>3.8%</td><td>33</td><td>Utah</td><td>161</td><td>0.9%</td></tr>
<tr><td>47</td><td>North Dakota</td><td>43</td><td>0.2%</td><td>34</td><td>Oregon</td><td>143</td><td>0.8%</td></tr>
<tr><td>6</td><td>Ohio</td><td>820</td><td>4.3%</td><td>35</td><td>New Mexico</td><td>120</td><td>0.6%</td></tr>
<tr><td>24</td><td>Oklahoma</td><td>267</td><td>1.4%</td><td>36</td><td>Nebraska</td><td>114</td><td>0.6%</td></tr>
<tr><td>34</td><td>Oregon</td><td>143</td><td>0.8%</td><td>37</td><td>Nevada</td><td>100</td><td>0.5%</td></tr>
<tr><td>7</td><td>Pennsylvania</td><td>731</td><td>3.9%</td><td>38</td><td>West Virginia</td><td>95</td><td>0.5%</td></tr>
<tr><td>42</td><td>Rhode Island</td><td>65</td><td>0.3%</td><td>39</td><td>Hawaii</td><td>89</td><td>0.5%</td></tr>
<tr><td>20</td><td>South Carolina</td><td>362</td><td>1.9%</td><td>39</td><td>Idaho</td><td>89</td><td>0.5%</td></tr>
<tr><td>45</td><td>South Dakota</td><td>47</td><td>0.2%</td><td>41</td><td>Delaware</td><td>73</td><td>0.4%</td></tr>
<tr><td>15</td><td>Tennessee</td><td>434</td><td>2.3%</td><td>42</td><td>Rhode Island</td><td>65</td><td>0.3%</td></tr>
<tr><td>2</td><td>Texas</td><td>1,363</td><td>7.2%</td><td>43</td><td>Maine</td><td>58</td><td>0.3%</td></tr>
<tr><td>33</td><td>Utah</td><td>161</td><td>0.9%</td><td>44</td><td>New Hampshire</td><td>49</td><td>0.3%</td></tr>
<tr><td>48</td><td>Vermont</td><td>38</td><td>0.2%</td><td>45</td><td>South Dakota</td><td>47</td><td>0.2%</td></tr>
<tr><td>12</td><td>Virginia</td><td>509</td><td>2.7%</td><td>46</td><td>Montana</td><td>45</td><td>0.2%</td></tr>
<tr><td>23</td><td>Washington</td><td>287</td><td>1.5%</td><td>47</td><td>North Dakota</td><td>43</td><td>0.2%</td></tr>
<tr><td>38</td><td>West Virginia</td><td>95</td><td>0.5%</td><td>48</td><td>Vermont</td><td>38</td><td>0.2%</td></tr>
<tr><td>21</td><td>Wisconsin</td><td>344</td><td>1.8%</td><td>49</td><td>Alaska</td><td>29</td><td>0.2%</td></tr>
<tr><td>50</td><td>Wyoming</td><td>28</td><td>0.1%</td><td>50</td><td>Wyoming</td><td>28</td><td>0.1%</td></tr>
<tr><td></td><td></td><td></td><td></td><td></td><td>District of Columbia</td><td>55</td><td>0.3%</td></tr>
</table>

Source: U.S. Department of Health and Human Services, National Center for Health Statistics
  "National Vital Statistics Reports" (Vol. 48, No. 11, July 24, 2000)
Final data. Deaths of infants under 28 days, exclusive of fetal deaths.

Neonatal Death Rate in 1998

National Rate = 4.8 Deaths per 1,000 Live Births*

RANK	STATE	RATE
2	Alabama	6.7
50	Alaska	2.9
26	Arizona	4.8
12	Arkansas	5.5
44	California	3.8
37	Colorado	4.4
20	Connecticut	5.1
1	Delaware	6.9
26	Florida	4.8
8	Georgia	5.8
20	Hawaii	5.1
29	Idaho	4.6
10	Illinois	5.6
18	Indiana	5.2
29	Iowa	4.6
29	Kansas	4.6
24	Kentucky	4.9
7	Louisiana	5.9
39	Maine	4.2
5	Maryland	6.2
43	Massachusetts	3.9
17	Michigan	5.3
41	Minnesota	4.0
5	Mississippi	6.2
24	Missouri	4.9
39	Montana	4.2
26	Nebraska	4.8
47	Nevada	3.5
48	New Hampshire	3.4
34	New Jersey	4.5
37	New Mexico	4.4
34	New York	4.5
4	North Carolina	6.4
13	North Dakota	5.4
13	Ohio	5.4
13	Oklahoma	5.4
49	Oregon	3.2
23	Pennsylvania	5.0
18	Rhode Island	5.2
2	South Carolina	6.7
29	South Dakota	4.6
10	Tennessee	5.6
41	Texas	4.0
45	Utah	3.6
8	Vermont	5.8
13	Virginia	5.4
45	Washington	3.6
29	West Virginia	4.6
20	Wisconsin	5.1
34	Wyoming	4.5

RANK	STATE	RATE
1	Delaware	6.9
2	Alabama	6.7
2	South Carolina	6.7
4	North Carolina	6.4
5	Maryland	6.2
5	Mississippi	6.2
7	Louisiana	5.9
8	Georgia	5.8
8	Vermont	5.8
10	Illinois	5.6
10	Tennessee	5.6
12	Arkansas	5.5
13	North Dakota	5.4
13	Ohio	5.4
13	Oklahoma	5.4
13	Virginia	5.4
17	Michigan	5.3
18	Indiana	5.2
18	Rhode Island	5.2
20	Connecticut	5.1
20	Hawaii	5.1
20	Wisconsin	5.1
23	Pennsylvania	5.0
24	Kentucky	4.9
24	Missouri	4.9
26	Arizona	4.8
26	Florida	4.8
26	Nebraska	4.8
29	Idaho	4.6
29	Iowa	4.6
29	Kansas	4.6
29	South Dakota	4.6
29	West Virginia	4.6
34	New Jersey	4.5
34	New York	4.5
34	Wyoming	4.5
37	Colorado	4.4
37	New Mexico	4.4
39	Maine	4.2
39	Montana	4.2
41	Minnesota	4.0
41	Texas	4.0
43	Massachusetts	3.9
44	California	3.8
45	Utah	3.6
45	Washington	3.6
47	Nevada	3.5
48	New Hampshire	3.4
49	Oregon	3.2
50	Alaska	2.9
	District of Columbia	7.2

Source: U.S. Department of Health and Human Services, National Center for Health Statistics
"National Vital Statistics Reports" (Vol. 48, No. 11, July 24, 2000)
Final data. Deaths of infants under 28 days, exclusive of fetal deaths.

White Neonatal Deaths in 1998

National Total = 12,406 Deaths*

ALPHA ORDER

RANK	STATE	DEATHS	% of USA
24	Alabama	188	1.5%
49	Alaska	19	0.2%
12	Arizona	308	2.5%
31	Arkansas	134	1.1%
1	California	1,525	12.3%
19	Colorado	231	1.9%
28	Connecticut	153	1.2%
47	Delaware	32	0.3%
6	Florida	567	4.6%
11	Georgia	311	2.5%
50	Hawaii	14	0.1%
37	Idaho	84	0.7%
4	Illinois	629	5.1%
10	Indiana	322	2.6%
29	Iowa	151	1.2%
26	Kansas	162	1.3%
21	Kentucky	218	1.8%
30	Louisiana	144	1.2%
40	Maine	56	0.5%
25	Maryland	170	1.4%
15	Massachusetts	258	2.1%
8	Michigan	430	3.5%
22	Minnesota	204	1.6%
38	Mississippi	76	0.6%
16	Missouri	247	2.0%
43	Montana	40	0.3%
35	Nebraska	94	0.8%
39	Nevada	68	0.5%
42	New Hampshire	46	0.4%
13	New Jersey	306	2.5%
34	New Mexico	98	0.8%
3	New York	716	5.8%
9	North Carolina	346	2.8%
44	North Dakota	39	0.3%
5	Ohio	612	4.9%
22	Oklahoma	204	1.6%
33	Oregon	131	1.1%
7	Pennsylvania	509	4.1%
41	Rhode Island	53	0.4%
32	South Carolina	133	1.1%
46	South Dakota	35	0.3%
18	Tennessee	245	2.0%
2	Texas	1,060	8.5%
27	Utah	154	1.2%
45	Vermont	37	0.3%
14	Virginia	261	2.1%
20	Washington	225	1.8%
36	West Virginia	88	0.7%
16	Wisconsin	247	2.0%
48	Wyoming	21	0.2%

RANK ORDER

RANK	STATE	DEATHS	% of USA
1	California	1,525	12.3%
2	Texas	1,060	8.5%
3	New York	716	5.8%
4	Illinois	629	5.1%
5	Ohio	612	4.9%
6	Florida	567	4.6%
7	Pennsylvania	509	4.1%
8	Michigan	430	3.5%
9	North Carolina	346	2.8%
10	Indiana	322	2.6%
11	Georgia	311	2.5%
12	Arizona	308	2.5%
13	New Jersey	306	2.5%
14	Virginia	261	2.1%
15	Massachusetts	258	2.1%
16	Missouri	247	2.0%
16	Wisconsin	247	2.0%
18	Tennessee	245	2.0%
19	Colorado	231	1.9%
20	Washington	225	1.8%
21	Kentucky	218	1.8%
22	Minnesota	204	1.6%
22	Oklahoma	204	1.6%
24	Alabama	188	1.5%
25	Maryland	170	1.4%
26	Kansas	162	1.3%
27	Utah	154	1.2%
28	Connecticut	153	1.2%
29	Iowa	151	1.2%
30	Louisiana	144	1.2%
31	Arkansas	134	1.1%
32	South Carolina	133	1.1%
33	Oregon	131	1.1%
34	New Mexico	98	0.8%
35	Nebraska	94	0.8%
36	West Virginia	88	0.7%
37	Idaho	84	0.7%
38	Mississippi	76	0.6%
39	Nevada	68	0.5%
40	Maine	56	0.5%
41	Rhode Island	53	0.4%
42	New Hampshire	46	0.4%
43	Montana	40	0.3%
44	North Dakota	39	0.3%
45	Vermont	37	0.3%
46	South Dakota	35	0.3%
47	Delaware	32	0.3%
48	Wyoming	21	0.2%
49	Alaska	19	0.2%
50	Hawaii	14	0.1%
	District of Columbia	5	0.0%

Source: U.S. Department of Health and Human Services, National Center for Health Statistics
  "National Vital Statistics Reports" (Vol. 48, No. 11, July 24, 2000)
*Final data. Deaths of infants under 28 days, exclusive of fetal deaths. Based on race of the mother.

White Neonatal Death Rate in 1998

National Rate = 4.0 White Neonatal Deaths per 1,000 White Live Births*

<table>
<tr><td colspan="3">ALPHA ORDER</td><td colspan="3">RANK ORDER</td></tr>
<tr><th>RANK</th><th>STATE</th><th>RATE</th><th>RANK</th><th>STATE</th><th>RATE</th></tr>
<tr><td>8</td><td>Alabama</td><td>4.5</td><td>1</td><td>Vermont</td><td>5.7</td></tr>
<tr><td>NA</td><td>Alaska**</td><td>NA</td><td>2</td><td>North Dakota</td><td>5.5</td></tr>
<tr><td>8</td><td>Arizona</td><td>4.5</td><td>3</td><td>Oklahoma</td><td>5.2</td></tr>
<tr><td>6</td><td>Arkansas</td><td>4.7</td><td>4</td><td>Ohio</td><td>4.8</td></tr>
<tr><td>38</td><td>California</td><td>3.6</td><td>4</td><td>Rhode Island</td><td>4.8</td></tr>
<tr><td>16</td><td>Colorado</td><td>4.3</td><td>6</td><td>Arkansas</td><td>4.7</td></tr>
<tr><td>20</td><td>Connecticut</td><td>4.2</td><td>6</td><td>Kansas</td><td>4.7</td></tr>
<tr><td>20</td><td>Delaware</td><td>4.2</td><td>8</td><td>Alabama</td><td>4.5</td></tr>
<tr><td>31</td><td>Florida</td><td>3.9</td><td>8</td><td>Arizona</td><td>4.5</td></tr>
<tr><td>29</td><td>Georgia</td><td>4.0</td><td>8</td><td>Idaho</td><td>4.5</td></tr>
<tr><td>NA</td><td>Hawaii**</td><td>NA</td><td>8</td><td>Illinois</td><td>4.5</td></tr>
<tr><td>8</td><td>Idaho</td><td>4.5</td><td>8</td><td>Kentucky</td><td>4.5</td></tr>
<tr><td>8</td><td>Illinois</td><td>4.5</td><td>13</td><td>Nebraska</td><td>4.4</td></tr>
<tr><td>16</td><td>Indiana</td><td>4.3</td><td>13</td><td>North Carolina</td><td>4.4</td></tr>
<tr><td>16</td><td>Iowa</td><td>4.3</td><td>13</td><td>West Virginia</td><td>4.4</td></tr>
<tr><td>6</td><td>Kansas</td><td>4.7</td><td>16</td><td>Colorado</td><td>4.3</td></tr>
<tr><td>8</td><td>Kentucky</td><td>4.5</td><td>16</td><td>Indiana</td><td>4.3</td></tr>
<tr><td>33</td><td>Louisiana</td><td>3.8</td><td>16</td><td>Iowa</td><td>4.3</td></tr>
<tr><td>20</td><td>Maine</td><td>4.2</td><td>16</td><td>New Mexico</td><td>4.3</td></tr>
<tr><td>33</td><td>Maryland</td><td>3.8</td><td>20</td><td>Connecticut</td><td>4.2</td></tr>
<tr><td>37</td><td>Massachusetts</td><td>3.7</td><td>20</td><td>Delaware</td><td>4.2</td></tr>
<tr><td>27</td><td>Michigan</td><td>4.1</td><td>20</td><td>Maine</td><td>4.2</td></tr>
<tr><td>38</td><td>Minnesota</td><td>3.6</td><td>20</td><td>Montana</td><td>4.2</td></tr>
<tr><td>44</td><td>Mississippi</td><td>3.3</td><td>20</td><td>Pennsylvania</td><td>4.2</td></tr>
<tr><td>29</td><td>Missouri</td><td>4.0</td><td>20</td><td>South Dakota</td><td>4.2</td></tr>
<tr><td>20</td><td>Montana</td><td>4.2</td><td>20</td><td>Wisconsin</td><td>4.2</td></tr>
<tr><td>13</td><td>Nebraska</td><td>4.4</td><td>27</td><td>Michigan</td><td>4.1</td></tr>
<tr><td>48</td><td>Nevada</td><td>2.8</td><td>27</td><td>Tennessee</td><td>4.1</td></tr>
<tr><td>44</td><td>New Hampshire</td><td>3.3</td><td>29</td><td>Georgia</td><td>4.0</td></tr>
<tr><td>38</td><td>New Jersey</td><td>3.6</td><td>29</td><td>Missouri</td><td>4.0</td></tr>
<tr><td>16</td><td>New Mexico</td><td>4.3</td><td>31</td><td>Florida</td><td>3.9</td></tr>
<tr><td>33</td><td>New York</td><td>3.8</td><td>31</td><td>South Carolina</td><td>3.9</td></tr>
<tr><td>13</td><td>North Carolina</td><td>4.4</td><td>33</td><td>Louisiana</td><td>3.8</td></tr>
<tr><td>2</td><td>North Dakota</td><td>5.5</td><td>33</td><td>Maryland</td><td>3.8</td></tr>
<tr><td>4</td><td>Ohio</td><td>4.8</td><td>33</td><td>New York</td><td>3.8</td></tr>
<tr><td>3</td><td>Oklahoma</td><td>5.2</td><td>33</td><td>Virginia</td><td>3.8</td></tr>
<tr><td>47</td><td>Oregon</td><td>3.1</td><td>37</td><td>Massachusetts</td><td>3.7</td></tr>
<tr><td>20</td><td>Pennsylvania</td><td>4.2</td><td>38</td><td>California</td><td>3.6</td></tr>
<tr><td>4</td><td>Rhode Island</td><td>4.8</td><td>38</td><td>Minnesota</td><td>3.6</td></tr>
<tr><td>31</td><td>South Carolina</td><td>3.9</td><td>38</td><td>New Jersey</td><td>3.6</td></tr>
<tr><td>20</td><td>South Dakota</td><td>4.2</td><td>38</td><td>Texas</td><td>3.6</td></tr>
<tr><td>27</td><td>Tennessee</td><td>4.1</td><td>38</td><td>Utah</td><td>3.6</td></tr>
<tr><td>38</td><td>Texas</td><td>3.6</td><td>38</td><td>Wyoming</td><td>3.6</td></tr>
<tr><td>38</td><td>Utah</td><td>3.6</td><td>44</td><td>Mississippi</td><td>3.3</td></tr>
<tr><td>1</td><td>Vermont</td><td>5.7</td><td>44</td><td>New Hampshire</td><td>3.3</td></tr>
<tr><td>33</td><td>Virginia</td><td>3.8</td><td>44</td><td>Washington</td><td>3.3</td></tr>
<tr><td>44</td><td>Washington</td><td>3.3</td><td>47</td><td>Oregon</td><td>3.1</td></tr>
<tr><td>13</td><td>West Virginia</td><td>4.4</td><td>48</td><td>Nevada</td><td>2.8</td></tr>
<tr><td>20</td><td>Wisconsin</td><td>4.2</td><td>NA</td><td>Alaska**</td><td>NA</td></tr>
<tr><td>38</td><td>Wyoming</td><td>3.6</td><td>NA</td><td>Hawaii**</td><td>NA</td></tr>
<tr><td></td><td></td><td></td><td></td><td>District of Columbia**</td><td>NA</td></tr>
</table>

Source: U.S. Department of Health and Human Services, National Center for Health Statistics
   "National Vital Statistics Reports" (Vol. 48, No. 11, July 24, 2000)
*Final data. Deaths of infants under 28 days, exclusive of fetal deaths. Based on race of the mother.
**Not available. Fewer than 20 white neonatal deaths.

Black Neonatal Deaths in 1998

National Total = 5,824 Deaths*

RANK	STATE	DEATHS	% of USA
13	Alabama	222	3.8%
47	Alaska	0	0.0%
28	Arizona	37	0.6%
22	Arkansas	68	1.2%
6	California	303	5.2%
30	Colorado	31	0.5%
22	Connecticut	68	1.2%
26	Delaware	41	0.7%
4	Florida	359	6.2%
2	Georgia	388	6.7%
40	Hawaii	4	0.1%
41	Idaho	2	0.0%
3	Illinois	375	6.4%
20	Indiana	111	1.9%
35	Iowa	13	0.2%
34	Kansas	15	0.3%
25	Kentucky	45	0.8%
10	Louisiana	251	4.3%
41	Maine	2	0.0%
9	Maryland	266	4.6%
24	Massachusetts	51	0.9%
8	Michigan	268	4.6%
29	Minnesota	32	0.5%
16	Mississippi	188	3.2%
19	Missouri	124	2.1%
44	Montana	1	0.0%
33	Nebraska	16	0.3%
32	Nevada	22	0.4%
41	New Hampshire	2	0.0%
16	New Jersey	188	3.2%
38	New Mexico	6	0.1%
1	New York	400	6.9%
5	North Carolina	356	6.1%
47	North Dakota	0	0.0%
15	Ohio	203	3.5%
27	Oklahoma	40	0.7%
38	Oregon	6	0.1%
14	Pennsylvania	210	3.6%
36	Rhode Island	11	0.2%
12	South Carolina	228	3.9%
44	South Dakota	1	0.0%
18	Tennessee	183	3.1%
7	Texas	274	4.7%
47	Utah	0	0.0%
47	Vermont	0	0.0%
11	Virginia	244	4.2%
31	Washington	27	0.5%
37	West Virginia	7	0.1%
21	Wisconsin	87	1.5%
44	Wyoming	1	0.0%

RANK	STATE	DEATHS	% of USA
1	New York	400	6.9%
2	Georgia	388	6.7%
3	Illinois	375	6.4%
4	Florida	359	6.2%
5	North Carolina	356	6.1%
6	California	303	5.2%
7	Texas	274	4.7%
8	Michigan	268	4.6%
9	Maryland	266	4.6%
10	Louisiana	251	4.3%
11	Virginia	244	4.2%
12	South Carolina	228	3.9%
13	Alabama	222	3.8%
14	Pennsylvania	210	3.6%
15	Ohio	203	3.5%
16	Mississippi	188	3.2%
16	New Jersey	188	3.2%
18	Tennessee	183	3.1%
19	Missouri	124	2.1%
20	Indiana	111	1.9%
21	Wisconsin	87	1.5%
22	Arkansas	68	1.2%
22	Connecticut	68	1.2%
24	Massachusetts	51	0.9%
25	Kentucky	45	0.8%
26	Delaware	41	0.7%
27	Oklahoma	40	0.7%
28	Arizona	37	0.6%
29	Minnesota	32	0.5%
30	Colorado	31	0.5%
31	Washington	27	0.5%
32	Nevada	22	0.4%
33	Nebraska	16	0.3%
34	Kansas	15	0.3%
35	Iowa	13	0.2%
36	Rhode Island	11	0.2%
37	West Virginia	7	0.1%
38	New Mexico	6	0.1%
38	Oregon	6	0.1%
40	Hawaii	4	0.1%
41	Idaho	2	0.0%
41	Maine	2	0.0%
41	New Hampshire	2	0.0%
44	Montana	1	0.0%
44	South Dakota	1	0.0%
44	Wyoming	1	0.0%
47	Alaska	0	0.0%
47	North Dakota	0	0.0%
47	Utah	0	0.0%
47	Vermont	0	0.0%
	District of Columbia	47	0.8%

Source: U.S. Department of Health and Human Services, National Center for Health Statistics
"National Vital Statistics Reports" (Vol. 48, No. 11, July 24, 2000)
Final data. Deaths of infants under 28 days, exclusive of fetal deaths. Based on race of the mother.

Black Neonatal Death Rate in 1998

National Rate = 9.5 Black Neonatal Deaths per 1,000 Black Live Births*

<table>
<tr><td colspan="3">ALPHA ORDER</td><td colspan="3">RANK ORDER</td></tr>
<tr><td>RANK</td><td>STATE</td><td>RATE</td><td>RANK</td><td>STATE</td><td>RATE</td></tr>
<tr><td>8</td><td>Alabama</td><td>11.1</td><td>1</td><td>Delaware</td><td>15.6</td></tr>
<tr><td>NA</td><td>Alaska**</td><td>NA</td><td>2</td><td>Arizona</td><td>13.9</td></tr>
<tr><td>2</td><td>Arizona</td><td>13.9</td><td>3</td><td>Wisconsin</td><td>13.3</td></tr>
<tr><td>26</td><td>Arkansas</td><td>8.5</td><td>4</td><td>North Carolina</td><td>12.6</td></tr>
<tr><td>28</td><td>California</td><td>8.2</td><td>5</td><td>Connecticut</td><td>12.5</td></tr>
<tr><td>13</td><td>Colorado</td><td>10.8</td><td>6</td><td>South Carolina</td><td>12.1</td></tr>
<tr><td>5</td><td>Connecticut</td><td>12.5</td><td>7</td><td>Indiana</td><td>12.0</td></tr>
<tr><td>1</td><td>Delaware</td><td>15.6</td><td>8</td><td>Alabama</td><td>11.1</td></tr>
<tr><td>29</td><td>Florida</td><td>8.1</td><td>8</td><td>Maryland</td><td>11.1</td></tr>
<tr><td>19</td><td>Georgia</td><td>9.4</td><td>8</td><td>Virginia</td><td>11.1</td></tr>
<tr><td>NA</td><td>Hawaii**</td><td>NA</td><td>11</td><td>Michigan</td><td>11.0</td></tr>
<tr><td>NA</td><td>Idaho**</td><td>NA</td><td>12</td><td>Missouri</td><td>10.9</td></tr>
<tr><td>15</td><td>Illinois</td><td>10.5</td><td>13</td><td>Colorado</td><td>10.8</td></tr>
<tr><td>7</td><td>Indiana</td><td>12.0</td><td>13</td><td>Tennessee</td><td>10.8</td></tr>
<tr><td>NA</td><td>Iowa**</td><td>NA</td><td>15</td><td>Illinois</td><td>10.5</td></tr>
<tr><td>NA</td><td>Kansas**</td><td>NA</td><td>16</td><td>Pennsylvania</td><td>10.1</td></tr>
<tr><td>20</td><td>Kentucky</td><td>9.3</td><td>17</td><td>Nevada</td><td>9.8</td></tr>
<tr><td>21</td><td>Louisiana</td><td>9.1</td><td>18</td><td>Mississippi</td><td>9.7</td></tr>
<tr><td>NA</td><td>Maine**</td><td>NA</td><td>19</td><td>Georgia</td><td>9.4</td></tr>
<tr><td>8</td><td>Maryland</td><td>11.1</td><td>20</td><td>Kentucky</td><td>9.3</td></tr>
<tr><td>32</td><td>Massachusetts</td><td>6.5</td><td>21</td><td>Louisiana</td><td>9.1</td></tr>
<tr><td>11</td><td>Michigan</td><td>11.0</td><td>22</td><td>Ohio</td><td>8.9</td></tr>
<tr><td>24</td><td>Minnesota</td><td>8.7</td><td>23</td><td>New Jersey</td><td>8.8</td></tr>
<tr><td>18</td><td>Mississippi</td><td>9.7</td><td>24</td><td>Minnesota</td><td>8.7</td></tr>
<tr><td>12</td><td>Missouri</td><td>10.9</td><td>24</td><td>Washington</td><td>8.7</td></tr>
<tr><td>NA</td><td>Montana**</td><td>NA</td><td>26</td><td>Arkansas</td><td>8.5</td></tr>
<tr><td>NA</td><td>Nebraska**</td><td>NA</td><td>27</td><td>Oklahoma</td><td>8.3</td></tr>
<tr><td>17</td><td>Nevada</td><td>9.8</td><td>28</td><td>California</td><td>8.2</td></tr>
<tr><td>NA</td><td>New Hampshire**</td><td>NA</td><td>29</td><td>Florida</td><td>8.1</td></tr>
<tr><td>23</td><td>New Jersey</td><td>8.8</td><td>30</td><td>New York</td><td>7.3</td></tr>
<tr><td>NA</td><td>New Mexico**</td><td>NA</td><td>31</td><td>Texas</td><td>6.8</td></tr>
<tr><td>30</td><td>New York</td><td>7.3</td><td>32</td><td>Massachusetts</td><td>6.5</td></tr>
<tr><td>4</td><td>North Carolina</td><td>12.6</td><td>NA</td><td>Alaska**</td><td>NA</td></tr>
<tr><td>NA</td><td>North Dakota**</td><td>NA</td><td>NA</td><td>Hawaii**</td><td>NA</td></tr>
<tr><td>22</td><td>Ohio</td><td>8.9</td><td>NA</td><td>Idaho**</td><td>NA</td></tr>
<tr><td>27</td><td>Oklahoma</td><td>8.3</td><td>NA</td><td>Iowa**</td><td>NA</td></tr>
<tr><td>NA</td><td>Oregon**</td><td>NA</td><td>NA</td><td>Kansas**</td><td>NA</td></tr>
<tr><td>16</td><td>Pennsylvania</td><td>10.1</td><td>NA</td><td>Maine**</td><td>NA</td></tr>
<tr><td>NA</td><td>Rhode Island**</td><td>NA</td><td>NA</td><td>Montana**</td><td>NA</td></tr>
<tr><td>6</td><td>South Carolina</td><td>12.1</td><td>NA</td><td>Nebraska**</td><td>NA</td></tr>
<tr><td>NA</td><td>South Dakota**</td><td>NA</td><td>NA</td><td>New Hampshire**</td><td>NA</td></tr>
<tr><td>13</td><td>Tennessee</td><td>10.8</td><td>NA</td><td>New Mexico**</td><td>NA</td></tr>
<tr><td>31</td><td>Texas</td><td>6.8</td><td>NA</td><td>North Dakota**</td><td>NA</td></tr>
<tr><td>NA</td><td>Utah**</td><td>NA</td><td>NA</td><td>Oregon**</td><td>NA</td></tr>
<tr><td>NA</td><td>Vermont**</td><td>NA</td><td>NA</td><td>Rhode Island**</td><td>NA</td></tr>
<tr><td>8</td><td>Virginia</td><td>11.1</td><td>NA</td><td>South Dakota**</td><td>NA</td></tr>
<tr><td>24</td><td>Washington</td><td>8.7</td><td>NA</td><td>Utah**</td><td>NA</td></tr>
<tr><td>NA</td><td>West Virginia**</td><td>NA</td><td>NA</td><td>Vermont**</td><td>NA</td></tr>
<tr><td>3</td><td>Wisconsin</td><td>13.3</td><td>NA</td><td>West Virginia**</td><td>NA</td></tr>
<tr><td>NA</td><td>Wyoming**</td><td>NA</td><td>NA</td><td>Wyoming**</td><td>NA</td></tr>
<tr><td></td><td></td><td></td><td></td><td>District of Columbia</td><td>8.6</td></tr>
</table>

Source: U.S. Department of Health and Human Services, National Center for Health Statistics
    "National Vital Statistics Reports" (Vol. 48, No. 11, July 24, 2000)
*Final data. Deaths of infants under 28 days, exclusive of fetal deaths. Based on race of the mother.
**Not available. Fewer than 20 black neonatal deaths.

Deaths by AIDS Through 1998

National Total = 324,029 Deaths*

RANK	STATE	DEATHS	% of USA
23	Alabama	2,748	0.8%
46	Alaska	176	0.1%
21	Arizona	3,276	1.0%
32	Arkansas	1,091	0.3%
2	California	53,837	16.6%
22	Colorado	3,186	1.0%
17	Connecticut	4,087	1.3%
36	Delaware	915	0.3%
3	Florida	31,219	9.6%
6	Georgia	11,394	3.5%
35	Hawaii	962	0.3%
44	Idaho	253	0.1%
7	Illinois	10,680	3.3%
24	Indiana	2,476	0.8%
39	Iowa	612	0.2%
33	Kansas	1,029	0.3%
31	Kentucky	1,325	0.4%
14	Louisiana	5,540	1.7%
42	Maine	493	0.2%
9	Maryland	8,404	2.6%
11	Massachusetts	6,480	2.0%
15	Michigan	5,484	1.7%
28	Minnesota	1,783	0.6%
26	Mississippi	1,895	0.6%
19	Missouri	3,544	1.1%
47	Montana	163	0.1%
40	Nebraska	503	0.2%
30	Nevada	1,442	0.4%
43	New Hampshire	341	0.1%
5	New Jersey	19,547	6.0%
34	New Mexico	965	0.3%
1	New York	63,062	19.5%
10	North Carolina	6,834	2.1%
50	North Dakota	63	0.0%
12	Ohio	5,877	1.8%
27	Oklahoma	1,805	0.6%
25	Oregon	2,096	0.6%
8	Pennsylvania	10,000	3.1%
37	Rhode Island	802	0.2%
18	South Carolina	4,023	1.2%
48	South Dakota	94	0.0%
20	Tennessee	3,280	1.0%
4	Texas	22,200	6.9%
38	Utah	627	0.2%
45	Vermont	187	0.1%
13	Virginia	5,660	1.7%
16	Washington	4,248	1.3%
41	West Virginia	500	0.2%
29	Wisconsin	1,662	0.5%
49	Wyoming	80	0.0%

RANK	STATE	DEATHS	% of USA
1	New York	63,062	19.5%
2	California	53,837	16.6%
3	Florida	31,219	9.6%
4	Texas	22,200	6.9%
5	New Jersey	19,547	6.0%
6	Georgia	11,394	3.5%
7	Illinois	10,680	3.3%
8	Pennsylvania	10,000	3.1%
9	Maryland	8,404	2.6%
10	North Carolina	6,834	2.1%
11	Massachusetts	6,480	2.0%
12	Ohio	5,877	1.8%
13	Virginia	5,660	1.7%
14	Louisiana	5,540	1.7%
15	Michigan	5,484	1.7%
16	Washington	4,248	1.3%
17	Connecticut	4,087	1.3%
18	South Carolina	4,023	1.2%
19	Missouri	3,544	1.1%
20	Tennessee	3,280	1.0%
21	Arizona	3,276	1.0%
22	Colorado	3,186	1.0%
23	Alabama	2,748	0.8%
24	Indiana	2,476	0.8%
25	Oregon	2,096	0.6%
26	Mississippi	1,895	0.6%
27	Oklahoma	1,805	0.6%
28	Minnesota	1,783	0.6%
29	Wisconsin	1,662	0.5%
30	Nevada	1,442	0.4%
31	Kentucky	1,325	0.4%
32	Arkansas	1,091	0.3%
33	Kansas	1,029	0.3%
34	New Mexico	965	0.3%
35	Hawaii	962	0.3%
36	Delaware	915	0.3%
37	Rhode Island	802	0.2%
38	Utah	627	0.2%
39	Iowa	612	0.2%
40	Nebraska	503	0.2%
41	West Virginia	500	0.2%
42	Maine	493	0.2%
43	New Hampshire	341	0.1%
44	Idaho	253	0.1%
45	Vermont	187	0.1%
46	Alaska	176	0.1%
47	Montana	163	0.1%
48	South Dakota	94	0.0%
49	Wyoming	80	0.0%
50	North Dakota	63	0.0%
	District of Columbia	5,079	1.6%

Source: U.S. Department of Health and Human Services, National Center for Health Statistics (http://wonder.cdc.gov/WONDER/)

Cumulative deaths through 1998. However, due to reporting delays, these totals should increase. AIDS is Acquired Immunodeficiency Syndrome. The definition of what is AIDS was expanded in 1985, 1987 and 1993. Of these deaths, 276,558 were male and 47,471 were female.

Deaths by AIDS in 1998

National Total = 13,426 Deaths*

RANK ORDER

ALPHA ORDER					RANK ORDER			
RANK	STATE		DEATHS	% of USA	RANK	STATE	DEATHS	% of USA
18	Alabama		175	1.3%	1	New York	2,195	16.3%
46	Alaska		6	0.0%	2	Florida	1,546	11.5%
22	Arizona		138	1.0%	3	California	1,444	10.8%
29	Arkansas		66	0.5%	4	Texas	938	7.0%
3	California		1,444	10.8%	5	New Jersey	730	5.4%
26	Colorado		84	0.6%	6	Georgia	692	5.2%
19	Connecticut		168	1.3%	7	Maryland	502	3.7%
32	Delaware		55	0.4%	8	Illinois	488	3.6%
2	Florida		1,546	11.5%	9	Pennsylvania	483	3.6%
6	Georgia		692	5.2%	10	North Carolina	436	3.2%
38	Hawaii		22	0.2%	11	Louisiana	361	2.7%
42	Idaho		13	0.1%	12	Virginia	307	2.3%
8	Illinois		488	3.6%	13	Michigan	271	2.0%
24	Indiana		98	0.7%	14	South Carolina	270	2.0%
44	Iowa		9	0.1%	15	Tennessee	231	1.7%
35	Kansas		26	0.2%	16	Ohio	220	1.6%
27	Kentucky		78	0.6%	17	Massachusetts	213	1.6%
11	Louisiana		361	2.7%	18	Alabama	175	1.3%
41	Maine		15	0.1%	19	Connecticut	168	1.3%
7	Maryland		502	3.7%	20	Missouri	146	1.1%
17	Massachusetts		213	1.6%	21	Mississippi	140	1.0%
13	Michigan		271	2.0%	22	Arizona	138	1.0%
32	Minnesota		55	0.4%	23	Washington	116	0.9%
21	Mississippi		140	1.0%	24	Indiana	98	0.7%
20	Missouri		146	1.1%	25	Oklahoma	85	0.6%
45	Montana		7	0.1%	26	Colorado	84	0.6%
37	Nebraska		24	0.2%	27	Kentucky	78	0.6%
28	Nevada		73	0.5%	28	Nevada	73	0.5%
42	New Hampshire		13	0.1%	29	Arkansas	66	0.5%
5	New Jersey		730	5.4%	30	Wisconsin	60	0.4%
34	New Mexico		41	0.3%	31	Oregon	57	0.4%
1	New York		2,195	16.3%	32	Delaware	55	0.4%
10	North Carolina		436	3.2%	32	Minnesota	55	0.4%
49	North Dakota		2	0.0%	34	New Mexico	41	0.3%
16	Ohio		220	1.6%	35	Kansas	26	0.2%
25	Oklahoma		85	0.6%	35	Rhode Island	26	0.2%
31	Oregon		57	0.4%	37	Nebraska	24	0.2%
9	Pennsylvania		483	3.6%	38	Hawaii	22	0.2%
35	Rhode Island		26	0.2%	39	West Virginia	20	0.1%
14	South Carolina		270	2.0%	40	Utah	17	0.1%
46	South Dakota		6	0.0%	41	Maine	15	0.1%
15	Tennessee		231	1.7%	42	Idaho	13	0.1%
4	Texas		938	7.0%	42	New Hampshire	13	0.1%
40	Utah		17	0.1%	44	Iowa	9	0.1%
46	Vermont		6	0.0%	45	Montana	7	0.1%
12	Virginia		307	2.3%	46	Alaska	6	0.0%
23	Washington		116	0.9%	46	South Dakota	6	0.0%
39	West Virginia		20	0.1%	46	Vermont	6	0.0%
30	Wisconsin		60	0.4%	49	North Dakota	2	0.0%
49	Wyoming		2	0.0%	49	Wyoming	2	0.0%
						District of Columbia	250	1.9%

Source: U.S. Department of Health and Human Services, National Center for Health Statistics
   "National Vital Statistics Reports" (Vol. 48, No. 11, July 24, 2000)
*AIDS is Acquired Immunodeficiency Syndrome. It is a specific group of diseases or conditions which are indicative
of severe immunosuppression related to infection with the Human Immunodeficiency Virus (HIV).

Death Rate by AIDS in 1998

National Rate = 5.0 Deaths per 100,000 Population*

	ALPHA ORDER				RANK ORDER	
RANK	STATE	RATE		RANK	STATE	RATE
18	Alabama	4.0		1	New York	12.1
NA	Alaska**	NA		2	Florida	10.4
21	Arizona	3.0		3	Maryland	9.8
24	Arkansas	2.6		4	Georgia	9.1
14	California	4.4		5	New Jersey	9.0
28	Colorado	2.1		6	Louisiana	8.3
10	Connecticut	5.1		7	Delaware	7.4
7	Delaware	7.4		8	South Carolina	7.0
2	Florida	10.4		9	North Carolina	5.8
4	Georgia	9.1		10	Connecticut	5.1
32	Hawaii	1.8		10	Mississippi	5.1
NA	Idaho**	NA		12	Texas	4.7
17	Illinois	4.1		13	Virginia	4.5
33	Indiana	1.7		14	California	4.4
NA	Iowa**	NA		15	Tennessee	4.3
39	Kansas	1.0		16	Nevada	4.2
29	Kentucky	2.0		17	Illinois	4.1
6	Louisiana	8.3		18	Alabama	4.0
NA	Maine**	NA		18	Pennsylvania	4.0
3	Maryland	9.8		20	Massachusetts	3.5
20	Massachusetts	3.5		21	Arizona	3.0
22	Michigan	2.8		22	Michigan	2.8
36	Minnesota	1.2		23	Missouri	2.7
10	Mississippi	5.1		24	Arkansas	2.6
23	Missouri	2.7		24	Rhode Island	2.6
NA	Montana**	NA		26	Oklahoma	2.5
35	Nebraska	1.4		27	New Mexico	2.4
16	Nevada	4.2		28	Colorado	2.1
NA	New Hampshire**	NA		29	Kentucky	2.0
5	New Jersey	9.0		29	Ohio	2.0
27	New Mexico	2.4		29	Washington	2.0
1	New York	12.1		32	Hawaii	1.8
9	North Carolina	5.8		33	Indiana	1.7
NA	North Dakota**	NA		33	Oregon	1.7
29	Ohio	2.0		35	Nebraska	1.4
26	Oklahoma	2.5		36	Minnesota	1.2
33	Oregon	1.7		37	West Virginia	1.1
18	Pennsylvania	4.0		37	Wisconsin	1.1
24	Rhode Island	2.6		39	Kansas	1.0
8	South Carolina	7.0		NA	Alaska**	NA
NA	South Dakota**	NA		NA	Idaho**	NA
15	Tennessee	4.3		NA	Iowa**	NA
12	Texas	4.7		NA	Maine**	NA
NA	Utah**	NA		NA	Montana**	NA
NA	Vermont**	NA		NA	New Hampshire**	NA
13	Virginia	4.5		NA	North Dakota**	NA
29	Washington	2.0		NA	South Dakota**	NA
37	West Virginia	1.1		NA	Utah**	NA
37	Wisconsin	1.1		NA	Vermont**	NA
NA	Wyoming**	NA		NA	Wyoming**	NA

District of Columbia   47.8

Source: U.S. Department of Health and Human Services, National Center for Health Statistics
    "National Vital Statistics Reports" (Vol. 48, No. 11, July 24, 2000)
*AIDS is Acquired Immunodeficiency Syndrome. It is a specific group of diseases or conditions which are indicative of severe immunosuppression related to infection with the Human Immunodeficiency Virus (HIV). Not age-adjusted.
**Insufficient data to determine a reliable rate.

Age-Adjusted Death Rate by AIDS in 1998

National Rate = 4.6 Deaths per 100,000 Population*

<table>
<tr><td colspan="3"><u>ALPHA ORDER</u></td><td colspan="3"><u>RANK ORDER</u></td></tr>
<tr><td>RANK</td><td>STATE</td><td>RATE</td><td>RANK</td><td>STATE</td><td>RATE</td></tr>
<tr><td>17</td><td>Alabama</td><td>3.8</td><td>1</td><td>New York</td><td>11.0</td></tr>
<tr><td>NA</td><td>Alaska**</td><td>NA</td><td>2</td><td>Florida</td><td>10.2</td></tr>
<tr><td>21</td><td>Arizona</td><td>2.9</td><td>3</td><td>Maryland</td><td>8.7</td></tr>
<tr><td>22</td><td>Arkansas</td><td>2.6</td><td>4</td><td>Georgia</td><td>8.2</td></tr>
<tr><td>13</td><td>California</td><td>4.1</td><td>4</td><td>Louisiana</td><td>8.2</td></tr>
<tr><td>28</td><td>Colorado</td><td>1.9</td><td>6</td><td>New Jersey</td><td>8.0</td></tr>
<tr><td>11</td><td>Connecticut</td><td>4.7</td><td>7</td><td>Delaware</td><td>6.6</td></tr>
<tr><td>7</td><td>Delaware</td><td>6.6</td><td>8</td><td>South Carolina</td><td>6.5</td></tr>
<tr><td>2</td><td>Florida</td><td>10.2</td><td>9</td><td>North Carolina</td><td>5.4</td></tr>
<tr><td>4</td><td>Georgia</td><td>8.2</td><td>10</td><td>Mississippi</td><td>5.0</td></tr>
<tr><td>32</td><td>Hawaii</td><td>1.8</td><td>11</td><td>Connecticut</td><td>4.7</td></tr>
<tr><td>NA</td><td>Idaho**</td><td>NA</td><td>12</td><td>Texas</td><td>4.6</td></tr>
<tr><td>17</td><td>Illinois</td><td>3.8</td><td>13</td><td>California</td><td>4.1</td></tr>
<tr><td>33</td><td>Indiana</td><td>1.6</td><td>14</td><td>Virginia</td><td>4.0</td></tr>
<tr><td>NA</td><td>Iowa**</td><td>NA</td><td>15</td><td>Nevada</td><td>3.9</td></tr>
<tr><td>38</td><td>Kansas</td><td>1.0</td><td>15</td><td>Tennessee</td><td>3.9</td></tr>
<tr><td>28</td><td>Kentucky</td><td>1.9</td><td>17</td><td>Alabama</td><td>3.8</td></tr>
<tr><td>4</td><td>Louisiana</td><td>8.2</td><td>17</td><td>Illinois</td><td>3.8</td></tr>
<tr><td>NA</td><td>Maine**</td><td>NA</td><td>17</td><td>Pennsylvania</td><td>3.8</td></tr>
<tr><td>3</td><td>Maryland</td><td>8.7</td><td>20</td><td>Massachusetts</td><td>3.1</td></tr>
<tr><td>20</td><td>Massachusetts</td><td>3.1</td><td>21</td><td>Arizona</td><td>2.9</td></tr>
<tr><td>25</td><td>Michigan</td><td>2.5</td><td>22</td><td>Arkansas</td><td>2.6</td></tr>
<tr><td>36</td><td>Minnesota</td><td>1.1</td><td>22</td><td>Missouri</td><td>2.6</td></tr>
<tr><td>10</td><td>Mississippi</td><td>5.0</td><td>22</td><td>Oklahoma</td><td>2.6</td></tr>
<tr><td>22</td><td>Missouri</td><td>2.6</td><td>25</td><td>Michigan</td><td>2.5</td></tr>
<tr><td>NA</td><td>Montana**</td><td>NA</td><td>26</td><td>New Mexico</td><td>2.4</td></tr>
<tr><td>35</td><td>Nebraska</td><td>1.4</td><td>27</td><td>Rhode Island</td><td>2.3</td></tr>
<tr><td>15</td><td>Nevada</td><td>3.9</td><td>28</td><td>Colorado</td><td>1.9</td></tr>
<tr><td>NA</td><td>New Hampshire**</td><td>NA</td><td>28</td><td>Kentucky</td><td>1.9</td></tr>
<tr><td>6</td><td>New Jersey</td><td>8.0</td><td>28</td><td>Ohio</td><td>1.9</td></tr>
<tr><td>26</td><td>New Mexico</td><td>2.4</td><td>28</td><td>Washington</td><td>1.9</td></tr>
<tr><td>1</td><td>New York</td><td>11.0</td><td>32</td><td>Hawaii</td><td>1.8</td></tr>
<tr><td>9</td><td>North Carolina</td><td>5.4</td><td>33</td><td>Indiana</td><td>1.6</td></tr>
<tr><td>NA</td><td>North Dakota**</td><td>NA</td><td>33</td><td>Oregon</td><td>1.6</td></tr>
<tr><td>28</td><td>Ohio</td><td>1.9</td><td>35</td><td>Nebraska</td><td>1.4</td></tr>
<tr><td>22</td><td>Oklahoma</td><td>2.6</td><td>36</td><td>Minnesota</td><td>1.1</td></tr>
<tr><td>33</td><td>Oregon</td><td>1.6</td><td>36</td><td>Wisconsin</td><td>1.1</td></tr>
<tr><td>17</td><td>Pennsylvania</td><td>3.8</td><td>38</td><td>Kansas</td><td>1.0</td></tr>
<tr><td>27</td><td>Rhode Island</td><td>2.3</td><td>38</td><td>West Virginia</td><td>1.0</td></tr>
<tr><td>8</td><td>South Carolina</td><td>6.5</td><td>NA</td><td>Alaska**</td><td>NA</td></tr>
<tr><td>NA</td><td>South Dakota**</td><td>NA</td><td>NA</td><td>Idaho**</td><td>NA</td></tr>
<tr><td>15</td><td>Tennessee</td><td>3.9</td><td>NA</td><td>Iowa**</td><td>NA</td></tr>
<tr><td>12</td><td>Texas</td><td>4.6</td><td>NA</td><td>Maine**</td><td>NA</td></tr>
<tr><td>NA</td><td>Utah**</td><td>NA</td><td>NA</td><td>Montana**</td><td>NA</td></tr>
<tr><td>NA</td><td>Vermont**</td><td>NA</td><td>NA</td><td>New Hampshire**</td><td>NA</td></tr>
<tr><td>14</td><td>Virginia</td><td>4.0</td><td>NA</td><td>North Dakota**</td><td>NA</td></tr>
<tr><td>28</td><td>Washington</td><td>1.9</td><td>NA</td><td>South Dakota**</td><td>NA</td></tr>
<tr><td>38</td><td>West Virginia</td><td>1.0</td><td>NA</td><td>Utah**</td><td>NA</td></tr>
<tr><td>36</td><td>Wisconsin</td><td>1.1</td><td>NA</td><td>Vermont**</td><td>NA</td></tr>
<tr><td>NA</td><td>Wyoming**</td><td>NA</td><td>NA</td><td>Wyoming**</td><td>NA</td></tr>
<tr><td></td><td></td><td></td><td></td><td>District of Columbia</td><td>41.3</td></tr>
</table>

Source: U.S. Department of Health and Human Services, National Center for Health Statistics
"National Vital Statistics Reports" (Vol. 48, No. 11, July 24, 2000)
*AIDS is Acquired Immunodeficiency Syndrome. It is a specific group of diseases or conditions which are indicative of severe immunosuppression related to infection with the Human Immunodeficiency Virus (HIV).
**Insufficient data to determine a reliable rate.

Estimated Deaths by Cancer in 2001

National Estimated Total = 553,400 Deaths

ALPHA ORDER

RANK	STATE	DEATHS	% of USA
20	Alabama	9,900	1.8%
50	Alaska	700	0.1%
22	Arizona	9,300	1.7%
31	Arkansas	6,100	1.1%
1	California	51,200	9.3%
30	Colorado	6,200	1.1%
28	Connecticut	7,000	1.3%
45	Delaware	1,800	0.3%
2	Florida	40,000	7.2%
12	Georgia	13,600	2.5%
43	Hawaii	2,000	0.4%
42	Idaho	2,200	0.4%
7	Illinois	24,800	4.5%
14	Indiana	12,800	2.3%
29	Iowa	6,500	1.2%
33	Kansas	5,300	1.0%
23	Kentucky	9,200	1.7%
21	Louisiana	9,500	1.7%
37	Maine	3,000	0.5%
19	Maryland	10,300	1.9%
11	Massachusetts	13,700	2.5%
8	Michigan	19,800	3.6%
24	Minnesota	9,000	1.6%
31	Mississippi	6,100	1.1%
16	Missouri	12,400	2.2%
44	Montana	1,900	0.3%
36	Nebraska	3,300	0.6%
35	Nevada	4,000	0.7%
39	New Hampshire	2,500	0.5%
9	New Jersey	18,000	3.3%
37	New Mexico	3,000	0.5%
3	New York	36,300	6.6%
10	North Carolina	16,300	2.9%
47	North Dakota	1,300	0.2%
6	Ohio	25,400	4.6%
26	Oklahoma	7,300	1.3%
26	Oregon	7,300	1.3%
5	Pennsylvania	29,800	5.4%
41	Rhode Island	2,400	0.4%
25	South Carolina	8,200	1.5%
46	South Dakota	1,600	0.3%
15	Tennessee	12,600	2.3%
4	Texas	34,400	6.2%
39	Utah	2,500	0.5%
48	Vermont	1,200	0.2%
13	Virginia	13,300	2.4%
18	Washington	10,800	2.0%
34	West Virginia	4,800	0.9%
17	Wisconsin	10,900	2.0%
49	Wyoming	1,000	0.2%

RANK ORDER

RANK	STATE	DEATHS	% of USA
1	California	51,200	9.3%
2	Florida	40,000	7.2%
3	New York	36,300	6.6%
4	Texas	34,400	6.2%
5	Pennsylvania	29,800	5.4%
6	Ohio	25,400	4.6%
7	Illinois	24,800	4.5%
8	Michigan	19,800	3.6%
9	New Jersey	18,000	3.3%
10	North Carolina	16,300	2.9%
11	Massachusetts	13,700	2.5%
12	Georgia	13,600	2.5%
13	Virginia	13,300	2.4%
14	Indiana	12,800	2.3%
15	Tennessee	12,600	2.3%
16	Missouri	12,400	2.2%
17	Wisconsin	10,900	2.0%
18	Washington	10,800	2.0%
19	Maryland	10,300	1.9%
20	Alabama	9,900	1.8%
21	Louisiana	9,500	1.7%
22	Arizona	9,300	1.7%
23	Kentucky	9,200	1.7%
24	Minnesota	9,000	1.6%
25	South Carolina	8,200	1.5%
26	Oklahoma	7,300	1.3%
26	Oregon	7,300	1.3%
28	Connecticut	7,000	1.3%
29	Iowa	6,500	1.2%
30	Colorado	6,200	1.1%
31	Arkansas	6,100	1.1%
31	Mississippi	6,100	1.1%
33	Kansas	5,300	1.0%
34	West Virginia	4,800	0.9%
35	Nevada	4,000	0.7%
36	Nebraska	3,300	0.6%
37	Maine	3,000	0.5%
37	New Mexico	3,000	0.5%
39	New Hampshire	2,500	0.5%
39	Utah	2,500	0.5%
41	Rhode Island	2,400	0.4%
42	Idaho	2,200	0.4%
43	Hawaii	2,000	0.4%
44	Montana	1,900	0.3%
45	Delaware	1,800	0.3%
46	South Dakota	1,600	0.3%
47	North Dakota	1,300	0.2%
48	Vermont	1,200	0.2%
49	Wyoming	1,000	0.2%
50	Alaska	700	0.1%
	District of Columbia	1,200	0.2%

Source: American Cancer Society
"Cancer Facts & Figures 2001" (Copyright 2001, Reprinted with permission from the American Cancer Society)

Estimated Death Rate by Cancer in 2001

National Estimated Rate = 196.6 Deaths per 100,000 Population*

ALPHA ORDER

RANK ORDER

RANK	STATE	RATE
10	Alabama	222.6
50	Alaska	111.7
41	Arizona	181.3
7	Arkansas	228.2
47	California	151.2
48	Colorado	144.1
23	Connecticut	205.5
5	Delaware	229.7
2	Florida	250.3
43	Georgia	166.1
44	Hawaii	165.1
42	Idaho	170.0
31	Illinois	199.7
22	Indiana	210.5
11	Iowa	222.1
33	Kansas	197.1
8	Kentucky	227.6
18	Louisiana	212.6
4	Maine	235.3
35	Maryland	194.5
14	Massachusetts	215.8
32	Michigan	199.2
40	Minnesota	182.9
15	Mississippi	214.4
12	Missouri	221.6
21	Montana	210.6
36	Nebraska	192.8
30	Nevada	200.2
29	New Hampshire	202.3
16	New Jersey	213.9
46	New Mexico	164.9
37	New York	191.3
26	North Carolina	202.5
28	North Dakota	202.4
9	Ohio	223.7
20	Oklahoma	211.6
17	Oregon	213.4
3	Pennsylvania	242.7
6	Rhode Island	228.9
24	South Carolina	204.4
19	South Dakota	212.0
13	Tennessee	221.5
45	Texas	165.0
49	Utah	111.9
33	Vermont	197.1
38	Virginia	187.9
39	Washington	183.2
1	West Virginia	265.4
25	Wisconsin	203.2
26	Wyoming	202.5

RANK	STATE	RATE
1	West Virginia	265.4
2	Florida	250.3
3	Pennsylvania	242.7
4	Maine	235.3
5	Delaware	229.7
6	Rhode Island	228.9
7	Arkansas	228.2
8	Kentucky	227.6
9	Ohio	223.7
10	Alabama	222.6
11	Iowa	222.1
12	Missouri	221.6
13	Tennessee	221.5
14	Massachusetts	215.8
15	Mississippi	214.4
16	New Jersey	213.9
17	Oregon	213.4
18	Louisiana	212.6
19	South Dakota	212.0
20	Oklahoma	211.6
21	Montana	210.6
22	Indiana	210.5
23	Connecticut	205.5
24	South Carolina	204.4
25	Wisconsin	203.2
26	North Carolina	202.5
26	Wyoming	202.5
28	North Dakota	202.4
29	New Hampshire	202.3
30	Nevada	200.2
31	Illinois	199.7
32	Michigan	199.2
33	Kansas	197.1
33	Vermont	197.1
35	Maryland	194.5
36	Nebraska	192.8
37	New York	191.3
38	Virginia	187.9
39	Washington	183.2
40	Minnesota	182.9
41	Arizona	181.3
42	Idaho	170.0
43	Georgia	166.1
44	Hawaii	165.1
45	Texas	165.0
46	New Mexico	164.9
47	California	151.2
48	Colorado	144.1
49	Utah	111.9
50	Alaska	111.7
	District of Columbia	209.8

Source: Morgan Quitno Press using data from American Cancer Society
   "Cancer Facts & Figures 2001" (Copyright 2001, Reprinted with permission from the American Cancer Society)
*Rates calculated using 2000 Census resident population figures. Not age-adjusted.

Estimated Deaths by Female Breast Cancer in 2001

National Estimated Total = 40,200 Deaths

ALPHA ORDER

RANK	STATE	DEATHS	% of USA
23	Alabama	600	1.5%
43	Alaska	100	0.2%
19	Arizona	700	1.7%
30	Arkansas	400	1.0%
1	California	3,900	9.7%
30	Colorado	400	1.0%
26	Connecticut	500	1.2%
43	Delaware	100	0.2%
3	Florida	2,600	6.5%
11	Georgia	1,000	2.5%
43	Hawaii	100	0.2%
35	Idaho	200	0.5%
6	Illinois	1,900	4.7%
14	Indiana	900	2.2%
26	Iowa	500	1.2%
30	Kansas	400	1.0%
23	Kentucky	600	1.5%
19	Louisiana	700	1.7%
35	Maine	200	0.5%
16	Maryland	800	2.0%
11	Massachusetts	1,000	2.5%
8	Michigan	1,400	3.5%
19	Minnesota	700	1.7%
30	Mississippi	400	1.0%
16	Missouri	800	2.0%
43	Montana	100	0.2%
35	Nebraska	200	0.5%
35	Nevada	200	0.5%
35	New Hampshire	200	0.5%
8	New Jersey	1,400	3.5%
35	New Mexico	200	0.5%
2	New York	3,000	7.5%
10	North Carolina	1,100	2.7%
43	North Dakota	100	0.2%
6	Ohio	1,900	4.7%
26	Oklahoma	500	1.2%
26	Oregon	500	1.2%
5	Pennsylvania	2,200	5.5%
35	Rhode Island	200	0.5%
23	South Carolina	600	1.5%
43	South Dakota	100	0.2%
14	Tennessee	900	2.2%
3	Texas	2,600	6.5%
35	Utah	200	0.5%
43	Vermont	100	0.2%
11	Virginia	1,000	2.5%
16	Washington	800	2.0%
34	West Virginia	300	0.7%
19	Wisconsin	700	1.7%
43	Wyoming	100	0.2%

RANK ORDER

RANK	STATE	DEATHS	% of USA
1	California	3,900	9.7%
2	New York	3,000	7.5%
3	Florida	2,600	6.5%
3	Texas	2,600	6.5%
5	Pennsylvania	2,200	5.5%
6	Illinois	1,900	4.7%
6	Ohio	1,900	4.7%
8	Michigan	1,400	3.5%
8	New Jersey	1,400	3.5%
10	North Carolina	1,100	2.7%
11	Georgia	1,000	2.5%
11	Massachusetts	1,000	2.5%
11	Virginia	1,000	2.5%
14	Indiana	900	2.2%
14	Tennessee	900	2.2%
16	Maryland	800	2.0%
16	Missouri	800	2.0%
16	Washington	800	2.0%
19	Arizona	700	1.7%
19	Louisiana	700	1.7%
19	Minnesota	700	1.7%
19	Wisconsin	700	1.7%
23	Alabama	600	1.5%
23	Kentucky	600	1.5%
23	South Carolina	600	1.5%
26	Connecticut	500	1.2%
26	Iowa	500	1.2%
26	Oklahoma	500	1.2%
26	Oregon	500	1.2%
30	Arkansas	400	1.0%
30	Colorado	400	1.0%
30	Kansas	400	1.0%
30	Mississippi	400	1.0%
34	West Virginia	300	0.7%
35	Idaho	200	0.5%
35	Maine	200	0.5%
35	Nebraska	200	0.5%
35	Nevada	200	0.5%
35	New Hampshire	200	0.5%
35	New Mexico	200	0.5%
35	Rhode Island	200	0.5%
35	Utah	200	0.5%
43	Alaska	100	0.2%
43	Delaware	100	0.2%
43	Hawaii	100	0.2%
43	Montana	100	0.2%
43	North Dakota	100	0.2%
43	South Dakota	100	0.2%
43	Vermont	100	0.2%
43	Wyoming	100	0.2%
	District of Columbia	100	0.2%

Source: American Cancer Society
   "Cancer Facts & Figures 2001" (Copyright 2001, Reprinted with permission from the American Cancer Society)

Estimated Death Rate by Female Breast Cancer in 2001

National Estimated Rate = 28.8 Deaths per 100,000 Female Population*

ALPHA ORDER

RANK	STATE	RATE
38	Alabama	26.4
4	Alaska	34.0
29	Arizona	29.0
20	Arkansas	30.3
43	California	23.5
48	Colorado	19.6
25	Connecticut	29.6
40	Delaware	25.8
6	Florida	33.4
42	Georgia	25.0
50	Hawaii	16.9
12	Idaho	31.9
19	Illinois	30.6
26	Indiana	29.5
4	Iowa	34.0
24	Kansas	29.7
26	Kentucky	29.5
18	Louisiana	30.9
17	Maine	31.2
21	Maryland	30.1
16	Massachusetts	31.3
35	Michigan	27.6
30	Minnesota	28.9
34	Mississippi	27.7
32	Missouri	28.4
46	Montana	22.5
43	Nebraska	23.5
46	Nevada	22.5
9	New Hampshire	32.8
6	New Jersey	33.4
45	New Mexico	22.6
13	New York	31.8
33	North Carolina	27.9
15	North Dakota	31.4
10	Ohio	32.7
28	Oklahoma	29.1
22	Oregon	29.8
3	Pennsylvania	35.3
2	Rhode Island	38.9
22	South Carolina	29.8
37	South Dakota	26.8
14	Tennessee	31.7
41	Texas	25.6
49	Utah	18.7
8	Vermont	33.2
31	Virginia	28.5
35	Washington	27.6
11	West Virginia	32.0
39	Wisconsin	26.2
1	Wyoming	41.9

RANK ORDER

RANK	STATE	RATE
1	Wyoming	41.9
2	Rhode Island	38.9
3	Pennsylvania	35.3
4	Alaska	34.0
4	Iowa	34.0
6	Florida	33.4
6	New Jersey	33.4
8	Vermont	33.2
9	New Hampshire	32.8
10	Ohio	32.7
11	West Virginia	32.0
12	Idaho	31.9
13	New York	31.8
14	Tennessee	31.7
15	North Dakota	31.4
16	Massachusetts	31.3
17	Maine	31.2
18	Louisiana	30.9
19	Illinois	30.6
20	Arkansas	30.3
21	Maryland	30.1
22	Oregon	29.8
22	South Carolina	29.8
24	Kansas	29.7
25	Connecticut	29.6
26	Indiana	29.5
26	Kentucky	29.5
28	Oklahoma	29.1
29	Arizona	29.0
30	Minnesota	28.9
31	Virginia	28.5
32	Missouri	28.4
33	North Carolina	27.9
34	Mississippi	27.7
35	Michigan	27.6
35	Washington	27.6
37	South Dakota	26.8
38	Alabama	26.4
39	Wisconsin	26.2
40	Delaware	25.8
41	Texas	25.6
42	Georgia	25.0
43	California	23.5
43	Nebraska	23.5
45	New Mexico	22.6
46	Montana	22.5
46	Nevada	22.5
48	Colorado	19.6
49	Utah	18.7
50	Hawaii	16.9
	District of Columbia	36.2

Source: Morgan Quitno Press using data from American Cancer Society
"Cancer Facts & Figures 2001" (Copyright 2001, Reprinted with permission from the American Cancer Society)
*Rates calculated using 1999 Census resident female population estimates. Not age-adjusted.

Estimated Deaths by Colon and Rectum Cancer in 2001

National Estimated Total = 56,700 Deaths

<u>ALPHA ORDER</u>

RANK	STATE	DEATHS	% of USA
24	Alabama	800	1.4%
48	Alaska	100	0.2%
21	Arizona	900	1.6%
30	Arkansas	600	1.1%
1	California	4,900	8.6%
30	Colorado	600	1.1%
27	Connecticut	700	1.2%
42	Delaware	200	0.4%
3	Florida	4,000	7.1%
15	Georgia	1,200	2.1%
42	Hawaii	200	0.4%
42	Idaho	200	0.4%
7	Illinois	2,600	4.6%
12	Indiana	1,400	2.5%
24	Iowa	800	1.4%
33	Kansas	500	0.9%
21	Kentucky	900	1.6%
19	Louisiana	1,000	1.8%
37	Maine	300	0.5%
17	Maryland	1,100	1.9%
11	Massachusetts	1,500	2.6%
8	Michigan	2,100	3.7%
21	Minnesota	900	1.6%
30	Mississippi	600	1.1%
14	Missouri	1,300	2.3%
42	Montana	200	0.4%
35	Nebraska	400	0.7%
35	Nevada	400	0.7%
37	New Hampshire	300	0.5%
9	New Jersey	1,900	3.4%
37	New Mexico	300	0.5%
2	New York	4,100	7.2%
10	North Carolina	1,700	3.0%
48	North Dakota	100	0.2%
6	Ohio	2,700	4.8%
27	Oklahoma	700	1.2%
27	Oregon	700	1.2%
5	Pennsylvania	3,300	5.8%
37	Rhode Island	300	0.5%
24	South Carolina	800	1.4%
42	South Dakota	200	0.4%
15	Tennessee	1,200	2.1%
4	Texas	3,600	6.3%
37	Utah	300	0.5%
42	Vermont	200	0.4%
12	Virginia	1,400	2.5%
19	Washington	1,000	1.8%
33	West Virginia	500	0.9%
17	Wisconsin	1,100	1.9%
48	Wyoming	100	0.2%

<u>RANK ORDER</u>

RANK	STATE	DEATHS	% of USA
1	California	4,900	8.6%
2	New York	4,100	7.2%
3	Florida	4,000	7.1%
4	Texas	3,600	6.3%
5	Pennsylvania	3,300	5.8%
6	Ohio	2,700	4.8%
7	Illinois	2,600	4.6%
8	Michigan	2,100	3.7%
9	New Jersey	1,900	3.4%
10	North Carolina	1,700	3.0%
11	Massachusetts	1,500	2.6%
12	Indiana	1,400	2.5%
12	Virginia	1,400	2.5%
14	Missouri	1,300	2.3%
15	Georgia	1,200	2.1%
15	Tennessee	1,200	2.1%
17	Maryland	1,100	1.9%
17	Wisconsin	1,100	1.9%
19	Louisiana	1,000	1.8%
19	Washington	1,000	1.8%
21	Arizona	900	1.6%
21	Kentucky	900	1.6%
21	Minnesota	900	1.6%
24	Alabama	800	1.4%
24	Iowa	800	1.4%
24	South Carolina	800	1.4%
27	Connecticut	700	1.2%
27	Oklahoma	700	1.2%
27	Oregon	700	1.2%
30	Arkansas	600	1.1%
30	Colorado	600	1.1%
30	Mississippi	600	1.1%
33	Kansas	500	0.9%
33	West Virginia	500	0.9%
35	Nebraska	400	0.7%
35	Nevada	400	0.7%
37	Maine	300	0.5%
37	New Hampshire	300	0.5%
37	New Mexico	300	0.5%
37	Rhode Island	300	0.5%
37	Utah	300	0.5%
42	Delaware	200	0.4%
42	Hawaii	200	0.4%
42	Idaho	200	0.4%
42	Montana	200	0.4%
42	South Dakota	200	0.4%
42	Vermont	200	0.4%
48	Alaska	100	0.2%
48	North Dakota	100	0.2%
48	Wyoming	100	0.2%
	District of Columbia	100	0.2%

Source: American Cancer Society
"Cancer Facts & Figures 2001" (Copyright 2001, Reprinted with permission from the American Cancer Society)

Estimated Death Rate by Colon and Rectum Cancer in 2001

National Estimated Rate = 20.1 Deaths per 100,000 Population*

ALPHA ORDER

RANK ORDER

RANK	STATE	RATE		RANK	STATE	RATE
38	Alabama	18.0		1	Vermont	32.9
44	Alaska	16.0		2	Rhode Island	28.6
39	Arizona	17.5		3	West Virginia	27.6
17	Arkansas	22.4		4	Iowa	27.3
48	California	14.5		5	Pennsylvania	26.9
49	Colorado	13.9		6	South Dakota	26.5
28	Connecticut	20.6		7	Delaware	25.5
7	Delaware	25.5		8	Florida	25.0
8	Florida	25.0		9	New Hampshire	24.3
47	Georgia	14.7		10	Ohio	23.8
42	Hawaii	16.5		11	Massachusetts	23.6
46	Idaho	15.5		12	Maine	23.5
26	Illinois	20.9		13	Nebraska	23.4
15	Indiana	23.0		14	Missouri	23.2
4	Iowa	27.3		15	Indiana	23.0
36	Kansas	18.6		16	New Jersey	22.6
19	Kentucky	22.3		17	Arkansas	22.4
17	Louisiana	22.4		17	Louisiana	22.4
12	Maine	23.5		19	Kentucky	22.3
27	Maryland	20.8		20	Montana	22.2
11	Massachusetts	23.6		21	New York	21.6
22	Michigan	21.1		22	Michigan	21.1
37	Minnesota	18.3		22	Mississippi	21.1
22	Mississippi	21.1		22	North Carolina	21.1
14	Missouri	23.2		22	Tennessee	21.1
20	Montana	22.2		26	Illinois	20.9
13	Nebraska	23.4		27	Maryland	20.8
33	Nevada	20.0		28	Connecticut	20.6
9	New Hampshire	24.3		29	Oregon	20.5
16	New Jersey	22.6		29	Wisconsin	20.5
42	New Mexico	16.5		31	Oklahoma	20.3
21	New York	21.6		31	Wyoming	20.3
22	North Carolina	21.1		33	Nevada	20.0
45	North Dakota	15.6		34	South Carolina	19.9
10	Ohio	23.8		35	Virginia	19.8
31	Oklahoma	20.3		36	Kansas	18.6
29	Oregon	20.5		37	Minnesota	18.3
5	Pennsylvania	26.9		38	Alabama	18.0
2	Rhode Island	28.6		39	Arizona	17.5
34	South Carolina	19.9		40	Texas	17.3
6	South Dakota	26.5		41	Washington	17.0
22	Tennessee	21.1		42	Hawaii	16.5
40	Texas	17.3		42	New Mexico	16.5
50	Utah	13.4		44	Alaska	16.0
1	Vermont	32.9		45	North Dakota	15.6
35	Virginia	19.8		46	Idaho	15.5
41	Washington	17.0		47	Georgia	14.7
3	West Virginia	27.6		48	California	14.5
29	Wisconsin	20.5		49	Colorado	13.9
31	Wyoming	20.3		50	Utah	13.4
					District of Columbia	17.5

Source: Morgan Quitno Press using data from American Cancer Society
   "Cancer Facts & Figures 2001" (Copyright 2001, Reprinted with permission from the American Cancer Society)
*Rates calculated using 2000 Census resident population figures. Not age-adjusted.

Estimated Deaths by Leukemia in 2001

National Estimated Total = 21,500 Deaths

ALPHA ORDER

ALPHA ORDER

RANK	STATE	DEATHS	% of USA
18	Alabama	400	1.9%
NA	Alaska*	NA	NA
22	Arizona	300	1.4%
31	Arkansas	200	0.9%
1	California	2,100	9.8%
22	Colorado	300	1.4%
22	Connecticut	300	1.4%
36	Delaware	100	0.5%
2	Florida	1,500	7.0%
11	Georgia	500	2.3%
36	Hawaii	100	0.5%
36	Idaho	100	0.5%
6	Illinois	1,000	4.7%
11	Indiana	500	2.3%
22	Iowa	300	1.4%
31	Kansas	200	0.9%
22	Kentucky	300	1.4%
22	Louisiana	300	1.4%
36	Maine	100	0.5%
18	Maryland	400	1.9%
11	Massachusetts	500	2.3%
9	Michigan	700	3.3%
18	Minnesota	400	1.9%
31	Mississippi	200	0.9%
11	Missouri	500	2.3%
36	Montana	100	0.5%
31	Nebraska	200	0.9%
36	Nevada	100	0.5%
36	New Hampshire	100	0.5%
8	New Jersey	800	3.7%
36	New Mexico	100	0.5%
3	New York	1,400	6.5%
10	North Carolina	600	2.8%
36	North Dakota	100	0.5%
6	Ohio	1,000	4.7%
22	Oklahoma	300	1.4%
22	Oregon	300	1.4%
5	Pennsylvania	1,100	5.1%
36	Rhode Island	100	0.5%
22	South Carolina	300	1.4%
36	South Dakota	100	0.5%
11	Tennessee	500	2.3%
3	Texas	1,400	6.5%
36	Utah	100	0.5%
NA	Vermont*	NA	NA
11	Virginia	500	2.3%
18	Washington	400	1.9%
31	West Virginia	200	0.9%
11	Wisconsin	500	2.3%
NA	Wyoming*	NA	NA

RANK ORDER

RANK	STATE	DEATHS	% of USA
1	California	2,100	9.8%
2	Florida	1,500	7.0%
3	New York	1,400	6.5%
3	Texas	1,400	6.5%
5	Pennsylvania	1,100	5.1%
6	Illinois	1,000	4.7%
6	Ohio	1,000	4.7%
8	New Jersey	800	3.7%
9	Michigan	700	3.3%
10	North Carolina	600	2.8%
11	Georgia	500	2.3%
11	Indiana	500	2.3%
11	Massachusetts	500	2.3%
11	Missouri	500	2.3%
11	Tennessee	500	2.3%
11	Virginia	500	2.3%
11	Wisconsin	500	2.3%
18	Alabama	400	1.9%
18	Maryland	400	1.9%
18	Minnesota	400	1.9%
18	Washington	400	1.9%
22	Arizona	300	1.4%
22	Colorado	300	1.4%
22	Connecticut	300	1.4%
22	Iowa	300	1.4%
22	Kentucky	300	1.4%
22	Louisiana	300	1.4%
22	Oklahoma	300	1.4%
22	Oregon	300	1.4%
22	South Carolina	300	1.4%
31	Arkansas	200	0.9%
31	Kansas	200	0.9%
31	Mississippi	200	0.9%
31	Nebraska	200	0.9%
31	West Virginia	200	0.9%
36	Delaware	100	0.5%
36	Hawaii	100	0.5%
36	Idaho	100	0.5%
36	Maine	100	0.5%
36	Montana	100	0.5%
36	Nevada	100	0.5%
36	New Hampshire	100	0.5%
36	New Mexico	100	0.5%
36	North Dakota	100	0.5%
36	Rhode Island	100	0.5%
36	South Dakota	100	0.5%
36	Utah	100	0.5%
NA	Alaska*	NA	NA
NA	Vermont*	NA	NA
NA	Wyoming*	NA	NA
	District of Columbia*	NA	NA

Source: American Cancer Society
   "Cancer Facts & Figures 2001" (Copyright 2001, Reprinted with permission from the American Cancer Society)
Fewer than 50 deaths.

Estimated Death Rate by Leukemia in 2001

National Estimated Rate = 7.6 Deaths per 100,000 Population*

ALPHA ORDER

RANK	STATE	RATE
12	Alabama	9.0
NA	Alaska**	NA
44	Arizona	5.8
29	Arkansas	7.5
42	California	6.2
36	Colorado	7.0
15	Connecticut	8.8
3	Delaware	12.8
10	Florida	9.4
43	Georgia	6.1
20	Hawaii	8.3
27	Idaho	7.7
22	Illinois	8.1
21	Indiana	8.2
7	Iowa	10.3
32	Kansas	7.4
32	Kentucky	7.4
40	Louisiana	6.7
26	Maine	7.8
28	Maryland	7.6
25	Massachusetts	7.9
36	Michigan	7.0
22	Minnesota	8.1
36	Mississippi	7.0
14	Missouri	8.9
5	Montana	11.1
4	Nebraska	11.7
46	Nevada	5.0
22	New Hampshire	8.1
8	New Jersey	9.5
45	New Mexico	5.5
32	New York	7.4
29	North Carolina	7.5
1	North Dakota	15.6
15	Ohio	8.8
19	Oklahoma	8.7
15	Oregon	8.8
12	Pennsylvania	9.0
8	Rhode Island	9.5
29	South Carolina	7.5
2	South Dakota	13.2
15	Tennessee	8.8
40	Texas	6.7
47	Utah	4.5
NA	Vermont**	NA
35	Virginia	7.1
39	Washington	6.8
5	West Virginia	11.1
11	Wisconsin	9.3
NA	Wyoming**	NA

RANK ORDER

RANK	STATE	RATE
1	North Dakota	15.6
2	South Dakota	13.2
3	Delaware	12.8
4	Nebraska	11.7
5	Montana	11.1
5	West Virginia	11.1
7	Iowa	10.3
8	New Jersey	9.5
8	Rhode Island	9.5
10	Florida	9.4
11	Wisconsin	9.3
12	Alabama	9.0
12	Pennsylvania	9.0
14	Missouri	8.9
15	Connecticut	8.8
15	Ohio	8.8
15	Oregon	8.8
15	Tennessee	8.8
19	Oklahoma	8.7
20	Hawaii	8.3
21	Indiana	8.2
22	Illinois	8.1
22	Minnesota	8.1
22	New Hampshire	8.1
25	Massachusetts	7.9
26	Maine	7.8
27	Idaho	7.7
28	Maryland	7.6
29	Arkansas	7.5
29	North Carolina	7.5
29	South Carolina	7.5
32	Kansas	7.4
32	Kentucky	7.4
32	New York	7.4
35	Virginia	7.1
36	Colorado	7.0
36	Michigan	7.0
36	Mississippi	7.0
39	Washington	6.8
40	Louisiana	6.7
40	Texas	6.7
42	California	6.2
43	Georgia	6.1
44	Arizona	5.8
45	New Mexico	5.5
46	Nevada	5.0
47	Utah	4.5
NA	Alaska**	NA
NA	Vermont**	NA
NA	Wyoming**	NA

District of Columbia** NA

Source: Morgan Quitno Press using data from American Cancer Society
    "Cancer Facts & Figures 2001" (Copyright 2001, Reprinted with permission from the American Cancer Society)
*Rates calculated using 2000 Census resident population figures. Not age-adjusted.
**Fewer than 50 deaths.

Estimated Deaths by Liver Cancer in 2001

National Estimated Total = 14,100 Deaths

<u>ALPHA ORDER</u>

RANK	STATE	DEATHS	% of USA
10	Alabama	300	2.1%
NA	Alaska*	NA	NA
20	Arizona	200	1.4%
20	Arkansas	200	1.4%
1	California	1,800	12.8%
30	Colorado	100	0.7%
20	Connecticut	200	1.4%
NA	Delaware*	NA	NA
3	Florida	1,000	7.1%
10	Georgia	300	2.1%
30	Hawaii	100	0.7%
NA	Idaho*	NA	NA
5	Illinois	700	5.0%
10	Indiana	300	2.1%
30	Iowa	100	0.7%
30	Kansas	100	0.7%
20	Kentucky	200	1.4%
10	Louisiana	300	2.1%
30	Maine	100	0.7%
20	Maryland	200	1.4%
10	Massachusetts	300	2.1%
7	Michigan	500	3.5%
20	Minnesota	200	1.4%
20	Mississippi	200	1.4%
10	Missouri	300	2.1%
NA	Montana*	NA	NA
30	Nebraska	100	0.7%
30	Nevada	100	0.7%
30	New Hampshire	100	0.7%
7	New Jersey	500	3.5%
30	New Mexico	100	0.7%
3	New York	1,000	7.1%
10	North Carolina	300	2.1%
NA	North Dakota*	NA	NA
7	Ohio	500	3.5%
20	Oklahoma	200	1.4%
30	Oregon	100	0.7%
5	Pennsylvania	700	5.0%
30	Rhode Island	100	0.7%
20	South Carolina	200	1.4%
NA	South Dakota*	NA	NA
10	Tennessee	300	2.1%
2	Texas	1,200	8.5%
30	Utah	100	0.7%
NA	Vermont*	NA	NA
10	Virginia	300	2.1%
10	Washington	300	2.1%
30	West Virginia	100	0.7%
20	Wisconsin	200	1.4%
NA	Wyoming*	NA	NA

<u>RANK ORDER</u>

RANK	STATE	DEATHS	% of USA
1	California	1,800	12.8%
2	Texas	1,200	8.5%
3	Florida	1,000	7.1%
3	New York	1,000	7.1%
5	Illinois	700	5.0%
5	Pennsylvania	700	5.0%
7	Michigan	500	3.5%
7	New Jersey	500	3.5%
7	Ohio	500	3.5%
10	Alabama	300	2.1%
10	Georgia	300	2.1%
10	Indiana	300	2.1%
10	Louisiana	300	2.1%
10	Massachusetts	300	2.1%
10	Missouri	300	2.1%
10	North Carolina	300	2.1%
10	Tennessee	300	2.1%
10	Virginia	300	2.1%
10	Washington	300	2.1%
20	Arizona	200	1.4%
20	Arkansas	200	1.4%
20	Connecticut	200	1.4%
20	Kentucky	200	1.4%
20	Maryland	200	1.4%
20	Minnesota	200	1.4%
20	Mississippi	200	1.4%
20	Oklahoma	200	1.4%
20	South Carolina	200	1.4%
20	Wisconsin	200	1.4%
30	Colorado	100	0.7%
30	Hawaii	100	0.7%
30	Iowa	100	0.7%
30	Kansas	100	0.7%
30	Maine	100	0.7%
30	Nebraska	100	0.7%
30	Nevada	100	0.7%
30	New Hampshire	100	0.7%
30	New Mexico	100	0.7%
30	Oregon	100	0.7%
30	Rhode Island	100	0.7%
30	Utah	100	0.7%
30	West Virginia	100	0.7%
NA	Alaska*	NA	NA
NA	Delaware*	NA	NA
NA	Idaho*	NA	NA
NA	Montana*	NA	NA
NA	North Dakota*	NA	NA
NA	South Dakota*	NA	NA
NA	Vermont*	NA	NA
NA	Wyoming*	NA	NA
	District of Columbia*	NA	NA

Source: American Cancer Society
"Cancer Facts & Figures 2001" (Copyright 2001, Reprinted with permission from the American Cancer Society)
Fewer than 50 deaths.

Estimate Death Rate by Liver Cancer in 2001

National Estimated Rate = 5.0 Deaths per 100,000 Population*

ALPHA ORDER

RANK	STATE	RATE
7	Alabama	6.7
NA	Alaska**	NA
34	Arizona	3.9
5	Arkansas	7.5
20	California	5.3
42	Colorado	2.3
10	Connecticut	5.9
NA	Delaware**	NA
9	Florida	6.3
36	Georgia	3.7
2	Hawaii	8.3
NA	Idaho**	NA
16	Illinois	5.6
27	Indiana	4.9
40	Iowa	3.4
36	Kansas	3.7
27	Kentucky	4.9
7	Louisiana	6.7
4	Maine	7.8
35	Maryland	3.8
29	Massachusetts	4.7
24	Michigan	5.0
33	Minnesota	4.1
6	Mississippi	7.0
19	Missouri	5.4
NA	Montana**	NA
12	Nebraska	5.8
24	Nevada	5.0
3	New Hampshire	8.1
10	New Jersey	5.9
17	New Mexico	5.5
20	New York	5.3
36	North Carolina	3.7
NA	North Dakota**	NA
31	Ohio	4.4
12	Oklahoma	5.8
41	Oregon	2.9
15	Pennsylvania	5.7
1	Rhode Island	9.5
24	South Carolina	5.0
NA	South Dakota**	NA
20	Tennessee	5.3
12	Texas	5.8
30	Utah	4.5
NA	Vermont**	NA
32	Virginia	4.2
23	Washington	5.1
17	West Virginia	5.5
36	Wisconsin	3.7
NA	Wyoming**	NA

RANK ORDER

RANK	STATE	RATE
1	Rhode Island	9.5
2	Hawaii	8.3
3	New Hampshire	8.1
4	Maine	7.8
5	Arkansas	7.5
6	Mississippi	7.0
7	Alabama	6.7
7	Louisiana	6.7
9	Florida	6.3
10	Connecticut	5.9
10	New Jersey	5.9
12	Nebraska	5.8
12	Oklahoma	5.8
12	Texas	5.8
15	Pennsylvania	5.7
16	Illinois	5.6
17	New Mexico	5.5
17	West Virginia	5.5
19	Missouri	5.4
20	California	5.3
20	New York	5.3
20	Tennessee	5.3
23	Washington	5.1
24	Michigan	5.0
24	Nevada	5.0
24	South Carolina	5.0
27	Indiana	4.9
27	Kentucky	4.9
29	Massachusetts	4.7
30	Utah	4.5
31	Ohio	4.4
32	Virginia	4.2
33	Minnesota	4.1
34	Arizona	3.9
35	Maryland	3.8
36	Georgia	3.7
36	Kansas	3.7
36	North Carolina	3.7
36	Wisconsin	3.7
40	Iowa	3.4
41	Oregon	2.9
42	Colorado	2.3
NA	Alaska**	NA
NA	Delaware**	NA
NA	Idaho**	NA
NA	Montana**	NA
NA	North Dakota**	NA
NA	South Dakota**	NA
NA	Vermont**	NA
NA	Wyoming**	NA
	District of Columbia**	NA

Source: Morgan Quitno Press using data from American Cancer Society
    "Cancer Facts & Figures 2001" (Copyright 2001, Reprinted with permission from the American Cancer Society)
*Rates calculated using 2000 Census resident population figures. Not age-adjusted.
**Fewer than 50 deaths.

117

Estimated Deaths by Lung Cancer in 2001

National Estimated Total = 157,400 Deaths

RANK	STATE	DEATHS	% of USA
20	Alabama	2,900	1.8%
49	Alaska	200	0.1%
23	Arizona	2,600	1.7%
28	Arkansas	2,000	1.3%
1	California	13,200	8.4%
32	Colorado	1,500	1.0%
29	Connecticut	1,900	1.2%
43	Delaware	500	0.3%
2	Florida	12,000	7.6%
11	Georgia	4,100	2.6%
41	Hawaii	600	0.4%
41	Idaho	600	0.4%
7	Illinois	6,900	4.4%
14	Indiana	3,900	2.5%
31	Iowa	1,800	1.1%
32	Kansas	1,500	1.0%
17	Kentucky	3,200	2.0%
22	Louisiana	2,700	1.7%
36	Maine	900	0.6%
19	Maryland	3,000	1.9%
16	Massachusetts	3,700	2.4%
8	Michigan	5,700	3.6%
26	Minnesota	2,300	1.5%
29	Mississippi	1,900	1.2%
12	Missouri	4,000	2.5%
43	Montana	500	0.3%
36	Nebraska	900	0.6%
35	Nevada	1,200	0.8%
38	New Hampshire	700	0.4%
10	New Jersey	4,600	2.9%
38	New Mexico	700	0.4%
4	New York	9,300	5.9%
9	North Carolina	5,000	3.2%
48	North Dakota	300	0.2%
6	Ohio	7,500	4.8%
24	Oklahoma	2,400	1.5%
27	Oregon	2,100	1.3%
5	Pennsylvania	8,200	5.2%
38	Rhode Island	700	0.4%
24	South Carolina	2,400	1.5%
45	South Dakota	400	0.3%
12	Tennessee	4,000	2.5%
3	Texas	10,200	6.5%
45	Utah	400	0.3%
45	Vermont	400	0.3%
14	Virginia	3,900	2.5%
18	Washington	3,100	2.0%
32	West Virginia	1,500	1.0%
21	Wisconsin	2,800	1.8%
49	Wyoming	200	0.1%

RANK	STATE	DEATHS	% of USA
1	California	13,200	8.4%
2	Florida	12,000	7.6%
3	Texas	10,200	6.5%
4	New York	9,300	5.9%
5	Pennsylvania	8,200	5.2%
6	Ohio	7,500	4.8%
7	Illinois	6,900	4.4%
8	Michigan	5,700	3.6%
9	North Carolina	5,000	3.2%
10	New Jersey	4,600	2.9%
11	Georgia	4,100	2.6%
12	Missouri	4,000	2.5%
12	Tennessee	4,000	2.5%
14	Indiana	3,900	2.5%
14	Virginia	3,900	2.5%
16	Massachusetts	3,700	2.4%
17	Kentucky	3,200	2.0%
18	Washington	3,100	2.0%
19	Maryland	3,000	1.9%
20	Alabama	2,900	1.8%
21	Wisconsin	2,800	1.8%
22	Louisiana	2,700	1.7%
23	Arizona	2,600	1.7%
24	Oklahoma	2,400	1.5%
24	South Carolina	2,400	1.5%
26	Minnesota	2,300	1.5%
27	Oregon	2,100	1.3%
28	Arkansas	2,000	1.3%
29	Connecticut	1,900	1.2%
29	Mississippi	1,900	1.2%
31	Iowa	1,800	1.1%
32	Colorado	1,500	1.0%
32	Kansas	1,500	1.0%
32	West Virginia	1,500	1.0%
35	Nevada	1,200	0.8%
36	Maine	900	0.6%
36	Nebraska	900	0.6%
38	New Hampshire	700	0.4%
38	New Mexico	700	0.4%
38	Rhode Island	700	0.4%
41	Hawaii	600	0.4%
41	Idaho	600	0.4%
43	Delaware	500	0.3%
43	Montana	500	0.3%
45	South Dakota	400	0.3%
45	Utah	400	0.3%
45	Vermont	400	0.3%
48	North Dakota	300	0.2%
49	Alaska	200	0.1%
49	Wyoming	200	0.1%
	District of Columbia	300	0.2%

Source: American Cancer Society
"Cancer Facts & Figures 2001" (Copyright 2001, Reprinted with permission from the American Cancer Society)

Estimated Death Rate by Lung Cancer in 2001

National Estimated Rate = 55.9 Deaths per 100,000 Population*

ALPHA ORDER

RANK ORDER

RANK	STATE	RATE		RANK	STATE	RATE
14	Alabama	65.2		1	West Virginia	82.9
49	Alaska	31.9		2	Kentucky	79.2
37	Arizona	50.7		3	Florida	75.1
4	Arkansas	74.8		4	Arkansas	74.8
46	California	39.0		5	Missouri	71.5
48	Colorado	34.9		6	Maine	70.6
27	Connecticut	55.8		7	Tennessee	70.3
16	Delaware	63.8		8	Oklahoma	69.6
3	Florida	75.1		9	Mississippi	66.8
38	Georgia	50.1		9	Pennsylvania	66.8
39	Hawaii	49.5		9	Rhode Island	66.8
44	Idaho	46.4		12	Ohio	66.1
29	Illinois	55.6		13	Vermont	65.7
15	Indiana	64.1		14	Alabama	65.2
18	Iowa	61.5		15	Indiana	64.1
27	Kansas	55.8		16	Delaware	63.8
2	Kentucky	79.2		17	North Carolina	62.1
20	Louisiana	60.4		18	Iowa	61.5
6	Maine	70.6		19	Oregon	61.4
25	Maryland	56.6		20	Louisiana	60.4
23	Massachusetts	58.3		21	Nevada	60.1
24	Michigan	57.4		22	South Carolina	59.8
42	Minnesota	46.8		23	Massachusetts	58.3
9	Mississippi	66.8		24	Michigan	57.4
5	Missouri	71.5		25	Maryland	56.6
30	Montana	55.4		25	New Hampshire	56.6
34	Nebraska	52.6		27	Connecticut	55.8
21	Nevada	60.1		27	Kansas	55.8
25	New Hampshire	56.6		29	Illinois	55.6
32	New Jersey	54.7		30	Montana	55.4
47	New Mexico	38.5		31	Virginia	55.1
40	New York	49.0		32	New Jersey	54.7
17	North Carolina	62.1		33	South Dakota	53.0
43	North Dakota	46.7		34	Nebraska	52.6
12	Ohio	66.1		34	Washington	52.6
8	Oklahoma	69.6		36	Wisconsin	52.2
19	Oregon	61.4		37	Arizona	50.7
9	Pennsylvania	66.8		38	Georgia	50.1
9	Rhode Island	66.8		39	Hawaii	49.5
22	South Carolina	59.8		40	New York	49.0
33	South Dakota	53.0		41	Texas	48.9
7	Tennessee	70.3		42	Minnesota	46.8
41	Texas	48.9		43	North Dakota	46.7
50	Utah	17.9		44	Idaho	46.4
13	Vermont	65.7		45	Wyoming	40.5
31	Virginia	55.1		46	California	39.0
34	Washington	52.6		47	New Mexico	38.5
1	West Virginia	82.9		48	Colorado	34.9
36	Wisconsin	52.2		49	Alaska	31.9
45	Wyoming	40.5		50	Utah	17.9

District of Columbia   52.4

Source: Morgan Quitno Press using data from American Cancer Society
   "Cancer Facts & Figures 2001" (Copyright 2001, Reprinted with permission from the American Cancer Society)
*Rates calculated using 2000 Census resident population figures. Not age-adjusted.

119

Estimated Deaths by Non-Hodgkin's Lymphoma in 2001

National Estimated Total = 26,300 Deaths

ALPHA ORDER

RANK	STATE	DEATHS	% of USA
21	Alabama	400	1.5%
NA	Alaska*	NA	NA
17	Arizona	500	1.9%
27	Arkansas	300	1.1%
1	California	2,500	9.5%
27	Colorado	300	1.1%
21	Connecticut	400	1.5%
39	Delaware	100	0.4%
2	Florida	2,000	7.6%
17	Georgia	500	1.9%
39	Hawaii	100	0.4%
39	Idaho	100	0.4%
7	Illinois	1,200	4.6%
12	Indiana	600	2.3%
27	Iowa	300	1.1%
32	Kansas	200	0.8%
21	Kentucky	400	1.5%
21	Louisiana	400	1.5%
32	Maine	200	0.8%
21	Maryland	400	1.5%
10	Massachusetts	700	2.7%
8	Michigan	1,000	3.8%
17	Minnesota	500	1.9%
32	Mississippi	200	0.8%
12	Missouri	600	2.3%
39	Montana	100	0.4%
32	Nebraska	200	0.8%
32	Nevada	200	0.8%
39	New Hampshire	100	0.4%
9	New Jersey	900	3.4%
39	New Mexico	100	0.4%
3	New York	1,700	6.5%
10	North Carolina	700	2.7%
39	North Dakota	100	0.4%
6	Ohio	1,300	4.9%
27	Oklahoma	300	1.1%
21	Oregon	400	1.5%
5	Pennsylvania	1,400	5.3%
39	Rhode Island	100	0.4%
27	South Carolina	300	1.1%
39	South Dakota	100	0.4%
12	Tennessee	600	2.3%
3	Texas	1,700	6.5%
32	Utah	200	0.8%
39	Vermont	100	0.4%
12	Virginia	600	2.3%
17	Washington	500	1.9%
32	West Virginia	200	0.8%
12	Wisconsin	600	2.3%
NA	Wyoming*	NA	NA

RANK ORDER

RANK	STATE	DEATHS	% of USA
1	California	2,500	9.5%
2	Florida	2,000	7.6%
3	New York	1,700	6.5%
3	Texas	1,700	6.5%
5	Pennsylvania	1,400	5.3%
6	Ohio	1,300	4.9%
7	Illinois	1,200	4.6%
8	Michigan	1,000	3.8%
9	New Jersey	900	3.4%
10	Massachusetts	700	2.7%
10	North Carolina	700	2.7%
12	Indiana	600	2.3%
12	Missouri	600	2.3%
12	Tennessee	600	2.3%
12	Virginia	600	2.3%
12	Wisconsin	600	2.3%
17	Arizona	500	1.9%
17	Georgia	500	1.9%
17	Minnesota	500	1.9%
17	Washington	500	1.9%
21	Alabama	400	1.5%
21	Connecticut	400	1.5%
21	Kentucky	400	1.5%
21	Louisiana	400	1.5%
21	Maryland	400	1.5%
21	Oregon	400	1.5%
27	Arkansas	300	1.1%
27	Colorado	300	1.1%
27	Iowa	300	1.1%
27	Oklahoma	300	1.1%
27	South Carolina	300	1.1%
32	Kansas	200	0.8%
32	Maine	200	0.8%
32	Mississippi	200	0.8%
32	Nebraska	200	0.8%
32	Nevada	200	0.8%
32	Utah	200	0.8%
32	West Virginia	200	0.8%
39	Delaware	100	0.4%
39	Hawaii	100	0.4%
39	Idaho	100	0.4%
39	Montana	100	0.4%
39	New Hampshire	100	0.4%
39	New Mexico	100	0.4%
39	North Dakota	100	0.4%
39	Rhode Island	100	0.4%
39	South Dakota	100	0.4%
39	Vermont	100	0.4%
NA	Alaska*	NA	NA
NA	Wyoming*	NA	NA
	District of Columbia*	NA	NA

Source: American Cancer Society
  "Cancer Facts & Figures 2001" (Copyright 2001, Reprinted with permission from the American Cancer Society)
*Fewer than 50 deaths.

Estimated Death Rate by Non-Hodgkin's Lymphoma in 2001

National Estimated Rate = 9.3 Deaths per 100,000 Population*

RANK	STATE	RATE
29	Alabama	9.0
NA	Alaska**	NA
26	Arizona	9.7
12	Arkansas	11.2
43	California	7.4
45	Colorado	7.0
7	Connecticut	11.7
5	Delaware	12.8
6	Florida	12.5
47	Georgia	6.1
37	Hawaii	8.3
40	Idaho	7.7
26	Illinois	9.7
24	Indiana	9.9
20	Iowa	10.3
43	Kansas	7.4
24	Kentucky	9.9
29	Louisiana	9.0
2	Maine	15.7
41	Maryland	7.6
16	Massachusetts	11.0
22	Michigan	10.1
21	Minnesota	10.2
45	Mississippi	7.0
17	Missouri	10.7
14	Montana	11.1
7	Nebraska	11.7
23	Nevada	10.0
39	New Hampshire	8.1
17	New Jersey	10.7
48	New Mexico	5.5
29	New York	9.0
33	North Carolina	8.7
3	North Dakota	15.6
10	Ohio	11.5
33	Oklahoma	8.7
7	Oregon	11.7
11	Pennsylvania	11.4
28	Rhode Island	9.5
42	South Carolina	7.5
4	South Dakota	13.2
19	Tennessee	10.5
38	Texas	8.2
29	Utah	9.0
1	Vermont	16.4
35	Virginia	8.5
35	Washington	8.5
14	West Virginia	11.1
12	Wisconsin	11.2
NA	Wyoming**	NA

RANK	STATE	RATE
1	Vermont	16.4
2	Maine	15.7
3	North Dakota	15.6
4	South Dakota	13.2
5	Delaware	12.8
6	Florida	12.5
7	Connecticut	11.7
7	Nebraska	11.7
7	Oregon	11.7
10	Ohio	11.5
11	Pennsylvania	11.4
12	Arkansas	11.2
12	Wisconsin	11.2
14	Montana	11.1
14	West Virginia	11.1
16	Massachusetts	11.0
17	Missouri	10.7
17	New Jersey	10.7
19	Tennessee	10.5
20	Iowa	10.3
21	Minnesota	10.2
22	Michigan	10.1
23	Nevada	10.0
24	Indiana	9.9
24	Kentucky	9.9
26	Arizona	9.7
26	Illinois	9.7
28	Rhode Island	9.5
29	Alabama	9.0
29	Louisiana	9.0
29	New York	9.0
29	Utah	9.0
33	North Carolina	8.7
33	Oklahoma	8.7
35	Virginia	8.5
35	Washington	8.5
37	Hawaii	8.3
38	Texas	8.2
39	New Hampshire	8.1
40	Idaho	7.7
41	Maryland	7.6
42	South Carolina	7.5
43	California	7.4
43	Kansas	7.4
45	Colorado	7.0
45	Mississippi	7.0
47	Georgia	6.1
48	New Mexico	5.5
NA	Alaska**	NA
NA	Wyoming**	NA
	District of Columbia**	NA

Source: Morgan Quitno Press using data from American Cancer Society
"Cancer Facts & Figures 2001" (Copyright 2001, Reprinted with permission from the American Cancer Society)
*Rates calculated using 2000 Census resident population figures. Not age-adjusted.
**Fewer than 50 deaths.

Estimated Deaths by Pancreatic Cancer in 2001

National Estimated Total = 28,900 Deaths

ALPHA ORDER

RANK	STATE	DEATHS	% of USA
20	Alabama	500	1.7%
NA	Alaska*	NA	NA
20	Arizona	500	1.7%
29	Arkansas	300	1.0%
1	California	2,800	9.7%
25	Colorado	400	1.4%
25	Connecticut	400	1.4%
39	Delaware	100	0.3%
3	Florida	2,100	7.3%
13	Georgia	600	2.1%
39	Hawaii	100	0.3%
39	Idaho	100	0.3%
6	Illinois	1,300	4.5%
13	Indiana	600	2.1%
29	Iowa	300	1.0%
29	Kansas	300	1.0%
25	Kentucky	400	1.4%
20	Louisiana	500	1.7%
34	Maine	200	0.7%
13	Maryland	600	2.1%
11	Massachusetts	700	2.4%
8	Michigan	1,100	3.8%
20	Minnesota	500	1.7%
29	Mississippi	300	1.0%
13	Missouri	600	2.1%
39	Montana	100	0.3%
34	Nebraska	200	0.7%
34	Nevada	200	0.7%
39	New Hampshire	100	0.3%
9	New Jersey	1,000	3.5%
34	New Mexico	200	0.7%
2	New York	2,200	7.6%
10	North Carolina	800	2.8%
39	North Dakota	100	0.3%
6	Ohio	1,300	4.5%
29	Oklahoma	300	1.0%
25	Oregon	400	1.4%
5	Pennsylvania	1,500	5.2%
39	Rhode Island	100	0.3%
20	South Carolina	500	1.7%
39	South Dakota	100	0.3%
13	Tennessee	600	2.1%
4	Texas	1,700	5.9%
39	Utah	100	0.3%
39	Vermont	100	0.3%
11	Virginia	700	2.4%
13	Washington	600	2.1%
34	West Virginia	200	0.7%
13	Wisconsin	600	2.1%
NA	Wyoming*	NA	NA

RANK ORDER

RANK	STATE	DEATHS	% of USA
1	California	2,800	9.7%
2	New York	2,200	7.6%
3	Florida	2,100	7.3%
4	Texas	1,700	5.9%
5	Pennsylvania	1,500	5.2%
6	Illinois	1,300	4.5%
6	Ohio	1,300	4.5%
8	Michigan	1,100	3.8%
9	New Jersey	1,000	3.5%
10	North Carolina	800	2.8%
11	Massachusetts	700	2.4%
11	Virginia	700	2.4%
13	Georgia	600	2.1%
13	Indiana	600	2.1%
13	Maryland	600	2.1%
13	Missouri	600	2.1%
13	Tennessee	600	2.1%
13	Washington	600	2.1%
13	Wisconsin	600	2.1%
20	Alabama	500	1.7%
20	Arizona	500	1.7%
20	Louisiana	500	1.7%
20	Minnesota	500	1.7%
20	South Carolina	500	1.7%
25	Colorado	400	1.4%
25	Connecticut	400	1.4%
25	Kentucky	400	1.4%
25	Oregon	400	1.4%
29	Arkansas	300	1.0%
29	Iowa	300	1.0%
29	Kansas	300	1.0%
29	Mississippi	300	1.0%
29	Oklahoma	300	1.0%
34	Maine	200	0.7%
34	Nebraska	200	0.7%
34	Nevada	200	0.7%
34	New Mexico	200	0.7%
34	West Virginia	200	0.7%
39	Delaware	100	0.3%
39	Hawaii	100	0.3%
39	Idaho	100	0.3%
39	Montana	100	0.3%
39	New Hampshire	100	0.3%
39	North Dakota	100	0.3%
39	Rhode Island	100	0.3%
39	South Dakota	100	0.3%
39	Utah	100	0.3%
39	Vermont	100	0.3%
NA	Alaska*	NA	NA
NA	Wyoming*	NA	NA
	District of Columbia	100	0.3%

Source: American Cancer Society
"Cancer Facts & Figures 2001" (Copyright 2001, Reprinted with permission from the American Cancer Society)
Fewer than 50 deaths.

Estimated Death Rate by Pancreatic Cancer in 2001

National Estimated Rate = 10.3 Deaths per 100,000 Population*

ALPHA ORDER

RANK	STATE	RATE
16	Alabama	11.2
NA	Alaska**	NA
38	Arizona	9.7
16	Arkansas	11.2
42	California	8.3
40	Colorado	9.3
10	Connecticut	11.7
6	Delaware	12.8
5	Florida	13.1
47	Georgia	7.3
42	Hawaii	8.3
46	Idaho	7.7
27	Illinois	10.5
34	Indiana	9.9
30	Iowa	10.3
16	Kansas	11.2
34	Kentucky	9.9
16	Louisiana	11.2
2	Maine	15.7
15	Maryland	11.3
24	Massachusetts	11.0
21	Michigan	11.1
31	Minnesota	10.2
27	Mississippi	10.5
26	Missouri	10.7
21	Montana	11.1
10	Nebraska	11.7
33	Nevada	10.0
45	New Hampshire	8.1
9	New Jersey	11.9
24	New Mexico	11.0
13	New York	11.6
34	North Carolina	9.9
3	North Dakota	15.6
14	Ohio	11.5
41	Oklahoma	8.7
10	Oregon	11.7
8	Pennsylvania	12.2
39	Rhode Island	9.5
7	South Carolina	12.5
4	South Dakota	13.2
27	Tennessee	10.5
44	Texas	8.2
48	Utah	4.5
1	Vermont	16.4
34	Virginia	9.9
31	Washington	10.2
21	West Virginia	11.1
16	Wisconsin	11.2
NA	Wyoming**	NA

RANK ORDER

RANK	STATE	RATE
1	Vermont	16.4
2	Maine	15.7
3	North Dakota	15.6
4	South Dakota	13.2
5	Florida	13.1
6	Delaware	12.8
7	South Carolina	12.5
8	Pennsylvania	12.2
9	New Jersey	11.9
10	Connecticut	11.7
10	Nebraska	11.7
10	Oregon	11.7
13	New York	11.6
14	Ohio	11.5
15	Maryland	11.3
16	Alabama	11.2
16	Arkansas	11.2
16	Kansas	11.2
16	Louisiana	11.2
16	Wisconsin	11.2
21	Michigan	11.1
21	Montana	11.1
21	West Virginia	11.1
24	Massachusetts	11.0
24	New Mexico	11.0
26	Missouri	10.7
27	Illinois	10.5
27	Mississippi	10.5
27	Tennessee	10.5
30	Iowa	10.3
31	Minnesota	10.2
31	Washington	10.2
33	Nevada	10.0
34	Indiana	9.9
34	Kentucky	9.9
34	North Carolina	9.9
34	Virginia	9.9
38	Arizona	9.7
39	Rhode Island	9.5
40	Colorado	9.3
41	Oklahoma	8.7
42	California	8.3
42	Hawaii	8.3
44	Texas	8.2
45	New Hampshire	8.1
46	Idaho	7.7
47	Georgia	7.3
48	Utah	4.5
NA	Alaska**	NA
NA	Wyoming**	NA
	District of Columbia	17.5

Source: Morgan Quitno Press using data from American Cancer Society
    "Cancer Facts & Figures 2001" (Copyright 2001, Reprinted with permission from the American Cancer Society)
*Rates calculated using 2000 Census resident population figures. Not age-adjusted.
**Fewer than 50 deaths.

Estimated Deaths by Prostate Cancer in 2001

National Estimated Total = 31,500 Deaths

ALPHA ORDER

RANK	STATE	DEATHS	% of USA
16	Alabama	600	1.9%
NA	Alaska*	NA	NA
16	Arizona	600	1.9%
26	Arkansas	400	1.3%
1	California	2,800	8.9%
31	Colorado	300	1.0%
26	Connecticut	400	1.3%
39	Delaware	100	0.3%
2	Florida	2,400	7.6%
11	Georgia	800	2.5%
39	Hawaii	100	0.3%
39	Idaho	100	0.3%
6	Illinois	1,400	4.4%
13	Indiana	700	2.2%
26	Iowa	400	1.3%
31	Kansas	300	1.0%
26	Kentucky	400	1.3%
16	Louisiana	600	1.9%
39	Maine	100	0.3%
16	Maryland	600	1.9%
13	Massachusetts	700	2.2%
8	Michigan	1,100	3.5%
16	Minnesota	600	1.9%
26	Mississippi	400	1.3%
16	Missouri	600	1.9%
39	Montana	100	0.3%
34	Nebraska	200	0.6%
34	Nevada	200	0.6%
39	New Hampshire	100	0.3%
9	New Jersey	1,000	3.2%
34	New Mexico	200	0.6%
3	New York	2,000	6.3%
10	North Carolina	900	2.9%
39	North Dakota	100	0.3%
6	Ohio	1,400	4.4%
31	Oklahoma	300	1.0%
23	Oregon	500	1.6%
5	Pennsylvania	1,700	5.4%
39	Rhode Island	100	0.3%
23	South Carolina	500	1.6%
39	South Dakota	100	0.3%
16	Tennessee	600	1.9%
3	Texas	2,000	6.3%
34	Utah	200	0.6%
39	Vermont	100	0.3%
11	Virginia	800	2.5%
23	Washington	500	1.6%
34	West Virginia	200	0.6%
13	Wisconsin	700	2.2%
39	Wyoming	100	0.3%

RANK ORDER

RANK	STATE	DEATHS	% of USA
1	California	2,800	8.9%
2	Florida	2,400	7.6%
3	New York	2,000	6.3%
3	Texas	2,000	6.3%
5	Pennsylvania	1,700	5.4%
6	Illinois	1,400	4.4%
6	Ohio	1,400	4.4%
8	Michigan	1,100	3.5%
9	New Jersey	1,000	3.2%
10	North Carolina	900	2.9%
11	Georgia	800	2.5%
11	Virginia	800	2.5%
13	Indiana	700	2.2%
13	Massachusetts	700	2.2%
13	Wisconsin	700	2.2%
16	Alabama	600	1.9%
16	Arizona	600	1.9%
16	Louisiana	600	1.9%
16	Maryland	600	1.9%
16	Minnesota	600	1.9%
16	Missouri	600	1.9%
16	Tennessee	600	1.9%
23	Oregon	500	1.6%
23	South Carolina	500	1.6%
23	Washington	500	1.6%
26	Arkansas	400	1.3%
26	Connecticut	400	1.3%
26	Iowa	400	1.3%
26	Kentucky	400	1.3%
26	Mississippi	400	1.3%
31	Colorado	300	1.0%
31	Kansas	300	1.0%
31	Oklahoma	300	1.0%
34	Nebraska	200	0.6%
34	Nevada	200	0.6%
34	New Mexico	200	0.6%
34	Utah	200	0.6%
34	West Virginia	200	0.6%
39	Delaware	100	0.3%
39	Hawaii	100	0.3%
39	Idaho	100	0.3%
39	Maine	100	0.3%
39	Montana	100	0.3%
39	New Hampshire	100	0.3%
39	North Dakota	100	0.3%
39	Rhode Island	100	0.3%
39	South Dakota	100	0.3%
39	Vermont	100	0.3%
39	Wyoming	100	0.3%
NA	Alaska*	NA	NA
	District of Columbia	100	0.3%

Source: American Cancer Society
"Cancer Facts & Figures 2001" (Copyright 2001, Reprinted with permission from the American Cancer Society)
*Fewer than 50 deaths.

Estimated Death Rate by Prostate Cancer in 2001

National Estimated Rate = 23.6 Deaths per 100,000 Male Population*

ALPHA ORDER

RANK	STATE	RATE
9	Alabama	28.6
NA	Alaska**	NA
18	Arizona	25.4
4	Arkansas	32.4
44	California	16.9
49	Colorado	14.9
20	Connecticut	25.1
13	Delaware	27.3
3	Florida	32.7
37	Georgia	21.1
44	Hawaii	16.9
48	Idaho	16.0
26	Illinois	23.7
23	Indiana	24.2
9	Iowa	28.6
29	Kansas	23.0
39	Kentucky	20.8
11	Louisiana	28.5
47	Maine	16.4
24	Maryland	23.9
27	Massachusetts	23.5
31	Michigan	22.9
17	Minnesota	25.5
7	Mississippi	30.1
35	Missouri	22.6
32	Montana	22.8
21	Nebraska	24.6
36	Nevada	21.7
44	New Hampshire	16.9
19	New Jersey	25.3
28	New Mexico	23.4
32	New York	22.8
22	North Carolina	24.3
5	North Dakota	31.7
16	Ohio	25.7
42	Oklahoma	18.3
6	Oregon	30.5
8	Pennsylvania	29.5
38	Rhode Island	21.0
15	South Carolina	26.7
12	South Dakota	27.7
34	Tennessee	22.7
40	Texas	20.2
41	Utah	18.9
2	Vermont	34.2
25	Virginia	23.8
43	Washington	17.5
29	West Virginia	23.0
14	Wisconsin	27.1
1	Wyoming	41.5

RANK ORDER

RANK	STATE	RATE
1	Wyoming	41.5
2	Vermont	34.2
3	Florida	32.7
4	Arkansas	32.4
5	North Dakota	31.7
6	Oregon	30.5
7	Mississippi	30.1
8	Pennsylvania	29.5
9	Alabama	28.6
9	Iowa	28.6
11	Louisiana	28.5
12	South Dakota	27.7
13	Delaware	27.3
14	Wisconsin	27.1
15	South Carolina	26.7
16	Ohio	25.7
17	Minnesota	25.5
18	Arizona	25.4
19	New Jersey	25.3
20	Connecticut	25.1
21	Nebraska	24.6
22	North Carolina	24.3
23	Indiana	24.2
24	Maryland	23.9
25	Virginia	23.8
26	Illinois	23.7
27	Massachusetts	23.5
28	New Mexico	23.4
29	Kansas	23.0
29	West Virginia	23.0
31	Michigan	22.9
32	Montana	22.8
32	New York	22.8
34	Tennessee	22.7
35	Missouri	22.6
36	Nevada	21.7
37	Georgia	21.1
38	Rhode Island	21.0
39	Kentucky	20.8
40	Texas	20.2
41	Utah	18.9
42	Oklahoma	18.3
43	Washington	17.5
44	California	16.9
44	Hawaii	16.9
44	New Hampshire	16.9
47	Maine	16.4
48	Idaho	16.0
49	Colorado	14.9
NA	Alaska**	NA
	District of Columbia	41.1

Source: Morgan Quitno Press using data from American Cancer Society
   "Cancer Facts & Figures 2001" (Copyright 2001, Reprinted with permission from the American Cancer Society)
*Rates calculated using 1999 Census resident male population estimates. Not age-adjusted.
**Fewer than 50 deaths.

Estimated Deaths by Ovarian Cancer in 2001

National Estimated Total = 13,900 Deaths

ALPHA ORDER

RANK	STATE	DEATHS	% of USA
11	Alabama	300	2.2%
NA	Alaska*	NA	NA
21	Arizona	200	1.4%
21	Arkansas	200	1.4%
1	California	1,400	10.1%
21	Colorado	200	1.4%
21	Connecticut	200	1.4%
NA	Delaware*	NA	NA
2	Florida	1,000	7.2%
11	Georgia	300	2.2%
NA	Hawaii*	NA	NA
32	Idaho	100	0.7%
6	Illinois	600	4.3%
11	Indiana	300	2.2%
21	Iowa	200	1.4%
32	Kansas	100	0.7%
21	Kentucky	200	1.4%
21	Louisiana	200	1.4%
32	Maine	100	0.7%
11	Maryland	300	2.2%
11	Massachusetts	300	2.2%
8	Michigan	500	3.6%
21	Minnesota	200	1.4%
32	Mississippi	100	0.7%
11	Missouri	300	2.2%
32	Montana	100	0.7%
32	Nebraska	100	0.7%
32	Nevada	100	0.7%
32	New Hampshire	100	0.7%
8	New Jersey	500	3.6%
32	New Mexico	100	0.7%
3	New York	900	6.5%
10	North Carolina	400	2.9%
NA	North Dakota*	NA	NA
6	Ohio	600	4.3%
21	Oklahoma	200	1.4%
21	Oregon	200	1.4%
5	Pennsylvania	700	5.0%
32	Rhode Island	100	0.7%
21	South Carolina	200	1.4%
NA	South Dakota*	NA	NA
11	Tennessee	300	2.2%
4	Texas	800	5.8%
32	Utah	100	0.7%
NA	Vermont*	NA	NA
11	Virginia	300	2.2%
11	Washington	300	2.2%
32	West Virginia	100	0.7%
11	Wisconsin	300	2.2%
NA	Wyoming*	NA	NA

RANK ORDER

RANK	STATE	DEATHS	% of USA
1	California	1,400	10.1%
2	Florida	1,000	7.2%
3	New York	900	6.5%
4	Texas	800	5.8%
5	Pennsylvania	700	5.0%
6	Illinois	600	4.3%
6	Ohio	600	4.3%
8	Michigan	500	3.6%
8	New Jersey	500	3.6%
10	North Carolina	400	2.9%
11	Alabama	300	2.2%
11	Georgia	300	2.2%
11	Indiana	300	2.2%
11	Maryland	300	2.2%
11	Massachusetts	300	2.2%
11	Missouri	300	2.2%
11	Tennessee	300	2.2%
11	Virginia	300	2.2%
11	Washington	300	2.2%
11	Wisconsin	300	2.2%
21	Arizona	200	1.4%
21	Arkansas	200	1.4%
21	Colorado	200	1.4%
21	Connecticut	200	1.4%
21	Iowa	200	1.4%
21	Kentucky	200	1.4%
21	Louisiana	200	1.4%
21	Minnesota	200	1.4%
21	Oklahoma	200	1.4%
21	Oregon	200	1.4%
21	South Carolina	200	1.4%
32	Idaho	100	0.7%
32	Kansas	100	0.7%
32	Maine	100	0.7%
32	Mississippi	100	0.7%
32	Montana	100	0.7%
32	Nebraska	100	0.7%
32	Nevada	100	0.7%
32	New Hampshire	100	0.7%
32	New Mexico	100	0.7%
32	Rhode Island	100	0.7%
32	Utah	100	0.7%
32	West Virginia	100	0.7%
NA	Alaska*	NA	NA
NA	Delaware*	NA	NA
NA	Hawaii*	NA	NA
NA	North Dakota*	NA	NA
NA	South Dakota*	NA	NA
NA	Vermont*	NA	NA
NA	Wyoming*	NA	NA
	District of Columbia*	NA	NA

Source: American Cancer Society
"Cancer Facts & Figures 2001" (Copyright 2001, Reprinted with permission from the American Cancer Society)
*Fewer than 50 deaths.

Estimated Death Rate by Ovarian Cancer in 2001

National Estimated Rate = 10.0 Deaths per 100,000 Female Population*

ALPHA ORDER

RANK	STATE	RATE
8	Alabama	13.2
NA	Alaska**	NA
38	Arizona	8.3
6	Arkansas	15.2
36	California	8.5
28	Colorado	9.8
12	Connecticut	11.8
NA	Delaware**	NA
9	Florida	12.9
41	Georgia	7.5
NA	Hawaii**	NA
4	Idaho	15.9
31	Illinois	9.7
28	Indiana	9.8
7	Iowa	13.6
42	Kansas	7.4
28	Kentucky	9.8
35	Louisiana	8.8
5	Maine	15.6
15	Maryland	11.3
33	Massachusetts	9.4
26	Michigan	9.9
38	Minnesota	8.3
43	Mississippi	6.9
21	Missouri	10.6
1	Montana	22.5
13	Nebraska	11.7
15	Nevada	11.3
3	New Hampshire	16.4
10	New Jersey	11.9
15	New Mexico	11.3
32	New York	9.5
25	North Carolina	10.2
NA	North Dakota**	NA
24	Ohio	10.3
14	Oklahoma	11.6
10	Oregon	11.9
18	Pennsylvania	11.2
2	Rhode Island	19.4
26	South Carolina	9.9
NA	South Dakota**	NA
21	Tennessee	10.6
40	Texas	7.9
34	Utah	9.3
NA	Vermont**	NA
36	Virginia	8.5
23	Washington	10.4
20	West Virginia	10.7
18	Wisconsin	11.2
NA	Wyoming**	NA

RANK ORDER

RANK	STATE	RATE
1	Montana	22.5
2	Rhode Island	19.4
3	New Hampshire	16.4
4	Idaho	15.9
5	Maine	15.6
6	Arkansas	15.2
7	Iowa	13.6
8	Alabama	13.2
9	Florida	12.9
10	New Jersey	11.9
10	Oregon	11.9
12	Connecticut	11.8
13	Nebraska	11.7
14	Oklahoma	11.6
15	Maryland	11.3
15	Nevada	11.3
15	New Mexico	11.3
18	Pennsylvania	11.2
18	Wisconsin	11.2
20	West Virginia	10.7
21	Missouri	10.6
21	Tennessee	10.6
23	Washington	10.4
24	Ohio	10.3
25	North Carolina	10.2
26	Michigan	9.9
26	South Carolina	9.9
28	Colorado	9.8
28	Indiana	9.8
28	Kentucky	9.8
31	Illinois	9.7
32	New York	9.5
33	Massachusetts	9.4
34	Utah	9.3
35	Louisiana	8.8
36	California	8.5
36	Virginia	8.5
38	Arizona	8.3
38	Minnesota	8.3
40	Texas	7.9
41	Georgia	7.5
42	Kansas	7.4
43	Mississippi	6.9
NA	Alaska**	NA
NA	Delaware**	NA
NA	Hawaii**	NA
NA	North Dakota**	NA
NA	South Dakota**	NA
NA	Vermont**	NA
NA	Wyoming**	NA
	District of Columbia**	NA

Source: Morgan Quitno Press using data from American Cancer Society
    "Cancer Facts & Figures 2001" (Copyright 2001, Reprinted with permission from the American Cancer Society)
*Rates calculated using 1999 Census resident female population estimates. Not age-adjusted.
**Fewer than 50 deaths.

Estimated Deaths by Brain Cancer in 2001

National Estimated Total = 13,100 Deaths

ALPHA ORDER

RANK	STATE	DEATHS	% of USA
19	Alabama	200	1.5%
NA	Alaska*	NA	NA
19	Arizona	200	1.5%
19	Arkansas	200	1.5%
1	California	1,500	11.5%
19	Colorado	200	1.5%
31	Connecticut	100	0.8%
NA	Delaware*	NA	NA
2	Florida	1,000	7.6%
10	Georgia	300	2.3%
NA	Hawaii*	NA	NA
31	Idaho	100	0.8%
7	Illinois	500	3.8%
10	Indiana	300	2.3%
19	Iowa	200	1.5%
31	Kansas	100	0.8%
19	Kentucky	200	1.5%
19	Louisiana	200	1.5%
31	Maine	100	0.8%
19	Maryland	200	1.5%
10	Massachusetts	300	2.3%
7	Michigan	500	3.8%
19	Minnesota	200	1.5%
19	Mississippi	200	1.5%
10	Missouri	300	2.3%
NA	Montana*	NA	NA
31	Nebraska	100	0.8%
31	Nevada	100	0.8%
31	New Hampshire	100	0.8%
10	New Jersey	300	2.3%
31	New Mexico	100	0.8%
4	New York	800	6.1%
9	North Carolina	400	3.1%
31	North Dakota	100	0.8%
5	Ohio	600	4.6%
31	Oklahoma	100	0.8%
19	Oregon	200	1.5%
5	Pennsylvania	600	4.6%
31	Rhode Island	100	0.8%
19	South Carolina	200	1.5%
NA	South Dakota*	NA	NA
10	Tennessee	300	2.3%
3	Texas	900	6.9%
31	Utah	100	0.8%
NA	Vermont*	NA	NA
10	Virginia	300	2.3%
10	Washington	300	2.3%
31	West Virginia	100	0.8%
10	Wisconsin	300	2.3%
NA	Wyoming*	NA	NA

RANK ORDER

RANK	STATE	DEATHS	% of USA
1	California	1,500	11.5%
2	Florida	1,000	7.6%
3	Texas	900	6.9%
4	New York	800	6.1%
5	Ohio	600	4.6%
5	Pennsylvania	600	4.6%
7	Illinois	500	3.8%
7	Michigan	500	3.8%
9	North Carolina	400	3.1%
10	Georgia	300	2.3%
10	Indiana	300	2.3%
10	Massachusetts	300	2.3%
10	Missouri	300	2.3%
10	New Jersey	300	2.3%
10	Tennessee	300	2.3%
10	Virginia	300	2.3%
10	Washington	300	2.3%
10	Wisconsin	300	2.3%
19	Alabama	200	1.5%
19	Arizona	200	1.5%
19	Arkansas	200	1.5%
19	Colorado	200	1.5%
19	Iowa	200	1.5%
19	Kentucky	200	1.5%
19	Louisiana	200	1.5%
19	Maryland	200	1.5%
19	Minnesota	200	1.5%
19	Mississippi	200	1.5%
19	Oregon	200	1.5%
19	South Carolina	200	1.5%
31	Connecticut	100	0.8%
31	Idaho	100	0.8%
31	Kansas	100	0.8%
31	Maine	100	0.8%
31	Nebraska	100	0.8%
31	Nevada	100	0.8%
31	New Hampshire	100	0.8%
31	New Mexico	100	0.8%
31	North Dakota	100	0.8%
31	Oklahoma	100	0.8%
31	Rhode Island	100	0.8%
31	Utah	100	0.8%
31	West Virginia	100	0.8%
NA	Alaska*	NA	NA
NA	Delaware*	NA	NA
NA	Hawaii*	NA	NA
NA	Montana*	NA	NA
NA	South Dakota*	NA	NA
NA	Vermont*	NA	NA
NA	Wyoming*	NA	NA
	District of Columbia*	NA	NA

Source: American Cancer Society
   "Cancer Facts & Figures 2001" (Copyright 2001, Reprinted with permission from the American Cancer Society)
*Fewer than 50 deaths.

Estimated Death Rate by Brain Cancer in 2001

National Estimated Rate = 4.7 Deaths per 100,000 Population*

ALPHA ORDER

RANK	STATE	RATE
28	Alabama	4.5
NA	Alaska**	NA
37	Arizona	3.9
6	Arkansas	7.5
31	California	4.4
27	Colorado	4.6
42	Connecticut	2.9
NA	Delaware**	NA
9	Florida	6.3
39	Georgia	3.7
NA	Hawaii**	NA
5	Idaho	7.7
36	Illinois	4.0
23	Indiana	4.9
8	Iowa	6.8
39	Kansas	3.7
23	Kentucky	4.9
28	Louisiana	4.5
4	Maine	7.8
38	Maryland	3.8
26	Massachusetts	4.7
19	Michigan	5.0
35	Minnesota	4.1
7	Mississippi	7.0
15	Missouri	5.4
NA	Montana**	NA
10	Nebraska	5.8
19	Nevada	5.0
3	New Hampshire	8.1
41	New Jersey	3.6
13	New Mexico	5.5
33	New York	4.2
19	North Carolina	5.0
1	North Dakota	15.6
16	Ohio	5.3
42	Oklahoma	2.9
10	Oregon	5.8
23	Pennsylvania	4.9
2	Rhode Island	9.5
19	South Carolina	5.0
NA	South Dakota**	NA
16	Tennessee	5.3
32	Texas	4.3
28	Utah	4.5
NA	Vermont**	NA
33	Virginia	4.2
18	Washington	5.1
13	West Virginia	5.5
12	Wisconsin	5.6
NA	Wyoming**	NA

RANK ORDER

RANK	STATE	RATE
1	North Dakota	15.6
2	Rhode Island	9.5
3	New Hampshire	8.1
4	Maine	7.8
5	Idaho	7.7
6	Arkansas	7.5
7	Mississippi	7.0
8	Iowa	6.8
9	Florida	6.3
10	Nebraska	5.8
10	Oregon	5.8
12	Wisconsin	5.6
13	New Mexico	5.5
13	West Virginia	5.5
15	Missouri	5.4
16	Ohio	5.3
16	Tennessee	5.3
18	Washington	5.1
19	Michigan	5.0
19	Nevada	5.0
19	North Carolina	5.0
19	South Carolina	5.0
23	Indiana	4.9
23	Kentucky	4.9
23	Pennsylvania	4.9
26	Massachusetts	4.7
27	Colorado	4.6
28	Alabama	4.5
28	Louisiana	4.5
28	Utah	4.5
31	California	4.4
32	Texas	4.3
33	New York	4.2
33	Virginia	4.2
35	Minnesota	4.1
36	Illinois	4.0
37	Arizona	3.9
38	Maryland	3.8
39	Georgia	3.7
39	Kansas	3.7
41	New Jersey	3.6
42	Connecticut	2.9
42	Oklahoma	2.9
NA	Alaska**	NA
NA	Delaware**	NA
NA	Hawaii**	NA
NA	Montana**	NA
NA	South Dakota**	NA
NA	Vermont**	NA
NA	Wyoming**	NA
	District of Columbia**	NA

Source: Morgan Quitno Press using data from American Cancer Society
"Cancer Facts & Figures 2001" (Copyright 2001, Reprinted with permission from the American Cancer Society)
*Rates calculated using 2000 Census resident population figures. Not age-adjusted.
**Fewer than 50 deaths.

Deaths by Alzheimer's Disease in 1998

National Total = 22,725 Deaths*

RANK	STATE	DEATHS	% of USA
20	Alabama	454	2.0%
50	Alaska	14	0.1%
18	Arizona	487	2.1%
32	Arkansas	231	1.0%
1	California	2,091	9.2%
25	Colorado	376	1.7%
30	Connecticut	262	1.2%
47	Delaware	56	0.2%
3	Florida	1,600	7.0%
13	Georgia	600	2.6%
48	Hawaii	54	0.2%
41	Idaho	117	0.5%
4	Illinois	1,120	4.9%
14	Indiana	587	2.6%
27	Iowa	325	1.4%
31	Kansas	250	1.1%
23	Kentucky	427	1.9%
22	Louisiana	435	1.9%
35	Maine	161	0.7%
26	Maryland	362	1.6%
8	Massachusetts	677	3.0%
10	Michigan	664	2.9%
19	Minnesota	460	2.0%
34	Mississippi	201	0.9%
16	Missouri	518	2.3%
43	Montana	107	0.5%
33	Nebraska	203	0.9%
42	Nevada	114	0.5%
40	New Hampshire	126	0.6%
11	New Jersey	650	2.9%
38	New Mexico	138	0.6%
9	New York	673	3.0%
7	North Carolina	748	3.3%
46	North Dakota	57	0.3%
5	Ohio	1,032	4.5%
29	Oklahoma	292	1.3%
24	Oregon	409	1.8%
6	Pennsylvania	954	4.2%
39	Rhode Island	127	0.6%
28	South Carolina	305	1.3%
44	South Dakota	73	0.3%
21	Tennessee	445	2.0%
2	Texas	1,612	7.1%
35	Utah	161	0.7%
45	Vermont	68	0.3%
15	Virginia	555	2.4%
12	Washington	605	2.7%
37	West Virginia	145	0.6%
17	Wisconsin	514	2.3%
49	Wyoming	43	0.2%

RANK	STATE	DEATHS	% of USA
1	California	2,091	9.2%
2	Texas	1,612	7.1%
3	Florida	1,600	7.0%
4	Illinois	1,120	4.9%
5	Ohio	1,032	4.5%
6	Pennsylvania	954	4.2%
7	North Carolina	748	3.3%
8	Massachusetts	677	3.0%
9	New York	673	3.0%
10	Michigan	664	2.9%
11	New Jersey	650	2.9%
12	Washington	605	2.7%
13	Georgia	600	2.6%
14	Indiana	587	2.6%
15	Virginia	555	2.4%
16	Missouri	518	2.3%
17	Wisconsin	514	2.3%
18	Arizona	487	2.1%
19	Minnesota	460	2.0%
20	Alabama	454	2.0%
21	Tennessee	445	2.0%
22	Louisiana	435	1.9%
23	Kentucky	427	1.9%
24	Oregon	409	1.8%
25	Colorado	376	1.7%
26	Maryland	362	1.6%
27	Iowa	325	1.4%
28	South Carolina	305	1.3%
29	Oklahoma	292	1.3%
30	Connecticut	262	1.2%
31	Kansas	250	1.1%
32	Arkansas	231	1.0%
33	Nebraska	203	0.9%
34	Mississippi	201	0.9%
35	Maine	161	0.7%
35	Utah	161	0.7%
37	West Virginia	145	0.6%
38	New Mexico	138	0.6%
39	Rhode Island	127	0.6%
40	New Hampshire	126	0.6%
41	Idaho	117	0.5%
42	Nevada	114	0.5%
43	Montana	107	0.5%
44	South Dakota	73	0.3%
45	Vermont	68	0.3%
46	North Dakota	57	0.3%
47	Delaware	56	0.2%
48	Hawaii	54	0.2%
49	Wyoming	43	0.2%
50	Alaska	14	0.1%
	District of Columbia	40	0.2%

Source: U.S. Department of Health and Human Services, National Center for Health Statistics "National Vital Statistics Reports" (Vol. 48, No. 11, July 24, 2000)
Final data by state of residence. A degenerative disease of the brain cells producing loss of memory and general intellectual impairment. It usually affects people over age 65. As the disease progresses, a variety of symptoms may become apparent, including confusion, irritability, and restlessness, as well as disorientation and impaired judgment and concentration.

Death Rate by Alzheimer's Disease in 1998

National Rate = 8.4 Deaths per 100,000 Population*

ALPHA ORDER

RANK	STATE	RATE
13	Alabama	10.4
NA	Alaska**	NA
13	Arizona	10.4
27	Arkansas	9.1
47	California	6.4
21	Colorado	9.5
34	Connecticut	8.0
42	Delaware	7.5
10	Florida	10.7
38	Georgia	7.9
48	Hawaii	4.5
21	Idaho	9.5
25	Illinois	9.3
15	Indiana	10.0
7	Iowa	11.4
21	Kansas	9.5
9	Kentucky	10.8
15	Louisiana	10.0
1	Maine	12.9
44	Maryland	7.0
8	Massachusetts	11.0
45	Michigan	6.8
20	Minnesota	9.7
43	Mississippi	7.3
21	Missouri	9.5
4	Montana	12.2
4	Nebraska	12.2
46	Nevada	6.5
11	New Hampshire	10.6
34	New Jersey	8.0
38	New Mexico	7.9
49	New York	3.7
17	North Carolina	9.9
28	North Dakota	8.9
26	Ohio	9.2
30	Oklahoma	8.7
3	Oregon	12.5
38	Pennsylvania	7.9
2	Rhode Island	12.8
34	South Carolina	8.0
17	South Dakota	9.9
31	Tennessee	8.2
31	Texas	8.2
41	Utah	7.7
6	Vermont	11.5
31	Virginia	8.2
11	Washington	10.6
34	West Virginia	8.0
19	Wisconsin	9.8
28	Wyoming	8.9

RANK ORDER

RANK	STATE	RATE
1	Maine	12.9
2	Rhode Island	12.8
3	Oregon	12.5
4	Montana	12.2
4	Nebraska	12.2
6	Vermont	11.5
7	Iowa	11.4
8	Massachusetts	11.0
9	Kentucky	10.8
10	Florida	10.7
11	New Hampshire	10.6
11	Washington	10.6
13	Alabama	10.4
13	Arizona	10.4
15	Indiana	10.0
15	Louisiana	10.0
17	North Carolina	9.9
17	South Dakota	9.9
19	Wisconsin	9.8
20	Minnesota	9.7
21	Colorado	9.5
21	Idaho	9.5
21	Kansas	9.5
21	Missouri	9.5
25	Illinois	9.3
26	Ohio	9.2
27	Arkansas	9.1
28	North Dakota	8.9
28	Wyoming	8.9
30	Oklahoma	8.7
31	Tennessee	8.2
31	Texas	8.2
31	Virginia	8.2
34	Connecticut	8.0
34	New Jersey	8.0
34	South Carolina	8.0
34	West Virginia	8.0
38	Georgia	7.9
38	New Mexico	7.9
38	Pennsylvania	7.9
41	Utah	7.7
42	Delaware	7.5
43	Mississippi	7.3
44	Maryland	7.0
45	Michigan	6.8
46	Nevada	6.5
47	California	6.4
48	Hawaii	4.5
49	New York	3.7
NA	Alaska**	NA
	District of Columbia	7.6

Source: U.S. Department of Health and Human Services, National Center for Health Statistics
"National Vital Statistics Reports" (Vol. 48, No. 11, July 24, 2000)
*Final data by state of residence. A degenerative disease of the brain cells producing loss of memory and general intellectual impairment. It usually affects people over age 65. As the disease progresses, a variety of symptoms may become apparent, including confusion, irritability, and restlessness, as well as disorientation and impaired judgment and concentration. Not age-adjusted. **Insufficient data to determine a reliable rate.

Age-Adjusted Death Rate by Alzheimer's Disease in 1998

National Rate = 2.6 Deaths per 100,000 Population*

ALPHA ORDER

RANK	STATE	RATE
8	Alabama	3.4
NA	Alaska**	NA
18	Arizona	3.1
26	Arkansas	2.7
41	California	2.3
2	Colorado	3.6
45	Connecticut	2.2
35	Delaware	2.6
41	Florida	2.3
8	Georgia	3.4
48	Hawaii	1.4
15	Idaho	3.2
21	Illinois	3.0
15	Indiana	3.2
35	Iowa	2.6
26	Kansas	2.7
2	Kentucky	3.6
1	Louisiana	3.8
14	Maine	3.3
37	Maryland	2.5
18	Massachusetts	3.1
41	Michigan	2.3
23	Minnesota	2.9
26	Mississippi	2.7
26	Missouri	2.7
21	Montana	3.0
15	Nebraska	3.2
26	Nevada	2.7
8	New Hampshire	3.4
39	New Jersey	2.4
25	New Mexico	2.8
49	New York	1.1
8	North Carolina	3.4
46	North Dakota	2.1
26	Ohio	2.7
26	Oklahoma	2.7
2	Oregon	3.6
47	Pennsylvania	2.0
37	Rhode Island	2.5
23	South Carolina	2.9
39	South Dakota	2.4
26	Tennessee	2.7
8	Texas	3.4
5	Utah	3.5
5	Vermont	3.5
18	Virginia	3.1
5	Washington	3.5
41	West Virginia	2.3
26	Wisconsin	2.7
8	Wyoming	3.4

RANK ORDER

RANK	STATE	RATE
1	Louisiana	3.8
2	Colorado	3.6
2	Kentucky	3.6
2	Oregon	3.6
5	Utah	3.5
5	Vermont	3.5
5	Washington	3.5
8	Alabama	3.4
8	Georgia	3.4
8	New Hampshire	3.4
8	North Carolina	3.4
8	Texas	3.4
8	Wyoming	3.4
14	Maine	3.3
15	Idaho	3.2
15	Indiana	3.2
15	Nebraska	3.2
18	Arizona	3.1
18	Massachusetts	3.1
18	Virginia	3.1
21	Illinois	3.0
21	Montana	3.0
23	Minnesota	2.9
23	South Carolina	2.9
25	New Mexico	2.8
26	Arkansas	2.7
26	Kansas	2.7
26	Mississippi	2.7
26	Missouri	2.7
26	Nevada	2.7
26	Ohio	2.7
26	Oklahoma	2.7
26	Tennessee	2.7
26	Wisconsin	2.7
35	Delaware	2.6
35	Iowa	2.6
37	Maryland	2.5
37	Rhode Island	2.5
39	New Jersey	2.4
39	South Dakota	2.4
41	California	2.3
41	Florida	2.3
41	Michigan	2.3
41	West Virginia	2.3
45	Connecticut	2.2
46	North Dakota	2.1
47	Pennsylvania	2.0
48	Hawaii	1.4
49	New York	1.1
NA	Alaska**	NA
	District of Columbia	2.0

Source: U.S. Department of Health and Human Services, National Center for Health Statistics
    "National Vital Statistics Reports" (Vol. 48, No. 11, July 24, 2000)
*Final data by state of residence. A degenerative disease of the brain cells producing loss of memory and general intellectual impairment. It usually affects people over age 65. As the disease progresses, a variety of symptoms may become apparent, including confusion, irritability, and restlessness, as well as disorientation and impaired judgment and concentration. **Insufficient data to determine a reliable rate.*

Deaths by Atherosclerosis in 1998

National Total = 15,279 Deaths*

ALPHA ORDER

RANK	STATE	DEATHS	% of USA
25	Alabama	234	1.5%
50	Alaska	11	0.1%
19	Arizona	295	1.9%
32	Arkansas	148	1.0%
1	California	1,951	12.8%
11	Colorado	414	2.7%
29	Connecticut	186	1.2%
46	Delaware	20	0.1%
2	Florida	1,109	7.3%
9	Georgia	486	3.2%
47	Hawaii	19	0.1%
44	Idaho	54	0.4%
8	Illinois	575	3.8%
13	Indiana	385	2.5%
16	Iowa	338	2.2%
22	Kansas	271	1.8%
30	Kentucky	167	1.1%
27	Louisiana	224	1.5%
42	Maine	65	0.4%
33	Maryland	132	0.9%
15	Massachusetts	344	2.3%
6	Michigan	655	4.3%
24	Minnesota	246	1.6%
36	Mississippi	86	0.6%
21	Missouri	275	1.8%
39	Montana	67	0.4%
28	Nebraska	207	1.4%
35	Nevada	87	0.6%
41	New Hampshire	66	0.4%
10	New Jersey	419	2.7%
36	New Mexico	86	0.6%
5	New York	692	4.5%
12	North Carolina	396	2.6%
43	North Dakota	63	0.4%
7	Ohio	608	4.0%
17	Oklahoma	336	2.2%
26	Oregon	225	1.5%
4	Pennsylvania	702	4.6%
39	Rhode Island	67	0.4%
34	South Carolina	114	0.7%
45	South Dakota	43	0.3%
14	Tennessee	350	2.3%
3	Texas	890	5.8%
38	Utah	74	0.5%
48	Vermont	16	0.1%
20	Virginia	280	1.8%
18	Washington	329	2.2%
31	West Virginia	165	1.1%
23	Wisconsin	260	1.7%
48	Wyoming	16	0.1%

RANK ORDER

RANK	STATE	DEATHS	% of USA
1	California	1,951	12.8%
2	Florida	1,109	7.3%
3	Texas	890	5.8%
4	Pennsylvania	702	4.6%
5	New York	692	4.5%
6	Michigan	655	4.3%
7	Ohio	608	4.0%
8	Illinois	575	3.8%
9	Georgia	486	3.2%
10	New Jersey	419	2.7%
11	Colorado	414	2.7%
12	North Carolina	396	2.6%
13	Indiana	385	2.5%
14	Tennessee	350	2.3%
15	Massachusetts	344	2.3%
16	Iowa	338	2.2%
17	Oklahoma	336	2.2%
18	Washington	329	2.2%
19	Arizona	295	1.9%
20	Virginia	280	1.8%
21	Missouri	275	1.8%
22	Kansas	271	1.8%
23	Wisconsin	260	1.7%
24	Minnesota	246	1.6%
25	Alabama	234	1.5%
26	Oregon	225	1.5%
27	Louisiana	224	1.5%
28	Nebraska	207	1.4%
29	Connecticut	186	1.2%
30	Kentucky	167	1.1%
31	West Virginia	165	1.1%
32	Arkansas	148	1.0%
33	Maryland	132	0.9%
34	South Carolina	114	0.7%
35	Nevada	87	0.6%
36	Mississippi	86	0.6%
36	New Mexico	86	0.6%
38	Utah	74	0.5%
39	Montana	67	0.4%
39	Rhode Island	67	0.4%
41	New Hampshire	66	0.4%
42	Maine	65	0.4%
43	North Dakota	63	0.4%
44	Idaho	54	0.4%
45	South Dakota	43	0.3%
46	Delaware	20	0.1%
47	Hawaii	19	0.1%
48	Vermont	16	0.1%
48	Wyoming	16	0.1%
50	Alaska	11	0.1%
	District of Columbia	31	0.2%

Source: U.S. Department of Health and Human Services, National Center for Health Statistics
(http://wonder.cdc.gov/WONDER/)
*Final data by state of residence. Atherosclerosis is a form of hardening of the arteries.

Death Rate by Atherosclerosis in 1998

National Rate = 5.7 Deaths per 100,000 Population*

ALPHA ORDER

RANK	STATE	RATE
25	Alabama	5.4
49	Alaska**	1.8
16	Arizona	6.3
19	Arkansas	5.8
17	California	6.0
3	Colorado	10.4
22	Connecticut	5.7
46	Delaware	2.7
9	Florida	7.4
14	Georgia	6.4
50	Hawaii**	1.6
38	Idaho	4.4
36	Illinois	4.8
13	Indiana	6.5
2	Iowa	11.8
4	Kansas	10.3
39	Kentucky	4.2
31	Louisiana	5.1
27	Maine	5.2
48	Maryland	2.6
23	Massachusetts	5.6
12	Michigan	6.7
27	Minnesota	5.2
44	Mississippi	3.1
31	Missouri	5.1
8	Montana	7.6
1	Nebraska	12.4
33	Nevada	5.0
23	New Hampshire	5.6
27	New Jersey	5.2
33	New Mexico	5.0
41	New York	3.8
27	North Carolina	5.2
6	North Dakota	9.9
25	Ohio	5.4
5	Oklahoma	10.0
10	Oregon	6.9
18	Pennsylvania	5.9
11	Rhode Island	6.8
45	South Carolina	3.0
19	South Dakota	5.8
14	Tennessee	6.4
37	Texas	4.5
42	Utah	3.5
46	Vermont**	2.7
40	Virginia	4.1
19	Washington	5.8
7	West Virginia	9.1
33	Wisconsin	5.0
43	Wyoming**	3.3

RANK ORDER

RANK	STATE	RATE
1	Nebraska	12.4
2	Iowa	11.8
3	Colorado	10.4
4	Kansas	10.3
5	Oklahoma	10.0
6	North Dakota	9.9
7	West Virginia	9.1
8	Montana	7.6
9	Florida	7.4
10	Oregon	6.9
11	Rhode Island	6.8
12	Michigan	6.7
13	Indiana	6.5
14	Georgia	6.4
14	Tennessee	6.4
16	Arizona	6.3
17	California	6.0
18	Pennsylvania	5.9
19	Arkansas	5.8
19	South Dakota	5.8
19	Washington	5.8
22	Connecticut	5.7
23	Massachusetts	5.6
23	New Hampshire	5.6
25	Alabama	5.4
25	Ohio	5.4
27	Maine	5.2
27	Minnesota	5.2
27	New Jersey	5.2
27	North Carolina	5.2
31	Louisiana	5.1
31	Missouri	5.1
33	Nevada	5.0
33	New Mexico	5.0
33	Wisconsin	5.0
36	Illinois	4.8
37	Texas	4.5
38	Idaho	4.4
39	Kentucky	4.2
40	Virginia	4.1
41	New York	3.8
42	Utah	3.5
43	Wyoming**	3.3
44	Mississippi	3.1
45	South Carolina	3.0
46	Delaware	2.7
46	Vermont**	2.7
48	Maryland	2.6
49	Alaska**	1.8
50	Hawaii**	1.6

	District of Columbia	5.9

Source: U.S. Department of Health and Human Services, National Center for Health Statistics (http://wonder.cdc.gov/WONDER/)

*Final data by state of residence. Atherosclerosis is a form of hardening of the arteries. Not age-adjusted.

**Due to low numbers of deaths, rates for these states should be interpreted with caution.

Age-Adjusted Death Rate by Atherosclerosis in 1998

National Rate = 1.9 Deaths per 100,000 Population*

ALPHA ORDER					RANK ORDER		
RANK	STATE	RATE			RANK	STATE	RATE
15	Alabama	2.2			1	Colorado	4.0
19	Alaska**	2.0			2	Oklahoma	3.6
15	Arizona	2.2			3	Nebraska	3.3
32	Arkansas	1.6			4	Georgia	3.1
11	California	2.3			5	Montana	2.9
1	Colorado	4.0			6	Iowa	2.7
32	Connecticut	1.6			7	Kansas	2.6
46	Delaware	1.2			7	West Virginia	2.6
26	Florida	1.8			9	Michigan	2.4
4	Georgia	3.1			9	Oregon	2.4
50	Hawaii**	0.6			11	California	2.3
40	Idaho	1.4			11	Nevada	2.3
32	Illinois	1.6			11	North Dakota	2.3
15	Indiana	2.2			11	Tennessee	2.3
6	Iowa	2.7			15	Alabama	2.2
7	Kansas	2.6			15	Arizona	2.2
40	Kentucky	1.4			15	Indiana	2.2
19	Louisiana	2.0			18	Washington	2.1
19	Maine	2.0			19	Alaska**	2.0
49	Maryland	0.8			19	Louisiana	2.0
32	Massachusetts	1.6			19	Maine	2.0
9	Michigan	2.4			19	New Hampshire	2.0
27	Minnesota	1.7			19	North Carolina	2.0
32	Mississippi	1.6			19	Texas	2.0
40	Missouri	1.4			25	Utah	1.9
5	Montana	2.9			26	Florida	1.8
3	Nebraska	3.3			27	Minnesota	1.7
11	Nevada	2.3			27	New Jersey	1.7
19	New Hampshire	2.0			27	New Mexico	1.7
27	New Jersey	1.7			27	Ohio	1.7
27	New Mexico	1.7			27	Virginia	1.7
44	New York	1.3			32	Arkansas	1.6
19	North Carolina	2.0			32	Connecticut	1.6
11	North Dakota	2.3			32	Illinois	1.6
27	Ohio	1.7			32	Massachusetts	1.6
2	Oklahoma	3.6			32	Mississippi	1.6
9	Oregon	2.4			32	Pennsylvania	1.6
32	Pennsylvania	1.6			32	Rhode Island	1.6
32	Rhode Island	1.6			39	Wisconsin	1.5
46	South Carolina	1.2			40	Idaho	1.4
44	South Dakota	1.3			40	Kentucky	1.4
11	Tennessee	2.3			40	Missouri	1.4
19	Texas	2.0			40	Vermont**	1.4
25	Utah	1.9			44	New York	1.3
40	Vermont**	1.4			44	South Dakota	1.3
27	Virginia	1.7			46	Delaware	1.2
18	Washington	2.1			46	South Carolina	1.2
7	West Virginia	2.6			46	Wyoming**	1.2
39	Wisconsin	1.5			49	Maryland	0.8
46	Wyoming**	1.2			50	Hawaii**	0.6
						District of Columbia	1.9

Source: U.S. Department of Health and Human Services, National Center for Health Statistics
(http://wonder.cdc.gov/WONDER/)

*Final data by state of residence. Atherosclerosis is a form of hardening of the arteries.

**Due to low numbers of deaths, rates for these states should be interpreted with caution.

Deaths by Cerebrovascular Diseases in 1998

National Total = 158,448 Deaths*

ALPHA ORDER

RANK	STATE	DEATHS	% of USA
19	Alabama	2,929	1.8%
50	Alaska	153	0.1%
26	Arizona	2,472	1.6%
27	Arkansas	2,355	1.5%
1	California	16,512	10.4%
33	Colorado	1,740	1.1%
30	Connecticut	1,947	1.2%
47	Delaware	367	0.2%
2	Florida	10,085	6.4%
10	Georgia	4,158	2.6%
41	Hawaii	658	0.4%
40	Idaho	704	0.4%
6	Illinois	7,172	4.5%
14	Indiana	3,892	2.5%
29	Iowa	2,208	1.4%
31	Kansas	1,831	1.2%
25	Kentucky	2,488	1.6%
24	Louisiana	2,526	1.6%
38	Maine	788	0.5%
22	Maryland	2,636	1.7%
18	Massachusetts	3,322	2.1%
8	Michigan	5,768	3.6%
21	Minnesota	2,858	1.8%
32	Mississippi	1,816	1.1%
13	Missouri	3,898	2.5%
44	Montana	579	0.4%
35	Nebraska	1,158	0.7%
36	Nevada	812	0.5%
42	New Hampshire	618	0.4%
11	New Jersey	4,094	2.6%
39	New Mexico	719	0.5%
5	New York	7,776	4.9%
9	North Carolina	5,439	3.4%
46	North Dakota	461	0.3%
7	Ohio	6,719	4.2%
28	Oklahoma	2,290	1.4%
23	Oregon	2,621	1.7%
4	Pennsylvania	8,224	5.2%
43	Rhode Island	591	0.4%
20	South Carolina	2,900	1.8%
45	South Dakota	538	0.3%
12	Tennessee	3,958	2.5%
3	Texas	9,827	6.2%
37	Utah	796	0.5%
48	Vermont	330	0.2%
15	Virginia	3,820	2.4%
17	Washington	3,428	2.2%
34	West Virginia	1,215	0.8%
16	Wisconsin	3,648	2.3%
49	Wyoming	289	0.2%

RANK ORDER

RANK	STATE	DEATHS	% of USA
1	California	16,512	10.4%
2	Florida	10,085	6.4%
3	Texas	9,827	6.2%
4	Pennsylvania	8,224	5.2%
5	New York	7,776	4.9%
6	Illinois	7,172	4.5%
7	Ohio	6,719	4.2%
8	Michigan	5,768	3.6%
9	North Carolina	5,439	3.4%
10	Georgia	4,158	2.6%
11	New Jersey	4,094	2.6%
12	Tennessee	3,958	2.5%
13	Missouri	3,898	2.5%
14	Indiana	3,892	2.5%
15	Virginia	3,820	2.4%
16	Wisconsin	3,648	2.3%
17	Washington	3,428	2.2%
18	Massachusetts	3,322	2.1%
19	Alabama	2,929	1.8%
20	South Carolina	2,900	1.8%
21	Minnesota	2,858	1.8%
22	Maryland	2,636	1.7%
23	Oregon	2,621	1.7%
24	Louisiana	2,526	1.6%
25	Kentucky	2,488	1.6%
26	Arizona	2,472	1.6%
27	Arkansas	2,355	1.5%
28	Oklahoma	2,290	1.4%
29	Iowa	2,208	1.4%
30	Connecticut	1,947	1.2%
31	Kansas	1,831	1.2%
32	Mississippi	1,816	1.1%
33	Colorado	1,740	1.1%
34	West Virginia	1,215	0.8%
35	Nebraska	1,158	0.7%
36	Nevada	812	0.5%
37	Utah	796	0.5%
38	Maine	788	0.5%
39	New Mexico	719	0.5%
40	Idaho	704	0.4%
41	Hawaii	658	0.4%
42	New Hampshire	618	0.4%
43	Rhode Island	591	0.4%
44	Montana	579	0.4%
45	South Dakota	538	0.3%
46	North Dakota	461	0.3%
47	Delaware	367	0.2%
48	Vermont	330	0.2%
49	Wyoming	289	0.2%
50	Alaska	153	0.1%
	District of Columbia	315	0.2%

Source: U.S. Department of Health and Human Services, National Center for Health Statistics
     "National Vital Statistics Reports" (Vol. 48, No. 11, July 24, 2000)
*Final data by state of residence. Cerebrovascular diseases include stroke and other disorders of the blood vessels of the brain.

Death Rate by Cerebrovascular Diseases in 1998

National Rate = 58.6 Deaths per 100,000 Population*

ALPHA ORDER

RANK	STATE	RATE
16	Alabama	67.3
50	Alaska	24.9
38	Arizona	52.9
1	Arkansas	92.8
41	California	50.5
46	Colorado	43.8
28	Connecticut	59.5
44	Delaware	49.4
15	Florida	67.6
36	Georgia	54.4
35	Hawaii	55.2
32	Idaho	57.3
28	Illinois	59.5
18	Indiana	66.0
3	Iowa	77.1
11	Kansas	69.6
22	Kentucky	63.2
31	Louisiana	57.8
21	Maine	63.3
40	Maryland	51.3
37	Massachusetts	54.0
30	Michigan	58.8
23	Minnesota	60.5
18	Mississippi	66.0
9	Missouri	71.7
20	Montana	65.8
11	Nebraska	69.6
45	Nevada	46.5
39	New Hampshire	52.1
42	New Jersey	50.4
48	New Mexico	41.4
47	New York	42.8
8	North Carolina	72.1
7	North Dakota	72.2
26	Ohio	59.9
14	Oklahoma	68.4
2	Oregon	79.9
13	Pennsylvania	68.5
27	Rhode Island	59.8
4	South Carolina	75.6
5	South Dakota	72.9
5	Tennessee	72.9
43	Texas	49.7
49	Utah	37.9
34	Vermont	55.8
33	Virginia	56.2
24	Washington	60.3
17	West Virginia	67.1
10	Wisconsin	69.8
25	Wyoming	60.1

RANK ORDER

RANK	STATE	RATE
1	Arkansas	92.8
2	Oregon	79.9
3	Iowa	77.1
4	South Carolina	75.6
5	South Dakota	72.9
5	Tennessee	72.9
7	North Dakota	72.2
8	North Carolina	72.1
9	Missouri	71.7
10	Wisconsin	69.8
11	Kansas	69.6
11	Nebraska	69.6
13	Pennsylvania	68.5
14	Oklahoma	68.4
15	Florida	67.6
16	Alabama	67.3
17	West Virginia	67.1
18	Indiana	66.0
18	Mississippi	66.0
20	Montana	65.8
21	Maine	63.3
22	Kentucky	63.2
23	Minnesota	60.5
24	Washington	60.3
25	Wyoming	60.1
26	Ohio	59.9
27	Rhode Island	59.8
28	Connecticut	59.5
28	Illinois	59.5
30	Michigan	58.8
31	Louisiana	57.8
32	Idaho	57.3
33	Virginia	56.2
34	Vermont	55.8
35	Hawaii	55.2
36	Georgia	54.4
37	Massachusetts	54.0
38	Arizona	52.9
39	New Hampshire	52.1
40	Maryland	51.3
41	California	50.5
42	New Jersey	50.4
43	Texas	49.7
44	Delaware	49.4
45	Nevada	46.5
46	Colorado	43.8
47	New York	42.8
48	New Mexico	41.4
49	Utah	37.9
50	Alaska	24.9

| | District of Columbia | 60.2 |

Source: U.S. Department of Health and Human Services, National Center for Health Statistics
   "National Vital Statistics Reports" (Vol. 48, No. 11, July 24, 2000)
*Final data by state of residence. Cerebrovascular diseases include stroke and other disorders of the blood vessels of the brain. Not age-adjusted.

Age-Adjusted Death Rate by Cerebrovascular Diseases in 1998

National Rate = 25.1 Deaths per 100,000 Population*

ALPHA ORDER

RANK	STATE	RATE
7	Alabama	30.6
22	Alaska	25.2
38	Arizona	22.5
2	Arkansas	35.3
25	California	25.0
43	Colorado	21.8
45	Connecticut	20.9
33	Delaware	23.2
40	Florida	22.0
6	Georgia	31.6
31	Hawaii	24.1
26	Idaho	24.7
20	Illinois	25.4
10	Indiana	28.1
36	Iowa	23.1
26	Kansas	24.7
12	Kentucky	27.6
8	Louisiana	30.0
37	Maine	22.6
24	Maryland	25.1
49	Massachusetts	18.6
18	Michigan	25.9
42	Minnesota	21.9
3	Mississippi	33.4
13	Missouri	27.3
33	Montana	23.2
22	Nebraska	25.2
21	Nevada	25.3
46	New Hampshire	20.5
44	New Jersey	21.1
48	New Mexico	19.6
50	New York	18.3
4	North Carolina	33.1
38	North Dakota	22.5
29	Ohio	24.3
11	Oklahoma	27.7
9	Oregon	29.0
32	Pennsylvania	23.5
47	Rhode Island	20.0
1	South Carolina	37.0
29	South Dakota	24.3
5	Tennessee	32.6
15	Texas	26.4
40	Utah	22.0
33	Vermont	23.2
14	Virginia	27.2
19	Washington	25.6
26	West Virginia	24.7
17	Wisconsin	26.0
16	Wyoming	26.2

RANK ORDER

RANK	STATE	RATE
1	South Carolina	37.0
2	Arkansas	35.3
3	Mississippi	33.4
4	North Carolina	33.1
5	Tennessee	32.6
6	Georgia	31.6
7	Alabama	30.6
8	Louisiana	30.0
9	Oregon	29.0
10	Indiana	28.1
11	Oklahoma	27.7
12	Kentucky	27.6
13	Missouri	27.3
14	Virginia	27.2
15	Texas	26.4
16	Wyoming	26.2
17	Wisconsin	26.0
18	Michigan	25.9
19	Washington	25.6
20	Illinois	25.4
21	Nevada	25.3
22	Alaska	25.2
22	Nebraska	25.2
24	Maryland	25.1
25	California	25.0
26	Idaho	24.7
26	Kansas	24.7
26	West Virginia	24.7
29	Ohio	24.3
29	South Dakota	24.3
31	Hawaii	24.1
32	Pennsylvania	23.5
33	Delaware	23.2
33	Montana	23.2
33	Vermont	23.2
36	Iowa	23.1
37	Maine	22.6
38	Arizona	22.5
38	North Dakota	22.5
40	Florida	22.0
40	Utah	22.0
42	Minnesota	21.9
43	Colorado	21.8
44	New Jersey	21.1
45	Connecticut	20.9
46	New Hampshire	20.5
47	Rhode Island	20.0
48	New Mexico	19.6
49	Massachusetts	18.6
50	New York	18.3
	District of Columbia	28.4

Source: U.S. Department of Health and Human Services, National Center for Health Statistics
"National Vital Statistics Reports" (Vol. 48, No. 11, July 24, 2000)
Final data by state of residence. Cerebrovascular diseases include stroke and other disorders of the blood vessels of the brain.

Deaths by Chronic Liver Disease and Cirrhosis in 1998

National Total = 25,192 Deaths*

ALPHA ORDER

RANK	STATE	DEATHS	% of USA
19	Alabama	400	1.6%
49	Alaska	50	0.2%
11	Arizona	586	2.3%
35	Arkansas	203	0.8%
1	California	3,512	13.9%
24	Colorado	348	1.4%
29	Connecticut	287	1.1%
45	Delaware	73	0.3%
3	Florida	1,883	7.5%
12	Georgia	579	2.3%
46	Hawaii	69	0.3%
42	Idaho	87	0.3%
6	Illinois	1,080	4.3%
16	Indiana	472	1.9%
34	Iowa	208	0.8%
36	Kansas	190	0.8%
25	Kentucky	331	1.3%
22	Louisiana	379	1.5%
39	Maine	103	0.4%
18	Maryland	438	1.7%
13	Massachusetts	575	2.3%
7	Michigan	972	3.9%
28	Minnesota	290	1.2%
32	Mississippi	233	0.9%
20	Missouri	393	1.6%
43	Montana	80	0.3%
41	Nebraska	91	0.4%
30	Nevada	270	1.1%
38	New Hampshire	105	0.4%
9	New Jersey	735	2.9%
31	New Mexico	268	1.1%
4	New York	1,531	6.1%
10	North Carolina	700	2.8%
48	North Dakota	51	0.2%
8	Ohio	964	3.8%
27	Oklahoma	302	1.2%
26	Oregon	318	1.3%
5	Pennsylvania	1,091	4.3%
40	Rhode Island	101	0.4%
23	South Carolina	375	1.5%
44	South Dakota	75	0.3%
14	Tennessee	541	2.1%
2	Texas	1,962	7.8%
37	Utah	116	0.5%
50	Vermont	45	0.2%
15	Virginia	527	2.1%
17	Washington	463	1.8%
33	West Virginia	219	0.9%
21	Wisconsin	387	1.5%
47	Wyoming	65	0.3%

RANK ORDER

RANK	STATE	DEATHS	% of USA
1	California	3,512	13.9%
2	Texas	1,962	7.8%
3	Florida	1,883	7.5%
4	New York	1,531	6.1%
5	Pennsylvania	1,091	4.3%
6	Illinois	1,080	4.3%
7	Michigan	972	3.9%
8	Ohio	964	3.8%
9	New Jersey	735	2.9%
10	North Carolina	700	2.8%
11	Arizona	586	2.3%
12	Georgia	579	2.3%
13	Massachusetts	575	2.3%
14	Tennessee	541	2.1%
15	Virginia	527	2.1%
16	Indiana	472	1.9%
17	Washington	463	1.8%
18	Maryland	438	1.7%
19	Alabama	400	1.6%
20	Missouri	393	1.6%
21	Wisconsin	387	1.5%
22	Louisiana	379	1.5%
23	South Carolina	375	1.5%
24	Colorado	348	1.4%
25	Kentucky	331	1.3%
26	Oregon	318	1.3%
27	Oklahoma	302	1.2%
28	Minnesota	290	1.2%
29	Connecticut	287	1.1%
30	Nevada	270	1.1%
31	New Mexico	268	1.1%
32	Mississippi	233	0.9%
33	West Virginia	219	0.9%
34	Iowa	208	0.8%
35	Arkansas	203	0.8%
36	Kansas	190	0.8%
37	Utah	116	0.5%
38	New Hampshire	105	0.4%
39	Maine	103	0.4%
40	Rhode Island	101	0.4%
41	Nebraska	91	0.4%
42	Idaho	87	0.3%
43	Montana	80	0.3%
44	South Dakota	75	0.3%
45	Delaware	73	0.3%
46	Hawaii	69	0.3%
47	Wyoming	65	0.3%
48	North Dakota	51	0.2%
49	Alaska	50	0.2%
50	Vermont	45	0.2%
	District of Columbia	69	0.3%

Source: U.S. Department of Health and Human Services, National Center for Health Statistics
    "National Vital Statistics Reports" (Vol. 48, No. 11, July 24, 2000)
*Final data by state of residence. Cirrhosis of the liver is characterized by the replacement of normal tissue with fibrous tissue and the loss of functional liver cells. It can result from alcohol abuse, nutritional deprivation, or infection especially by the hepatitis virus.

Death Rate by Chronic Liver Disease and Cirrhosis in 1998

National Rate = 9.3 Deaths per 100,000 Population*

ALPHA ORDER

RANK	STATE	RATE
18	Alabama	9.2
34	Alaska	8.1
4	Arizona	12.6
36	Arkansas	8.0
7	California	10.8
25	Colorado	8.8
25	Connecticut	8.8
13	Delaware	9.8
4	Florida	12.6
40	Georgia	7.6
48	Hawaii	5.8
46	Idaho	7.1
22	Illinois	9.0
36	Indiana	8.0
43	Iowa	7.3
44	Kansas	7.2
31	Kentucky	8.4
27	Louisiana	8.7
33	Maine	8.3
29	Maryland	8.5
16	Massachusetts	9.4
11	Michigan	9.9
47	Minnesota	6.1
29	Mississippi	8.5
44	Missouri	7.2
19	Montana	9.1
49	Nebraska	5.5
1	Nevada	15.5
24	New Hampshire	8.9
19	New Jersey	9.1
2	New Mexico	15.4
31	New York	8.4
17	North Carolina	9.3
36	North Dakota	8.0
28	Ohio	8.6
22	Oklahoma	9.0
15	Oregon	9.7
19	Pennsylvania	9.1
8	Rhode Island	10.2
13	South Carolina	9.8
8	South Dakota	10.2
10	Tennessee	10.0
11	Texas	9.9
49	Utah	5.5
40	Vermont	7.6
39	Virginia	7.8
34	Washington	8.1
6	West Virginia	12.1
42	Wisconsin	7.4
3	Wyoming	13.5

RANK ORDER

RANK	STATE	RATE
1	Nevada	15.5
2	New Mexico	15.4
3	Wyoming	13.5
4	Arizona	12.6
4	Florida	12.6
6	West Virginia	12.1
7	California	10.8
8	Rhode Island	10.2
8	South Dakota	10.2
10	Tennessee	10.0
11	Michigan	9.9
11	Texas	9.9
13	Delaware	9.8
13	South Carolina	9.8
15	Oregon	9.7
16	Massachusetts	9.4
17	North Carolina	9.3
18	Alabama	9.2
19	Montana	9.1
19	New Jersey	9.1
19	Pennsylvania	9.1
22	Illinois	9.0
22	Oklahoma	9.0
24	New Hampshire	8.9
25	Colorado	8.8
25	Connecticut	8.8
27	Louisiana	8.7
28	Ohio	8.6
29	Maryland	8.5
29	Mississippi	8.5
31	Kentucky	8.4
31	New York	8.4
33	Maine	8.3
34	Alaska	8.1
34	Washington	8.1
36	Arkansas	8.0
36	Indiana	8.0
36	North Dakota	8.0
39	Virginia	7.8
40	Georgia	7.6
40	Vermont	7.6
42	Wisconsin	7.4
43	Iowa	7.3
44	Kansas	7.2
44	Missouri	7.2
46	Idaho	7.1
47	Minnesota	6.1
48	Hawaii	5.8
49	Nebraska	5.5
49	Utah	5.5

District of Columbia	13.2

Source: U.S. Department of Health and Human Services, National Center for Health Statistics
"National Vital Statistics Reports" (Vol. 48, No. 11, July 24, 2000)
*Final data by state of residence. Cirrhosis of the liver is characterized by the replacement of normal tissue with fibrous tissue and the loss of functional liver cells. It can result from alcohol abuse, nutritional deprivation, or infection especially by the hepatitis virus. Not age-adjusted.

Age-Adjusted Death Rate by Chronic Liver Disease and Cirrhosis in 1998

National Rate = 7.2 Deaths per 100,000 Population*

ALPHA ORDER

RANK	STATE	RATE
25	Alabama	6.7
9	Alaska	8.0
4	Arizona	10.1
38	Arkansas	5.9
5	California	9.4
15	Colorado	7.1
33	Connecticut	6.2
14	Delaware	7.2
6	Florida	8.5
30	Georgia	6.4
50	Hawaii	4.0
36	Idaho	6.0
15	Illinois	7.1
35	Indiana	6.1
48	Iowa	4.7
41	Kansas	5.7
31	Kentucky	6.3
21	Louisiana	6.9
41	Maine	5.7
25	Maryland	6.7
23	Massachusetts	6.8
11	Michigan	7.9
47	Minnesota	4.8
18	Mississippi	7.0
43	Missouri	5.5
23	Montana	6.8
49	Nebraska	4.3
2	Nevada	12.6
27	New Hampshire	6.6
29	New Jersey	6.5
1	New Mexico	13.0
31	New York	6.3
18	North Carolina	7.0
40	North Dakota	5.8
33	Ohio	6.2
18	Oklahoma	7.0
21	Oregon	6.9
38	Pennsylvania	5.9
15	Rhode Island	7.1
12	South Carolina	7.6
8	South Dakota	8.3
12	Tennessee	7.6
6	Texas	8.5
43	Utah	5.5
46	Vermont	5.3
36	Virginia	6.0
27	Washington	6.6
9	West Virginia	8.0
45	Wisconsin	5.4
3	Wyoming	10.9

RANK ORDER

RANK	STATE	RATE
1	New Mexico	13.0
2	Nevada	12.6
3	Wyoming	10.9
4	Arizona	10.1
5	California	9.4
6	Florida	8.5
6	Texas	8.5
8	South Dakota	8.3
9	Alaska	8.0
9	West Virginia	8.0
11	Michigan	7.9
12	South Carolina	7.6
12	Tennessee	7.6
14	Delaware	7.2
15	Colorado	7.1
15	Illinois	7.1
15	Rhode Island	7.1
18	Mississippi	7.0
18	North Carolina	7.0
18	Oklahoma	7.0
21	Louisiana	6.9
21	Oregon	6.9
23	Massachusetts	6.8
23	Montana	6.8
25	Alabama	6.7
25	Maryland	6.7
27	New Hampshire	6.6
27	Washington	6.6
29	New Jersey	6.5
30	Georgia	6.4
31	Kentucky	6.3
31	New York	6.3
33	Connecticut	6.2
33	Ohio	6.2
35	Indiana	6.1
36	Idaho	6.0
36	Virginia	6.0
38	Arkansas	5.9
38	Pennsylvania	5.9
40	North Dakota	5.8
41	Kansas	5.7
41	Maine	5.7
43	Missouri	5.5
43	Utah	5.5
45	Wisconsin	5.4
46	Vermont	5.3
47	Minnesota	4.8
48	Iowa	4.7
49	Nebraska	4.3
50	Hawaii	4.0
	District of Columbia	10.5

Source: U.S. Department of Health and Human Services, National Center for Health Statistics
    "National Vital Statistics Reports" (Vol. 48, No. 11, July 24, 2000)
*Final data by state of residence. Cirrhosis of the liver is characterized by the replacement of normal tissue with fibrous tissue and the loss of functional liver cells. It can result from alcohol abuse, nutritional deprivation, or infection especially by the hepatitis virus.

141

Deaths by Chronic Obstructive Pulmonary Diseases in 1998

National Total = 112,584 Deaths*

ALPHA ORDER

RANK ORDER

RANK	STATE	DEATHS	% of USA
20	Alabama	1,985	1.8%
50	Alaska	112	0.1%
18	Arizona	2,401	2.1%
30	Arkansas	1,244	1.1%
1	California	12,341	11.0%
22	Colorado	1,836	1.6%
31	Connecticut	1,243	1.1%
44	Delaware	327	0.3%
2	Florida	8,188	7.3%
12	Georgia	2,744	2.4%
47	Hawaii	266	0.2%
40	Idaho	540	0.5%
7	Illinois	4,542	4.0%
11	Indiana	2,762	2.5%
29	Iowa	1,439	1.3%
32	Kansas	1,198	1.1%
21	Kentucky	1,963	1.7%
28	Louisiana	1,566	1.4%
37	Maine	769	0.7%
25	Maryland	1,708	1.5%
15	Massachusetts	2,546	2.3%
8	Michigan	3,813	3.4%
24	Minnesota	1,745	1.5%
34	Mississippi	1,141	1.0%
13	Missouri	2,725	2.4%
41	Montana	505	0.4%
36	Nebraska	784	0.7%
35	Nevada	947	0.8%
39	New Hampshire	572	0.5%
10	New Jersey	2,794	2.5%
38	New Mexico	764	0.7%
4	New York	6,430	5.7%
9	North Carolina	3,204	2.8%
46	North Dakota	272	0.2%
6	Ohio	5,404	4.8%
23	Oklahoma	1,750	1.6%
26	Oregon	1,612	1.4%
5	Pennsylvania	5,596	5.0%
43	Rhode Island	454	0.4%
27	South Carolina	1,568	1.4%
45	South Dakota	317	0.3%
14	Tennessee	2,641	2.3%
3	Texas	6,603	5.9%
42	Utah	483	0.4%
48	Vermont	250	0.2%
16	Virginia	2,481	2.2%
17	Washington	2,403	2.1%
33	West Virginia	1,146	1.0%
19	Wisconsin	2,062	1.8%
49	Wyoming	240	0.2%

RANK	STATE	DEATHS	% of USA
1	California	12,341	11.0%
2	Florida	8,188	7.3%
3	Texas	6,603	5.9%
4	New York	6,430	5.7%
5	Pennsylvania	5,596	5.0%
6	Ohio	5,404	4.8%
7	Illinois	4,542	4.0%
8	Michigan	3,813	3.4%
9	North Carolina	3,204	2.8%
10	New Jersey	2,794	2.5%
11	Indiana	2,762	2.5%
12	Georgia	2,744	2.4%
13	Missouri	2,725	2.4%
14	Tennessee	2,641	2.3%
15	Massachusetts	2,546	2.3%
16	Virginia	2,481	2.2%
17	Washington	2,403	2.1%
18	Arizona	2,401	2.1%
19	Wisconsin	2,062	1.8%
20	Alabama	1,985	1.8%
21	Kentucky	1,963	1.7%
22	Colorado	1,836	1.6%
23	Oklahoma	1,750	1.6%
24	Minnesota	1,745	1.5%
25	Maryland	1,708	1.5%
26	Oregon	1,612	1.4%
27	South Carolina	1,568	1.4%
28	Louisiana	1,566	1.4%
29	Iowa	1,439	1.3%
30	Arkansas	1,244	1.1%
31	Connecticut	1,243	1.1%
32	Kansas	1,198	1.1%
33	West Virginia	1,146	1.0%
34	Mississippi	1,141	1.0%
35	Nevada	947	0.8%
36	Nebraska	784	0.7%
37	Maine	769	0.7%
38	New Mexico	764	0.7%
39	New Hampshire	572	0.5%
40	Idaho	540	0.5%
41	Montana	505	0.4%
42	Utah	483	0.4%
43	Rhode Island	454	0.4%
44	Delaware	327	0.3%
45	South Dakota	317	0.3%
46	North Dakota	272	0.2%
47	Hawaii	266	0.2%
48	Vermont	250	0.2%
49	Wyoming	240	0.2%
50	Alaska	112	0.1%
	District of Columbia	158	0.1%

Source: U.S. Department of Health and Human Services, National Center for Health Statistics
    "National Vital Statistics Reports" (Vol. 48, No. 11, July 24, 2000)
*Final data by state of residence. Chronic obstructive pulmonary diseases are diseases of the lungs including bronchitis, emphysema and asthma. Includes allied conditions.

Death Rate by Chronic Obstructive Pulmonary Diseases in 1998

National Rate = 41.7 Deaths per 100,000 Population*

<u>ALPHA ORDER</u>

RANK	STATE	RATE
22	Alabama	45.6
50	Alaska	18.2
7	Arizona	51.4
13	Arkansas	49.0
38	California	37.8
20	Colorado	46.2
37	Connecticut	38.0
24	Delaware	44.0
4	Florida	54.9
42	Georgia	35.9
49	Hawaii	22.3
26	Idaho	43.9
39	Illinois	37.7
18	Indiana	46.8
8	Iowa	50.3
22	Kansas	45.6
10	Kentucky	49.9
43	Louisiana	35.8
2	Maine	61.8
47	Maryland	33.3
33	Massachusetts	41.4
36	Michigan	38.8
40	Minnesota	36.9
32	Mississippi	41.5
9	Missouri	50.1
3	Montana	57.4
17	Nebraska	47.2
5	Nevada	54.2
15	New Hampshire	48.3
45	New Jersey	34.4
24	New Mexico	44.0
44	New York	35.4
29	North Carolina	42.5
28	North Dakota	42.6
16	Ohio	48.2
6	Oklahoma	52.3
12	Oregon	49.1
19	Pennsylvania	46.6
21	Rhode Island	45.9
34	South Carolina	40.9
27	South Dakota	42.9
14	Tennessee	48.6
46	Texas	33.4
48	Utah	23.0
30	Vermont	42.3
41	Virginia	36.5
31	Washington	42.2
1	West Virginia	63.3
35	Wisconsin	39.5
10	Wyoming	49.9

<u>RANK ORDER</u>

RANK	STATE	RATE
1	West Virginia	63.3
2	Maine	61.8
3	Montana	57.4
4	Florida	54.9
5	Nevada	54.2
6	Oklahoma	52.3
7	Arizona	51.4
8	Iowa	50.3
9	Missouri	50.1
10	Kentucky	49.9
10	Wyoming	49.9
12	Oregon	49.1
13	Arkansas	49.0
14	Tennessee	48.6
15	New Hampshire	48.3
16	Ohio	48.2
17	Nebraska	47.2
18	Indiana	46.8
19	Pennsylvania	46.6
20	Colorado	46.2
21	Rhode Island	45.9
22	Alabama	45.6
22	Kansas	45.6
24	Delaware	44.0
24	New Mexico	44.0
26	Idaho	43.9
27	South Dakota	42.9
28	North Dakota	42.6
29	North Carolina	42.5
30	Vermont	42.3
31	Washington	42.2
32	Mississippi	41.5
33	Massachusetts	41.4
34	South Carolina	40.9
35	Wisconsin	39.5
36	Michigan	38.8
37	Connecticut	38.0
38	California	37.8
39	Illinois	37.7
40	Minnesota	36.9
41	Virginia	36.5
42	Georgia	35.9
43	Louisiana	35.8
44	New York	35.4
45	New Jersey	34.4
46	Texas	33.4
47	Maryland	33.3
48	Utah	23.0
49	Hawaii	22.3
50	Alaska	18.2
	District of Columbia	30.2

Source: U.S. Department of Health and Human Services, National Center for Health Statistics
   "National Vital Statistics Reports" (Vol. 48, No. 11, July 24, 2000)
*Final data by state of residence. Chronic obstructive pulmonary diseases are diseases of the lungs including bronchitis, emphysema and asthma. Includes allied conditions. Not age-adjusted.

Age-Adjusted Death Rate by Chronic Obstructive Pulmonary Diseases in 1998

National Rate = 21.3 Deaths per 100,000 Population*

ALPHA ORDER

RANK	STATE	RATE
20	Alabama	23.6
33	Alaska	20.8
11	Arizona	25.4
20	Arkansas	23.6
28	California	21.5
2	Colorado	28.5
48	Connecticut	16.0
29	Delaware	21.2
36	Florida	20.2
15	Georgia	23.8
50	Hawaii	10.8
12	Idaho	25.1
37	Illinois	19.9
13	Indiana	24.6
31	Iowa	21.0
25	Kansas	22.3
6	Kentucky	26.7
32	Louisiana	20.9
5	Maine	26.9
44	Maryland	18.1
42	Massachusetts	18.4
35	Michigan	20.7
45	Minnesota	17.9
15	Mississippi	23.8
14	Missouri	24.4
6	Montana	26.7
26	Nebraska	21.8
1	Nevada	32.1
10	New Hampshire	26.1
49	New Jersey	15.6
19	New Mexico	23.7
47	New York	17.1
23	North Carolina	23.3
43	North Dakota	18.3
20	Ohio	23.6
8	Oklahoma	26.4
15	Oregon	23.8
38	Pennsylvania	19.1
38	Rhode Island	19.1
15	South Carolina	23.8
40	South Dakota	18.7
9	Tennessee	26.3
30	Texas	21.1
46	Utah	17.3
26	Vermont	21.8
33	Virginia	20.8
24	Washington	22.9
4	West Virginia	27.6
41	Wisconsin	18.5
3	Wyoming	28.4

RANK ORDER

RANK	STATE	RATE
1	Nevada	32.1
2	Colorado	28.5
3	Wyoming	28.4
4	West Virginia	27.6
5	Maine	26.9
6	Kentucky	26.7
6	Montana	26.7
8	Oklahoma	26.4
9	Tennessee	26.3
10	New Hampshire	26.1
11	Arizona	25.4
12	Idaho	25.1
13	Indiana	24.6
14	Missouri	24.4
15	Georgia	23.8
15	Mississippi	23.8
15	Oregon	23.8
15	South Carolina	23.8
19	New Mexico	23.7
20	Alabama	23.6
20	Arkansas	23.6
20	Ohio	23.6
23	North Carolina	23.3
24	Washington	22.9
25	Kansas	22.3
26	Nebraska	21.8
26	Vermont	21.8
28	California	21.5
29	Delaware	21.2
30	Texas	21.1
31	Iowa	21.0
32	Louisiana	20.9
33	Alaska	20.8
33	Virginia	20.8
35	Michigan	20.7
36	Florida	20.2
37	Illinois	19.9
38	Pennsylvania	19.1
38	Rhode Island	19.1
40	South Dakota	18.7
41	Wisconsin	18.5
42	Massachusetts	18.4
43	North Dakota	18.3
44	Maryland	18.1
45	Minnesota	17.9
46	Utah	17.3
47	New York	17.1
48	Connecticut	16.0
49	New Jersey	15.6
50	Hawaii	10.8

District of Columbia	15.7

Source: U.S. Department of Health and Human Services, National Center for Health Statistics
    "National Vital Statistics Reports" (Vol. 48, No. 11, July 24, 2000)
*Final data by state of residence. Chronic obstructive pulmonary diseases are diseases of the lungs including
bronchitis, emphysema and asthma. Includes allied conditions.

Deaths by Diabetes Mellitus in 1998

National Total = 64,751 Deaths*

ALPHA ORDER

RANK	STATE	DEATHS	% of USA
19	Alabama	1,312	2.0%
50	Alaska	64	0.1%
24	Arizona	1,010	1.6%
31	Arkansas	648	1.0%
1	California	5,846	9.0%
34	Colorado	566	0.9%
29	Connecticut	664	1.0%
42	Delaware	232	0.4%
3	Florida	4,034	6.2%
16	Georgia	1,389	2.1%
45	Hawaii	202	0.3%
41	Idaho	238	0.4%
7	Illinois	2,740	4.2%
13	Indiana	1,426	2.2%
30	Iowa	657	1.0%
32	Kansas	641	1.0%
23	Kentucky	1,093	1.7%
11	Louisiana	1,826	2.8%
38	Maine	333	0.5%
12	Maryland	1,444	2.2%
14	Massachusetts	1,402	2.2%
8	Michigan	2,435	3.8%
22	Minnesota	1,097	1.7%
33	Mississippi	635	1.0%
15	Missouri	1,394	2.2%
46	Montana	197	0.3%
37	Nebraska	338	0.5%
42	Nevada	232	0.4%
39	New Hampshire	266	0.4%
9	New Jersey	2,320	3.6%
36	New Mexico	422	0.7%
4	New York	3,606	5.6%
10	North Carolina	1,966	3.0%
47	North Dakota	190	0.3%
6	Ohio	3,455	5.3%
26	Oklahoma	927	1.4%
27	Oregon	858	1.3%
5	Pennsylvania	3,507	5.4%
40	Rhode Island	261	0.4%
25	South Carolina	990	1.5%
44	South Dakota	206	0.3%
17	Tennessee	1,347	2.1%
2	Texas	4,894	7.6%
35	Utah	469	0.7%
48	Vermont	133	0.2%
18	Virginia	1,332	2.1%
21	Washington	1,199	1.9%
28	West Virginia	723	1.1%
20	Wisconsin	1,277	2.0%
49	Wyoming	115	0.2%

RANK ORDER

RANK	STATE	DEATHS	% of USA
1	California	5,846	9.0%
2	Texas	4,894	7.6%
3	Florida	4,034	6.2%
4	New York	3,606	5.6%
5	Pennsylvania	3,507	5.4%
6	Ohio	3,455	5.3%
7	Illinois	2,740	4.2%
8	Michigan	2,435	3.8%
9	New Jersey	2,320	3.6%
10	North Carolina	1,966	3.0%
11	Louisiana	1,826	2.8%
12	Maryland	1,444	2.2%
13	Indiana	1,426	2.2%
14	Massachusetts	1,402	2.2%
15	Missouri	1,394	2.2%
16	Georgia	1,389	2.1%
17	Tennessee	1,347	2.1%
18	Virginia	1,332	2.1%
19	Alabama	1,312	2.0%
20	Wisconsin	1,277	2.0%
21	Washington	1,199	1.9%
22	Minnesota	1,097	1.7%
23	Kentucky	1,093	1.7%
24	Arizona	1,010	1.6%
25	South Carolina	990	1.5%
26	Oklahoma	927	1.4%
27	Oregon	858	1.3%
28	West Virginia	723	1.1%
29	Connecticut	664	1.0%
30	Iowa	657	1.0%
31	Arkansas	648	1.0%
32	Kansas	641	1.0%
33	Mississippi	635	1.0%
34	Colorado	566	0.9%
35	Utah	469	0.7%
36	New Mexico	422	0.7%
37	Nebraska	338	0.5%
38	Maine	333	0.5%
39	New Hampshire	266	0.4%
40	Rhode Island	261	0.4%
41	Idaho	238	0.4%
42	Delaware	232	0.4%
42	Nevada	232	0.4%
44	South Dakota	206	0.3%
45	Hawaii	202	0.3%
46	Montana	197	0.3%
47	North Dakota	190	0.3%
48	Vermont	133	0.2%
49	Wyoming	115	0.2%
50	Alaska	64	0.1%
	District of Columbia	193	0.3%

Source: U.S. Department of Health and Human Services, National Center for Health Statistics
"National Vital Statistics Reports" (Vol. 48, No. 11, July 24, 2000)
*Final data by state of residence. A severe, chronic form of diabetes caused by insufficient production of insulin and resulting in abnormal metabolism of carbohydrates, fats, and proteins. The disease, which typically appears in childhood or adolescence, is characterized by increased sugar levels in the blood and urine, excessive thirst and frequent urination.

Death Rate by Diabetes Mellitus in 1998

National Rate = 24.0 Deaths per 100,000 Population*

ALPHA ORDER

RANK	STATE	RATE
5	Alabama	30.1
50	Alaska	10.4
38	Arizona	21.6
20	Arkansas	25.5
46	California	17.9
48	Colorado	14.3
40	Connecticut	20.3
3	Delaware	31.2
13	Florida	27.0
45	Georgia	18.2
47	Hawaii	16.9
44	Idaho	19.4
33	Illinois	22.7
27	Indiana	24.2
31	Iowa	23.0
24	Kansas	24.4
11	Kentucky	27.8
1	Louisiana	41.8
14	Maine	26.8
9	Maryland	28.1
32	Massachusetts	22.8
21	Michigan	24.8
29	Minnesota	23.2
30	Mississippi	23.1
19	Missouri	25.6
35	Montana	22.4
40	Nebraska	20.3
49	Nevada	13.3
35	New Hampshire	22.4
8	New Jersey	28.6
26	New Mexico	24.3
42	New York	19.8
16	North Carolina	26.1
6	North Dakota	29.8
4	Ohio	30.8
12	Oklahoma	27.7
16	Oregon	26.1
7	Pennsylvania	29.2
15	Rhode Island	26.4
18	South Carolina	25.8
10	South Dakota	27.9
21	Tennessee	24.8
21	Texas	24.8
37	Utah	22.3
34	Vermont	22.5
43	Virginia	19.6
39	Washington	21.1
2	West Virginia	39.9
24	Wisconsin	24.4
28	Wyoming	23.9

RANK ORDER

RANK	STATE	RATE
1	Louisiana	41.8
2	West Virginia	39.9
3	Delaware	31.2
4	Ohio	30.8
5	Alabama	30.1
6	North Dakota	29.8
7	Pennsylvania	29.2
8	New Jersey	28.6
9	Maryland	28.1
10	South Dakota	27.9
11	Kentucky	27.8
12	Oklahoma	27.7
13	Florida	27.0
14	Maine	26.8
15	Rhode Island	26.4
16	North Carolina	26.1
16	Oregon	26.1
18	South Carolina	25.8
19	Missouri	25.6
20	Arkansas	25.5
21	Michigan	24.8
21	Tennessee	24.8
21	Texas	24.8
24	Kansas	24.4
24	Wisconsin	24.4
26	New Mexico	24.3
27	Indiana	24.2
28	Wyoming	23.9
29	Minnesota	23.2
30	Mississippi	23.1
31	Iowa	23.0
32	Massachusetts	22.8
33	Illinois	22.7
34	Vermont	22.5
35	Montana	22.4
35	New Hampshire	22.4
37	Utah	22.3
38	Arizona	21.6
39	Washington	21.1
40	Connecticut	20.3
40	Nebraska	20.3
42	New York	19.8
43	Virginia	19.6
44	Idaho	19.4
45	Georgia	18.2
46	California	17.9
47	Hawaii	16.9
48	Colorado	14.3
49	Nevada	13.3
50	Alaska	10.4

District of Columbia 36.9

Source: U.S. Department of Health and Human Services, National Center for Health Statistics
"National Vital Statistics Reports" (Vol. 48, No. 11, July 24, 2000)
Final data by state of residence. A severe, chronic form of diabetes caused by insufficient production of insulin and resulting in abnormal metabolism of carbohydrates, fats, and proteins. The disease, which typically appears in childhood or adolescence, is characterized by increased sugar levels in the blood and urine, excessive thirst and frequent urination. Not age-adjusted.

Age-Adjusted Death Rate by Diabetes Mellitus in 1998

National Rate = 13.6 Deaths per 100,000 Population*

ALPHA ORDER

RANK	STATE	RATE
5	Alabama	16.8
42	Alaska	11.5
26	Arizona	13.1
23	Arkansas	13.4
38	California	12.0
49	Colorado	9.5
48	Connecticut	9.8
5	Delaware	16.8
35	Florida	12.3
28	Georgia	12.8
47	Hawaii	9.9
40	Idaho	11.9
28	Illinois	12.8
23	Indiana	13.4
46	Iowa	10.2
32	Kansas	12.6
12	Kentucky	15.4
1	Louisiana	25.8
19	Maine	13.7
3	Maryland	17.1
41	Massachusetts	11.6
18	Michigan	14.2
37	Minnesota	12.2
16	Mississippi	14.5
21	Missouri	13.6
43	Montana	11.2
45	Nebraska	10.3
50	Nevada	8.6
28	New Hampshire	12.8
13	New Jersey	15.2
14	New Mexico	15.1
44	New York	10.8
10	North Carolina	15.6
25	North Dakota	13.3
7	Ohio	16.6
11	Oklahoma	15.5
19	Oregon	13.7
22	Pennsylvania	13.5
32	Rhode Island	12.6
9	South Carolina	16.2
15	South Dakota	14.9
16	Tennessee	14.5
3	Texas	17.1
8	Utah	16.4
38	Vermont	12.0
35	Virginia	12.3
31	Washington	12.7
2	West Virginia	18.9
32	Wisconsin	12.6
27	Wyoming	13.0

RANK ORDER

RANK	STATE	RATE
1	Louisiana	25.8
2	West Virginia	18.9
3	Maryland	17.1
3	Texas	17.1
5	Alabama	16.8
5	Delaware	16.8
7	Ohio	16.6
8	Utah	16.4
9	South Carolina	16.2
10	North Carolina	15.6
11	Oklahoma	15.5
12	Kentucky	15.4
13	New Jersey	15.2
14	New Mexico	15.1
15	South Dakota	14.9
16	Mississippi	14.5
16	Tennessee	14.5
18	Michigan	14.2
19	Maine	13.7
19	Oregon	13.7
21	Missouri	13.6
22	Pennsylvania	13.5
23	Arkansas	13.4
23	Indiana	13.4
25	North Dakota	13.3
26	Arizona	13.1
27	Wyoming	13.0
28	Georgia	12.8
28	Illinois	12.8
28	New Hampshire	12.8
31	Washington	12.7
32	Kansas	12.6
32	Rhode Island	12.6
32	Wisconsin	12.6
35	Florida	12.3
35	Virginia	12.3
37	Minnesota	12.2
38	California	12.0
38	Vermont	12.0
40	Idaho	11.9
41	Massachusetts	11.6
42	Alaska	11.5
43	Montana	11.2
44	New York	10.8
45	Nebraska	10.3
46	Iowa	10.2
47	Hawaii	9.9
48	Connecticut	9.8
49	Colorado	9.5
50	Nevada	8.6

District of Columbia — 20.7

Source: U.S. Department of Health and Human Services, National Center for Health Statistics
"National Vital Statistics Reports" (Vol. 48, No. 11, July 24, 2000)
*Final data by state of residence. A severe, chronic form of diabetes caused by insufficient production of insulin and resulting in abnormal metabolism of carbohydrates, fats, and proteins. The disease, which typically appears in childhood or adolescence, is characterized by increased sugar levels in the blood and urine, excessive thirst and frequent urination.

Deaths by Diseases of the Heart in 1998

National Total = 724,859 Deaths*

ALPHA ORDER

RANK	STATE	DEATHS	% of USA
18	Alabama	13,480	1.9%
50	Alaska	564	0.1%
24	Arizona	10,543	1.5%
30	Arkansas	8,461	1.2%
1	California	69,747	9.6%
34	Colorado	6,644	0.9%
26	Connecticut	9,639	1.3%
46	Delaware	1,917	0.3%
3	Florida	51,131	7.1%
12	Georgia	17,964	2.5%
42	Hawaii	2,458	0.3%
43	Idaho	2,422	0.3%
7	Illinois	32,816	4.5%
14	Indiana	16,483	2.3%
29	Iowa	9,148	1.3%
32	Kansas	7,207	1.0%
20	Kentucky	11,924	1.6%
21	Louisiana	11,866	1.6%
37	Maine	3,562	0.5%
19	Maryland	11,939	1.6%
16	Massachusetts	16,007	2.2%
8	Michigan	28,005	3.9%
28	Minnesota	9,372	1.3%
27	Mississippi	9,539	1.3%
11	Missouri	17,968	2.5%
45	Montana	2,006	0.3%
35	Nebraska	4,733	0.7%
36	Nevada	4,120	0.6%
41	New Hampshire	2,833	0.4%
9	New Jersey	23,384	3.2%
38	New Mexico	3,221	0.4%
2	New York	59,531	8.2%
10	North Carolina	19,489	2.7%
47	North Dakota	1,738	0.2%
6	Ohio	33,355	4.6%
23	Oklahoma	11,297	1.6%
31	Oregon	7,290	1.0%
5	Pennsylvania	41,413	5.7%
39	Rhode Island	3,070	0.4%
25	South Carolina	10,026	1.4%
44	South Dakota	2,108	0.3%
13	Tennessee	16,516	2.3%
4	Texas	42,788	5.9%
40	Utah	2,881	0.4%
48	Vermont	1,434	0.2%
15	Virginia	16,022	2.2%
22	Washington	11,517	1.6%
33	West Virginia	6,883	0.9%
17	Wisconsin	13,685	1.9%
49	Wyoming	1,051	0.1%

RANK ORDER

RANK	STATE	DEATHS	% of USA
1	California	69,747	9.6%
2	New York	59,531	8.2%
3	Florida	51,131	7.1%
4	Texas	42,788	5.9%
5	Pennsylvania	41,413	5.7%
6	Ohio	33,355	4.6%
7	Illinois	32,816	4.5%
8	Michigan	28,005	3.9%
9	New Jersey	23,384	3.2%
10	North Carolina	19,489	2.7%
11	Missouri	17,968	2.5%
12	Georgia	17,964	2.5%
13	Tennessee	16,516	2.3%
14	Indiana	16,483	2.3%
15	Virginia	16,022	2.2%
16	Massachusetts	16,007	2.2%
17	Wisconsin	13,685	1.9%
18	Alabama	13,480	1.9%
19	Maryland	11,939	1.6%
20	Kentucky	11,924	1.6%
21	Louisiana	11,866	1.6%
22	Washington	11,517	1.6%
23	Oklahoma	11,297	1.6%
24	Arizona	10,543	1.5%
25	South Carolina	10,026	1.4%
26	Connecticut	9,639	1.3%
27	Mississippi	9,539	1.3%
28	Minnesota	9,372	1.3%
29	Iowa	9,148	1.3%
30	Arkansas	8,461	1.2%
31	Oregon	7,290	1.0%
32	Kansas	7,207	1.0%
33	West Virginia	6,883	0.9%
34	Colorado	6,644	0.9%
35	Nebraska	4,733	0.7%
36	Nevada	4,120	0.6%
37	Maine	3,562	0.5%
38	New Mexico	3,221	0.4%
39	Rhode Island	3,070	0.4%
40	Utah	2,881	0.4%
41	New Hampshire	2,833	0.4%
42	Hawaii	2,458	0.3%
43	Idaho	2,422	0.3%
44	South Dakota	2,108	0.3%
45	Montana	2,006	0.3%
46	Delaware	1,917	0.3%
47	North Dakota	1,738	0.2%
48	Vermont	1,434	0.2%
49	Wyoming	1,051	0.1%
50	Alaska	564	0.1%
	District of Columbia	1,662	0.2%

Source: U.S. Department of Health and Human Services, National Center for Health Statistics
     "National Vital Statistics Reports" (Vol. 48, No. 11, July 24, 2000)
*Final data by state of residence.

Death Rate by Diseases of the Heart in 1998

National Rate = 268.2 Deaths per 100,000 Population*

ALPHA ORDER				RANK ORDER		
RANK	STATE	RATE		RANK	STATE	RATE
11	Alabama	309.7		1	West Virginia	380.0
50	Alaska	91.9		2	Mississippi	346.6
38	Arizona	225.8		3	Pennsylvania	345.1
6	Arkansas	333.3		4	Florida	342.8
42	California	213.5		5	Oklahoma	337.6
48	Colorado	167.3		6	Arkansas	333.3
15	Connecticut	294.4		7	Missouri	330.4
30	Delaware	257.8		8	New York	327.5
4	Florida	342.8		9	Iowa	319.6
35	Georgia	235.1		10	Rhode Island	310.6
43	Hawaii	206.0		11	Alabama	309.7
46	Idaho	197.1		12	Tennessee	304.1
23	Illinois	272.4		13	Kentucky	302.9
21	Indiana	279.4		14	Ohio	297.6
9	Iowa	319.6		15	Connecticut	294.4
22	Kansas	274.1		16	New Jersey	288.2
13	Kentucky	302.9		17	Maine	286.3
25	Louisiana	271.6		18	South Dakota	285.6
17	Maine	286.3		19	Michigan	285.3
36	Maryland	232.5		20	Nebraska	284.7
28	Massachusetts	260.4		21	Indiana	279.4
19	Michigan	285.3		22	Kansas	274.1
45	Minnesota	198.3		23	Illinois	272.4
2	Mississippi	346.6		24	North Dakota	272.3
7	Missouri	330.4		25	Louisiana	271.6
37	Montana	227.8		26	Wisconsin	262.0
20	Nebraska	284.7		27	South Carolina	261.4
34	Nevada	235.8		28	Massachusetts	260.4
32	New Hampshire	239.1		29	North Carolina	258.3
16	New Jersey	288.2		30	Delaware	257.8
47	New Mexico	185.4		31	Vermont	242.7
8	New York	327.5		32	New Hampshire	239.1
29	North Carolina	258.3		33	Virginia	235.9
24	North Dakota	272.3		34	Nevada	235.8
14	Ohio	297.6		35	Georgia	235.1
5	Oklahoma	337.6		36	Maryland	232.5
39	Oregon	222.1		37	Montana	227.8
3	Pennsylvania	345.1		38	Arizona	225.8
10	Rhode Island	310.6		39	Oregon	222.1
27	South Carolina	261.4		40	Wyoming	218.5
18	South Dakota	285.6		41	Texas	216.5
12	Tennessee	304.1		42	California	213.5
41	Texas	216.5		43	Hawaii	206.0
49	Utah	137.2		44	Washington	202.4
31	Vermont	242.7		45	Minnesota	198.3
33	Virginia	235.9		46	Idaho	197.1
44	Washington	202.4		47	New Mexico	185.4
1	West Virginia	380.0		48	Colorado	167.3
26	Wisconsin	262.0		49	Utah	137.2
40	Wyoming	218.5		50	Alaska	91.9
					District of Columbia	317.7

Source: U.S. Department of Health and Human Services, National Center for Health Statistics
   "National Vital Statistics Reports" (Vol. 48, No. 11, July 24, 2000)
*Final data by state of residence. Not age-adjusted.

Age-Adjusted Death Rate by Diseases of the Heart in 1998

National Rate = 126.6 Deaths per 100,000 Population*

ALPHA ORDER

RANK	STATE	RATE
4	Alabama	152.3
46	Alaska	96.5
37	Arizona	109.2
8	Arkansas	147.6
33	California	113.1
48	Colorado	92.9
29	Connecticut	115.9
22	Delaware	127.4
26	Florida	118.0
9	Georgia	147.2
42	Hawaii	100.4
44	Idaho	96.8
19	Illinois	131.5
16	Indiana	134.5
28	Iowa	117.4
30	Kansas	114.8
7	Kentucky	148.7
6	Louisiana	150.0
25	Maine	118.1
23	Maryland	124.2
39	Massachusetts	106.6
13	Michigan	138.8
49	Minnesota	88.4
1	Mississippi	181.4
11	Missouri	142.7
43	Montana	100.2
36	Nebraska	111.5
12	Nevada	139.7
30	New Hampshire	114.8
24	New Jersey	121.4
45	New Mexico	96.6
13	New York	138.8
17	North Carolina	132.9
38	North Dakota	107.5
15	Ohio	136.5
5	Oklahoma	150.8
46	Oregon	96.5
18	Pennsylvania	132.3
27	Rhode Island	117.7
10	South Carolina	143.0
32	South Dakota	114.3
3	Tennessee	153.5
21	Texas	127.9
50	Utah	87.4
40	Vermont	105.2
20	Virginia	128.0
41	Washington	100.7
2	West Virginia	160.9
34	Wisconsin	112.9
35	Wyoming	111.6

RANK ORDER

RANK	STATE	RATE
1	Mississippi	181.4
2	West Virginia	160.9
3	Tennessee	153.5
4	Alabama	152.3
5	Oklahoma	150.8
6	Louisiana	150.0
7	Kentucky	148.7
8	Arkansas	147.6
9	Georgia	147.2
10	South Carolina	143.0
11	Missouri	142.7
12	Nevada	139.7
13	Michigan	138.8
13	New York	138.8
15	Ohio	136.5
16	Indiana	134.5
17	North Carolina	132.9
18	Pennsylvania	132.3
19	Illinois	131.5
20	Virginia	128.0
21	Texas	127.9
22	Delaware	127.4
23	Maryland	124.2
24	New Jersey	121.4
25	Maine	118.1
26	Florida	118.0
27	Rhode Island	117.7
28	Iowa	117.4
29	Connecticut	115.9
30	Kansas	114.8
30	New Hampshire	114.8
32	South Dakota	114.3
33	California	113.1
34	Wisconsin	112.9
35	Wyoming	111.6
36	Nebraska	111.5
37	Arizona	109.2
38	North Dakota	107.5
39	Massachusetts	106.6
40	Vermont	105.2
41	Washington	100.7
42	Hawaii	100.4
43	Montana	100.2
44	Idaho	96.8
45	New Mexico	96.6
46	Alaska	96.5
46	Oregon	96.5
48	Colorado	92.9
49	Minnesota	88.4
50	Utah	87.4
	District of Columbia	161.5

Source: U.S. Department of Health and Human Services, National Center for Health Statistics
    "National Vital Statistics Reports" (Vol. 48, No. 11, July 24, 2000)
Final data by state of residence.

Deaths by Malignant Neoplasms in 1998

National Total = 541,532 Deaths*

ALPHA ORDER

RANK	STATE	DEATHS	% of USA
20	Alabama	9,680	1.8%
50	Alaska	651	0.1%
24	Arizona	8,477	1.6%
30	Arkansas	5,961	1.1%
1	California	51,428	9.5%
32	Colorado	5,814	1.1%
27	Connecticut	7,106	1.3%
45	Delaware	1,652	0.3%
2	Florida	38,171	7.0%
12	Georgia	13,128	2.4%
43	Hawaii	1,969	0.4%
42	Idaho	2,089	0.4%
7	Illinois	24,637	4.5%
14	Indiana	12,652	2.3%
29	Iowa	6,429	1.2%
33	Kansas	5,110	0.9%
22	Kentucky	8,875	1.6%
21	Louisiana	9,358	1.7%
37	Maine	2,919	0.5%
19	Maryland	10,199	1.9%
11	Massachusetts	13,811	2.6%
8	Michigan	19,398	3.6%
23	Minnesota	8,798	1.6%
31	Mississippi	5,958	1.1%
15	Missouri	12,338	2.3%
44	Montana	1,825	0.3%
36	Nebraska	3,277	0.6%
35	Nevada	3,523	0.7%
40	New Hampshire	2,434	0.4%
9	New Jersey	18,032	3.3%
38	New Mexico	2,741	0.5%
3	New York	36,914	6.8%
10	North Carolina	15,357	2.8%
47	North Dakota	1,339	0.2%
6	Ohio	24,946	4.6%
26	Oklahoma	7,109	1.3%
28	Oregon	6,970	1.3%
5	Pennsylvania	29,821	5.5%
39	Rhode Island	2,480	0.5%
25	South Carolina	7,705	1.4%
46	South Dakota	1,564	0.3%
16	Tennessee	11,990	2.2%
4	Texas	32,315	6.0%
41	Utah	2,371	0.4%
48	Vermont	1,213	0.2%
13	Virginia	12,891	2.4%
18	Washington	10,277	1.9%
34	West Virginia	4,724	0.9%
17	Wisconsin	10,904	2.0%
49	Wyoming	845	0.2%

RANK ORDER

RANK	STATE	DEATHS	% of USA
1	California	51,428	9.5%
2	Florida	38,171	7.0%
3	New York	36,914	6.8%
4	Texas	32,315	6.0%
5	Pennsylvania	29,821	5.5%
6	Ohio	24,946	4.6%
7	Illinois	24,637	4.5%
8	Michigan	19,398	3.6%
9	New Jersey	18,032	3.3%
10	North Carolina	15,357	2.8%
11	Massachusetts	13,811	2.6%
12	Georgia	13,128	2.4%
13	Virginia	12,891	2.4%
14	Indiana	12,652	2.3%
15	Missouri	12,338	2.3%
16	Tennessee	11,990	2.2%
17	Wisconsin	10,904	2.0%
18	Washington	10,277	1.9%
19	Maryland	10,199	1.9%
20	Alabama	9,680	1.8%
21	Louisiana	9,358	1.7%
22	Kentucky	8,875	1.6%
23	Minnesota	8,798	1.6%
24	Arizona	8,477	1.6%
25	South Carolina	7,705	1.4%
26	Oklahoma	7,109	1.3%
27	Connecticut	7,106	1.3%
28	Oregon	6,970	1.3%
29	Iowa	6,429	1.2%
30	Arkansas	5,961	1.1%
31	Mississippi	5,958	1.1%
32	Colorado	5,814	1.1%
33	Kansas	5,110	0.9%
34	West Virginia	4,724	0.9%
35	Nevada	3,523	0.7%
36	Nebraska	3,277	0.6%
37	Maine	2,919	0.5%
38	New Mexico	2,741	0.5%
39	Rhode Island	2,480	0.5%
40	New Hampshire	2,434	0.4%
41	Utah	2,371	0.4%
42	Idaho	2,089	0.4%
43	Hawaii	1,969	0.4%
44	Montana	1,825	0.3%
45	Delaware	1,652	0.3%
46	South Dakota	1,564	0.3%
47	North Dakota	1,339	0.2%
48	Vermont	1,213	0.2%
49	Wyoming	845	0.2%
50	Alaska	651	0.1%
	District of Columbia	1,357	0.3%

Source: U.S. Department of Health and Human Services, National Center for Health Statistics
"National Vital Statistics Reports" (Vol. 48, No. 11, July 24, 2000)
*Final data by state of residence. Neoplasms are abnormal tissue, tumors. Includes many cancers.

Death Rate by Malignant Neoplasms in 1998

National Rate = 200.3 Deaths per 100,000 Population*

ALPHA ORDER				RANK ORDER		
RANK	STATE	RATE		RANK	STATE	RATE
12	Alabama	222.4		1	West Virginia	260.8
50	Alaska	106.0		2	Florida	255.9
39	Arizona	181.6		3	Rhode Island	250.9
5	Arkansas	234.8		4	Pennsylvania	248.5
47	California	157.4		5	Arkansas	234.8
48	Colorado	146.4		6	Maine	234.6
16	Connecticut	217.0		7	Missouri	226.9
13	Delaware	222.2		8	Kentucky	225.5
2	Florida	255.9		9	Massachusetts	224.7
42	Georgia	171.8		10	Iowa	224.6
44	Hawaii	165.0		11	Ohio	222.5
43	Idaho	170.0		12	Alabama	222.4
28	Illinois	204.5		13	Delaware	222.2
18	Indiana	214.5		13	New Jersey	222.2
10	Iowa	224.6		15	Tennessee	220.8
36	Kansas	194.4		16	Connecticut	217.0
8	Kentucky	225.5		17	Mississippi	216.5
19	Louisiana	214.2		18	Indiana	214.5
6	Maine	234.6		19	Louisiana	214.2
33	Maryland	198.6		20	Oklahoma	212.4
9	Massachusetts	224.7		20	Oregon	212.4
34	Michigan	197.6		22	South Dakota	211.9
38	Minnesota	186.2		23	North Dakota	209.8
17	Mississippi	216.5		24	Wisconsin	208.7
7	Missouri	226.9		25	Montana	207.3
25	Montana	207.3		26	New Hampshire	205.4
35	Nebraska	197.1		27	Vermont	205.3
31	Nevada	201.7		28	Illinois	204.5
26	New Hampshire	205.4		29	North Carolina	203.5
13	New Jersey	222.2		30	New York	203.1
46	New Mexico	157.8		31	Nevada	201.7
30	New York	203.1		32	South Carolina	200.9
29	North Carolina	203.5		33	Maryland	198.6
23	North Dakota	209.8		34	Michigan	197.6
11	Ohio	222.5		35	Nebraska	197.1
20	Oklahoma	212.4		36	Kansas	194.4
20	Oregon	212.4		37	Virginia	189.8
4	Pennsylvania	248.5		38	Minnesota	186.2
3	Rhode Island	250.9		39	Arizona	181.6
32	South Carolina	200.9		40	Washington	180.6
22	South Dakota	211.9		41	Wyoming	175.7
15	Tennessee	220.8		42	Georgia	171.8
45	Texas	163.5		43	Idaho	170.0
49	Utah	112.9		44	Hawaii	165.0
27	Vermont	205.3		45	Texas	163.5
37	Virginia	189.8		46	New Mexico	157.8
40	Washington	180.6		47	California	157.4
1	West Virginia	260.8		48	Colorado	146.4
24	Wisconsin	208.7		49	Utah	112.9
41	Wyoming	175.7		50	Alaska	106.0
					District of Columbia	259.4

Source: U.S. Department of Health and Human Services, National Center for Health Statistics
    "National Vital Statistics Reports" (Vol. 48, No. 11, July 24, 2000)
*Final data by state of residence. Neoplasms are abnormal tissue, tumors. Includes many cancers. Not age-adjusted.

Age-Adjusted Death Rate by Malignant Neoplasms in 1998

National Rate = 123.6 Deaths per 100,000 Population*

ALPHA ORDER

RANK	STATE	RATE
7	Alabama	135.6
37	Alaska	116.6
44	Arizona	110.6
11	Arkansas	133.2
44	California	110.6
48	Colorado	101.9
33	Connecticut	119.1
5	Delaware	138.9
29	Florida	122.6
18	Georgia	129.8
49	Hawaii	100.5
46	Idaho	110.4
20	Illinois	128.4
10	Indiana	133.4
35	Iowa	117.4
40	Kansas	112.9
2	Kentucky	141.9
1	Louisiana	143.9
16	Maine	130.8
15	Maryland	131.3
25	Massachusetts	126.1
27	Michigan	124.7
41	Minnesota	112.7
3	Mississippi	141.3
12	Missouri	132.9
43	Montana	112.2
38	Nebraska	114.0
9	Nevada	133.9
8	New Hampshire	134.2
22	New Jersey	126.8
47	New Mexico	104.3
32	New York	119.8
19	North Carolina	128.6
39	North Dakota	113.3
14	Ohio	131.5
24	Oklahoma	126.4
28	Oregon	123.4
21	Pennsylvania	127.8
13	Rhode Island	132.0
17	South Carolina	130.5
36	South Dakota	116.7
5	Tennessee	138.9
31	Texas	120.2
50	Utah	93.5
26	Vermont	124.9
22	Virginia	126.8
34	Washington	117.9
4	West Virginia	139.1
30	Wisconsin	121.3
42	Wyoming	112.3

RANK ORDER

RANK	STATE	RATE
1	Louisiana	143.9
2	Kentucky	141.9
3	Mississippi	141.3
4	West Virginia	139.1
5	Delaware	138.9
5	Tennessee	138.9
7	Alabama	135.6
8	New Hampshire	134.2
9	Nevada	133.9
10	Indiana	133.4
11	Arkansas	133.2
12	Missouri	132.9
13	Rhode Island	132.0
14	Ohio	131.5
15	Maryland	131.3
16	Maine	130.8
17	South Carolina	130.5
18	Georgia	129.8
19	North Carolina	128.6
20	Illinois	128.4
21	Pennsylvania	127.8
22	New Jersey	126.8
22	Virginia	126.8
24	Oklahoma	126.4
25	Massachusetts	126.1
26	Vermont	124.9
27	Michigan	124.7
28	Oregon	123.4
29	Florida	122.6
30	Wisconsin	121.3
31	Texas	120.2
32	New York	119.8
33	Connecticut	119.1
34	Washington	117.9
35	Iowa	117.4
36	South Dakota	116.7
37	Alaska	116.6
38	Nebraska	114.0
39	North Dakota	113.3
40	Kansas	112.9
41	Minnesota	112.7
42	Wyoming	112.3
43	Montana	112.2
44	Arizona	110.6
44	California	110.6
46	Idaho	110.4
47	New Mexico	104.3
48	Colorado	101.9
49	Hawaii	100.5
50	Utah	93.5

District of Columbia   154.3

Source: U.S. Department of Health and Human Services, National Center for Health Statistics
    "National Vital Statistics Reports" (Vol. 48, No. 11, July 24, 2000)
Final data by state of residence. Neoplasms are abnormal tissue, tumors. Includes many cancers.

Deaths by Pneumonia and Influenza in 1998

National Total = 91,871 Deaths*

ALPHA ORDER

RANK	STATE	DEATHS	% of USA
20	Alabama	1,518	1.7%
50	Alaska	52	0.1%
22	Arizona	1,444	1.6%
28	Arkansas	1,101	1.2%
1	California	13,378	14.6%
31	Colorado	1,037	1.1%
26	Connecticut	1,225	1.3%
47	Delaware	248	0.3%
5	Florida	4,111	4.5%
13	Georgia	2,264	2.5%
40	Hawaii	391	0.4%
42	Idaho	376	0.4%
6	Illinois	3,974	4.3%
17	Indiana	1,822	2.0%
24	Iowa	1,364	1.5%
33	Kansas	990	1.1%
21	Kentucky	1,474	1.6%
27	Louisiana	1,105	1.2%
37	Maine	468	0.5%
19	Maryland	1,641	1.8%
9	Massachusetts	2,895	3.2%
8	Michigan	3,083	3.4%
23	Minnesota	1,412	1.5%
30	Mississippi	1,071	1.2%
11	Missouri	2,422	2.6%
43	Montana	372	0.4%
35	Nebraska	610	0.7%
39	Nevada	403	0.4%
45	New Hampshire	277	0.3%
12	New Jersey	2,356	2.6%
38	New Mexico	455	0.5%
2	New York	6,853	7.5%
10	North Carolina	2,692	2.9%
46	North Dakota	257	0.3%
7	Ohio	3,789	4.1%
25	Oklahoma	1,348	1.5%
32	Oregon	1,016	1.1%
4	Pennsylvania	4,534	4.9%
41	Rhode Island	382	0.4%
29	South Carolina	1,095	1.2%
44	South Dakota	285	0.3%
14	Tennessee	2,243	2.4%
3	Texas	4,594	5.0%
36	Utah	487	0.5%
48	Vermont	237	0.3%
15	Virginia	2,048	2.2%
18	Washington	1,714	1.9%
34	West Virginia	697	0.8%
16	Wisconsin	1,907	2.1%
49	Wyoming	150	0.2%

RANK ORDER

RANK	STATE	DEATHS	% of USA
1	California	13,378	14.6%
2	New York	6,853	7.5%
3	Texas	4,594	5.0%
4	Pennsylvania	4,534	4.9%
5	Florida	4,111	4.5%
6	Illinois	3,974	4.3%
7	Ohio	3,789	4.1%
8	Michigan	3,083	3.4%
9	Massachusetts	2,895	3.2%
10	North Carolina	2,692	2.9%
11	Missouri	2,422	2.6%
12	New Jersey	2,356	2.6%
13	Georgia	2,264	2.5%
14	Tennessee	2,243	2.4%
15	Virginia	2,048	2.2%
16	Wisconsin	1,907	2.1%
17	Indiana	1,822	2.0%
18	Washington	1,714	1.9%
19	Maryland	1,641	1.8%
20	Alabama	1,518	1.7%
21	Kentucky	1,474	1.6%
22	Arizona	1,444	1.6%
23	Minnesota	1,412	1.5%
24	Iowa	1,364	1.5%
25	Oklahoma	1,348	1.5%
26	Connecticut	1,225	1.3%
27	Louisiana	1,105	1.2%
28	Arkansas	1,101	1.2%
29	South Carolina	1,095	1.2%
30	Mississippi	1,071	1.2%
31	Colorado	1,037	1.1%
32	Oregon	1,016	1.1%
33	Kansas	990	1.1%
34	West Virginia	697	0.8%
35	Nebraska	610	0.7%
36	Utah	487	0.5%
37	Maine	468	0.5%
38	New Mexico	455	0.5%
39	Nevada	403	0.4%
40	Hawaii	391	0.4%
41	Rhode Island	382	0.4%
42	Idaho	376	0.4%
43	Montana	372	0.4%
44	South Dakota	285	0.3%
45	New Hampshire	277	0.3%
46	North Dakota	257	0.3%
47	Delaware	248	0.3%
48	Vermont	237	0.3%
49	Wyoming	150	0.2%
50	Alaska	52	0.1%
	District of Columbia	204	0.2%

Source: U.S. Department of Health and Human Services, National Center for Health Statistics
    "National Vital Statistics Reports" (Vol. 48, No. 11, July 24, 2000)
*Final data by state of residence.

Death Rate by Pneumonia and Influenza in 1998

National Rate = 34.0 Deaths per 100,000 Population*

ALPHA ORDER

RANK	STATE	RATE
24	Alabama	34.9
50	Alaska	8.5
33	Arizona	30.9
4	Arkansas	43.4
7	California	41.0
44	Colorado	26.1
19	Connecticut	37.4
26	Delaware	33.4
42	Florida	27.6
39	Georgia	29.6
28	Hawaii	32.8
35	Idaho	30.6
27	Illinois	33.0
33	Indiana	30.9
1	Iowa	47.7
16	Kansas	37.7
19	Kentucky	37.4
45	Louisiana	25.3
18	Maine	37.6
29	Maryland	32.0
2	Massachusetts	47.1
30	Michigan	31.4
38	Minnesota	29.9
11	Mississippi	38.9
3	Missouri	44.5
5	Montana	42.3
21	Nebraska	36.7
49	Nevada	23.1
46	New Hampshire	23.4
40	New Jersey	29.0
43	New Mexico	26.2
16	New York	37.7
23	North Carolina	35.7
8	North Dakota	40.3
25	Ohio	33.8
8	Oklahoma	40.3
32	Oregon	31.0
15	Pennsylvania	37.8
12	Rhode Island	38.6
41	South Carolina	28.5
12	South Dakota	38.6
6	Tennessee	41.3
47	Texas	23.2
47	Utah	23.2
10	Vermont	40.1
36	Virginia	30.2
37	Washington	30.1
14	West Virginia	38.5
22	Wisconsin	36.5
31	Wyoming	31.2

RANK ORDER

RANK	STATE	RATE
1	Iowa	47.7
2	Massachusetts	47.1
3	Missouri	44.5
4	Arkansas	43.4
5	Montana	42.3
6	Tennessee	41.3
7	California	41.0
8	North Dakota	40.3
8	Oklahoma	40.3
10	Vermont	40.1
11	Mississippi	38.9
12	Rhode Island	38.6
12	South Dakota	38.6
14	West Virginia	38.5
15	Pennsylvania	37.8
16	Kansas	37.7
16	New York	37.7
18	Maine	37.6
19	Connecticut	37.4
19	Kentucky	37.4
21	Nebraska	36.7
22	Wisconsin	36.5
23	North Carolina	35.7
24	Alabama	34.9
25	Ohio	33.8
26	Delaware	33.4
27	Illinois	33.0
28	Hawaii	32.8
29	Maryland	32.0
30	Michigan	31.4
31	Wyoming	31.2
32	Oregon	31.0
33	Arizona	30.9
33	Indiana	30.9
35	Idaho	30.6
36	Virginia	30.2
37	Washington	30.1
38	Minnesota	29.9
39	Georgia	29.6
40	New Jersey	29.0
41	South Carolina	28.5
42	Florida	27.6
43	New Mexico	26.2
44	Colorado	26.1
45	Louisiana	25.3
46	New Hampshire	23.4
47	Texas	23.2
47	Utah	23.2
49	Nevada	23.1
50	Alaska	8.5
	District of Columbia	39.0

Source: U.S. Department of Health and Human Services, National Center for Health Statistics
"National Vital Statistics Reports" (Vol. 48, No. 11, July 24, 2000)
*Final data by state of residence. Not age-adjusted.

Age-Adjusted Death Rate by Pneumonia and Influenza in 1998

National Rate = 13.2 Deaths per 100,000 Population*

ALPHA ORDER

RANK	STATE	RATE
14	Alabama	13.8
50	Alaska	8.4
22	Arizona	13.1
5	Arkansas	15.6
1	California	17.7
32	Colorado	12.0
42	Connecticut	11.4
11	Delaware	14.2
48	Florida	8.7
4	Georgia	15.9
19	Hawaii	13.3
36	Idaho	11.7
17	Illinois	13.4
28	Indiana	12.2
26	Iowa	12.6
34	Kansas	11.8
9	Kentucky	14.8
41	Louisiana	11.5
28	Maine	12.2
10	Maryland	14.3
12	Massachusetts	14.1
23	Michigan	13.0
47	Minnesota	9.2
2	Mississippi	17.2
7	Missouri	14.9
20	Montana	13.2
43	Nebraska	11.2
25	Nevada	12.8
49	New Hampshire	8.5
45	New Jersey	10.7
39	New Mexico	11.6
12	New York	14.1
6	North Carolina	15.3
43	North Dakota	11.2
26	Ohio	12.6
7	Oklahoma	14.9
46	Oregon	10.5
31	Pennsylvania	12.1
39	Rhode Island	11.6
20	South Carolina	13.2
33	South Dakota	11.9
3	Tennessee	16.8
36	Texas	11.7
28	Utah	12.2
16	Vermont	13.5
17	Virginia	13.4
36	Washington	11.7
15	West Virginia	13.6
34	Wisconsin	11.8
24	Wyoming	12.9

RANK ORDER

RANK	STATE	RATE
1	California	17.7
2	Mississippi	17.2
3	Tennessee	16.8
4	Georgia	15.9
5	Arkansas	15.6
6	North Carolina	15.3
7	Missouri	14.9
7	Oklahoma	14.9
9	Kentucky	14.8
10	Maryland	14.3
11	Delaware	14.2
12	Massachusetts	14.1
12	New York	14.1
14	Alabama	13.8
15	West Virginia	13.6
16	Vermont	13.5
17	Illinois	13.4
17	Virginia	13.4
19	Hawaii	13.3
20	Montana	13.2
20	South Carolina	13.2
22	Arizona	13.1
23	Michigan	13.0
24	Wyoming	12.9
25	Nevada	12.8
26	Iowa	12.6
26	Ohio	12.6
28	Indiana	12.2
28	Maine	12.2
28	Utah	12.2
31	Pennsylvania	12.1
32	Colorado	12.0
33	South Dakota	11.9
34	Kansas	11.8
34	Wisconsin	11.8
36	Idaho	11.7
36	Texas	11.7
36	Washington	11.7
39	New Mexico	11.6
39	Rhode Island	11.6
41	Louisiana	11.5
42	Connecticut	11.4
43	Nebraska	11.2
43	North Dakota	11.2
45	New Jersey	10.7
46	Oregon	10.5
47	Minnesota	9.2
48	Florida	8.7
49	New Hampshire	8.5
50	Alaska	8.4

District of Columbia   15.6

Source: U.S. Department of Health and Human Services, National Center for Health Statistics
"National Vital Statistics Reports" (Vol. 48, No. 11, July 24, 2000)
*Final data by state of residence.

Deaths by Complications of Pregnancy and Childbirth in 1998

National Total = 281 Deaths*

ALPHA ORDER

RANK	STATE	DEATHS	% of USA
11	Alabama	8	2.8%
40	Alaska	1	0.4%
31	Arizona	2	0.7%
21	Arkansas	3	1.1%
1	California	40	14.2%
8	Colorado	9	3.2%
31	Connecticut	2	0.7%
31	Delaware	2	0.7%
3	Florida	18	6.4%
8	Georgia	9	3.2%
31	Hawaii	2	0.7%
31	Idaho	2	0.7%
4	Illinois	16	5.7%
31	Indiana	2	0.7%
21	Iowa	3	1.1%
21	Kansas	3	1.1%
21	Kentucky	3	1.1%
21	Louisiana	3	1.1%
40	Maine	1	0.4%
7	Maryland	10	3.6%
31	Massachusetts	2	0.7%
8	Michigan	9	3.2%
21	Minnesota	3	1.1%
18	Mississippi	4	1.4%
11	Missouri	8	2.8%
40	Montana	1	0.4%
40	Nebraska	1	0.4%
40	Nevada	1	0.4%
31	New Hampshire	2	0.7%
31	New Jersey	2	0.7%
40	New Mexico	1	0.4%
2	New York	29	10.3%
16	North Carolina	5	1.8%
40	North Dakota	1	0.4%
13	Ohio	7	2.5%
16	Oklahoma	5	1.8%
18	Oregon	4	1.4%
6	Pennsylvania	12	4.3%
49	Rhode Island	0	0.0%
18	South Carolina	4	1.4%
21	South Dakota	3	1.1%
14	Tennessee	6	2.1%
5	Texas	15	5.3%
21	Utah	3	1.1%
40	Vermont	1	0.4%
21	Virginia	3	1.1%
21	Washington	3	1.1%
40	West Virginia	1	0.4%
14	Wisconsin	6	2.1%
49	Wyoming	0	0.0%

RANK ORDER

RANK	STATE	DEATHS	% of USA
1	California	40	14.2%
2	New York	29	10.3%
3	Florida	18	6.4%
4	Illinois	16	5.7%
5	Texas	15	5.3%
6	Pennsylvania	12	4.3%
7	Maryland	10	3.6%
8	Colorado	9	3.2%
8	Georgia	9	3.2%
8	Michigan	9	3.2%
11	Alabama	8	2.8%
11	Missouri	8	2.8%
13	Ohio	7	2.5%
14	Tennessee	6	2.1%
14	Wisconsin	6	2.1%
16	North Carolina	5	1.8%
16	Oklahoma	5	1.8%
18	Mississippi	4	1.4%
18	Oregon	4	1.4%
18	South Carolina	4	1.4%
21	Arkansas	3	1.1%
21	Iowa	3	1.1%
21	Kansas	3	1.1%
21	Kentucky	3	1.1%
21	Louisiana	3	1.1%
21	Minnesota	3	1.1%
21	South Dakota	3	1.1%
21	Utah	3	1.1%
21	Virginia	3	1.1%
21	Washington	3	1.1%
31	Arizona	2	0.7%
31	Connecticut	2	0.7%
31	Delaware	2	0.7%
31	Hawaii	2	0.7%
31	Idaho	2	0.7%
31	Indiana	2	0.7%
31	Massachusetts	2	0.7%
31	New Hampshire	2	0.7%
31	New Jersey	2	0.7%
40	Alaska	1	0.4%
40	Maine	1	0.4%
40	Montana	1	0.4%
40	Nebraska	1	0.4%
40	Nevada	1	0.4%
40	New Mexico	1	0.4%
40	North Dakota	1	0.4%
40	Vermont	1	0.4%
40	West Virginia	1	0.4%
49	Rhode Island	0	0.0%
49	Wyoming	0	0.0%
	District of Columbia	0	0.0%

Source: U.S. Department of Health and Human Services, National Center for Health Statistics
    (http://wonder.cdc.gov/WONDER/)
*By state of residence.

Death Rate by Complications of Pregnancy and Childbirth in 1998

National Rate = 0.20 Deaths per 100,000 Female Population*

ALPHA ORDER				RANK ORDER		
RANK	**STATE**	**RATE**		**RANK**	**STATE**	**RATE**
5	Alabama	0.35		1	South Dakota	0.80
6	Alaska	0.34		2	Delaware	0.52
45	Arizona	0.08		3	Colorado	0.45
20	Arkansas	0.23		4	Maryland	0.38
18	California	0.24		5	Alabama	0.35
3	Colorado	0.45		6	Alaska	0.34
37	Connecticut	0.12		6	Hawaii	0.34
2	Delaware	0.52		8	New Hampshire	0.33
20	Florida	0.23		8	Vermont	0.33
20	Georgia	0.23		10	Idaho	0.32
6	Hawaii	0.34		11	New York	0.31
10	Idaho	0.32		11	North Dakota	0.31
17	Illinois	0.26		13	Missouri	0.29
46	Indiana	0.07		13	Oklahoma	0.29
27	Iowa	0.20		15	Mississippi	0.28
25	Kansas	0.22		15	Utah	0.28
32	Kentucky	0.15		17	Illinois	0.26
34	Louisiana	0.13		18	California	0.24
31	Maine	0.16		18	Oregon	0.24
4	Maryland	0.38		20	Arkansas	0.23
47	Massachusetts	0.06		20	Florida	0.23
30	Michigan	0.18		20	Georgia	0.23
34	Minnesota	0.13		20	Montana	0.23
15	Mississippi	0.28		20	Wisconsin	0.23
13	Missouri	0.29		25	Kansas	0.22
20	Montana	0.23		26	Tennessee	0.21
37	Nebraska	0.12		27	Iowa	0.20
37	Nevada	0.12		27	South Carolina	0.20
8	New Hampshire	0.33		29	Pennsylvania	0.19
48	New Jersey	0.05		30	Michigan	0.18
41	New Mexico	0.11		31	Maine	0.16
11	New York	0.31		32	Kentucky	0.15
34	North Carolina	0.13		32	Texas	0.15
11	North Dakota	0.31		34	Louisiana	0.13
37	Ohio	0.12		34	Minnesota	0.13
13	Oklahoma	0.29		34	North Carolina	0.13
18	Oregon	0.24		37	Connecticut	0.12
29	Pennsylvania	0.19		37	Nebraska	0.12
49	Rhode Island	0.00		37	Nevada	0.12
27	South Carolina	0.20		37	Ohio	0.12
1	South Dakota	0.80		41	New Mexico	0.11
26	Tennessee	0.21		41	West Virginia	0.11
32	Texas	0.15		43	Washington	0.10
15	Utah	0.28		44	Virginia	0.09
8	Vermont	0.33		45	Arizona	0.08
44	Virginia	0.09		46	Indiana	0.07
43	Washington	0.10		47	Massachusetts	0.06
41	West Virginia	0.11		48	New Jersey	0.05
20	Wisconsin	0.23		49	Rhode Island	0.00
49	Wyoming	0.00		49	Wyoming	0.00
					District of Columbia	0.00

Source: U.S. Department of Health and Human Services, National Center for Health Statistics
 (http://wonder.cdc.gov/WONDER/)
*By state of residence. Not-age adjusted. Due to low numbers of deaths, rates for all states should be interpreted with caution.

Age-Adjusted Death Rate by Complications of Pregnancy and Childbirth in 1998

National Rate = 0.2 Deaths per 100,000 Female Population*

ALPHA ORDER

RANK	STATE	RATE
5	Alabama	0.4
5	Alaska	0.4
34	Arizona	0.1
12	Arkansas	0.3
12	California	0.3
2	Colorado	0.5
34	Connecticut	0.1
2	Delaware	0.5
12	Florida	0.3
27	Georgia	0.2
5	Hawaii	0.4
12	Idaho	0.3
12	Illinois	0.3
34	Indiana	0.1
12	Iowa	0.3
12	Kansas	0.3
27	Kentucky	0.2
34	Louisiana	0.1
34	Maine	0.1
5	Maryland	0.4
34	Massachusetts	0.1
27	Michigan	0.2
34	Minnesota	0.1
12	Mississippi	0.3
12	Missouri	0.3
12	Montana	0.3
34	Nebraska	0.1
34	Nevada	0.1
5	New Hampshire	0.4
34	New Jersey	0.1
34	New Mexico	0.1
12	New York	0.3
27	North Carolina	0.2
5	North Dakota	0.4
34	Ohio	0.1
5	Oklahoma	0.4
12	Oregon	0.3
27	Pennsylvania	0.2
49	Rhode Island	0.0
27	South Carolina	0.2
1	South Dakota	1.1
12	Tennessee	0.3
27	Texas	0.2
12	Utah	0.3
2	Vermont	0.5
34	Virginia	0.1
34	Washington	0.1
34	West Virginia	0.1
12	Wisconsin	0.3
49	Wyoming	0.0

RANK ORDER

RANK	STATE	RATE
1	South Dakota	1.1
2	Colorado	0.5
2	Delaware	0.5
2	Vermont	0.5
5	Alabama	0.4
5	Alaska	0.4
5	Hawaii	0.4
5	Maryland	0.4
5	New Hampshire	0.4
5	North Dakota	0.4
5	Oklahoma	0.4
12	Arkansas	0.3
12	California	0.3
12	Florida	0.3
12	Idaho	0.3
12	Illinois	0.3
12	Iowa	0.3
12	Kansas	0.3
12	Mississippi	0.3
12	Missouri	0.3
12	Montana	0.3
12	New York	0.3
12	Oregon	0.3
12	Tennessee	0.3
12	Utah	0.3
12	Wisconsin	0.3
27	Georgia	0.2
27	Kentucky	0.2
27	Michigan	0.2
27	North Carolina	0.2
27	Pennsylvania	0.2
27	South Carolina	0.2
27	Texas	0.2
34	Arizona	0.1
34	Connecticut	0.1
34	Indiana	0.1
34	Louisiana	0.1
34	Maine	0.1
34	Massachusetts	0.1
34	Minnesota	0.1
34	Nebraska	0.1
34	Nevada	0.1
34	New Jersey	0.1
34	New Mexico	0.1
34	Ohio	0.1
34	Virginia	0.1
34	Washington	0.1
34	West Virginia	0.1
49	Rhode Island	0.0
49	Wyoming	0.0
	District of Columbia	0.0

Source: U.S. Department of Health and Human Services, National Center for Health Statistics
(http://wonder.cdc.gov/WONDER/)
*By state of residence. Due to low numbers of deaths, rates for all states should be interpreted with caution.

Deaths by Tuberculosis in 1998

National Total = 1,112 Deaths*

ALPHA ORDER					RANK ORDER			
RANK	STATE		DEATHS	% of USA	RANK	STATE	DEATHS	% of USA
14	Alabama		28	2.5%	1	California	168	15.1%
46	Alaska		1	0.1%	2	Texas	108	9.7%
15	Arizona		24	2.2%	3	New York	81	7.3%
18	Arkansas		18	1.6%	4	Florida	72	6.5%
1	California		168	15.1%	5	Illinois	64	5.8%
24	Colorado		14	1.3%	6	North Carolina	45	4.0%
29	Connecticut		11	1.0%	7	Georgia	35	3.1%
37	Delaware		3	0.3%	7	Ohio	35	3.1%
4	Florida		72	6.5%	9	Michigan	33	3.0%
7	Georgia		35	3.1%	10	Louisiana	32	2.9%
40	Hawaii		2	0.2%	11	New Jersey	31	2.8%
46	Idaho		1	0.1%	11	Pennsylvania	31	2.8%
5	Illinois		64	5.8%	13	Tennessee	30	2.7%
16	Indiana		23	2.1%	14	Alabama	28	2.5%
30	Iowa		9	0.8%	15	Arizona	24	2.2%
32	Kansas		5	0.4%	16	Indiana	23	2.1%
21	Kentucky		15	1.3%	17	Virginia	21	1.9%
10	Louisiana		32	2.9%	18	Arkansas	18	1.6%
40	Maine		2	0.2%	18	Missouri	18	1.6%
27	Maryland		13	1.2%	18	South Carolina	18	1.6%
27	Massachusetts		13	1.2%	21	Kentucky	15	1.3%
9	Michigan		33	3.0%	21	Mississippi	15	1.3%
33	Minnesota		4	0.4%	21	Wisconsin	15	1.3%
21	Mississippi		15	1.3%	24	Colorado	14	1.3%
18	Missouri		18	1.6%	24	Oklahoma	14	1.3%
33	Montana		4	0.4%	24	Washington	14	1.3%
46	Nebraska		1	0.1%	27	Maryland	13	1.2%
37	Nevada		3	0.3%	27	Massachusetts	13	1.2%
40	New Hampshire		2	0.2%	29	Connecticut	11	1.0%
11	New Jersey		31	2.8%	30	Iowa	9	0.8%
37	New Mexico		3	0.3%	30	Oregon	9	0.8%
3	New York		81	7.3%	32	Kansas	5	0.4%
6	North Carolina		45	4.0%	33	Minnesota	4	0.4%
46	North Dakota		1	0.1%	33	Montana	4	0.4%
7	Ohio		35	3.1%	33	South Dakota	4	0.4%
24	Oklahoma		14	1.3%	33	West Virginia	4	0.4%
30	Oregon		9	0.8%	37	Delaware	3	0.3%
11	Pennsylvania		31	2.8%	37	Nevada	3	0.3%
40	Rhode Island		2	0.2%	37	New Mexico	3	0.3%
18	South Carolina		18	1.6%	40	Hawaii	2	0.2%
33	South Dakota		4	0.4%	40	Maine	2	0.2%
13	Tennessee		30	2.7%	40	New Hampshire	2	0.2%
2	Texas		108	9.7%	40	Rhode Island	2	0.2%
40	Utah		2	0.2%	40	Utah	2	0.2%
40	Vermont		2	0.2%	40	Vermont	2	0.2%
17	Virginia		21	1.9%	46	Alaska	1	0.1%
24	Washington		14	1.3%	46	Idaho	1	0.1%
33	West Virginia		4	0.4%	46	Nebraska	1	0.1%
21	Wisconsin		15	1.3%	46	North Dakota	1	0.1%
50	Wyoming		0	0.0%	50	Wyoming	0	0.0%
						District of Columbia	9	0.8%

Source: U.S. Department of Health and Human Services, National Center for Health Statistics
(http://wonder.cdc.gov/WONDER/)
*By state of residence.

Death Rate by Tuberculosis in 1998

National Rate = 0.41 Deaths per 100,000 Population*

ALPHA ORDER				RANK ORDER		
RANK	STATE	RATE		RANK	STATE	RATE
3	Alabama	0.64		1	Louisiana	0.73
43	Alaska	0.16		2	Arkansas	0.71
10	Arizona	0.51		3	Alabama	0.64
2	Arkansas	0.71		4	North Carolina	0.60
10	California	0.51		5	Tennessee	0.55
22	Colorado	0.35		5	Texas	0.55
23	Connecticut	0.34		7	Mississippi	0.54
18	Delaware	0.40		7	South Dakota	0.54
12	Florida	0.48		9	Illinois	0.53
14	Georgia	0.46		10	Arizona	0.51
39	Hawaii	0.17		10	California	0.51
47	Idaho	0.08		12	Florida	0.48
9	Illinois	0.53		13	South Carolina	0.47
19	Indiana	0.39		14	Georgia	0.46
27	Iowa	0.31		15	Montana	0.45
38	Kansas	0.19		15	New York	0.45
20	Kentucky	0.38		17	Oklahoma	0.42
1	Louisiana	0.73		18	Delaware	0.40
43	Maine	0.16		19	Indiana	0.39
33	Maryland	0.25		20	Kentucky	0.38
36	Massachusetts	0.21		20	New Jersey	0.38
23	Michigan	0.34		22	Colorado	0.35
47	Minnesota	0.08		23	Connecticut	0.34
7	Mississippi	0.54		23	Michigan	0.34
26	Missouri	0.33		23	Vermont	0.34
15	Montana	0.45		26	Missouri	0.33
49	Nebraska	0.06		27	Iowa	0.31
39	Nevada	0.17		27	Ohio	0.31
39	New Hampshire	0.17		27	Virginia	0.31
20	New Jersey	0.38		30	Wisconsin	0.29
39	New Mexico	0.17		31	Oregon	0.27
15	New York	0.45		32	Pennsylvania	0.26
4	North Carolina	0.60		33	Maryland	0.25
43	North Dakota	0.16		33	Washington	0.25
27	Ohio	0.31		35	West Virginia	0.22
17	Oklahoma	0.42		36	Massachusetts	0.21
31	Oregon	0.27		37	Rhode Island	0.20
32	Pennsylvania	0.26		38	Kansas	0.19
37	Rhode Island	0.20		39	Hawaii	0.17
13	South Carolina	0.47		39	Nevada	0.17
7	South Dakota	0.54		39	New Hampshire	0.17
5	Tennessee	0.55		39	New Mexico	0.17
5	Texas	0.55		43	Alaska	0.16
46	Utah	0.10		43	Maine	0.16
23	Vermont	0.34		43	North Dakota	0.16
27	Virginia	0.31		46	Utah	0.10
33	Washington	0.25		47	Idaho	0.08
35	West Virginia	0.22		47	Minnesota	0.08
30	Wisconsin	0.29		49	Nebraska	0.06
50	Wyoming	0.00		50	Wyoming	0.00
					District of Columbia	1.72

Source: U.S. Department of Health and Human Services, National Center for Health Statistics
    (http://wonder.cdc.gov/WONDER/)
*By state of residence. Not age-adjusted. Due to low numbers of deaths, rates for all states should be interpreted
with caution.

Age-Adjusted Death Rate by Tuberculosis in 1998

National Rate = 0.3 Deaths per 100,000 Population*

<u>ALPHA ORDER</u>

RANK	STATE	RATE
2	Alabama	0.4
19	Alaska	0.2
8	Arizona	0.3
8	Arkansas	0.3
2	California	0.4
19	Colorado	0.2
19	Connecticut	0.2
19	Delaware	0.2
8	Florida	0.3
8	Georgia	0.3
35	Hawaii	0.1
47	Idaho	0.0
2	Illinois	0.4
19	Indiana	0.2
19	Iowa	0.2
35	Kansas	0.1
19	Kentucky	0.2
1	Louisiana	0.5
35	Maine	0.1
19	Maryland	0.2
35	Massachusetts	0.1
19	Michigan	0.2
35	Minnesota	0.1
8	Mississippi	0.3
19	Missouri	0.2
8	Montana	0.3
47	Nebraska	0.0
35	Nevada	0.1
35	New Hampshire	0.1
19	New Jersey	0.2
35	New Mexico	0.1
8	New York	0.3
2	North Carolina	0.4
47	North Dakota	0.0
19	Ohio	0.2
8	Oklahoma	0.3
35	Oregon	0.1
19	Pennsylvania	0.2
35	Rhode Island	0.1
8	South Carolina	0.3
2	South Dakota	0.4
8	Tennessee	0.3
2	Texas	0.4
35	Utah	0.1
8	Vermont	0.3
19	Virginia	0.2
19	Washington	0.2
35	West Virginia	0.1
19	Wisconsin	0.2
47	Wyoming	0.0

<u>RANK ORDER</u>

RANK	STATE	RATE
1	Louisiana	0.5
2	Alabama	0.4
2	California	0.4
2	Illinois	0.4
2	North Carolina	0.4
2	South Dakota	0.4
2	Texas	0.4
8	Arizona	0.3
8	Arkansas	0.3
8	Florida	0.3
8	Georgia	0.3
8	Mississippi	0.3
8	Montana	0.3
8	New York	0.3
8	Oklahoma	0.3
8	South Carolina	0.3
8	Tennessee	0.3
8	Vermont	0.3
19	Alaska	0.2
19	Colorado	0.2
19	Connecticut	0.2
19	Delaware	0.2
19	Indiana	0.2
19	Iowa	0.2
19	Kentucky	0.2
19	Maryland	0.2
19	Michigan	0.2
19	Missouri	0.2
19	New Jersey	0.2
19	Ohio	0.2
19	Pennsylvania	0.2
19	Virginia	0.2
19	Washington	0.2
19	Wisconsin	0.2
35	Hawaii	0.1
35	Kansas	0.1
35	Maine	0.1
35	Massachusetts	0.1
35	Minnesota	0.1
35	Nevada	0.1
35	New Hampshire	0.1
35	New Mexico	0.1
35	Oregon	0.1
35	Rhode Island	0.1
35	Utah	0.1
35	West Virginia	0.1
47	Idaho	0.0
47	Nebraska	0.0
47	North Dakota	0.0
47	Wyoming	0.0
	District of Columbia	1.0

Source: U.S. Department of Health and Human Services, National Center for Health Statistics
   (http://wonder.cdc.gov/WONDER/)
By state of residence. Due to low numbers of deaths, rates for all states should be interpreted with caution.

Deaths by Injury in 1998

National Total = 150,445 Deaths*

RANK	STATE	DEATHS	% of USA
16	Alabama	3,272	2.2%
45	Alaska	432	0.3%
14	Arizona	3,556	2.4%
30	Arkansas	1,936	1.3%
1	California	15,346	10.2%
26	Colorado	2,417	1.6%
33	Connecticut	1,486	1.0%
47	Delaware	391	0.3%
3	Florida	9,249	6.1%
10	Georgia	4,738	3.1%
44	Hawaii	478	0.3%
39	Idaho	818	0.5%
6	Illinois	6,160	4.1%
15	Indiana	3,383	2.2%
32	Iowa	1,501	1.0%
31	Kansas	1,649	1.1%
23	Kentucky	2,521	1.7%
18	Louisiana	3,082	2.0%
40	Maine	676	0.4%
20	Maryland	2,980	2.0%
25	Massachusetts	2,424	1.6%
8	Michigan	5,022	3.3%
27	Minnesota	2,361	1.6%
24	Mississippi	2,427	1.6%
13	Missouri	3,611	2.4%
41	Montana	662	0.4%
38	Nebraska	950	0.6%
35	Nevada	1,319	0.9%
42	New Hampshire	524	0.3%
17	New Jersey	3,201	2.1%
34	New Mexico	1,464	1.0%
4	New York	7,155	4.8%
9	North Carolina	4,846	3.2%
48	North Dakota	384	0.3%
7	Ohio	5,152	3.4%
28	Oklahoma	2,352	1.6%
29	Oregon	2,146	1.4%
5	Pennsylvania	6,767	4.5%
46	Rhode Island	406	0.3%
22	South Carolina	2,617	1.7%
43	South Dakota	491	0.3%
11	Tennessee	3,929	2.6%
2	Texas	11,173	7.4%
36	Utah	1,262	0.8%
50	Vermont	315	0.2%
12	Virginia	3,633	2.4%
19	Washington	2,989	2.0%
37	West Virginia	1,203	0.8%
21	Wisconsin	2,761	1.8%
49	Wyoming	340	0.2%

RANK	STATE	DEATHS	% of USA
1	California	15,346	10.2%
2	Texas	11,173	7.4%
3	Florida	9,249	6.1%
4	New York	7,155	4.8%
5	Pennsylvania	6,767	4.5%
6	Illinois	6,160	4.1%
7	Ohio	5,152	3.4%
8	Michigan	5,022	3.3%
9	North Carolina	4,846	3.2%
10	Georgia	4,738	3.1%
11	Tennessee	3,929	2.6%
12	Virginia	3,633	2.4%
13	Missouri	3,611	2.4%
14	Arizona	3,556	2.4%
15	Indiana	3,383	2.2%
16	Alabama	3,272	2.2%
17	New Jersey	3,201	2.1%
18	Louisiana	3,082	2.0%
19	Washington	2,989	2.0%
20	Maryland	2,980	2.0%
21	Wisconsin	2,761	1.8%
22	South Carolina	2,617	1.7%
23	Kentucky	2,521	1.7%
24	Mississippi	2,427	1.6%
25	Massachusetts	2,424	1.6%
26	Colorado	2,417	1.6%
27	Minnesota	2,361	1.6%
28	Oklahoma	2,352	1.6%
29	Oregon	2,146	1.4%
30	Arkansas	1,936	1.3%
31	Kansas	1,649	1.1%
32	Iowa	1,501	1.0%
33	Connecticut	1,486	1.0%
34	New Mexico	1,464	1.0%
35	Nevada	1,319	0.9%
36	Utah	1,262	0.8%
37	West Virginia	1,203	0.8%
38	Nebraska	950	0.6%
39	Idaho	818	0.5%
40	Maine	676	0.4%
41	Montana	662	0.4%
42	New Hampshire	524	0.3%
43	South Dakota	491	0.3%
44	Hawaii	478	0.3%
45	Alaska	432	0.3%
46	Rhode Island	406	0.3%
47	Delaware	391	0.3%
48	North Dakota	384	0.3%
49	Wyoming	340	0.2%
50	Vermont	315	0.2%
	District of Columbia	488	0.3%

Source: U.S. Department of Health and Human Services, National Center for Health Statistics
(http://wonder.cdc.gov/WONDER/)
*By state of residence. Injury as used here includes Accidents (including motor vehicle), Suicides, Homicides and "Other" undetermined.

Death Rate by Injury in 1998

National Rate = 55.6 Deaths per 100,000 Population*

<table>
<tr><td colspan="3">ALPHA ORDER</td><td colspan="3">RANK ORDER</td></tr>
<tr><td>RANK</td><td>STATE</td><td>RATE</td><td>RANK</td><td>STATE</td><td>RATE</td></tr>
<tr><td>7</td><td>Alabama</td><td>75.1</td><td>1</td><td>Mississippi</td><td>88.1</td></tr>
<tr><td>11</td><td>Alaska</td><td>70.3</td><td>2</td><td>New Mexico</td><td>84.2</td></tr>
<tr><td>4</td><td>Arizona</td><td>76.1</td><td>3</td><td>Arkansas</td><td>76.2</td></tr>
<tr><td>3</td><td>Arkansas</td><td>76.2</td><td>4</td><td>Arizona</td><td>76.1</td></tr>
<tr><td>42</td><td>California</td><td>47.0</td><td>5</td><td>Nevada</td><td>75.4</td></tr>
<tr><td>24</td><td>Colorado</td><td>60.8</td><td>6</td><td>Montana</td><td>75.2</td></tr>
<tr><td>44</td><td>Connecticut</td><td>45.4</td><td>7</td><td>Alabama</td><td>75.1</td></tr>
<tr><td>36</td><td>Delaware</td><td>52.5</td><td>8</td><td>Tennessee</td><td>72.3</td></tr>
<tr><td>22</td><td>Florida</td><td>62.0</td><td>9</td><td>Wyoming</td><td>70.7</td></tr>
<tr><td>23</td><td>Georgia</td><td>61.9</td><td>10</td><td>Louisiana</td><td>70.5</td></tr>
<tr><td>47</td><td>Hawaii</td><td>40.0</td><td>11</td><td>Alaska</td><td>70.3</td></tr>
<tr><td>14</td><td>Idaho</td><td>66.5</td><td>12</td><td>Oklahoma</td><td>70.2</td></tr>
<tr><td>39</td><td>Illinois</td><td>51.1</td><td>13</td><td>South Carolina</td><td>68.2</td></tr>
<tr><td>28</td><td>Indiana</td><td>57.3</td><td>14</td><td>Idaho</td><td>66.5</td></tr>
<tr><td>38</td><td>Iowa</td><td>52.4</td><td>14</td><td>South Dakota</td><td>66.5</td></tr>
<tr><td>21</td><td>Kansas</td><td>62.7</td><td>16</td><td>Missouri</td><td>66.4</td></tr>
<tr><td>20</td><td>Kentucky</td><td>64.0</td><td>17</td><td>West Virginia</td><td>66.3</td></tr>
<tr><td>10</td><td>Louisiana</td><td>70.5</td><td>18</td><td>Oregon</td><td>65.3</td></tr>
<tr><td>32</td><td>Maine</td><td>54.3</td><td>19</td><td>North Carolina</td><td>64.2</td></tr>
<tr><td>27</td><td>Maryland</td><td>58.0</td><td>20</td><td>Kentucky</td><td>64.0</td></tr>
<tr><td>48</td><td>Massachusetts</td><td>39.4</td><td>21</td><td>Kansas</td><td>62.7</td></tr>
<tr><td>39</td><td>Michigan</td><td>51.1</td><td>22</td><td>Florida</td><td>62.0</td></tr>
<tr><td>41</td><td>Minnesota</td><td>49.9</td><td>23</td><td>Georgia</td><td>61.9</td></tr>
<tr><td>1</td><td>Mississippi</td><td>88.1</td><td>24</td><td>Colorado</td><td>60.8</td></tr>
<tr><td>16</td><td>Missouri</td><td>66.4</td><td>25</td><td>North Dakota</td><td>60.2</td></tr>
<tr><td>6</td><td>Montana</td><td>75.2</td><td>26</td><td>Utah</td><td>60.0</td></tr>
<tr><td>29</td><td>Nebraska</td><td>57.1</td><td>27</td><td>Maryland</td><td>58.0</td></tr>
<tr><td>5</td><td>Nevada</td><td>75.4</td><td>28</td><td>Indiana</td><td>57.3</td></tr>
<tr><td>45</td><td>New Hampshire</td><td>44.2</td><td>29</td><td>Nebraska</td><td>57.1</td></tr>
<tr><td>48</td><td>New Jersey</td><td>39.4</td><td>30</td><td>Texas</td><td>56.5</td></tr>
<tr><td>2</td><td>New Mexico</td><td>84.2</td><td>31</td><td>Pennsylvania</td><td>56.4</td></tr>
<tr><td>48</td><td>New York</td><td>39.4</td><td>32</td><td>Maine</td><td>54.3</td></tr>
<tr><td>19</td><td>North Carolina</td><td>64.2</td><td>33</td><td>Virginia</td><td>53.5</td></tr>
<tr><td>25</td><td>North Dakota</td><td>60.2</td><td>34</td><td>Vermont</td><td>53.3</td></tr>
<tr><td>43</td><td>Ohio</td><td>45.9</td><td>35</td><td>Wisconsin</td><td>52.8</td></tr>
<tr><td>12</td><td>Oklahoma</td><td>70.2</td><td>36</td><td>Delaware</td><td>52.5</td></tr>
<tr><td>18</td><td>Oregon</td><td>65.3</td><td>36</td><td>Washington</td><td>52.5</td></tr>
<tr><td>31</td><td>Pennsylvania</td><td>56.4</td><td>38</td><td>Iowa</td><td>52.4</td></tr>
<tr><td>46</td><td>Rhode Island</td><td>41.1</td><td>39</td><td>Illinois</td><td>51.1</td></tr>
<tr><td>13</td><td>South Carolina</td><td>68.2</td><td>39</td><td>Michigan</td><td>51.1</td></tr>
<tr><td>14</td><td>South Dakota</td><td>66.5</td><td>41</td><td>Minnesota</td><td>49.9</td></tr>
<tr><td>8</td><td>Tennessee</td><td>72.3</td><td>42</td><td>California</td><td>47.0</td></tr>
<tr><td>30</td><td>Texas</td><td>56.5</td><td>43</td><td>Ohio</td><td>45.9</td></tr>
<tr><td>26</td><td>Utah</td><td>60.0</td><td>44</td><td>Connecticut</td><td>45.4</td></tr>
<tr><td>34</td><td>Vermont</td><td>53.3</td><td>45</td><td>New Hampshire</td><td>44.2</td></tr>
<tr><td>33</td><td>Virginia</td><td>53.5</td><td>46</td><td>Rhode Island</td><td>41.1</td></tr>
<tr><td>36</td><td>Washington</td><td>52.5</td><td>47</td><td>Hawaii</td><td>40.0</td></tr>
<tr><td>17</td><td>West Virginia</td><td>66.3</td><td>48</td><td>Massachusetts</td><td>39.4</td></tr>
<tr><td>35</td><td>Wisconsin</td><td>52.8</td><td>48</td><td>New Jersey</td><td>39.4</td></tr>
<tr><td>9</td><td>Wyoming</td><td>70.7</td><td>48</td><td>New York</td><td>39.4</td></tr>
<tr><td></td><td></td><td></td><td></td><td>District of Columbia</td><td>93.0</td></tr>
</table>

Source: U.S. Department of Health and Human Services, National Center for Health Statistics
(http://wonder.cdc.gov/WONDER/)
*By state of residence. Injury as used here includes Accidents (including motor vehicle), Suicides, Homicides and "Other" undetermined. Not age-adjusted.

Age-Adjusted Death Rate by Injury in 1998

National Rate = 49.1 Deaths per 100,000 Population*

RANK	STATE	RATE
7	Alabama	67.0
4	Alaska	71.3
5	Arizona	68.9
6	Arkansas	68.2
39	California	43.4
24	Colorado	54.1
45	Connecticut	37.4
36	Delaware	44.4
23	Florida	54.6
19	Georgia	55.9
46	Hawaii	35.4
14	Idaho	58.2
32	Illinois	46.9
28	Indiana	50.4
41	Iowa	41.1
25	Kansas	53.9
20	Kentucky	55.8
8	Louisiana	66.1
37	Maine	44.3
26	Maryland	52.6
50	Massachusetts	32.2
33	Michigan	46.1
42	Minnesota	39.7
1	Mississippi	79.8
18	Missouri	56.9
11	Montana	63.7
29	Nebraska	47.7
3	Nevada	71.6
44	New Hampshire	38.0
49	New Jersey	33.4
2	New Mexico	78.0
47	New York	33.9
17	North Carolina	57.1
31	North Dakota	47.1
43	Ohio	38.6
13	Oklahoma	61.0
20	Oregon	55.8
30	Pennsylvania	47.2
48	Rhode Island	33.5
12	South Carolina	61.7
16	South Dakota	57.5
9	Tennessee	64.2
27	Texas	52.5
15	Utah	57.9
38	Vermont	43.8
34	Virginia	45.8
35	Washington	45.7
22	West Virginia	55.7
40	Wisconsin	43.3
9	Wyoming	64.2

RANK	STATE	RATE
1	Mississippi	79.8
2	New Mexico	78.0
3	Nevada	71.6
4	Alaska	71.3
5	Arizona	68.9
6	Arkansas	68.2
7	Alabama	67.0
8	Louisiana	66.1
9	Tennessee	64.2
9	Wyoming	64.2
11	Montana	63.7
12	South Carolina	61.7
13	Oklahoma	61.0
14	Idaho	58.2
15	Utah	57.9
16	South Dakota	57.5
17	North Carolina	57.1
18	Missouri	56.9
19	Georgia	55.9
20	Kentucky	55.8
20	Oregon	55.8
22	West Virginia	55.7
23	Florida	54.6
24	Colorado	54.1
25	Kansas	53.9
26	Maryland	52.6
27	Texas	52.5
28	Indiana	50.4
29	Nebraska	47.7
30	Pennsylvania	47.2
31	North Dakota	47.1
32	Illinois	46.9
33	Michigan	46.1
34	Virginia	45.8
35	Washington	45.7
36	Delaware	44.4
37	Maine	44.3
38	Vermont	43.8
39	California	43.4
40	Wisconsin	43.3
41	Iowa	41.1
42	Minnesota	39.7
43	Ohio	38.6
44	New Hampshire	38.0
45	Connecticut	37.4
46	Hawaii	35.4
47	New York	33.9
48	Rhode Island	33.5
49	New Jersey	33.4
50	Massachusetts	32.2
	District of Columbia	88.1

Source: U.S. Department of Health and Human Services, National Center for Health Statistics
(http://wonder.cdc.gov/WONDER/)
*By state of residence. Injury as used here includes Accidents (including motor vehicle), Suicides, Homicides and "Other" undetermined.

Deaths by Accidents in 1998

National Total = 97,835 Deaths*

ALPHA ORDER

RANK ORDER

RANK	STATE	DEATHS	% of USA		RANK	STATE	DEATHS	% of USA
16	Alabama	2,204	2.3%		1	California	9,264	9.5%
47	Alaska	251	0.3%		2	Texas	7,421	7.6%
14	Arizona	2,228	2.3%		3	Florida	5,877	6.0%
30	Arkansas	1,287	1.3%		4	New York	4,676	4.8%
1	California	9,264	9.5%		5	Pennsylvania	4,573	4.7%
26	Colorado	1,530	1.6%		6	Illinois	3,891	4.0%
33	Connecticut	1,067	1.1%		7	Ohio	3,546	3.6%
46	Delaware	289	0.3%		8	North Carolina	3,278	3.4%
3	Florida	5,877	6.0%		9	Georgia	3,156	3.2%
9	Georgia	3,156	3.2%		10	Michigan	3,133	3.2%
44	Hawaii	299	0.3%		11	Tennessee	2,627	2.7%
39	Idaho	571	0.6%		12	Missouri	2,455	2.5%
6	Illinois	3,891	4.0%		13	Virginia	2,334	2.4%
17	Indiana	2,199	2.2%		14	Arizona	2,228	2.3%
32	Iowa	1,094	1.1%		15	New Jersey	2,215	2.3%
31	Kansas	1,152	1.2%		16	Alabama	2,204	2.3%
24	Kentucky	1,715	1.8%		17	Indiana	2,199	2.2%
19	Louisiana	1,939	2.0%		18	Washington	1,950	2.0%
41	Maine	448	0.5%		19	Louisiana	1,939	2.0%
28	Maryland	1,398	1.4%		20	Wisconsin	1,924	2.0%
29	Massachusetts	1,336	1.4%		21	South Carolina	1,803	1.8%
10	Michigan	3,133	3.2%		22	Minnesota	1,728	1.8%
22	Minnesota	1,728	1.8%		23	Mississippi	1,716	1.8%
23	Mississippi	1,716	1.8%		24	Kentucky	1,715	1.8%
12	Missouri	2,455	2.5%		25	Oklahoma	1,610	1.6%
40	Montana	461	0.5%		26	Colorado	1,530	1.6%
37	Nebraska	676	0.7%		27	Oregon	1,405	1.4%
38	Nevada	665	0.7%		28	Maryland	1,398	1.4%
43	New Hampshire	343	0.4%		29	Massachusetts	1,336	1.4%
15	New Jersey	2,215	2.3%		30	Arkansas	1,287	1.3%
34	New Mexico	996	1.0%		31	Kansas	1,152	1.2%
4	New York	4,676	4.8%		32	Iowa	1,094	1.1%
8	North Carolina	3,278	3.4%		33	Connecticut	1,067	1.1%
45	North Dakota	296	0.3%		34	New Mexico	996	1.0%
7	Ohio	3,546	3.6%		35	West Virginia	840	0.9%
25	Oklahoma	1,610	1.6%		36	Utah	713	0.7%
27	Oregon	1,405	1.4%		37	Nebraska	676	0.7%
5	Pennsylvania	4,573	4.7%		38	Nevada	665	0.7%
48	Rhode Island	242	0.2%		39	Idaho	571	0.6%
21	South Carolina	1,803	1.8%		40	Montana	461	0.5%
42	South Dakota	360	0.4%		41	Maine	448	0.5%
11	Tennessee	2,627	2.7%		42	South Dakota	360	0.4%
2	Texas	7,421	7.6%		43	New Hampshire	343	0.4%
36	Utah	713	0.7%		44	Hawaii	299	0.3%
50	Vermont	216	0.2%		45	North Dakota	296	0.3%
13	Virginia	2,334	2.4%		46	Delaware	289	0.3%
18	Washington	1,950	2.0%		47	Alaska	251	0.3%
35	West Virginia	840	0.9%		48	Rhode Island	242	0.2%
20	Wisconsin	1,924	2.0%		49	Wyoming	231	0.2%
49	Wyoming	231	0.2%		50	Vermont	216	0.2%
						District of Columbia	207	0.2%

Source: U.S. Department of Health and Human Services, National Center for Health Statistics
    "National Vital Statistics Reports" (Vol. 48, No. 11, July 24, 2000)
*Final data by state of residence. Includes motor vehicle deaths, poisoning, falls, drowning and other accidents.

Death Rate by Accidents in 1998

National Rate = 36.2 Deaths per 100,000 Population*

ALPHA ORDER				RANK ORDER		
RANK	STATE	RATE		RANK	STATE	RATE
5	Alabama	50.6		1	Mississippi	62.4
22	Alaska	40.9		2	New Mexico	57.3
10	Arizona	47.7		3	Montana	52.4
4	Arkansas	50.7		4	Arkansas	50.7
44	California	28.4		5	Alabama	50.6
26	Colorado	38.5		6	South Dakota	48.8
39	Connecticut	32.6		7	Tennessee	48.4
25	Delaware	38.9		8	Oklahoma	48.1
24	Florida	39.4		9	Wyoming	48.0
21	Georgia	41.3		10	Arizona	47.7
48	Hawaii	25.1		11	South Carolina	47.0
12	Idaho	46.5		12	Idaho	46.5
40	Illinois	32.3		13	North Dakota	46.4
31	Indiana	37.3		13	West Virginia	46.4
27	Iowa	38.2		15	Missouri	45.1
17	Kansas	43.8		16	Louisiana	44.4
18	Kentucky	43.6		17	Kansas	43.8
16	Louisiana	44.4		18	Kentucky	43.6
35	Maine	36.0		19	North Carolina	43.4
46	Maryland	27.2		20	Oregon	42.8
50	Massachusetts	21.7		21	Georgia	41.3
41	Michigan	31.9		22	Alaska	40.9
33	Minnesota	36.6		23	Nebraska	40.7
1	Mississippi	62.4		24	Florida	39.4
15	Missouri	45.1		25	Delaware	38.9
3	Montana	52.4		26	Colorado	38.5
23	Nebraska	40.7		27	Iowa	38.2
28	Nevada	38.1		28	Nevada	38.1
43	New Hampshire	28.9		28	Pennsylvania	38.1
45	New Jersey	27.3		30	Texas	37.6
2	New Mexico	57.3		31	Indiana	37.3
47	New York	25.7		32	Wisconsin	36.8
19	North Carolina	43.4		33	Minnesota	36.6
13	North Dakota	46.4		33	Vermont	36.6
42	Ohio	31.6		35	Maine	36.0
8	Oklahoma	48.1		36	Virginia	34.4
20	Oregon	42.8		37	Washington	34.3
28	Pennsylvania	38.1		38	Utah	34.0
49	Rhode Island	24.5		39	Connecticut	32.6
11	South Carolina	47.0		40	Illinois	32.3
6	South Dakota	48.8		41	Michigan	31.9
7	Tennessee	48.4		42	Ohio	31.6
30	Texas	37.6		43	New Hampshire	28.9
38	Utah	34.0		44	California	28.4
33	Vermont	36.6		45	New Jersey	27.3
36	Virginia	34.4		46	Maryland	27.2
37	Washington	34.3		47	New York	25.7
13	West Virginia	46.4		48	Hawaii	25.1
32	Wisconsin	36.8		49	Rhode Island	24.5
9	Wyoming	48.0		50	Massachusetts	21.7
					District of Columbia	39.6

Source: U.S. Department of Health and Human Services, National Center for Health Statistics
    "National Vital Statistics Reports" (Vol. 48, No. 11, July 24, 2000)
*Final data by state of residence. Includes motor vehicle deaths, poisoning, falls, drowning and other accidents.
Not age-adjusted.*

Age-Adjusted Death Rate by Accidents in 1998

National Rate = 30.1 Deaths per 100,000 Population*

ALPHA ORDER

RANK	STATE	RATE
3	Alabama	43.2
9	Alaska	40.7
9	Arizona	40.7
5	Arkansas	42.3
41	California	25.2
26	Colorado	32.8
43	Connecticut	24.5
27	Delaware	31.8
25	Florida	33.3
18	Georgia	35.9
47	Hawaii	21.0
14	Idaho	39.4
37	Illinois	27.5
29	Indiana	30.7
36	Iowa	27.6
21	Kansas	34.9
16	Kentucky	36.9
11	Louisiana	39.9
39	Maine	27.1
45	Maryland	22.2
50	Massachusetts	15.5
38	Michigan	27.2
40	Minnesota	26.4
1	Mississippi	54.4
19	Missouri	35.8
6	Montana	42.1
28	Nebraska	31.6
20	Nevada	35.1
44	New Hampshire	23.3
46	New Jersey	21.7
2	New Mexico	51.2
48	New York	20.4
16	North Carolina	36.9
23	North Dakota	34.0
42	Ohio	24.9
13	Oklahoma	39.5
21	Oregon	34.9
31	Pennsylvania	29.2
49	Rhode Island	17.3
7	South Carolina	41.2
12	South Dakota	39.8
8	Tennessee	40.9
24	Texas	33.7
30	Utah	30.6
31	Vermont	29.2
34	Virginia	27.7
33	Washington	28.5
15	West Virginia	37.1
34	Wisconsin	27.7
4	Wyoming	42.5

RANK ORDER

RANK	STATE	RATE
1	Mississippi	54.4
2	New Mexico	51.2
3	Alabama	43.2
4	Wyoming	42.5
5	Arkansas	42.3
6	Montana	42.1
7	South Carolina	41.2
8	Tennessee	40.9
9	Alaska	40.7
9	Arizona	40.7
11	Louisiana	39.9
12	South Dakota	39.8
13	Oklahoma	39.5
14	Idaho	39.4
15	West Virginia	37.1
16	Kentucky	36.9
16	North Carolina	36.9
18	Georgia	35.9
19	Missouri	35.8
20	Nevada	35.1
21	Kansas	34.9
21	Oregon	34.9
23	North Dakota	34.0
24	Texas	33.7
25	Florida	33.3
26	Colorado	32.8
27	Delaware	31.8
28	Nebraska	31.6
29	Indiana	30.7
30	Utah	30.6
31	Pennsylvania	29.2
31	Vermont	29.2
33	Washington	28.5
34	Virginia	27.7
34	Wisconsin	27.7
36	Iowa	27.6
37	Illinois	27.5
38	Michigan	27.2
39	Maine	27.1
40	Minnesota	26.4
41	California	25.2
42	Ohio	24.9
43	Connecticut	24.5
44	New Hampshire	23.3
45	Maryland	22.2
46	New Jersey	21.7
47	Hawaii	21.0
48	New York	20.4
49	Rhode Island	17.3
50	Massachusetts	15.5
	District of Columbia	31.5

Source: U.S. Department of Health and Human Services, National Center for Health Statistics
    "National Vital Statistics Reports" (Vol. 48, No. 11, July 24, 2000)
*Final data by state of residence. Includes motor vehicle deaths, poisoning, falls, drowning and other accidents.

Deaths by Motor Vehicle Accidents in 1998

National Total = 43,501 Deaths*

ALPHA ORDER

RANK	STATE	DEATHS	% of USA
13	Alabama	1,103	2.5%
50	Alaska	72	0.2%
19	Arizona	941	2.2%
25	Arkansas	680	1.6%
1	California	3,779	8.7%
27	Colorado	663	1.5%
38	Connecticut	341	0.8%
47	Delaware	116	0.3%
3	Florida	2,941	6.8%
7	Georgia	1,657	3.8%
45	Hawaii	124	0.3%
39	Idaho	269	0.6%
8	Illinois	1,521	3.5%
14	Indiana	1,046	2.4%
32	Iowa	462	1.1%
29	Kansas	550	1.3%
20	Kentucky	823	1.9%
16	Louisiana	983	2.3%
41	Maine	180	0.4%
28	Maryland	647	1.5%
31	Massachusetts	485	1.1%
9	Michigan	1,472	3.4%
26	Minnesota	674	1.5%
17	Mississippi	963	2.2%
12	Missouri	1,147	2.6%
40	Montana	219	0.5%
37	Nebraska	346	0.8%
36	Nevada	349	0.8%
43	New Hampshire	140	0.3%
21	New Jersey	783	1.8%
34	New Mexico	385	0.9%
4	New York	1,686	3.9%
5	North Carolina	1,672	3.8%
46	North Dakota	118	0.3%
10	Ohio	1,451	3.3%
22	Oklahoma	777	1.8%
29	Oregon	550	1.3%
6	Pennsylvania	1,661	3.8%
48	Rhode Island	86	0.2%
15	South Carolina	992	2.3%
42	South Dakota	165	0.4%
11	Tennessee	1,223	2.8%
2	Texas	3,769	8.7%
33	Utah	395	0.9%
49	Vermont	82	0.2%
18	Virginia	942	2.2%
24	Washington	750	1.7%
35	West Virginia	375	0.9%
23	Wisconsin	755	1.7%
44	Wyoming	135	0.3%

RANK ORDER

RANK	STATE	DEATHS	% of USA
1	California	3,779	8.7%
2	Texas	3,769	8.7%
3	Florida	2,941	6.8%
4	New York	1,686	3.9%
5	North Carolina	1,672	3.8%
6	Pennsylvania	1,661	3.8%
7	Georgia	1,657	3.8%
8	Illinois	1,521	3.5%
9	Michigan	1,472	3.4%
10	Ohio	1,451	3.3%
11	Tennessee	1,223	2.8%
12	Missouri	1,147	2.6%
13	Alabama	1,103	2.5%
14	Indiana	1,046	2.4%
15	South Carolina	992	2.3%
16	Louisiana	983	2.3%
17	Mississippi	963	2.2%
18	Virginia	942	2.2%
19	Arizona	941	2.2%
20	Kentucky	823	1.9%
21	New Jersey	783	1.8%
22	Oklahoma	777	1.8%
23	Wisconsin	755	1.7%
24	Washington	750	1.7%
25	Arkansas	680	1.6%
26	Minnesota	674	1.5%
27	Colorado	663	1.5%
28	Maryland	647	1.5%
29	Kansas	550	1.3%
29	Oregon	550	1.3%
31	Massachusetts	485	1.1%
32	Iowa	462	1.1%
33	Utah	395	0.9%
34	New Mexico	385	0.9%
35	West Virginia	375	0.9%
36	Nevada	349	0.8%
37	Nebraska	346	0.8%
38	Connecticut	341	0.8%
39	Idaho	269	0.6%
40	Montana	219	0.5%
41	Maine	180	0.4%
42	South Dakota	165	0.4%
43	New Hampshire	140	0.3%
44	Wyoming	135	0.3%
45	Hawaii	124	0.3%
46	North Dakota	118	0.3%
47	Delaware	116	0.3%
48	Rhode Island	86	0.2%
49	Vermont	82	0.2%
50	Alaska	72	0.2%
	District of Columbia	56	0.1%

Source: U.S. Department of Health and Human Services, National Center for Health Statistics
"National Vital Statistics Reports" (Vol. 48, No. 11, July 24, 2000)
*Final data by state of residence. These numbers are compiled from death certificates by the Centers for Disease Control and Prevention. They may differ from motor vehicle deaths collected by the U.S. Department of Transportation from other sources.

Death Rate by Motor Vehicle Accidents in 1998

National Rate = 16.1 Deaths per 100,000 Population*

<u>ALPHA ORDER</u>

RANK	STATE	RATE
5	Alabama	25.3
43	Alaska	11.7
20	Arizona	20.2
3	Arkansas	26.8
44	California	11.6
28	Colorado	16.7
45	Connecticut	10.4
30	Delaware	15.6
22	Florida	19.7
14	Georgia	21.7
45	Hawaii	10.4
13	Idaho	21.9
40	Illinois	12.6
26	Indiana	17.7
29	Iowa	16.1
16	Kansas	20.9
16	Kentucky	20.9
8	Louisiana	22.5
32	Maine	14.5
40	Maryland	12.6
50	Massachusetts	7.9
31	Michigan	15.0
34	Minnesota	14.3
1	Mississippi	35.0
15	Missouri	21.1
6	Montana	24.9
18	Nebraska	20.8
21	Nevada	20.0
42	New Hampshire	11.8
47	New Jersey	9.6
11	New Mexico	22.2
48	New York	9.3
11	North Carolina	22.2
25	North Dakota	18.5
39	Ohio	12.9
7	Oklahoma	23.2
27	Oregon	16.8
37	Pennsylvania	13.8
49	Rhode Island	8.7
4	South Carolina	25.9
10	South Dakota	22.4
8	Tennessee	22.5
23	Texas	19.1
24	Utah	18.8
35	Vermont	13.9
35	Virginia	13.9
38	Washington	13.2
19	West Virginia	20.7
32	Wisconsin	14.5
2	Wyoming	28.1

<u>RANK ORDER</u>

RANK	STATE	RATE
1	Mississippi	35.0
2	Wyoming	28.1
3	Arkansas	26.8
4	South Carolina	25.9
5	Alabama	25.3
6	Montana	24.9
7	Oklahoma	23.2
8	Louisiana	22.5
8	Tennessee	22.5
10	South Dakota	22.4
11	New Mexico	22.2
11	North Carolina	22.2
13	Idaho	21.9
14	Georgia	21.7
15	Missouri	21.1
16	Kansas	20.9
16	Kentucky	20.9
18	Nebraska	20.8
19	West Virginia	20.7
20	Arizona	20.2
21	Nevada	20.0
22	Florida	19.7
23	Texas	19.1
24	Utah	18.8
25	North Dakota	18.5
26	Indiana	17.7
27	Oregon	16.8
28	Colorado	16.7
29	Iowa	16.1
30	Delaware	15.6
31	Michigan	15.0
32	Maine	14.5
32	Wisconsin	14.5
34	Minnesota	14.3
35	Vermont	13.9
35	Virginia	13.9
37	Pennsylvania	13.8
38	Washington	13.2
39	Ohio	12.9
40	Illinois	12.6
40	Maryland	12.6
42	New Hampshire	11.8
43	Alaska	11.7
44	California	11.6
45	Connecticut	10.4
45	Hawaii	10.4
47	New Jersey	9.6
48	New York	9.3
49	Rhode Island	8.7
50	Massachusetts	7.9
	District of Columbia	10.7

Source: U.S. Department of Health and Human Services, National Center for Health Statistics "National Vital Statistics Reports" (Vol. 48, No. 11, July 24, 2000)

*Final data by state of residence. These numbers are compiled from death certificates by the Centers for Disease Control and Prevention. They may differ from motor vehicle deaths collected by the U.S. Department of Transportation from other sources. Not age-adjusted.

Age-Adjusted Death Rate by Motor Vehicle Accidents in 1998

National Rate = 15.6 Deaths per 100,000 Population*

ALPHA ORDER

RANK ORDER

RANK	STATE	RATE
5	Alabama	24.6
42	Alaska	12.0
20	Arizona	19.8
3	Arkansas	26.0
44	California	11.3
27	Colorado	16.8
46	Connecticut	10.1
29	Delaware	15.2
22	Florida	19.0
14	Georgia	21.0
45	Hawaii	10.6
13	Idaho	21.3
40	Illinois	12.6
26	Indiana	17.4
29	Iowa	15.2
18	Kansas	20.1
16	Kentucky	20.2
10	Louisiana	22.1
34	Maine	13.4
41	Maryland	12.3
50	Massachusetts	7.7
31	Michigan	14.5
33	Minnesota	13.6
1	Mississippi	34.3
15	Missouri	20.6
6	Montana	23.6
21	Nebraska	19.6
19	Nevada	20.0
43	New Hampshire	11.9
47	New Jersey	9.3
9	New Mexico	22.3
48	New York	8.7
12	North Carolina	21.9
25	North Dakota	18.2
39	Ohio	12.8
7	Oklahoma	22.5
28	Oregon	16.3
36	Pennsylvania	13.3
48	Rhode Island	8.7
4	South Carolina	25.2
8	South Dakota	22.4
10	Tennessee	22.1
23	Texas	18.9
24	Utah	18.3
34	Vermont	13.4
37	Virginia	13.2
38	Washington	13.1
16	West Virginia	20.2
32	Wisconsin	13.9
2	Wyoming	27.6

RANK	STATE	RATE
1	Mississippi	34.3
2	Wyoming	27.6
3	Arkansas	26.0
4	South Carolina	25.2
5	Alabama	24.6
6	Montana	23.6
7	Oklahoma	22.5
8	South Dakota	22.4
9	New Mexico	22.3
10	Louisiana	22.1
10	Tennessee	22.1
12	North Carolina	21.9
13	Idaho	21.3
14	Georgia	21.0
15	Missouri	20.6
16	Kentucky	20.2
16	West Virginia	20.2
18	Kansas	20.1
19	Nevada	20.0
20	Arizona	19.8
21	Nebraska	19.6
22	Florida	19.0
23	Texas	18.9
24	Utah	18.3
25	North Dakota	18.2
26	Indiana	17.4
27	Colorado	16.8
28	Oregon	16.3
29	Delaware	15.2
29	Iowa	15.2
31	Michigan	14.5
32	Wisconsin	13.9
33	Minnesota	13.6
34	Maine	13.4
34	Vermont	13.4
36	Pennsylvania	13.3
37	Virginia	13.2
38	Washington	13.1
39	Ohio	12.8
40	Illinois	12.6
41	Maryland	12.3
42	Alaska	12.0
43	New Hampshire	11.9
44	California	11.3
45	Hawaii	10.6
46	Connecticut	10.1
47	New Jersey	9.3
48	New York	8.7
48	Rhode Island	8.7
50	Massachusetts	7.7

District of Columbia   9.8

Source: U.S. Department of Health and Human Services, National Center for Health Statistics
   "National Vital Statistics Reports" (Vol. 48, No. 11, July 24, 2000)
*Final data by state of residence. These numbers are compiled from death certificates by the Centers for Disease
Control and Prevention. They may differ from motor vehicle deaths collected by the U.S. Department of
Transportation from other sources.

Deaths by Homicide in 1998

National Total = 18,272 Homicides*

ALPHA ORDER

RANK	STATE	HOMICIDES	% of USA
13	Alabama	457	2.5%
39	Alaska	49	0.3%
16	Arizona	444	2.4%
24	Arkansas	234	1.3%
1	California	2,401	13.1%
27	Colorado	188	1.0%
32	Connecticut	145	0.8%
41	Delaware	30	0.2%
4	Florida	1,083	5.9%
8	Georgia	669	3.7%
42	Hawaii	28	0.2%
40	Idaho	34	0.2%
3	Illinois	1,113	6.1%
18	Indiana	410	2.2%
36	Iowa	67	0.4%
30	Kansas	158	0.9%
22	Kentucky	253	1.4%
10	Louisiana	596	3.3%
42	Maine	28	0.2%
11	Maryland	580	3.2%
33	Massachusetts	124	0.7%
6	Michigan	774	4.2%
34	Minnesota	119	0.7%
19	Mississippi	358	2.0%
17	Missouri	428	2.3%
44	Montana	27	0.1%
38	Nebraska	56	0.3%
28	Nevada	172	0.9%
46	New Hampshire	19	0.1%
21	New Jersey	333	1.8%
29	New Mexico	168	0.9%
5	New York	974	5.3%
7	North Carolina	672	3.7%
48	North Dakota	11	0.1%
14	Ohio	446	2.4%
25	Oklahoma	232	1.3%
31	Oregon	146	0.8%
9	Pennsylvania	637	3.5%
45	Rhode Island	24	0.1%
20	South Carolina	354	1.9%
49	South Dakota	10	0.1%
12	Tennessee	492	2.7%
2	Texas	1,453	8.0%
37	Utah	64	0.4%
49	Vermont	10	0.1%
14	Virginia	446	2.4%
23	Washington	235	1.3%
35	West Virginia	89	0.5%
26	Wisconsin	194	1.1%
46	Wyoming	19	0.1%

RANK ORDER

RANK	STATE	HOMICIDES	% of USA
1	California	2,401	13.1%
2	Texas	1,453	8.0%
3	Illinois	1,113	6.1%
4	Florida	1,083	5.9%
5	New York	974	5.3%
6	Michigan	774	4.2%
7	North Carolina	672	3.7%
8	Georgia	669	3.7%
9	Pennsylvania	637	3.5%
10	Louisiana	596	3.3%
11	Maryland	580	3.2%
12	Tennessee	492	2.7%
13	Alabama	457	2.5%
14	Ohio	446	2.4%
14	Virginia	446	2.4%
16	Arizona	444	2.4%
17	Missouri	428	2.3%
18	Indiana	410	2.2%
19	Mississippi	358	2.0%
20	South Carolina	354	1.9%
21	New Jersey	333	1.8%
22	Kentucky	253	1.4%
23	Washington	235	1.3%
24	Arkansas	234	1.3%
25	Oklahoma	232	1.3%
26	Wisconsin	194	1.1%
27	Colorado	188	1.0%
28	Nevada	172	0.9%
29	New Mexico	168	0.9%
30	Kansas	158	0.9%
31	Oregon	146	0.8%
32	Connecticut	145	0.8%
33	Massachusetts	124	0.7%
34	Minnesota	119	0.7%
35	West Virginia	89	0.5%
36	Iowa	67	0.4%
37	Utah	64	0.4%
38	Nebraska	56	0.3%
39	Alaska	49	0.3%
40	Idaho	34	0.2%
41	Delaware	30	0.2%
42	Hawaii	28	0.2%
42	Maine	28	0.2%
44	Montana	27	0.1%
45	Rhode Island	24	0.1%
46	New Hampshire	19	0.1%
46	Wyoming	19	0.1%
48	North Dakota	11	0.1%
49	South Dakota	10	0.1%
49	Vermont	10	0.1%
	District of Columbia	219	1.2%

Source: U.S. Department of Health and Human Services, National Center for Health Statistics
"National Vital Statistics Reports" (Vol. 48, No. 11, July 24, 2000)
*By state of residence. Includes legal intervention. Homicide data shown here are collected by the Centers for Disease Control and Prevention based on death certificates and differ from murder data collected by the F.B.I. from other sources.

Death Rate by Homicide in 1998

National Rate = 6.8 Deaths per 100,000 Population*

RANK	STATE	RATE	RANK	STATE	RATE
4	Alabama	10.5	1	Louisiana	13.6
14	Alaska	8.0	2	Mississippi	13.0
7	Arizona	9.5	3	Maryland	11.3
8	Arkansas	9.2	4	Alabama	10.5
17	California	7.4	5	Nevada	9.8
28	Colorado	4.7	6	New Mexico	9.7
29	Connecticut	4.4	7	Arizona	9.5
33	Delaware	4.0	8	Arkansas	9.2
19	Florida	7.3	8	Illinois	9.2
13	Georgia	8.8	8	South Carolina	9.2
42	Hawaii	2.3	11	Tennessee	9.1
39	Idaho	2.8	12	North Carolina	8.9
8	Illinois	9.2	13	Georgia	8.8
20	Indiana	7.0	14	Alaska	8.0
42	Iowa	2.3	15	Michigan	7.9
24	Kansas	6.0	15	Missouri	7.9
23	Kentucky	6.4	17	California	7.4
1	Louisiana	13.6	17	Texas	7.4
42	Maine	2.3	19	Florida	7.3
3	Maryland	11.3	20	Indiana	7.0
45	Massachusetts	2.0	21	Oklahoma	6.9
15	Michigan	7.9	22	Virginia	6.6
40	Minnesota	2.5	23	Kentucky	6.4
2	Mississippi	13.0	24	Kansas	6.0
15	Missouri	7.9	25	New York	5.4
37	Montana	3.1	26	Pennsylvania	5.3
36	Nebraska	3.4	27	West Virginia	4.9
5	Nevada	9.8	28	Colorado	4.7
NA	New Hampshire**	NA	29	Connecticut	4.4
31	New Jersey	4.1	29	Oregon	4.4
6	New Mexico	9.7	31	New Jersey	4.1
25	New York	5.4	31	Washington	4.1
12	North Carolina	8.9	33	Delaware	4.0
NA	North Dakota**	NA	33	Ohio	4.0
33	Ohio	4.0	35	Wisconsin	3.7
21	Oklahoma	6.9	36	Nebraska	3.4
29	Oregon	4.4	37	Montana	3.1
26	Pennsylvania	5.3	38	Utah	3.0
41	Rhode Island	2.4	39	Idaho	2.8
8	South Carolina	9.2	40	Minnesota	2.5
NA	South Dakota**	NA	41	Rhode Island	2.4
11	Tennessee	9.1	42	Hawaii	2.3
17	Texas	7.4	42	Iowa	2.3
38	Utah	3.0	42	Maine	2.3
NA	Vermont**	NA	45	Massachusetts	2.0
22	Virginia	6.6	NA	New Hampshire**	NA
31	Washington	4.1	NA	North Dakota**	NA
27	West Virginia	4.9	NA	South Dakota**	NA
35	Wisconsin	3.7	NA	Vermont**	NA
NA	Wyoming**	NA	NA	Wyoming**	NA
				District of Columbia	41.9

ALPHA ORDER — RANK ORDER

Source: U.S. Department of Health and Human Services, National Center for Health Statistics
  "National Vital Statistics Reports" (Vol. 48, No. 11, July 24, 2000)
By state of residence. Includes legal intervention. Homicide data shown here are collected by the Centers for Disease Control and Prevention based on death certificates and differ from murder data collected by the F.B.I. from other sources. Not age-adjusted.
  **Insufficient data to determine a reliable rate.*

Age-Adjusted Death Rate by Homicide in 1998

National Rate = 7.3 Deaths per 100,000 Population*

RANK	STATE	RATE		RANK	STATE	RATE
	ALPHA ORDER				RANK ORDER	
4	Alabama	10.9		1	Louisiana	14.5
16	Alaska	8.1		2	Mississippi	13.2
6	Arizona	10.5		3	Maryland	12.6
9	Arkansas	10.0		4	Alabama	10.9
18	California	7.9		5	Nevada	10.6
27	Colorado	5.2		6	Arizona	10.5
28	Connecticut	5.1		6	Illinois	10.5
34	Delaware	4.1		8	New Mexico	10.3
17	Florida	8.0		9	Arkansas	10.0
13	Georgia	8.9		10	South Carolina	9.6
42	Hawaii	2.5		11	Tennessee	9.5
40	Idaho	2.7		12	North Carolina	9.4
6	Illinois	10.5		13	Georgia	8.9
20	Indiana	7.3		14	Missouri	8.5
42	Iowa	2.5		15	Michigan	8.4
23	Kansas	6.6		16	Alaska	8.1
24	Kentucky	6.5		17	Florida	8.0
1	Louisiana	14.5		18	California	7.9
44	Maine	2.4		19	Texas	7.6
3	Maryland	12.6		20	Indiana	7.3
45	Massachusetts	2.3		20	Oklahoma	7.3
15	Michigan	8.4		22	Virginia	6.7
40	Minnesota	2.7		23	Kansas	6.6
2	Mississippi	13.2		24	Kentucky	6.5
14	Missouri	8.5		25	Pennsylvania	6.1
37	Montana	3.3		26	New York	5.9
36	Nebraska	3.7		27	Colorado	5.2
5	Nevada	10.6		28	Connecticut	5.1
NA	New Hampshire**	NA		29	West Virginia	5.0
31	New Jersey	4.5		30	Oregon	4.7
8	New Mexico	10.3		31	New Jersey	4.5
26	New York	5.9		32	Washington	4.4
12	North Carolina	9.4		33	Ohio	4.3
NA	North Dakota**	NA		34	Delaware	4.1
33	Ohio	4.3		35	Wisconsin	4.0
20	Oklahoma	7.3		36	Nebraska	3.7
30	Oregon	4.7		37	Montana	3.3
25	Pennsylvania	6.1		38	Utah	3.1
39	Rhode Island	2.8		39	Rhode Island	2.8
10	South Carolina	9.6		40	Idaho	2.7
NA	South Dakota**	NA		40	Minnesota	2.7
11	Tennessee	9.5		42	Hawaii	2.5
19	Texas	7.6		42	Iowa	2.5
38	Utah	3.1		44	Maine	2.4
NA	Vermont**	NA		45	Massachusetts	2.3
22	Virginia	6.7		NA	New Hampshire**	NA
32	Washington	4.4		NA	North Dakota**	NA
29	West Virginia	5.0		NA	South Dakota**	NA
35	Wisconsin	4.0		NA	Vermont**	NA
NA	Wyoming**	NA		NA	Wyoming**	NA
					District of Columbia	46.7

Source: U.S. Department of Health and Human Services, National Center for Health Statistics
   "National Vital Statistics Reports" (Vol. 48, No. 11, July 24, 2000)
*By state of residence. Includes legal intervention. Homicide data shown here are collected by the Centers for Disease Control and Prevention based on death certificates and differ from murder data collected by the F.B.I. from other sources.
**Insufficient data to determine a reliable rate.

Deaths by Suicide in 1998

National Total = 30,575 Suicides*

ALPHA ORDER

RANK ORDER

RANK	STATE	SUICIDES	% of USA		RANK	STATE	SUICIDES	% of USA
20	Alabama	569	1.9%		1	California	3,415	11.2%
43	Alaska	129	0.4%		2	Florida	2,172	7.1%
12	Arizona	804	2.6%		3	Texas	2,133	7.0%
30	Arkansas	344	1.1%		4	Pennsylvania	1,370	4.5%
1	California	3,415	11.2%		5	New York	1,364	4.5%
17	Colorado	611	2.0%		6	Ohio	1,108	3.6%
36	Connecticut	257	0.8%		7	Illinois	1,036	3.4%
50	Delaware	68	0.2%		8	Michigan	969	3.2%
2	Florida	2,172	7.1%		9	North Carolina	857	2.8%
11	Georgia	822	2.7%		10	Virginia	827	2.7%
44	Hawaii	116	0.4%		11	Georgia	822	2.7%
39	Idaho	201	0.7%		12	Arizona	804	2.6%
7	Illinois	1,036	3.4%		13	Tennessee	744	2.4%
15	Indiana	699	2.3%		14	Washington	708	2.3%
32	Iowa	329	1.1%		15	Indiana	699	2.3%
34	Kansas	325	1.1%		16	Missouri	698	2.3%
22	Kentucky	526	1.7%		17	Colorado	611	2.0%
25	Louisiana	480	1.6%		18	Wisconsin	594	1.9%
40	Maine	196	0.6%		19	New Jersey	581	1.9%
24	Maryland	497	1.6%		20	Alabama	569	1.9%
23	Massachusetts	506	1.7%		21	Oregon	545	1.8%
8	Michigan	969	3.2%		22	Kentucky	526	1.7%
27	Minnesota	459	1.5%		23	Massachusetts	506	1.7%
32	Mississippi	329	1.1%		24	Maryland	497	1.6%
16	Missouri	698	2.3%		25	Louisiana	480	1.6%
41	Montana	158	0.5%		26	Oklahoma	471	1.5%
38	Nebraska	204	0.7%		27	Minnesota	459	1.5%
29	Nevada	397	1.3%		28	South Carolina	449	1.5%
42	New Hampshire	154	0.5%		29	Nevada	397	1.3%
19	New Jersey	581	1.9%		30	Arkansas	344	1.1%
35	New Mexico	297	1.0%		31	Utah	336	1.1%
5	New York	1,364	4.5%		32	Iowa	329	1.1%
9	North Carolina	857	2.8%		32	Mississippi	329	1.1%
49	North Dakota	72	0.2%		34	Kansas	325	1.1%
6	Ohio	1,108	3.6%		35	New Mexico	297	1.0%
26	Oklahoma	471	1.5%		36	Connecticut	257	0.8%
21	Oregon	545	1.8%		37	West Virginia	232	0.8%
4	Pennsylvania	1,370	4.5%		38	Nebraska	204	0.7%
47	Rhode Island	86	0.3%		39	Idaho	201	0.7%
28	South Carolina	449	1.5%		40	Maine	196	0.6%
45	South Dakota	115	0.4%		41	Montana	158	0.5%
13	Tennessee	744	2.4%		42	New Hampshire	154	0.5%
3	Texas	2,133	7.0%		43	Alaska	129	0.4%
31	Utah	336	1.1%		44	Hawaii	116	0.4%
47	Vermont	86	0.3%		45	South Dakota	115	0.4%
10	Virginia	827	2.7%		46	Wyoming	87	0.3%
14	Washington	708	2.3%		47	Rhode Island	86	0.3%
37	West Virginia	232	0.8%		47	Vermont	86	0.3%
18	Wisconsin	594	1.9%		49	North Dakota	72	0.2%
46	Wyoming	87	0.3%		50	Delaware	68	0.2%
						District of Columbia	43	0.1%

Source: U.S. Department of Health and Human Services, National Center for Health Statistics
   "National Vital Statistics Reports" (Vol. 48, No. 11, July 24, 2000)
*Final data by state of residence.

Death Rate by Suicide in 1998

National Rate = 11.3 Suicides per 100,000 Population*

ALPHA ORDER

RANK	STATE	RATE
19	Alabama	13.1
2	Alaska	21.0
5	Arizona	17.2
17	Arkansas	13.6
38	California	10.5
12	Colorado	15.4
48	Connecticut	7.8
44	Delaware	9.1
13	Florida	14.6
36	Georgia	10.8
41	Hawaii	9.7
8	Idaho	16.4
46	Illinois	8.6
28	Indiana	11.8
30	Iowa	11.5
23	Kansas	12.4
18	Kentucky	13.4
35	Louisiana	11.0
10	Maine	15.8
41	Maryland	9.7
47	Massachusetts	8.2
39	Michigan	9.9
41	Minnesota	9.7
27	Mississippi	12.0
21	Missouri	12.8
4	Montana	17.9
25	Nebraska	12.3
1	Nevada	22.7
20	New Hampshire	13.0
50	New Jersey	7.2
6	New Mexico	17.1
49	New York	7.5
31	North Carolina	11.4
34	North Dakota	11.3
39	Ohio	9.9
15	Oklahoma	14.1
7	Oregon	16.6
31	Pennsylvania	11.4
45	Rhode Island	8.7
29	South Carolina	11.7
11	South Dakota	15.6
16	Tennessee	13.7
36	Texas	10.8
9	Utah	16.0
13	Vermont	14.6
26	Virginia	12.2
23	Washington	12.4
21	West Virginia	12.8
31	Wisconsin	11.4
3	Wyoming	18.1

RANK ORDER

RANK	STATE	RATE
1	Nevada	22.7
2	Alaska	21.0
3	Wyoming	18.1
4	Montana	17.9
5	Arizona	17.2
6	New Mexico	17.1
7	Oregon	16.6
8	Idaho	16.4
9	Utah	16.0
10	Maine	15.8
11	South Dakota	15.6
12	Colorado	15.4
13	Florida	14.6
13	Vermont	14.6
15	Oklahoma	14.1
16	Tennessee	13.7
17	Arkansas	13.6
18	Kentucky	13.4
19	Alabama	13.1
20	New Hampshire	13.0
21	Missouri	12.8
21	West Virginia	12.8
23	Kansas	12.4
23	Washington	12.4
25	Nebraska	12.3
26	Virginia	12.2
27	Mississippi	12.0
28	Indiana	11.8
29	South Carolina	11.7
30	Iowa	11.5
31	North Carolina	11.4
31	Pennsylvania	11.4
31	Wisconsin	11.4
34	North Dakota	11.3
35	Louisiana	11.0
36	Georgia	10.8
36	Texas	10.8
38	California	10.5
39	Michigan	9.9
39	Ohio	9.9
41	Hawaii	9.7
41	Maryland	9.7
41	Minnesota	9.7
44	Delaware	9.1
45	Rhode Island	8.7
46	Illinois	8.6
47	Massachusetts	8.2
48	Connecticut	7.8
49	New York	7.5
50	New Jersey	7.2

District of Columbia	8.2

Source: U.S. Department of Health and Human Services, National Center for Health Statistics
   "National Vital Statistics Reports" (Vol. 48, No. 11, July 24, 2000)
*Final data by state of residence. Not age-adjusted.

Age-Adjusted Death Rate by Suicide in 1998

National Rate = 10.4 Suicides per 100,000 Population*

<table>
<tr><td colspan="3">ALPHA ORDER</td><td colspan="3">RANK ORDER</td></tr>
<tr><th>RANK</th><th>STATE</th><th>RATE</th><th>RANK</th><th>STATE</th><th>RATE</th></tr>
<tr><td>20</td><td>Alabama</td><td>12.0</td><td>1</td><td>Alaska</td><td>22.1</td></tr>
<tr><td>1</td><td>Alaska</td><td>22.1</td><td>2</td><td>Nevada</td><td>21.2</td></tr>
<tr><td>7</td><td>Arizona</td><td>16.0</td><td>3</td><td>Wyoming</td><td>16.8</td></tr>
<tr><td>13</td><td>Arkansas</td><td>13.1</td><td>4</td><td>Utah</td><td>16.6</td></tr>
<tr><td>38</td><td>California</td><td>9.6</td><td>5</td><td>New Mexico</td><td>16.4</td></tr>
<tr><td>12</td><td>Colorado</td><td>14.2</td><td>6</td><td>Montana</td><td>16.3</td></tr>
<tr><td>48</td><td>Connecticut</td><td>7.2</td><td>7</td><td>Arizona</td><td>16.0</td></tr>
<tr><td>46</td><td>Delaware</td><td>8.0</td><td>8</td><td>South Dakota</td><td>15.4</td></tr>
<tr><td>17</td><td>Florida</td><td>12.6</td><td>9</td><td>Idaho</td><td>15.2</td></tr>
<tr><td>37</td><td>Georgia</td><td>10.0</td><td>10</td><td>Oregon</td><td>14.8</td></tr>
<tr><td>40</td><td>Hawaii</td><td>9.2</td><td>11</td><td>Maine</td><td>14.5</td></tr>
<tr><td>9</td><td>Idaho</td><td>15.2</td><td>12</td><td>Colorado</td><td>14.2</td></tr>
<tr><td>44</td><td>Illinois</td><td>8.1</td><td>13</td><td>Arkansas</td><td>13.1</td></tr>
<tr><td>27</td><td>Indiana</td><td>11.1</td><td>13</td><td>Oklahoma</td><td>13.1</td></tr>
<tr><td>29</td><td>Iowa</td><td>10.7</td><td>15</td><td>Vermont</td><td>12.9</td></tr>
<tr><td>21</td><td>Kansas</td><td>11.9</td><td>16</td><td>New Hampshire</td><td>12.7</td></tr>
<tr><td>22</td><td>Kentucky</td><td>11.8</td><td>17</td><td>Florida</td><td>12.6</td></tr>
<tr><td>33</td><td>Louisiana</td><td>10.4</td><td>17</td><td>Tennessee</td><td>12.6</td></tr>
<tr><td>11</td><td>Maine</td><td>14.5</td><td>19</td><td>Missouri</td><td>12.1</td></tr>
<tr><td>43</td><td>Maryland</td><td>8.9</td><td>20</td><td>Alabama</td><td>12.0</td></tr>
<tr><td>47</td><td>Massachusetts</td><td>7.5</td><td>21</td><td>Kansas</td><td>11.9</td></tr>
<tr><td>41</td><td>Michigan</td><td>9.1</td><td>22</td><td>Kentucky</td><td>11.8</td></tr>
<tr><td>39</td><td>Minnesota</td><td>9.4</td><td>23</td><td>Nebraska</td><td>11.6</td></tr>
<tr><td>24</td><td>Mississippi</td><td>11.5</td><td>24</td><td>Mississippi</td><td>11.5</td></tr>
<tr><td>19</td><td>Missouri</td><td>12.1</td><td>24</td><td>West Virginia</td><td>11.5</td></tr>
<tr><td>6</td><td>Montana</td><td>16.3</td><td>26</td><td>Washington</td><td>11.4</td></tr>
<tr><td>23</td><td>Nebraska</td><td>11.6</td><td>27</td><td>Indiana</td><td>11.1</td></tr>
<tr><td>2</td><td>Nevada</td><td>21.2</td><td>28</td><td>Virginia</td><td>11.0</td></tr>
<tr><td>16</td><td>New Hampshire</td><td>12.7</td><td>29</td><td>Iowa</td><td>10.7</td></tr>
<tr><td>50</td><td>New Jersey</td><td>6.4</td><td>29</td><td>South Carolina</td><td>10.7</td></tr>
<tr><td>5</td><td>New Mexico</td><td>16.4</td><td>29</td><td>Wisconsin</td><td>10.7</td></tr>
<tr><td>49</td><td>New York</td><td>6.9</td><td>32</td><td>North Dakota</td><td>10.6</td></tr>
<tr><td>33</td><td>North Carolina</td><td>10.4</td><td>33</td><td>Louisiana</td><td>10.4</td></tr>
<tr><td>32</td><td>North Dakota</td><td>10.6</td><td>33</td><td>North Carolina</td><td>10.4</td></tr>
<tr><td>42</td><td>Ohio</td><td>9.0</td><td>33</td><td>Pennsylvania</td><td>10.4</td></tr>
<tr><td>13</td><td>Oklahoma</td><td>13.1</td><td>36</td><td>Texas</td><td>10.3</td></tr>
<tr><td>10</td><td>Oregon</td><td>14.8</td><td>37</td><td>Georgia</td><td>10.0</td></tr>
<tr><td>33</td><td>Pennsylvania</td><td>10.4</td><td>38</td><td>California</td><td>9.6</td></tr>
<tr><td>44</td><td>Rhode Island</td><td>8.1</td><td>39</td><td>Minnesota</td><td>9.4</td></tr>
<tr><td>29</td><td>South Carolina</td><td>10.7</td><td>40</td><td>Hawaii</td><td>9.2</td></tr>
<tr><td>8</td><td>South Dakota</td><td>15.4</td><td>41</td><td>Michigan</td><td>9.1</td></tr>
<tr><td>17</td><td>Tennessee</td><td>12.6</td><td>42</td><td>Ohio</td><td>9.0</td></tr>
<tr><td>36</td><td>Texas</td><td>10.3</td><td>43</td><td>Maryland</td><td>8.9</td></tr>
<tr><td>4</td><td>Utah</td><td>16.6</td><td>44</td><td>Illinois</td><td>8.1</td></tr>
<tr><td>15</td><td>Vermont</td><td>12.9</td><td>44</td><td>Rhode Island</td><td>8.1</td></tr>
<tr><td>28</td><td>Virginia</td><td>11.0</td><td>46</td><td>Delaware</td><td>8.0</td></tr>
<tr><td>26</td><td>Washington</td><td>11.4</td><td>47</td><td>Massachusetts</td><td>7.5</td></tr>
<tr><td>24</td><td>West Virginia</td><td>11.5</td><td>48</td><td>Connecticut</td><td>7.2</td></tr>
<tr><td>29</td><td>Wisconsin</td><td>10.7</td><td>49</td><td>New York</td><td>6.9</td></tr>
<tr><td>3</td><td>Wyoming</td><td>16.8</td><td>50</td><td>New Jersey</td><td>6.4</td></tr>
<tr><td></td><td></td><td></td><td></td><td>District of Columbia</td><td>7.3</td></tr>
</table>

Source: U.S. Department of Health and Human Services, National Center for Health Statistics
   "National Vital Statistics Reports" (Vol. 48, No. 11, July 24, 2000)
*Final data by state of residence.

Years Lost by Premature Death in 1998

National Average = 7,455 Years Lost per 100,000 Population*

ALPHA ORDER

RANK	STATE	YEARS
3	Alabama	9,623
20	Alaska	7,547
15	Arizona	8,015
5	Arkansas	9,253
34	California	6,649
38	Colorado	6,419
37	Connecticut	6,459
18	Delaware	7,878
14	Florida	8,046
7	Georgia	8,743
45	Hawaii	6,058
35	Idaho	6,568
19	Illinois	7,744
21	Indiana	7,520
44	Iowa	6,132
31	Kansas	7,043
12	Kentucky	8,113
2	Louisiana	9,814
42	Maine	6,142
13	Maryland	8,108
48	Massachusetts	5,841
23	Michigan	7,461
50	Minnesota	5,590
1	Mississippi	10,583
16	Missouri	8,005
30	Montana	7,051
36	Nebraska	6,556
9	Nevada	8,588
49	New Hampshire	5,759
32	New Jersey	6,934
17	New Mexico	7,931
28	New York	7,152
10	North Carolina	8,469
46	North Dakota	6,054
26	Ohio	7,186
8	Oklahoma	8,595
33	Oregon	6,765
24	Pennsylvania	7,378
39	Rhode Island	6,270
4	South Carolina	9,365
29	South Dakota	7,065
6	Tennessee	8,941
22	Texas	7,468
43	Utah	6,137
47	Vermont	6,023
25	Virginia	7,194
41	Washington	6,259
11	West Virginia	8,262
39	Wisconsin	6,270
27	Wyoming	7,169

RANK ORDER

RANK	STATE	YEARS
1	Mississippi	10,583
2	Louisiana	9,814
3	Alabama	9,623
4	South Carolina	9,365
5	Arkansas	9,253
6	Tennessee	8,941
7	Georgia	8,743
8	Oklahoma	8,595
9	Nevada	8,588
10	North Carolina	8,469
11	West Virginia	8,262
12	Kentucky	8,113
13	Maryland	8,108
14	Florida	8,046
15	Arizona	8,015
16	Missouri	8,005
17	New Mexico	7,931
18	Delaware	7,878
19	Illinois	7,744
20	Alaska	7,547
21	Indiana	7,520
22	Texas	7,468
23	Michigan	7,461
24	Pennsylvania	7,378
25	Virginia	7,194
26	Ohio	7,186
27	Wyoming	7,169
28	New York	7,152
29	South Dakota	7,065
30	Montana	7,051
31	Kansas	7,043
32	New Jersey	6,934
33	Oregon	6,765
34	California	6,649
35	Idaho	6,568
36	Nebraska	6,556
37	Connecticut	6,459
38	Colorado	6,419
39	Rhode Island	6,270
39	Wisconsin	6,270
41	Washington	6,259
42	Maine	6,142
43	Utah	6,137
44	Iowa	6,132
45	Hawaii	6,058
46	North Dakota	6,054
47	Vermont	6,023
48	Massachusetts	5,841
49	New Hampshire	5,759
50	Minnesota	5,590
	District of Columbia	16,100

Source: U.S. Department of Health and Human Services, National Center for Health Statistics
     unpublished data

*Age-adjusted years of potential life lost due to death before age 75.

Years Lost by Premature Death from Cancer in 1998

National Average = 1,490 Years Lost per 100,000 Population*

ALPHA ORDER			RANK ORDER		
RANK	STATE	YEARS	RANK	STATE	YEARS
7	Alabama	1,678	1	Mississippi	1,781
44	Alaska	1,297	2	Louisiana	1,776
38	Arizona	1,362	3	Delaware	1,751
9	Arkansas	1,669	4	West Virginia	1,722
39	California	1,359	5	Kentucky	1,717
49	Colorado	1,136	6	Tennessee	1,715
33	Connecticut	1,407	7	Alabama	1,678
3	Delaware	1,751	8	South Carolina	1,670
13	Florida	1,594	9	Arkansas	1,669
12	Georgia	1,597	10	New Hampshire	1,648
43	Hawaii	1,299	11	Missouri	1,614
46	Idaho	1,247	12	Georgia	1,597
21	Illinois	1,542	13	Florida	1,594
16	Indiana	1,559	14	Oklahoma	1,587
35	Iowa	1,397	15	North Carolina	1,574
42	Kansas	1,319	16	Indiana	1,559
5	Kentucky	1,717	17	Ohio	1,558
2	Louisiana	1,776	18	Rhode Island	1,556
20	Maine	1,543	19	Maryland	1,551
19	Maryland	1,551	20	Maine	1,543
30	Massachusetts	1,448	21	Illinois	1,542
25	Michigan	1,486	22	Pennsylvania	1,512
45	Minnesota	1,280	23	Nevada	1,499
1	Mississippi	1,781	24	New Jersey	1,494
11	Missouri	1,614	25	Michigan	1,486
48	Montana	1,155	25	Virginia	1,486
40	Nebraska	1,349	27	Vermont	1,473
23	Nevada	1,499	28	New York	1,466
10	New Hampshire	1,648	29	Oregon	1,450
24	New Jersey	1,494	30	Massachusetts	1,448
47	New Mexico	1,194	31	Texas	1,435
28	New York	1,466	32	South Dakota	1,411
15	North Carolina	1,574	33	Connecticut	1,407
36	North Dakota	1,387	34	Wisconsin	1,403
17	Ohio	1,558	35	Iowa	1,397
14	Oklahoma	1,587	36	North Dakota	1,387
29	Oregon	1,450	37	Washington	1,365
22	Pennsylvania	1,512	38	Arizona	1,362
18	Rhode Island	1,556	39	California	1,359
8	South Carolina	1,670	40	Nebraska	1,349
32	South Dakota	1,411	41	Wyoming	1,339
6	Tennessee	1,715	42	Kansas	1,319
31	Texas	1,435	43	Hawaii	1,299
50	Utah	1,076	44	Alaska	1,297
27	Vermont	1,473	45	Minnesota	1,280
25	Virginia	1,486	46	Idaho	1,247
37	Washington	1,365	47	New Mexico	1,194
4	West Virginia	1,722	48	Montana	1,155
34	Wisconsin	1,403	49	Colorado	1,136
41	Wyoming	1,339	50	Utah	1,076
				District of Columbia	2,042

Source: U.S. Department of Health and Human Services, National Center for Health Statistics
    unpublished data
*Age-adjusted years of potential life lost due to death before age 75.

Years Lost by Premature Death from Heart Disease in 1998

National Average = 1,155 Years Lost per 100,000 Population*

ALPHA ORDER

RANK	STATE	YEARS
3	Alabama	1,585
41	Alaska	893
26	Arizona	1,038
7	Arkansas	1,493
35	California	976
48	Colorado	777
32	Connecticut	987
14	Delaware	1,270
24	Florida	1,133
8	Georgia	1,438
29	Hawaii	1,016
47	Idaho	793
16	Illinois	1,252
18	Indiana	1,209
30	Iowa	1,009
28	Kansas	1,017
10	Kentucky	1,425
4	Louisiana	1,546
38	Maine	950
22	Maryland	1,163
39	Massachusetts	921
15	Michigan	1,259
49	Minnesota	766
1	Mississippi	1,941
12	Missouri	1,325
42	Montana	880
34	Nebraska	983
13	Nevada	1,291
40	New Hampshire	904
31	New Jersey	993
45	New Mexico	817
23	New York	1,142
11	North Carolina	1,337
36	North Dakota	964
17	Ohio	1,220
9	Oklahoma	1,437
44	Oregon	830
21	Pennsylvania	1,165
27	Rhode Island	1,020
6	South Carolina	1,502
25	South Dakota	1,101
5	Tennessee	1,516
20	Texas	1,172
50	Utah	737
46	Vermont	810
19	Virginia	1,198
43	Washington	856
2	West Virginia	1,613
37	Wisconsin	962
33	Wyoming	985

RANK ORDER

RANK	STATE	YEARS
1	Mississippi	1,941
2	West Virginia	1,613
3	Alabama	1,585
4	Louisiana	1,546
5	Tennessee	1,516
6	South Carolina	1,502
7	Arkansas	1,493
8	Georgia	1,438
9	Oklahoma	1,437
10	Kentucky	1,425
11	North Carolina	1,337
12	Missouri	1,325
13	Nevada	1,291
14	Delaware	1,270
15	Michigan	1,259
16	Illinois	1,252
17	Ohio	1,220
18	Indiana	1,209
19	Virginia	1,198
20	Texas	1,172
21	Pennsylvania	1,165
22	Maryland	1,163
23	New York	1,142
24	Florida	1,133
25	South Dakota	1,101
26	Arizona	1,038
27	Rhode Island	1,020
28	Kansas	1,017
29	Hawaii	1,016
30	Iowa	1,009
31	New Jersey	993
32	Connecticut	987
33	Wyoming	985
34	Nebraska	983
35	California	976
36	North Dakota	964
37	Wisconsin	962
38	Maine	950
39	Massachusetts	921
40	New Hampshire	904
41	Alaska	893
42	Montana	880
43	Washington	856
44	Oregon	830
45	New Mexico	817
46	Vermont	810
47	Idaho	793
48	Colorado	777
49	Minnesota	766
50	Utah	737

District of Columbia   1,872

Source: U.S. Department of Health and Human Services, National Center for Health Statistics
unpublished data
*Age-adjusted years of potential life lost due to death before age 75.

Years Lost by Premature Death from Homicide in 1998

National Average = 331 Years Lost per 100,000 Population*

ALPHA ORDER

RANK	STATE	YEARS
7	Alabama	474
21	Alaska	314
6	Arizona	477
9	Arkansas	443
16	California	365
27	Colorado	251
28	Connecticut	237
35	Delaware	176
17	Florida	348
13	Georgia	399
45	Hawaii	94
41	Idaho	118
4	Illinois	509
19	Indiana	331
44	Iowa	108
20	Kansas	323
26	Kentucky	272
1	Louisiana	655
43	Maine	112
2	Maryland	602
42	Massachusetts	113
15	Michigan	392
38	Minnesota	136
3	Mississippi	562
14	Missouri	393
37	Montana	149
36	Nebraska	171
5	Nevada	490
NA	New Hampshire**	NA
30	New Jersey	207
8	New Mexico	453
25	New York	277
11	North Carolina	421
NA	North Dakota**	NA
31	Ohio	201
22	Oklahoma	303
33	Oregon	195
24	Pennsylvania	290
39	Rhode Island	133
12	South Carolina	409
NA	South Dakota**	NA
10	Tennessee	424
18	Texas	340
40	Utah	126
NA	Vermont**	NA
23	Virginia	296
32	Washington	199
29	West Virginia	216
34	Wisconsin	193
NA	Wyoming**	NA

RANK ORDER

RANK	STATE	YEARS
1	Louisiana	655
2	Maryland	602
3	Mississippi	562
4	Illinois	509
5	Nevada	490
6	Arizona	477
7	Alabama	474
8	New Mexico	453
9	Arkansas	443
10	Tennessee	424
11	North Carolina	421
12	South Carolina	409
13	Georgia	399
14	Missouri	393
15	Michigan	392
16	California	365
17	Florida	348
18	Texas	340
19	Indiana	331
20	Kansas	323
21	Alaska	314
22	Oklahoma	303
23	Virginia	296
24	Pennsylvania	290
25	New York	277
26	Kentucky	272
27	Colorado	251
28	Connecticut	237
29	West Virginia	216
30	New Jersey	207
31	Ohio	201
32	Washington	199
33	Oregon	195
34	Wisconsin	193
35	Delaware	176
36	Nebraska	171
37	Montana	149
38	Minnesota	136
39	Rhode Island	133
40	Utah	126
41	Idaho	118
42	Massachusetts	113
43	Maine	112
44	Iowa	108
45	Hawaii	94
NA	New Hampshire**	NA
NA	North Dakota**	NA
NA	South Dakota**	NA
NA	Vermont**	NA
NA	Wyoming**	NA

District of Columbia   2,191

Source: U.S. Department of Health and Human Services, National Center for Health Statistics
    unpublished data
*Age-adjusted years of potential life lost due to death before age 75.
**Data for states with fewer than 20 deaths from homicide for persons under 75 years of age are considered unreliable and are not shown.

Years Lost by Premature Death from Suicide in 1998

National Average = 371 Years Lost per 100,000 Population*

ALPHA ORDER				RANK ORDER		
RANK	STATE	YEARS		RANK	STATE	YEARS
25	Alabama	413		1	Alaska	891
1	Alaska	891		2	Nevada	741
8	Arizona	582		3	Utah	607
14	Arkansas	494		4	Montana	606
42	California	317		5	New Mexico	604
12	Colorado	509		6	Wyoming	603
47	Connecticut	275		7	South Dakota	602
48	Delaware	264		8	Arizona	582
20	Florida	431		9	Idaho	559
39	Georgia	352		10	Maine	554
38	Hawaii	354		11	Oregon	524
9	Idaho	559		12	Colorado	509
44	Illinois	295		13	New Hampshire	500
26	Indiana	401		14	Arkansas	494
29	Iowa	397		15	Oklahoma	478
16	Kansas	458		16	Kansas	458
27	Kentucky	400		17	Tennessee	450
32	Louisiana	382		18	Missouri	447
10	Maine	554		19	Vermont	444
43	Maryland	311		20	Florida	431
45	Massachusetts	279		21	Nebraska	430
40	Michigan	331		22	North Dakota	426
36	Minnesota	366		23	West Virginia	422
24	Mississippi	421		24	Mississippi	421
18	Missouri	447		25	Alabama	413
4	Montana	606		26	Indiana	401
21	Nebraska	430		27	Kentucky	400
2	Nevada	741		27	Washington	400
13	New Hampshire	500		29	Iowa	397
50	New Jersey	221		30	Wisconsin	389
5	New Mexico	604		31	Virginia	386
49	New York	244		32	Louisiana	382
37	North Carolina	362		32	South Carolina	382
22	North Dakota	426		34	Pennsylvania	378
41	Ohio	321		35	Texas	368
15	Oklahoma	478		36	Minnesota	366
11	Oregon	524		37	North Carolina	362
34	Pennsylvania	378		38	Hawaii	354
45	Rhode Island	279		39	Georgia	352
32	South Carolina	382		40	Michigan	331
7	South Dakota	602		41	Ohio	321
17	Tennessee	450		42	California	317
35	Texas	368		43	Maryland	311
3	Utah	607		44	Illinois	295
19	Vermont	444		45	Massachusetts	279
31	Virginia	386		45	Rhode Island	279
27	Washington	400		47	Connecticut	275
23	West Virginia	422		48	Delaware	264
30	Wisconsin	389		49	New York	244
6	Wyoming	603		50	New Jersey	221
					District of Columbia	269

Source: U.S. Department of Health and Human Services, National Center for Health Statistics unpublished data

*Age-adjusted years of potential life lost due to death before age 75.

Years Lost by Premature Death from Unintentional Injuries in 1998

National Average = 1,103 Years Lost per 100,000 Population*

<table>
<tr><td colspan="3">ALPHA ORDER</td><td colspan="3">RANK ORDER</td></tr>
<tr><td>RANK</td><td>STATE</td><td>YEARS</td><td>RANK</td><td>STATE</td><td>YEARS</td></tr>
<tr><td>3</td><td>Alabama</td><td>1,640</td><td>1</td><td>Mississippi</td><td>2,053</td></tr>
<tr><td>8</td><td>Alaska</td><td>1,544</td><td>2</td><td>New Mexico</td><td>1,866</td></tr>
<tr><td>13</td><td>Arizona</td><td>1,492</td><td>3</td><td>Alabama</td><td>1,640</td></tr>
<tr><td>5</td><td>Arkansas</td><td>1,622</td><td>4</td><td>Wyoming</td><td>1,630</td></tr>
<tr><td>41</td><td>California</td><td>896</td><td>5</td><td>Arkansas</td><td>1,622</td></tr>
<tr><td>26</td><td>Colorado</td><td>1,178</td><td>6</td><td>South Dakota</td><td>1,572</td></tr>
<tr><td>43</td><td>Connecticut</td><td>857</td><td>7</td><td>South Carolina</td><td>1,546</td></tr>
<tr><td>28</td><td>Delaware</td><td>1,148</td><td>8</td><td>Alaska</td><td>1,544</td></tr>
<tr><td>22</td><td>Florida</td><td>1,301</td><td>9</td><td>Montana</td><td>1,521</td></tr>
<tr><td>23</td><td>Georgia</td><td>1,278</td><td>9</td><td>Tennessee</td><td>1,521</td></tr>
<tr><td>45</td><td>Hawaii</td><td>777</td><td>11</td><td>Louisiana</td><td>1,520</td></tr>
<tr><td>12</td><td>Idaho</td><td>1,500</td><td>12</td><td>Idaho</td><td>1,500</td></tr>
<tr><td>36</td><td>Illinois</td><td>999</td><td>13</td><td>Arizona</td><td>1,492</td></tr>
<tr><td>27</td><td>Indiana</td><td>1,164</td><td>14</td><td>Oklahoma</td><td>1,469</td></tr>
<tr><td>35</td><td>Iowa</td><td>1,006</td><td>15</td><td>West Virginia</td><td>1,382</td></tr>
<tr><td>21</td><td>Kansas</td><td>1,305</td><td>16</td><td>Kentucky</td><td>1,380</td></tr>
<tr><td>16</td><td>Kentucky</td><td>1,380</td><td>16</td><td>North Carolina</td><td>1,380</td></tr>
<tr><td>11</td><td>Louisiana</td><td>1,520</td><td>18</td><td>Nevada</td><td>1,352</td></tr>
<tr><td>38</td><td>Maine</td><td>947</td><td>19</td><td>Missouri</td><td>1,326</td></tr>
<tr><td>47</td><td>Maryland</td><td>763</td><td>20</td><td>Oregon</td><td>1,313</td></tr>
<tr><td>50</td><td>Massachusetts</td><td>531</td><td>21</td><td>Kansas</td><td>1,305</td></tr>
<tr><td>33</td><td>Michigan</td><td>1,017</td><td>22</td><td>Florida</td><td>1,301</td></tr>
<tr><td>42</td><td>Minnesota</td><td>882</td><td>23</td><td>Georgia</td><td>1,278</td></tr>
<tr><td>1</td><td>Mississippi</td><td>2,053</td><td>24</td><td>North Dakota</td><td>1,263</td></tr>
<tr><td>19</td><td>Missouri</td><td>1,326</td><td>25</td><td>Texas</td><td>1,254</td></tr>
<tr><td>9</td><td>Montana</td><td>1,521</td><td>26</td><td>Colorado</td><td>1,178</td></tr>
<tr><td>29</td><td>Nebraska</td><td>1,140</td><td>27</td><td>Indiana</td><td>1,164</td></tr>
<tr><td>18</td><td>Nevada</td><td>1,352</td><td>28</td><td>Delaware</td><td>1,148</td></tr>
<tr><td>44</td><td>New Hampshire</td><td>796</td><td>29</td><td>Nebraska</td><td>1,140</td></tr>
<tr><td>46</td><td>New Jersey</td><td>774</td><td>30</td><td>Vermont</td><td>1,089</td></tr>
<tr><td>2</td><td>New Mexico</td><td>1,866</td><td>31</td><td>Utah</td><td>1,072</td></tr>
<tr><td>48</td><td>New York</td><td>707</td><td>32</td><td>Pennsylvania</td><td>1,062</td></tr>
<tr><td>16</td><td>North Carolina</td><td>1,380</td><td>33</td><td>Michigan</td><td>1,017</td></tr>
<tr><td>24</td><td>North Dakota</td><td>1,263</td><td>34</td><td>Washington</td><td>1,015</td></tr>
<tr><td>40</td><td>Ohio</td><td>897</td><td>35</td><td>Iowa</td><td>1,006</td></tr>
<tr><td>14</td><td>Oklahoma</td><td>1,469</td><td>36</td><td>Illinois</td><td>999</td></tr>
<tr><td>20</td><td>Oregon</td><td>1,313</td><td>37</td><td>Wisconsin</td><td>972</td></tr>
<tr><td>32</td><td>Pennsylvania</td><td>1,062</td><td>38</td><td>Maine</td><td>947</td></tr>
<tr><td>49</td><td>Rhode Island</td><td>623</td><td>39</td><td>Virginia</td><td>946</td></tr>
<tr><td>7</td><td>South Carolina</td><td>1,546</td><td>40</td><td>Ohio</td><td>897</td></tr>
<tr><td>6</td><td>South Dakota</td><td>1,572</td><td>41</td><td>California</td><td>896</td></tr>
<tr><td>9</td><td>Tennessee</td><td>1,521</td><td>42</td><td>Minnesota</td><td>882</td></tr>
<tr><td>25</td><td>Texas</td><td>1,254</td><td>43</td><td>Connecticut</td><td>857</td></tr>
<tr><td>31</td><td>Utah</td><td>1,072</td><td>44</td><td>New Hampshire</td><td>796</td></tr>
<tr><td>30</td><td>Vermont</td><td>1,089</td><td>45</td><td>Hawaii</td><td>777</td></tr>
<tr><td>39</td><td>Virginia</td><td>946</td><td>46</td><td>New Jersey</td><td>774</td></tr>
<tr><td>34</td><td>Washington</td><td>1,015</td><td>47</td><td>Maryland</td><td>763</td></tr>
<tr><td>15</td><td>West Virginia</td><td>1,382</td><td>48</td><td>New York</td><td>707</td></tr>
<tr><td>37</td><td>Wisconsin</td><td>972</td><td>49</td><td>Rhode Island</td><td>623</td></tr>
<tr><td>4</td><td>Wyoming</td><td>1,630</td><td>50</td><td>Massachusetts</td><td>531</td></tr>
<tr><td></td><td></td><td></td><td></td><td>District of Columbia</td><td>1,064</td></tr>
</table>

Source: U.S. Department of Health and Human Services, National Center for Health Statistics
    unpublished data

*Age-adjusted years of potential life lost due to death before age 75. Includes such subcategories as falls, drowning, fires/burns, poisonings and motor vehicle injuries.

Average Annual Deaths Due to Smoking: 1990-1994

National Estimated Total = 430,741 Deaths*

ALPHA ORDER					RANK ORDER			

RANK	STATE	DEATHS	% of USA		RANK	STATE	DEATHS	% of USA
22	Alabama	7,055	1.6%		1	California	41,883	9.7%
50	Alaska	421	0.1%		2	New York	30,741	7.1%
25	Arizona	5,912	1.4%		3	Florida	29,060	6.7%
27	Arkansas	5,271	1.2%		4	Texas	24,789	5.8%
1	California	41,883	9.7%		5	Pennsylvania	23,170	5.4%
32	Colorado	4,467	1.0%		6	Ohio	19,527	4.5%
28	Connecticut	5,251	1.2%		7	Illinois	19,016	4.4%
43	Delaware	1,248	0.3%		8	Michigan	15,786	3.7%
3	Florida	29,060	6.7%		9	New Jersey	12,831	3.0%
14	Georgia	9,666	2.2%		10	North Carolina	11,642	2.7%
45	Hawaii	1,163	0.3%		11	Indiana	10,373	2.4%
42	Idaho	1,404	0.3%		12	Massachusetts	10,242	2.4%
7	Illinois	19,016	4.4%		13	Missouri	9,960	2.3%
11	Indiana	10,373	2.4%		14	Georgia	9,666	2.2%
30	Iowa	4,962	1.2%		15	Virginia	9,530	2.2%
34	Kansas	4,215	1.0%		16	Tennessee	9,359	2.2%
17	Kentucky	7,953	1.8%		17	Kentucky	7,953	1.8%
21	Louisiana	7,075	1.6%		18	Washington	7,892	1.8%
37	Maine	2,326	0.5%		19	Wisconsin	7,853	1.8%
20	Maryland	7,180	1.7%		20	Maryland	7,180	1.7%
12	Massachusetts	10,242	2.4%		21	Louisiana	7,075	1.6%
8	Michigan	15,786	3.7%		22	Alabama	7,055	1.6%
24	Minnesota	6,150	1.4%		23	Oklahoma	6,255	1.5%
31	Mississippi	4,762	1.1%		24	Minnesota	6,150	1.4%
13	Missouri	9,960	2.3%		25	Arizona	5,912	1.4%
41	Montana	1,434	0.3%		26	South Carolina	5,887	1.4%
36	Nebraska	2,623	0.6%		27	Arkansas	5,271	1.2%
35	Nevada	2,665	0.6%		28	Connecticut	5,251	1.2%
40	New Hampshire	1,777	0.4%		29	Oregon	5,210	1.2%
9	New Jersey	12,831	3.0%		30	Iowa	4,962	1.2%
38	New Mexico	1,871	0.4%		31	Mississippi	4,762	1.1%
2	New York	30,741	7.1%		32	Colorado	4,467	1.0%
10	North Carolina	11,642	2.7%		33	West Virginia	4,229	1.0%
47	North Dakota	968	0.2%		34	Kansas	4,215	1.0%
6	Ohio	19,527	4.5%		35	Nevada	2,665	0.6%
23	Oklahoma	6,255	1.5%		36	Nebraska	2,623	0.6%
29	Oregon	5,210	1.2%		37	Maine	2,326	0.5%
5	Pennsylvania	23,170	5.4%		38	New Mexico	1,871	0.4%
39	Rhode Island	1,849	0.4%		39	Rhode Island	1,849	0.4%
26	South Carolina	5,887	1.4%		40	New Hampshire	1,777	0.4%
44	South Dakota	1,198	0.3%		41	Montana	1,434	0.3%
16	Tennessee	9,359	2.2%		42	Idaho	1,404	0.3%
4	Texas	24,789	5.8%		43	Delaware	1,248	0.3%
46	Utah	1,133	0.3%		44	South Dakota	1,198	0.3%
48	Vermont	914	0.2%		45	Hawaii	1,163	0.3%
15	Virginia	9,530	2.2%		46	Utah	1,133	0.3%
18	Washington	7,892	1.8%		47	North Dakota	968	0.2%
33	West Virginia	4,229	1.0%		48	Vermont	914	0.2%
19	Wisconsin	7,853	1.8%		49	Wyoming	712	0.2%
49	Wyoming	712	0.2%		50	Alaska	421	0.1%
						District of Columbia	929	0.2%

Source: Centers for Disease Control and Prevention, Office on Smoking and Health
  "State and National Tobacco Control Highlights" (http://www.cdc.gov/nccdphp/osh/statehi/statehi.htm)
*Estimates.

Average Annual Death Rate Due to Smoking: 1990-1994

National Rate = 358 Deaths per 100,000 Population*

ALPHA ORDER				RANK ORDER		
RANK	STATE	RATE		RANK	STATE	RATE
23	Alabama	353		1	Nevada	469
15	Alaska	367		2	Kentucky	444
38	Arizona	325		3	West Virginia	424
4	Arkansas	405		4	Arkansas	405
32	California	343		5	Delaware	400
35	Colorado	331		6	Mississippi	392
41	Connecticut	310		7	Tennessee	390
5	Delaware	400		8	Louisiana	388
27	Florida	350		9	Indiana	387
17	Georgia	364		9	Oklahoma	387
49	Hawaii	237		11	South Carolina	378
45	Idaho	296		12	Maine	371
30	Illinois	347		13	Michigan	368
9	Indiana	387		13	North Carolina	368
43	Iowa	308		15	Alaska	367
39	Kansas	319		15	Missouri	367
2	Kentucky	444		17	Georgia	364
8	Louisiana	388		17	Ohio	364
12	Maine	371		19	New Hampshire	361
24	Maryland	351		20	Virginia	360
35	Massachusetts	331		21	Texas	358
13	Michigan	368		22	Wyoming	357
47	Minnesota	287		23	Alabama	353
6	Mississippi	392		24	Maryland	351
15	Missouri	367		24	Vermont	351
28	Montana	348		24	Washington	351
43	Nebraska	308		27	Florida	350
1	Nevada	469		28	Montana	348
19	New Hampshire	361		28	Oregon	348
37	New Jersey	327		30	Illinois	347
46	New Mexico	289		31	Pennsylvania	346
32	New York	343		32	California	343
13	North Carolina	368		32	New York	343
48	North Dakota	280		34	Rhode Island	340
17	Ohio	364		35	Colorado	331
9	Oklahoma	387		35	Massachusetts	331
28	Oregon	348		37	New Jersey	327
31	Pennsylvania	346		38	Arizona	325
34	Rhode Island	340		39	Kansas	319
11	South Carolina	378		40	Wisconsin	313
42	South Dakota	309		41	Connecticut	310
7	Tennessee	390		42	South Dakota	309
21	Texas	358		43	Iowa	308
50	Utah	188		43	Nebraska	308
24	Vermont	351		45	Idaho	296
20	Virginia	360		46	New Mexico	289
24	Washington	351		47	Minnesota	287
3	West Virginia	424		48	North Dakota	280
40	Wisconsin	313		49	Hawaii	237
22	Wyoming	357		50	Utah	188
					District of Columbia	327

Source: Centers for Disease Control and Prevention, Office on Smoking and Health
   "State and National Tobacco Control Highlights" (http://www.cdc.gov/nccdphp/osh/statehi/statehi.htm)
Estimates.

Alcohol-Induced Deaths in 1998

National Total = 19,515 Deaths*

RANK	STATE	DEATHS	% of USA
29	Alabama	247	1.3%
40	Alaska	83	0.4%
11	Arizona	468	2.4%
37	Arkansas	109	0.6%
1	California	3,423	17.5%
17	Colorado	371	1.9%
33	Connecticut	159	0.8%
45	Delaware	67	0.3%
2	Florida	1,346	6.9%
10	Georgia	480	2.5%
48	Hawaii	47	0.2%
42	Idaho	81	0.4%
5	Illinois	668	3.4%
22	Indiana	321	1.6%
34	Iowa	149	0.8%
32	Kansas	160	0.8%
30	Kentucky	233	1.2%
26	Louisiana	274	1.4%
39	Maine	99	0.5%
27	Maryland	266	1.4%
19	Massachusetts	354	1.8%
7	Michigan	631	3.2%
23	Minnesota	298	1.5%
31	Mississippi	169	0.9%
18	Missouri	357	1.8%
42	Montana	81	0.4%
40	Nebraska	83	0.4%
24	Nevada	293	1.5%
38	New Hampshire	108	0.6%
12	New Jersey	447	2.3%
25	New Mexico	284	1.5%
3	New York	1,297	6.6%
6	North Carolina	637	3.3%
49	North Dakota	43	0.2%
8	Ohio	585	3.0%
28	Oklahoma	262	1.3%
20	Oregon	351	1.8%
12	Pennsylvania	447	2.3%
46	Rhode Island	59	0.3%
14	South Carolina	407	2.1%
44	South Dakota	72	0.4%
15	Tennessee	389	2.0%
4	Texas	1,125	5.8%
35	Utah	126	0.6%
50	Vermont	32	0.2%
20	Virginia	351	1.8%
9	Washington	531	2.7%
36	West Virginia	124	0.6%
16	Wisconsin	380	1.9%
47	Wyoming	58	0.3%

RANK	STATE	DEATHS	% of USA
1	California	3,423	17.5%
2	Florida	1,346	6.9%
3	New York	1,297	6.6%
4	Texas	1,125	5.8%
5	Illinois	668	3.4%
6	North Carolina	637	3.3%
7	Michigan	631	3.2%
8	Ohio	585	3.0%
9	Washington	531	2.7%
10	Georgia	480	2.5%
11	Arizona	468	2.4%
12	New Jersey	447	2.3%
12	Pennsylvania	447	2.3%
14	South Carolina	407	2.1%
15	Tennessee	389	2.0%
16	Wisconsin	380	1.9%
17	Colorado	371	1.9%
18	Missouri	357	1.8%
19	Massachusetts	354	1.8%
20	Oregon	351	1.8%
20	Virginia	351	1.8%
22	Indiana	321	1.6%
23	Minnesota	298	1.5%
24	Nevada	293	1.5%
25	New Mexico	284	1.5%
26	Louisiana	274	1.4%
27	Maryland	266	1.4%
28	Oklahoma	262	1.3%
29	Alabama	247	1.3%
30	Kentucky	233	1.2%
31	Mississippi	169	0.9%
32	Kansas	160	0.8%
33	Connecticut	159	0.8%
34	Iowa	149	0.8%
35	Utah	126	0.6%
36	West Virginia	124	0.6%
37	Arkansas	109	0.6%
38	New Hampshire	108	0.6%
39	Maine	99	0.5%
40	Alaska	83	0.4%
40	Nebraska	83	0.4%
42	Idaho	81	0.4%
42	Montana	81	0.4%
44	South Dakota	72	0.4%
45	Delaware	67	0.3%
46	Rhode Island	59	0.3%
47	Wyoming	58	0.3%
48	Hawaii	47	0.2%
49	North Dakota	43	0.2%
50	Vermont	32	0.2%
	District of Columbia	83	0.4%

Source: U.S. Department of Health and Human Services, National Center for Health Statistics (http://wonder.cdc.gov/WONDER/)

*By state of residence. Includes excessive blood level of alcohol, accidental poisoning by alcohol and the following alcohol-related causes: psychoses, dependence syndrome, polyneuropathy, cardiomyopathy, gastritis, chronic liver disease and cirrhosis. Excludes accidents, homicides and other causes indirectly related to alcohol use.

Death Rate from Alcohol-Induced Deaths in 1998

National Rate = 7.2 Deaths per 100,000 Population*

ALPHA ORDER

RANK	STATE	RATE
36	Alabama	5.7
3	Alaska	13.5
8	Arizona	10.0
48	Arkansas	4.3
7	California	10.5
10	Colorado	9.3
47	Connecticut	4.9
14	Delaware	9.0
14	Florida	9.0
27	Georgia	6.3
49	Hawaii	3.9
24	Idaho	6.6
38	Illinois	5.5
40	Indiana	5.4
42	Iowa	5.2
30	Kansas	6.1
34	Kentucky	5.9
27	Louisiana	6.3
17	Maine	8.0
42	Maryland	5.2
35	Massachusetts	5.8
26	Michigan	6.4
27	Minnesota	6.3
30	Mississippi	6.1
24	Missouri	6.6
12	Montana	9.2
46	Nebraska	5.0
1	Nevada	16.8
13	New Hampshire	9.1
38	New Jersey	5.5
2	New Mexico	16.3
21	New York	7.1
16	North Carolina	8.4
23	North Dakota	6.7
42	Ohio	5.2
18	Oklahoma	7.8
5	Oregon	10.7
50	Pennsylvania	3.7
32	Rhode Island	6.0
6	South Carolina	10.6
9	South Dakota	9.8
20	Tennessee	7.2
36	Texas	5.7
32	Utah	6.0
40	Vermont	5.4
42	Virginia	5.2
10	Washington	9.3
22	West Virginia	6.8
19	Wisconsin	7.3
4	Wyoming	12.1

RANK ORDER

RANK	STATE	RATE
1	Nevada	16.8
2	New Mexico	16.3
3	Alaska	13.5
4	Wyoming	12.1
5	Oregon	10.7
6	South Carolina	10.6
7	California	10.5
8	Arizona	10.0
9	South Dakota	9.8
10	Colorado	9.3
10	Washington	9.3
12	Montana	9.2
13	New Hampshire	9.1
14	Delaware	9.0
14	Florida	9.0
16	North Carolina	8.4
17	Maine	8.0
18	Oklahoma	7.8
19	Wisconsin	7.3
20	Tennessee	7.2
21	New York	7.1
22	West Virginia	6.8
23	North Dakota	6.7
24	Idaho	6.6
24	Missouri	6.6
26	Michigan	6.4
27	Georgia	6.3
27	Louisiana	6.3
27	Minnesota	6.3
30	Kansas	6.1
30	Mississippi	6.1
32	Rhode Island	6.0
32	Utah	6.0
34	Kentucky	5.9
35	Massachusetts	5.8
36	Alabama	5.7
36	Texas	5.7
38	Illinois	5.5
38	New Jersey	5.5
40	Indiana	5.4
40	Vermont	5.4
42	Iowa	5.2
42	Maryland	5.2
42	Ohio	5.2
42	Virginia	5.2
46	Nebraska	5.0
47	Connecticut	4.9
48	Arkansas	4.3
49	Hawaii	3.9
50	Pennsylvania	3.7

District of Columbia	15.8

Source: U.S. Department of Health and Human Services, National Center for Health Statistics
   (http://wonder.cdc.gov/WONDER/)
*By state of residence. Includes excessive blood level of alcohol, accidental poisoning by alcohol and the
following alcohol-related causes: psychoses, dependence syndrome, polyneuropathy, cardiomyopathy, gastritis,
chronic liver disease and cirrhosis. Excludes accidents, homicides and other causes indirectly related to alcohol
use. Not age-adjusted.

Age-Adjusted Death Rate from Alcohol-Induced Deaths in 1998

National Rate = 6.1 Deaths per 100,000 Population*

ALPHA ORDER

RANK	STATE	RATE
37	Alabama	4.8
3	Alaska	13.0
7	Arizona	8.8
48	Arkansas	3.7
5	California	9.5
10	Colorado	7.8
47	Connecticut	4.0
12	Delaware	7.3
15	Florida	7.1
24	Georgia	5.7
49	Hawaii	3.0
23	Idaho	5.8
34	Illinois	4.9
39	Indiana	4.7
45	Iowa	4.2
31	Kansas	5.3
34	Kentucky	4.9
28	Louisiana	5.5
19	Maine	6.2
41	Maryland	4.4
37	Massachusetts	4.8
25	Michigan	5.6
30	Minnesota	5.4
25	Mississippi	5.6
28	Missouri	5.5
12	Montana	7.3
45	Nebraska	4.2
2	Nevada	14.1
12	New Hampshire	7.3
40	New Jersey	4.5
1	New Mexico	14.7
22	New York	5.9
15	North Carolina	7.1
25	North Dakota	5.6
43	Ohio	4.3
17	Oklahoma	6.6
9	Oregon	8.3
50	Pennsylvania	2.9
34	Rhode Island	4.9
7	South Carolina	8.8
6	South Dakota	9.0
21	Tennessee	6.0
32	Texas	5.2
18	Utah	6.5
43	Vermont	4.3
41	Virginia	4.4
10	Washington	7.8
33	West Virginia	5.1
20	Wisconsin	6.1
4	Wyoming	9.8

RANK ORDER

RANK	STATE	RATE
1	New Mexico	14.7
2	Nevada	14.1
3	Alaska	13.0
4	Wyoming	9.8
5	California	9.5
6	South Dakota	9.0
7	Arizona	8.8
7	South Carolina	8.8
9	Oregon	8.3
10	Colorado	7.8
10	Washington	7.8
12	Delaware	7.3
12	Montana	7.3
12	New Hampshire	7.3
15	Florida	7.1
15	North Carolina	7.1
17	Oklahoma	6.6
18	Utah	6.5
19	Maine	6.2
20	Wisconsin	6.1
21	Tennessee	6.0
22	New York	5.9
23	Idaho	5.8
24	Georgia	5.7
25	Michigan	5.6
25	Mississippi	5.6
25	North Dakota	5.6
28	Louisiana	5.5
28	Missouri	5.5
30	Minnesota	5.4
31	Kansas	5.3
32	Texas	5.2
33	West Virginia	5.1
34	Illinois	4.9
34	Kentucky	4.9
34	Rhode Island	4.9
37	Alabama	4.8
37	Massachusetts	4.8
39	Indiana	4.7
40	New Jersey	4.5
41	Maryland	4.4
41	Virginia	4.4
43	Ohio	4.3
43	Vermont	4.3
45	Iowa	4.2
45	Nebraska	4.2
47	Connecticut	4.0
48	Arkansas	3.7
49	Hawaii	3.0
50	Pennsylvania	2.9
	District of Columbia	13.4

Source: U.S. Department of Health and Human Services, National Center for Health Statistics
  (http://wonder.cdc.gov/WONDER/)
*By state of residence. Includes excessive blood level of alcohol, accidental poisoning by alcohol and the
following alcohol-related causes: psychoses, dependence syndrome, polyneuropathy, cardiomyopathy, gastritis,
chronic liver disease and cirrhosis. Excludes accidents, homicides and other causes indirectly related to alcohol use.

Drug-Induced Deaths in 1998

National Total = 16,926 Deaths*

ALPHA ORDER

RANK	STATE	DEATHS	% of USA
29	Alabama	151	0.9%
45	Alaska	42	0.2%
11	Arizona	489	2.9%
33	Arkansas	94	0.6%
1	California	2,956	17.5%
18	Colorado	279	1.6%
23	Connecticut	224	1.3%
38	Delaware	63	0.4%
4	Florida	973	5.7%
16	Georgia	319	1.9%
35	Hawaii	79	0.5%
43	Idaho	48	0.3%
6	Illinois	731	4.3%
25	Indiana	217	1.3%
40	Iowa	58	0.3%
34	Kansas	86	0.5%
28	Kentucky	185	1.1%
26	Louisiana	212	1.3%
42	Maine	57	0.3%
9	Maryland	596	3.5%
10	Massachusetts	539	3.2%
7	Michigan	656	3.9%
32	Minnesota	126	0.7%
35	Mississippi	79	0.5%
22	Missouri	227	1.3%
46	Montana	39	0.2%
44	Nebraska	43	0.3%
24	Nevada	218	1.3%
37	New Hampshire	67	0.4%
8	New Jersey	633	3.7%
20	New Mexico	261	1.5%
3	New York	1,082	6.4%
15	North Carolina	323	1.9%
50	North Dakota	12	0.1%
13	Ohio	400	2.4%
30	Oklahoma	145	0.9%
14	Oregon	325	1.9%
5	Pennsylvania	915	5.4%
40	Rhode Island	58	0.3%
31	South Carolina	128	0.8%
49	South Dakota	20	0.1%
17	Tennessee	303	1.8%
2	Texas	1,093	6.5%
27	Utah	191	1.1%
47	Vermont	29	0.2%
19	Virginia	276	1.6%
12	Washington	477	2.8%
39	West Virginia	61	0.4%
21	Wisconsin	230	1.4%
48	Wyoming	25	0.1%

RANK ORDER

RANK	STATE	DEATHS	% of USA
1	California	2,956	17.5%
2	Texas	1,093	6.5%
3	New York	1,082	6.4%
4	Florida	973	5.7%
5	Pennsylvania	915	5.4%
6	Illinois	731	4.3%
7	Michigan	656	3.9%
8	New Jersey	633	3.7%
9	Maryland	596	3.5%
10	Massachusetts	539	3.2%
11	Arizona	489	2.9%
12	Washington	477	2.8%
13	Ohio	400	2.4%
14	Oregon	325	1.9%
15	North Carolina	323	1.9%
16	Georgia	319	1.9%
17	Tennessee	303	1.8%
18	Colorado	279	1.6%
19	Virginia	276	1.6%
20	New Mexico	261	1.5%
21	Wisconsin	230	1.4%
22	Missouri	227	1.3%
23	Connecticut	224	1.3%
24	Nevada	218	1.3%
25	Indiana	217	1.3%
26	Louisiana	212	1.3%
27	Utah	191	1.1%
28	Kentucky	185	1.1%
29	Alabama	151	0.9%
30	Oklahoma	145	0.9%
31	South Carolina	128	0.8%
32	Minnesota	126	0.7%
33	Arkansas	94	0.6%
34	Kansas	86	0.5%
35	Hawaii	79	0.5%
35	Mississippi	79	0.5%
37	New Hampshire	67	0.4%
38	Delaware	63	0.4%
39	West Virginia	61	0.4%
40	Iowa	58	0.3%
40	Rhode Island	58	0.3%
42	Maine	57	0.3%
43	Idaho	48	0.3%
44	Nebraska	43	0.3%
45	Alaska	42	0.2%
46	Montana	39	0.2%
47	Vermont	29	0.2%
48	Wyoming	25	0.1%
49	South Dakota	20	0.1%
50	North Dakota	12	0.1%
	District of Columbia	86	0.5%

Source: U.S. Department of Health and Human Services, National Center for Health Statistics
   (http://wonder.cdc.gov/WONDER/)
*By state of residence. Includes drug psychoses, drug dependence, nondependent use excluding alcohol and tobacco, accidental poisoning or suicide by drugs, medicaments and biologicals. Excludes accidents, homicides and other causes indirectly related to drug use.

Death Rate from Drug-Induced Deaths in 1998

National Rate = 6.3 Deaths per 100,000 Population*

ALPHA ORDER

RANK	STATE	RATE
41	Alabama	3.5
14	Alaska	6.8
4	Arizona	10.5
38	Arkansas	3.7
6	California	9.1
13	Colorado	7.0
14	Connecticut	6.8
9	Delaware	8.5
18	Florida	6.5
34	Georgia	4.2
17	Hawaii	6.6
37	Idaho	3.9
19	Illinois	6.1
38	Indiana	3.7
49	Iowa	2.0
43	Kansas	3.3
28	Kentucky	4.7
26	Louisiana	4.9
29	Maine	4.6
3	Maryland	11.6
8	Massachusetts	8.8
16	Michigan	6.7
46	Minnesota	2.7
45	Mississippi	2.9
34	Missouri	4.2
30	Montana	4.4
48	Nebraska	2.6
2	Nevada	12.5
22	New Hampshire	5.7
11	New Jersey	7.8
1	New Mexico	15.0
20	New York	6.0
32	North Carolina	4.3
50	North Dakota**	1.9
40	Ohio	3.6
32	Oklahoma	4.3
5	Oregon	9.9
12	Pennsylvania	7.6
21	Rhode Island	5.9
43	South Carolina	3.3
46	South Dakota	2.7
23	Tennessee	5.6
24	Texas	5.5
6	Utah	9.1
26	Vermont	4.9
36	Virginia	4.1
10	Washington	8.4
42	West Virginia	3.4
30	Wisconsin	4.4
25	Wyoming	5.2

RANK ORDER

RANK	STATE	RATE
1	New Mexico	15.0
2	Nevada	12.5
3	Maryland	11.6
4	Arizona	10.5
5	Oregon	9.9
6	California	9.1
6	Utah	9.1
8	Massachusetts	8.8
9	Delaware	8.5
10	Washington	8.4
11	New Jersey	7.8
12	Pennsylvania	7.6
13	Colorado	7.0
14	Alaska	6.8
14	Connecticut	6.8
16	Michigan	6.7
17	Hawaii	6.6
18	Florida	6.5
19	Illinois	6.1
20	New York	6.0
21	Rhode Island	5.9
22	New Hampshire	5.7
23	Tennessee	5.6
24	Texas	5.5
25	Wyoming	5.2
26	Louisiana	4.9
26	Vermont	4.9
28	Kentucky	4.7
29	Maine	4.6
30	Montana	4.4
30	Wisconsin	4.4
32	North Carolina	4.3
32	Oklahoma	4.3
34	Georgia	4.2
34	Missouri	4.2
36	Virginia	4.1
37	Idaho	3.9
38	Arkansas	3.7
38	Indiana	3.7
40	Ohio	3.6
41	Alabama	3.5
42	West Virginia	3.4
43	Kansas	3.3
43	South Carolina	3.3
45	Mississippi	2.9
46	Minnesota	2.7
46	South Dakota	2.7
48	Nebraska	2.6
49	Iowa	2.0
50	North Dakota**	1.9
	District of Columbia	16.4

Source: U.S. Department of Health and Human Services, National Center for Health Statistics (http://wonder.cdc.gov/WONDER/)

By state of residence. Includes drug psychoses, drug dependence, nondependent use excluding alcohol and tobacco, accidental poisoning or suicide by drugs, medicaments and biologicals. Excludes accidents, homicides and other causes indirectly related to drug use. Not age-adjusted.

**Due to low numbers of deaths, rates for this state should be interpreted with caution.*

Age-Adjusted Death Rate from Drug-Induced Deaths in 1998

National Rate = 5.9 Deaths per 100,000 Population*

ALPHA ORDER

RANK ORDER

RANK	STATE	RATE		RANK	STATE	RATE
40	Alabama	3.3		1	New Mexico	15.1
14	Alaska	6.4		2	Nevada	11.6
4	Arizona	10.3		3	Maryland	10.4
36	Arkansas	3.7		4	Arizona	10.3
7	California	8.4		5	Utah	9.9
14	Colorado	6.4		6	Oregon	9.6
13	Connecticut	6.5		7	California	8.4
9	Delaware	7.5		8	Massachusetts	8.0
16	Florida	6.3		9	Delaware	7.5
35	Georgia	3.8		9	New Jersey	7.5
18	Hawaii	6.1		9	Washington	7.5
36	Idaho	3.7		12	Pennsylvania	7.3
19	Illinois	5.8		13	Connecticut	6.5
38	Indiana	3.5		14	Alaska	6.4
49	Iowa	2.0		14	Colorado	6.4
40	Kansas	3.3		16	Florida	6.3
27	Kentucky	4.5		17	Michigan	6.2
26	Louisiana	4.7		18	Hawaii	6.1
28	Maine	4.3		19	Illinois	5.8
3	Maryland	10.4		20	Rhode Island	5.6
8	Massachusetts	8.0		21	New York	5.5
17	Michigan	6.2		22	Texas	5.3
47	Minnesota	2.4		23	New Hampshire	5.2
45	Mississippi	2.7		23	Tennessee	5.2
32	Missouri	3.9		25	Wyoming	5.1
30	Montana	4.0		26	Louisiana	4.7
46	Nebraska	2.5		27	Kentucky	4.5
2	Nevada	11.6		28	Maine	4.3
23	New Hampshire	5.2		29	Vermont	4.2
9	New Jersey	7.5		30	Montana	4.0
1	New Mexico	15.1		30	Wisconsin	4.0
21	New York	5.5		32	Missouri	3.9
32	North Carolina	3.9		32	North Carolina	3.9
50	North Dakota**	1.8		32	Oklahoma	3.9
42	Ohio	3.2		35	Georgia	3.8
32	Oklahoma	3.9		36	Arkansas	3.7
6	Oregon	9.6		36	Idaho	3.7
12	Pennsylvania	7.3		38	Indiana	3.5
20	Rhode Island	5.6		38	Virginia	3.5
44	South Carolina	3.0		40	Alabama	3.3
48	South Dakota	2.3		40	Kansas	3.3
23	Tennessee	5.2		42	Ohio	3.2
22	Texas	5.3		42	West Virginia	3.2
5	Utah	9.9		44	South Carolina	3.0
29	Vermont	4.2		45	Mississippi	2.7
38	Virginia	3.5		46	Nebraska	2.5
9	Washington	7.5		47	Minnesota	2.4
42	West Virginia	3.2		48	South Dakota	2.3
30	Wisconsin	4.0		49	Iowa	2.0
25	Wyoming	5.1		50	North Dakota**	1.8
					District of Columbia	14.3

Source: U.S. Department of Health and Human Services, National Center for Health Statistics
    (http://wonder.cdc.gov/WONDER/)
*By state of residence. Includes drug psychoses, drug dependence, nondependent use excluding alcohol and tobacco, accidental poisoning or suicide by drugs, medicaments and biologicals. Excludes accidents, homicides and other causes indirectly related to drug use.
**Due to low numbers of deaths, rates for this state should be interpreted with caution.

Occupational Fatalities in 1999

National Total = 6,055 Deaths*

ALPHA ORDER

RANK	STATE	DEATHS	% of USA
16	Alabama	135	2.2%
41	Alaska	43	0.7%
29	Arizona	74	1.2%
25	Arkansas	86	1.4%
1	California	626	10.3%
27	Colorado	77	1.3%
35	Connecticut	57	0.9%
50	Delaware	11	0.2%
3	Florida	384	6.3%
8	Georgia	202	3.3%
48	Hawaii	12	0.2%
38	Idaho	51	0.8%
7	Illinois	216	3.6%
13	Indiana	155	2.6%
31	Iowa	68	1.1%
22	Kansas	98	1.6%
17	Kentucky	117	1.9%
12	Louisiana	159	2.6%
44	Maine	26	0.4%
26	Maryland	78	1.3%
40	Massachusetts	44	0.7%
10	Michigan	179	3.0%
24	Minnesota	88	1.5%
18	Mississippi	113	1.9%
15	Missouri	145	2.4%
34	Montana	58	1.0%
37	Nebraska	56	0.9%
33	Nevada	60	1.0%
46	New Hampshire	23	0.4%
21	New Jersey	103	1.7%
39	New Mexico	48	0.8%
4	New York	243	4.0%
6	North Carolina	228	3.8%
45	North Dakota	24	0.4%
9	Ohio	186	3.1%
28	Oklahoma	75	1.2%
30	Oregon	72	1.2%
5	Pennsylvania	235	3.9%
48	Rhode Island	12	0.2%
20	South Carolina	111	1.8%
43	South Dakota	28	0.5%
14	Tennessee	150	2.5%
2	Texas	523	8.6%
32	Utah	67	1.1%
47	Vermont	16	0.3%
11	Virginia	177	2.9%
18	Washington	113	1.9%
35	West Virginia	57	0.9%
23	Wisconsin	97	1.6%
42	Wyoming	33	0.5%

RANK ORDER

RANK	STATE	DEATHS	% of USA
1	California	626	10.3%
2	Texas	523	8.6%
3	Florida	384	6.3%
4	New York	243	4.0%
5	Pennsylvania	235	3.9%
6	North Carolina	228	3.8%
7	Illinois	216	3.6%
8	Georgia	202	3.3%
9	Ohio	186	3.1%
10	Michigan	179	3.0%
11	Virginia	177	2.9%
12	Louisiana	159	2.6%
13	Indiana	155	2.6%
14	Tennessee	150	2.5%
15	Missouri	145	2.4%
16	Alabama	135	2.2%
17	Kentucky	117	1.9%
18	Mississippi	113	1.9%
18	Washington	113	1.9%
20	South Carolina	111	1.8%
21	New Jersey	103	1.7%
22	Kansas	98	1.6%
23	Wisconsin	97	1.6%
24	Minnesota	88	1.5%
25	Arkansas	86	1.4%
26	Maryland	78	1.3%
27	Colorado	77	1.3%
28	Oklahoma	75	1.2%
29	Arizona	74	1.2%
30	Oregon	72	1.2%
31	Iowa	68	1.1%
32	Utah	67	1.1%
33	Nevada	60	1.0%
34	Montana	58	1.0%
35	Connecticut	57	0.9%
35	West Virginia	57	0.9%
37	Nebraska	56	0.9%
38	Idaho	51	0.8%
39	New Mexico	48	0.8%
40	Massachusetts	44	0.7%
41	Alaska	43	0.7%
42	Wyoming	33	0.5%
43	South Dakota	28	0.5%
44	Maine	26	0.4%
45	North Dakota	24	0.4%
46	New Hampshire	23	0.4%
47	Vermont	16	0.3%
48	Hawaii	12	0.2%
48	Rhode Island	12	0.2%
50	Delaware	11	0.2%
	District of Columbia	13	0.2%

Source: Morgan Quitno Press using data from U.S. Department of Labor, Bureau of Labor Statistics
"National Census of Fatal Occupational Injuries, 1999" (press release, August 17, 2000)
*Includes three fatalities that occurred outside the 50 states and the District of Columbia.

Occupational Fatality Rate in 1999

National Rate = 4.5 Deaths per 100,000 Workers*

ALPHA ORDER

RANK ORDER

RANK	STATE	RATE
16	Alabama	6.0
1	Alaska	14.2
41	Arizona	3.1
12	Arkansas	6.5
36	California	3.8
30	Colorado	4.5
48	Connecticut	2.3
37	Delaware	3.7
28	Florida	4.9
19	Georgia	5.8
21	Hawaii	5.7
10	Idaho	6.9
40	Illinois	3.4
21	Indiana	5.7
24	Iowa	5.2
19	Kansas	5.8
13	Kentucky	6.4
9	Louisiana	7.2
27	Maine	5.0
41	Maryland	3.1
46	Massachusetts	2.6
37	Michigan	3.7
45	Minnesota	2.7
5	Mississippi	10.6
16	Missouri	6.0
4	Montana	10.9
8	Nebraska	7.3
14	Nevada	6.3
50	New Hampshire	2.2
46	New Jersey	2.6
26	New Mexico	5.1
44	New York	2.9
18	North Carolina	5.9
11	North Dakota	6.8
34	Ohio	4.0
15	Oklahoma	6.2
33	Oregon	4.2
35	Pennsylvania	3.9
48	Rhode Island	2.3
7	South Carolina	7.4
3	South Dakota	11.6
21	Tennessee	5.7
29	Texas	4.8
24	Utah	5.2
32	Vermont	4.3
30	Virginia	4.5
43	Washington	3.0
6	West Virginia	7.5
37	Wisconsin	3.7
2	Wyoming	12.9

RANK	STATE	RATE
1	Alaska	14.2
2	Wyoming	12.9
3	South Dakota	11.6
4	Montana	10.9
5	Mississippi	10.6
6	West Virginia	7.5
7	South Carolina	7.4
8	Nebraska	7.3
9	Louisiana	7.2
10	Idaho	6.9
11	North Dakota	6.8
12	Arkansas	6.5
13	Kentucky	6.4
14	Nevada	6.3
15	Oklahoma	6.2
16	Alabama	6.0
16	Missouri	6.0
18	North Carolina	5.9
19	Georgia	5.8
19	Kansas	5.8
21	Hawaii	5.7
21	Indiana	5.7
21	Tennessee	5.7
24	Iowa	5.2
24	Utah	5.2
26	New Mexico	5.1
27	Maine	5.0
28	Florida	4.9
29	Texas	4.8
30	Colorado	4.5
30	Virginia	4.5
32	Vermont	4.3
33	Oregon	4.2
34	Ohio	4.0
35	Pennsylvania	3.9
36	California	3.8
37	Delaware	3.7
37	Michigan	3.7
37	Wisconsin	3.7
40	Illinois	3.4
41	Arizona	3.1
41	Maryland	3.1
43	Washington	3.0
44	New York	2.9
45	Minnesota	2.7
46	Massachusetts	2.6
46	New Jersey	2.6
48	Connecticut	2.3
48	Rhode Island	2.3
50	New Hampshire	2.2

District of Columbia   5.3

Source: Morgan Quitno Press using data from U.S. Department of Labor, Bureau of Labor Statistics
"National Census of Fatal Occupational Injuries, 1999" (press release, August 17, 2000)
*Based on employed civilian labor force. Does not include fatalities occurring outside the territorial boundaries of the United States.

III. FACILITIES

Community Hospitals in 1999

National Total = 4,956 Hospitals*

ALPHA ORDER

RANK	STATE	HOSPITALS	% of USA
19	Alabama	109	2.2%
47	Alaska	17	0.3%
31	Arizona	61	1.2%
26	Arkansas	83	1.7%
2	California	395	8.0%
29	Colorado	67	1.4%
42	Connecticut	35	0.7%
50	Delaware	6	0.1%
5	Florida	203	4.1%
8	Georgia	154	3.1%
45	Hawaii	22	0.4%
37	Idaho	42	0.8%
6	Illinois	198	4.0%
18	Indiana	111	2.2%
16	Iowa	115	2.3%
11	Kansas	131	2.6%
21	Kentucky	105	2.1%
13	Louisiana	122	2.5%
40	Maine	37	0.7%
35	Maryland	49	1.0%
28	Massachusetts	79	1.6%
9	Michigan	145	2.9%
10	Minnesota	134	2.7%
22	Mississippi	96	1.9%
15	Missouri	118	2.4%
34	Montana	53	1.1%
25	Nebraska	85	1.7%
45	Nevada	22	0.4%
43	New Hampshire	28	0.6%
27	New Jersey	81	1.6%
41	New Mexico	36	0.7%
3	New York	218	4.4%
17	North Carolina	114	2.3%
39	North Dakota	41	0.8%
7	Ohio	167	3.4%
19	Oklahoma	109	2.2%
32	Oregon	59	1.2%
4	Pennsylvania	210	4.2%
49	Rhode Island	11	0.2%
30	South Carolina	64	1.3%
36	South Dakota	48	1.0%
14	Tennessee	121	2.4%
1	Texas	408	8.2%
37	Utah	42	0.8%
48	Vermont	14	0.3%
23	Virginia	89	1.8%
24	Washington	86	1.7%
33	West Virginia	58	1.2%
12	Wisconsin	123	2.5%
44	Wyoming	23	0.5%

RANK ORDER

RANK	STATE	HOSPITALS	% of USA
1	Texas	408	8.2%
2	California	395	8.0%
3	New York	218	4.4%
4	Pennsylvania	210	4.2%
5	Florida	203	4.1%
6	Illinois	198	4.0%
7	Ohio	167	3.4%
8	Georgia	154	3.1%
9	Michigan	145	2.9%
10	Minnesota	134	2.7%
11	Kansas	131	2.6%
12	Wisconsin	123	2.5%
13	Louisiana	122	2.5%
14	Tennessee	121	2.4%
15	Missouri	118	2.4%
16	Iowa	115	2.3%
17	North Carolina	114	2.3%
18	Indiana	111	2.2%
19	Alabama	109	2.2%
19	Oklahoma	109	2.2%
21	Kentucky	105	2.1%
22	Mississippi	96	1.9%
23	Virginia	89	1.8%
24	Washington	86	1.7%
25	Nebraska	85	1.7%
26	Arkansas	83	1.7%
27	New Jersey	81	1.6%
28	Massachusetts	79	1.6%
29	Colorado	67	1.4%
30	South Carolina	64	1.3%
31	Arizona	61	1.2%
32	Oregon	59	1.2%
33	West Virginia	58	1.2%
34	Montana	53	1.1%
35	Maryland	49	1.0%
36	South Dakota	48	1.0%
37	Idaho	42	0.8%
37	Utah	42	0.8%
39	North Dakota	41	0.8%
40	Maine	37	0.7%
41	New Mexico	36	0.7%
42	Connecticut	35	0.7%
43	New Hampshire	28	0.6%
44	Wyoming	23	0.5%
45	Hawaii	22	0.4%
45	Nevada	22	0.4%
47	Alaska	17	0.3%
48	Vermont	14	0.3%
49	Rhode Island	11	0.2%
50	Delaware	6	0.1%
	District of Columbia	12	0.2%

Source: American Hospital Association (Chicago, IL)
    "Hospital Statistics" (2001 edition)
*Community hospitals are all nonfederal, short-term, general and special hospitals whose facilities and services are available to the public.

Rate of Community Hospitals in 1999

National Rate = 1.8 Community Hospitals per 100,000 Population*

ALPHA ORDER

RANK	STATE	RATE
18	Alabama	2.5
16	Alaska	2.7
39	Arizona	1.3
10	Arkansas	3.3
43	California	1.2
32	Colorado	1.7
46	Connecticut	1.1
50	Delaware	0.8
39	Florida	1.3
25	Georgia	2.0
28	Hawaii	1.9
9	Idaho	3.4
33	Illinois	1.6
28	Indiana	1.9
7	Iowa	4.0
5	Kansas	4.9
16	Kentucky	2.7
14	Louisiana	2.8
13	Maine	3.0
49	Maryland	0.9
39	Massachusetts	1.3
35	Michigan	1.5
14	Minnesota	2.8
8	Mississippi	3.5
22	Missouri	2.2
3	Montana	6.0
4	Nebraska	5.1
43	Nevada	1.2
20	New Hampshire	2.3
48	New Jersey	1.0
24	New Mexico	2.1
43	New York	1.2
35	North Carolina	1.5
1	North Dakota	6.5
35	Ohio	1.5
11	Oklahoma	3.2
30	Oregon	1.8
30	Pennsylvania	1.8
46	Rhode Island	1.1
33	South Carolina	1.6
1	South Dakota	6.5
22	Tennessee	2.2
25	Texas	2.0
25	Utah	2.0
19	Vermont	2.4
39	Virginia	1.3
35	Washington	1.5
11	West Virginia	3.2
20	Wisconsin	2.3
6	Wyoming	4.8

RANK ORDER

RANK	STATE	RATE
1	North Dakota	6.5
1	South Dakota	6.5
3	Montana	6.0
4	Nebraska	5.1
5	Kansas	4.9
6	Wyoming	4.8
7	Iowa	4.0
8	Mississippi	3.5
9	Idaho	3.4
10	Arkansas	3.3
11	Oklahoma	3.2
11	West Virginia	3.2
13	Maine	3.0
14	Louisiana	2.8
14	Minnesota	2.8
16	Alaska	2.7
16	Kentucky	2.7
18	Alabama	2.5
19	Vermont	2.4
20	New Hampshire	2.3
20	Wisconsin	2.3
22	Missouri	2.2
22	Tennessee	2.2
24	New Mexico	2.1
25	Georgia	2.0
25	Texas	2.0
25	Utah	2.0
28	Hawaii	1.9
28	Indiana	1.9
30	Oregon	1.8
30	Pennsylvania	1.8
32	Colorado	1.7
33	Illinois	1.6
33	South Carolina	1.6
35	Michigan	1.5
35	North Carolina	1.5
35	Ohio	1.5
35	Washington	1.5
39	Arizona	1.3
39	Florida	1.3
39	Massachusetts	1.3
39	Virginia	1.3
43	California	1.2
43	Nevada	1.2
43	New York	1.2
46	Connecticut	1.1
46	Rhode Island	1.1
48	New Jersey	1.0
49	Maryland	0.9
50	Delaware	0.8
	District of Columbia	2.3

Source: Morgan Quitno Press using data from American Hospital Association (Chicago, IL)
"Hospital Statistics" (2001 edition)
*Community hospitals are all nonfederal, short-term, general and special hospitals whose facilities and services are available to the public.

Community Hospitals per 1,000 Square Miles in 1999

National Rate = 1.3 Community Hospitals*

ALPHA ORDER

RANK	STATE	RATE
22	Alabama	2.1
50	Alaska**	0.0
43	Arizona	0.5
29	Arkansas	1.6
17	California	2.5
39	Colorado	0.6
4	Connecticut	6.3
17	Delaware	2.5
9	Florida	3.4
15	Georgia	2.6
9	Hawaii	3.4
43	Idaho	0.5
9	Illinois	3.4
12	Indiana	3.0
25	Iowa	2.0
29	Kansas	1.6
15	Kentucky	2.6
17	Louisiana	2.5
37	Maine	1.1
6	Maryland	4.0
3	Massachusetts	8.5
32	Michigan	1.5
32	Minnesota	1.5
25	Mississippi	2.0
28	Missouri	1.7
46	Montana	0.4
37	Nebraska	1.1
48	Nevada	0.2
12	New Hampshire	3.0
1	New Jersey	9.9
47	New Mexico	0.3
6	New York	4.0
21	North Carolina	2.2
39	North Dakota	0.6
8	Ohio	3.7
29	Oklahoma	1.6
39	Oregon	0.6
5	Pennsylvania	4.6
2	Rhode Island	8.9
22	South Carolina	2.1
39	South Dakota	0.6
14	Tennessee	2.9
32	Texas	1.5
43	Utah	0.5
32	Vermont	1.5
22	Virginia	2.1
36	Washington	1.2
20	West Virginia	2.4
27	Wisconsin	1.9
48	Wyoming	0.2

RANK ORDER

RANK	STATE	RATE
1	New Jersey	9.9
2	Rhode Island	8.9
3	Massachusetts	8.5
4	Connecticut	6.3
5	Pennsylvania	4.6
6	Maryland	4.0
6	New York	4.0
8	Ohio	3.7
9	Florida	3.4
9	Hawaii	3.4
9	Illinois	3.4
12	Indiana	3.0
12	New Hampshire	3.0
14	Tennessee	2.9
15	Georgia	2.6
15	Kentucky	2.6
17	California	2.5
17	Delaware	2.5
17	Louisiana	2.5
20	West Virginia	2.4
21	North Carolina	2.2
22	Alabama	2.1
22	South Carolina	2.1
22	Virginia	2.1
25	Iowa	2.0
25	Mississippi	2.0
27	Wisconsin	1.9
28	Missouri	1.7
29	Arkansas	1.6
29	Kansas	1.6
29	Oklahoma	1.6
32	Michigan	1.5
32	Minnesota	1.5
32	Texas	1.5
32	Vermont	1.5
36	Washington	1.2
37	Maine	1.1
37	Nebraska	1.1
39	Colorado	0.6
39	North Dakota	0.6
39	Oregon	0.6
39	South Dakota	0.6
43	Arizona	0.5
43	Idaho	0.5
43	Utah	0.5
46	Montana	0.4
47	New Mexico	0.3
48	Nevada	0.2
48	Wyoming	0.2
50	Alaska**	0.0
	District of Columbia***	NA

Source: Morgan Quitno Press using data from American Hospital Association (Chicago, IL)
"Hospital Statistics" (2001 edition)

*Based on 1990 Census land and water area figures. Community hospitals are nonfederal short-term general and other special hospitals, whose facilities and services are available to the public.

**Alaska has 17 community hospitals for its 615,230 square miles.

***The District of Columbia has 12 community hospitals for its 68 square miles.

Community Hospitals in Urban Areas in 1999

National Total = 2,767 Hospitals*

RANK	STATE	HOSPITALS	% of USA
16	Alabama	57	2.1%
48	Alaska	2	0.1%
21	Arizona	45	1.6%
29	Arkansas	28	1.0%
1	California	354	12.8%
27	Colorado	32	1.2%
28	Connecticut	29	1.0%
46	Delaware	4	0.1%
4	Florida	172	6.2%
11	Georgia	68	2.5%
39	Hawaii	12	0.4%
43	Idaho	7	0.3%
6	Illinois	125	4.5%
13	Indiana	65	2.3%
32	Iowa	21	0.8%
31	Kansas	26	0.9%
26	Kentucky	33	1.2%
10	Louisiana	74	2.7%
42	Maine	8	0.3%
24	Maryland	40	1.4%
11	Massachusetts	68	2.5%
8	Michigan	87	3.1%
22	Minnesota	44	1.6%
33	Mississippi	20	0.7%
14	Missouri	60	2.2%
47	Montana	3	0.1%
37	Nebraska	13	0.5%
36	Nevada	14	0.5%
40	New Hampshire	10	0.4%
9	New Jersey	81	2.9%
37	New Mexico	13	0.5%
3	New York	182	6.6%
19	North Carolina	52	1.9%
44	North Dakota	6	0.2%
7	Ohio	114	4.1%
23	Oklahoma	41	1.5%
30	Oregon	27	1.0%
5	Pennsylvania	165	6.0%
40	Rhode Island	10	0.4%
25	South Carolina	36	1.3%
45	South Dakota	5	0.2%
15	Tennessee	58	2.1%
2	Texas	245	8.9%
33	Utah	20	0.7%
48	Vermont	2	0.1%
18	Virginia	54	2.0%
20	Washington	46	1.7%
35	West Virginia	18	0.7%
16	Wisconsin	57	2.1%
48	Wyoming	2	0.1%

RANK	STATE	HOSPITALS	% of USA
1	California	354	12.8%
2	Texas	245	8.9%
3	New York	182	6.6%
4	Florida	172	6.2%
5	Pennsylvania	165	6.0%
6	Illinois	125	4.5%
7	Ohio	114	4.1%
8	Michigan	87	3.1%
9	New Jersey	81	2.9%
10	Louisiana	74	2.7%
11	Georgia	68	2.5%
11	Massachusetts	68	2.5%
13	Indiana	65	2.3%
14	Missouri	60	2.2%
15	Tennessee	58	2.1%
16	Alabama	57	2.1%
16	Wisconsin	57	2.1%
18	Virginia	54	2.0%
19	North Carolina	52	1.9%
20	Washington	46	1.7%
21	Arizona	45	1.6%
22	Minnesota	44	1.6%
23	Oklahoma	41	1.5%
24	Maryland	40	1.4%
25	South Carolina	36	1.3%
26	Kentucky	33	1.2%
27	Colorado	32	1.2%
28	Connecticut	29	1.0%
29	Arkansas	28	1.0%
30	Oregon	27	1.0%
31	Kansas	26	0.9%
32	Iowa	21	0.8%
33	Mississippi	20	0.7%
33	Utah	20	0.7%
35	West Virginia	18	0.7%
36	Nevada	14	0.5%
37	Nebraska	13	0.5%
37	New Mexico	13	0.5%
39	Hawaii	12	0.4%
40	New Hampshire	10	0.4%
40	Rhode Island	10	0.4%
42	Maine	8	0.3%
43	Idaho	7	0.3%
44	North Dakota	6	0.2%
45	South Dakota	5	0.2%
46	Delaware	4	0.1%
47	Montana	3	0.1%
48	Alaska	2	0.1%
48	Vermont	2	0.1%
48	Wyoming	2	0.1%
	District of Columbia	12	0.4%

*Source: American Hospital Association (Chicago, IL)
"Hospital Statistics" (2001 edition)*

Community hospitals are all nonfederal, short-term, general and special hospitals whose facilities and services are available to the public. Urban is defined as any area inside a metropolitan statistical area as defined by the U.S. Office of Management and Budget.

Percent of Community Hospitals in Urban Areas in 1999

National Percent = 55.8% of Community Hospitals*

RANK	STATE	PERCENT
23	Alabama	52.3
47	Alaska	11.8
10	Arizona	73.8
35	Arkansas	33.7
3	California	89.6
26	Colorado	47.8
7	Connecticut	82.9
12	Delaware	66.7
5	Florida	84.7
31	Georgia	44.2
21	Hawaii	54.5
43	Idaho	16.7
14	Illinois	63.1
19	Indiana	58.6
42	Iowa	18.3
41	Kansas	19.8
37	Kentucky	31.4
15	Louisiana	60.7
39	Maine	21.6
8	Maryland	81.6
4	Massachusetts	86.1
17	Michigan	60.0
36	Minnesota	32.8
40	Mississippi	20.8
24	Missouri	50.8
50	Montana	5.7
44	Nebraska	15.3
13	Nevada	63.6
34	New Hampshire	35.7
1	New Jersey	100.0
33	New Mexico	36.1
6	New York	83.5
30	North Carolina	45.6
45	North Dakota	14.6
11	Ohio	68.3
32	Oklahoma	37.6
29	Oregon	45.8
9	Pennsylvania	78.6
2	Rhode Island	90.9
20	South Carolina	56.3
48	South Dakota	10.4
25	Tennessee	47.9
17	Texas	60.0
27	Utah	47.6
46	Vermont	14.3
15	Virginia	60.7
22	Washington	53.5
38	West Virginia	31.0
28	Wisconsin	46.3
49	Wyoming	8.7

RANK	STATE	PERCENT
1	New Jersey	100.0
2	Rhode Island	90.9
3	California	89.6
4	Massachusetts	86.1
5	Florida	84.7
6	New York	83.5
7	Connecticut	82.9
8	Maryland	81.6
9	Pennsylvania	78.6
10	Arizona	73.8
11	Ohio	68.3
12	Delaware	66.7
13	Nevada	63.6
14	Illinois	63.1
15	Louisiana	60.7
15	Virginia	60.7
17	Michigan	60.0
17	Texas	60.0
19	Indiana	58.6
20	South Carolina	56.3
21	Hawaii	54.5
22	Washington	53.5
23	Alabama	52.3
24	Missouri	50.8
25	Tennessee	47.9
26	Colorado	47.8
27	Utah	47.6
28	Wisconsin	46.3
29	Oregon	45.8
30	North Carolina	45.6
31	Georgia	44.2
32	Oklahoma	37.6
33	New Mexico	36.1
34	New Hampshire	35.7
35	Arkansas	33.7
36	Minnesota	32.8
37	Kentucky	31.4
38	West Virginia	31.0
39	Maine	21.6
40	Mississippi	20.8
41	Kansas	19.8
42	Iowa	18.3
43	Idaho	16.7
44	Nebraska	15.3
45	North Dakota	14.6
46	Vermont	14.3
47	Alaska	11.8
48	South Dakota	10.4
49	Wyoming	8.7
50	Montana	5.7

District of Columbia	100.0

Source: Morgan Quitno Press using data from American Hospital Association (Chicago, IL)
"Hospital Statistics" (2001 edition)

*Community hospitals are all nonfederal, short-term, general and special hospitals whose facilities and services are available to the public. Urban is defined as any area inside a metropolitan statistical area as defined by the U.S. Office of Management and Budget.

Community Hospitals in Rural Areas in 1999

National Total = 2,189 Hospitals*

ALPHA ORDER

RANK	STATE	HOSPITALS	% of USA
18	Alabama	52	2.4%
41	Alaska	15	0.7%
40	Arizona	16	0.7%
16	Arkansas	55	2.5%
24	California	41	1.9%
28	Colorado	35	1.6%
47	Connecticut	6	0.3%
48	Delaware	2	0.1%
33	Florida	31	1.4%
5	Georgia	86	3.9%
44	Hawaii	10	0.5%
28	Idaho	35	1.6%
7	Illinois	73	3.3%
21	Indiana	46	2.1%
3	Iowa	94	4.3%
2	Kansas	105	4.8%
8	Kentucky	72	3.3%
20	Louisiana	48	2.2%
34	Maine	29	1.3%
45	Maryland	9	0.4%
43	Massachusetts	11	0.5%
14	Michigan	58	2.6%
4	Minnesota	90	4.1%
6	Mississippi	76	3.5%
14	Missouri	58	2.6%
19	Montana	50	2.3%
8	Nebraska	72	3.3%
46	Nevada	8	0.4%
39	New Hampshire	18	0.8%
50	New Jersey	0	0.0%
36	New Mexico	23	1.1%
27	New York	36	1.6%
13	North Carolina	62	2.8%
28	North Dakota	35	1.6%
17	Ohio	53	2.4%
10	Oklahoma	68	3.1%
32	Oregon	32	1.5%
22	Pennsylvania	45	2.1%
49	Rhode Island	1	0.0%
35	South Carolina	28	1.3%
23	South Dakota	43	2.0%
12	Tennessee	63	2.9%
1	Texas	163	7.4%
37	Utah	22	1.0%
42	Vermont	12	0.5%
28	Virginia	35	1.6%
25	Washington	40	1.8%
25	West Virginia	40	1.8%
11	Wisconsin	66	3.0%
38	Wyoming	21	1.0%

RANK ORDER

RANK	STATE	HOSPITALS	% of USA
1	Texas	163	7.4%
2	Kansas	105	4.8%
3	Iowa	94	4.3%
4	Minnesota	90	4.1%
5	Georgia	86	3.9%
6	Mississippi	76	3.5%
7	Illinois	73	3.3%
8	Kentucky	72	3.3%
8	Nebraska	72	3.3%
10	Oklahoma	68	3.1%
11	Wisconsin	66	3.0%
12	Tennessee	63	2.9%
13	North Carolina	62	2.8%
14	Michigan	58	2.6%
14	Missouri	58	2.6%
16	Arkansas	55	2.5%
17	Ohio	53	2.4%
18	Alabama	52	2.4%
19	Montana	50	2.3%
20	Louisiana	48	2.2%
21	Indiana	46	2.1%
22	Pennsylvania	45	2.1%
23	South Dakota	43	2.0%
24	California	41	1.9%
25	Washington	40	1.8%
25	West Virginia	40	1.8%
27	New York	36	1.6%
28	Colorado	35	1.6%
28	Idaho	35	1.6%
28	North Dakota	35	1.6%
28	Virginia	35	1.6%
32	Oregon	32	1.5%
33	Florida	31	1.4%
34	Maine	29	1.3%
35	South Carolina	28	1.3%
36	New Mexico	23	1.1%
37	Utah	22	1.0%
38	Wyoming	21	1.0%
39	New Hampshire	18	0.8%
40	Arizona	16	0.7%
41	Alaska	15	0.7%
42	Vermont	12	0.5%
43	Massachusetts	11	0.5%
44	Hawaii	10	0.5%
45	Maryland	9	0.4%
46	Nevada	8	0.4%
47	Connecticut	6	0.3%
48	Delaware	2	0.1%
49	Rhode Island	1	0.0%
50	New Jersey	0	0.0%
	District of Columbia	0	0.0%

Source: American Hospital Association (Chicago, IL)
   "Hospital Statistics" (2001 edition)

*Community hospitals are all nonfederal, short-term, general and special hospitals whose facilities and services are available to the public. Rural is defined as any area outside a metropolitan statistical area as defined by the U.S. Office of Management and Budget.

Percent of Community Hospitals in Rural Areas in 1999

National Percent = 44.2% of Community Hospitals*

ALPHA ORDER

RANK	STATE	PERCENT
28	Alabama	47.7
4	Alaska	88.2
41	Arizona	26.2
16	Arkansas	66.3
48	California	10.4
25	Colorado	52.2
44	Connecticut	17.1
39	Delaware	33.3
46	Florida	15.3
20	Georgia	55.8
30	Hawaii	45.5
8	Idaho	83.3
37	Illinois	36.9
32	Indiana	41.4
9	Iowa	81.7
10	Kansas	80.2
14	Kentucky	68.6
35	Louisiana	39.3
12	Maine	78.4
43	Maryland	18.4
47	Massachusetts	13.9
33	Michigan	40.0
15	Minnesota	67.2
11	Mississippi	79.2
27	Missouri	49.2
1	Montana	94.3
7	Nebraska	84.7
38	Nevada	36.4
17	New Hampshire	64.3
50	New Jersey	0.0
18	New Mexico	63.9
45	New York	16.5
21	North Carolina	54.4
6	North Dakota	85.4
40	Ohio	31.7
19	Oklahoma	62.4
22	Oregon	54.2
42	Pennsylvania	21.4
49	Rhode Island	9.1
31	South Carolina	43.8
3	South Dakota	89.6
26	Tennessee	52.1
33	Texas	40.0
24	Utah	52.4
5	Vermont	85.7
35	Virginia	39.3
29	Washington	46.5
13	West Virginia	69.0
23	Wisconsin	53.7
2	Wyoming	91.3

RANK ORDER

RANK	STATE	PERCENT
1	Montana	94.3
2	Wyoming	91.3
3	South Dakota	89.6
4	Alaska	88.2
5	Vermont	85.7
6	North Dakota	85.4
7	Nebraska	84.7
8	Idaho	83.3
9	Iowa	81.7
10	Kansas	80.2
11	Mississippi	79.2
12	Maine	78.4
13	West Virginia	69.0
14	Kentucky	68.6
15	Minnesota	67.2
16	Arkansas	66.3
17	New Hampshire	64.3
18	New Mexico	63.9
19	Oklahoma	62.4
20	Georgia	55.8
21	North Carolina	54.4
22	Oregon	54.2
23	Wisconsin	53.7
24	Utah	52.4
25	Colorado	52.2
26	Tennessee	52.1
27	Missouri	49.2
28	Alabama	47.7
29	Washington	46.5
30	Hawaii	45.5
31	South Carolina	43.8
32	Indiana	41.4
33	Michigan	40.0
33	Texas	40.0
35	Louisiana	39.3
35	Virginia	39.3
37	Illinois	36.9
38	Nevada	36.4
39	Delaware	33.3
40	Ohio	31.7
41	Arizona	26.2
42	Pennsylvania	21.4
43	Maryland	18.4
44	Connecticut	17.1
45	New York	16.5
46	Florida	15.3
47	Massachusetts	13.9
48	California	10.4
49	Rhode Island	9.1
50	New Jersey	0.0

District of Columbia   0.0

Source: Morgan Quitno Press using data from American Hospital Association (Chicago, IL)
"Hospital Statistics" (2001 edition)

*Community hospitals are all nonfederal, short-term, general and special hospitals whose facilities and services are available to the public. Rural is defined as any area outside a metropolitan statistical area as defined by the U.S. Office of Management and Budget.

Nongovernment Not-For-Profit Hospitals in 1999

National Total = 3,012 Hospitals*

ALPHA ORDER

RANK	STATE	HOSPITALS	% of USA
29	Alabama	40	1.3%
47	Alaska	9	0.3%
29	Arizona	40	1.3%
22	Arkansas	48	1.6%
1	California	222	7.4%
36	Colorado	32	1.1%
34	Connecticut	33	1.1%
48	Delaware	6	0.2%
10	Florida	86	2.9%
17	Georgia	63	2.1%
44	Hawaii	13	0.4%
45	Idaho	11	0.4%
4	Illinois	161	5.3%
21	Indiana	54	1.8%
19	Iowa	56	1.9%
18	Kansas	61	2.0%
12	Kentucky	73	2.4%
37	Louisiana	30	1.0%
34	Maine	33	1.1%
23	Maryland	47	1.6%
15	Massachusetts	69	2.3%
7	Michigan	122	4.1%
9	Minnesota	92	3.1%
38	Mississippi	28	0.9%
14	Missouri	71	2.4%
27	Montana	41	1.4%
25	Nebraska	43	1.4%
48	Nevada	6	0.2%
39	New Hampshire	24	0.8%
11	New Jersey	77	2.6%
40	New Mexico	20	0.7%
3	New York	185	6.1%
13	North Carolina	72	2.4%
32	North Dakota	39	1.3%
6	Ohio	139	4.6%
24	Oklahoma	44	1.5%
27	Oregon	41	1.4%
2	Pennsylvania	199	6.6%
45	Rhode Island	11	0.4%
40	South Carolina	20	0.7%
29	South Dakota	40	1.3%
19	Tennessee	56	1.9%
5	Texas	143	4.7%
40	Utah	20	0.7%
43	Vermont	14	0.5%
16	Virginia	68	2.3%
25	Washington	43	1.4%
33	West Virginia	34	1.1%
8	Wisconsin	120	4.0%
50	Wyoming	5	0.2%

RANK ORDER

RANK	STATE	HOSPITALS	% of USA
1	California	222	7.4%
2	Pennsylvania	199	6.6%
3	New York	185	6.1%
4	Illinois	161	5.3%
5	Texas	143	4.7%
6	Ohio	139	4.6%
7	Michigan	122	4.1%
8	Wisconsin	120	4.0%
9	Minnesota	92	3.1%
10	Florida	86	2.9%
11	New Jersey	77	2.6%
12	Kentucky	73	2.4%
13	North Carolina	72	2.4%
14	Missouri	71	2.4%
15	Massachusetts	69	2.3%
16	Virginia	68	2.3%
17	Georgia	63	2.1%
18	Kansas	61	2.0%
19	Iowa	56	1.9%
19	Tennessee	56	1.9%
21	Indiana	54	1.8%
22	Arkansas	48	1.6%
23	Maryland	47	1.6%
24	Oklahoma	44	1.5%
25	Nebraska	43	1.4%
25	Washington	43	1.4%
27	Montana	41	1.4%
27	Oregon	41	1.4%
29	Alabama	40	1.3%
29	Arizona	40	1.3%
29	South Dakota	40	1.3%
32	North Dakota	39	1.3%
33	West Virginia	34	1.1%
34	Connecticut	33	1.1%
34	Maine	33	1.1%
36	Colorado	32	1.1%
37	Louisiana	30	1.0%
38	Mississippi	28	0.9%
39	New Hampshire	24	0.8%
40	New Mexico	20	0.7%
40	South Carolina	20	0.7%
40	Utah	20	0.7%
43	Vermont	14	0.5%
44	Hawaii	13	0.4%
45	Idaho	11	0.4%
45	Rhode Island	11	0.4%
47	Alaska	9	0.3%
48	Delaware	6	0.2%
48	Nevada	6	0.2%
50	Wyoming	5	0.2%
	District of Columbia	8	0.3%

Source: American Hospital Association (Chicago, IL)
   "Hospital Statistics" (2001 edition)
*Nongovernment not-for-profit hospitals are a subset of community hospitals.

Investor-Owned (For-Profit) Hospitals in 1999

National Total = 747 Hospitals*

ALPHA ORDER

RANK	STATE	HOSPITALS	% of USA
7	Alabama	26	3.5%
38	Alaska	1	0.1%
13	Arizona	15	2.0%
10	Arkansas	19	2.5%
2	California	100	13.4%
21	Colorado	8	1.1%
43	Connecticut	0	0.0%
43	Delaware	0	0.0%
3	Florida	93	12.4%
6	Georgia	36	4.8%
38	Hawaii	1	0.1%
31	Idaho	3	0.4%
24	Illinois	7	0.9%
17	Indiana	12	1.6%
43	Iowa	0	0.0%
24	Kansas	7	0.9%
11	Kentucky	18	2.4%
5	Louisiana	37	5.0%
38	Maine	1	0.1%
35	Maryland	2	0.3%
26	Massachusetts	6	0.8%
29	Michigan	4	0.5%
43	Minnesota	0	0.0%
8	Mississippi	22	2.9%
17	Missouri	12	1.6%
43	Montana	0	0.0%
38	Nebraska	1	0.1%
21	Nevada	8	1.1%
29	New Hampshire	4	0.5%
35	New Jersey	2	0.3%
27	New Mexico	5	0.7%
21	New York	8	1.1%
20	North Carolina	9	1.2%
35	North Dakota	2	0.3%
27	Ohio	5	0.7%
13	Oklahoma	15	2.0%
31	Oregon	3	0.4%
19	Pennsylvania	10	1.3%
43	Rhode Island	0	0.0%
9	South Carolina	20	2.7%
43	South Dakota	0	0.0%
4	Tennessee	38	5.1%
1	Texas	134	17.9%
16	Utah	13	1.7%
43	Vermont	0	0.0%
12	Virginia	16	2.1%
31	Washington	3	0.4%
15	West Virginia	14	1.9%
38	Wisconsin	1	0.1%
31	Wyoming	3	0.4%

RANK ORDER

RANK	STATE	HOSPITALS	% of USA
1	Texas	134	17.9%
2	California	100	13.4%
3	Florida	93	12.4%
4	Tennessee	38	5.1%
5	Louisiana	37	5.0%
6	Georgia	36	4.8%
7	Alabama	26	3.5%
8	Mississippi	22	2.9%
9	South Carolina	20	2.7%
10	Arkansas	19	2.5%
11	Kentucky	18	2.4%
12	Virginia	16	2.1%
13	Arizona	15	2.0%
13	Oklahoma	15	2.0%
15	West Virginia	14	1.9%
16	Utah	13	1.7%
17	Indiana	12	1.6%
17	Missouri	12	1.6%
19	Pennsylvania	10	1.3%
20	North Carolina	9	1.2%
21	Colorado	8	1.1%
21	Nevada	8	1.1%
21	New York	8	1.1%
24	Illinois	7	0.9%
24	Kansas	7	0.9%
26	Massachusetts	6	0.8%
27	New Mexico	5	0.7%
27	Ohio	5	0.7%
29	Michigan	4	0.5%
29	New Hampshire	4	0.5%
31	Idaho	3	0.4%
31	Oregon	3	0.4%
31	Washington	3	0.4%
31	Wyoming	3	0.4%
35	Maryland	2	0.3%
35	New Jersey	2	0.3%
35	North Dakota	2	0.3%
38	Alaska	1	0.1%
38	Hawaii	1	0.1%
38	Maine	1	0.1%
38	Nebraska	1	0.1%
38	Wisconsin	1	0.1%
43	Connecticut	0	0.0%
43	Delaware	0	0.0%
43	Iowa	0	0.0%
43	Minnesota	0	0.0%
43	Montana	0	0.0%
43	Rhode Island	0	0.0%
43	South Dakota	0	0.0%
43	Vermont	0	0.0%
	District of Columbia	3	0.4%

Source: American Hospital Association (Chicago, IL)
   "Hospital Statistics" (2001 edition)
Investor-owned (for-profit) hospitals are a subset of community hospitals.

State and Local Government-Owned Hospitals in 1999

National Total = 1,197 Hospitals*

<table>
<tr><td colspan="4">ALPHA ORDER</td><td colspan="4">RANK ORDER</td></tr>
<tr><td>RANK</td><td>STATE</td><td>HOSPITALS</td><td>% of USA</td><td>RANK</td><td>STATE</td><td>HOSPITALS</td><td>% of USA</td></tr>
<tr><td>10</td><td>Alabama</td><td>43</td><td>3.6%</td><td>1</td><td>Texas</td><td>131</td><td>10.9%</td></tr>
<tr><td>36</td><td>Alaska</td><td>7</td><td>0.6%</td><td>2</td><td>California</td><td>73</td><td>6.1%</td></tr>
<tr><td>37</td><td>Arizona</td><td>6</td><td>0.5%</td><td>3</td><td>Kansas</td><td>63</td><td>5.3%</td></tr>
<tr><td>25</td><td>Arkansas</td><td>16</td><td>1.3%</td><td>4</td><td>Iowa</td><td>59</td><td>4.9%</td></tr>
<tr><td>2</td><td>California</td><td>73</td><td>6.1%</td><td>5</td><td>Georgia</td><td>55</td><td>4.6%</td></tr>
<tr><td>18</td><td>Colorado</td><td>27</td><td>2.3%</td><td>5</td><td>Louisiana</td><td>55</td><td>4.6%</td></tr>
<tr><td>41</td><td>Connecticut</td><td>2</td><td>0.2%</td><td>7</td><td>Oklahoma</td><td>50</td><td>4.2%</td></tr>
<tr><td>45</td><td>Delaware</td><td>0</td><td>0.0%</td><td>8</td><td>Mississippi</td><td>46</td><td>3.8%</td></tr>
<tr><td>21</td><td>Florida</td><td>24</td><td>2.0%</td><td>9</td><td>Indiana</td><td>45</td><td>3.8%</td></tr>
<tr><td>5</td><td>Georgia</td><td>55</td><td>4.6%</td><td>10</td><td>Alabama</td><td>43</td><td>3.6%</td></tr>
<tr><td>33</td><td>Hawaii</td><td>8</td><td>0.7%</td><td>11</td><td>Minnesota</td><td>42</td><td>3.5%</td></tr>
<tr><td>17</td><td>Idaho</td><td>28</td><td>2.3%</td><td>12</td><td>Nebraska</td><td>41</td><td>3.4%</td></tr>
<tr><td>16</td><td>Illinois</td><td>30</td><td>2.5%</td><td>13</td><td>Washington</td><td>40</td><td>3.3%</td></tr>
<tr><td>9</td><td>Indiana</td><td>45</td><td>3.8%</td><td>14</td><td>Missouri</td><td>35</td><td>2.9%</td></tr>
<tr><td>4</td><td>Iowa</td><td>59</td><td>4.9%</td><td>15</td><td>North Carolina</td><td>33</td><td>2.8%</td></tr>
<tr><td>3</td><td>Kansas</td><td>63</td><td>5.3%</td><td>16</td><td>Illinois</td><td>30</td><td>2.5%</td></tr>
<tr><td>28</td><td>Kentucky</td><td>14</td><td>1.2%</td><td>17</td><td>Idaho</td><td>28</td><td>2.3%</td></tr>
<tr><td>5</td><td>Louisiana</td><td>55</td><td>4.6%</td><td>18</td><td>Colorado</td><td>27</td><td>2.3%</td></tr>
<tr><td>40</td><td>Maine</td><td>3</td><td>0.3%</td><td>18</td><td>Tennessee</td><td>27</td><td>2.3%</td></tr>
<tr><td>45</td><td>Maryland</td><td>0</td><td>0.0%</td><td>20</td><td>New York</td><td>25</td><td>2.1%</td></tr>
<tr><td>39</td><td>Massachusetts</td><td>4</td><td>0.3%</td><td>21</td><td>Florida</td><td>24</td><td>2.0%</td></tr>
<tr><td>24</td><td>Michigan</td><td>19</td><td>1.6%</td><td>21</td><td>South Carolina</td><td>24</td><td>2.0%</td></tr>
<tr><td>11</td><td>Minnesota</td><td>42</td><td>3.5%</td><td>23</td><td>Ohio</td><td>23</td><td>1.9%</td></tr>
<tr><td>8</td><td>Mississippi</td><td>46</td><td>3.8%</td><td>24</td><td>Michigan</td><td>19</td><td>1.6%</td></tr>
<tr><td>14</td><td>Missouri</td><td>35</td><td>2.9%</td><td>25</td><td>Arkansas</td><td>16</td><td>1.3%</td></tr>
<tr><td>29</td><td>Montana</td><td>12</td><td>1.0%</td><td>26</td><td>Oregon</td><td>15</td><td>1.3%</td></tr>
<tr><td>12</td><td>Nebraska</td><td>41</td><td>3.4%</td><td>26</td><td>Wyoming</td><td>15</td><td>1.3%</td></tr>
<tr><td>33</td><td>Nevada</td><td>8</td><td>0.7%</td><td>28</td><td>Kentucky</td><td>14</td><td>1.2%</td></tr>
<tr><td>45</td><td>New Hampshire</td><td>0</td><td>0.0%</td><td>29</td><td>Montana</td><td>12</td><td>1.0%</td></tr>
<tr><td>41</td><td>New Jersey</td><td>2</td><td>0.2%</td><td>30</td><td>New Mexico</td><td>11</td><td>0.9%</td></tr>
<tr><td>30</td><td>New Mexico</td><td>11</td><td>0.9%</td><td>31</td><td>West Virginia</td><td>10</td><td>0.8%</td></tr>
<tr><td>20</td><td>New York</td><td>25</td><td>2.1%</td><td>32</td><td>Utah</td><td>9</td><td>0.8%</td></tr>
<tr><td>15</td><td>North Carolina</td><td>33</td><td>2.8%</td><td>33</td><td>Hawaii</td><td>8</td><td>0.7%</td></tr>
<tr><td>45</td><td>North Dakota</td><td>0</td><td>0.0%</td><td>33</td><td>Nevada</td><td>8</td><td>0.7%</td></tr>
<tr><td>23</td><td>Ohio</td><td>23</td><td>1.9%</td><td>33</td><td>South Dakota</td><td>8</td><td>0.7%</td></tr>
<tr><td>7</td><td>Oklahoma</td><td>50</td><td>4.2%</td><td>36</td><td>Alaska</td><td>7</td><td>0.6%</td></tr>
<tr><td>26</td><td>Oregon</td><td>15</td><td>1.3%</td><td>37</td><td>Arizona</td><td>6</td><td>0.5%</td></tr>
<tr><td>44</td><td>Pennsylvania</td><td>1</td><td>0.1%</td><td>38</td><td>Virginia</td><td>5</td><td>0.4%</td></tr>
<tr><td>45</td><td>Rhode Island</td><td>0</td><td>0.0%</td><td>39</td><td>Massachusetts</td><td>4</td><td>0.3%</td></tr>
<tr><td>21</td><td>South Carolina</td><td>24</td><td>2.0%</td><td>40</td><td>Maine</td><td>3</td><td>0.3%</td></tr>
<tr><td>33</td><td>South Dakota</td><td>8</td><td>0.7%</td><td>41</td><td>Connecticut</td><td>2</td><td>0.2%</td></tr>
<tr><td>18</td><td>Tennessee</td><td>27</td><td>2.3%</td><td>41</td><td>New Jersey</td><td>2</td><td>0.2%</td></tr>
<tr><td>1</td><td>Texas</td><td>131</td><td>10.9%</td><td>41</td><td>Wisconsin</td><td>2</td><td>0.2%</td></tr>
<tr><td>32</td><td>Utah</td><td>9</td><td>0.8%</td><td>44</td><td>Pennsylvania</td><td>1</td><td>0.1%</td></tr>
<tr><td>45</td><td>Vermont</td><td>0</td><td>0.0%</td><td>45</td><td>Delaware</td><td>0</td><td>0.0%</td></tr>
<tr><td>38</td><td>Virginia</td><td>5</td><td>0.4%</td><td>45</td><td>Maryland</td><td>0</td><td>0.0%</td></tr>
<tr><td>13</td><td>Washington</td><td>40</td><td>3.3%</td><td>45</td><td>New Hampshire</td><td>0</td><td>0.0%</td></tr>
<tr><td>31</td><td>West Virginia</td><td>10</td><td>0.8%</td><td>45</td><td>North Dakota</td><td>0</td><td>0.0%</td></tr>
<tr><td>41</td><td>Wisconsin</td><td>2</td><td>0.2%</td><td>45</td><td>Rhode Island</td><td>0</td><td>0.0%</td></tr>
<tr><td>26</td><td>Wyoming</td><td>15</td><td>1.3%</td><td>45</td><td>Vermont</td><td>0</td><td>0.0%</td></tr>
<tr><td></td><td></td><td></td><td></td><td></td><td>District of Columbia</td><td>1</td><td>0.1%</td></tr>
</table>

Source: American Hospital Association (Chicago, IL)
   "Hospital Statistics" (2001 edition)
*State and local government-owned hospitals are a subset of community hospitals.

Beds in Community Hospitals in 1999

National Total = 829,575 Beds*

ALPHA ORDER

RANK	STATE	BEDS	% of USA
19	Alabama	16,306	2.0%
50	Alaska	1,250	0.2%
29	Arizona	10,576	1.3%
30	Arkansas	10,051	1.2%
1	California	73,672	8.9%
31	Colorado	9,349	1.1%
34	Connecticut	7,872	0.9%
47	Delaware	2,000	0.2%
4	Florida	49,434	6.0%
9	Georgia	24,784	3.0%
45	Hawaii	2,913	0.4%
42	Idaho	3,499	0.4%
6	Illinois	37,658	4.5%
14	Indiana	19,225	2.3%
23	Iowa	11,838	1.4%
26	Kansas	11,615	1.4%
21	Kentucky	14,956	1.8%
16	Louisiana	16,782	2.0%
41	Maine	3,691	0.4%
24	Maryland	11,629	1.4%
18	Massachusetts	16,309	2.0%
8	Michigan	26,144	3.2%
17	Minnesota	16,458	2.0%
22	Mississippi	13,217	1.6%
13	Missouri	20,253	2.4%
36	Montana	4,668	0.6%
32	Nebraska	8,326	1.0%
40	Nevada	3,706	0.4%
44	New Hampshire	2,974	0.4%
10	New Jersey	24,570	3.0%
43	New Mexico	3,370	0.4%
2	New York	68,924	8.3%
11	North Carolina	23,391	2.8%
39	North Dakota	3,884	0.5%
7	Ohio	34,164	4.1%
28	Oklahoma	11,075	1.3%
35	Oregon	6,643	0.8%
5	Pennsylvania	42,999	5.2%
46	Rhode Island	2,400	0.3%
24	South Carolina	11,629	1.4%
37	South Dakota	4,344	0.5%
12	Tennessee	20,627	2.5%
3	Texas	56,824	6.8%
38	Utah	4,170	0.5%
49	Vermont	1,669	0.2%
15	Virginia	17,295	2.1%
27	Washington	11,092	1.3%
33	West Virginia	8,109	1.0%
20	Wisconsin	15,870	1.9%
48	Wyoming	1,830	0.2%

RANK ORDER

RANK	STATE	BEDS	% of USA
1	California	73,672	8.9%
2	New York	68,924	8.3%
3	Texas	56,824	6.8%
4	Florida	49,434	6.0%
5	Pennsylvania	42,999	5.2%
6	Illinois	37,658	4.5%
7	Ohio	34,164	4.1%
8	Michigan	26,144	3.2%
9	Georgia	24,784	3.0%
10	New Jersey	24,570	3.0%
11	North Carolina	23,391	2.8%
12	Tennessee	20,627	2.5%
13	Missouri	20,253	2.4%
14	Indiana	19,225	2.3%
15	Virginia	17,295	2.1%
16	Louisiana	16,782	2.0%
17	Minnesota	16,458	2.0%
18	Massachusetts	16,309	2.0%
19	Alabama	16,306	2.0%
20	Wisconsin	15,870	1.9%
21	Kentucky	14,956	1.8%
22	Mississippi	13,217	1.6%
23	Iowa	11,838	1.4%
24	Maryland	11,629	1.4%
24	South Carolina	11,629	1.4%
26	Kansas	11,615	1.4%
27	Washington	11,092	1.3%
28	Oklahoma	11,075	1.3%
29	Arizona	10,576	1.3%
30	Arkansas	10,051	1.2%
31	Colorado	9,349	1.1%
32	Nebraska	8,326	1.0%
33	West Virginia	8,109	1.0%
34	Connecticut	7,872	0.9%
35	Oregon	6,643	0.8%
36	Montana	4,668	0.6%
37	South Dakota	4,344	0.5%
38	Utah	4,170	0.5%
39	North Dakota	3,884	0.5%
40	Nevada	3,706	0.4%
41	Maine	3,691	0.4%
42	Idaho	3,499	0.4%
43	New Mexico	3,370	0.4%
44	New Hampshire	2,974	0.4%
45	Hawaii	2,913	0.4%
46	Rhode Island	2,400	0.3%
47	Delaware	2,000	0.2%
48	Wyoming	1,830	0.2%
49	Vermont	1,669	0.2%
50	Alaska	1,250	0.2%
	District of Columbia	3,541	0.4%

Source: American Hospital Association (Chicago, IL)
"Hospital Statistics" (2001 edition)
*All nonfederal short-term general and other special hospitals, whose facilities and services are available to the public. Includes beds in hospital and nursing home units.

Rate of Beds in Community Hospitals in 1999

National Rate = 304 Beds per 100,000 Population*

ALPHA ORDER

RANK	STATE	RATE
15	Alabama	373
46	Alaska	202
44	Arizona	221
9	Arkansas	394
43	California	222
41	Colorado	230
40	Connecticut	240
33	Delaware	265
20	Florida	327
22	Georgia	318
38	Hawaii	246
32	Idaho	280
23	Illinois	310
21	Indiana	323
8	Iowa	413
7	Kansas	438
13	Kentucky	378
10	Louisiana	384
29	Maine	295
42	Maryland	225
35	Massachusetts	264
33	Michigan	265
18	Minnesota	345
5	Mississippi	477
16	Missouri	370
3	Montana	529
4	Nebraska	500
45	Nevada	205
37	New Hampshire	248
26	New Jersey	302
49	New Mexico	194
12	New York	379
24	North Carolina	306
1	North Dakota	613
25	Ohio	304
19	Oklahoma	330
47	Oregon	200
17	Pennsylvania	359
39	Rhode Island	242
28	South Carolina	299
2	South Dakota	593
14	Tennessee	376
30	Texas	283
48	Utah	196
31	Vermont	281
36	Virginia	252
50	Washington	193
6	West Virginia	449
26	Wisconsin	302
11	Wyoming	382

RANK ORDER

RANK	STATE	RATE
1	North Dakota	613
2	South Dakota	593
3	Montana	529
4	Nebraska	500
5	Mississippi	477
6	West Virginia	449
7	Kansas	438
8	Iowa	413
9	Arkansas	394
10	Louisiana	384
11	Wyoming	382
12	New York	379
13	Kentucky	378
14	Tennessee	376
15	Alabama	373
16	Missouri	370
17	Pennsylvania	359
18	Minnesota	345
19	Oklahoma	330
20	Florida	327
21	Indiana	323
22	Georgia	318
23	Illinois	310
24	North Carolina	306
25	Ohio	304
26	New Jersey	302
26	Wisconsin	302
28	South Carolina	299
29	Maine	295
30	Texas	283
31	Vermont	281
32	Idaho	280
33	Delaware	265
33	Michigan	265
35	Massachusetts	264
36	Virginia	252
37	New Hampshire	248
38	Hawaii	246
39	Rhode Island	242
40	Connecticut	240
41	Colorado	230
42	Maryland	225
43	California	222
44	Arizona	221
45	Nevada	205
46	Alaska	202
47	Oregon	200
48	Utah	196
49	New Mexico	194
50	Washington	193

District of Columbia   682

Source: Morgan Quitno Press using data from American Hospital Association (Chicago, IL)
"Hospital Statistics" (2001 edition)
*All nonfederal short-term general and other special hospitals, whose facilities and services are available to the public. Includes beds in hospital and nursing home units.

Average Number of Beds per Community Hospital in 1999

National Average = 167 Beds per Community Hospital*

ALPHA ORDER

RANK	STATE	BEDS
23	Alabama	150
50	Alaska	74
17	Arizona	173
34	Arkansas	121
14	California	187
25	Colorado	140
6	Connecticut	225
1	Delaware	333
4	Florida	244
22	Georgia	161
30	Hawaii	132
48	Idaho	83
13	Illinois	190
17	Indiana	173
38	Iowa	103
46	Kansas	89
24	Kentucky	142
28	Louisiana	138
40	Maine	100
5	Maryland	237
8	Massachusetts	206
16	Michigan	180
33	Minnesota	123
28	Mississippi	138
19	Missouri	172
47	Montana	88
42	Nebraska	98
21	Nevada	168
37	New Hampshire	106
3	New Jersey	303
44	New Mexico	94
2	New York	316
9	North Carolina	205
43	North Dakota	95
9	Ohio	205
39	Oklahoma	102
36	Oregon	113
9	Pennsylvania	205
7	Rhode Island	218
15	South Carolina	182
45	South Dakota	91
20	Tennessee	170
27	Texas	139
41	Utah	99
35	Vermont	119
12	Virginia	194
31	Washington	129
25	West Virginia	140
31	Wisconsin	129
49	Wyoming	80

RANK ORDER

RANK	STATE	BEDS
1	Delaware	333
2	New York	316
3	New Jersey	303
4	Florida	244
5	Maryland	237
6	Connecticut	225
7	Rhode Island	218
8	Massachusetts	206
9	North Carolina	205
9	Ohio	205
9	Pennsylvania	205
12	Virginia	194
13	Illinois	190
14	California	187
15	South Carolina	182
16	Michigan	180
17	Arizona	173
17	Indiana	173
19	Missouri	172
20	Tennessee	170
21	Nevada	168
22	Georgia	161
23	Alabama	150
24	Kentucky	142
25	Colorado	140
25	West Virginia	140
27	Texas	139
28	Louisiana	138
28	Mississippi	138
30	Hawaii	132
31	Washington	129
31	Wisconsin	129
33	Minnesota	123
34	Arkansas	121
35	Vermont	119
36	Oregon	113
37	New Hampshire	106
38	Iowa	103
39	Oklahoma	102
40	Maine	100
41	Utah	99
42	Nebraska	98
43	North Dakota	95
44	New Mexico	94
45	South Dakota	91
46	Kansas	89
47	Montana	88
48	Idaho	83
49	Wyoming	80
50	Alaska	74

| | District of Columbia | 295 |

Source: Morgan Quitno Press using data from American Hospital Association (Chicago, IL)
     "Hospital Statistics" (2001 edition)

*All nonfederal short-term general and other special hospitals, whose facilities and services are available to the public. Includes beds in hospital and nursing home units.

Admissions to Community Hospitals in 1999

National Total = 32,359,042 Admissions*

ALPHA ORDER

RANK	STATE	ADMISSIONS	% of USA
17	Alabama	670,059	2.1%
50	Alaska	40,785	0.1%
23	Arizona	511,084	1.6%
29	Arkansas	375,297	1.2%
1	California	3,244,086	10.0%
28	Colorado	383,283	1.2%
31	Connecticut	337,821	1.0%
46	Delaware	87,200	0.3%
4	Florida	2,020,073	6.2%
11	Georgia	824,376	2.5%
43	Hawaii	99,191	0.3%
40	Idaho	119,928	0.4%
6	Illinois	1,508,816	4.7%
16	Indiana	683,264	2.1%
30	Iowa	359,142	1.1%
32	Kansas	326,352	1.0%
20	Kentucky	569,792	1.8%
18	Louisiana	626,801	1.9%
39	Maine	146,378	0.5%
19	Maryland	576,551	1.8%
14	Massachusetts	739,375	2.3%
8	Michigan	1,084,277	3.4%
22	Minnesota	534,692	1.7%
26	Mississippi	415,776	1.3%
13	Missouri	742,867	2.3%
44	Montana	97,875	0.3%
35	Nebraska	199,471	0.6%
36	Nevada	197,501	0.6%
42	New Hampshire	109,110	0.3%
9	New Jersey	1,068,664	3.3%
38	New Mexico	163,700	0.5%
2	New York	2,406,327	7.4%
10	North Carolina	930,747	2.9%
47	North Dakota	86,931	0.3%
7	Ohio	1,358,662	4.2%
27	Oklahoma	411,025	1.3%
33	Oregon	317,808	1.0%
5	Pennsylvania	1,755,029	5.4%
41	Rhode Island	117,163	0.4%
25	South Carolina	478,936	1.5%
45	South Dakota	97,316	0.3%
12	Tennessee	751,523	2.3%
3	Texas	2,302,892	7.1%
37	Utah	189,430	0.6%
48	Vermont	50,820	0.2%
15	Virginia	723,803	2.2%
24	Washington	490,659	1.5%
34	West Virginia	289,427	0.9%
21	Wisconsin	553,337	1.7%
49	Wyoming	45,212	0.1%

RANK ORDER

RANK	STATE	ADMISSIONS	% of USA
1	California	3,244,086	10.0%
2	New York	2,406,327	7.4%
3	Texas	2,302,892	7.1%
4	Florida	2,020,073	6.2%
5	Pennsylvania	1,755,029	5.4%
6	Illinois	1,508,816	4.7%
7	Ohio	1,358,662	4.2%
8	Michigan	1,084,277	3.4%
9	New Jersey	1,068,664	3.3%
10	North Carolina	930,747	2.9%
11	Georgia	824,376	2.5%
12	Tennessee	751,523	2.3%
13	Missouri	742,867	2.3%
14	Massachusetts	739,375	2.3%
15	Virginia	723,803	2.2%
16	Indiana	683,264	2.1%
17	Alabama	670,059	2.1%
18	Louisiana	626,801	1.9%
19	Maryland	576,551	1.8%
20	Kentucky	569,792	1.8%
21	Wisconsin	553,337	1.7%
22	Minnesota	534,692	1.7%
23	Arizona	511,084	1.6%
24	Washington	490,659	1.5%
25	South Carolina	478,936	1.5%
26	Mississippi	415,776	1.3%
27	Oklahoma	411,025	1.3%
28	Colorado	383,283	1.2%
29	Arkansas	375,297	1.2%
30	Iowa	359,142	1.1%
31	Connecticut	337,821	1.0%
32	Kansas	326,352	1.0%
33	Oregon	317,808	1.0%
34	West Virginia	289,427	0.9%
35	Nebraska	199,471	0.6%
36	Nevada	197,501	0.6%
37	Utah	189,430	0.6%
38	New Mexico	163,700	0.5%
39	Maine	146,378	0.5%
40	Idaho	119,928	0.4%
41	Rhode Island	117,163	0.4%
42	New Hampshire	109,110	0.3%
43	Hawaii	99,191	0.3%
44	Montana	97,875	0.3%
45	South Dakota	97,316	0.3%
46	Delaware	87,200	0.3%
47	North Dakota	86,931	0.3%
48	Vermont	50,820	0.2%
49	Wyoming	45,212	0.1%
50	Alaska	40,785	0.1%
	District of Columbia	138,408	0.4%

Source: American Hospital Association (Chicago, IL)
   "Hospital Statistics" (2001 edition)
Admissions to all nonfederal short-term general and other special hospitals, whose facilities and services are available to the public. Includes admissions to hospital and nursing home units.

Inpatient Days in Community Hospitals in 1999

National Total = 191,824,270 Inpatient Days*

ALPHA ORDER

RANK	STATE	DAYS	% of USA
18	Alabama	3,603,498	1.9%
50	Alaska	246,872	0.1%
26	Arizona	2,383,512	1.2%
30	Arkansas	2,195,965	1.1%
2	California	17,090,813	8.9%
32	Colorado	1,947,693	1.0%
31	Connecticut	2,070,480	1.1%
47	Delaware	492,551	0.3%
4	Florida	11,135,544	5.8%
11	Georgia	5,625,261	2.9%
42	Hawaii	769,824	0.4%
44	Idaho	694,361	0.4%
6	Illinois	8,267,158	4.3%
17	Indiana	3,998,799	2.1%
25	Iowa	2,498,984	1.3%
29	Kansas	2,232,737	1.2%
21	Kentucky	3,296,591	1.7%
19	Louisiana	3,472,409	1.8%
39	Maine	872,635	0.5%
22	Maryland	3,023,508	1.6%
14	Massachusetts	4,210,454	2.2%
8	Michigan	6,295,931	3.3%
16	Minnesota	4,046,050	2.1%
23	Mississippi	2,916,549	1.5%
13	Missouri	4,247,921	2.2%
36	Montana	1,161,334	0.6%
33	Nebraska	1,821,925	0.9%
38	Nevada	1,000,369	0.5%
46	New Hampshire	599,777	0.3%
9	New Jersey	6,150,912	3.2%
43	New Mexico	725,713	0.4%
1	New York	19,349,127	10.1%
10	North Carolina	5,726,618	3.0%
41	North Dakota	852,457	0.4%
7	Ohio	7,362,468	3.8%
28	Oklahoma	2,273,850	1.2%
35	Oregon	1,409,906	0.7%
5	Pennsylvania	10,652,791	5.6%
45	Rhode Island	623,306	0.3%
24	South Carolina	2,816,481	1.5%
37	South Dakota	1,052,039	0.5%
12	Tennessee	4,296,679	2.2%
3	Texas	12,015,612	6.3%
40	Utah	871,864	0.5%
48	Vermont	394,752	0.2%
15	Virginia	4,133,834	2.2%
27	Washington	2,375,711	1.2%
34	West Virginia	1,792,038	0.9%
20	Wisconsin	3,394,502	1.8%
49	Wyoming	350,011	0.2%

RANK ORDER

RANK	STATE	DAYS	% of USA
1	New York	19,349,127	10.1%
2	California	17,090,813	8.9%
3	Texas	12,015,612	6.3%
4	Florida	11,135,544	5.8%
5	Pennsylvania	10,652,791	5.6%
6	Illinois	8,267,158	4.3%
7	Ohio	7,362,468	3.8%
8	Michigan	6,295,931	3.3%
9	New Jersey	6,150,912	3.2%
10	North Carolina	5,726,618	3.0%
11	Georgia	5,625,261	2.9%
12	Tennessee	4,296,679	2.2%
13	Missouri	4,247,921	2.2%
14	Massachusetts	4,210,454	2.2%
15	Virginia	4,133,834	2.2%
16	Minnesota	4,046,050	2.1%
17	Indiana	3,998,799	2.1%
18	Alabama	3,603,498	1.9%
19	Louisiana	3,472,409	1.8%
20	Wisconsin	3,394,502	1.8%
21	Kentucky	3,296,591	1.7%
22	Maryland	3,023,508	1.6%
23	Mississippi	2,916,549	1.5%
24	South Carolina	2,816,481	1.5%
25	Iowa	2,498,984	1.3%
26	Arizona	2,383,512	1.2%
27	Washington	2,375,711	1.2%
28	Oklahoma	2,273,850	1.2%
29	Kansas	2,232,737	1.2%
30	Arkansas	2,195,965	1.1%
31	Connecticut	2,070,480	1.1%
32	Colorado	1,947,693	1.0%
33	Nebraska	1,821,925	0.9%
34	West Virginia	1,792,038	0.9%
35	Oregon	1,409,906	0.7%
36	Montana	1,161,334	0.6%
37	South Dakota	1,052,039	0.5%
38	Nevada	1,000,369	0.5%
39	Maine	872,635	0.5%
40	Utah	871,864	0.5%
41	North Dakota	852,457	0.4%
42	Hawaii	769,824	0.4%
43	New Mexico	725,713	0.4%
44	Idaho	694,361	0.4%
45	Rhode Island	623,306	0.3%
46	New Hampshire	599,777	0.3%
47	Delaware	492,551	0.3%
48	Vermont	394,752	0.2%
49	Wyoming	350,011	0.2%
50	Alaska	246,872	0.1%
	District of Columbia	984,094	0.5%

Source: American Hospital Association (Chicago, IL)
    "Hospital Statistics" (2001 edition)
*Inpatient days in all nonfederal short-term general and other special hospitals, whose facilities and services are available to the public. Includes days in hospital and nursing home units.

Average Daily Census in Community Hospitals in 1999

National Average = 525,546 Inpatients*

ALPHA ORDER

RANK	STATE	INPATIENTS	% of USA
18	Alabama	9,873	1.9%
50	Alaska	676	0.1%
26	Arizona	6,530	1.2%
30	Arkansas	6,016	1.1%
2	California	46,824	8.9%
32	Colorado	5,336	1.0%
31	Connecticut	5,673	1.1%
47	Delaware	1,349	0.3%
4	Florida	30,508	5.8%
11	Georgia	15,412	2.9%
42	Hawaii	2,109	0.4%
44	Idaho	1,902	0.4%
6	Illinois	22,650	4.3%
17	Indiana	10,956	2.1%
25	Iowa	6,847	1.3%
29	Kansas	6,117	1.2%
21	Kentucky	9,032	1.7%
19	Louisiana	9,513	1.8%
39	Maine	2,391	0.5%
22	Maryland	8,284	1.6%
14	Massachusetts	11,535	2.2%
8	Michigan	17,249	3.3%
16	Minnesota	11,085	2.1%
23	Mississippi	7,991	1.5%
13	Missouri	11,638	2.2%
36	Montana	3,182	0.6%
33	Nebraska	4,992	0.9%
38	Nevada	2,741	0.5%
46	New Hampshire	1,643	0.3%
9	New Jersey	16,852	3.2%
43	New Mexico	1,988	0.4%
1	New York	53,011	10.1%
10	North Carolina	15,689	3.0%
41	North Dakota	2,335	0.4%
7	Ohio	20,171	3.8%
28	Oklahoma	6,230	1.2%
35	Oregon	3,863	0.7%
5	Pennsylvania	29,186	5.6%
45	Rhode Island	1,708	0.3%
24	South Carolina	7,716	1.5%
37	South Dakota	2,882	0.5%
12	Tennessee	11,772	2.2%
3	Texas	32,919	6.3%
40	Utah	2,389	0.5%
48	Vermont	1,082	0.2%
15	Virginia	11,326	2.2%
27	Washington	6,509	1.2%
34	West Virginia	4,910	0.9%
20	Wisconsin	9,300	1.8%
49	Wyoming	959	0.2%

RANK ORDER

RANK	STATE	INPATIENTS	% of USA
1	New York	53,011	10.1%
2	California	46,824	8.9%
3	Texas	32,919	6.3%
4	Florida	30,508	5.8%
5	Pennsylvania	29,186	5.6%
6	Illinois	22,650	4.3%
7	Ohio	20,171	3.8%
8	Michigan	17,249	3.3%
9	New Jersey	16,852	3.2%
10	North Carolina	15,689	3.0%
11	Georgia	15,412	2.9%
12	Tennessee	11,772	2.2%
13	Missouri	11,638	2.2%
14	Massachusetts	11,535	2.2%
15	Virginia	11,326	2.2%
16	Minnesota	11,085	2.1%
17	Indiana	10,956	2.1%
18	Alabama	9,873	1.9%
19	Louisiana	9,513	1.8%
20	Wisconsin	9,300	1.8%
21	Kentucky	9,032	1.7%
22	Maryland	8,284	1.6%
23	Mississippi	7,991	1.5%
24	South Carolina	7,716	1.5%
25	Iowa	6,847	1.3%
26	Arizona	6,530	1.2%
27	Washington	6,509	1.2%
28	Oklahoma	6,230	1.2%
29	Kansas	6,117	1.2%
30	Arkansas	6,016	1.1%
31	Connecticut	5,673	1.1%
32	Colorado	5,336	1.0%
33	Nebraska	4,992	0.9%
34	West Virginia	4,910	0.9%
35	Oregon	3,863	0.7%
36	Montana	3,182	0.6%
37	South Dakota	2,882	0.5%
38	Nevada	2,741	0.5%
39	Maine	2,391	0.5%
40	Utah	2,389	0.5%
41	North Dakota	2,335	0.4%
42	Hawaii	2,109	0.4%
43	New Mexico	1,988	0.4%
44	Idaho	1,902	0.4%
45	Rhode Island	1,708	0.3%
46	New Hampshire	1,643	0.3%
47	Delaware	1,349	0.3%
48	Vermont	1,082	0.2%
49	Wyoming	959	0.2%
50	Alaska	676	0.1%
	District of Columbia	2,696	0.5%

Source: Morgan Quitno Press using data from American Hospital Association (Chicago, IL)
       "Hospital Statistics" (2001 edition)
*Average total of inpatients receiving care in all nonfederal short-term general and other special hospitals, whose facilities and services are available to the public. Excludes newborns.

Average Stay in Community Hospitals in 1999

National Average = 5.9 Days*

RANK	STATE	DAYS
38	Alabama	5.4
16	Alaska	6.1
47	Arizona	4.7
21	Arkansas	5.9
40	California	5.3
44	Colorado	5.1
16	Connecticut	6.1
32	Delaware	5.6
33	Florida	5.5
12	Georgia	6.8
6	Hawaii	7.8
24	Idaho	5.8
33	Illinois	5.5
21	Indiana	5.9
10	Iowa	7.0
12	Kansas	6.8
24	Kentucky	5.8
33	Louisiana	5.5
20	Maine	6.0
42	Maryland	5.2
28	Massachusetts	5.7
24	Michigan	5.8
9	Minnesota	7.6
10	Mississippi	7.0
28	Missouri	5.7
1	Montana	11.9
4	Nebraska	9.1
44	Nevada	5.1
33	New Hampshire	5.5
24	New Jersey	5.8
49	New Mexico	4.4
5	New York	8.0
14	North Carolina	6.2
3	North Dakota	9.8
38	Ohio	5.4
33	Oklahoma	5.5
49	Oregon	4.4
16	Pennsylvania	6.1
40	Rhode Island	5.3
21	South Carolina	5.9
2	South Dakota	10.8
28	Tennessee	5.7
42	Texas	5.2
48	Utah	4.6
6	Vermont	7.8
28	Virginia	5.7
46	Washington	4.8
14	West Virginia	6.2
16	Wisconsin	6.1
8	Wyoming	7.7

RANK	STATE	DAYS
1	Montana	11.9
2	South Dakota	10.8
3	North Dakota	9.8
4	Nebraska	9.1
5	New York	8.0
6	Hawaii	7.8
6	Vermont	7.8
8	Wyoming	7.7
9	Minnesota	7.6
10	Iowa	7.0
10	Mississippi	7.0
12	Georgia	6.8
12	Kansas	6.8
14	North Carolina	6.2
14	West Virginia	6.2
16	Alaska	6.1
16	Connecticut	6.1
16	Pennsylvania	6.1
16	Wisconsin	6.1
20	Maine	6.0
21	Arkansas	5.9
21	Indiana	5.9
21	South Carolina	5.9
24	Idaho	5.8
24	Kentucky	5.8
24	Michigan	5.8
24	New Jersey	5.8
28	Massachusetts	5.7
28	Missouri	5.7
28	Tennessee	5.7
28	Virginia	5.7
32	Delaware	5.6
33	Florida	5.5
33	Illinois	5.5
33	Louisiana	5.5
33	New Hampshire	5.5
33	Oklahoma	5.5
38	Alabama	5.4
38	Ohio	5.4
40	California	5.3
40	Rhode Island	5.3
42	Maryland	5.2
42	Texas	5.2
44	Colorado	5.1
44	Nevada	5.1
46	Washington	4.8
47	Arizona	4.7
48	Utah	4.6
49	New Mexico	4.4
49	Oregon	4.4
	District of Columbia	7.1

Source: American Hospital Association (Chicago, IL)
    "Hospital Statistics" (2001 edition)
*All nonfederal short-term general and other special hospitals, whose facilities and services are available to the public.

Occupancy Rate in Community Hospitals in 1999

National Rate = 63.4% of Community Hospital Beds Occupied*

ALPHA ORDER

RANK	STATE	PERCENT
25	Alabama	60.5
48	Alaska	54.1
22	Arizona	61.7
31	Arkansas	59.9
20	California	63.6
41	Colorado	57.1
4	Connecticut	72.1
11	Delaware	67.5
22	Florida	61.7
21	Georgia	62.2
3	Hawaii	72.4
47	Idaho	54.4
28	Illinois	60.1
43	Indiana	57.0
38	Iowa	57.8
49	Kansas	52.7
27	Kentucky	60.4
44	Louisiana	56.7
18	Maine	64.8
5	Maryland	71.2
7	Massachusetts	70.7
16	Michigan	66.0
12	Minnesota	67.4
25	Mississippi	60.5
39	Missouri	57.5
9	Montana	68.2
30	Nebraska	60.0
2	Nevada	74.0
46	New Hampshire	55.2
8	New Jersey	68.6
32	New Mexico	59.0
1	New York	76.9
13	North Carolina	67.1
28	North Dakota	60.1
32	Ohio	59.0
45	Oklahoma	56.3
36	Oregon	58.2
10	Pennsylvania	67.9
5	Rhode Island	71.2
14	South Carolina	66.4
15	South Dakota	66.3
41	Tennessee	57.1
37	Texas	57.9
40	Utah	57.3
18	Vermont	64.8
17	Virginia	65.5
34	Washington	58.7
24	West Virginia	60.6
35	Wisconsin	58.6
50	Wyoming	52.4

RANK ORDER

RANK	STATE	PERCENT
1	New York	76.9
2	Nevada	74.0
3	Hawaii	72.4
4	Connecticut	72.1
5	Maryland	71.2
5	Rhode Island	71.2
7	Massachusetts	70.7
8	New Jersey	68.6
9	Montana	68.2
10	Pennsylvania	67.9
11	Delaware	67.5
12	Minnesota	67.4
13	North Carolina	67.1
14	South Carolina	66.4
15	South Dakota	66.3
16	Michigan	66.0
17	Virginia	65.5
18	Maine	64.8
18	Vermont	64.8
20	California	63.6
21	Georgia	62.2
22	Arizona	61.7
22	Florida	61.7
24	West Virginia	60.6
25	Alabama	60.5
25	Mississippi	60.5
27	Kentucky	60.4
28	Illinois	60.1
28	North Dakota	60.1
30	Nebraska	60.0
31	Arkansas	59.9
32	New Mexico	59.0
32	Ohio	59.0
34	Washington	58.7
35	Wisconsin	58.6
36	Oregon	58.2
37	Texas	57.9
38	Iowa	57.8
39	Missouri	57.5
40	Utah	57.3
41	Colorado	57.1
41	Tennessee	57.1
43	Indiana	57.0
44	Louisiana	56.7
45	Oklahoma	56.3
46	New Hampshire	55.2
47	Idaho	54.4
48	Alaska	54.1
49	Kansas	52.7
50	Wyoming	52.4

District of Columbia	76.1

Source: Morgan Quitno Press using data from American Hospital Association (Chicago, IL)
   "Hospital Statistics" (2001 edition)
*Average daily census compared to number of community hospital beds.

Outpatient Visits to Community Hospitals in 1999

National Total = 495,346,286 Visits*

ALPHA ORDER					RANK ORDER			

RANK	STATE	VISITS	% of USA
22	Alabama	7,835,488	1.6%
49	Alaska	1,032,283	0.2%
31	Arizona	4,942,953	1.0%
34	Arkansas	3,955,872	0.8%
2	California	44,779,061	9.0%
26	Colorado	6,439,511	1.3%
23	Connecticut	6,818,177	1.4%
48	Delaware	1,347,313	0.3%
8	Florida	19,699,490	4.0%
14	Georgia	10,838,910	2.2%
40	Hawaii	2,436,652	0.5%
42	Idaho	2,182,313	0.4%
6	Illinois	23,916,001	4.8%
12	Indiana	13,113,838	2.6%
20	Iowa	8,563,256	1.7%
30	Kansas	5,024,380	1.0%
21	Kentucky	7,981,840	1.6%
17	Louisiana	9,513,994	1.9%
38	Maine	2,777,399	0.6%
28	Maryland	5,943,083	1.2%
10	Massachusetts	15,708,869	3.2%
7	Michigan	22,372,164	4.5%
25	Minnesota	6,450,624	1.3%
35	Mississippi	3,457,477	0.7%
11	Missouri	14,643,361	3.0%
39	Montana	2,539,413	0.5%
37	Nebraska	3,001,824	0.6%
43	Nevada	2,126,489	0.4%
41	New Hampshire	2,400,776	0.5%
9	New Jersey	16,126,169	3.3%
36	New Mexico	3,134,970	0.6%
1	New York	45,742,573	9.2%
13	North Carolina	11,540,402	2.3%
45	North Dakota	1,631,439	0.3%
5	Ohio	24,886,214	5.0%
32	Oklahoma	4,624,837	0.9%
24	Oregon	6,657,630	1.3%
3	Pennsylvania	29,269,126	5.9%
44	Rhode Island	1,911,557	0.4%
27	South Carolina	6,360,072	1.3%
46	South Dakota	1,553,753	0.3%
18	Tennessee	9,479,866	1.9%
4	Texas	28,258,876	5.7%
33	Utah	4,365,726	0.9%
47	Vermont	1,413,834	0.3%
19	Virginia	8,730,884	1.8%
16	Washington	9,959,994	2.0%
29	West Virginia	5,095,446	1.0%
15	Wisconsin	10,511,079	2.1%
50	Wyoming	865,679	0.2%

RANK	STATE	VISITS	% of USA
1	New York	45,742,573	9.2%
2	California	44,779,061	9.0%
3	Pennsylvania	29,269,126	5.9%
4	Texas	28,258,876	5.7%
5	Ohio	24,886,214	5.0%
6	Illinois	23,916,001	4.8%
7	Michigan	22,372,164	4.5%
8	Florida	19,699,490	4.0%
9	New Jersey	16,126,169	3.3%
10	Massachusetts	15,708,869	3.2%
11	Missouri	14,643,361	3.0%
12	Indiana	13,113,838	2.6%
13	North Carolina	11,540,402	2.3%
14	Georgia	10,838,910	2.2%
15	Wisconsin	10,511,079	2.1%
16	Washington	9,959,994	2.0%
17	Louisiana	9,513,994	1.9%
18	Tennessee	9,479,866	1.9%
19	Virginia	8,730,884	1.8%
20	Iowa	8,563,256	1.7%
21	Kentucky	7,981,840	1.6%
22	Alabama	7,835,488	1.6%
23	Connecticut	6,818,177	1.4%
24	Oregon	6,657,630	1.3%
25	Minnesota	6,450,624	1.3%
26	Colorado	6,439,511	1.3%
27	South Carolina	6,360,072	1.3%
28	Maryland	5,943,083	1.2%
29	West Virginia	5,095,446	1.0%
30	Kansas	5,024,380	1.0%
31	Arizona	4,942,953	1.0%
32	Oklahoma	4,624,837	0.9%
33	Utah	4,365,726	0.9%
34	Arkansas	3,955,872	0.8%
35	Mississippi	3,457,477	0.7%
36	New Mexico	3,134,970	0.6%
37	Nebraska	3,001,824	0.6%
38	Maine	2,777,399	0.6%
39	Montana	2,539,413	0.5%
40	Hawaii	2,436,652	0.5%
41	New Hampshire	2,400,776	0.5%
42	Idaho	2,182,313	0.4%
43	Nevada	2,126,489	0.4%
44	Rhode Island	1,911,557	0.4%
45	North Dakota	1,631,439	0.3%
46	South Dakota	1,553,753	0.3%
47	Vermont	1,413,834	0.3%
48	Delaware	1,347,313	0.3%
49	Alaska	1,032,283	0.2%
50	Wyoming	865,679	0.2%
	District of Columbia	1,383,349	0.3%

Source: American Hospital Association (Chicago, IL)
     "Hospital Statistics" (2001 edition)
*All nonfederal short-term general and other special hospitals, whose facilities and services are available to the public. Includes emergency and other visits.

Emergency Outpatient Visits to Community Hospitals in 1999

National Total = 99,484,462 Visits*

ALPHA ORDER

RANK	STATE	VISITS	% of USA
19	Alabama	1,969,275	2.0%
50	Alaska	164,113	0.2%
27	Arizona	1,340,258	1.3%
30	Arkansas	1,073,440	1.1%
1	California	9,294,157	9.3%
28	Colorado	1,324,504	1.3%
26	Connecticut	1,344,816	1.4%
43	Delaware	285,276	0.3%
4	Florida	5,488,609	5.5%
10	Georgia	2,854,136	2.9%
46	Hawaii	239,560	0.2%
42	Idaho	414,388	0.4%
7	Illinois	4,420,908	4.4%
17	Indiana	2,120,329	2.1%
31	Iowa	1,051,682	1.1%
34	Kansas	921,066	0.9%
18	Kentucky	1,990,266	2.0%
16	Louisiana	2,182,109	2.2%
36	Maine	579,803	0.6%
23	Maryland	1,667,655	1.7%
12	Massachusetts	2,726,113	2.7%
8	Michigan	3,528,497	3.5%
25	Minnesota	1,364,802	1.4%
24	Mississippi	1,429,819	1.4%
14	Missouri	2,411,820	2.4%
44	Montana	263,239	0.3%
40	Nebraska	491,438	0.5%
37	Nevada	527,219	0.5%
39	New Hampshire	491,840	0.5%
9	New Jersey	2,882,031	2.9%
38	New Mexico	512,645	0.5%
2	New York	7,141,070	7.2%
11	North Carolina	2,844,680	2.9%
45	North Dakota	249,955	0.3%
5	Ohio	4,906,178	4.9%
29	Oklahoma	1,172,259	1.2%
33	Oregon	921,414	0.9%
6	Pennsylvania	4,615,588	4.6%
41	Rhode Island	421,667	0.4%
22	South Carolina	1,675,252	1.7%
48	South Dakota	192,035	0.2%
13	Tennessee	2,589,171	2.6%
3	Texas	7,071,236	7.1%
35	Utah	687,822	0.7%
47	Vermont	220,500	0.2%
15	Virginia	2,291,867	2.3%
20	Washington	1,887,881	1.9%
32	West Virginia	1,002,071	1.0%
21	Wisconsin	1,723,490	1.7%
49	Wyoming	184,370	0.2%

RANK ORDER

RANK	STATE	VISITS	% of USA
1	California	9,294,157	9.3%
2	New York	7,141,070	7.2%
3	Texas	7,071,236	7.1%
4	Florida	5,488,609	5.5%
5	Ohio	4,906,178	4.9%
6	Pennsylvania	4,615,588	4.6%
7	Illinois	4,420,908	4.4%
8	Michigan	3,528,497	3.5%
9	New Jersey	2,882,031	2.9%
10	Georgia	2,854,136	2.9%
11	North Carolina	2,844,680	2.9%
12	Massachusetts	2,726,113	2.7%
13	Tennessee	2,589,171	2.6%
14	Missouri	2,411,820	2.4%
15	Virginia	2,291,867	2.3%
16	Louisiana	2,182,109	2.2%
17	Indiana	2,120,329	2.1%
18	Kentucky	1,990,266	2.0%
19	Alabama	1,969,275	2.0%
20	Washington	1,887,881	1.9%
21	Wisconsin	1,723,490	1.7%
22	South Carolina	1,675,252	1.7%
23	Maryland	1,667,655	1.7%
24	Mississippi	1,429,819	1.4%
25	Minnesota	1,364,802	1.4%
26	Connecticut	1,344,816	1.4%
27	Arizona	1,340,258	1.3%
28	Colorado	1,324,504	1.3%
29	Oklahoma	1,172,259	1.2%
30	Arkansas	1,073,440	1.1%
31	Iowa	1,051,682	1.1%
32	West Virginia	1,002,071	1.0%
33	Oregon	921,414	0.9%
34	Kansas	921,066	0.9%
35	Utah	687,822	0.7%
36	Maine	579,803	0.6%
37	Nevada	527,219	0.5%
38	New Mexico	512,645	0.5%
39	New Hampshire	491,840	0.5%
40	Nebraska	491,438	0.5%
41	Rhode Island	421,667	0.4%
42	Idaho	414,388	0.4%
43	Delaware	285,276	0.3%
44	Montana	263,239	0.3%
45	North Dakota	249,955	0.3%
46	Hawaii	239,560	0.2%
47	Vermont	220,500	0.2%
48	South Dakota	192,035	0.2%
49	Wyoming	184,370	0.2%
50	Alaska	164,113	0.2%
	District of Columbia	330,143	0.3%

Source: American Hospital Association (Chicago, IL)
   "Hospital Statistics" (2001 edition)
All nonfederal short-term general and other special hospitals, whose facilities and services are available to the public.

Surgical Operations in Community Hospitals in 1999

National Total = 25,385,085 Surgical Operations*

ALPHA ORDER

RANK	STATE	OPERATIONS	% of USA
20	Alabama	476,210	1.9%
49	Alaska	38,402	0.2%
26	Arizona	357,621	1.4%
34	Arkansas	259,004	1.0%
1	California	2,024,816	8.0%
27	Colorado	329,153	1.3%
30	Connecticut	290,592	1.1%
42	Delaware	93,529	0.4%
5	Florida	1,373,837	5.4%
11	Georgia	686,690	2.7%
45	Hawaii	75,329	0.3%
41	Idaho	99,231	0.4%
7	Illinois	1,041,433	4.1%
15	Indiana	598,571	2.4%
24	Iowa	386,215	1.5%
31	Kansas	267,634	1.1%
18	Kentucky	497,987	2.0%
21	Louisiana	446,903	1.8%
39	Maine	140,698	0.6%
19	Maryland	496,532	2.0%
12	Massachusetts	654,967	2.6%
8	Michigan	985,303	3.9%
22	Minnesota	426,315	1.7%
33	Mississippi	266,256	1.0%
16	Missouri	563,168	2.2%
47	Montana	68,947	0.3%
36	Nebraska	181,060	0.7%
35	Nevada	190,429	0.8%
43	New Hampshire	93,471	0.4%
9	New Jersey	721,974	2.8%
38	New Mexico	143,670	0.6%
2	New York	1,886,290	7.4%
10	North Carolina	721,916	2.8%
46	North Dakota	72,259	0.3%
6	Ohio	1,156,191	4.6%
28	Oklahoma	310,389	1.2%
32	Oregon	266,309	1.0%
4	Pennsylvania	1,525,262	6.0%
40	Rhode Island	121,899	0.5%
25	South Carolina	370,571	1.5%
44	South Dakota	78,692	0.3%
14	Tennessee	614,944	2.4%
3	Texas	1,728,743	6.8%
37	Utah	177,023	0.7%
48	Vermont	49,333	0.2%
13	Virginia	615,563	2.4%
23	Washington	412,212	1.6%
29	West Virginia	297,114	1.2%
17	Wisconsin	508,465	2.0%
50	Wyoming	38,121	0.2%

RANK ORDER

RANK	STATE	OPERATIONS	% of USA
1	California	2,024,816	8.0%
2	New York	1,886,290	7.4%
3	Texas	1,728,743	6.8%
4	Pennsylvania	1,525,262	6.0%
5	Florida	1,373,837	5.4%
6	Ohio	1,156,191	4.6%
7	Illinois	1,041,433	4.1%
8	Michigan	985,303	3.9%
9	New Jersey	721,974	2.8%
10	North Carolina	721,916	2.8%
11	Georgia	686,690	2.7%
12	Massachusetts	654,967	2.6%
13	Virginia	615,563	2.4%
14	Tennessee	614,944	2.4%
15	Indiana	598,571	2.4%
16	Missouri	563,168	2.2%
17	Wisconsin	508,465	2.0%
18	Kentucky	497,987	2.0%
19	Maryland	496,532	2.0%
20	Alabama	476,210	1.9%
21	Louisiana	446,903	1.8%
22	Minnesota	426,315	1.7%
23	Washington	412,212	1.6%
24	Iowa	386,215	1.5%
25	South Carolina	370,571	1.5%
26	Arizona	357,621	1.4%
27	Colorado	329,153	1.3%
28	Oklahoma	310,389	1.2%
29	West Virginia	297,114	1.2%
30	Connecticut	290,592	1.1%
31	Kansas	267,634	1.1%
32	Oregon	266,309	1.0%
33	Mississippi	266,256	1.0%
34	Arkansas	259,004	1.0%
35	Nevada	190,429	0.8%
36	Nebraska	181,060	0.7%
37	Utah	177,023	0.7%
38	New Mexico	143,670	0.6%
39	Maine	140,698	0.6%
40	Rhode Island	121,899	0.5%
41	Idaho	99,231	0.4%
42	Delaware	93,529	0.4%
43	New Hampshire	93,471	0.4%
44	South Dakota	78,692	0.3%
45	Hawaii	75,329	0.3%
46	North Dakota	72,259	0.3%
47	Montana	68,947	0.3%
48	Vermont	49,333	0.2%
49	Alaska	38,402	0.2%
50	Wyoming	38,121	0.2%
	District of Columbia	157,842	0.6%

Source: American Hospital Association (Chicago, IL)
    "Hospital Statistics" (2001 edition)
*Includes inpatient and outpatient surgeries.

Medicare and Medicaid Certified Facilities in 2001

National Total = 225,171 Facilities*

<table>
<tr><td colspan="4">ALPHA ORDER</td><td colspan="4">RANK ORDER</td></tr>
<tr><td>RANK</td><td>STATE</td><td>FACILITIES</td><td>% of USA</td><td>RANK</td><td>STATE</td><td>FACILITIES</td><td>% of USA</td></tr>
<tr><td>19</td><td>Alabama</td><td>3,876</td><td>1.7%</td><td>1</td><td>California</td><td>21,838</td><td>9.7%</td></tr>
<tr><td>49</td><td>Alaska</td><td>513</td><td>0.2%</td><td>2</td><td>Texas</td><td>18,217</td><td>8.1%</td></tr>
<tr><td>27</td><td>Arizona</td><td>3,185</td><td>1.4%</td><td>3</td><td>Florida</td><td>13,796</td><td>6.1%</td></tr>
<tr><td>31</td><td>Arkansas</td><td>2,662</td><td>1.2%</td><td>4</td><td>New York</td><td>12,309</td><td>5.5%</td></tr>
<tr><td>1</td><td>California</td><td>21,838</td><td>9.7%</td><td>5</td><td>Ohio</td><td>10,882</td><td>4.8%</td></tr>
<tr><td>30</td><td>Colorado</td><td>2,901</td><td>1.3%</td><td>6</td><td>Illinois</td><td>9,724</td><td>4.3%</td></tr>
<tr><td>28</td><td>Connecticut</td><td>3,162</td><td>1.4%</td><td>7</td><td>Pennsylvania</td><td>9,486</td><td>4.2%</td></tr>
<tr><td>47</td><td>Delaware</td><td>679</td><td>0.3%</td><td>8</td><td>Michigan</td><td>7,263</td><td>3.2%</td></tr>
<tr><td>3</td><td>Florida</td><td>13,796</td><td>6.1%</td><td>9</td><td>Georgia</td><td>6,711</td><td>3.0%</td></tr>
<tr><td>9</td><td>Georgia</td><td>6,711</td><td>3.0%</td><td>10</td><td>North Carolina</td><td>6,514</td><td>2.9%</td></tr>
<tr><td>45</td><td>Hawaii</td><td>916</td><td>0.4%</td><td>11</td><td>Indiana</td><td>6,065</td><td>2.7%</td></tr>
<tr><td>40</td><td>Idaho</td><td>1,068</td><td>0.5%</td><td>12</td><td>New Jersey</td><td>5,746</td><td>2.6%</td></tr>
<tr><td>6</td><td>Illinois</td><td>9,724</td><td>4.3%</td><td>13</td><td>Missouri</td><td>5,535</td><td>2.5%</td></tr>
<tr><td>11</td><td>Indiana</td><td>6,065</td><td>2.7%</td><td>14</td><td>Louisiana</td><td>5,053</td><td>2.2%</td></tr>
<tr><td>24</td><td>Iowa</td><td>3,491</td><td>1.6%</td><td>15</td><td>Virginia</td><td>5,018</td><td>2.2%</td></tr>
<tr><td>29</td><td>Kansas</td><td>3,158</td><td>1.4%</td><td>16</td><td>Tennessee</td><td>4,962</td><td>2.2%</td></tr>
<tr><td>26</td><td>Kentucky</td><td>3,446</td><td>1.5%</td><td>17</td><td>Massachusetts</td><td>4,547</td><td>2.0%</td></tr>
<tr><td>14</td><td>Louisiana</td><td>5,053</td><td>2.2%</td><td>18</td><td>Maryland</td><td>4,086</td><td>1.8%</td></tr>
<tr><td>37</td><td>Maine</td><td>1,316</td><td>0.6%</td><td>19</td><td>Alabama</td><td>3,876</td><td>1.7%</td></tr>
<tr><td>18</td><td>Maryland</td><td>4,086</td><td>1.8%</td><td>20</td><td>Oklahoma</td><td>3,736</td><td>1.7%</td></tr>
<tr><td>17</td><td>Massachusetts</td><td>4,547</td><td>2.0%</td><td>21</td><td>Minnesota</td><td>3,591</td><td>1.6%</td></tr>
<tr><td>8</td><td>Michigan</td><td>7,263</td><td>3.2%</td><td>22</td><td>Washington</td><td>3,539</td><td>1.6%</td></tr>
<tr><td>21</td><td>Minnesota</td><td>3,591</td><td>1.6%</td><td>23</td><td>Wisconsin</td><td>3,515</td><td>1.6%</td></tr>
<tr><td>32</td><td>Mississippi</td><td>2,580</td><td>1.1%</td><td>24</td><td>Iowa</td><td>3,491</td><td>1.6%</td></tr>
<tr><td>13</td><td>Missouri</td><td>5,535</td><td>2.5%</td><td>25</td><td>South Carolina</td><td>3,459</td><td>1.5%</td></tr>
<tr><td>43</td><td>Montana</td><td>932</td><td>0.4%</td><td>26</td><td>Kentucky</td><td>3,446</td><td>1.5%</td></tr>
<tr><td>35</td><td>Nebraska</td><td>1,795</td><td>0.8%</td><td>27</td><td>Arizona</td><td>3,185</td><td>1.4%</td></tr>
<tr><td>39</td><td>Nevada</td><td>1,155</td><td>0.5%</td><td>28</td><td>Connecticut</td><td>3,162</td><td>1.4%</td></tr>
<tr><td>41</td><td>New Hampshire</td><td>1,028</td><td>0.5%</td><td>29</td><td>Kansas</td><td>3,158</td><td>1.4%</td></tr>
<tr><td>12</td><td>New Jersey</td><td>5,746</td><td>2.6%</td><td>30</td><td>Colorado</td><td>2,901</td><td>1.3%</td></tr>
<tr><td>36</td><td>New Mexico</td><td>1,470</td><td>0.7%</td><td>31</td><td>Arkansas</td><td>2,662</td><td>1.2%</td></tr>
<tr><td>4</td><td>New York</td><td>12,309</td><td>5.5%</td><td>32</td><td>Mississippi</td><td>2,580</td><td>1.1%</td></tr>
<tr><td>10</td><td>North Carolina</td><td>6,514</td><td>2.9%</td><td>33</td><td>Oregon</td><td>2,450</td><td>1.1%</td></tr>
<tr><td>46</td><td>North Dakota</td><td>847</td><td>0.4%</td><td>34</td><td>West Virginia</td><td>2,052</td><td>0.9%</td></tr>
<tr><td>5</td><td>Ohio</td><td>10,882</td><td>4.8%</td><td>35</td><td>Nebraska</td><td>1,795</td><td>0.8%</td></tr>
<tr><td>20</td><td>Oklahoma</td><td>3,736</td><td>1.7%</td><td>36</td><td>New Mexico</td><td>1,470</td><td>0.7%</td></tr>
<tr><td>33</td><td>Oregon</td><td>2,450</td><td>1.1%</td><td>37</td><td>Maine</td><td>1,316</td><td>0.6%</td></tr>
<tr><td>7</td><td>Pennsylvania</td><td>9,486</td><td>4.2%</td><td>38</td><td>Utah</td><td>1,301</td><td>0.6%</td></tr>
<tr><td>42</td><td>Rhode Island</td><td>944</td><td>0.4%</td><td>39</td><td>Nevada</td><td>1,155</td><td>0.5%</td></tr>
<tr><td>25</td><td>South Carolina</td><td>3,459</td><td>1.5%</td><td>40</td><td>Idaho</td><td>1,068</td><td>0.5%</td></tr>
<tr><td>44</td><td>South Dakota</td><td>924</td><td>0.4%</td><td>41</td><td>New Hampshire</td><td>1,028</td><td>0.5%</td></tr>
<tr><td>16</td><td>Tennessee</td><td>4,962</td><td>2.2%</td><td>42</td><td>Rhode Island</td><td>944</td><td>0.4%</td></tr>
<tr><td>2</td><td>Texas</td><td>18,217</td><td>8.1%</td><td>43</td><td>Montana</td><td>932</td><td>0.4%</td></tr>
<tr><td>38</td><td>Utah</td><td>1,301</td><td>0.6%</td><td>44</td><td>South Dakota</td><td>924</td><td>0.4%</td></tr>
<tr><td>48</td><td>Vermont</td><td>530</td><td>0.2%</td><td>45</td><td>Hawaii</td><td>916</td><td>0.4%</td></tr>
<tr><td>15</td><td>Virginia</td><td>5,018</td><td>2.2%</td><td>46</td><td>North Dakota</td><td>847</td><td>0.4%</td></tr>
<tr><td>22</td><td>Washington</td><td>3,539</td><td>1.6%</td><td>47</td><td>Delaware</td><td>679</td><td>0.3%</td></tr>
<tr><td>34</td><td>West Virginia</td><td>2,052</td><td>0.9%</td><td>48</td><td>Vermont</td><td>530</td><td>0.2%</td></tr>
<tr><td>23</td><td>Wisconsin</td><td>3,515</td><td>1.6%</td><td>49</td><td>Alaska</td><td>513</td><td>0.2%</td></tr>
<tr><td>50</td><td>Wyoming</td><td>508</td><td>0.2%</td><td>50</td><td>Wyoming</td><td>508</td><td>0.2%</td></tr>
<tr><td></td><td></td><td></td><td></td><td></td><td>District of Columbia</td><td>690</td><td>0.3%</td></tr>
</table>

Source: U.S. Department of Health and Human Services, Health Care Financing Administration
OSCAR Report 10 (February 2, 2001)

*Certified by HCFA to participate in the Medicare/Medicaid programs. All provider groups including hospitals, home health agencies, rural health centers, community mental health centers, nursing facilities, outpatient physical therapy facilities and hospices. Also includes 168,814 laboratories. National total does not include 1,250 certified facilities in U.S. territories.

Medicare and Medicaid Certified Hospitals in 2001

National Total = 5,970 Hospitals*

ALPHA ORDER					RANK ORDER			
RANK	STATE	HOSPITALS	% of USA		RANK	STATE	HOSPITALS	% of USA
19	Alabama	123	2.1%		1	Texas	482	8.1%
47	Alaska	24	0.4%		2	California	463	7.8%
29	Arizona	84	1.4%		3	New York	266	4.5%
26	Arkansas	98	1.6%		4	Pennsylvania	253	4.2%
2	California	463	7.8%		5	Florida	235	3.9%
30	Colorado	82	1.4%		6	Illinois	218	3.7%
40	Connecticut	47	0.8%		7	Ohio	203	3.4%
50	Delaware	11	0.2%		8	Georgia	182	3.0%
5	Florida	235	3.9%		9	Louisiana	177	3.0%
8	Georgia	182	3.0%		10	Michigan	174	2.9%
45	Hawaii	27	0.5%		11	Oklahoma	151	2.5%
40	Idaho	47	0.8%		12	Indiana	150	2.5%
6	Illinois	218	3.7%		12	Minnesota	150	2.5%
12	Indiana	150	2.5%		14	Kansas	149	2.5%
20	Iowa	120	2.0%		15	Tennessee	148	2.5%
14	Kansas	149	2.5%		16	Missouri	141	2.4%
23	Kentucky	114	1.9%		17	Wisconsin	139	2.3%
9	Louisiana	177	3.0%		18	North Carolina	135	2.3%
43	Maine	41	0.7%		19	Alabama	123	2.1%
32	Maryland	67	1.1%		20	Iowa	120	2.0%
21	Massachusetts	117	2.0%		21	Massachusetts	117	2.0%
10	Michigan	174	2.9%		21	Virginia	117	2.0%
12	Minnesota	150	2.5%		23	Kentucky	114	1.9%
25	Mississippi	105	1.8%		24	New Jersey	107	1.8%
16	Missouri	141	2.4%		25	Mississippi	105	1.8%
36	Montana	62	1.0%		26	Arkansas	98	1.6%
27	Nebraska	96	1.6%		27	Nebraska	96	1.6%
42	Nevada	42	0.7%		27	Washington	96	1.6%
44	New Hampshire	30	0.5%		29	Arizona	84	1.4%
24	New Jersey	107	1.8%		30	Colorado	82	1.4%
38	New Mexico	51	0.9%		31	South Carolina	76	1.3%
3	New York	266	4.5%		32	Maryland	67	1.1%
18	North Carolina	135	2.3%		33	West Virginia	66	1.1%
37	North Dakota	52	0.9%		34	Oregon	63	1.1%
7	Ohio	203	3.4%		34	South Dakota	63	1.1%
11	Oklahoma	151	2.5%		36	Montana	62	1.0%
34	Oregon	63	1.1%		37	North Dakota	52	0.9%
4	Pennsylvania	253	4.2%		38	New Mexico	51	0.9%
48	Rhode Island	17	0.3%		39	Utah	50	0.8%
31	South Carolina	76	1.3%		40	Connecticut	47	0.8%
34	South Dakota	63	1.1%		40	Idaho	47	0.8%
15	Tennessee	148	2.5%		42	Nevada	42	0.7%
1	Texas	482	8.1%		43	Maine	41	0.7%
39	Utah	50	0.8%		44	New Hampshire	30	0.5%
49	Vermont	16	0.3%		45	Hawaii	27	0.5%
21	Virginia	117	2.0%		45	Wyoming	27	0.5%
27	Washington	96	1.6%		47	Alaska	24	0.4%
33	West Virginia	66	1.1%		48	Rhode Island	17	0.3%
17	Wisconsin	139	2.3%		49	Vermont	16	0.3%
45	Wyoming	27	0.5%		50	Delaware	11	0.2%
						District of Columbia	16	0.3%

Source: U.S. Department of Health and Human Services, Health Care Financing Administration
    OSCAR Report 10 (February 2, 2001)
*Certified by HCFA to participate in the Medicare/Medicaid programs. Excludes licensed facilities that do not accept federal funding and facilities managed by the Department of Veterans Affairs. National total does not include 62 certified hospitals in U.S. territories.

Beds in Medicare and Medicaid Certified Hospitals in 2001

National Total = 968,661 Beds*

ALPHA ORDER

RANK ORDER

RANK	STATE	BEDS	% of USA	RANK	STATE	BEDS	% of USA
17	Alabama	20,591	2.1%	1	California	83,555	8.6%
50	Alaska	1,524	0.2%	2	New York	82,121	8.5%
31	Arizona	11,304	1.2%	3	Texas	57,749	6.0%
29	Arkansas	11,982	1.2%	4	Florida	53,475	5.5%
1	California	83,555	8.6%	5	Illinois	49,477	5.1%
30	Colorado	11,436	1.2%	6	Ohio	48,187	5.0%
32	Connecticut	10,771	1.1%	7	Pennsylvania	44,165	4.6%
47	Delaware	2,325	0.2%	8	New Jersey	31,970	3.3%
4	Florida	53,475	5.5%	9	Michigan	31,902	3.3%
10	Georgia	26,438	2.7%	10	Georgia	26,438	2.7%
46	Hawaii	2,777	0.3%	11	North Carolina	26,347	2.7%
44	Idaho	2,876	0.3%	12	Missouri	26,116	2.7%
5	Illinois	49,477	5.1%	13	Tennessee	26,048	2.7%
16	Indiana	21,206	2.2%	14	Virginia	22,461	2.3%
27	Iowa	12,307	1.3%	15	Louisiana	22,110	2.3%
28	Kansas	12,103	1.2%	16	Indiana	21,206	2.2%
20	Kentucky	17,716	1.8%	17	Alabama	20,591	2.1%
15	Louisiana	22,110	2.3%	18	Massachusetts	20,220	2.1%
40	Maine	4,188	0.4%	19	Wisconsin	19,982	2.1%
22	Maryland	16,675	1.7%	20	Kentucky	17,716	1.8%
18	Massachusetts	20,220	2.1%	21	Minnesota	17,156	1.8%
9	Michigan	31,902	3.3%	22	Maryland	16,675	1.7%
21	Minnesota	17,156	1.8%	23	Oklahoma	14,661	1.5%
25	Mississippi	12,521	1.3%	24	Washington	13,888	1.4%
12	Missouri	26,116	2.7%	25	Mississippi	12,521	1.3%
45	Montana	2,864	0.3%	26	South Carolina	12,497	1.3%
35	Nebraska	6,892	0.7%	27	Iowa	12,307	1.3%
38	Nevada	4,768	0.5%	28	Kansas	12,103	1.2%
41	New Hampshire	3,442	0.4%	29	Arkansas	11,982	1.2%
8	New Jersey	31,970	3.3%	30	Colorado	11,436	1.2%
37	New Mexico	4,957	0.5%	31	Arizona	11,304	1.2%
2	New York	82,121	8.5%	32	Connecticut	10,771	1.1%
11	North Carolina	26,347	2.7%	33	West Virginia	9,674	1.0%
42	North Dakota	3,430	0.4%	34	Oregon	8,063	0.8%
6	Ohio	48,187	5.0%	35	Nebraska	6,892	0.7%
23	Oklahoma	14,661	1.5%	36	Utah	5,351	0.6%
34	Oregon	8,063	0.8%	37	New Mexico	4,957	0.5%
7	Pennsylvania	44,165	4.6%	38	Nevada	4,768	0.5%
39	Rhode Island	4,220	0.4%	39	Rhode Island	4,220	0.4%
26	South Carolina	12,497	1.3%	40	Maine	4,188	0.4%
43	South Dakota	3,341	0.3%	41	New Hampshire	3,442	0.4%
13	Tennessee	26,048	2.7%	42	North Dakota	3,430	0.4%
3	Texas	57,749	6.0%	43	South Dakota	3,341	0.3%
36	Utah	5,351	0.6%	44	Idaho	2,876	0.3%
48	Vermont	2,095	0.2%	45	Montana	2,864	0.3%
14	Virginia	22,461	2.3%	46	Hawaii	2,777	0.3%
24	Washington	13,888	1.4%	47	Delaware	2,325	0.2%
33	West Virginia	9,674	1.0%	48	Vermont	2,095	0.2%
19	Wisconsin	19,982	2.1%	49	Wyoming	1,632	0.2%
49	Wyoming	1,632	0.2%	50	Alaska	1,524	0.2%
					District of Columbia	5,105	0.5%

Source: U.S. Department of Health and Human Services, Health Care Financing Administration
OSCAR Database (February 16, 2001)

*Beds in hospitals certified by HCFA to participate in the Medicare/Medicaid programs. Excludes licensed facilities that do not accept federal funding and facilities managed by the Department of Veterans Affairs. National total does not include 11,072 beds in U.S. territories.

Medicare and Medicaid Certified Children's Hospitals in 2001

National Total = 72 Hospitals*

ALPHA ORDER

RANK ORDER

RANK	STATE	HOSPITALS	% of USA
17	Alabama	1	1.4%
33	Alaska	0	0.0%
17	Arizona	1	1.4%
17	Arkansas	1	1.4%
1	California	9	12.5%
17	Colorado	1	1.4%
17	Connecticut	1	1.4%
17	Delaware	1	1.4%
6	Florida	2	2.8%
6	Georgia	2	2.8%
17	Hawaii	1	1.4%
33	Idaho	0	0.0%
6	Illinois	2	2.8%
17	Indiana	1	1.4%
33	Iowa	0	0.0%
17	Kansas	1	1.4%
33	Kentucky	0	0.0%
17	Louisiana	1	1.4%
33	Maine	0	0.0%
6	Maryland	2	2.8%
6	Massachusetts	2	2.8%
17	Michigan	1	1.4%
5	Minnesota	3	4.2%
33	Mississippi	0	0.0%
6	Missouri	2	2.8%
33	Montana	0	0.0%
6	Nebraska	2	2.8%
33	Nevada	0	0.0%
33	New Hampshire	0	0.0%
17	New Jersey	1	1.4%
17	New Mexico	1	1.4%
17	New York	1	1.4%
33	North Carolina	0	0.0%
33	North Dakota	0	0.0%
2	Ohio	8	11.1%
6	Oklahoma	2	2.8%
33	Oregon	0	0.0%
4	Pennsylvania	5	6.9%
33	Rhode Island	0	0.0%
33	South Carolina	0	0.0%
33	South Dakota	0	0.0%
6	Tennessee	2	2.8%
2	Texas	8	11.1%
17	Utah	1	1.4%
33	Vermont	0	0.0%
6	Virginia	2	2.8%
6	Washington	2	2.8%
33	West Virginia	0	0.0%
17	Wisconsin	1	1.4%
33	Wyoming	0	0.0%

RANK	STATE	HOSPITALS	% of USA
1	California	9	12.5%
2	Ohio	8	11.1%
2	Texas	8	11.1%
4	Pennsylvania	5	6.9%
5	Minnesota	3	4.2%
6	Florida	2	2.8%
6	Georgia	2	2.8%
6	Illinois	2	2.8%
6	Maryland	2	2.8%
6	Massachusetts	2	2.8%
6	Missouri	2	2.8%
6	Nebraska	2	2.8%
6	Oklahoma	2	2.8%
6	Tennessee	2	2.8%
6	Virginia	2	2.8%
6	Washington	2	2.8%
17	Alabama	1	1.4%
17	Arizona	1	1.4%
17	Arkansas	1	1.4%
17	Colorado	1	1.4%
17	Connecticut	1	1.4%
17	Delaware	1	1.4%
17	Hawaii	1	1.4%
17	Indiana	1	1.4%
17	Kansas	1	1.4%
17	Louisiana	1	1.4%
17	Michigan	1	1.4%
17	New Jersey	1	1.4%
17	New Mexico	1	1.4%
17	New York	1	1.4%
17	Utah	1	1.4%
17	Wisconsin	1	1.4%
33	Alaska	0	0.0%
33	Idaho	0	0.0%
33	Iowa	0	0.0%
33	Kentucky	0	0.0%
33	Maine	0	0.0%
33	Mississippi	0	0.0%
33	Montana	0	0.0%
33	Nevada	0	0.0%
33	New Hampshire	0	0.0%
33	North Carolina	0	0.0%
33	North Dakota	0	0.0%
33	Oregon	0	0.0%
33	Rhode Island	0	0.0%
33	South Carolina	0	0.0%
33	South Dakota	0	0.0%
33	Vermont	0	0.0%
33	West Virginia	0	0.0%
33	Wyoming	0	0.0%
	District of Columbia	1	1.4%

Source: U.S. Department of Health and Human Services, Health Care Financing Administration
   OSCAR Report 10 (February 2, 2001)
*Certified by HCFA to participate in the Medicare/Medicaid programs. National total does not include one facility in U.S. territories. Excludes licensed facilities that do not accept federal funding and facilities managed by the Department of Veterans Affairs.

Beds in Medicare and Medicaid Certified Children's Hospitals in 2001

National Total = 11,271 Beds*

RANK	STATE	BEDS	% of USA
17	Alabama	225	2.0%
33	Alaska	0	0.0%
32	Arizona	15	0.1%
13	Arkansas	280	2.5%
2	California	1,329	11.8%
15	Colorado	253	2.2%
25	Connecticut	97	0.9%
25	Delaware	97	0.9%
9	Florida	376	3.3%
8	Georgia	400	3.5%
19	Hawaii	201	1.8%
33	Idaho	0	0.0%
10	Illinois	351	3.1%
31	Indiana	20	0.2%
33	Iowa	0	0.0%
30	Kansas	34	0.3%
33	Kentucky	0	0.0%
21	Louisiana	188	1.7%
33	Maine	0	0.0%
23	Maryland	165	1.5%
5	Massachusetts	425	3.8%
16	Michigan	228	2.0%
11	Minnesota	329	2.9%
33	Mississippi	0	0.0%
7	Missouri	402	3.6%
33	Montana	0	0.0%
24	Nebraska	150	1.3%
33	Nevada	0	0.0%
33	New Hampshire	0	0.0%
27	New Jersey	73	0.6%
29	New Mexico	37	0.3%
6	New York	405	3.6%
33	North Carolina	0	0.0%
33	North Dakota	0	0.0%
1	Ohio	1,809	16.1%
28	Oklahoma	68	0.6%
33	Oregon	0	0.0%
4	Pennsylvania	641	5.7%
33	Rhode Island	0	0.0%
33	South Carolina	0	0.0%
33	South Dakota	0	0.0%
22	Tennessee	175	1.6%
3	Texas	1,277	11.3%
20	Utah	194	1.7%
33	Vermont	0	0.0%
12	Virginia	286	2.5%
14	Washington	276	2.4%
33	West Virginia	0	0.0%
18	Wisconsin	222	2.0%
33	Wyoming	0	0.0%

RANK ORDER

RANK	STATE	BEDS	% of USA
1	Ohio	1,809	16.1%
2	California	1,329	11.8%
3	Texas	1,277	11.3%
4	Pennsylvania	641	5.7%
5	Massachusetts	425	3.8%
6	New York	405	3.6%
7	Missouri	402	3.6%
8	Georgia	400	3.5%
9	Florida	376	3.3%
10	Illinois	351	3.1%
11	Minnesota	329	2.9%
12	Virginia	286	2.5%
13	Arkansas	280	2.5%
14	Washington	276	2.4%
15	Colorado	253	2.2%
16	Michigan	228	2.0%
17	Alabama	225	2.0%
18	Wisconsin	222	2.0%
19	Hawaii	201	1.8%
20	Utah	194	1.7%
21	Louisiana	188	1.7%
22	Tennessee	175	1.6%
23	Maryland	165	1.5%
24	Nebraska	150	1.3%
25	Connecticut	97	0.9%
25	Delaware	97	0.9%
27	New Jersey	73	0.6%
28	Oklahoma	68	0.6%
29	New Mexico	37	0.3%
30	Kansas	34	0.3%
31	Indiana	20	0.2%
32	Arizona	15	0.1%
33	Alaska	0	0.0%
33	Idaho	0	0.0%
33	Iowa	0	0.0%
33	Kentucky	0	0.0%
33	Maine	0	0.0%
33	Mississippi	0	0.0%
33	Montana	0	0.0%
33	Nevada	0	0.0%
33	New Hampshire	0	0.0%
33	North Carolina	0	0.0%
33	North Dakota	0	0.0%
33	Oregon	0	0.0%
33	Rhode Island	0	0.0%
33	South Carolina	0	0.0%
33	South Dakota	0	0.0%
33	Vermont	0	0.0%
33	West Virginia	0	0.0%
33	Wyoming	0	0.0%
	District of Columbia	243	2.2%

Source: U.S. Department of Health and Human Services, Health Care Financing Administration OSCAR Database (February 16, 2001)

*Beds in hospitals certified by HCFA to participate in the Medicare/Medicaid programs. Excludes licensed facilities that do not accept federal funding and facilities managed by the Department of Veterans Affairs. National total does not include 215 beds in U.S. territories.

Medicare and Medicaid Certified Rehabilitation Hospitals in 2001

National Total = 204 Hospitals*

ALPHA ORDER

RANK ORDER

RANK	STATE	HOSPITALS	% of USA	RANK	STATE	HOSPITALS	% of USA
10	Alabama	5	2.5%	1	Texas	34	16.7%
43	Alaska	0	0.0%	2	Louisiana	19	9.3%
21	Arizona	3	1.5%	3	Pennsylvania	18	8.8%
8	Arkansas	6	2.9%	4	Florida	13	6.4%
5	California	9	4.4%	5	California	9	4.4%
25	Colorado	2	1.0%	6	Massachusetts	7	3.4%
25	Connecticut	2	1.0%	6	New Jersey	7	3.4%
31	Delaware	1	0.5%	8	Arkansas	6	2.9%
4	Florida	13	6.4%	8	West Virginia	6	2.9%
25	Georgia	2	1.0%	10	Alabama	5	2.5%
31	Hawaii	1	0.5%	10	Indiana	5	2.5%
31	Idaho	1	0.5%	10	Michigan	5	2.5%
21	Illinois	3	1.5%	10	Virginia	5	2.5%
10	Indiana	5	2.5%	14	Kansas	4	2.0%
43	Iowa	0	0.0%	14	Kentucky	4	2.0%
14	Kansas	4	2.0%	14	Nevada	4	2.0%
14	Kentucky	4	2.0%	14	New Mexico	4	2.0%
2	Louisiana	19	9.3%	14	New York	4	2.0%
31	Maine	1	0.5%	14	South Carolina	4	2.0%
25	Maryland	2	1.0%	14	Tennessee	4	2.0%
6	Massachusetts	7	3.4%	21	Arizona	3	1.5%
10	Michigan	5	2.5%	21	Illinois	3	1.5%
31	Minnesota	1	0.5%	21	Missouri	3	1.5%
31	Mississippi	1	0.5%	21	Oklahoma	3	1.5%
21	Missouri	3	1.5%	25	Colorado	2	1.0%
43	Montana	0	0.0%	25	Connecticut	2	1.0%
31	Nebraska	1	0.5%	25	Georgia	2	1.0%
14	Nevada	4	2.0%	25	Maryland	2	1.0%
25	New Hampshire	2	1.0%	25	New Hampshire	2	1.0%
6	New Jersey	7	3.4%	25	North Carolina	2	1.0%
14	New Mexico	4	2.0%	31	Delaware	1	0.5%
14	New York	4	2.0%	31	Hawaii	1	0.5%
25	North Carolina	2	1.0%	31	Idaho	1	0.5%
43	North Dakota	0	0.0%	31	Maine	1	0.5%
31	Ohio	1	0.5%	31	Minnesota	1	0.5%
21	Oklahoma	3	1.5%	31	Mississippi	1	0.5%
43	Oregon	0	0.0%	31	Nebraska	1	0.5%
3	Pennsylvania	18	8.8%	31	Ohio	1	0.5%
31	Rhode Island	1	0.5%	31	Rhode Island	1	0.5%
14	South Carolina	4	2.0%	31	Utah	1	0.5%
43	South Dakota	0	0.0%	31	Washington	1	0.5%
14	Tennessee	4	2.0%	31	Wisconsin	1	0.5%
1	Texas	34	16.7%	43	Alaska	0	0.0%
31	Utah	1	0.5%	43	Iowa	0	0.0%
43	Vermont	0	0.0%	43	Montana	0	0.0%
10	Virginia	5	2.5%	43	North Dakota	0	0.0%
31	Washington	1	0.5%	43	Oregon	0	0.0%
8	West Virginia	6	2.9%	43	South Dakota	0	0.0%
31	Wisconsin	1	0.5%	43	Vermont	0	0.0%
43	Wyoming	0	0.0%	43	Wyoming	0	0.0%
					District of Columbia	1	0.5%

Source: U.S. Department of Health and Human Services, Health Care Financing Administration
   OSCAR Report 10 (February 2, 2001)
*Certified by HCFA to participate in the Medicare/Medicaid programs. Excludes licensed facilities that do not accept federal funding and facilities managed by the Department of Veterans Affairs. National total does not include one certified hospital in U.S. territories.

Beds in Medicare and Medicaid Certified Rehabilitation Hospitals in 2001

National Total = 13,187 Beds*

ALPHA ORDER				RANK ORDER			
RANK	STATE	BEDS	% of USA	RANK	STATE	BEDS	% of USA
13	Alabama	296	2.2%	1	Texas	1,763	13.4%
43	Alaska	0	0.0%	2	Pennsylvania	1,658	12.6%
25	Arizona	165	1.3%	3	Florida	823	6.2%
7	Arkansas	452	3.4%	4	Massachusetts	739	5.6%
8	California	449	3.4%	5	New Jersey	666	5.1%
21	Colorado	202	1.5%	6	Louisiana	550	4.2%
34	Connecticut	84	0.6%	7	Arkansas	452	3.4%
38	Delaware	60	0.5%	8	California	449	3.4%
3	Florida	823	6.2%	9	New York	428	3.2%
30	Georgia	108	0.8%	10	Illinois	371	2.8%
32	Hawaii	100	0.8%	11	Indiana	349	2.6%
39	Idaho	52	0.4%	12	Michigan	315	2.4%
10	Illinois	371	2.8%	13	Alabama	296	2.2%
11	Indiana	349	2.6%	14	Tennessee	290	2.2%
43	Iowa	0	0.0%	15	Virginia	281	2.1%
16	Kansas	257	1.9%	16	Kansas	257	1.9%
17	Kentucky	248	1.9%	17	Kentucky	248	1.9%
6	Louisiana	550	4.2%	18	West Virginia	246	1.9%
32	Maine	100	0.8%	19	South Carolina	239	1.8%
37	Maryland	66	0.5%	20	North Carolina	223	1.7%
4	Massachusetts	739	5.6%	21	Colorado	202	1.5%
12	Michigan	315	2.4%	22	Nevada	185	1.4%
42	Minnesota	15	0.1%	23	Missouri	180	1.4%
28	Mississippi	124	0.9%	24	Oklahoma	167	1.3%
23	Missouri	180	1.4%	25	Arizona	165	1.3%
43	Montana	0	0.0%	26	New Hampshire	152	1.2%
41	Nebraska	40	0.3%	27	New Mexico	149	1.1%
22	Nevada	185	1.4%	28	Mississippi	124	0.9%
26	New Hampshire	152	1.2%	29	Ohio	120	0.9%
5	New Jersey	666	5.1%	30	Georgia	108	0.8%
27	New Mexico	149	1.1%	31	Washington	102	0.8%
9	New York	428	3.2%	32	Hawaii	100	0.8%
20	North Carolina	223	1.7%	32	Maine	100	0.8%
43	North Dakota	0	0.0%	34	Connecticut	84	0.6%
29	Ohio	120	0.9%	35	Rhode Island	82	0.6%
24	Oklahoma	167	1.3%	36	Wisconsin	81	0.6%
43	Oregon	0	0.0%	37	Maryland	66	0.5%
2	Pennsylvania	1,658	12.6%	38	Delaware	60	0.5%
35	Rhode Island	82	0.6%	39	Idaho	52	0.4%
19	South Carolina	239	1.8%	40	Utah	50	0.4%
43	South Dakota	0	0.0%	41	Nebraska	40	0.3%
14	Tennessee	290	2.2%	42	Minnesota	15	0.1%
1	Texas	1,763	13.4%	43	Alaska	0	0.0%
40	Utah	50	0.4%	43	Iowa	0	0.0%
43	Vermont	0	0.0%	43	Montana	0	0.0%
15	Virginia	281	2.1%	43	North Dakota	0	0.0%
31	Washington	102	0.8%	43	Oregon	0	0.0%
18	West Virginia	246	1.9%	43	South Dakota	0	0.0%
36	Wisconsin	81	0.6%	43	Vermont	0	0.0%
43	Wyoming	0	0.0%	43	Wyoming	0	0.0%
					District of Columbia	160	1.2%

Source: U.S. Department of Health and Human Services, Health Care Financing Administration
OSCAR Database (February 16, 2001)
Beds in hospitals certified by HCFA to participate in the Medicare/Medicaid programs. Excludes licensed facilities
that do not accept federal funding and facilities managed by the Department of Veterans Affairs. National total
does not include 30 beds in U.S. territories.

Medicare and Medicaid Certified Psychiatric Hospitals in 2001

National Total = 511 Psychiatric Hospitals*

ALPHA ORDER

ALPHA ORDER

RANK ORDER

RANK	STATE	HOSPITALS	% of USA
22	Alabama	9	1.8%
44	Alaska	2	0.4%
24	Arizona	8	1.6%
22	Arkansas	9	1.8%
1	California	38	7.4%
28	Colorado	6	1.2%
24	Connecticut	8	1.6%
39	Delaware	3	0.6%
4	Florida	26	5.1%
13	Georgia	15	2.9%
49	Hawaii	1	0.2%
31	Idaho	4	0.8%
7	Illinois	17	3.3%
6	Indiana	20	3.9%
31	Iowa	4	0.8%
29	Kansas	5	1.0%
16	Kentucky	12	2.3%
9	Louisiana	16	3.1%
31	Maine	4	0.8%
20	Maryland	11	2.2%
7	Massachusetts	17	3.3%
21	Michigan	10	2.0%
26	Minnesota	7	1.4%
39	Mississippi	3	0.6%
13	Missouri	15	2.9%
44	Montana	2	0.4%
31	Nebraska	4	0.8%
31	Nevada	4	0.8%
44	New Hampshire	2	0.4%
9	New Jersey	16	3.1%
39	New Mexico	3	0.6%
2	New York	35	6.8%
16	North Carolina	12	2.3%
39	North Dakota	3	0.6%
9	Ohio	16	3.1%
16	Oklahoma	12	2.3%
31	Oregon	4	0.8%
4	Pennsylvania	26	5.1%
39	Rhode Island	3	0.6%
26	South Carolina	7	1.4%
49	South Dakota	1	0.2%
16	Tennessee	12	2.3%
3	Texas	30	5.9%
31	Utah	4	0.8%
44	Vermont	2	0.4%
9	Virginia	16	3.1%
29	Washington	5	1.0%
31	West Virginia	4	0.8%
15	Wisconsin	13	2.5%
44	Wyoming	2	0.4%

RANK	STATE	HOSPITALS	% of USA
1	California	38	7.4%
2	New York	35	6.8%
3	Texas	30	5.9%
4	Florida	26	5.1%
4	Pennsylvania	26	5.1%
6	Indiana	20	3.9%
7	Illinois	17	3.3%
7	Massachusetts	17	3.3%
9	Louisiana	16	3.1%
9	New Jersey	16	3.1%
9	Ohio	16	3.1%
9	Virginia	16	3.1%
13	Georgia	15	2.9%
13	Missouri	15	2.9%
15	Wisconsin	13	2.5%
16	Kentucky	12	2.3%
16	North Carolina	12	2.3%
16	Oklahoma	12	2.3%
16	Tennessee	12	2.3%
20	Maryland	11	2.2%
21	Michigan	10	2.0%
22	Alabama	9	1.8%
22	Arkansas	9	1.8%
24	Arizona	8	1.6%
24	Connecticut	8	1.6%
26	Minnesota	7	1.4%
26	South Carolina	7	1.4%
28	Colorado	6	1.2%
29	Kansas	5	1.0%
29	Washington	5	1.0%
31	Idaho	4	0.8%
31	Iowa	4	0.8%
31	Maine	4	0.8%
31	Nebraska	4	0.8%
31	Nevada	4	0.8%
31	Oregon	4	0.8%
31	Utah	4	0.8%
31	West Virginia	4	0.8%
39	Delaware	3	0.6%
39	Mississippi	3	0.6%
39	New Mexico	3	0.6%
39	North Dakota	3	0.6%
39	Rhode Island	3	0.6%
44	Alaska	2	0.4%
44	Montana	2	0.4%
44	New Hampshire	2	0.4%
44	Vermont	2	0.4%
44	Wyoming	2	0.4%
49	Hawaii	1	0.2%
49	South Dakota	1	0.2%
	District of Columbia	3	0.6%

Source: U.S. Department of Health and Human Services, Health Care Financing Administration
    OSCAR Report 10 (February 2, 2001)
Certified by HCFA to participate in the Medicare/Medicaid programs. Excludes licensed facilities that do not accept federal funding and facilities managed by the Department of Veterans Affairs. National total does not include four certified psychiatric hospitals in U.S. territories.

Beds in Medicare and Medicaid Certified Psychiatric Hospitals in 2001

National Total = 67,944 Beds*

ALPHA ORDER

RANK	STATE	BEDS	% of USA
29	Alabama	693	1.0%
45	Alaska	188	0.3%
31	Arizona	539	0.8%
27	Arkansas	803	1.2%
6	California	2,746	4.0%
24	Colorado	991	1.5%
22	Connecticut	1,127	1.7%
40	Delaware	241	0.4%
9	Florida	2,007	3.0%
10	Georgia	1,979	2.9%
48	Hawaii	88	0.1%
46	Idaho	145	0.2%
12	Illinois	1,730	2.5%
20	Indiana	1,266	1.9%
34	Iowa	363	0.5%
28	Kansas	716	1.1%
13	Kentucky	1,656	2.4%
11	Louisiana	1,841	2.7%
37	Maine	344	0.5%
5	Maryland	2,750	4.0%
18	Massachusetts	1,312	1.9%
7	Michigan	2,432	3.6%
17	Minnesota	1,368	2.0%
41	Mississippi	233	0.3%
23	Missouri	1,033	1.5%
50	Montana	30	0.0%
30	Nebraska	626	0.9%
36	Nevada	353	0.5%
38	New Hampshire	323	0.5%
4	New Jersey	2,918	4.3%
39	New Mexico	245	0.4%
1	New York	12,568	18.5%
3	North Carolina	3,035	4.5%
43	North Dakota	217	0.3%
16	Ohio	1,500	2.2%
25	Oklahoma	844	1.2%
35	Oregon	362	0.5%
2	Pennsylvania	5,310	7.8%
42	Rhode Island	219	0.3%
26	South Carolina	831	1.2%
47	South Dakota	133	0.2%
19	Tennessee	1,293	1.9%
8	Texas	2,355	3.5%
33	Utah	474	0.7%
44	Vermont	205	0.3%
14	Virginia	1,564	2.3%
21	Washington	1,142	1.7%
32	West Virginia	485	0.7%
15	Wisconsin	1,508	2.2%
49	Wyoming	80	0.1%

RANK ORDER

RANK	STATE	BEDS	% of USA
1	New York	12,568	18.5%
2	Pennsylvania	5,310	7.8%
3	North Carolina	3,035	4.5%
4	New Jersey	2,918	4.3%
5	Maryland	2,750	4.0%
6	California	2,746	4.0%
7	Michigan	2,432	3.6%
8	Texas	2,355	3.5%
9	Florida	2,007	3.0%
10	Georgia	1,979	2.9%
11	Louisiana	1,841	2.7%
12	Illinois	1,730	2.5%
13	Kentucky	1,656	2.4%
14	Virginia	1,564	2.3%
15	Wisconsin	1,508	2.2%
16	Ohio	1,500	2.2%
17	Minnesota	1,368	2.0%
18	Massachusetts	1,312	1.9%
19	Tennessee	1,293	1.9%
20	Indiana	1,266	1.9%
21	Washington	1,142	1.7%
22	Connecticut	1,127	1.7%
23	Missouri	1,033	1.5%
24	Colorado	991	1.5%
25	Oklahoma	844	1.2%
26	South Carolina	831	1.2%
27	Arkansas	803	1.2%
28	Kansas	716	1.1%
29	Alabama	693	1.0%
30	Nebraska	626	0.9%
31	Arizona	539	0.8%
32	West Virginia	485	0.7%
33	Utah	474	0.7%
34	Iowa	363	0.5%
35	Oregon	362	0.5%
36	Nevada	353	0.5%
37	Maine	344	0.5%
38	New Hampshire	323	0.5%
39	New Mexico	245	0.4%
40	Delaware	241	0.4%
41	Mississippi	233	0.3%
42	Rhode Island	219	0.3%
43	North Dakota	217	0.3%
44	Vermont	205	0.3%
45	Alaska	188	0.3%
46	Idaho	145	0.2%
47	South Dakota	133	0.2%
48	Hawaii	88	0.1%
49	Wyoming	80	0.1%
50	Montana	30	0.0%
	District of Columbia	733	1.1%

Source: U.S. Department of Health and Human Services, Health Care Financing Administration
  OSCAR Database (February 16, 2001)
*Beds in hospitals certified by HCFA to participate in the Medicare/Medicaid programs. Excludes licensed facilities
that do not accept federal funding and facilities managed by the Department of Veterans Affairs. National total
does not include 903 beds in U.S. territories.

Medicare and Medicaid Certified Community Mental Health Centers in 2001

National Total = 757 Centers*

ALPHA ORDER

RANK	STATE	CENTERS	% of USA
2	Alabama	78	10.3%
44	Alaska	0	0.0%
33	Arizona	4	0.5%
17	Arkansas	14	1.8%
11	California	21	2.8%
17	Colorado	14	1.8%
30	Connecticut	5	0.7%
44	Delaware	0	0.0%
1	Florida	111	14.7%
25	Georgia	9	1.2%
44	Hawaii	0	0.0%
44	Idaho	0	0.0%
13	Illinois	19	2.5%
22	Indiana	11	1.5%
23	Iowa	10	1.3%
14	Kansas	18	2.4%
17	Kentucky	14	1.8%
4	Louisiana	39	5.2%
34	Maine	3	0.4%
29	Maryland	6	0.8%
15	Massachusetts	16	2.1%
23	Michigan	10	1.3%
20	Minnesota	13	1.7%
30	Mississippi	5	0.7%
11	Missouri	21	2.8%
38	Montana	2	0.3%
42	Nebraska	1	0.1%
38	Nevada	2	0.3%
38	New Hampshire	2	0.3%
4	New Jersey	39	5.2%
16	New Mexico	15	2.0%
25	New York	9	1.2%
7	North Carolina	27	3.6%
44	North Dakota	0	0.0%
8	Ohio	24	3.2%
25	Oklahoma	9	1.2%
21	Oregon	12	1.6%
9	Pennsylvania	23	3.0%
44	Rhode Island	0	0.0%
28	South Carolina	7	0.9%
38	South Dakota	2	0.3%
10	Tennessee	22	2.9%
3	Texas	76	10.0%
34	Utah	3	0.4%
44	Vermont	0	0.0%
30	Virginia	5	0.7%
6	Washington	29	3.8%
34	West Virginia	3	0.4%
42	Wisconsin	1	0.1%
34	Wyoming	3	0.4%

RANK ORDER

RANK	STATE	CENTERS	% of USA
1	Florida	111	14.7%
2	Alabama	78	10.3%
3	Texas	76	10.0%
4	Louisiana	39	5.2%
4	New Jersey	39	5.2%
6	Washington	29	3.8%
7	North Carolina	27	3.6%
8	Ohio	24	3.2%
9	Pennsylvania	23	3.0%
10	Tennessee	22	2.9%
11	California	21	2.8%
11	Missouri	21	2.8%
13	Illinois	19	2.5%
14	Kansas	18	2.4%
15	Massachusetts	16	2.1%
16	New Mexico	15	2.0%
17	Arkansas	14	1.8%
17	Colorado	14	1.8%
17	Kentucky	14	1.8%
20	Minnesota	13	1.7%
21	Oregon	12	1.6%
22	Indiana	11	1.5%
23	Iowa	10	1.3%
23	Michigan	10	1.3%
25	Georgia	9	1.2%
25	New York	9	1.2%
25	Oklahoma	9	1.2%
28	South Carolina	7	0.9%
29	Maryland	6	0.8%
30	Connecticut	5	0.7%
30	Mississippi	5	0.7%
30	Virginia	5	0.7%
33	Arizona	4	0.5%
34	Maine	3	0.4%
34	Utah	3	0.4%
34	West Virginia	3	0.4%
34	Wyoming	3	0.4%
38	Montana	2	0.3%
38	Nevada	2	0.3%
38	New Hampshire	2	0.3%
38	South Dakota	2	0.3%
42	Nebraska	1	0.1%
42	Wisconsin	1	0.1%
44	Alaska	0	0.0%
44	Delaware	0	0.0%
44	Hawaii	0	0.0%
44	Idaho	0	0.0%
44	North Dakota	0	0.0%
44	Rhode Island	0	0.0%
44	Vermont	0	0.0%
	District of Columbia	0	0.0%

Source: U.S. Department of Health and Human Services, Health Care Financing Administration
OSCAR Report 10 (February 2, 2001)
Certified by HCFA to participate in the Medicare/Medicaid programs. Excludes licensed facilities that do not accept federal funding and facilities managed by the Department of Veterans Affairs. National total does not include nine certified mental health centers in U.S. territories.

Medicare and Medicaid Certified Outpatient Physical Therapy Facilities in 2001

National Total = 2,881 Facilities*

ALPHA ORDER

RANK	STATE	FACILITIES	% of USA
34	Alabama	20	0.7%
36	Alaska	16	0.6%
26	Arizona	36	1.2%
28	Arkansas	31	1.1%
2	California	231	8.0%
20	Colorado	51	1.8%
24	Connecticut	38	1.3%
33	Delaware	21	0.7%
1	Florida	252	8.7%
7	Georgia	126	4.4%
40	Hawaii	11	0.4%
38	Idaho	12	0.4%
12	Illinois	84	2.9%
16	Indiana	58	2.0%
24	Iowa	38	1.3%
31	Kansas	27	0.9%
14	Kentucky	62	2.2%
19	Louisiana	55	1.9%
32	Maine	22	0.8%
10	Maryland	90	3.1%
36	Massachusetts	16	0.6%
4	Michigan	202	7.0%
17	Minnesota	57	2.0%
23	Mississippi	46	1.6%
15	Missouri	61	2.1%
42	Montana	10	0.3%
42	Nebraska	10	0.3%
38	Nevada	12	0.4%
40	New Hampshire	11	0.4%
9	New Jersey	103	3.6%
27	New Mexico	34	1.2%
29	New York	28	1.0%
22	North Carolina	49	1.7%
47	North Dakota	5	0.2%
5	Ohio	134	4.7%
21	Oklahoma	50	1.7%
35	Oregon	19	0.7%
6	Pennsylvania	132	4.6%
48	Rhode Island	4	0.1%
17	South Carolina	57	2.0%
48	South Dakota	4	0.1%
11	Tennessee	89	3.1%
2	Texas	231	8.0%
44	Utah	9	0.3%
50	Vermont	2	0.1%
8	Virginia	113	3.9%
29	Washington	28	1.0%
45	West Virginia	6	0.2%
13	Wisconsin	70	2.4%
45	Wyoming	6	0.2%

RANK ORDER

RANK	STATE	FACILITIES	% of USA
1	Florida	252	8.7%
2	California	231	8.0%
2	Texas	231	8.0%
4	Michigan	202	7.0%
5	Ohio	134	4.7%
6	Pennsylvania	132	4.6%
7	Georgia	126	4.4%
8	Virginia	113	3.9%
9	New Jersey	103	3.6%
10	Maryland	90	3.1%
11	Tennessee	89	3.1%
12	Illinois	84	2.9%
13	Wisconsin	70	2.4%
14	Kentucky	62	2.2%
15	Missouri	61	2.1%
16	Indiana	58	2.0%
17	Minnesota	57	2.0%
17	South Carolina	57	2.0%
19	Louisiana	55	1.9%
20	Colorado	51	1.8%
21	Oklahoma	50	1.7%
22	North Carolina	49	1.7%
23	Mississippi	46	1.6%
24	Connecticut	38	1.3%
24	Iowa	38	1.3%
26	Arizona	36	1.2%
27	New Mexico	34	1.2%
28	Arkansas	31	1.1%
29	New York	28	1.0%
29	Washington	28	1.0%
31	Kansas	27	0.9%
32	Maine	22	0.8%
33	Delaware	21	0.7%
34	Alabama	20	0.7%
35	Oregon	19	0.7%
36	Alaska	16	0.6%
36	Massachusetts	16	0.6%
38	Idaho	12	0.4%
38	Nevada	12	0.4%
40	Hawaii	11	0.4%
40	New Hampshire	11	0.4%
42	Montana	10	0.3%
42	Nebraska	10	0.3%
44	Utah	9	0.3%
45	West Virginia	6	0.2%
45	Wyoming	6	0.2%
47	North Dakota	5	0.2%
48	Rhode Island	4	0.1%
48	South Dakota	4	0.1%
50	Vermont	2	0.1%
	District of Columbia	2	0.1%

Source: U.S. Department of Health and Human Services, Health Care Financing Administration
   OSCAR Report 10 (February 2, 2001)
*Certified by HCFA to participate in the Medicare/Medicaid programs. Excludes licensed facilities that do not accept federal funding and facilities managed by the Department of Veterans Affairs. National total does not include two certified outpatient physical therapy facilities in U.S. territories.

Medicare and Medicaid Certified Rural Health Clinics in 2001

National Total = 3,344 Rural Health Clinics*

ALPHA ORDER

RANK	STATE	CLINICS	% of USA
23	Alabama	57	1.7%
40	Alaska	11	0.3%
42	Arizona	8	0.2%
13	Arkansas	80	2.4%
2	California	226	6.8%
29	Colorado	44	1.3%
46	Connecticut	0	0.0%
46	Delaware	0	0.0%
7	Florida	133	4.0%
11	Georgia	120	3.6%
44	Hawaii	1	0.0%
30	Idaho	35	1.0%
3	Illinois	196	5.9%
25	Indiana	53	1.6%
8	Iowa	132	3.9%
5	Kansas	155	4.6%
16	Kentucky	74	2.2%
28	Louisiana	49	1.5%
26	Maine	52	1.6%
46	Maryland	0	0.0%
46	Massachusetts	0	0.0%
6	Michigan	153	4.6%
21	Minnesota	60	1.8%
8	Mississippi	132	3.9%
4	Missouri	163	4.9%
32	Montana	32	1.0%
15	Nebraska	76	2.3%
43	Nevada	2	0.1%
35	New Hampshire	21	0.6%
46	New Jersey	0	0.0%
39	New Mexico	14	0.4%
41	New York	10	0.3%
10	North Carolina	123	3.7%
13	North Dakota	80	2.4%
36	Ohio	19	0.6%
20	Oklahoma	61	1.8%
33	Oregon	29	0.9%
27	Pennsylvania	51	1.5%
44	Rhode Island	1	0.0%
12	South Carolina	96	2.9%
24	South Dakota	55	1.6%
31	Tennessee	33	1.0%
1	Texas	394	11.8%
38	Utah	15	0.4%
34	Vermont	23	0.7%
22	Virginia	59	1.8%
19	Washington	64	1.9%
17	West Virginia	69	2.1%
18	Wisconsin	65	1.9%
37	Wyoming	18	0.5%

RANK ORDER

RANK	STATE	CLINICS	% of USA
1	Texas	394	11.8%
2	California	226	6.8%
3	Illinois	196	5.9%
4	Missouri	163	4.9%
5	Kansas	155	4.6%
6	Michigan	153	4.6%
7	Florida	133	4.0%
8	Iowa	132	3.9%
8	Mississippi	132	3.9%
10	North Carolina	123	3.7%
11	Georgia	120	3.6%
12	South Carolina	96	2.9%
13	Arkansas	80	2.4%
13	North Dakota	80	2.4%
15	Nebraska	76	2.3%
16	Kentucky	74	2.2%
17	West Virginia	69	2.1%
18	Wisconsin	65	1.9%
19	Washington	64	1.9%
20	Oklahoma	61	1.8%
21	Minnesota	60	1.8%
22	Virginia	59	1.8%
23	Alabama	57	1.7%
24	South Dakota	55	1.6%
25	Indiana	53	1.6%
26	Maine	52	1.6%
27	Pennsylvania	51	1.5%
28	Louisiana	49	1.5%
29	Colorado	44	1.3%
30	Idaho	35	1.0%
31	Tennessee	33	1.0%
32	Montana	32	1.0%
33	Oregon	29	0.9%
34	Vermont	23	0.7%
35	New Hampshire	21	0.6%
36	Ohio	19	0.6%
37	Wyoming	18	0.5%
38	Utah	15	0.4%
39	New Mexico	14	0.4%
40	Alaska	11	0.3%
41	New York	10	0.3%
42	Arizona	8	0.2%
43	Nevada	2	0.1%
44	Hawaii	1	0.0%
44	Rhode Island	1	0.0%
46	Connecticut	0	0.0%
46	Delaware	0	0.0%
46	Maryland	0	0.0%
46	Massachusetts	0	0.0%
46	New Jersey	0	0.0%
	District of Columbia	0	0.0%

Source: U.S. Department of Health and Human Services, Health Care Financing Administration
OSCAR Report 10 (February 2, 2001)

Certified by HCFA to participate in the Medicare/Medicaid programs. Excludes licensed facilities that do not accept federal funding and facilities managed by the Department of Veterans Affairs. There are no certified rural health centers in U.S. territories.

Medicare and Medicaid Certified Home Health Agencies in 2001

National Total = 7,084 Home Health Agencies*

ALPHA ORDER

RANK	STATE	AGENCIES	% of USA
19	Alabama	143	2.0%
48	Alaska	16	0.2%
30	Arizona	67	0.9%
12	Arkansas	182	2.6%
2	California	578	8.2%
22	Colorado	131	1.8%
26	Connecticut	81	1.1%
48	Delaware	16	0.2%
5	Florida	320	4.5%
25	Georgia	98	1.4%
47	Hawaii	19	0.3%
37	Idaho	53	0.7%
6	Illinois	290	4.1%
13	Indiana	179	2.5%
13	Iowa	179	2.5%
19	Kansas	143	2.0%
24	Kentucky	111	1.6%
7	Louisiana	253	3.6%
42	Maine	36	0.5%
35	Maryland	54	0.8%
21	Massachusetts	132	1.9%
10	Michigan	194	2.7%
8	Minnesota	250	3.5%
32	Mississippi	61	0.9%
15	Missouri	170	2.4%
38	Montana	51	0.7%
28	Nebraska	70	1.0%
42	Nevada	36	0.5%
44	New Hampshire	35	0.5%
35	New Jersey	54	0.8%
30	New Mexico	67	0.9%
9	New York	211	3.0%
17	North Carolina	163	2.3%
44	North Dakota	35	0.5%
3	Ohio	350	4.9%
11	Oklahoma	188	2.7%
34	Oregon	60	0.8%
4	Pennsylvania	326	4.6%
46	Rhode Island	24	0.3%
27	South Carolina	76	1.1%
39	South Dakota	46	0.6%
18	Tennessee	153	2.2%
1	Texas	847	12.0%
40	Utah	42	0.6%
50	Vermont	13	0.2%
16	Virginia	164	2.3%
32	Washington	61	0.9%
29	West Virginia	69	1.0%
22	Wisconsin	131	1.8%
41	Wyoming	39	0.6%

RANK ORDER

RANK	STATE	AGENCIES	% of USA
1	Texas	847	12.0%
2	California	578	8.2%
3	Ohio	350	4.9%
4	Pennsylvania	326	4.6%
5	Florida	320	4.5%
6	Illinois	290	4.1%
7	Louisiana	253	3.6%
8	Minnesota	250	3.5%
9	New York	211	3.0%
10	Michigan	194	2.7%
11	Oklahoma	188	2.7%
12	Arkansas	182	2.6%
13	Indiana	179	2.5%
13	Iowa	179	2.5%
15	Missouri	170	2.4%
16	Virginia	164	2.3%
17	North Carolina	163	2.3%
18	Tennessee	153	2.2%
19	Alabama	143	2.0%
19	Kansas	143	2.0%
21	Massachusetts	132	1.9%
22	Colorado	131	1.8%
22	Wisconsin	131	1.8%
24	Kentucky	111	1.6%
25	Georgia	98	1.4%
26	Connecticut	81	1.1%
27	South Carolina	76	1.1%
28	Nebraska	70	1.0%
29	West Virginia	69	1.0%
30	Arizona	67	0.9%
30	New Mexico	67	0.9%
32	Mississippi	61	0.9%
32	Washington	61	0.9%
34	Oregon	60	0.8%
35	Maryland	54	0.8%
35	New Jersey	54	0.8%
37	Idaho	53	0.7%
38	Montana	51	0.7%
39	South Dakota	46	0.6%
40	Utah	42	0.6%
41	Wyoming	39	0.6%
42	Maine	36	0.5%
42	Nevada	36	0.5%
44	New Hampshire	35	0.5%
44	North Dakota	35	0.5%
46	Rhode Island	24	0.3%
47	Hawaii	19	0.3%
48	Alaska	16	0.2%
48	Delaware	16	0.2%
50	Vermont	13	0.2%
	District of Columbia	17	0.2%

Source: U.S. Department of Health and Human Services, Health Care Financing Administration
OSCAR Report 10 (February 2, 2001)

Certified by HCFA to participate in the Medicare/Medicaid programs. Excludes agencies that do not accept federal funding. National total does not include 49 certified home health agencies in U.S. territories. A home health agency provides health services to individuals in their homes for the purpose of promoting, maintaining or restoring health or maximizing the level of independence, while minimizing the effects of disability and illness.

Medicare and Medicaid Certified Hospices in 2001

National Total = 2,249 Hospices*

ALPHA ORDER

RANK	STATE	HOSPICES	% of USA
10	Alabama	69	3.1%
50	Alaska	2	0.1%
26	Arizona	35	1.6%
19	Arkansas	47	2.1%
1	California	175	7.8%
26	Colorado	35	1.6%
33	Connecticut	28	1.2%
49	Delaware	5	0.2%
24	Florida	40	1.8%
7	Georgia	79	3.5%
46	Hawaii	7	0.3%
36	Idaho	25	1.1%
5	Illinois	87	3.9%
12	Indiana	63	2.8%
14	Iowa	61	2.7%
26	Kansas	35	1.6%
35	Kentucky	26	1.2%
21	Louisiana	43	1.9%
41	Maine	16	0.7%
30	Maryland	30	1.3%
23	Massachusetts	41	1.8%
6	Michigan	83	3.7%
12	Minnesota	63	2.8%
20	Mississippi	44	2.0%
11	Missouri	66	2.9%
37	Montana	21	0.9%
31	Nebraska	29	1.3%
46	Nevada	7	0.3%
39	New Hampshire	19	0.8%
24	New Jersey	40	1.8%
33	New Mexico	28	1.2%
15	New York	54	2.4%
9	North Carolina	74	3.3%
43	North Dakota	15	0.7%
4	Ohio	96	4.3%
8	Oklahoma	76	3.4%
22	Oregon	42	1.9%
3	Pennsylvania	115	5.1%
46	Rhode Island	7	0.3%
29	South Carolina	32	1.4%
43	South Dakota	15	0.7%
18	Tennessee	48	2.1%
2	Texas	125	5.6%
39	Utah	19	0.8%
45	Vermont	9	0.4%
17	Virginia	50	2.2%
31	Washington	29	1.3%
38	West Virginia	20	0.9%
15	Wisconsin	54	2.4%
41	Wyoming	16	0.7%

RANK ORDER

RANK	STATE	HOSPICES	% of USA
1	California	175	7.8%
2	Texas	125	5.6%
3	Pennsylvania	115	5.1%
4	Ohio	96	4.3%
5	Illinois	87	3.9%
6	Michigan	83	3.7%
7	Georgia	79	3.5%
8	Oklahoma	76	3.4%
9	North Carolina	74	3.3%
10	Alabama	69	3.1%
11	Missouri	66	2.9%
12	Indiana	63	2.8%
12	Minnesota	63	2.8%
14	Iowa	61	2.7%
15	New York	54	2.4%
15	Wisconsin	54	2.4%
17	Virginia	50	2.2%
18	Tennessee	48	2.1%
19	Arkansas	47	2.1%
20	Mississippi	44	2.0%
21	Louisiana	43	1.9%
22	Oregon	42	1.9%
23	Massachusetts	41	1.8%
24	Florida	40	1.8%
24	New Jersey	40	1.8%
26	Arizona	35	1.6%
26	Colorado	35	1.6%
26	Kansas	35	1.6%
29	South Carolina	32	1.4%
30	Maryland	30	1.3%
31	Nebraska	29	1.3%
31	Washington	29	1.3%
33	Connecticut	28	1.2%
33	New Mexico	28	1.2%
35	Kentucky	26	1.2%
36	Idaho	25	1.1%
37	Montana	21	0.9%
38	West Virginia	20	0.9%
39	New Hampshire	19	0.8%
39	Utah	19	0.8%
41	Maine	16	0.7%
41	Wyoming	16	0.7%
43	North Dakota	15	0.7%
43	South Dakota	15	0.7%
45	Vermont	9	0.4%
46	Hawaii	7	0.3%
46	Nevada	7	0.3%
46	Rhode Island	7	0.3%
49	Delaware	5	0.2%
50	Alaska	2	0.1%
	District of Columbia	4	0.2%

Source: U.S. Department of Health and Human Services, Health Care Financing Administration
    OSCAR Report 10 (February 2, 2001)
*Certified by HCFA to participate in the Medicare/Medicaid programs. Excludes licensed facilities that do not accept federal funding and facilities managed by the Department of Veterans Affairs. National total does not include 32 certified hospices in U.S. territories. An hospice provides specialized services for terminally ill people and their families.

Hospice Patients in Residential Facilities in 2001

National Total = 20,232 Patients*

ALPHA ORDER

RANK ORDER

RANK	STATE	PATIENTS	% of USA		RANK	STATE	PATIENTS	% of USA
26	Alabama	150	0.7%		1	Pennsylvania	4,101	20.3%
48	Alaska	0	0.0%		2	Florida	2,371	11.7%
19	Arizona	276	1.4%		3	Texas	1,321	6.5%
31	Arkansas	104	0.5%		4	Michigan	1,302	6.4%
6	California	887	4.4%		5	Ohio	1,071	5.3%
18	Colorado	303	1.5%		6	California	887	4.4%
30	Connecticut	132	0.7%		7	Illinois	884	4.4%
44	Delaware	7	0.0%		8	Indiana	868	4.3%
2	Florida	2,371	11.7%		9	Oklahoma	804	4.0%
12	Georgia	510	2.5%		10	Missouri	534	2.6%
46	Hawaii	3	0.0%		11	New York	528	2.6%
43	Idaho	12	0.1%		12	Georgia	510	2.5%
7	Illinois	884	4.4%		13	Washington	444	2.2%
8	Indiana	868	4.3%		14	Kansas	380	1.9%
22	Iowa	240	1.2%		15	Oregon	353	1.7%
14	Kansas	380	1.9%		16	Kentucky	306	1.5%
16	Kentucky	306	1.5%		16	Wisconsin	306	1.5%
29	Louisiana	136	0.7%		18	Colorado	303	1.5%
39	Maine	28	0.1%		19	Arizona	276	1.4%
25	Maryland	165	0.8%		20	New Jersey	263	1.3%
23	Massachusetts	239	1.2%		21	North Carolina	250	1.2%
4	Michigan	1,302	6.4%		22	Iowa	240	1.2%
27	Minnesota	146	0.7%		23	Massachusetts	239	1.2%
33	Mississippi	57	0.3%		24	Nebraska	173	0.9%
10	Missouri	534	2.6%		25	Maryland	165	0.8%
38	Montana	35	0.2%		26	Alabama	150	0.7%
24	Nebraska	173	0.9%		27	Minnesota	146	0.7%
34	Nevada	50	0.2%		28	South Carolina	144	0.7%
48	New Hampshire	0	0.0%		29	Louisiana	136	0.7%
20	New Jersey	263	1.3%		30	Connecticut	132	0.7%
39	New Mexico	28	0.1%		31	Arkansas	104	0.5%
11	New York	528	2.6%		32	Tennessee	97	0.5%
21	North Carolina	250	1.2%		33	Mississippi	57	0.3%
35	North Dakota	42	0.2%		34	Nevada	50	0.2%
5	Ohio	1,071	5.3%		35	North Dakota	42	0.2%
9	Oklahoma	804	4.0%		36	Vermont	38	0.2%
15	Oregon	353	1.7%		37	Utah	37	0.2%
1	Pennsylvania	4,101	20.3%		38	Montana	35	0.2%
48	Rhode Island	0	0.0%		39	Maine	28	0.1%
28	South Carolina	144	0.7%		39	New Mexico	28	0.1%
45	South Dakota	4	0.0%		39	Virginia	28	0.1%
32	Tennessee	97	0.5%		42	West Virginia	26	0.1%
3	Texas	1,321	6.5%		43	Idaho	12	0.1%
37	Utah	37	0.2%		44	Delaware	7	0.0%
36	Vermont	38	0.2%		45	South Dakota	4	0.0%
39	Virginia	28	0.1%		46	Hawaii	3	0.0%
13	Washington	444	2.2%		46	Wyoming	3	0.0%
42	West Virginia	26	0.1%		48	Alaska	0	0.0%
16	Wisconsin	306	1.5%		48	New Hampshire	0	0.0%
46	Wyoming	3	0.0%		48	Rhode Island	0	0.0%
						District of Columbia	46	0.2%

Source: U.S. Department of Health and Human Services, Health Care Financing Administration
   OSCAR Database (February 16, 2001)
*Patients in facilities certified by HCFA to participate in the Medicare/Medicaid programs. Excludes licensed facilities that do not accept federal funding and facilities managed by the Department of Veterans Affairs. National total does not include seven patients in U.S. territories. An hospice provides specialized services for terminally ill people and their families.

Medicare and Medicaid Certified Nursing Care Facilities in 2001

National Total = 16,894 Nursing Care Facilities*

ALPHA ORDER

RANK ORDER

RANK	STATE	FACILITIES	% of USA	RANK	STATE	FACILITIES	% of USA
29	Alabama	225	1.3%	1	California	1,367	8.1%
50	Alaska	15	0.1%	2	Texas	1,209	7.2%
34	Arizona	146	0.9%	3	Ohio	1,011	6.0%
26	Arkansas	256	1.5%	4	Illinois	868	5.1%
1	California	1,367	8.1%	5	Pennsylvania	768	4.5%
29	Colorado	225	1.3%	6	Florida	729	4.3%
25	Connecticut	259	1.5%	7	New York	664	3.9%
47	Delaware	43	0.3%	8	Indiana	567	3.4%
6	Florida	729	4.3%	9	Missouri	554	3.3%
19	Georgia	361	2.1%	10	Massachusetts	524	3.1%
46	Hawaii	45	0.3%	11	Iowa	470	2.8%
42	Idaho	84	0.5%	12	Michigan	436	2.6%
4	Illinois	868	5.1%	13	Minnesota	432	2.6%
8	Indiana	567	3.4%	14	Wisconsin	421	2.5%
11	Iowa	470	2.8%	15	North Carolina	415	2.5%
17	Kansas	390	2.3%	16	Oklahoma	392	2.3%
22	Kentucky	305	1.8%	17	Kansas	390	2.3%
21	Louisiana	337	2.0%	18	New Jersey	362	2.1%
36	Maine	126	0.7%	19	Georgia	361	2.1%
27	Maryland	255	1.5%	20	Tennessee	354	2.1%
10	Massachusetts	524	3.1%	21	Louisiana	337	2.0%
12	Michigan	436	2.6%	22	Kentucky	305	1.8%
13	Minnesota	432	2.6%	23	Virginia	286	1.7%
31	Mississippi	198	1.2%	24	Washington	277	1.6%
9	Missouri	554	3.3%	25	Connecticut	259	1.5%
38	Montana	104	0.6%	26	Arkansas	256	1.5%
28	Nebraska	236	1.4%	27	Maryland	255	1.5%
45	Nevada	51	0.3%	28	Nebraska	236	1.4%
43	New Hampshire	83	0.5%	29	Alabama	225	1.3%
18	New Jersey	362	2.1%	29	Colorado	225	1.3%
44	New Mexico	80	0.5%	31	Mississippi	198	1.2%
7	New York	664	3.9%	32	South Carolina	178	1.1%
15	North Carolina	415	2.5%	33	Oregon	149	0.9%
41	North Dakota	88	0.5%	34	Arizona	146	0.9%
3	Ohio	1,011	6.0%	35	West Virginia	140	0.8%
16	Oklahoma	392	2.3%	36	Maine	126	0.7%
33	Oregon	149	0.9%	37	South Dakota	114	0.7%
5	Pennsylvania	768	4.5%	38	Montana	104	0.6%
39	Rhode Island	99	0.6%	39	Rhode Island	99	0.6%
32	South Carolina	178	1.1%	40	Utah	93	0.6%
37	South Dakota	114	0.7%	41	North Dakota	88	0.5%
20	Tennessee	354	2.1%	42	Idaho	84	0.5%
2	Texas	1,209	7.2%	43	New Hampshire	83	0.5%
40	Utah	93	0.6%	44	New Mexico	80	0.5%
47	Vermont	43	0.3%	45	Nevada	51	0.3%
23	Virginia	286	1.7%	46	Hawaii	45	0.3%
24	Washington	277	1.6%	47	Delaware	43	0.3%
35	West Virginia	140	0.8%	47	Vermont	43	0.3%
14	Wisconsin	421	2.5%	49	Wyoming	40	0.2%
49	Wyoming	40	0.2%	50	Alaska	15	0.1%
					District of Columbia	20	0.1%

Source: U.S. Department of Health and Human Services, Health Care Financing Administration
    OSCAR Report 10 (February 2, 2001)
*Certified by HCFA to participate in the Medicare/Medicaid programs. Excludes licensed facilities that do not accept federal funding and facilities managed by the Department of Veterans Affairs. National total does not include nine certified nursing facilities in U.S. territories.

Beds in Medicare and Medicaid Certified Nursing Care Facilities in 2001

National Total = 1,721,387 Beds*

ALPHA ORDER				RANK ORDER			
RANK	STATE	BEDS	% of USA	RANK	STATE	BEDS	% of USA
24	Alabama	25,181	1.5%	1	California	126,369	7.3%
50	Alaska	729	0.0%	2	New York	119,929	7.0%
33	Arizona	16,858	1.0%	3	Texas	111,778	6.5%
25	Arkansas	25,049	1.5%	4	Illinois	100,298	5.8%
1	California	126,369	7.3%	5	Pennsylvania	94,473	5.5%
29	Colorado	19,576	1.1%	6	Ohio	93,058	5.4%
21	Connecticut	31,542	1.8%	7	Florida	80,709	4.7%
46	Delaware	4,472	0.3%	8	Indiana	55,143	3.2%
7	Florida	80,709	4.7%	9	Massachusetts	55,066	3.2%
16	Georgia	39,669	2.3%	10	New Jersey	51,514	3.0%
47	Hawaii	3,963	0.2%	11	Missouri	50,408	2.9%
44	Idaho	6,234	0.4%	12	Michigan	48,079	2.8%
4	Illinois	100,298	5.8%	13	Wisconsin	46,457	2.7%
8	Indiana	55,143	3.2%	14	Minnesota	41,245	2.4%
19	Iowa	34,614	2.0%	15	North Carolina	41,179	2.4%
27	Kansas	24,938	1.4%	16	Georgia	39,669	2.3%
28	Kentucky	24,681	1.4%	17	Tennessee	38,355	2.2%
18	Louisiana	37,622	2.2%	18	Louisiana	37,622	2.2%
37	Maine	8,195	0.5%	19	Iowa	34,614	2.0%
23	Maryland	29,542	1.7%	20	Oklahoma	33,079	1.9%
9	Massachusetts	55,066	3.2%	21	Connecticut	31,542	1.8%
12	Michigan	48,079	2.8%	22	Virginia	30,429	1.8%
14	Minnesota	41,245	2.4%	23	Maryland	29,542	1.7%
30	Mississippi	17,582	1.0%	24	Alabama	25,181	1.5%
11	Missouri	50,408	2.9%	25	Arkansas	25,049	1.5%
40	Montana	7,642	0.4%	26	Washington	25,028	1.5%
32	Nebraska	16,995	1.0%	27	Kansas	24,938	1.4%
45	Nevada	5,519	0.3%	28	Kentucky	24,681	1.4%
38	New Hampshire	7,794	0.5%	29	Colorado	19,576	1.1%
10	New Jersey	51,514	3.0%	30	Mississippi	17,582	1.0%
43	New Mexico	6,860	0.4%	31	South Carolina	17,268	1.0%
2	New York	119,929	7.0%	32	Nebraska	16,995	1.0%
15	North Carolina	41,179	2.4%	33	Arizona	16,858	1.0%
42	North Dakota	6,954	0.4%	34	Oregon	12,674	0.7%
6	Ohio	93,058	5.4%	35	West Virginia	11,363	0.7%
20	Oklahoma	33,079	1.9%	36	Rhode Island	10,057	0.6%
34	Oregon	12,674	0.7%	37	Maine	8,195	0.5%
5	Pennsylvania	94,473	5.5%	38	New Hampshire	7,794	0.5%
36	Rhode Island	10,057	0.6%	39	South Dakota	7,723	0.4%
31	South Carolina	17,268	1.0%	40	Montana	7,642	0.4%
39	South Dakota	7,723	0.4%	41	Utah	7,626	0.4%
17	Tennessee	38,355	2.2%	42	North Dakota	6,954	0.4%
3	Texas	111,778	6.5%	43	New Mexico	6,860	0.4%
41	Utah	7,626	0.4%	44	Idaho	6,234	0.4%
48	Vermont	3,702	0.2%	45	Nevada	5,519	0.3%
22	Virginia	30,429	1.8%	46	Delaware	4,472	0.3%
26	Washington	25,028	1.5%	47	Hawaii	3,963	0.2%
35	West Virginia	11,363	0.7%	48	Vermont	3,702	0.2%
13	Wisconsin	46,457	2.7%	49	Wyoming	3,111	0.2%
49	Wyoming	3,111	0.2%	50	Alaska	729	0.0%
					District of Columbia	3,056	0.2%

Source: U.S. Department of Health and Human Services, Health Care Financing Administration
OSCAR Database (February 16, 2001)
*Beds in nursing care facilities certified by HCFA to participate in the Medicare/Medicaid programs. National total does not include 340 beds in U.S. territories.

Rate of Beds in Medicare and Medicaid Certified Nursing Care Facilities in 2001

National Rate = 412 Beds per 1,000 Population 85 Years and Older*

ALPHA ORDER

RANK	STATE	RATE
31	Alabama	388
44	Alaska	304
47	Arizona	256
4	Arkansas	563
46	California	298
28	Colorado	411
9	Connecticut	499
24	Delaware	441
48	Florida	252
22	Georgia	465
49	Hawaii	229
40	Idaho	348
7	Illinois	521
2	Indiana	611
5	Iowa	537
16	Kansas	483
26	Kentucky	430
1	Louisiana	673
36	Maine	369
23	Maryland	445
19	Massachusetts	477
42	Michigan	333
13	Minnesota	488
27	Mississippi	428
8	Missouri	514
9	Montana	499
11	Nebraska	495
41	Nevada	338
25	New Hampshire	436
33	New Jersey	386
43	New Mexico	317
32	New York	387
30	North Carolina	393
21	North Dakota	471
6	Ohio	527
3	Oklahoma	578
50	Oregon	225
29	Pennsylvania	407
20	Rhode Island	476
35	South Carolina	370
14	South Dakota	486
14	Tennessee	486
18	Texas	479
39	Utah	355
34	Vermont	382
37	Virginia	362
45	Washington	303
38	West Virginia	356
12	Wisconsin	491
17	Wyoming	481

RANK ORDER

RANK	STATE	RATE
1	Louisiana	673
2	Indiana	611
3	Oklahoma	578
4	Arkansas	563
5	Iowa	537
6	Ohio	527
7	Illinois	521
8	Missouri	514
9	Connecticut	499
9	Montana	499
11	Nebraska	495
12	Wisconsin	491
13	Minnesota	488
14	South Dakota	486
14	Tennessee	486
16	Kansas	483
17	Wyoming	481
18	Texas	479
19	Massachusetts	477
20	Rhode Island	476
21	North Dakota	471
22	Georgia	465
23	Maryland	445
24	Delaware	441
25	New Hampshire	436
26	Kentucky	430
27	Mississippi	428
28	Colorado	411
29	Pennsylvania	407
30	North Carolina	393
31	Alabama	388
32	New York	387
33	New Jersey	386
34	Vermont	382
35	South Carolina	370
36	Maine	369
37	Virginia	362
38	West Virginia	356
39	Utah	355
40	Idaho	348
41	Nevada	338
42	Michigan	333
43	New Mexico	317
44	Alaska	304
45	Washington	303
46	California	298
47	Arizona	256
48	Florida	252
49	Hawaii	229
50	Oregon	225

District of Columbia 331

Source: Morgan Quitno Press using data from U.S. Dept. of Health & Human Services, Health Care Financing Admin.
OSCAR Database (February 16, 2001)
*Beds in nursing care facilities certified by HCFA to participate in the Medicare/Medicaid programs. National rate does not include beds or population in U.S. territories. Calculated using 1999 Census population estimates.

Nursing Home Occupancy Rate in 1998

National Rate = 83.5% of Beds in Nursing Homes Occupied

ALPHA ORDER

RANK	STATE	RATE
5	Alabama	92.5
44	Alaska	76.3
42	Arizona	77.5
40	Arkansas	78.3
34	California	81.2
28	Colorado	83.8
10	Connecticut	91.6
46	Delaware	74.7
29	Florida	83.4
8	Georgia	92.2
9	Hawaii	92.0
45	Idaho	75.7
41	Illinois	77.8
49	Indiana	71.2
36	Iowa	80.2
35	Kansas	81.0
20	Kentucky	89.1
36	Louisiana	80.2
23	Maine	86.4
31	Maryland	82.4
19	Massachusetts	89.5
24	Michigan	85.4
11	Minnesota	91.3
2	Mississippi	93.1
47	Missouri	72.8
33	Montana	81.8
25	Nebraska	84.9
30	Nevada	83.2
7	New Hampshire	92.4
13	New Jersey	90.9
26	New Mexico	84.2
1	New York	94.4
5	North Carolina	92.5
3	North Dakota	92.9
38	Ohio	79.5
48	Oklahoma	72.6
39	Oregon	79.1
17	Pennsylvania	89.8
14	Rhode Island	90.3
22	South Carolina	87.1
4	South Dakota	92.8
18	Tennessee	89.7
50	Texas	68.5
43	Utah	77.4
16	Vermont	90.0
15	Virginia	90.2
32	Washington	82.1
12	West Virginia	91.2
21	Wisconsin	87.5
27	Wyoming	83.9

RANK ORDER

RANK	STATE	RATE
1	New York	94.4
2	Mississippi	93.1
3	North Dakota	92.9
4	South Dakota	92.8
5	Alabama	92.5
5	North Carolina	92.5
7	New Hampshire	92.4
8	Georgia	92.2
9	Hawaii	92.0
10	Connecticut	91.6
11	Minnesota	91.3
12	West Virginia	91.2
13	New Jersey	90.9
14	Rhode Island	90.3
15	Virginia	90.2
16	Vermont	90.0
17	Pennsylvania	89.8
18	Tennessee	89.7
19	Massachusetts	89.5
20	Kentucky	89.1
21	Wisconsin	87.5
22	South Carolina	87.1
23	Maine	86.4
24	Michigan	85.4
25	Nebraska	84.9
26	New Mexico	84.2
27	Wyoming	83.9
28	Colorado	83.8
29	Florida	83.4
30	Nevada	83.2
31	Maryland	82.4
32	Washington	82.1
33	Montana	81.8
34	California	81.2
35	Kansas	81.0
36	Iowa	80.2
36	Louisiana	80.2
38	Ohio	79.5
39	Oregon	79.1
40	Arkansas	78.3
41	Illinois	77.8
42	Arizona	77.5
43	Utah	77.4
44	Alaska	76.3
45	Idaho	75.7
46	Delaware	74.7
47	Missouri	72.8
48	Oklahoma	72.6
49	Indiana	71.2
50	Texas	68.5
	District of Columbia	95.0

Source: U.S. Department of Health and Human Services, Health Care Financing Administration
"Health, United States, 2000"

Nursing Home Resident Rate in 1998

National Rate = 373.6 Residents per 1,000 Population Age 85 and Older*

ALPHA ORDER

RANK	STATE	RATE
33	Alabama	363.4
44	Alaska	273.4
48	Arizona	218.7
8	Arkansas	462.3
45	California	265.9
29	Colorado	373.1
4	Connecticut	489.9
25	Delaware	396.1
47	Florida	221.9
17	Georgia	442.1
49	Hawaii	217.4
42	Idaho	283.1
14	Illinois	458.6
3	Indiana	496.8
6	Iowa	477.6
15	Kansas	456.0
24	Kentucky	400.8
1	Louisiana	551.2
32	Maine	364.3
23	Maryland	405.8
9	Massachusetts	462.0
39	Michigan	316.0
2	Minnesota	499.2
26	Mississippi	394.5
22	Missouri	415.8
19	Montana	423.7
10	Nebraska	461.1
46	Nevada	244.3
21	New Hampshire	420.9
35	New Jersey	358.9
40	New Mexico	294.1
30	New York	370.8
31	North Carolina	366.7
11	North Dakota	459.4
5	Ohio	485.0
18	Oklahoma	441.6
50	Oregon	206.8
27	Pennsylvania	387.5
12	Rhode Island	459.1
37	South Carolina	339.6
7	South Dakota	477.5
13	Tennessee	458.9
28	Texas	385.4
43	Utah	283.0
34	Vermont	362.9
36	Virginia	340.7
41	Washington	283.8
38	West Virginia	332.8
16	Wisconsin	450.9
20	Wyoming	422.9

RANK ORDER

RANK	STATE	RATE
1	Louisiana	551.2
2	Minnesota	499.2
3	Indiana	496.8
4	Connecticut	489.9
5	Ohio	485.0
6	Iowa	477.6
7	South Dakota	477.5
8	Arkansas	462.3
9	Massachusetts	462.0
10	Nebraska	461.1
11	North Dakota	459.4
12	Rhode Island	459.1
13	Tennessee	458.9
14	Illinois	458.6
15	Kansas	456.0
16	Wisconsin	450.9
17	Georgia	442.1
18	Oklahoma	441.6
19	Montana	423.7
20	Wyoming	422.9
21	New Hampshire	420.9
22	Missouri	415.8
23	Maryland	405.8
24	Kentucky	400.8
25	Delaware	396.1
26	Mississippi	394.5
27	Pennsylvania	387.5
28	Texas	385.4
29	Colorado	373.1
30	New York	370.8
31	North Carolina	366.7
32	Maine	364.3
33	Alabama	363.4
34	Vermont	362.9
35	New Jersey	358.9
36	Virginia	340.7
37	South Carolina	339.6
38	West Virginia	332.8
39	Michigan	316.0
40	New Mexico	294.1
41	Washington	283.8
42	Idaho	283.1
43	Utah	283.0
44	Alaska	273.4
45	California	265.9
46	Nevada	244.3
47	Florida	221.9
48	Arizona	218.7
49	Hawaii	217.4
50	Oregon	206.8
	District of Columbia	324.5

Source: U.S. Department of Health and Human Services, Health Care Financing Administration
    "Health, United States, 2000"
*Number of nursing home residents (all ages) per 1,000 resident population 85 years of age and over.

Nursing Home Population 85 Years Old and Older in 1998

National Total = 1,513,000*

ALPHA ORDER

RANK	STATE	POPULATION	% of USA
24	Alabama	23,000	1.5%
50	Alaska	1,000	0.1%
33	Arizona	14,000	0.9%
28	Arkansas	20,000	1.3%
2	California	109,000	7.2%
29	Colorado	17,000	1.1%
18	Connecticut	30,000	2.0%
45	Delaware	4,000	0.3%
7	Florida	68,000	4.5%
16	Georgia	36,000	2.4%
45	Hawaii	4,000	0.3%
44	Idaho	5,000	0.3%
5	Illinois	86,000	5.7%
10	Indiana	44,000	2.9%
18	Iowa	30,000	2.0%
24	Kansas	23,000	1.5%
24	Kentucky	23,000	1.5%
18	Louisiana	30,000	2.0%
37	Maine	8,000	0.5%
22	Maryland	26,000	1.7%
8	Massachusetts	52,000	3.4%
10	Michigan	44,000	2.9%
13	Minnesota	41,000	2.7%
30	Mississippi	16,000	1.1%
14	Missouri	40,000	2.6%
41	Montana	6,000	0.4%
30	Nebraska	16,000	1.1%
45	Nevada	4,000	0.3%
38	New Hampshire	7,000	0.5%
9	New Jersey	46,000	3.0%
41	New Mexico	6,000	0.4%
1	New York	112,000	7.4%
15	North Carolina	37,000	2.4%
38	North Dakota	7,000	0.5%
6	Ohio	83,000	5.5%
23	Oklahoma	25,000	1.7%
34	Oregon	11,000	0.7%
3	Pennsylvania	87,000	5.8%
36	Rhode Island	9,000	0.6%
32	South Carolina	15,000	1.0%
38	South Dakota	7,000	0.5%
17	Tennessee	35,000	2.3%
3	Texas	87,000	5.8%
41	Utah	6,000	0.4%
48	Vermont	3,000	0.2%
21	Virginia	28,000	1.9%
27	Washington	22,000	1.5%
35	West Virginia	10,000	0.7%
12	Wisconsin	42,000	2.8%
48	Wyoming	3,000	0.2%

RANK ORDER

RANK	STATE	POPULATION	% of USA
1	New York	112,000	7.4%
2	California	109,000	7.2%
3	Pennsylvania	87,000	5.8%
3	Texas	87,000	5.8%
5	Illinois	86,000	5.7%
6	Ohio	83,000	5.5%
7	Florida	68,000	4.5%
8	Massachusetts	52,000	3.4%
9	New Jersey	46,000	3.0%
10	Indiana	44,000	2.9%
10	Michigan	44,000	2.9%
12	Wisconsin	42,000	2.8%
13	Minnesota	41,000	2.7%
14	Missouri	40,000	2.6%
15	North Carolina	37,000	2.4%
16	Georgia	36,000	2.4%
17	Tennessee	35,000	2.3%
18	Connecticut	30,000	2.0%
18	Iowa	30,000	2.0%
18	Louisiana	30,000	2.0%
21	Virginia	28,000	1.9%
22	Maryland	26,000	1.7%
23	Oklahoma	25,000	1.7%
24	Alabama	23,000	1.5%
24	Kansas	23,000	1.5%
24	Kentucky	23,000	1.5%
27	Washington	22,000	1.5%
28	Arkansas	20,000	1.3%
29	Colorado	17,000	1.1%
30	Mississippi	16,000	1.1%
30	Nebraska	16,000	1.1%
32	South Carolina	15,000	1.0%
33	Arizona	14,000	0.9%
34	Oregon	11,000	0.7%
35	West Virginia	10,000	0.7%
36	Rhode Island	9,000	0.6%
37	Maine	8,000	0.5%
38	New Hampshire	7,000	0.5%
38	North Dakota	7,000	0.5%
38	South Dakota	7,000	0.5%
41	Montana	6,000	0.4%
41	New Mexico	6,000	0.4%
41	Utah	6,000	0.4%
44	Idaho	5,000	0.3%
45	Delaware	4,000	0.3%
45	Hawaii	4,000	0.3%
45	Nevada	4,000	0.3%
48	Vermont	3,000	0.2%
48	Wyoming	3,000	0.2%
50	Alaska	1,000	0.1%
	District of Columbia	3,000	0.2%

Source: Morgan Quitno Press using data from U.S. Dept. of Health & Human Services, Health Care Financing Admin. "Health, United States, 2000"

Estimated using nursing home resident rate and population 85 years old and older.

Health Care Establishments in 1998

National Total = 524,910 Establishments*

ALPHA ORDER

RANK	STATE	ESTABLISH'S	% of USA
27	Alabama	6,717	1.3%
48	Alaska	1,202	0.2%
20	Arizona	9,022	1.7%
32	Arkansas	4,571	0.9%
1	California	67,407	12.8%
21	Colorado	8,428	1.6%
24	Connecticut	7,390	1.4%
46	Delaware	1,377	0.3%
4	Florida	34,651	6.6%
10	Georgia	13,001	2.5%
40	Hawaii	2,455	0.5%
41	Idaho	2,428	0.5%
6	Illinois	21,273	4.1%
16	Indiana	10,008	1.9%
30	Iowa	5,346	1.0%
31	Kansas	4,935	0.9%
26	Kentucky	6,734	1.3%
22	Louisiana	8,105	1.5%
39	Maine	2,823	0.5%
15	Maryland	10,672	2.0%
11	Massachusetts	12,869	2.5%
8	Michigan	19,006	3.6%
23	Minnesota	8,101	1.5%
33	Mississippi	3,848	0.7%
18	Missouri	9,900	1.9%
44	Montana	1,954	0.4%
38	Nebraska	2,909	0.6%
36	Nevada	3,251	0.6%
42	New Hampshire	2,278	0.4%
9	New Jersey	18,571	3.5%
37	New Mexico	2,997	0.6%
2	New York	37,909	7.2%
12	North Carolina	12,029	2.3%
49	North Dakota	1,073	0.2%
7	Ohio	20,868	4.0%
28	Oklahoma	6,645	1.3%
25	Oregon	7,295	1.4%
5	Pennsylvania	25,748	4.9%
43	Rhode Island	2,199	0.4%
29	South Carolina	5,867	1.1%
45	South Dakota	1,411	0.3%
17	Tennessee	9,917	1.9%
3	Texas	36,315	6.9%
34	Utah	3,824	0.7%
47	Vermont	1,267	0.2%
14	Virginia	11,459	2.2%
13	Washington	11,505	2.2%
35	West Virginia	3,559	0.7%
19	Wisconsin	9,235	1.8%
50	Wyoming	1,020	0.2%

RANK ORDER

RANK	STATE	ESTABLISH'S	% of USA
1	California	67,407	12.8%
2	New York	37,909	7.2%
3	Texas	36,315	6.9%
4	Florida	34,651	6.6%
5	Pennsylvania	25,748	4.9%
6	Illinois	21,273	4.1%
7	Ohio	20,868	4.0%
8	Michigan	19,006	3.6%
9	New Jersey	18,571	3.5%
10	Georgia	13,001	2.5%
11	Massachusetts	12,869	2.5%
12	North Carolina	12,029	2.3%
13	Washington	11,505	2.2%
14	Virginia	11,459	2.2%
15	Maryland	10,672	2.0%
16	Indiana	10,008	1.9%
17	Tennessee	9,917	1.9%
18	Missouri	9,900	1.9%
19	Wisconsin	9,235	1.8%
20	Arizona	9,022	1.7%
21	Colorado	8,428	1.6%
22	Louisiana	8,105	1.5%
23	Minnesota	8,101	1.5%
24	Connecticut	7,390	1.4%
25	Oregon	7,295	1.4%
26	Kentucky	6,734	1.3%
27	Alabama	6,717	1.3%
28	Oklahoma	6,645	1.3%
29	South Carolina	5,867	1.1%
30	Iowa	5,346	1.0%
31	Kansas	4,935	0.9%
32	Arkansas	4,571	0.9%
33	Mississippi	3,848	0.7%
34	Utah	3,824	0.7%
35	West Virginia	3,559	0.7%
36	Nevada	3,251	0.6%
37	New Mexico	2,997	0.6%
38	Nebraska	2,909	0.6%
39	Maine	2,823	0.5%
40	Hawaii	2,455	0.5%
41	Idaho	2,428	0.5%
42	New Hampshire	2,278	0.4%
43	Rhode Island	2,199	0.4%
44	Montana	1,954	0.4%
45	South Dakota	1,411	0.3%
46	Delaware	1,377	0.3%
47	Vermont	1,267	0.2%
48	Alaska	1,202	0.2%
49	North Dakota	1,073	0.2%
50	Wyoming	1,020	0.2%
	District of Columbia	1,491	0.3%

Source: U.S. Bureau of the Census
    "County Business Patterns 1998 (NACIS)" (http://tier2.census.gov/cbp_naics/index.html)
*Includes establishments exempt from as well as subject to the federal income tax. Includes those establishments within the North American Industry Classification System (NACIS) classifications 621 (ambulatory health care services), 622 (hospitals) and 623 (nursing and residential care facilities).

236

Offices and Clinics of Doctors of Medicine in 1997

National Total = 185,094 Establishments*

ALPHA ORDER					RANK ORDER			
RANK	STATE	ESTABLISH'S	% of USA		RANK	STATE	ESTABLISH'S	% of USA
21	Alabama	2,694	1.5%		1	California	24,079	13.0%
47	Alaska	356	0.2%		2	New York	15,137	8.2%
17	Arizona	3,269	1.8%		3	Texas	14,041	7.6%
29	Arkansas	1,645	0.9%		4	Florida	13,784	7.4%
1	California	24,079	13.0%		5	Pennsylvania	9,078	4.9%
23	Colorado	2,586	1.4%		6	New Jersey	7,644	4.1%
22	Connecticut	2,661	1.4%		7	Ohio	7,573	4.1%
45	Delaware	572	0.3%		8	Illinois	7,440	4.0%
4	Florida	13,784	7.4%		9	Michigan	6,234	3.4%
10	Georgia	5,081	2.7%		10	Georgia	5,081	2.7%
37	Hawaii	1,022	0.6%		11	Maryland	4,343	2.3%
42	Idaho	752	0.4%		12	Virginia	4,277	2.3%
8	Illinois	7,440	4.0%		13	North Carolina	3,858	2.1%
16	Indiana	3,387	1.8%		14	Massachusetts	3,844	2.1%
34	Iowa	1,283	0.7%		15	Tennessee	3,620	2.0%
32	Kansas	1,368	0.7%		16	Indiana	3,387	1.8%
24	Kentucky	2,474	1.3%		17	Arizona	3,269	1.8%
20	Louisiana	3,051	1.6%		18	Missouri	3,160	1.7%
39	Maine	838	0.5%		19	Washington	3,058	1.7%
11	Maryland	4,343	2.3%		20	Louisiana	3,051	1.6%
14	Massachusetts	3,844	2.1%		21	Alabama	2,694	1.5%
9	Michigan	6,234	3.4%		22	Connecticut	2,661	1.4%
36	Minnesota	1,217	0.7%		23	Colorado	2,586	1.4%
30	Mississippi	1,520	0.8%		24	Kentucky	2,474	1.3%
18	Missouri	3,160	1.7%		25	South Carolina	2,216	1.2%
44	Montana	586	0.3%		26	Wisconsin	2,198	1.2%
40	Nebraska	774	0.4%		27	Oklahoma	2,189	1.2%
33	Nevada	1,335	0.7%		28	Oregon	2,040	1.1%
43	New Hampshire	656	0.4%		29	Arkansas	1,645	0.9%
6	New Jersey	7,644	4.1%		30	Mississippi	1,520	0.8%
38	New Mexico	941	0.5%		31	West Virginia	1,415	0.8%
2	New York	15,137	8.2%		32	Kansas	1,368	0.7%
13	North Carolina	3,858	2.1%		33	Nevada	1,335	0.7%
50	North Dakota	191	0.1%		34	Iowa	1,283	0.7%
7	Ohio	7,573	4.1%		35	Utah	1,219	0.7%
27	Oklahoma	2,189	1.2%		36	Minnesota	1,217	0.7%
28	Oregon	2,040	1.1%		37	Hawaii	1,022	0.6%
5	Pennsylvania	9,078	4.9%		38	New Mexico	941	0.5%
41	Rhode Island	764	0.4%		39	Maine	838	0.5%
25	South Carolina	2,216	1.2%		40	Nebraska	774	0.4%
49	South Dakota	332	0.2%		41	Rhode Island	764	0.4%
15	Tennessee	3,620	2.0%		42	Idaho	752	0.4%
3	Texas	14,041	7.6%		43	New Hampshire	656	0.4%
35	Utah	1,219	0.7%		44	Montana	586	0.3%
46	Vermont	360	0.2%		45	Delaware	572	0.3%
12	Virginia	4,277	2.3%		46	Vermont	360	0.2%
19	Washington	3,058	1.7%		47	Alaska	356	0.2%
31	West Virginia	1,415	0.8%		48	Wyoming	345	0.2%
26	Wisconsin	2,198	1.2%		49	South Dakota	332	0.2%
48	Wyoming	345	0.2%		50	North Dakota	191	0.1%
						District of Columbia	587	0.3%

Source: U.S. Bureau of the Census
   "1997 Economic Census, Health Care and Social Assistance" (EC97562A, October 1999)
*Includes only establishments subject to the federal income tax.

Offices and Clinics of Dentists in 1997

National Total = 114,178 Establishments*

ALPHA ORDER

RANK	STATE	ESTABLISH'S	% of USA
27	Alabama	1,356	1.2%
45	Alaska	292	0.3%
24	Arizona	1,641	1.4%
33	Arkansas	898	0.8%
1	California	16,269	14.2%
20	Colorado	2,042	1.8%
22	Connecticut	1,774	1.6%
49	Delaware	218	0.2%
4	Florida	6,182	5.4%
13	Georgia	2,547	2.3%
36	Hawaii	657	0.6%
41	Idaho	502	0.4%
6	Illinois	5,383	4.7%
16	Indiana	2,208	1.9%
30	Iowa	1,113	1.0%
32	Kansas	1,012	0.9%
26	Kentucky	1,516	1.3%
25	Louisiana	1,541	1.3%
42	Maine	462	0.4%
14	Maryland	2,371	2.1%
10	Massachusetts	2,929	2.6%
8	Michigan	4,352	3.8%
21	Minnesota	2,002	1.8%
34	Mississippi	780	0.7%
18	Missouri	2,052	1.8%
43	Montana	419	0.4%
35	Nebraska	754	0.7%
38	Nevada	575	0.5%
40	New Hampshire	533	0.5%
9	New Jersey	4,272	3.7%
39	New Mexico	557	0.5%
2	New York	8,694	7.6%
15	North Carolina	2,323	2.0%
48	North Dakota	246	0.2%
7	Ohio	4,519	4.0%
28	Oklahoma	1,268	1.1%
23	Oregon	1,680	1.5%
5	Pennsylvania	5,433	4.8%
44	Rhode Island	410	0.4%
29	South Carolina	1,216	1.1%
46	South Dakota	267	0.2%
19	Tennessee	2,050	1.8%
3	Texas	6,691	5.9%
31	Utah	1,088	1.0%
47	Vermont	256	0.2%
12	Virginia	2,645	2.3%
11	Washington	2,827	2.5%
37	West Virginia	588	0.5%
17	Wisconsin	2,203	1.9%
50	Wyoming	209	0.2%

RANK ORDER

RANK	STATE	ESTABLISH'S	% of USA
1	California	16,269	14.2%
2	New York	8,694	7.6%
3	Texas	6,691	5.9%
4	Florida	6,182	5.4%
5	Pennsylvania	5,433	4.8%
6	Illinois	5,383	4.7%
7	Ohio	4,519	4.0%
8	Michigan	4,352	3.8%
9	New Jersey	4,272	3.7%
10	Massachusetts	2,929	2.6%
11	Washington	2,827	2.5%
12	Virginia	2,645	2.3%
13	Georgia	2,574	2.3%
14	Maryland	2,371	2.1%
15	North Carolina	2,323	2.0%
16	Indiana	2,208	1.9%
17	Wisconsin	2,203	1.9%
18	Missouri	2,052	1.8%
19	Tennessee	2,050	1.8%
20	Colorado	2,042	1.8%
21	Minnesota	2,002	1.8%
22	Connecticut	1,774	1.6%
23	Oregon	1,680	1.5%
24	Arizona	1,641	1.4%
25	Louisiana	1,541	1.3%
26	Kentucky	1,516	1.3%
27	Alabama	1,356	1.2%
28	Oklahoma	1,268	1.1%
29	South Carolina	1,216	1.1%
30	Iowa	1,113	1.0%
31	Utah	1,088	1.0%
32	Kansas	1,012	0.9%
33	Arkansas	898	0.8%
34	Mississippi	780	0.7%
35	Nebraska	754	0.7%
36	Hawaii	657	0.6%
37	West Virginia	588	0.5%
38	Nevada	575	0.5%
39	New Mexico	557	0.5%
40	New Hampshire	533	0.5%
41	Idaho	502	0.4%
42	Maine	462	0.4%
43	Montana	419	0.4%
44	Rhode Island	410	0.4%
45	Alaska	292	0.3%
46	South Dakota	267	0.2%
47	Vermont	256	0.2%
48	North Dakota	246	0.2%
49	Delaware	218	0.2%
50	Wyoming	209	0.2%
	District of Columbia	329	0.3%

Source: U.S. Bureau of the Census
   "1997 Economic Census, Health Care and Social Assistance" (EC97562A, October 1999)
*Includes only establishments subject to the federal income tax.

IV. FINANCE

IV. FINANCE (Continued)

Personal Health Care Expenditures in 1998

National Total = $1,016,383,000,000*

ALPHA ORDER

RANK	STATE	EXPENDITURES	% of USA
22	Alabama	$16,056,000,000	1.6%
48	Alaska	2,299,000,000	0.2%
24	Arizona	14,782,000,000	1.5%
33	Arkansas	8,463,000,000	0.8%
1	California	110,057,000,000	10.8%
26	Colorado	13,669,000,000	1.3%
23	Connecticut	15,221,000,000	1.5%
44	Delaware	3,106,000,000	0.3%
4	Florida	59,724,000,000	5.9%
12	Georgia	27,219,000,000	2.7%
40	Hawaii	4,658,000,000	0.5%
43	Idaho	3,397,000,000	0.3%
6	Illinois	44,305,000,000	4.4%
15	Indiana	21,259,000,000	2.1%
30	Iowa	10,198,000,000	1.0%
31	Kansas	9,394,000,000	0.9%
25	Kentucky	14,414,000,000	1.4%
21	Louisiana	16,500,000,000	1.6%
39	Maine	4,925,000,000	0.5%
19	Maryland	19,646,000,000	1.9%
10	Massachusetts	30,039,000,000	3.0%
8	Michigan	35,647,000,000	3.5%
17	Minnesota	20,313,000,000	2.0%
32	Mississippi	8,882,000,000	0.9%
16	Missouri	20,911,000,000	2.1%
46	Montana	2,838,000,000	0.3%
35	Nebraska	6,095,000,000	0.6%
37	Nevada	5,606,000,000	0.6%
40	New Hampshire	4,658,000,000	0.5%
9	New Jersey	32,695,000,000	3.2%
38	New Mexico	5,344,000,000	0.5%
2	New York	85,785,000,000	8.4%
11	North Carolina	27,327,000,000	2.7%
47	North Dakota	2,680,000,000	0.3%
7	Ohio	42,581,000,000	4.2%
28	Oklahoma	10,988,000,000	1.1%
29	Oregon	10,840,000,000	1.1%
5	Pennsylvania	51,322,000,000	5.0%
42	Rhode Island	4,515,000,000	0.4%
27	South Carolina	13,204,000,000	1.3%
45	South Dakota	2,842,000,000	0.3%
14	Tennessee	22,021,000,000	2.2%
3	Texas	67,750,000,000	6.7%
36	Utah	5,944,000,000	0.6%
49	Vermont	2,066,000,000	0.2%
13	Virginia	22,261,000,000	2.2%
20	Washington	19,292,000,000	1.9%
34	West Virginia	7,037,000,000	0.7%
18	Wisconsin	19,945,000,000	2.0%
50	Wyoming	1,407,000,000	0.1%

RANK ORDER

RANK	STATE	EXPENDITURES	% of USA
1	California	$110,057,000,000	10.8%
2	New York	85,785,000,000	8.4%
3	Texas	67,750,000,000	6.7%
4	Florida	59,724,000,000	5.9%
5	Pennsylvania	51,322,000,000	5.0%
6	Illinois	44,305,000,000	4.4%
7	Ohio	42,581,000,000	4.2%
8	Michigan	35,647,000,000	3.5%
9	New Jersey	32,695,000,000	3.2%
10	Massachusetts	30,039,000,000	3.0%
11	North Carolina	27,327,000,000	2.7%
12	Georgia	27,219,000,000	2.7%
13	Virginia	22,261,000,000	2.2%
14	Tennessee	22,021,000,000	2.2%
15	Indiana	21,259,000,000	2.1%
16	Missouri	20,911,000,000	2.1%
17	Minnesota	20,313,000,000	2.0%
18	Wisconsin	19,945,000,000	2.0%
19	Maryland	19,646,000,000	1.9%
20	Washington	19,292,000,000	1.9%
21	Louisiana	16,500,000,000	1.6%
22	Alabama	16,056,000,000	1.6%
23	Connecticut	15,221,000,000	1.5%
24	Arizona	14,782,000,000	1.5%
25	Kentucky	14,414,000,000	1.4%
26	Colorado	13,669,000,000	1.3%
27	South Carolina	13,204,000,000	1.3%
28	Oklahoma	10,988,000,000	1.1%
29	Oregon	10,840,000,000	1.1%
30	Iowa	10,198,000,000	1.0%
31	Kansas	9,394,000,000	0.9%
32	Mississippi	8,882,000,000	0.9%
33	Arkansas	8,463,000,000	0.8%
34	West Virginia	7,037,000,000	0.7%
35	Nebraska	6,095,000,000	0.6%
36	Utah	5,944,000,000	0.6%
37	Nevada	5,606,000,000	0.6%
38	New Mexico	5,344,000,000	0.5%
39	Maine	4,925,000,000	0.5%
40	Hawaii	4,658,000,000	0.5%
40	New Hampshire	4,658,000,000	0.5%
42	Rhode Island	4,515,000,000	0.4%
43	Idaho	3,397,000,000	0.3%
44	Delaware	3,106,000,000	0.3%
45	South Dakota	2,842,000,000	0.3%
46	Montana	2,838,000,000	0.3%
47	North Dakota	2,680,000,000	0.3%
48	Alaska	2,299,000,000	0.2%
49	Vermont	2,066,000,000	0.2%
50	Wyoming	1,407,000,000	0.1%
	District of Columbia	4,258,000,000	0.4%

Source: U.S. Department of Health and Human Services, Health Care Financing Administration
    "State Health Care Expenditures" (http://www.hcfa.gov/stats/nhe-oact/stateestimates/)
*By state of provider. Includes hospital care, physician services, dental services, home health care, drugs, vision products, nursing home care and other personal health care services and products.

239

Health Care Expenditures as a Percent of Gross State Product in 1998

National Percent = 11.6% of Total Gross State Product*

ALPHA ORDER			RANK ORDER		
RANK	STATE	PERCENT	RANK	STATE	PERCENT
5	Alabama	14.6	1	West Virginia	17.6
47	Alaska	9.5	2	North Dakota	15.6
34	Arizona	11.0	3	Maine	15.2
11	Arkansas	13.7	4	Rhode Island	14.8
44	California	9.8	5	Alabama	14.6
45	Colorado	9.6	6	Florida	14.3
36	Connecticut	10.7	6	Mississippi	14.3
48	Delaware	9.2	6	Montana	14.3
6	Florida	14.3	9	Pennsylvania	14.1
36	Georgia	10.7	10	Tennessee	13.8
30	Hawaii	11.7	11	Arkansas	13.7
34	Idaho	11.0	12	Kentucky	13.5
39	Illinois	10.4	12	Oklahoma	13.5
23	Indiana	12.2	14	South Dakota	13.4
25	Iowa	12.1	15	South Carolina	13.2
23	Kansas	12.2	16	Louisiana	12.8
12	Kentucky	13.5	16	Missouri	12.8
16	Louisiana	12.8	18	Vermont	12.7
3	Maine	15.2	19	Minnesota	12.6
28	Maryland	11.9	19	Wisconsin	12.6
21	Massachusetts	12.5	21	Massachusetts	12.5
25	Michigan	12.1	21	Ohio	12.5
19	Minnesota	12.6	23	Indiana	12.2
6	Mississippi	14.3	23	Kansas	12.2
16	Missouri	12.8	25	Iowa	12.1
6	Montana	14.3	25	Michigan	12.1
29	Nebraska	11.8	25	New York	12.1
49	Nevada	8.9	28	Maryland	11.9
32	New Hampshire	11.3	29	Nebraska	11.8
41	New Jersey	10.2	30	Hawaii	11.7
33	New Mexico	11.2	31	North Carolina	11.6
25	New York	12.1	32	New Hampshire	11.3
31	North Carolina	11.6	33	New Mexico	11.2
2	North Dakota	15.6	34	Arizona	11.0
21	Ohio	12.5	34	Idaho	11.0
12	Oklahoma	13.5	36	Connecticut	10.7
40	Oregon	10.3	36	Georgia	10.7
9	Pennsylvania	14.1	38	Texas	10.5
4	Rhode Island	14.8	39	Illinois	10.4
15	South Carolina	13.2	40	Oregon	10.3
14	South Dakota	13.4	41	New Jersey	10.2
10	Tennessee	13.8	42	Utah	10.0
38	Texas	10.5	42	Washington	10.0
42	Utah	10.0	44	California	9.8
18	Vermont	12.7	45	Colorado	9.6
45	Virginia	9.6	45	Virginia	9.6
42	Washington	10.0	47	Alaska	9.5
1	West Virginia	17.6	48	Delaware	9.2
19	Wisconsin	12.6	49	Nevada	8.9
50	Wyoming	8.0	50	Wyoming	8.0
				District of Columbia	7.9

Source: Morgan Quitno Press using data from U.S. Dept of Health & Human Services, Health Care Financing Admin.
"State Health Care Expenditures" (http://www.hcfa.gov/stats/nhe-oact/stateestimates/)
*By state of provider. Includes hospital care, physician services, dental services, home health care, drugs, vision products, nursing home care and other personal health care services and products.

Percent Change in Personal Health Care Expenditures: 1990 to 1998

National Percent Change = 66.0% Increase*

ALPHA ORDER

RANK	STATE	PERCENT CHANGE
21	Alabama	75.2
30	Alaska	70.7
26	Arizona	72.6
28	Arkansas	71.8
50	California	48.0
19	Colorado	76.6
49	Connecticut	52.0
14	Delaware	79.7
37	Florida	66.9
16	Georgia	77.9
31	Hawaii	69.7
1	Idaho	100.2
44	Illinois	60.4
35	Indiana	67.5
33	Iowa	68.1
32	Kansas	69.6
7	Kentucky	84.3
39	Louisiana	65.4
10	Maine	82.7
36	Maryland	67.1
47	Massachusetts	57.9
43	Michigan	61.1
18	Minnesota	77.2
5	Mississippi	87.8
40	Missouri	64.8
22	Montana	74.3
26	Nebraska	72.6
2	Nevada	99.8
11	New Hampshire	82.1
42	New Jersey	62.1
9	New Mexico	83.2
45	New York	59.1
3	North Carolina	98.8
41	North Dakota	63.5
46	Ohio	58.3
25	Oklahoma	72.8
24	Oregon	73.5
48	Pennsylvania	57.3
38	Rhode Island	65.5
4	South Carolina	94.0
5	South Dakota	87.8
12	Tennessee	80.3
13	Texas	79.8
8	Utah	83.9
20	Vermont	76.3
34	Virginia	68.0
29	Washington	71.1
15	West Virginia	79.1
22	Wisconsin	74.3
17	Wyoming	77.4

RANK ORDER

RANK	STATE	PERCENT CHANGE
1	Idaho	100.2
2	Nevada	99.8
3	North Carolina	98.8
4	South Carolina	94.0
5	Mississippi	87.8
5	South Dakota	87.8
7	Kentucky	84.3
8	Utah	83.9
9	New Mexico	83.2
10	Maine	82.7
11	New Hampshire	82.1
12	Tennessee	80.3
13	Texas	79.8
14	Delaware	79.7
15	West Virginia	79.1
16	Georgia	77.9
17	Wyoming	77.4
18	Minnesota	77.2
19	Colorado	76.6
20	Vermont	76.3
21	Alabama	75.2
22	Montana	74.3
22	Wisconsin	74.3
24	Oregon	73.5
25	Oklahoma	72.8
26	Arizona	72.6
26	Nebraska	72.6
28	Arkansas	71.8
29	Washington	71.1
30	Alaska	70.7
31	Hawaii	69.7
32	Kansas	69.6
33	Iowa	68.1
34	Virginia	68.0
35	Indiana	67.5
36	Maryland	67.1
37	Florida	66.9
38	Rhode Island	65.5
39	Louisiana	65.4
40	Missouri	64.8
41	North Dakota	63.5
42	New Jersey	62.1
43	Michigan	61.1
44	Illinois	60.4
45	New York	59.1
46	Ohio	58.3
47	Massachusetts	57.9
48	Pennsylvania	57.3
49	Connecticut	52.0
50	California	48.0
	District of Columbia	19.5

Source: Morgan Quitno Press using data from U.S. Dept of Health & Human Services, Health Care Financing Admin.
"State Health Care Expenditures" (http://www.hcfa.gov/stats/nhe-oact/stateestimates/)
*By state of provider. Includes hospital care, physician services, dental services, home health care, drugs, vision products, nursing home care and other personal health care services and products.

Average Annual Change in Expenditures for Personal Health Care: 1990 to 1998
National Percent Change = 13.9% Average Annual Increase*

ALPHA ORDER

RANK	STATE	PERCENT CHANGE
19	Alabama	14.3
22	Alaska	14.1
3	Arizona	17.0
26	Arkansas	13.8
26	California	13.8
22	Colorado	14.1
8	Connecticut	15.6
12	Delaware	15.1
1	Florida	17.6
4	Georgia	16.4
15	Hawaii	14.6
33	Idaho	13.3
48	Illinois	11.4
30	Indiana	13.6
50	Iowa	11.2
45	Kansas	11.8
22	Kentucky	14.1
28	Louisiana	13.7
19	Maine	14.3
21	Maryland	14.2
22	Massachusetts	14.1
49	Michigan	11.3
33	Minnesota	13.3
35	Mississippi	13.1
38	Missouri	12.9
39	Montana	12.8
46	Nebraska	11.7
4	Nevada	16.4
1	New Hampshire	17.6
10	New Jersey	15.3
8	New Mexico	15.6
32	New York	13.4
6	North Carolina	16.0
40	North Dakota	12.7
36	Ohio	13.0
44	Oklahoma	11.9
36	Oregon	13.0
30	Pennsylvania	13.6
28	Rhode Island	13.7
7	South Carolina	15.8
40	South Dakota	12.7
14	Tennessee	14.7
15	Texas	14.6
11	Utah	15.2
15	Vermont	14.6
13	Virginia	15.0
18	Washington	14.5
43	West Virginia	12.0
42	Wisconsin	12.6
46	Wyoming	11.7

RANK ORDER

RANK	STATE	PERCENT CHANGE
1	Florida	17.6
1	New Hampshire	17.6
3	Arizona	17.0
4	Georgia	16.4
4	Nevada	16.4
6	North Carolina	16.0
7	South Carolina	15.8
8	Connecticut	15.6
8	New Mexico	15.6
10	New Jersey	15.3
11	Utah	15.2
12	Delaware	15.1
13	Virginia	15.0
14	Tennessee	14.7
15	Hawaii	14.6
15	Texas	14.6
15	Vermont	14.6
18	Washington	14.5
19	Alabama	14.3
19	Maine	14.3
21	Maryland	14.2
22	Alaska	14.1
22	Colorado	14.1
22	Kentucky	14.1
22	Massachusetts	14.1
26	Arkansas	13.8
26	California	13.8
28	Louisiana	13.7
28	Rhode Island	13.7
30	Indiana	13.6
30	Pennsylvania	13.6
32	New York	13.4
33	Idaho	13.3
33	Minnesota	13.3
35	Mississippi	13.1
36	Ohio	13.0
36	Oregon	13.0
38	Missouri	12.9
39	Montana	12.8
40	North Dakota	12.7
40	South Dakota	12.7
42	Wisconsin	12.6
43	West Virginia	12.0
44	Oklahoma	11.9
45	Kansas	11.8
46	Nebraska	11.7
46	Wyoming	11.7
48	Illinois	11.4
49	Michigan	11.3
50	Iowa	11.2

District of Columbia	12.5

*Source: U.S. Department of Health and Human Services, Health Care Financing Administration
"State Health Care Expenditures" (http://www.hcfa.gov/stats/nhe-oact/stateestimates/)*
By state of provider. Includes hospital care, physician services, dental services, home health care, drugs, vision products, nursing home care and other personal health care services and products.

Per Capita Personal Health Care Expenditures in 1998

National Per Capita = $3,761*

ALPHA ORDER				RANK ORDER		
RANK	STATE	PER CAPITA		RANK	STATE	PER CAPITA
23	Alabama	$3,690		1	Massachusetts	$4,889
22	Alaska	3,737		2	New York	4,724
46	Arizona	3,167		3	Connecticut	4,651
39	Arkansas	3,334		4	Rhode Island	4,571
38	California	3,367		5	Minnesota	4,298
34	Colorado	3,444		6	Pennsylvania	4,276
3	Connecticut	4,651		7	North Dakota	4,202
8	Delaware	4,174		8	Delaware	4,174
11	Florida	4,006		9	Tennessee	4,053
30	Georgia	3,564		10	New Jersey	4,039
14	Hawaii	3,913		11	Florida	4,006
50	Idaho	2,760		12	Maine	3,948
24	Illinois	3,671		13	New Hampshire	3,928
29	Indiana	3,599		14	Hawaii	3,913
30	Iowa	3,564		15	South Dakota	3,889
32	Kansas	3,560		16	West Virginia	3,884
26	Kentucky	3,664		17	Missouri	3,846
21	Louisiana	3,782		18	Maryland	3,830
12	Maine	3,948		19	Wisconsin	3,819
18	Maryland	3,830		20	Ohio	3,789
1	Massachusetts	4,889		21	Louisiana	3,782
27	Michigan	3,630		22	Alaska	3,737
5	Minnesota	4,298		23	Alabama	3,690
43	Mississippi	3,228		24	Illinois	3,671
17	Missouri	3,846		25	Nebraska	3,670
44	Montana	3,227		26	Kentucky	3,664
25	Nebraska	3,670		27	Michigan	3,630
45	Nevada	3,215		28	North Carolina	3,621
13	New Hampshire	3,928		29	Indiana	3,599
10	New Jersey	4,039		30	Georgia	3,564
47	New Mexico	3,083		30	Iowa	3,564
2	New York	4,724		32	Kansas	3,560
28	North Carolina	3,621		33	Vermont	3,498
7	North Dakota	4,202		34	Colorado	3,444
20	Ohio	3,789		35	South Carolina	3,439
41	Oklahoma	3,290		36	Texas	3,437
40	Oregon	3,303		37	Washington	3,392
6	Pennsylvania	4,276		38	California	3,367
4	Rhode Island	4,571		39	Arkansas	3,334
35	South Carolina	3,439		40	Oregon	3,303
15	South Dakota	3,889		41	Oklahoma	3,290
9	Tennessee	4,053		42	Virginia	3,279
36	Texas	3,437		43	Mississippi	3,228
49	Utah	2,830		44	Montana	3,227
33	Vermont	3,498		45	Nevada	3,215
42	Virginia	3,279		46	Arizona	3,167
37	Washington	3,392		47	New Mexico	3,083
16	West Virginia	3,884		48	Wyoming	2,931
19	Wisconsin	3,819		49	Utah	2,830
48	Wyoming	2,931		50	Idaho	2,760
					District of Columbia	8,166

Source: Morgan Quitno Press using data from U.S. Dept of Health & Human Services, Health Care Financing Admin. "State Health Care Expenditures" (http://www.hcfa.gov/stats/nhe-oact/stateestimates/)
By state of provider. Per capita calculated using resident population. These figures may be skewed due to residents crossing state borders for care. Includes hospital care, physician services, dental services, home health care, drugs, vision products, nursing home care and other personal health care services and products.

Percent Change in Per Capita Expenditures for
Personal Health Care: 1990 to 1998
National Percent Change = 53.3% Increase*

RANK	STATE	PERCENT CHANGE
18	Alabama	63.1
37	Alaska	53.5
49	Arizona	36.1
24	Arkansas	59.4
50	California	35.6
46	Colorado	47.0
39	Connecticut	52.8
21	Delaware	61.6
47	Florida	45.7
42	Georgia	51.5
26	Hawaii	58.6
12	Idaho	64.6
41	Illinois	52.1
29	Indiana	57.5
17	Iowa	63.3
24	Kansas	59.4
7	Kentucky	73.0
23	Louisiana	60.0
1	Maine	80.4
30	Maryland	56.3
35	Massachusetts	54.7
40	Michigan	52.7
13	Minnesota	64.5
5	Mississippi	75.9
33	Missouri	55.4
26	Montana	58.6
14	Nebraska	64.3
48	Nevada	39.6
8	New Hampshire	70.7
34	New Jersey	55.3
22	New Mexico	60.7
28	New York	57.7
6	North Carolina	75.4
16	North Dakota	63.4
38	Ohio	53.0
19	Oklahoma	62.9
44	Oregon	51.2
31	Pennsylvania	55.9
10	Rhode Island	68.4
4	South Carolina	76.8
2	South Dakota	79.1
20	Tennessee	62.3
32	Texas	55.5
43	Utah	51.4
9	Vermont	68.5
36	Virginia	53.7
45	Washington	47.4
3	West Virginia	77.2
15	Wisconsin	63.6
11	Wyoming	67.6

RANK	STATE	PERCENT CHANGE
1	Maine	80.4
2	South Dakota	79.1
3	West Virginia	77.2
4	South Carolina	76.8
5	Mississippi	75.9
6	North Carolina	75.4
7	Kentucky	73.0
8	New Hampshire	70.7
9	Vermont	68.5
10	Rhode Island	68.4
11	Wyoming	67.6
12	Idaho	64.6
13	Minnesota	64.5
14	Nebraska	64.3
15	Wisconsin	63.6
16	North Dakota	63.4
17	Iowa	63.3
18	Alabama	63.1
19	Oklahoma	62.9
20	Tennessee	62.3
21	Delaware	61.6
22	New Mexico	60.7
23	Louisiana	60.0
24	Arkansas	59.4
24	Kansas	59.4
26	Hawaii	58.6
26	Montana	58.6
28	New York	57.7
29	Indiana	57.5
30	Maryland	56.3
31	Pennsylvania	55.9
32	Texas	55.5
33	Missouri	55.4
34	New Jersey	55.3
35	Massachusetts	54.7
36	Virginia	53.7
37	Alaska	53.5
38	Ohio	53.0
39	Connecticut	52.8
40	Michigan	52.7
41	Illinois	52.1
42	Georgia	51.5
43	Utah	51.4
44	Oregon	51.2
45	Washington	47.4
46	Colorado	47.0
47	Florida	45.7
48	Nevada	39.6
49	Arizona	36.1
50	California	35.6

| | District of Columbia | 38.4 |

Source: Morgan Quitno Press using data from U.S. Dept of Health & Human Services, Health Care Financing Admin.
"State Health Care Expenditures" (http://www.hcfa.gov/stats/nhe-oact/stateestimates/)
By state of provider. Per capita calculated using resident population. These figures may be skewed due to residents crossing state borders for care. Includes hospital care, physician services, dental services, home health care, drugs, vision products, nursing home care and other personal health care services and products.

Average Annual Change in Per Capita Expenditures
For Personal Health Care: 1990 to 1998
National Percent Change = 5.5% Average Annual Increase*

ALPHA ORDER

RANK ORDER

RANK	STATE	PERCENT CHANGE		RANK	STATE	PERCENT CHANGE
15	Alabama	6.3		1	Maine	7.7
36	Alaska	5.5		2	South Dakota	7.6
49	Arizona	3.9		3	South Carolina	7.4
23	Arkansas	6.0		3	West Virginia	7.4
49	California	3.9		5	Mississippi	7.3
46	Colorado	4.9		5	North Carolina	7.3
39	Connecticut	5.4		7	Kentucky	7.1
20	Delaware	6.2		8	New Hampshire	6.9
47	Florida	4.8		9	Rhode Island	6.7
42	Georgia	5.3		9	Vermont	6.7
26	Hawaii	5.9		9	Wyoming	6.7
12	Idaho	6.4		12	Idaho	6.4
39	Illinois	5.4		12	Minnesota	6.4
29	Indiana	5.8		12	Nebraska	6.4
15	Iowa	6.3		15	Alabama	6.3
23	Kansas	6.0		15	Iowa	6.3
7	Kentucky	7.1		15	North Dakota	6.3
23	Louisiana	6.0		15	Oklahoma	6.3
1	Maine	7.7		15	Wisconsin	6.3
30	Maryland	5.7		20	Delaware	6.2
35	Massachusetts	5.6		20	Tennessee	6.2
39	Michigan	5.4		22	New Mexico	6.1
12	Minnesota	6.4		23	Arkansas	6.0
5	Mississippi	7.3		23	Kansas	6.0
30	Missouri	5.7		23	Louisiana	6.0
26	Montana	5.9		26	Hawaii	5.9
12	Nebraska	6.4		26	Montana	5.9
48	Nevada	4.3		26	New York	5.9
8	New Hampshire	6.9		29	Indiana	5.8
30	New Jersey	5.7		30	Maryland	5.7
22	New Mexico	6.1		30	Missouri	5.7
26	New York	5.9		30	New Jersey	5.7
5	North Carolina	7.3		30	Pennsylvania	5.7
15	North Dakota	6.3		30	Texas	5.7
36	Ohio	5.5		35	Massachusetts	5.6
15	Oklahoma	6.3		36	Alaska	5.5
42	Oregon	5.3		36	Ohio	5.5
30	Pennsylvania	5.7		36	Virginia	5.5
9	Rhode Island	6.7		39	Connecticut	5.4
3	South Carolina	7.4		39	Illinois	5.4
2	South Dakota	7.6		39	Michigan	5.4
20	Tennessee	6.2		42	Georgia	5.3
30	Texas	5.7		42	Oregon	5.3
42	Utah	5.3		42	Utah	5.3
9	Vermont	6.7		45	Washington	5.0
36	Virginia	5.5		46	Colorado	4.9
45	Washington	5.0		47	Florida	4.8
3	West Virginia	7.4		48	Nevada	4.3
15	Wisconsin	6.3		49	Arizona	3.9
9	Wyoming	6.7		49	California	3.9
					District of Columbia	4.1

Source: Morgan Quitno Press using data from U.S. Dept of Health & Human Services, Health Care Financing Admin.
"State Health Care Expenditures" (http://www.hcfa.gov/stats/nhe-oact/stateestimates/)
*By state of provider. Per capita calculated using resident population. These figures may be skewed due to residents crossing state borders for care. Includes hospital care, physician services, dental services, home health care, drugs, vision products, nursing home care and other personal health care services and products.

Per Capita Medicare Expenditures for Personal Health Care in 1998

National Per Capita = $775*

ALPHA ORDER				RANK ORDER		
RANK	STATE	PER CAPITA		RANK	STATE	PER CAPITA
12	Alabama	$817		1	Florida	$1,138
50	Alaska	289		2	Pennsylvania	1,077
28	Arizona	679		3	Massachusetts	1,047
17	Arkansas	777		4	Rhode Island	1,040
24	California	705		5	Louisiana	1,009
44	Colorado	553		6	Connecticut	937
6	Connecticut	937		7	New York	926
33	Delaware	638		8	Missouri	864
1	Florida	1,138		9	Tennessee	848
36	Georgia	605		10	West Virginia	846
48	Hawaii	426		11	New Jersey	832
46	Idaho	467		12	Alabama	817
25	Illinois	692		13	Mississippi	812
23	Indiana	718		14	Michigan	789
34	Iowa	626		15	Ohio	784
31	Kansas	658		16	Oklahoma	781
21	Kentucky	735		17	Arkansas	777
5	Louisiana	1,009		18	Maryland	750
19	Maine	741		19	Maine	741
18	Maryland	750		20	North Dakota	738
3	Massachusetts	1,047		21	Kentucky	735
14	Michigan	789		22	Texas	732
40	Minnesota	586		23	Indiana	718
13	Mississippi	812		24	California	705
8	Missouri	864		25	Illinois	692
37	Montana	595		26	Nevada	690
32	Nebraska	650		27	North Carolina	688
26	Nevada	690		28	Arizona	679
39	New Hampshire	589		29	South Dakota	673
11	New Jersey	832		30	South Carolina	662
45	New Mexico	515		31	Kansas	658
7	New York	926		32	Nebraska	650
27	North Carolina	688		33	Delaware	638
20	North Dakota	738		34	Iowa	626
15	Ohio	784		35	Wisconsin	611
16	Oklahoma	781		36	Georgia	605
38	Oregon	593		37	Montana	595
2	Pennsylvania	1,077		38	Oregon	593
4	Rhode Island	1,040		39	New Hampshire	589
30	South Carolina	662		40	Minnesota	586
29	South Dakota	673		41	Vermont	567
9	Tennessee	848		42	Virginia	565
22	Texas	732		43	Washington	562
49	Utah	410		44	Colorado	553
41	Vermont	567		45	New Mexico	515
42	Virginia	565		46	Idaho	467
43	Washington	562		47	Wyoming	433
10	West Virginia	846		48	Hawaii	426
35	Wisconsin	611		49	Utah	410
47	Wyoming	433		50	Alaska	289
					District of Columbia	1,552

Source: Morgan Quitno Press using data from U.S. Dept of Health & Human Services, Health Care Financing Admin.
"State Health Care Expenditures" (http://www.hcfa.gov/stats/nhe-oact/stateestimates/)
*By state of provider. Per capita calculated using resident population. These figures may be skewed due to residents crossing state borders for care. Includes hospital care, physician services, dental services, home health care, drugs, vision products, nursing home care and other personal health care services and products.

Per Capita Medicaid Expenditures for Personal Health Care in 1998

National Per Capita = $589*

ALPHA ORDER			RANK ORDER		
RANK	STATE	PER CAPITA	RANK	STATE	PER CAPITA
35	Alabama	$474	1	New York	$1,486
18	Alaska	582	2	Rhode Island	973
46	Arizona	371	3	Massachusetts	928
23	Arkansas	548	4	Maine	849
37	California	436	5	Connecticut	816
45	Colorado	379	6	Louisiana	717
5	Connecticut	816	7	West Virginia	700
29	Delaware	531	8	Pennsylvania	680
41	Florida	421	9	Tennessee	660
38	Georgia	428	10	Vermont	657
28	Hawaii	535	11	Kentucky	627
47	Idaho	367	12	Minnesota	614
21	Illinois	560	13	North Carolina	599
39	Indiana	426	14	New Hampshire	598
19	Iowa	579	15	New Jersey	590
44	Kansas	400	16	South Carolina	587
11	Kentucky	627	17	Ohio	585
6	Louisiana	717	18	Alaska	582
4	Maine	849	19	Iowa	579
34	Maryland	490	20	New Mexico	568
3	Massachusetts	928	21	Illinois	560
25	Michigan	546	22	Mississippi	550
12	Minnesota	614	23	Arkansas	548
22	Mississippi	550	23	Washington	548
26	Missouri	540	25	Michigan	546
36	Montana	458	26	Missouri	540
30	Nebraska	523	27	North Dakota	538
50	Nevada	286	28	Hawaii	535
14	New Hampshire	598	29	Delaware	531
15	New Jersey	590	30	Nebraska	523
20	New Mexico	568	31	Wisconsin	516
1	New York	1,486	32	Oregon	510
13	North Carolina	599	33	South Dakota	494
27	North Dakota	538	34	Maryland	490
17	Ohio	585	35	Alabama	474
43	Oklahoma	401	36	Montana	458
32	Oregon	510	37	California	436
8	Pennsylvania	680	38	Georgia	428
2	Rhode Island	973	39	Indiana	426
16	South Carolina	587	39	Texas	426
33	South Dakota	494	41	Florida	421
9	Tennessee	660	42	Wyoming	419
39	Texas	426	43	Oklahoma	401
49	Utah	322	44	Kansas	400
10	Vermont	657	45	Colorado	379
48	Virginia	325	46	Arizona	371
23	Washington	548	47	Idaho	367
7	West Virginia	700	48	Virginia	325
31	Wisconsin	516	49	Utah	322
42	Wyoming	419	50	Nevada	286
				District of Columbia	1,365

Source: Morgan Quitno Press using data from U.S. Dept of Health & Human Services, Health Care Financing Admin. "State Health Care Expenditures" (http://www.hcfa.gov/stats/nhe-oact/stateestimates/)
By state of provider. Per capita calculated using resident population. These figures may be skewed due to residents crossing state borders for care. Includes hospital care, physician services, dental services, home health care, drugs, vision products, nursing home care and other personal health care services and products.

Expenditures for Hospital Care in 1998

National Total = $380,050,000,000*

ALPHA ORDER				RANK ORDER			
RANK	STATE	EXPENDITURES	% of USA	RANK	STATE	EXPENDITURES	% of USA
20	Alabama	$6,618,000,000	1.7%	1	California	$34,948,000,000	9.2%
48	Alaska	986,000,000	0.3%	2	New York	32,636,000,000	8.6%
25	Arizona	4,977,000,000	1.3%	3	Texas	25,322,000,000	6.7%
33	Arkansas	3,324,000,000	0.9%	4	Pennsylvania	20,213,000,000	5.3%
1	California	34,948,000,000	9.2%	5	Florida	19,742,000,000	5.2%
26	Colorado	4,850,000,000	1.3%	6	Illinois	17,996,000,000	4.7%
27	Connecticut	4,686,000,000	1.2%	7	Ohio	16,763,000,000	4.4%
47	Delaware	1,166,000,000	0.3%	8	Michigan	14,641,000,000	3.9%
5	Florida	19,742,000,000	5.2%	9	Massachusetts	11,305,000,000	3.0%
12	Georgia	10,396,000,000	2.7%	10	New Jersey	11,191,000,000	2.9%
40	Hawaii	1,775,000,000	0.5%	11	North Carolina	10,987,000,000	2.9%
45	Idaho	1,236,000,000	0.3%	12	Georgia	10,396,000,000	2.7%
6	Illinois	17,996,000,000	4.7%	13	Missouri	8,828,000,000	2.3%
15	Indiana	8,515,000,000	2.2%	14	Virginia	8,689,000,000	2.3%
29	Iowa	4,084,000,000	1.1%	15	Indiana	8,515,000,000	2.2%
31	Kansas	3,580,000,000	0.9%	16	Tennessee	8,276,000,000	2.2%
23	Kentucky	5,731,000,000	1.5%	17	Maryland	7,313,000,000	1.9%
19	Louisiana	7,139,000,000	1.9%	18	Wisconsin	7,252,000,000	1.9%
39	Maine	1,846,000,000	0.5%	19	Louisiana	7,139,000,000	1.9%
17	Maryland	7,313,000,000	1.9%	20	Alabama	6,618,000,000	1.7%
9	Massachusetts	11,305,000,000	3.0%	21	Minnesota	6,540,000,000	1.7%
8	Michigan	14,641,000,000	3.9%	22	Washington	6,362,000,000	1.7%
21	Minnesota	6,540,000,000	1.7%	23	Kentucky	5,731,000,000	1.5%
30	Mississippi	3,848,000,000	1.0%	24	South Carolina	5,597,000,000	1.5%
13	Missouri	8,828,000,000	2.3%	25	Arizona	4,977,000,000	1.3%
46	Montana	1,224,000,000	0.3%	26	Colorado	4,850,000,000	1.3%
35	Nebraska	2,597,000,000	0.7%	27	Connecticut	4,686,000,000	1.2%
38	Nevada	1,865,000,000	0.5%	28	Oklahoma	4,218,000,000	1.1%
42	New Hampshire	1,559,000,000	0.4%	29	Iowa	4,084,000,000	1.1%
10	New Jersey	11,191,000,000	2.9%	30	Mississippi	3,848,000,000	1.0%
36	New Mexico	2,317,000,000	0.6%	31	Kansas	3,580,000,000	0.9%
2	New York	32,636,000,000	8.6%	32	Oregon	3,545,000,000	0.9%
11	North Carolina	10,987,000,000	2.9%	33	Arkansas	3,324,000,000	0.9%
43	North Dakota	1,282,000,000	0.3%	34	West Virginia	2,955,000,000	0.8%
7	Ohio	16,763,000,000	4.4%	35	Nebraska	2,597,000,000	0.7%
28	Oklahoma	4,218,000,000	1.1%	36	New Mexico	2,317,000,000	0.6%
32	Oregon	3,545,000,000	0.9%	37	Utah	2,290,000,000	0.6%
4	Pennsylvania	20,213,000,000	5.3%	38	Nevada	1,865,000,000	0.5%
41	Rhode Island	1,702,000,000	0.4%	39	Maine	1,846,000,000	0.5%
24	South Carolina	5,597,000,000	1.5%	40	Hawaii	1,775,000,000	0.5%
44	South Dakota	1,257,000,000	0.3%	41	Rhode Island	1,702,000,000	0.4%
16	Tennessee	8,276,000,000	2.2%	42	New Hampshire	1,559,000,000	0.4%
3	Texas	25,322,000,000	6.7%	43	North Dakota	1,282,000,000	0.3%
37	Utah	2,290,000,000	0.6%	44	South Dakota	1,257,000,000	0.3%
49	Vermont	712,000,000	0.2%	45	Idaho	1,236,000,000	0.3%
14	Virginia	8,689,000,000	2.3%	46	Montana	1,224,000,000	0.3%
22	Washington	6,362,000,000	1.7%	47	Delaware	1,166,000,000	0.3%
34	West Virginia	2,955,000,000	0.8%	48	Alaska	986,000,000	0.3%
18	Wisconsin	7,252,000,000	1.9%	49	Vermont	712,000,000	0.2%
50	Wyoming	582,000,000	0.2%	50	Wyoming	582,000,000	0.2%
					District of Columbia	2,585,000,000	0.7%

Source: U.S. Department of Health and Human Services, Health Care Financing Administration
"State Health Care Expenditures" (http://www.hcfa.gov/stats/nhe-oact/stateestimates/)
By state of provider.

Percent of Total Personal Health Care Expenditures
Spent on Hospital Care in 1998
National Percent = 37.4%*

ALPHA ORDER

RANK	STATE	PERCENT
13	Alabama	41.2
7	Alaska	42.9
42	Arizona	33.7
22	Arkansas	39.3
49	California	31.8
39	Colorado	35.5
50	Connecticut	30.8
33	Delaware	37.5
45	Florida	33.1
26	Georgia	38.2
27	Hawaii	38.1
37	Idaho	36.4
15	Illinois	40.6
17	Indiana	40.1
18	Iowa	40.0
27	Kansas	38.1
19	Kentucky	39.8
4	Louisiana	43.3
33	Maine	37.5
36	Maryland	37.2
31	Massachusetts	37.6
14	Michigan	41.1
48	Minnesota	32.2
4	Mississippi	43.3
10	Missouri	42.2
6	Montana	43.1
8	Nebraska	42.6
44	Nevada	33.3
43	New Hampshire	33.5
41	New Jersey	34.2
3	New Mexico	43.4
29	New York	38.0
16	North Carolina	40.2
1	North Dakota	47.8
20	Ohio	39.4
25	Oklahoma	38.4
47	Oregon	32.7
20	Pennsylvania	39.4
30	Rhode Island	37.7
9	South Carolina	42.4
2	South Dakota	44.2
31	Tennessee	37.6
35	Texas	37.4
24	Utah	38.5
40	Vermont	34.5
23	Virginia	39.0
46	Washington	33.0
11	West Virginia	42.0
37	Wisconsin	36.4
12	Wyoming	41.4

RANK ORDER

RANK	STATE	PERCENT
1	North Dakota	47.8
2	South Dakota	44.2
3	New Mexico	43.4
4	Louisiana	43.3
4	Mississippi	43.3
6	Montana	43.1
7	Alaska	42.9
8	Nebraska	42.6
9	South Carolina	42.4
10	Missouri	42.2
11	West Virginia	42.0
12	Wyoming	41.4
13	Alabama	41.2
14	Michigan	41.1
15	Illinois	40.6
16	North Carolina	40.2
17	Indiana	40.1
18	Iowa	40.0
19	Kentucky	39.8
20	Ohio	39.4
20	Pennsylvania	39.4
22	Arkansas	39.3
23	Virginia	39.0
24	Utah	38.5
25	Oklahoma	38.4
26	Georgia	38.2
27	Hawaii	38.1
27	Kansas	38.1
29	New York	38.0
30	Rhode Island	37.7
31	Massachusetts	37.6
31	Tennessee	37.6
33	Delaware	37.5
33	Maine	37.5
35	Texas	37.4
36	Maryland	37.2
37	Idaho	36.4
37	Wisconsin	36.4
39	Colorado	35.5
40	Vermont	34.5
41	New Jersey	34.2
42	Arizona	33.7
43	New Hampshire	33.5
44	Nevada	33.3
45	Florida	33.1
46	Washington	33.0
47	Oregon	32.7
48	Minnesota	32.2
49	California	31.8
50	Connecticut	30.8

District of Columbia	60.7

*Source: Morgan Quitno Press using data from U.S. Dept of Health & Human Services, Health Care Financing Admin.
"State Health Care Expenditures" (http://www.hcfa.gov/stats/nhe-oact/stateestimates/)*
*By state of provider.

Percent Change in Expenditures for Hospital Care: 1990 to 1998

National Percent Change = 49.6% Increase*

ALPHA ORDER

RANK	STATE	PERCENT CHANGE
16	Alabama	64.9
8	Alaska	76.7
33	Arizona	54.7
26	Arkansas	57.7
50	California	25.0
28	Colorado	56.3
49	Connecticut	28.1
18	Delaware	64.7
43	Florida	46.7
30	Georgia	55.6
37	Hawaii	54.1
2	Idaho	86.1
44	Illinois	45.2
20	Indiana	61.2
32	Iowa	55.2
29	Kansas	55.8
13	Kentucky	67.0
35	Louisiana	54.4
15	Maine	65.3
27	Maryland	57.0
47	Massachusetts	38.7
36	Michigan	54.2
22	Minnesota	60.2
9	Mississippi	75.9
40	Missouri	47.8
4	Montana	80.5
19	Nebraska	63.7
6	Nevada	78.8
40	New Hampshire	47.8
46	New Jersey	42.5
11	New Mexico	69.9
45	New York	43.7
1	North Carolina	86.3
6	North Dakota	78.8
42	Ohio	46.9
25	Oklahoma	57.8
34	Oregon	54.5
48	Pennsylvania	36.0
31	Rhode Island	55.4
5	South Carolina	80.0
3	South Dakota	81.1
39	Tennessee	50.3
24	Texas	58.9
10	Utah	72.8
23	Vermont	59.3
38	Virginia	53.4
21	Washington	60.5
12	West Virginia	67.8
14	Wisconsin	65.7
16	Wyoming	64.9

RANK ORDER

RANK	STATE	PERCENT CHANGE
1	North Carolina	86.3
2	Idaho	86.1
3	South Dakota	81.1
4	Montana	80.5
5	South Carolina	80.0
6	Nevada	78.8
6	North Dakota	78.8
8	Alaska	76.7
9	Mississippi	75.9
10	Utah	72.8
11	New Mexico	69.9
12	West Virginia	67.8
13	Kentucky	67.0
14	Wisconsin	65.7
15	Maine	65.3
16	Alabama	64.9
16	Wyoming	64.9
18	Delaware	64.7
19	Nebraska	63.7
20	Indiana	61.2
21	Washington	60.5
22	Minnesota	60.2
23	Vermont	59.3
24	Texas	58.9
25	Oklahoma	57.8
26	Arkansas	57.7
27	Maryland	57.0
28	Colorado	56.3
29	Kansas	55.8
30	Georgia	55.6
31	Rhode Island	55.4
32	Iowa	55.2
33	Arizona	54.7
34	Oregon	54.5
35	Louisiana	54.4
36	Michigan	54.2
37	Hawaii	54.1
38	Virginia	53.4
39	Tennessee	50.3
40	Missouri	47.8
40	New Hampshire	47.8
42	Ohio	46.9
43	Florida	46.7
44	Illinois	45.2
45	New York	43.7
46	New Jersey	42.5
47	Massachusetts	38.7
48	Pennsylvania	36.0
49	Connecticut	28.1
50	California	25.0

District of Columbia	21.0

Source: Morgan Quitno Press using data from U.S. Dept of Health & Human Services, Health Care Financing Admin.
"State Health Care Expenditures" (http://www.hcfa.gov/stats/nhe-oact/stateestimates/)
*By state of provider.

Average Annual Change in Expenditures for Hospital Care: 1990 to 1998

National Percent Change = 5.2% Average Annual Increase*

ALPHA ORDER

RANK	STATE	PERCENT CHANGE
16	Alabama	6.4
8	Alaska	7.4
32	Arizona	5.6
25	Arkansas	5.9
50	California	2.8
28	Colorado	5.7
49	Connecticut	3.1
16	Delaware	6.4
42	Florida	4.9
28	Georgia	5.7
32	Hawaii	5.6
1	Idaho	8.1
44	Illinois	4.8
20	Indiana	6.1
32	Iowa	5.6
28	Kansas	5.7
13	Kentucky	6.6
32	Louisiana	5.6
14	Maine	6.5
27	Maryland	5.8
47	Massachusetts	4.2
32	Michigan	5.6
20	Minnesota	6.1
9	Mississippi	7.3
40	Missouri	5.0
3	Montana	7.7
16	Nebraska	6.4
6	Nevada	7.5
40	New Hampshire	5.0
46	New Jersey	4.5
11	New Mexico	6.8
45	New York	4.6
1	North Carolina	8.1
6	North Dakota	7.5
42	Ohio	4.9
25	Oklahoma	5.9
32	Oregon	5.6
48	Pennsylvania	3.9
28	Rhode Island	5.7
5	South Carolina	7.6
3	South Dakota	7.7
39	Tennessee	5.2
23	Texas	6.0
10	Utah	7.1
23	Vermont	6.0
38	Virginia	5.5
20	Washington	6.1
12	West Virginia	6.7
14	Wisconsin	6.5
16	Wyoming	6.4

RANK ORDER

RANK	STATE	PERCENT CHANGE
1	Idaho	8.1
1	North Carolina	8.1
3	Montana	7.7
3	South Dakota	7.7
5	South Carolina	7.6
6	Nevada	7.5
6	North Dakota	7.5
8	Alaska	7.4
9	Mississippi	7.3
10	Utah	7.1
11	New Mexico	6.8
12	West Virginia	6.7
13	Kentucky	6.6
14	Maine	6.5
14	Wisconsin	6.5
16	Alabama	6.4
16	Delaware	6.4
16	Nebraska	6.4
16	Wyoming	6.4
20	Indiana	6.1
20	Minnesota	6.1
20	Washington	6.1
23	Texas	6.0
23	Vermont	6.0
25	Arkansas	5.9
25	Oklahoma	5.9
27	Maryland	5.8
28	Colorado	5.7
28	Georgia	5.7
28	Kansas	5.7
28	Rhode Island	5.7
32	Arizona	5.6
32	Hawaii	5.6
32	Iowa	5.6
32	Louisiana	5.6
32	Michigan	5.6
32	Oregon	5.6
38	Virginia	5.5
39	Tennessee	5.2
40	Missouri	5.0
40	New Hampshire	5.0
42	Florida	4.9
42	Ohio	4.9
44	Illinois	4.8
45	New York	4.6
46	New Jersey	4.5
47	Massachusetts	4.2
48	Pennsylvania	3.9
49	Connecticut	3.1
50	California	2.8
	District of Columbia	2.4

Source: U.S. Department of Health and Human Services, Health Care Financing Administration
"State Health Care Expenditures" (http://www.hcfa.gov/stats/nhe-oact/stateestimates/)
*By state of provider.

Per Capita Expenditures for Hospital Care in 1998

National Per Capita = $1,406*

ALPHA ORDER			RANK ORDER		
RANK	STATE	PER CAPITA	RANK	STATE	PER CAPITA
14	Alabama	$1,521	1	North Dakota	$2,010
10	Alaska	1,603	2	Massachusetts	1,840
49	Arizona	1,066	3	New York	1,797
37	Arkansas	1,310	4	Rhode Island	1,723
48	California	1,069	5	South Dakota	1,720
41	Colorado	1,222	6	Pennsylvania	1,684
24	Connecticut	1,432	7	Louisiana	1,636
11	Delaware	1,567	8	West Virginia	1,631
35	Florida	1,324	9	Missouri	1,624
32	Georgia	1,361	10	Alaska	1,603
16	Hawaii	1,491	11	Delaware	1,567
50	Idaho	1,004	12	Nebraska	1,564
16	Illinois	1,491	13	Tennessee	1,523
23	Indiana	1,441	14	Alabama	1,521
25	Iowa	1,427	15	Ohio	1,492
33	Kansas	1,357	16	Hawaii	1,491
21	Kentucky	1,457	16	Illinois	1,491
7	Louisiana	1,636	16	Michigan	1,491
19	Maine	1,480	19	Maine	1,480
26	Maryland	1,426	20	South Carolina	1,458
2	Massachusetts	1,840	21	Kentucky	1,457
16	Michigan	1,491	22	North Carolina	1,456
30	Minnesota	1,384	23	Indiana	1,441
27	Mississippi	1,399	24	Connecticut	1,432
9	Missouri	1,624	25	Iowa	1,427
28	Montana	1,392	26	Maryland	1,426
12	Nebraska	1,564	27	Mississippi	1,399
47	Nevada	1,070	28	Montana	1,392
36	New Hampshire	1,315	29	Wisconsin	1,389
31	New Jersey	1,382	30	Minnesota	1,384
34	New Mexico	1,337	31	New Jersey	1,382
3	New York	1,797	32	Georgia	1,361
22	North Carolina	1,456	33	Kansas	1,357
1	North Dakota	2,010	34	New Mexico	1,337
15	Ohio	1,492	35	Florida	1,324
40	Oklahoma	1,263	36	New Hampshire	1,315
46	Oregon	1,080	37	Arkansas	1,310
6	Pennsylvania	1,684	38	Texas	1,285
4	Rhode Island	1,723	39	Virginia	1,280
20	South Carolina	1,458	40	Oklahoma	1,263
5	South Dakota	1,720	41	Colorado	1,222
13	Tennessee	1,523	42	Wyoming	1,212
38	Texas	1,285	43	Vermont	1,206
45	Utah	1,090	44	Washington	1,119
43	Vermont	1,206	45	Utah	1,090
39	Virginia	1,280	46	Oregon	1,080
44	Washington	1,119	47	Nevada	1,070
8	West Virginia	1,631	48	California	1,069
29	Wisconsin	1,389	49	Arizona	1,066
42	Wyoming	1,212	50	Idaho	1,004
				District of Columbia	4,958

Source: Morgan Quitno Press using data from U.S. Dept of Health & Human Services, Health Care Financing Admin. "State Health Care Expenditures" (http://www.hcfa.gov/stats/nhe-oact/stateestimates/)

By state of provider. Per capita calculated using resident population. These figures may be skewed due to residents crossing state borders for care.

Percent Change in Per Capita Expenditures for Hospital Care: 1990 to 1998

National Percent Change = 38.0% Increase*

ALPHA ORDER			RANK ORDER		
RANK	STATE	PERCENT CHANGE	RANK	STATE	PERCENT CHANGE
15	Alabama	53.5	1	North Dakota	78.7
9	Alaska	58.9	2	South Dakota	72.7
49	Arizona	22.0	3	West Virginia	66.1
27	Arkansas	46.4	4	Mississippi	64.8
50	California	14.6	5	North Carolina	64.3
45	Colorado	30.1	6	Montana	64.2
46	Connecticut	28.8	7	South Carolina	64.0
24	Delaware	48.1	8	Maine	63.2
47	Florida	28.0	9	Alaska	58.9
44	Georgia	32.5	10	Rhode Island	58.1
29	Hawaii	44.1	11	Kentucky	56.8
16	Idaho	53.0	12	Nebraska	55.9
37	Illinois	37.8	13	Wyoming	55.6
18	Indiana	51.5	14	Wisconsin	55.5
19	Iowa	50.7	15	Alabama	53.5
26	Kansas	46.5	16	Idaho	53.0
11	Kentucky	56.8	17	Vermont	52.3
20	Louisiana	49.3	18	Indiana	51.5
8	Maine	63.2	19	Iowa	50.7
25	Maryland	46.9	20	Louisiana	49.3
40	Massachusetts	35.8	21	New Mexico	49.1
28	Michigan	46.2	22	Oklahoma	48.8
23	Minnesota	48.7	23	Minnesota	48.7
4	Mississippi	64.8	24	Delaware	48.1
34	Missouri	39.4	25	Maryland	46.9
6	Montana	64.2	26	Kansas	46.5
12	Nebraska	55.9	27	Arkansas	46.4
48	Nevada	25.0	28	Michigan	46.2
35	New Hampshire	38.6	29	Hawaii	44.1
39	New Jersey	36.6	30	New York	42.4
21	New Mexico	49.1	31	Utah	42.3
30	New York	42.4	32	Ohio	42.0
5	North Carolina	64.3	33	Virginia	40.5
1	North Dakota	78.7	34	Missouri	39.4
32	Ohio	42.0	35	New Hampshire	38.6
22	Oklahoma	48.8	36	Washington	38.3
43	Oregon	34.5	37	Illinois	37.8
42	Pennsylvania	34.8	38	Texas	37.4
10	Rhode Island	58.1	39	New Jersey	36.6
7	South Carolina	64.0	40	Massachusetts	35.8
2	South Dakota	72.7	41	Tennessee	35.3
41	Tennessee	35.3	42	Pennsylvania	34.8
38	Texas	37.4	43	Oregon	34.5
31	Utah	42.3	44	Georgia	32.5
17	Vermont	52.3	45	Colorado	30.1
33	Virginia	40.5	46	Connecticut	28.8
36	Washington	38.3	47	Florida	28.0
3	West Virginia	66.1	48	Nevada	25.0
14	Wisconsin	55.5	49	Arizona	22.0
13	Wyoming	55.6	50	California	14.6
				District of Columbia	40.1

Source: Morgan Quitno Press using data from U.S. Dept of Health & Human Services, Health Care Financing Admin.
    "State Health Care Expenditures" (http://www.hcfa.gov/stats/nhe-oact/stateestimates/)
*By state of provider. Per capita calculated using resident population. These figures may be skewed due to residents crossing state borders for care.

Average Annual Change in Per Capita Expenditures
For Hospital Care: 1990 to 1998
National Percent Change = 4.1% Average Annual Increase*

ALPHA ORDER				RANK ORDER		
RANK	STATE	PERCENT CHANGE		RANK	STATE	PERCENT CHANGE
15	Alabama	5.5		1	North Dakota	7.5
9	Alaska	6.0		2	South Dakota	7.1
49	Arizona	2.5		3	West Virginia	6.5
25	Arkansas	4.9		4	Mississippi	6.4
50	California	1.7		4	Montana	6.4
45	Colorado	3.3		4	North Carolina	6.4
46	Connecticut	3.2		4	South Carolina	6.4
24	Delaware	5.0		8	Maine	6.3
47	Florida	3.1		9	Alaska	6.0
44	Georgia	3.6		10	Rhode Island	5.9
29	Hawaii	4.7		11	Kentucky	5.8
15	Idaho	5.5		12	Nebraska	5.7
36	Illinois	4.1		12	Wisconsin	5.7
18	Indiana	5.3		12	Wyoming	5.7
18	Iowa	5.3		15	Alabama	5.5
25	Kansas	4.9		15	Idaho	5.5
11	Kentucky	5.8		17	Vermont	5.4
20	Louisiana	5.1		18	Indiana	5.3
8	Maine	6.3		18	Iowa	5.3
25	Maryland	4.9		20	Louisiana	5.1
40	Massachusetts	3.9		20	Minnesota	5.1
25	Michigan	4.9		20	New Mexico	5.1
20	Minnesota	5.1		20	Oklahoma	5.1
4	Mississippi	6.4		24	Delaware	5.0
34	Missouri	4.2		25	Arkansas	4.9
4	Montana	6.4		25	Kansas	4.9
12	Nebraska	5.7		25	Maryland	4.9
48	Nevada	2.8		25	Michigan	4.9
34	New Hampshire	4.2		29	Hawaii	4.7
39	New Jersey	4.0		30	New York	4.5
20	New Mexico	5.1		30	Ohio	4.5
30	New York	4.5		30	Utah	4.5
4	North Carolina	6.4		33	Virginia	4.3
1	North Dakota	7.5		34	Missouri	4.2
30	Ohio	4.5		34	New Hampshire	4.2
20	Oklahoma	5.1		36	Illinois	4.1
41	Oregon	3.8		36	Texas	4.1
41	Pennsylvania	3.8		36	Washington	4.1
10	Rhode Island	5.9		39	New Jersey	4.0
4	South Carolina	6.4		40	Massachusetts	3.9
2	South Dakota	7.1		41	Oregon	3.8
41	Tennessee	3.8		41	Pennsylvania	3.8
36	Texas	4.1		41	Tennessee	3.8
30	Utah	4.5		44	Georgia	3.6
17	Vermont	5.4		45	Colorado	3.3
33	Virginia	4.3		46	Connecticut	3.2
36	Washington	4.1		47	Florida	3.1
3	West Virginia	6.5		48	Nevada	2.8
12	Wisconsin	5.7		49	Arizona	2.5
12	Wyoming	5.7		50	California	1.7
				District of Columbia		4.3

Source: Morgan Quitno Press using data from U.S. Dept of Health & Human Services, Health Care Financing Admin.
"State Health Care Expenditures" (http://www.hcfa.gov/stats/nhe-oact/stateestimates/)
*By state of provider. Per capita calculated using resident population. These figures may be skewed due to residents crossing state borders for care.

Per Capita Medicare Expenditures for Hospital Care in 1998

National Per Capita = $457*

RANK	STATE	PER CAPITA	RANK	STATE	PER CAPITA
15	Alabama	$483	1	Pennsylvania	$648
50	Alaska	218	2	Massachusetts	626
41	Arizona	347	3	Louisiana	612
14	Arkansas	494	4	Rhode Island	586
33	California	385	5	West Virginia	579
44	Colorado	317	6	Florida	578
12	Connecticut	496	7	Missouri	564
35	Delaware	371	8	New York	559
6	Florida	578	9	North Dakota	530
38	Georgia	360	10	Mississippi	517
47	Hawaii	272	11	Tennessee	508
46	Idaho	285	12	Connecticut	496
24	Illinois	438	13	New Jersey	495
19	Indiana	460	14	Arkansas	494
27	Iowa	418	15	Alabama	483
30	Kansas	407	16	Michigan	479
17	Kentucky	474	17	Kentucky	474
3	Louisiana	612	18	Oklahoma	468
24	Maine	438	19	Indiana	460
22	Maryland	444	19	Ohio	460
2	Massachusetts	626	21	South Dakota	457
16	Michigan	479	22	Maryland	444
34	Minnesota	382	23	Nebraska	440
10	Mississippi	517	24	Illinois	438
7	Missouri	564	24	Maine	438
32	Montana	391	26	North Carolina	428
23	Nebraska	440	27	Iowa	418
31	Nevada	395	28	South Carolina	414
37	New Hampshire	362	29	Texas	408
13	New Jersey	495	30	Kansas	407
45	New Mexico	299	31	Nevada	395
8	New York	559	32	Montana	391
26	North Carolina	428	33	California	385
9	North Dakota	530	34	Minnesota	382
19	Ohio	460	35	Delaware	371
18	Oklahoma	468	36	Wisconsin	367
39	Oregon	353	37	New Hampshire	362
1	Pennsylvania	648	38	Georgia	360
4	Rhode Island	586	39	Oregon	353
28	South Carolina	414	40	Virginia	352
21	South Dakota	457	41	Arizona	347
11	Tennessee	508	42	Vermont	337
29	Texas	408	43	Washington	327
49	Utah	252	44	Colorado	317
42	Vermont	337	45	New Mexico	299
40	Virginia	352	46	Idaho	285
43	Washington	327	47	Hawaii	272
5	West Virginia	579	48	Wyoming	267
36	Wisconsin	367	49	Utah	252
48	Wyoming	267	50	Alaska	218

District of Columbia 1,105

Source: Morgan Quitno Press using data from U.S. Dept of Health & Human Services, Health Care Financing Admin.
"State Health Care Expenditures" (http://www.hcfa.gov/stats/nhe-oact/stateestimates/)
*By state of provider. Per capita calculated using resident population. These figures may be skewed due to residents crossing state borders for care.

Per Capita Medicaid Expenditures for Hospital Care in 1998

National Per Capita = $224*

RANK	STATE	PER CAPITA
32	Alabama	$158
16	Alaska	218
8	Arizona	242
27	Arkansas	177
15	California	225
39	Colorado	141
24	Connecticut	195
43	Delaware	125
35	Florida	151
28	Georgia	176
20	Hawaii	205
47	Idaho	106
7	Illinois	266
36	Indiana	146
22	Iowa	199
49	Kansas	100
10	Kentucky	234
2	Louisiana	340
6	Maine	273
17	Maryland	213
4	Massachusetts	302
17	Michigan	213
30	Minnesota	162
13	Mississippi	226
26	Missouri	189
25	Montana	193
37	Nebraska	142
42	Nevada	129
44	New Hampshire	121
13	New Jersey	226
19	New Mexico	209
1	New York	565
12	North Carolina	227
32	North Dakota	158
11	Ohio	229
45	Oklahoma	117
34	Oregon	157
21	Pennsylvania	200
3	Rhode Island	325
9	South Carolina	238
37	South Dakota	142
5	Tennessee	277
31	Texas	161
48	Utah	102
41	Vermont	130
40	Virginia	132
29	Washington	163
23	West Virginia	197
46	Wisconsin	110
50	Wyoming	90

RANK	STATE	PER CAPITA
1	New York	$565
2	Louisiana	340
3	Rhode Island	325
4	Massachusetts	302
5	Tennessee	277
6	Maine	273
7	Illinois	266
8	Arizona	242
9	South Carolina	238
10	Kentucky	234
11	Ohio	229
12	North Carolina	227
13	Mississippi	226
13	New Jersey	226
15	California	225
16	Alaska	218
17	Maryland	213
17	Michigan	213
19	New Mexico	209
20	Hawaii	205
21	Pennsylvania	200
22	Iowa	199
23	West Virginia	197
24	Connecticut	195
25	Montana	193
26	Missouri	189
27	Arkansas	177
28	Georgia	176
29	Washington	163
30	Minnesota	162
31	Texas	161
32	Alabama	158
32	North Dakota	158
34	Oregon	157
35	Florida	151
36	Indiana	146
37	Nebraska	142
37	South Dakota	142
39	Colorado	141
40	Virginia	132
41	Vermont	130
42	Nevada	129
43	Delaware	125
44	New Hampshire	121
45	Oklahoma	117
46	Wisconsin	110
47	Idaho	106
48	Utah	102
49	Kansas	100
50	Wyoming	90

District of Columbia 669

Source: Morgan Quitno Press using data from U.S. Dept of Health & Human Services, Health Care Financing Admin. "State Health Care Expenditures" (http://www.hcfa.gov/stats/nhe-oact/stateestimates/)
By state of provider. Per capita calculated using resident population. These figures may be skewed due to residents crossing state borders for care.

Expenditures for Physician and Other Professional Services in 1998

National Total = $296,102,000,000*

RANK	STATE	EXPENDITURES	% of USA
22	Alabama	$4,609,000,000	1.6%
48	Alaska	568,000,000	0.2%
21	Arizona	5,135,000,000	1.7%
32	Arkansas	2,225,000,000	0.8%
1	California	44,239,000,000	14.9%
23	Colorado	4,314,000,000	1.5%
24	Connecticut	4,292,000,000	1.4%
44	Delaware	792,000,000	0.3%
4	Florida	18,985,000,000	6.4%
10	Georgia	8,510,000,000	2.9%
37	Hawaii	1,594,000,000	0.5%
43	Idaho	935,000,000	0.3%
6	Illinois	11,975,000,000	4.0%
19	Indiana	5,613,000,000	1.9%
31	Iowa	2,457,000,000	0.8%
30	Kansas	2,538,000,000	0.9%
26	Kentucky	3,785,000,000	1.3%
25	Louisiana	4,249,000,000	1.4%
41	Maine	1,219,000,000	0.4%
16	Maryland	5,978,000,000	2.0%
11	Massachusetts	8,322,000,000	2.8%
9	Michigan	9,186,000,000	3.1%
12	Minnesota	7,183,000,000	2.4%
33	Mississippi	2,212,000,000	0.7%
20	Missouri	5,310,000,000	1.8%
46	Montana	695,000,000	0.2%
40	Nebraska	1,367,000,000	0.5%
34	Nevada	1,918,000,000	0.6%
39	New Hampshire	1,405,000,000	0.5%
8	New Jersey	9,506,000,000	3.2%
38	New Mexico	1,415,000,000	0.5%
2	New York	20,103,000,000	6.8%
13	North Carolina	7,106,000,000	2.4%
47	North Dakota	612,000,000	0.2%
7	Ohio	11,024,000,000	3.7%
29	Oklahoma	2,978,000,000	1.0%
27	Oregon	3,285,000,000	1.1%
5	Pennsylvania	13,434,000,000	4.5%
42	Rhode Island	1,095,000,000	0.4%
28	South Carolina	3,254,000,000	1.1%
45	South Dakota	747,000,000	0.3%
14	Tennessee	6,719,000,000	2.3%
3	Texas	20,071,000,000	6.8%
36	Utah	1,648,000,000	0.6%
49	Vermont	563,000,000	0.2%
15	Virginia	6,265,000,000	2.1%
17	Washington	5,908,000,000	2.0%
35	West Virginia	1,793,000,000	0.6%
18	Wisconsin	5,844,000,000	2.0%
50	Wyoming	343,000,000	0.1%

RANK	STATE	EXPENDITURES	% of USA
1	California	$44,239,000,000	14.9%
2	New York	20,103,000,000	6.8%
3	Texas	20,071,000,000	6.8%
4	Florida	18,985,000,000	6.4%
5	Pennsylvania	13,434,000,000	4.5%
6	Illinois	11,975,000,000	4.0%
7	Ohio	11,024,000,000	3.7%
8	New Jersey	9,506,000,000	3.2%
9	Michigan	9,186,000,000	3.1%
10	Georgia	8,510,000,000	2.9%
11	Massachusetts	8,322,000,000	2.8%
12	Minnesota	7,183,000,000	2.4%
13	North Carolina	7,106,000,000	2.4%
14	Tennessee	6,719,000,000	2.3%
15	Virginia	6,265,000,000	2.1%
16	Maryland	5,978,000,000	2.0%
17	Washington	5,908,000,000	2.0%
18	Wisconsin	5,844,000,000	2.0%
19	Indiana	5,613,000,000	1.9%
20	Missouri	5,310,000,000	1.8%
21	Arizona	5,135,000,000	1.7%
22	Alabama	4,609,000,000	1.6%
23	Colorado	4,314,000,000	1.5%
24	Connecticut	4,292,000,000	1.4%
25	Louisiana	4,249,000,000	1.4%
26	Kentucky	3,785,000,000	1.3%
27	Oregon	3,285,000,000	1.1%
28	South Carolina	3,254,000,000	1.1%
29	Oklahoma	2,978,000,000	1.0%
30	Kansas	2,538,000,000	0.9%
31	Iowa	2,457,000,000	0.8%
32	Arkansas	2,225,000,000	0.8%
33	Mississippi	2,212,000,000	0.7%
34	Nevada	1,918,000,000	0.6%
35	West Virginia	1,793,000,000	0.6%
36	Utah	1,648,000,000	0.6%
37	Hawaii	1,594,000,000	0.5%
38	New Mexico	1,415,000,000	0.5%
39	New Hampshire	1,405,000,000	0.5%
40	Nebraska	1,367,000,000	0.5%
41	Maine	1,219,000,000	0.4%
42	Rhode Island	1,095,000,000	0.4%
43	Idaho	935,000,000	0.3%
44	Delaware	792,000,000	0.3%
45	South Dakota	747,000,000	0.3%
46	Montana	695,000,000	0.2%
47	North Dakota	612,000,000	0.2%
48	Alaska	568,000,000	0.2%
49	Vermont	563,000,000	0.2%
50	Wyoming	343,000,000	0.1%
	District of Columbia	781,000,000	0.3%

Source: U.S. Department of Health and Human Services, Health Care Financing Administration
"State Health Care Expenditures" (http://www.hcfa.gov/stats/nhe-oact/stateestimates/)
*By state of provider. Includes "other professional services" previously listed as a separate category. These include services of licensed professionals such as chiropractors, optometrists, podiatrists and independently practicing nurses. Also includes specialty clinics, independently billing laboratories and Medicare ambulance services.

Percent of Total Personal Health Care Expenditures
Spent on Physician and Other Professional Services in 1998
National Percent = 29.1%*

ALPHA ORDER				RANK ORDER		
RANK	STATE	PERCENT		RANK	STATE	PERCENT
17	Alabama	28.7		1	California	40.2
42	Alaska	24.7		2	Minnesota	35.4
3	Arizona	34.7		3	Arizona	34.7
29	Arkansas	26.3		4	Hawaii	34.2
1	California	40.2		4	Nevada	34.2
7	Colorado	31.6		6	Florida	31.8
18	Connecticut	28.2		7	Colorado	31.6
37	Delaware	25.5		8	Georgia	31.3
6	Florida	31.8		9	Washington	30.6
8	Georgia	31.3		10	Tennessee	30.5
4	Hawaii	34.2		11	Maryland	30.4
22	Idaho	27.5		12	Oregon	30.3
25	Illinois	27.0		13	New Hampshire	30.2
28	Indiana	26.4		14	Texas	29.6
47	Iowa	24.1		15	Wisconsin	29.3
25	Kansas	27.0		16	New Jersey	29.1
29	Kentucky	26.3		17	Alabama	28.7
35	Louisiana	25.8		18	Connecticut	28.2
41	Maine	24.8		19	Virginia	28.1
11	Maryland	30.4		20	Massachusetts	27.7
20	Massachusetts	27.7		20	Utah	27.7
35	Michigan	25.8		22	Idaho	27.5
2	Minnesota	35.4		23	Vermont	27.3
40	Mississippi	24.9		24	Oklahoma	27.1
39	Missouri	25.4		25	Illinois	27.0
44	Montana	24.5		25	Kansas	27.0
50	Nebraska	22.4		27	New Mexico	26.5
4	Nevada	34.2		28	Indiana	26.4
13	New Hampshire	30.2		29	Arkansas	26.3
16	New Jersey	29.1		29	Kentucky	26.3
27	New Mexico	26.5		29	South Dakota	26.3
48	New York	23.4		32	Pennsylvania	26.2
33	North Carolina	26.0		33	North Carolina	26.0
49	North Dakota	22.8		34	Ohio	25.9
34	Ohio	25.9		35	Louisiana	25.8
24	Oklahoma	27.1		35	Michigan	25.8
12	Oregon	30.3		37	Delaware	25.5
32	Pennsylvania	26.2		37	West Virginia	25.5
46	Rhode Island	24.3		39	Missouri	25.4
43	South Carolina	24.6		40	Mississippi	24.9
29	South Dakota	26.3		41	Maine	24.8
10	Tennessee	30.5		42	Alaska	24.7
14	Texas	29.6		43	South Carolina	24.6
20	Utah	27.7		44	Montana	24.5
23	Vermont	27.3		45	Wyoming	24.4
19	Virginia	28.1		46	Rhode Island	24.3
9	Washington	30.6		47	Iowa	24.1
37	West Virginia	25.5		48	New York	23.4
15	Wisconsin	29.3		49	North Dakota	22.8
45	Wyoming	24.4		50	Nebraska	22.4
					District of Columbia	18.3

Source: Morgan Quitno Press using data from U.S. Dept of Health & Human Services, Health Care Financing Admin.
"State Health Care Expenditures" (http://www.hcfa.gov/stats/nhe-oact/stateestimates/)
*By state of provider. Includes "other professional services" previously listed as a separate category. These include services of licensed professionals such as chiropractors, optometrists, podiatrists and independently practicing nurses. Also includes specialty clinics, independently billing laboratories and Medicare ambulance services.

Percent Change in Expenditures for Physician and Other Professional Services: 1990 to 1998
National Percent Change = 63.6% Increase*

ALPHA ORDER				RANK ORDER		
RANK	STATE	PERCENT CHANGE		RANK	STATE	PERCENT CHANGE
22	Alabama	67.1		1	South Dakota	102.4
42	Alaska	57.8		2	Hawaii	102.0
26	Arizona	62.6		3	New Hampshire	100.1
42	Arkansas	57.8		4	Tennessee	96.8
44	California	56.6		5	Minnesota	95.9
18	Colorado	75.1		6	Idaho	95.6
46	Connecticut	52.3		7	South Carolina	92.9
31	Delaware	61.0		8	Mississippi	88.7
48	Florida	48.9		9	Maine	86.1
11	Georgia	84.2		9	North Carolina	86.1
2	Hawaii	102.0		11	Georgia	84.2
6	Idaho	95.6		12	New Mexico	83.1
37	Illinois	59.9		13	Nevada	82.7
33	Indiana	60.7		14	Vermont	81.0
28	Iowa	62.3		15	Wisconsin	79.4
35	Kansas	60.6		16	Kentucky	79.1
16	Kentucky	79.1		17	Utah	77.8
45	Louisiana	55.9		18	Colorado	75.1
9	Maine	86.1		19	Texas	74.2
27	Maryland	62.4		20	Wyoming	71.5
21	Massachusetts	69.6		21	Massachusetts	69.6
47	Michigan	51.8		22	Alabama	67.1
5	Minnesota	95.9		23	Oklahoma	67.0
8	Mississippi	88.7		24	West Virginia	63.7
30	Missouri	61.1		25	Montana	62.8
25	Montana	62.8		26	Arizona	62.6
39	Nebraska	59.0		27	Maryland	62.4
13	Nevada	82.7		28	Iowa	62.3
3	New Hampshire	100.1		29	Oregon	61.9
33	New Jersey	60.7		30	Missouri	61.1
12	New Mexico	83.1		31	Delaware	61.0
35	New York	60.6		32	Washington	60.8
9	North Carolina	86.1		33	Indiana	60.7
50	North Dakota	36.9		33	New Jersey	60.7
49	Ohio	44.6		35	Kansas	60.6
23	Oklahoma	67.0		35	New York	60.6
29	Oregon	61.9		37	Illinois	59.9
38	Pennsylvania	59.4		38	Pennsylvania	59.4
41	Rhode Island	58.0		39	Nebraska	59.0
7	South Carolina	92.9		40	Virginia	58.8
1	South Dakota	102.4		41	Rhode Island	58.0
4	Tennessee	96.8		42	Alaska	57.8
19	Texas	74.2		42	Arkansas	57.8
17	Utah	77.8		44	California	56.6
14	Vermont	81.0		45	Louisiana	55.9
40	Virginia	58.8		46	Connecticut	52.3
32	Washington	60.8		47	Michigan	51.8
24	West Virginia	63.7		48	Florida	48.9
15	Wisconsin	79.4		49	Ohio	44.6
20	Wyoming	71.5		50	North Dakota	36.9

District of Columbia (11.5)

Source: Morgan Quitno Press using data from U.S. Dept of Health & Human Services, Health Care Financing Admin. "State Health Care Expenditures" (http://www.hcfa.gov/stats/nhe-oact/stateestimates/)

By state of provider. Includes "other professional services" previously listed as a separate category. These include services of licensed professionals such as chiropractors, optometrists, podiatrists and independently practicing nurses. Also includes specialty clinics, independently billing laboratories and Medicare ambulance services.

Average Annual Change in Expenditures for Physician and Other Professional Services: 1990 to 1998
National Percent Change = 6.3% Average Annual Increase*

ALPHA ORDER

RANK	STATE	PERCENT CHANGE
22	Alabama	6.6
41	Alaska	5.9
25	Arizona	6.3
41	Arkansas	5.9
44	California	5.8
18	Colorado	7.3
46	Connecticut	5.4
30	Delaware	6.1
48	Florida	5.1
11	Georgia	7.9
1	Hawaii	9.2
6	Idaho	8.7
37	Illinois	6.0
30	Indiana	6.1
27	Iowa	6.2
30	Kansas	6.1
15	Kentucky	7.6
45	Louisiana	5.7
9	Maine	8.1
27	Maryland	6.2
21	Massachusetts	6.8
46	Michigan	5.4
4	Minnesota	8.8
8	Mississippi	8.3
30	Missouri	6.1
25	Montana	6.3
37	Nebraska	6.0
13	Nevada	7.8
3	New Hampshire	9.1
30	New Jersey	6.1
11	New Mexico	7.9
30	New York	6.1
9	North Carolina	8.1
50	North Dakota	4.0
49	Ohio	4.7
22	Oklahoma	6.6
27	Oregon	6.2
37	Pennsylvania	6.0
41	Rhode Island	5.9
7	South Carolina	8.6
1	South Dakota	9.2
4	Tennessee	8.8
19	Texas	7.2
17	Utah	7.5
14	Vermont	7.7
37	Virginia	6.0
30	Washington	6.1
24	West Virginia	6.4
15	Wisconsin	7.6
20	Wyoming	7.0

RANK ORDER

RANK	STATE	PERCENT CHANGE
1	Hawaii	9.2
1	South Dakota	9.2
3	New Hampshire	9.1
4	Minnesota	8.8
4	Tennessee	8.8
6	Idaho	8.7
7	South Carolina	8.6
8	Mississippi	8.3
9	Maine	8.1
9	North Carolina	8.1
11	Georgia	7.9
11	New Mexico	7.9
13	Nevada	7.8
14	Vermont	7.7
15	Kentucky	7.6
15	Wisconsin	7.6
17	Utah	7.5
18	Colorado	7.3
19	Texas	7.2
20	Wyoming	7.0
21	Massachusetts	6.8
22	Alabama	6.6
22	Oklahoma	6.6
24	West Virginia	6.4
25	Arizona	6.3
25	Montana	6.3
27	Iowa	6.2
27	Maryland	6.2
27	Oregon	6.2
30	Delaware	6.1
30	Indiana	6.1
30	Kansas	6.1
30	Missouri	6.1
30	New Jersey	6.1
30	New York	6.1
30	Washington	6.1
37	Illinois	6.0
37	Nebraska	6.0
37	Pennsylvania	6.0
37	Virginia	6.0
41	Alaska	5.9
41	Arkansas	5.9
41	Rhode Island	5.9
44	California	5.8
45	Louisiana	5.7
46	Connecticut	5.4
46	Michigan	5.4
48	Florida	5.1
49	Ohio	4.7
50	North Dakota	4.0

District of Columbia (1.5)

Source: U.S. Department of Health and Human Services, Health Care Financing Administration "State Health Care Expenditures" (http://www.hcfa.gov/stats/nhe-oact/stateestimates/)
By state of provider. Includes "other professional services" previously listed as a separate category. These include services of licensed professionals such as chiropractors, optometrists, podiatrists and independently practicing nurses. Also includes specialty clinics, independently billing laboratories and Medicare ambulance services.

Per Capita Expenditures for Physician and Other Professional Services in 1998

National Per Capita = $1,096*

ALPHA ORDER				RANK ORDER		
RANK	STATE	PER CAPITA		RANK	STATE	PER CAPITA
20	Alabama	$1,059		1	Minnesota	$1,520
38	Alaska	923		2	California	1,354
16	Arizona	1,100		2	Massachusetts	1,354
41	Arkansas	877		4	Hawaii	1,339
2	California	1,354		5	Connecticut	1,312
18	Colorado	1,087		6	Florida	1,273
5	Connecticut	1,312		7	Tennessee	1,237
19	Delaware	1,064		8	New Hampshire	1,185
6	Florida	1,273		9	New Jersey	1,174
13	Georgia	1,114		10	Maryland	1,165
4	Hawaii	1,339		11	Pennsylvania	1,119
49	Idaho	760		11	Wisconsin	1,119
25	Illinois	992		13	Georgia	1,114
35	Indiana	950		14	Rhode Island	1,109
42	Iowa	859		15	New York	1,107
31	Kansas	962		16	Arizona	1,100
31	Kentucky	962		16	Nevada	1,100
30	Louisiana	974		18	Colorado	1,087
28	Maine	977		19	Delaware	1,064
10	Maryland	1,165		20	Alabama	1,059
2	Massachusetts	1,354		21	Washington	1,039
37	Michigan	935		22	South Dakota	1,022
1	Minnesota	1,520		23	Texas	1,018
46	Mississippi	804		24	Oregon	1,001
28	Missouri	977		25	Illinois	992
47	Montana	790		26	West Virginia	990
44	Nebraska	823		27	Ohio	981
16	Nevada	1,100		28	Maine	977
8	New Hampshire	1,185		28	Missouri	977
9	New Jersey	1,174		30	Louisiana	974
45	New Mexico	816		31	Kansas	962
15	New York	1,107		31	Kentucky	962
36	North Carolina	942		33	North Dakota	960
33	North Dakota	960		34	Vermont	953
27	Ohio	981		35	Indiana	950
40	Oklahoma	892		36	North Carolina	942
24	Oregon	1,001		37	Michigan	935
11	Pennsylvania	1,119		38	Alaska	923
14	Rhode Island	1,109		38	Virginia	923
43	South Carolina	847		40	Oklahoma	892
22	South Dakota	1,022		41	Arkansas	877
7	Tennessee	1,237		42	Iowa	859
23	Texas	1,018		43	South Carolina	847
48	Utah	785		44	Nebraska	823
34	Vermont	953		45	New Mexico	816
38	Virginia	923		46	Mississippi	804
21	Washington	1,039		47	Montana	790
26	West Virginia	990		48	Utah	785
11	Wisconsin	1,119		49	Idaho	760
50	Wyoming	715		50	Wyoming	715
					District of Columbia	1,498

Source: Morgan Quitno Press using data from U.S. Dept of Health & Human Services, Health Care Financing Admin.
"State Health Care Expenditures" (http://www.hcfa.gov/stats/nhe-oact/stateestimates/)
*By state of provider. Per capita calculated using resident population. These figures may be skewed due to residents crossing state borders for care. Includes "other professional services" previously listed as a separate category. Services include licensed professionals such as chiropractors, optometrists, podiatrists and independently practicing nurses. Includes specialty clinics, independently billing laboratories and Medicare ambulance services.

Percent Change in Per Capita Expenditures for Physician and Other Professional Services: 1990 to 1998
National Percent Change = 51.0% Increase*

ALPHA ORDER

RANK	STATE	PERCENT CHANGE
24	Alabama	55.5
43	Alaska	41.8
49	Arizona	28.2
37	Arkansas	46.4
42	California	43.6
38	Colorado	45.7
26	Connecticut	53.1
40	Delaware	44.8
48	Florida	30.0
23	Georgia	56.9
2	Hawaii	88.9
16	Idaho	61.0
29	Illinois	51.7
31	Indiana	51.0
21	Iowa	57.6
31	Kansas	51.0
11	Kentucky	68.2
33	Louisiana	50.8
4	Maine	83.6
27	Maryland	51.9
12	Massachusetts	66.1
41	Michigan	43.8
5	Minnesota	81.8
7	Mississippi	76.7
27	Missouri	51.9
35	Montana	47.9
30	Nebraska	51.3
50	Nevada	27.6
3	New Hampshire	87.8
25	New Jersey	53.9
18	New Mexico	60.3
19	New York	59.3
13	North Carolina	64.1
47	North Dakota	36.9
45	Ohio	39.7
22	Oklahoma	57.3
44	Oregon	41.0
20	Pennsylvania	57.8
17	Rhode Island	60.7
8	South Carolina	75.7
1	South Dakota	92.8
6	Tennessee	77.2
34	Texas	50.6
36	Utah	46.5
9	Vermont	73.0
39	Virginia	45.4
46	Washington	38.5
15	West Virginia	62.0
10	Wisconsin	68.3
14	Wyoming	62.1

RANK ORDER

RANK	STATE	PERCENT CHANGE
1	South Dakota	92.8
2	Hawaii	88.9
3	New Hampshire	87.8
4	Maine	83.6
5	Minnesota	81.8
6	Tennessee	77.2
7	Mississippi	76.7
8	South Carolina	75.7
9	Vermont	73.0
10	Wisconsin	68.3
11	Kentucky	68.2
12	Massachusetts	66.1
13	North Carolina	64.1
14	Wyoming	62.1
15	West Virginia	62.0
16	Idaho	61.0
17	Rhode Island	60.7
18	New Mexico	60.3
19	New York	59.3
20	Pennsylvania	57.8
21	Iowa	57.6
22	Oklahoma	57.3
23	Georgia	56.9
24	Alabama	55.5
25	New Jersey	53.9
26	Connecticut	53.1
27	Maryland	51.9
27	Missouri	51.9
29	Illinois	51.7
30	Nebraska	51.3
31	Indiana	51.0
31	Kansas	51.0
33	Louisiana	50.8
34	Texas	50.6
35	Montana	47.9
36	Utah	46.5
37	Arkansas	46.4
38	Colorado	45.7
39	Virginia	45.4
40	Delaware	44.8
41	Michigan	43.8
42	California	43.6
43	Alaska	41.8
44	Oregon	41.0
45	Ohio	39.7
46	Washington	38.5
47	North Dakota	36.9
48	Florida	30.0
49	Arizona	28.2
50	Nevada	27.6

District of Columbia   2.5

Source: Morgan Quitno Press using data from U.S. Dept of Health & Human Services, Health Care Financing Admin.
"State Health Care Expenditures" (http://www.hcfa.gov/stats/nhe-oact/stateestimates/)
*By state of provider. Per capita calculated using resident population. These figures may be skewed due to residents crossing state borders for care. Includes "other professional services" previously listed as a separate category. Services include licensed professionals such as chiropractors, optometrists, podiatrists and independently practicing nurses. Includes specialty clinics, independently billing laboratories and Medicare ambulance services.

Average Annual Change in Per Capita Expenditures
For Physician Services: 1990 to 1998
National Percent Change = 5.3% Average Annual Increase*

ALPHA ORDER

RANK	STATE	PERCENT CHANGE
24	Alabama	5.7
43	Alaska	4.5
49	Arizona	3.2
36	Arkansas	4.9
41	California	4.6
38	Colorado	4.8
25	Connecticut	5.5
40	Delaware	4.7
48	Florida	3.3
22	Georgia	5.8
2	Hawaii	8.3
16	Idaho	6.1
29	Illinois	5.3
29	Indiana	5.3
20	Iowa	5.9
29	Kansas	5.3
10	Kentucky	6.7
29	Louisiana	5.3
4	Maine	7.9
27	Maryland	5.4
12	Massachusetts	6.6
41	Michigan	4.6
5	Minnesota	7.8
6	Mississippi	7.4
27	Missouri	5.4
35	Montana	5.0
29	Nebraska	5.3
50	Nevada	3.1
3	New Hampshire	8.2
25	New Jersey	5.5
16	New Mexico	6.1
19	New York	6.0
13	North Carolina	6.4
47	North Dakota	4.0
45	Ohio	4.3
22	Oklahoma	5.8
44	Oregon	4.4
20	Pennsylvania	5.9
16	Rhode Island	6.1
8	South Carolina	7.3
1	South Dakota	8.6
6	Tennessee	7.4
29	Texas	5.3
36	Utah	4.9
9	Vermont	7.1
38	Virginia	4.8
46	Washington	4.2
14	West Virginia	6.2
10	Wisconsin	6.7
14	Wyoming	6.2

RANK ORDER

RANK	STATE	PERCENT CHANGE
1	South Dakota	8.6
2	Hawaii	8.3
3	New Hampshire	8.2
4	Maine	7.9
5	Minnesota	7.8
6	Mississippi	7.4
6	Tennessee	7.4
8	South Carolina	7.3
9	Vermont	7.1
10	Kentucky	6.7
10	Wisconsin	6.7
12	Massachusetts	6.6
13	North Carolina	6.4
14	West Virginia	6.2
14	Wyoming	6.2
16	Idaho	6.1
16	New Mexico	6.1
16	Rhode Island	6.1
19	New York	6.0
20	Iowa	5.9
20	Pennsylvania	5.9
22	Georgia	5.8
22	Oklahoma	5.8
24	Alabama	5.7
25	Connecticut	5.5
25	New Jersey	5.5
27	Maryland	5.4
27	Missouri	5.4
29	Illinois	5.3
29	Indiana	5.3
29	Kansas	5.3
29	Louisiana	5.3
29	Nebraska	5.3
29	Texas	5.3
35	Montana	5.0
36	Arkansas	4.9
36	Utah	4.9
38	Colorado	4.8
38	Virginia	4.8
40	Delaware	4.7
41	California	4.6
41	Michigan	4.6
43	Alaska	4.5
44	Oregon	4.4
45	Ohio	4.3
46	Washington	4.2
47	North Dakota	4.0
48	Florida	3.3
49	Arizona	3.2
50	Nevada	3.1

District of Columbia   0.3

Source: Morgan Quitno Press using data from U.S. Dept of Health & Human Services, Health Care Financing Admin.
    "State Health Care Expenditures" (http://www.hcfa.gov/stats/nhe-oact/stateestimates/)
*By state of provider. Per capita calculated using resident population. These figures may be skewed due to residents crossing state borders for care. Includes "other professional services" previously listed as a separate category. Services include licensed professionals such as chiropractors, optometrists, podiatrists and independently practicing nurses. Includes specialty clinics, independently billing laboratories and Medicare ambulance services.

Per Capita Medicare Expenditures for Physician Services in 1998

National Per Capita = $181*

ALPHA ORDER

RANK	STATE	PER CAPITA
14	Alabama	$179
50	Alaska	42
9	Arizona	199
18	Arkansas	160
8	California	204
30	Colorado	137
7	Connecticut	206
23	Delaware	146
1	Florida	339
37	Georgia	128
44	Hawaii	111
47	Idaho	89
20	Illinois	152
29	Indiana	138
39	Iowa	126
22	Kansas	150
25	Kentucky	145
14	Louisiana	179
32	Maine	135
12	Maryland	187
5	Massachusetts	214
16	Michigan	174
39	Minnesota	126
35	Mississippi	130
13	Missouri	182
41	Montana	118
32	Nebraska	135
10	Nevada	197
45	New Hampshire	108
6	New Jersey	210
41	New Mexico	118
4	New York	227
30	North Carolina	137
21	North Dakota	151
11	Ohio	192
28	Oklahoma	144
18	Oregon	160
2	Pennsylvania	255
3	Rhode Island	233
37	South Carolina	128
34	South Dakota	131
17	Tennessee	166
25	Texas	145
48	Utah	81
46	Vermont	97
41	Virginia	118
25	Washington	145
23	West Virginia	146
36	Wisconsin	129
49	Wyoming	77

RANK ORDER

RANK	STATE	PER CAPITA
1	Florida	$339
2	Pennsylvania	255
3	Rhode Island	233
4	New York	227
5	Massachusetts	214
6	New Jersey	210
7	Connecticut	206
8	California	204
9	Arizona	199
10	Nevada	197
11	Ohio	192
12	Maryland	187
13	Missouri	182
14	Alabama	179
14	Louisiana	179
16	Michigan	174
17	Tennessee	166
18	Arkansas	160
18	Oregon	160
20	Illinois	152
21	North Dakota	151
22	Kansas	150
23	Delaware	146
23	West Virginia	146
25	Kentucky	145
25	Texas	145
25	Washington	145
28	Oklahoma	144
29	Indiana	138
30	Colorado	137
30	North Carolina	137
32	Maine	135
32	Nebraska	135
34	South Dakota	131
35	Mississippi	130
36	Wisconsin	129
37	Georgia	128
37	South Carolina	128
39	Iowa	126
39	Minnesota	126
41	Montana	118
41	New Mexico	118
41	Virginia	118
44	Hawaii	111
45	New Hampshire	108
46	Vermont	97
47	Idaho	89
48	Utah	81
49	Wyoming	77
50	Alaska	42
	District of Columbia	293

Source: Morgan Quitno Press using data from U.S. Dept of Health & Human Services, Health Care Financing Admin.
     "State Health Care Expenditures" (http://www.hcfa.gov/stats/nhe-oact/stateestimates/)
*By state of provider. Per capita calculated using resident population. These figures may be skewed due to residents crossing state borders for care.

Per Capita Medicaid Expenditures for Physician Services in 1998

National Per Capita = $55.39*

ALPHA ORDER

RANK	STATE	PER CAPITA
16	Alabama	$72.86
1	Alaska	144.67
6	Arizona	88.27
4	Arkansas	98.10
23	California	56.21
28	Colorado	48.12
48	Connecticut	24.45
22	Delaware	60.48
33	Florida	38.37
19	Georgia	66.52
13	Hawaii	74.76
32	Idaho	39.00
43	Illinois	29.25
45	Indiana	27.76
39	Iowa	34.25
49	Kansas	17.05
11	Kentucky	82.61
21	Louisiana	64.64
25	Maine	53.71
36	Maryland	35.48
12	Massachusetts	78.77
15	Michigan	73.32
41	Minnesota	33.64
20	Mississippi	66.15
46	Missouri	27.40
34	Montana	37.52
29	Nebraska	43.96
38	Nevada	34.41
7	New Hampshire	86.02
42	New Jersey	32.12
17	New Mexico	68.65
3	New York	101.27
8	North Carolina	85.88
30	North Dakota	43.90
27	Ohio	49.39
44	Oklahoma	27.85
31	Oregon	39.91
37	Pennsylvania	34.49
50	Rhode Island	15.19
10	South Carolina	84.64
26	South Dakota	50.63
2	Tennessee	102.16
35	Texas	36.58
14	Utah	74.27
18	Vermont	67.73
40	Virginia	33.73
9	Washington	84.92
5	West Virginia	91.63
47	Wisconsin	26.43
24	Wyoming	54.16

RANK ORDER

RANK	STATE	PER CAPITA
1	Alaska	$144.67
2	Tennessee	102.16
3	New York	101.27
4	Arkansas	98.10
5	West Virginia	91.63
6	Arizona	88.27
7	New Hampshire	86.02
8	North Carolina	85.88
9	Washington	84.92
10	South Carolina	84.64
11	Kentucky	82.61
12	Massachusetts	78.77
13	Hawaii	74.76
14	Utah	74.27
15	Michigan	73.32
16	Alabama	72.86
17	New Mexico	68.65
18	Vermont	67.73
19	Georgia	66.52
20	Mississippi	66.15
21	Louisiana	64.64
22	Delaware	60.48
23	California	56.21
24	Wyoming	54.16
25	Maine	53.71
26	South Dakota	50.63
27	Ohio	49.39
28	Colorado	48.12
29	Nebraska	43.96
30	North Dakota	43.90
31	Oregon	39.91
32	Idaho	39.00
33	Florida	38.37
34	Montana	37.52
35	Texas	36.58
36	Maryland	35.48
37	Pennsylvania	34.49
38	Nevada	34.41
39	Iowa	34.25
40	Virginia	33.73
41	Minnesota	33.64
42	New Jersey	32.12
43	Illinois	29.25
44	Oklahoma	27.85
45	Indiana	27.76
46	Missouri	27.40
47	Wisconsin	26.43
48	Connecticut	24.45
49	Kansas	17.05
50	Rhode Island	15.19

District of Columbia   140.00

Source: Morgan Quitno Press using data from U.S. Dept of Health & Human Services, Health Care Financing Admin.
"State Health Care Expenditures" (http://www.hcfa.gov/stats/nhe-oact/stateestimates/)
*By state of provider. Per capita calculated using resident population. These figures may be skewed due to residents crossing state borders for care.

Expenditures for Prescription Drugs in 1998

National Total = $90,648,000,000*

ALPHA ORDER

RANK	STATE	EXPENDITURES	% of USA
21	Alabama	$1,552,000,000	1.7%
49	Alaska	133,000,000	0.1%
24	Arizona	1,397,000,000	1.5%
32	Arkansas	903,000,000	1.0%
1	California	7,537,000,000	8.3%
28	Colorado	970,000,000	1.1%
25	Connecticut	1,354,000,000	1.5%
44	Delaware	300,000,000	0.3%
3	Florida	6,204,000,000	6.8%
11	Georgia	2,460,000,000	2.7%
43	Hawaii	311,000,000	0.3%
42	Idaho	334,000,000	0.4%
6	Illinois	3,964,000,000	4.4%
15	Indiana	2,058,000,000	2.3%
30	Iowa	945,000,000	1.0%
33	Kansas	854,000,000	0.9%
20	Kentucky	1,564,000,000	1.7%
22	Louisiana	1,507,000,000	1.7%
38	Maine	456,000,000	0.5%
18	Maryland	1,678,000,000	1.9%
12	Massachusetts	2,172,000,000	2.4%
8	Michigan	3,885,000,000	4.3%
23	Minnesota	1,491,000,000	1.6%
29	Mississippi	962,000,000	1.1%
16	Missouri	1,814,000,000	2.0%
45	Montana	234,000,000	0.3%
35	Nebraska	626,000,000	0.7%
37	Nevada	478,000,000	0.5%
41	New Hampshire	391,000,000	0.4%
9	New Jersey	3,545,000,000	3.9%
39	New Mexico	402,000,000	0.4%
2	New York	7,122,000,000	7.9%
10	North Carolina	2,566,000,000	2.8%
47	North Dakota	192,000,000	0.2%
7	Ohio	3,898,000,000	4.3%
27	Oklahoma	1,056,000,000	1.2%
31	Oregon	918,000,000	1.0%
5	Pennsylvania	5,035,000,000	5.6%
40	Rhode Island	400,000,000	0.4%
26	South Carolina	1,315,000,000	1.5%
46	South Dakota	201,000,000	0.2%
14	Tennessee	2,129,000,000	2.3%
4	Texas	6,023,000,000	6.6%
36	Utah	564,000,000	0.6%
48	Vermont	183,000,000	0.2%
13	Virginia	2,130,000,000	2.3%
19	Washington	1,603,000,000	1.8%
34	West Virginia	776,000,000	0.9%
17	Wisconsin	1,745,000,000	1.9%
49	Wyoming	133,000,000	0.1%

RANK ORDER

RANK	STATE	EXPENDITURES	% of USA
1	California	$7,537,000,000	8.3%
2	New York	7,122,000,000	7.9%
3	Florida	6,204,000,000	6.8%
4	Texas	6,023,000,000	6.6%
5	Pennsylvania	5,035,000,000	5.6%
6	Illinois	3,964,000,000	4.4%
7	Ohio	3,898,000,000	4.3%
8	Michigan	3,885,000,000	4.3%
9	New Jersey	3,545,000,000	3.9%
10	North Carolina	2,566,000,000	2.8%
11	Georgia	2,460,000,000	2.7%
12	Massachusetts	2,172,000,000	2.4%
13	Virginia	2,130,000,000	2.3%
14	Tennessee	2,129,000,000	2.3%
15	Indiana	2,058,000,000	2.3%
16	Missouri	1,814,000,000	2.0%
17	Wisconsin	1,745,000,000	1.9%
18	Maryland	1,678,000,000	1.9%
19	Washington	1,603,000,000	1.8%
20	Kentucky	1,564,000,000	1.7%
21	Alabama	1,552,000,000	1.7%
22	Louisiana	1,507,000,000	1.7%
23	Minnesota	1,491,000,000	1.6%
24	Arizona	1,397,000,000	1.5%
25	Connecticut	1,354,000,000	1.5%
26	South Carolina	1,315,000,000	1.5%
27	Oklahoma	1,056,000,000	1.2%
28	Colorado	970,000,000	1.1%
29	Mississippi	962,000,000	1.1%
30	Iowa	945,000,000	1.0%
31	Oregon	918,000,000	1.0%
32	Arkansas	903,000,000	1.0%
33	Kansas	854,000,000	0.9%
34	West Virginia	776,000,000	0.9%
35	Nebraska	626,000,000	0.7%
36	Utah	564,000,000	0.6%
37	Nevada	478,000,000	0.5%
38	Maine	456,000,000	0.5%
39	New Mexico	402,000,000	0.4%
40	Rhode Island	400,000,000	0.4%
41	New Hampshire	391,000,000	0.4%
42	Idaho	334,000,000	0.4%
43	Hawaii	311,000,000	0.3%
44	Delaware	300,000,000	0.3%
45	Montana	234,000,000	0.3%
46	South Dakota	201,000,000	0.2%
47	North Dakota	192,000,000	0.2%
48	Vermont	183,000,000	0.2%
49	Alaska	133,000,000	0.1%
49	Wyoming	133,000,000	0.1%
	District of Columbia	180,000,000	0.2%

Source: U.S. Department of Health and Human Services, Health Care Financing Administration
    "State Health Care Expenditures" (http://www.hcfa.gov/stats/nhe-oact/stateestimates/)
*Purchases in retail outlets. By state of outlet.

Percent of Total Personal Health Care Expenditures
Spent on Prescription Drugs in 1998
National Percent = 8.9%*

ALPHA ORDER

RANK	STATE	PERCENT
12	Alabama	9.7
50	Alaska	5.8
18	Arizona	9.5
6	Arkansas	10.7
48	California	6.8
46	Colorado	7.1
28	Connecticut	8.9
12	Delaware	9.7
7	Florida	10.4
27	Georgia	9.0
49	Hawaii	6.7
10	Idaho	9.8
28	Illinois	8.9
12	Indiana	9.7
22	Iowa	9.3
25	Kansas	9.1
2	Kentucky	10.9
25	Louisiana	9.1
22	Maine	9.3
35	Maryland	8.5
44	Massachusetts	7.2
2	Michigan	10.9
43	Minnesota	7.3
4	Mississippi	10.8
33	Missouri	8.7
41	Montana	8.2
8	Nebraska	10.3
35	Nevada	8.5
38	New Hampshire	8.4
4	New Jersey	10.8
42	New Mexico	7.5
39	New York	8.3
21	North Carolina	9.4
44	North Dakota	7.2
24	Ohio	9.2
16	Oklahoma	9.6
35	Oregon	8.5
10	Pennsylvania	9.8
28	Rhode Island	8.9
9	South Carolina	10.0
46	South Dakota	7.1
12	Tennessee	9.7
28	Texas	8.9
18	Utah	9.5
28	Vermont	8.9
16	Virginia	9.6
39	Washington	8.3
1	West Virginia	11.0
33	Wisconsin	8.7
18	Wyoming	9.5

RANK ORDER

RANK	STATE	PERCENT
1	West Virginia	11.0
2	Kentucky	10.9
2	Michigan	10.9
4	Mississippi	10.8
4	New Jersey	10.8
6	Arkansas	10.7
7	Florida	10.4
8	Nebraska	10.3
9	South Carolina	10.0
10	Idaho	9.8
10	Pennsylvania	9.8
12	Alabama	9.7
12	Delaware	9.7
12	Indiana	9.7
12	Tennessee	9.7
16	Oklahoma	9.6
16	Virginia	9.6
18	Arizona	9.5
18	Utah	9.5
18	Wyoming	9.5
21	North Carolina	9.4
22	Iowa	9.3
22	Maine	9.3
24	Ohio	9.2
25	Kansas	9.1
25	Louisiana	9.1
27	Georgia	9.0
28	Connecticut	8.9
28	Illinois	8.9
28	Rhode Island	8.9
28	Texas	8.9
28	Vermont	8.9
33	Missouri	8.7
33	Wisconsin	8.7
35	Maryland	8.5
35	Nevada	8.5
35	Oregon	8.5
38	New Hampshire	8.4
39	New York	8.3
39	Washington	8.3
41	Montana	8.2
42	New Mexico	7.5
43	Minnesota	7.3
44	Massachusetts	7.2
44	North Dakota	7.2
46	Colorado	7.1
46	South Dakota	7.1
48	California	6.8
49	Hawaii	6.7
50	Alaska	5.8

District of Columbia   4.2

Source: Morgan Quitno Press using data from U.S. Dept of Health & Human Services, Health Care Financing Admin.
"State Health Care Expenditures" (http://www.hcfa.gov/stats/nhe-oact/stateestimates/)
*Purchases in retail outlets. By state of outlet.

Percent Change in Expenditures for Prescription Drugs: 1990 to 1998

National Percent Change = 140.6% Increase*

ALPHA ORDER			RANK ORDER		
RANK	STATE	PERCENT CHANGE	RANK	STATE	PERCENT CHANGE
37	Alabama	129.6	1	Nevada	236.6
25	Alaska	141.8	2	Delaware	200.0
4	Arizona	180.0	3	Florida	198.1
30	Arkansas	134.5	4	Arizona	180.0
49	California	98.2	5	Oregon	179.9
8	Colorado	161.5	6	South Carolina	166.7
19	Connecticut	144.8	7	Maine	165.1
2	Delaware	200.0	8	Colorado	161.5
3	Florida	198.1	9	Idaho	160.9
15	Georgia	152.6	10	Minnesota	158.9
50	Hawaii	84.0	11	Utah	157.5
9	Idaho	160.9	12	North Carolina	156.9
46	Illinois	122.9	13	New Jersey	155.6
40	Indiana	127.7	14	New York	152.8
34	Iowa	131.6	15	Georgia	152.6
43	Kansas	124.7	16	Nebraska	152.4
23	Kentucky	142.1	17	Montana	148.9
47	Louisiana	120.3	18	Pennsylvania	146.6
7	Maine	165.1	19	Connecticut	144.8
42	Maryland	125.5	20	Tennessee	144.7
28	Massachusetts	136.6	21	New Hampshire	144.4
27	Michigan	137.0	22	Texas	142.5
10	Minnesota	158.9	23	Kentucky	142.1
29	Mississippi	135.2	23	Washington	142.1
45	Missouri	124.0	25	Alaska	141.8
17	Montana	148.9	26	Wisconsin	141.0
16	Nebraska	152.4	27	Michigan	137.0
1	Nevada	236.6	28	Massachusetts	136.6
21	New Hampshire	144.4	29	Mississippi	135.2
13	New Jersey	155.6	30	Arkansas	134.5
44	New Mexico	124.6	31	Oklahoma	134.1
14	New York	152.8	32	Virginia	133.6
12	North Carolina	156.9	33	Rhode Island	132.6
48	North Dakota	111.0	34	Iowa	131.6
36	Ohio	129.8	35	West Virginia	131.0
31	Oklahoma	134.1	36	Ohio	129.8
5	Oregon	179.9	37	Alabama	129.6
18	Pennsylvania	146.6	38	Wyoming	129.3
33	Rhode Island	132.6	39	Vermont	128.8
6	South Carolina	166.7	40	Indiana	127.7
41	South Dakota	125.8	41	South Dakota	125.8
20	Tennessee	144.7	42	Maryland	125.5
22	Texas	142.5	43	Kansas	124.7
11	Utah	157.5	44	New Mexico	124.6
39	Vermont	128.8	45	Missouri	124.0
32	Virginia	133.6	46	Illinois	122.9
23	Washington	142.1	47	Louisiana	120.3
35	West Virginia	131.0	48	North Dakota	111.0
26	Wisconsin	141.0	49	California	98.2
38	Wyoming	129.3	50	Hawaii	84.0
				District of Columbia	125.0

Source: Morgan Quitno Press using data from U.S. Dept of Health & Human Services, Health Care Financing Admin.
"State Health Care Expenditures" (http://www.hcfa.gov/stats/nhe-oact/stateestimates/)
*Purchases in retail outlets. By state of outlet.

Average Annual Change in Expenditures for Prescription Drugs: 1990 to 1998

National Percent Change = 11.6% Average Annual Increase*

ALPHA ORDER				RANK ORDER		
RANK	STATE	PERCENT CHANGE		RANK	STATE	PERCENT CHANGE
37	Alabama	10.9		1	Nevada	16.4
22	Alaska	11.7		2	Delaware	14.7
4	Arizona	13.7		3	Florida	14.6
30	Arkansas	11.2		4	Arizona	13.7
49	California	8.9		4	Oregon	13.7
8	Colorado	12.8		6	Maine	13.0
19	Connecticut	11.8		6	South Carolina	13.0
2	Delaware	14.7		8	Colorado	12.8
3	Florida	14.6		9	Idaho	12.7
14	Georgia	12.3		10	Minnesota	12.6
50	Hawaii	7.9		10	Utah	12.6
9	Idaho	12.7		12	North Carolina	12.5
46	Illinois	10.5		13	New Jersey	12.4
40	Indiana	10.8		14	Georgia	12.3
33	Iowa	11.1		14	Nebraska	12.3
41	Kansas	10.7		14	New York	12.3
22	Kentucky	11.7		17	Montana	12.1
47	Louisiana	10.4		18	Pennsylvania	11.9
6	Maine	13.0		19	Connecticut	11.8
41	Maryland	10.7		19	New Hampshire	11.8
27	Massachusetts	11.4		19	Tennessee	11.8
27	Michigan	11.4		22	Alaska	11.7
10	Minnesota	12.6		22	Kentucky	11.7
29	Mississippi	11.3		22	Texas	11.7
44	Missouri	10.6		22	Washington	11.7
17	Montana	12.1		26	Wisconsin	11.6
14	Nebraska	12.3		27	Massachusetts	11.4
1	Nevada	16.4		27	Michigan	11.4
19	New Hampshire	11.8		29	Mississippi	11.3
13	New Jersey	12.4		30	Arkansas	11.2
44	New Mexico	10.6		30	Oklahoma	11.2
14	New York	12.3		30	Virginia	11.2
12	North Carolina	12.5		33	Iowa	11.1
48	North Dakota	9.8		33	Rhode Island	11.1
35	Ohio	11.0		35	Ohio	11.0
30	Oklahoma	11.2		35	West Virginia	11.0
4	Oregon	13.7		37	Alabama	10.9
18	Pennsylvania	11.9		37	Vermont	10.9
33	Rhode Island	11.1		37	Wyoming	10.9
6	South Carolina	13.0		40	Indiana	10.8
41	South Dakota	10.7		41	Kansas	10.7
19	Tennessee	11.8		41	Maryland	10.7
22	Texas	11.7		41	South Dakota	10.7
10	Utah	12.6		44	Missouri	10.6
37	Vermont	10.9		44	New Mexico	10.6
30	Virginia	11.2		46	Illinois	10.5
22	Washington	11.7		47	Louisiana	10.4
35	West Virginia	11.0		48	North Dakota	9.8
26	Wisconsin	11.6		49	California	8.9
37	Wyoming	10.9		50	Hawaii	7.9
					District of Columbia	10.7

Source: U.S. Department of Health and Human Services, Health Care Financing Administration
"State Health Care Expenditures" (http://www.hcfa.gov/stats/nhe-oact/stateestimates/)
*Purchases in retail outlets. By state of outlet.

Per Capita Expenditures for Prescription Drugs in 1998

National Per Capita = $335*

ALPHA ORDER

RANK	STATE	PER CAPITA
14	Alabama	$357
50	Alaska	216
37	Arizona	299
15	Arkansas	356
49	California	231
47	Colorado	244
5	Connecticut	414
7	Delaware	403
4	Florida	416
30	Georgia	322
46	Hawaii	261
43	Idaho	271
27	Illinois	328
18	Indiana	348
25	Iowa	330
29	Kansas	324
8	Kentucky	398
20	Louisiana	345
13	Maine	366
28	Maryland	327
16	Massachusetts	353
9	Michigan	396
32	Minnesota	315
17	Mississippi	350
23	Missouri	334
45	Montana	266
12	Nebraska	377
42	Nevada	274
25	New Hampshire	330
1	New Jersey	438
48	New Mexico	232
10	New York	392
22	North Carolina	340
36	North Dakota	301
19	Ohio	347
31	Oklahoma	316
39	Oregon	280
3	Pennsylvania	420
6	Rhode Island	405
21	South Carolina	342
41	South Dakota	275
10	Tennessee	392
35	Texas	306
44	Utah	268
34	Vermont	310
33	Virginia	314
38	Washington	282
2	West Virginia	428
23	Wisconsin	334
40	Wyoming	277

RANK ORDER

RANK	STATE	PER CAPITA
1	New Jersey	$438
2	West Virginia	428
3	Pennsylvania	420
4	Florida	416
5	Connecticut	414
6	Rhode Island	405
7	Delaware	403
8	Kentucky	398
9	Michigan	396
10	New York	392
10	Tennessee	392
12	Nebraska	377
13	Maine	366
14	Alabama	357
15	Arkansas	356
16	Massachusetts	353
17	Mississippi	350
18	Indiana	348
19	Ohio	347
20	Louisiana	345
21	South Carolina	342
22	North Carolina	340
23	Missouri	334
23	Wisconsin	334
25	Iowa	330
25	New Hampshire	330
27	Illinois	328
28	Maryland	327
29	Kansas	324
30	Georgia	322
31	Oklahoma	316
32	Minnesota	315
33	Virginia	314
34	Vermont	310
35	Texas	306
36	North Dakota	301
37	Arizona	299
38	Washington	282
39	Oregon	280
40	Wyoming	277
41	South Dakota	275
42	Nevada	274
43	Idaho	271
44	Utah	268
45	Montana	266
46	Hawaii	261
47	Colorado	244
48	New Mexico	232
49	California	231
50	Alaska	216

District of Columbia   345

Source: Morgan Quitno Press using data from U.S. Dept of Health & Human Services, Health Care Financing Admin.
"State Health Care Expenditures" (http://www.hcfa.gov/stats/nhe-oact/stateestimates/)
*Purchases in retail outlets. By state of outlet.

Percent Change in Per Capita Expenditures for Prescription Drugs: 1990 to 1998

National Percent Change = 121.9% Increase*

ALPHA ORDER

RANK	STATE	PERCENT CHANGE
36	Alabama	113.8
29	Alaska	118.2
27	Arizona	119.9
31	Arkansas	117.1
49	California	81.9
30	Colorado	117.9
5	Connecticut	146.4
1	Delaware	170.5
3	Florida	160.0
35	Georgia	114.7
50	Hawaii	71.7
33	Idaho	115.1
41	Illinois	111.6
38	Indiana	113.5
22	Iowa	124.5
40	Kansas	111.8
17	Kentucky	127.4
39	Louisiana	113.0
2	Maine	161.4
43	Maryland	111.0
14	Massachusetts	130.7
21	Michigan	125.0
10	Minnesota	140.5
26	Mississippi	120.1
42	Missouri	111.4
20	Montana	125.4
11	Nebraska	140.1
13	Nevada	134.2
15	New Hampshire	129.2
6	New Jersey	144.7
48	New Mexico	96.6
4	New York	151.3
18	North Carolina	126.7
45	North Dakota	110.5
23	Ohio	122.4
24	Oklahoma	121.0
8	Oregon	143.5
7	Pennsylvania	144.2
12	Rhode Island	136.8
9	South Carolina	142.6
34	South Dakota	114.8
25	Tennessee	120.2
46	Texas	109.6
43	Utah	111.0
28	Vermont	118.3
37	Virginia	113.6
47	Washington	108.9
16	West Virginia	128.9
19	Wisconsin	125.7
32	Wyoming	116.4

RANK ORDER

RANK	STATE	PERCENT CHANGE
1	Delaware	170.5
2	Maine	161.4
3	Florida	160.0
4	New York	151.3
5	Connecticut	146.4
6	New Jersey	144.7
7	Pennsylvania	144.2
8	Oregon	143.5
9	South Carolina	142.6
10	Minnesota	140.5
11	Nebraska	140.1
12	Rhode Island	136.8
13	Nevada	134.2
14	Massachusetts	130.7
15	New Hampshire	129.2
16	West Virginia	128.9
17	Kentucky	127.4
18	North Carolina	126.7
19	Wisconsin	125.7
20	Montana	125.4
21	Michigan	125.0
22	Iowa	124.5
23	Ohio	122.4
24	Oklahoma	121.0
25	Tennessee	120.2
26	Mississippi	120.1
27	Arizona	119.9
28	Vermont	118.3
29	Alaska	118.2
30	Colorado	117.9
31	Arkansas	117.1
32	Wyoming	116.4
33	Idaho	115.1
34	South Dakota	114.8
35	Georgia	114.7
36	Alabama	113.8
37	Virginia	113.6
38	Indiana	113.5
39	Louisiana	113.0
40	Kansas	111.8
41	Illinois	111.6
42	Missouri	111.4
43	Maryland	111.0
43	Utah	111.0
45	North Dakota	110.5
46	Texas	109.6
47	Washington	108.9
48	New Mexico	96.6
49	California	81.9
50	Hawaii	71.7

District of Columbia   161.4

Source: Morgan Quitno Press using data from U.S. Dept of Health & Human Services, Health Care Financing Admin.
"State Health Care Expenditures" (http://www.hcfa.gov/stats/nhe-oact/stateestimates/)
*Purchases in retail outlets. By state of outlet.

Average Annual Change in Per Capita Expenditures
For Prescription Drugs: 1990 to 1998
National Percent Change = 10.5% Average Annual Increase*

ALPHA ORDER				RANK ORDER		
RANK	STATE	PERCENT CHANGE		RANK	STATE	PERCENT CHANGE
33	Alabama	10.0		1	Delaware	13.2
29	Alaska	10.2		2	Maine	12.8
27	Arizona	10.3		3	Florida	12.7
29	Arkansas	10.2		4	New York	12.2
49	California	7.8		5	Connecticut	11.9
29	Colorado	10.2		6	New Jersey	11.8
5	Connecticut	11.9		6	Oregon	11.8
1	Delaware	13.2		6	Pennsylvania	11.8
3	Florida	12.7		9	South Carolina	11.7
33	Georgia	10.0		10	Minnesota	11.6
50	Hawaii	7.0		10	Nebraska	11.6
33	Idaho	10.0		12	Rhode Island	11.4
40	Illinois	9.8		13	Nevada	11.2
38	Indiana	9.9		14	Massachusetts	11.0
22	Iowa	10.6		15	New Hampshire	10.9
40	Kansas	9.8		15	West Virginia	10.9
17	Kentucky	10.8		17	Kentucky	10.8
38	Louisiana	9.9		17	North Carolina	10.8
2	Maine	12.8		19	Michigan	10.7
40	Maryland	9.8		19	Montana	10.7
14	Massachusetts	11.0		19	Wisconsin	10.7
19	Michigan	10.7		22	Iowa	10.6
10	Minnesota	11.6		23	Ohio	10.5
24	Mississippi	10.4		24	Mississippi	10.4
40	Missouri	9.8		24	Oklahoma	10.4
19	Montana	10.7		24	Tennessee	10.4
10	Nebraska	11.6		27	Arizona	10.3
13	Nevada	11.2		27	Vermont	10.3
15	New Hampshire	10.9		29	Alaska	10.2
6	New Jersey	11.8		29	Arkansas	10.2
48	New Mexico	8.8		29	Colorado	10.2
4	New York	12.2		32	Wyoming	10.1
17	North Carolina	10.8		33	Alabama	10.0
45	North Dakota	9.7		33	Georgia	10.0
23	Ohio	10.5		33	Idaho	10.0
24	Oklahoma	10.4		33	South Dakota	10.0
6	Oregon	11.8		33	Virginia	10.0
6	Pennsylvania	11.8		38	Indiana	9.9
12	Rhode Island	11.4		38	Louisiana	9.9
9	South Carolina	11.7		40	Illinois	9.8
33	South Dakota	10.0		40	Kansas	9.8
24	Tennessee	10.4		40	Maryland	9.8
45	Texas	9.7		40	Missouri	9.8
40	Utah	9.8		40	Utah	9.8
27	Vermont	10.3		45	North Dakota	9.7
33	Virginia	10.0		45	Texas	9.7
47	Washington	9.6		47	Washington	9.6
15	West Virginia	10.9		48	New Mexico	8.8
19	Wisconsin	10.7		49	California	7.8
32	Wyoming	10.1		50	Hawaii	7.0
					District of Columbia	12.8

Source: Morgan Quitno Press using data from U.S. Dept of Health & Human Services, Health Care Financing Admin.
"State Health Care Expenditures" (http://www.hcfa.gov/stats/nhe-oact/stateestimates/)
*Purchases in retail outlets. By state of outlet.

Expenditures for Dental Services in 1998

National Total = $53,829,000,000*

ALPHA ORDER

RANK	STATE	EXPENDITURES	% of USA
26	Alabama	$652,000,000	1.2%
44	Alaska	173,000,000	0.3%
24	Arizona	867,000,000	1.6%
33	Arkansas	392,000,000	0.7%
1	California	7,999,000,000	14.9%
19	Colorado	944,000,000	1.8%
22	Connecticut	896,000,000	1.7%
45	Delaware	155,000,000	0.3%
4	Florida	2,957,000,000	5.5%
12	Georgia	1,381,000,000	2.6%
36	Hawaii	284,000,000	0.5%
40	Idaho	253,000,000	0.5%
5	Illinois	2,283,000,000	4.2%
18	Indiana	1,021,000,000	1.9%
31	Iowa	482,000,000	0.9%
30	Kansas	484,000,000	0.9%
28	Kentucky	533,000,000	1.0%
25	Louisiana	703,000,000	1.3%
41	Maine	233,000,000	0.4%
17	Maryland	1,047,000,000	1.9%
11	Massachusetts	1,472,000,000	2.7%
7	Michigan	2,141,000,000	4.0%
16	Minnesota	1,052,000,000	2.0%
35	Mississippi	317,000,000	0.6%
23	Missouri	877,000,000	1.6%
46	Montana	151,000,000	0.3%
38	Nebraska	274,000,000	0.5%
34	Nevada	391,000,000	0.7%
37	New Hampshire	283,000,000	0.5%
9	New Jersey	1,917,000,000	3.6%
39	New Mexico	268,000,000	0.5%
2	New York	3,698,000,000	6.9%
13	North Carolina	1,323,000,000	2.5%
49	North Dakota	110,000,000	0.2%
8	Ohio	1,978,000,000	3.7%
29	Oklahoma	505,000,000	0.9%
21	Oregon	902,000,000	1.7%
6	Pennsylvania	2,237,000,000	4.2%
43	Rhode Island	217,000,000	0.4%
27	South Carolina	591,000,000	1.1%
48	South Dakota	121,000,000	0.2%
20	Tennessee	927,000,000	1.7%
3	Texas	3,218,000,000	6.0%
32	Utah	461,000,000	0.9%
47	Vermont	127,000,000	0.2%
14	Virginia	1,272,000,000	2.4%
10	Washington	1,722,000,000	3.2%
42	West Virginia	221,000,000	0.4%
15	Wisconsin	1,089,000,000	2.0%
50	Wyoming	76,000,000	0.1%

RANK ORDER

RANK	STATE	EXPENDITURES	% of USA
1	California	$7,999,000,000	14.9%
2	New York	3,698,000,000	6.9%
3	Texas	3,218,000,000	6.0%
4	Florida	2,957,000,000	5.5%
5	Illinois	2,283,000,000	4.2%
6	Pennsylvania	2,237,000,000	4.2%
7	Michigan	2,141,000,000	4.0%
8	Ohio	1,978,000,000	3.7%
9	New Jersey	1,917,000,000	3.6%
10	Washington	1,722,000,000	3.2%
11	Massachusetts	1,472,000,000	2.7%
12	Georgia	1,381,000,000	2.6%
13	North Carolina	1,323,000,000	2.5%
14	Virginia	1,272,000,000	2.4%
15	Wisconsin	1,089,000,000	2.0%
16	Minnesota	1,052,000,000	2.0%
17	Maryland	1,047,000,000	1.9%
18	Indiana	1,021,000,000	1.9%
19	Colorado	944,000,000	1.8%
20	Tennessee	927,000,000	1.7%
21	Oregon	902,000,000	1.7%
22	Connecticut	896,000,000	1.7%
23	Missouri	877,000,000	1.6%
24	Arizona	867,000,000	1.6%
25	Louisiana	703,000,000	1.3%
26	Alabama	652,000,000	1.2%
27	South Carolina	591,000,000	1.1%
28	Kentucky	533,000,000	1.0%
29	Oklahoma	505,000,000	0.9%
30	Kansas	484,000,000	0.9%
31	Iowa	482,000,000	0.9%
32	Utah	461,000,000	0.9%
33	Arkansas	392,000,000	0.7%
34	Nevada	391,000,000	0.7%
35	Mississippi	317,000,000	0.6%
36	Hawaii	284,000,000	0.5%
37	New Hampshire	283,000,000	0.5%
38	Nebraska	274,000,000	0.5%
39	New Mexico	268,000,000	0.5%
40	Idaho	253,000,000	0.5%
41	Maine	233,000,000	0.4%
42	West Virginia	221,000,000	0.4%
43	Rhode Island	217,000,000	0.4%
44	Alaska	173,000,000	0.3%
45	Delaware	155,000,000	0.3%
46	Montana	151,000,000	0.3%
47	Vermont	127,000,000	0.2%
48	South Dakota	121,000,000	0.2%
49	North Dakota	110,000,000	0.2%
50	Wyoming	76,000,000	0.1%
	District of Columbia	151,000,000	0.3%

Source: U.S. Department of Health and Human Services, Health Care Financing Administration
"State Health Care Expenditures" (http://www.hcfa.gov/stats/nhe-oact/stateestimates/)
*By state of provider.

Percent of Total Personal Health Care Expenditures
Spent on Dental Services in 1998
National Percent = 5.3%*

ALPHA ORDER

RANK	STATE	PERCENT
46	Alabama	4.1
4	Alaska	7.5
13	Arizona	5.9
35	Arkansas	4.6
6	California	7.3
8	Colorado	6.9
13	Connecticut	5.9
25	Delaware	5.0
25	Florida	5.0
24	Georgia	5.1
9	Hawaii	6.1
5	Idaho	7.4
21	Illinois	5.2
29	Indiana	4.8
32	Iowa	4.7
21	Kansas	5.2
48	Kentucky	3.7
41	Louisiana	4.3
32	Maine	4.7
19	Maryland	5.3
28	Massachusetts	4.9
12	Michigan	6.0
21	Minnesota	5.2
49	Mississippi	3.6
44	Missouri	4.2
19	Montana	5.3
38	Nebraska	4.5
7	Nevada	7.0
9	New Hampshire	6.1
13	New Jersey	5.9
25	New Mexico	5.0
41	New York	4.3
29	North Carolina	4.8
46	North Dakota	4.1
35	Ohio	4.6
35	Oklahoma	4.6
2	Oregon	8.3
40	Pennsylvania	4.4
29	Rhode Island	4.8
38	South Carolina	4.5
41	South Dakota	4.3
44	Tennessee	4.2
32	Texas	4.7
3	Utah	7.8
9	Vermont	6.1
16	Virginia	5.7
1	Washington	8.9
50	West Virginia	3.1
17	Wisconsin	5.5
18	Wyoming	5.4

RANK ORDER

RANK	STATE	PERCENT
1	Washington	8.9
2	Oregon	8.3
3	Utah	7.8
4	Alaska	7.5
5	Idaho	7.4
6	California	7.3
7	Nevada	7.0
8	Colorado	6.9
9	Hawaii	6.1
9	New Hampshire	6.1
9	Vermont	6.1
12	Michigan	6.0
13	Arizona	5.9
13	Connecticut	5.9
13	New Jersey	5.9
16	Virginia	5.7
17	Wisconsin	5.5
18	Wyoming	5.4
19	Maryland	5.3
19	Montana	5.3
21	Illinois	5.2
21	Kansas	5.2
21	Minnesota	5.2
24	Georgia	5.1
25	Delaware	5.0
25	Florida	5.0
25	New Mexico	5.0
28	Massachusetts	4.9
29	Indiana	4.8
29	North Carolina	4.8
29	Rhode Island	4.8
32	Iowa	4.7
32	Maine	4.7
32	Texas	4.7
35	Arkansas	4.6
35	Ohio	4.6
35	Oklahoma	4.6
38	Nebraska	4.5
38	South Carolina	4.5
40	Pennsylvania	4.4
41	Louisiana	4.3
41	New York	4.3
41	South Dakota	4.3
44	Missouri	4.2
44	Tennessee	4.2
46	Alabama	4.1
46	North Dakota	4.1
48	Kentucky	3.7
49	Mississippi	3.6
50	West Virginia	3.1

District of Columbia   3.5

Source: Morgan Quitno Press using data from U.S. Dept of Health & Human Services, Health Care Financing Admin.
"State Health Care Expenditures" (http://www.hcfa.gov/stats/nhe-oact/stateestimates/)
*By state of provider.

Average Annual Change in Expenditures for Dental Services: 1990 to 1998

National Percent Change = 6.9% Average Annual Increase*

ALPHA ORDER				RANK ORDER		
RANK	STATE	PERCENT CHANGE		RANK	STATE	PERCENT CHANGE
26	Alabama	7.4		1	Nevada	11.1
20	Alaska	7.8		2	Idaho	9.3
6	Arizona	8.6		3	North Carolina	9.0
11	Arkansas	8.4		3	Utah	9.0
39	California	6.5		5	Louisiana	8.8
6	Colorado	8.6		6	Arizona	8.6
50	Connecticut	4.3		6	Colorado	8.6
12	Delaware	8.3		6	Oregon	8.6
28	Florida	7.3		6	Texas	8.6
17	Georgia	7.9		10	New Mexico	8.5
49	Hawaii	4.8		11	Arkansas	8.4
2	Idaho	9.3		12	Delaware	8.3
39	Illinois	6.5		12	Kentucky	8.3
14	Indiana	8.2		14	Indiana	8.2
28	Iowa	7.3		15	Washington	8.1
24	Kansas	7.5		16	South Carolina	8.0
12	Kentucky	8.3		17	Georgia	7.9
5	Louisiana	8.8		17	Mississippi	7.9
31	Maine	7.2		17	Tennessee	7.9
37	Maryland	6.6		20	Alaska	7.8
42	Massachusetts	6.3		20	Montana	7.8
43	Michigan	6.1		20	New Hampshire	7.8
37	Minnesota	6.6		23	South Dakota	7.7
17	Mississippi	7.9		24	Kansas	7.5
35	Missouri	6.9		24	Vermont	7.5
20	Montana	7.8		26	Alabama	7.4
33	Nebraska	7.0		26	Virginia	7.4
1	Nevada	11.1		28	Florida	7.3
20	New Hampshire	7.8		28	Iowa	7.3
45	New Jersey	5.4		28	Wisconsin	7.3
10	New Mexico	8.5		31	Maine	7.2
47	New York	5.0		31	North Dakota	7.2
3	North Carolina	9.0		33	Nebraska	7.0
31	North Dakota	7.2		33	West Virginia	7.0
39	Ohio	6.5		35	Missouri	6.9
36	Oklahoma	6.8		36	Oklahoma	6.8
6	Oregon	8.6		37	Maryland	6.6
48	Pennsylvania	4.9		37	Minnesota	6.6
46	Rhode Island	5.1		39	California	6.5
16	South Carolina	8.0		39	Illinois	6.5
23	South Dakota	7.7		39	Ohio	6.5
17	Tennessee	7.9		42	Massachusetts	6.3
6	Texas	8.6		43	Michigan	6.1
3	Utah	9.0		44	Wyoming	5.6
24	Vermont	7.5		45	New Jersey	5.4
26	Virginia	7.4		46	Rhode Island	5.1
15	Washington	8.1		47	New York	5.0
33	West Virginia	7.0		48	Pennsylvania	4.9
28	Wisconsin	7.3		49	Hawaii	4.8
44	Wyoming	5.6		50	Connecticut	4.3
					District of Columbia	5.3

Source: U.S. Department of Health and Human Services, Health Care Financing Administration
"State Health Care Expenditures" (http://www.hcfa.gov/stats/nhe-oact/stateestimates/)
*Purchases in retail outlets. By state of outlet. Includes over-the-counter drugs and sundries.

Per Capita Expenditures for Dental Services in 1998

National Per Capita = $199*

ALPHA ORDER			RANK ORDER		
RANK	STATE	PER CAPITA	RANK	STATE	PER CAPITA
47	Alabama	$150	1	Washington	$303
2	Alaska	281	2	Alaska	281
26	Arizona	186	3	Oregon	275
44	Arkansas	154	4	Connecticut	274
5	California	245	5	California	245
9	Colorado	238	6	Massachusetts	240
4	Connecticut	274	7	Hawaii	239
18	Delaware	208	7	New Hampshire	239
22	Florida	198	9	Colorado	238
29	Georgia	181	10	New Jersey	237
7	Hawaii	239	11	Nevada	224
19	Idaho	206	12	Minnesota	223
23	Illinois	189	13	Rhode Island	220
32	Indiana	173	14	Utah	219
36	Iowa	168	15	Michigan	218
28	Kansas	183	16	Vermont	215
48	Kentucky	135	17	Wisconsin	209
40	Louisiana	161	18	Delaware	208
24	Maine	187	19	Idaho	206
20	Maryland	204	20	Maryland	204
6	Massachusetts	240	20	New York	204
15	Michigan	218	22	Florida	198
12	Minnesota	223	23	Illinois	189
50	Mississippi	115	24	Maine	187
40	Missouri	161	24	Virginia	187
33	Montana	172	26	Arizona	186
38	Nebraska	165	26	Pennsylvania	186
11	Nevada	224	28	Kansas	183
7	New Hampshire	239	29	Georgia	181
10	New Jersey	237	30	Ohio	176
43	New Mexico	155	31	North Carolina	175
20	New York	204	32	Indiana	173
31	North Carolina	175	33	Montana	172
33	North Dakota	172	33	North Dakota	172
30	Ohio	176	35	Tennessee	171
46	Oklahoma	151	36	Iowa	168
3	Oregon	275	37	South Dakota	166
26	Pennsylvania	186	38	Nebraska	165
13	Rhode Island	220	39	Texas	163
44	South Carolina	154	40	Louisiana	161
37	South Dakota	166	40	Missouri	161
35	Tennessee	171	42	Wyoming	158
39	Texas	163	43	New Mexico	155
14	Utah	219	44	Arkansas	154
16	Vermont	215	44	South Carolina	154
24	Virginia	187	46	Oklahoma	151
1	Washington	303	47	Alabama	150
49	West Virginia	122	48	Kentucky	135
17	Wisconsin	209	49	West Virginia	122
42	Wyoming	158	50	Mississippi	115

District of Columbia   290

Source: Morgan Quitno Press using data from U.S. Dept of Health & Human Services, Health Care Financing Admin.
"State Health Care Expenditures" (http://www.hcfa.gov/stats/nhe-oact/stateestimates/)

By state of provider. Per capita calculated using resident population. These figures may be skewed due to residents crossing state borders for care.

Per Capita Medicaid Expenditures for Dental Services in 1998

National Per Capita = $7.37*

ALPHA ORDER

RANK	STATE	PER CAPITA
40	Alabama	$2.99
5	Alaska	13.00
6	Arizona	12.43
31	Arkansas	4.33
1	California	20.47
39	Colorado	3.02
42	Connecticut	2.75
35	Delaware	4.03
25	Florida	4.96
29	Georgia	4.58
49	Hawaii	0.84
12	Idaho	8.12
41	Illinois	2.90
30	Indiana	4.57
9	Iowa	9.44
37	Kansas	3.79
10	Kentucky	8.64
34	Louisiana	4.13
18	Maine	6.41
50	Maryland	0.39
3	Massachusetts	14.00
22	Michigan	5.50
27	Minnesota	4.65
48	Mississippi	1.09
43	Missouri	2.39
14	Montana	7.96
15	Nebraska	7.83
13	Nevada	8.03
32	New Hampshire	4.22
44	New Jersey	2.22
28	New Mexico	4.61
17	New York	6.61
20	North Carolina	5.96
19	North Dakota	6.27
36	Ohio	3.83
45	Oklahoma	2.10
47	Oregon	1.52
24	Pennsylvania	5.17
7	Rhode Island	12.15
26	South Carolina	4.69
23	South Dakota	5.47
21	Tennessee	5.89
16	Texas	6.90
11	Utah	8.57
4	Vermont	13.55
46	Virginia	1.91
2	Washington	20.22
8	West Virginia	11.59
38	Wisconsin	3.64
33	Wyoming	4.17

RANK ORDER

RANK	STATE	PER CAPITA
1	California	$20.47
2	Washington	20.22
3	Massachusetts	14.00
4	Vermont	13.55
5	Alaska	13.00
6	Arizona	12.43
7	Rhode Island	12.15
8	West Virginia	11.59
9	Iowa	9.44
10	Kentucky	8.64
11	Utah	8.57
12	Idaho	8.12
13	Nevada	8.03
14	Montana	7.96
15	Nebraska	7.83
16	Texas	6.90
17	New York	6.61
18	Maine	6.41
19	North Dakota	6.27
20	North Carolina	5.96
21	Tennessee	5.89
22	Michigan	5.50
23	South Dakota	5.47
24	Pennsylvania	5.17
25	Florida	4.96
26	South Carolina	4.69
27	Minnesota	4.65
28	New Mexico	4.61
29	Georgia	4.58
30	Indiana	4.57
31	Arkansas	4.33
32	New Hampshire	4.22
33	Wyoming	4.17
34	Louisiana	4.13
35	Delaware	4.03
36	Ohio	3.83
37	Kansas	3.79
38	Wisconsin	3.64
39	Colorado	3.02
40	Alabama	2.99
41	Illinois	2.90
42	Connecticut	2.75
43	Missouri	2.39
44	New Jersey	2.22
45	Oklahoma	2.10
46	Virginia	1.91
47	Oregon	1.52
48	Mississippi	1.09
49	Hawaii	0.84
50	Maryland	0.39
	District of Columbia	3.84

Source: Morgan Quitno Press using data from U.S. Dept of Health & Human Services, Health Care Financing Admin.
"State Health Care Expenditures" (http://www.hcfa.gov/stats/nhe-oact/stateestimates/)
*By state of provider. Per capita calculated using resident population. These figures may be skewed due to residents crossing state borders for care.

Expenditures for Other Personal Health Care Services in 1998

National Total = $31,917,000,000*

ALPHA ORDER				RANK ORDER			
RANK	STATE	EXPENDITURES	% of USA	RANK	STATE	EXPENDITURES	% of USA
26	Alabama	$407,000,000	1.3%	1	New York	$4,431,000,000	13.9%
35	Alaska	262,000,000	0.8%	2	Texas	2,083,000,000	6.5%
34	Arizona	300,000,000	0.9%	3	California	2,033,000,000	6.4%
36	Arkansas	240,000,000	0.8%	4	Pennsylvania	1,596,000,000	5.0%
3	California	2,033,000,000	6.4%	5	Florida	1,525,000,000	4.8%
22	Colorado	464,000,000	1.5%	6	Illinois	1,320,000,000	4.1%
21	Connecticut	548,000,000	1.7%	7	Massachusetts	1,144,000,000	3.6%
43	Delaware	153,000,000	0.5%	8	Ohio	940,000,000	2.9%
5	Florida	1,525,000,000	4.8%	9	North Carolina	880,000,000	2.8%
13	Georgia	778,000,000	2.4%	10	Michigan	868,000,000	2.7%
44	Hawaii	149,000,000	0.5%	11	Minnesota	808,000,000	2.5%
46	Idaho	116,000,000	0.4%	12	New Jersey	793,000,000	2.5%
6	Illinois	1,320,000,000	4.1%	13	Georgia	778,000,000	2.4%
28	Indiana	381,000,000	1.2%	14	Washington	732,000,000	2.3%
31	Iowa	344,000,000	1.1%	15	Virginia	666,000,000	2.1%
24	Kansas	437,000,000	1.4%	16	Wisconsin	656,000,000	2.1%
25	Kentucky	425,000,000	1.3%	17	Missouri	644,000,000	2.0%
32	Louisiana	342,000,000	1.1%	18	Maryland	598,000,000	1.9%
30	Maine	345,000,000	1.1%	19	South Carolina	576,000,000	1.8%
18	Maryland	598,000,000	1.9%	20	Oregon	563,000,000	1.8%
7	Massachusetts	1,144,000,000	3.6%	21	Connecticut	548,000,000	1.7%
10	Michigan	868,000,000	2.7%	22	Colorado	464,000,000	1.5%
11	Minnesota	808,000,000	2.5%	23	Tennessee	459,000,000	1.4%
39	Mississippi	211,000,000	0.7%	24	Kansas	437,000,000	1.4%
17	Missouri	644,000,000	2.0%	25	Kentucky	425,000,000	1.3%
48	Montana	99,000,000	0.3%	26	Alabama	407,000,000	1.3%
40	Nebraska	179,000,000	0.6%	27	Oklahoma	383,000,000	1.2%
45	Nevada	140,000,000	0.4%	28	Indiana	381,000,000	1.2%
38	New Hampshire	234,000,000	0.7%	29	Rhode Island	358,000,000	1.1%
12	New Jersey	793,000,000	2.5%	30	Maine	345,000,000	1.1%
37	New Mexico	238,000,000	0.7%	31	Iowa	344,000,000	1.1%
1	New York	4,431,000,000	13.9%	32	Louisiana	342,000,000	1.1%
9	North Carolina	880,000,000	2.8%	33	West Virginia	331,000,000	1.0%
49	North Dakota	83,000,000	0.3%	34	Arizona	300,000,000	0.9%
8	Ohio	940,000,000	2.9%	35	Alaska	262,000,000	0.8%
27	Oklahoma	383,000,000	1.2%	36	Arkansas	240,000,000	0.8%
20	Oregon	563,000,000	1.8%	37	New Mexico	238,000,000	0.7%
4	Pennsylvania	1,596,000,000	5.0%	38	New Hampshire	234,000,000	0.7%
29	Rhode Island	358,000,000	1.1%	39	Mississippi	211,000,000	0.7%
19	South Carolina	576,000,000	1.8%	40	Nebraska	179,000,000	0.6%
47	South Dakota	113,000,000	0.4%	41	Utah	160,000,000	0.5%
23	Tennessee	459,000,000	1.4%	42	Vermont	155,000,000	0.5%
2	Texas	2,083,000,000	6.5%	43	Delaware	153,000,000	0.5%
41	Utah	160,000,000	0.5%	44	Hawaii	149,000,000	0.5%
42	Vermont	155,000,000	0.5%	45	Nevada	140,000,000	0.4%
15	Virginia	666,000,000	2.1%	46	Idaho	116,000,000	0.4%
14	Washington	732,000,000	2.3%	47	South Dakota	113,000,000	0.4%
33	West Virginia	331,000,000	1.0%	48	Montana	99,000,000	0.3%
16	Wisconsin	656,000,000	2.1%	49	North Dakota	83,000,000	0.3%
50	Wyoming	69,000,000	0.2%	50	Wyoming	69,000,000	0.2%
					District of Columbia	161,000,000	0.5%

Source: U.S. Department of Health and Human Services, Health Care Financing Administration
"State Health Care Expenditures" (http://www.hcfa.gov/stats/nhe-oact/stateestimates/)
*By state of provider. Includes on-site services provided by employers for the health care needs of their employees.
Also includes shipboard facilities and field stations operated by the U.S. Department of Defense; certain state and local maternal and child health programs; school health programs and federal agency programs targeting veterans, military personnel, Native Americans and persons with dependency and mental-health-related problems.

Percent of Total Personal Health Care Expenditures
Spent on Other Personal Health Care Services in 1998
National Percent = 3.1%*

ALPHA ORDER				RANK ORDER		
RANK	**STATE**	**PERCENT**		**RANK**	**STATE**	**PERCENT**
40	Alabama	2.5		1	Alaska	11.4
1	Alaska	11.4		2	Rhode Island	7.9
48	Arizona	2.0		3	Vermont	7.5
37	Arkansas	2.8		4	Maine	7.0
49	California	1.8		5	New York	5.2
21	Colorado	3.4		5	Oregon	5.2
18	Connecticut	3.6		7	New Hampshire	5.0
8	Delaware	4.9		8	Delaware	4.9
39	Florida	2.6		8	Wyoming	4.9
34	Georgia	2.9		10	Kansas	4.7
25	Hawaii	3.2		10	West Virginia	4.7
21	Idaho	3.4		12	New Mexico	4.5
31	Illinois	3.0		13	South Carolina	4.4
49	Indiana	1.8		14	Minnesota	4.0
21	Iowa	3.4		14	South Dakota	4.0
10	Kansas	4.7		16	Massachusetts	3.8
34	Kentucky	2.9		16	Washington	3.8
46	Louisiana	2.1		18	Connecticut	3.6
4	Maine	7.0		19	Montana	3.5
31	Maryland	3.0		19	Oklahoma	3.5
16	Massachusetts	3.8		21	Colorado	3.4
42	Michigan	2.4		21	Idaho	3.4
14	Minnesota	4.0		21	Iowa	3.4
42	Mississippi	2.4		24	Wisconsin	3.3
27	Missouri	3.1		25	Hawaii	3.2
19	Montana	3.5		25	North Carolina	3.2
34	Nebraska	2.9		27	Missouri	3.1
40	Nevada	2.5		27	North Dakota	3.1
7	New Hampshire	5.0		27	Pennsylvania	3.1
42	New Jersey	2.4		27	Texas	3.1
12	New Mexico	4.5		31	Illinois	3.0
5	New York	5.2		31	Maryland	3.0
25	North Carolina	3.2		31	Virginia	3.0
27	North Dakota	3.1		34	Georgia	2.9
45	Ohio	2.2		34	Kentucky	2.9
19	Oklahoma	3.5		34	Nebraska	2.9
5	Oregon	5.2		37	Arkansas	2.8
27	Pennsylvania	3.1		38	Utah	2.7
2	Rhode Island	7.9		39	Florida	2.6
13	South Carolina	4.4		40	Alabama	2.5
14	South Dakota	4.0		40	Nevada	2.5
46	Tennessee	2.1		42	Michigan	2.4
27	Texas	3.1		42	Mississippi	2.4
38	Utah	2.7		42	New Jersey	2.4
3	Vermont	7.5		45	Ohio	2.2
31	Virginia	3.0		46	Louisiana	2.1
16	Washington	3.8		46	Tennessee	2.1
10	West Virginia	4.7		48	Arizona	2.0
24	Wisconsin	3.3		49	California	1.8
8	Wyoming	4.9		49	Indiana	1.8
					District of Columbia	3.8

Source: Morgan Quitno Press using data from U.S. Dept of Health & Human Services, Health Care Financing Admin.
"State Health Care Expenditures" (http://www.hcfa.gov/stats/nhe-oact/stateestimates/)
*By state of provider. Includes on-site services provided by employers for the health care needs of their employees. Also includes shipboard facilities and field stations operated by the U.S. Department of Defense; certain state and local maternal and child health programs; school health programs and federal agency programs targeting veterans, military personnel, Native Americans and persons with dependency and mental-health-related problems.

Average Annual Change in Expenditures for Other Personal Health Care Services: 1990 to 1998
National Percent Change = 14.1% Average Annual Increase*

ALPHA ORDER

RANK	STATE	PERCENT CHANGE
44	Alabama	10.1
48	Alaska	7.9
42	Arizona	11.1
11	Arkansas	17.5
50	California	6.9
34	Colorado	12.7
31	Connecticut	12.9
15	Delaware	16.5
29	Florida	13.1
40	Georgia	11.6
45	Hawaii	9.3
26	Idaho	14.2
20	Illinois	15.0
46	Indiana	9.1
7	Iowa	19.4
1	Kansas	22.7
25	Kentucky	14.4
43	Louisiana	10.8
2	Maine	22.3
34	Maryland	12.7
24	Massachusetts	14.8
37	Michigan	12.1
14	Minnesota	16.9
41	Mississippi	11.2
13	Missouri	17.0
48	Montana	7.9
28	Nebraska	13.3
16	Nevada	15.9
16	New Hampshire	15.9
47	New Jersey	8.2
19	New Mexico	15.3
5	New York	20.2
9	North Carolina	18.1
38	North Dakota	11.8
39	Ohio	11.7
8	Oklahoma	19.2
11	Oregon	17.5
20	Pennsylvania	15.0
3	Rhode Island	21.8
23	South Carolina	14.9
32	South Dakota	12.8
27	Tennessee	13.6
18	Texas	15.7
32	Utah	12.8
9	Vermont	18.1
30	Virginia	13.0
20	Washington	15.0
4	West Virginia	20.4
36	Wisconsin	12.2
6	Wyoming	20.0

RANK ORDER

RANK	STATE	PERCENT CHANGE
1	Kansas	22.7
2	Maine	22.3
3	Rhode Island	21.8
4	West Virginia	20.4
5	New York	20.2
6	Wyoming	20.0
7	Iowa	19.4
8	Oklahoma	19.2
9	North Carolina	18.1
9	Vermont	18.1
11	Arkansas	17.5
11	Oregon	17.5
13	Missouri	17.0
14	Minnesota	16.9
15	Delaware	16.5
16	Nevada	15.9
16	New Hampshire	15.9
18	Texas	15.7
19	New Mexico	15.3
20	Illinois	15.0
20	Pennsylvania	15.0
20	Washington	15.0
23	South Carolina	14.9
24	Massachusetts	14.8
25	Kentucky	14.4
26	Idaho	14.2
27	Tennessee	13.6
28	Nebraska	13.3
29	Florida	13.1
30	Virginia	13.0
31	Connecticut	12.9
32	South Dakota	12.8
32	Utah	12.8
34	Colorado	12.7
34	Maryland	12.7
36	Wisconsin	12.2
37	Michigan	12.1
38	North Dakota	11.8
39	Ohio	11.7
40	Georgia	11.6
41	Mississippi	11.2
42	Arizona	11.1
43	Louisiana	10.8
44	Alabama	10.1
45	Hawaii	9.3
46	Indiana	9.1
47	New Jersey	8.2
48	Alaska	7.9
48	Montana	7.9
50	California	6.9

| | District of Columbia | 7.1 |

Source: U.S. Department of Health and Human Services, Health Care Financing Administration
"State Health Care Expenditures" (http://www.hcfa.gov/stats/nhe-oact/stateestimates/)
*By state of provider. Includes on-site services provided by employers for the health care needs of their employees. Also includes shipboard facilities and field stations operated by the U.S. Department of Defense; certain state and local maternal and child health programs; school health programs and federal agency programs targeting veterans, military personnel, Native Americans and persons with dependency and mental-health-related problems.

Per Capita Expenditures for Other Personal Health Care Services in 1998

National Per Capita = $118*

ALPHA ORDER

RANK	STATE	PER CAPITA
39	Alabama	$94
1	Alaska	426
48	Arizona	64
38	Arkansas	95
50	California	62
25	Colorado	117
12	Connecticut	167
6	Delaware	206
34	Florida	102
34	Georgia	102
22	Hawaii	125
39	Idaho	94
30	Illinois	109
48	Indiana	64
23	Iowa	120
13	Kansas	166
31	Kentucky	108
45	Louisiana	78
3	Maine	277
25	Maryland	117
8	Massachusetts	186
41	Michigan	88
11	Minnesota	171
46	Mississippi	77
24	Missouri	118
29	Montana	113
31	Nebraska	108
44	Nevada	80
7	New Hampshire	197
36	New Jersey	98
17	New Mexico	137
5	New York	244
25	North Carolina	117
19	North Dakota	130
42	Ohio	84
28	Oklahoma	115
10	Oregon	172
18	Pennsylvania	133
2	Rhode Island	362
15	South Carolina	150
14	South Dakota	155
42	Tennessee	84
33	Texas	106
47	Utah	76
4	Vermont	262
36	Virginia	98
20	Washington	129
9	West Virginia	183
21	Wisconsin	126
16	Wyoming	144

RANK ORDER

RANK	STATE	PER CAPITA
1	Alaska	$426
2	Rhode Island	362
3	Maine	277
4	Vermont	262
5	New York	244
6	Delaware	206
7	New Hampshire	197
8	Massachusetts	186
9	West Virginia	183
10	Oregon	172
11	Minnesota	171
12	Connecticut	167
13	Kansas	166
14	South Dakota	155
15	South Carolina	150
16	Wyoming	144
17	New Mexico	137
18	Pennsylvania	133
19	North Dakota	130
20	Washington	129
21	Wisconsin	126
22	Hawaii	125
23	Iowa	120
24	Missouri	118
25	Colorado	117
25	Maryland	117
25	North Carolina	117
28	Oklahoma	115
29	Montana	113
30	Illinois	109
31	Kentucky	108
31	Nebraska	108
33	Texas	106
34	Florida	102
34	Georgia	102
36	New Jersey	98
36	Virginia	98
38	Arkansas	95
39	Alabama	94
39	Idaho	94
41	Michigan	88
42	Ohio	84
42	Tennessee	84
44	Nevada	80
45	Louisiana	78
46	Mississippi	77
47	Utah	76
48	Arizona	64
48	Indiana	64
50	California	62

District of Columbia 309

Source: Morgan Quitno Press using data from U.S. Dept of Health & Human Services, Health Care Financing Admin. "State Health Care Expenditures" (http://www.hcfa.gov/stats/nhe-oact/stateestimates/)

By state of provider. Includes on-site services provided by employers for the health care needs of their employees. Also includes shipboard facilities and field stations operated by the U.S. Department of Defense; certain state and local maternal and child health programs; school health programs and federal agency programs targeting veterans, military personnel, Native Americans and persons with dependency and mental-health-related problems.

Expenditures for Home Health Care in 1998

National Total = $29,255,000,000*

ALPHA ORDER

RANK	STATE	EXPENDITURES	% of USA
19	Alabama	$470,000,000	1.6%
50	Alaska	9,000,000	0.0%
27	Arizona	331,000,000	1.1%
31	Arkansas	242,000,000	0.8%
4	California	1,951,000,000	6.7%
28	Colorado	324,000,000	1.1%
15	Connecticut	599,000,000	2.0%
41	Delaware	110,000,000	0.4%
3	Florida	2,225,000,000	7.6%
12	Georgia	810,000,000	2.8%
44	Hawaii	60,000,000	0.2%
44	Idaho	60,000,000	0.2%
8	Illinois	972,000,000	3.3%
21	Indiana	415,000,000	1.4%
30	Iowa	248,000,000	0.8%
32	Kansas	220,000,000	0.8%
17	Kentucky	506,000,000	1.7%
13	Louisiana	629,000,000	2.2%
33	Maine	188,000,000	0.6%
25	Maryland	390,000,000	1.3%
7	Massachusetts	999,000,000	3.4%
11	Michigan	841,000,000	2.9%
20	Minnesota	419,000,000	1.4%
29	Mississippi	293,000,000	1.0%
16	Missouri	567,000,000	1.9%
46	Montana	56,000,000	0.2%
42	Nebraska	71,000,000	0.2%
35	Nevada	180,000,000	0.6%
37	New Hampshire	145,000,000	0.5%
9	New Jersey	938,000,000	3.2%
38	New Mexico	143,000,000	0.5%
1	New York	4,292,000,000	14.7%
10	North Carolina	934,000,000	3.2%
48	North Dakota	20,000,000	0.1%
5	Ohio	1,224,000,000	4.2%
23	Oklahoma	391,000,000	1.3%
36	Oregon	151,000,000	0.5%
6	Pennsylvania	1,109,000,000	3.8%
40	Rhode Island	134,000,000	0.5%
23	South Carolina	391,000,000	1.3%
49	South Dakota	11,000,000	0.0%
14	Tennessee	617,000,000	2.1%
2	Texas	2,862,000,000	9.8%
39	Utah	136,000,000	0.5%
43	Vermont	68,000,000	0.2%
18	Virginia	484,000,000	1.7%
26	Washington	365,000,000	1.2%
34	West Virginia	187,000,000	0.6%
22	Wisconsin	393,000,000	1.3%
47	Wyoming	24,000,000	0.1%

RANK ORDER

RANK	STATE	EXPENDITURES	% of USA
1	New York	$4,292,000,000	14.7%
2	Texas	2,862,000,000	9.8%
3	Florida	2,225,000,000	7.6%
4	California	1,951,000,000	6.7%
5	Ohio	1,224,000,000	4.2%
6	Pennsylvania	1,109,000,000	3.8%
7	Massachusetts	999,000,000	3.4%
8	Illinois	972,000,000	3.3%
9	New Jersey	938,000,000	3.2%
10	North Carolina	934,000,000	3.2%
11	Michigan	841,000,000	2.9%
12	Georgia	810,000,000	2.8%
13	Louisiana	629,000,000	2.2%
14	Tennessee	617,000,000	2.1%
15	Connecticut	599,000,000	2.0%
16	Missouri	567,000,000	1.9%
17	Kentucky	506,000,000	1.7%
18	Virginia	484,000,000	1.7%
19	Alabama	470,000,000	1.6%
20	Minnesota	419,000,000	1.4%
21	Indiana	415,000,000	1.4%
22	Wisconsin	393,000,000	1.3%
23	Oklahoma	391,000,000	1.3%
23	South Carolina	391,000,000	1.3%
25	Maryland	390,000,000	1.3%
26	Washington	365,000,000	1.2%
27	Arizona	331,000,000	1.1%
28	Colorado	324,000,000	1.1%
29	Mississippi	293,000,000	1.0%
30	Iowa	248,000,000	0.8%
31	Arkansas	242,000,000	0.8%
32	Kansas	220,000,000	0.8%
33	Maine	188,000,000	0.6%
34	West Virginia	187,000,000	0.6%
35	Nevada	180,000,000	0.6%
36	Oregon	151,000,000	0.5%
37	New Hampshire	145,000,000	0.5%
38	New Mexico	143,000,000	0.5%
39	Utah	136,000,000	0.5%
40	Rhode Island	134,000,000	0.5%
41	Delaware	110,000,000	0.4%
42	Nebraska	71,000,000	0.2%
43	Vermont	68,000,000	0.2%
44	Hawaii	60,000,000	0.2%
44	Idaho	60,000,000	0.2%
46	Montana	56,000,000	0.2%
47	Wyoming	24,000,000	0.1%
48	North Dakota	20,000,000	0.1%
49	South Dakota	11,000,000	0.0%
50	Alaska	9,000,000	0.0%
	District of Columbia	54,000,000	0.2%

Source: U.S. Department of Health and Human Services, Health Care Financing Administration
"State Health Care Expenditures" (http://www.hcfa.gov/stats/nhe-oact/stateestimates/)
*By state of provider. Includes spending for services and products by public and private freestanding home health agencies. Excludes home health care services provided by hospital-based agencies which are included in hospital expenditures.

Percent of Total Personal Health Care Expenditures
Spent on Home Health Care in 1998
National Percent = 2.9%*

ALPHA ORDER

RANK	STATE	PERCENT
19	Alabama	2.9
49	Alaska	0.4
32	Arizona	2.2
19	Arkansas	2.9
42	California	1.8
27	Colorado	2.4
3	Connecticut	3.9
8	Delaware	3.5
6	Florida	3.7
16	Georgia	3.0
46	Hawaii	1.3
42	Idaho	1.8
32	Illinois	2.2
37	Indiana	2.0
27	Iowa	2.4
30	Kansas	2.3
8	Kentucky	3.5
4	Louisiana	3.8
4	Maine	3.8
37	Maryland	2.0
11	Massachusetts	3.3
27	Michigan	2.4
36	Minnesota	2.1
11	Mississippi	3.3
24	Missouri	2.7
37	Montana	2.0
47	Nebraska	1.2
14	Nevada	3.2
15	New Hampshire	3.1
19	New Jersey	2.9
24	New Mexico	2.7
1	New York	5.0
10	North Carolina	3.4
48	North Dakota	0.7
19	Ohio	2.9
7	Oklahoma	3.6
45	Oregon	1.4
32	Pennsylvania	2.2
16	Rhode Island	3.0
16	South Carolina	3.0
49	South Dakota	0.4
23	Tennessee	2.8
2	Texas	4.2
30	Utah	2.3
11	Vermont	3.3
32	Virginia	2.2
41	Washington	1.9
24	West Virginia	2.7
37	Wisconsin	2.0
44	Wyoming	1.7

RANK ORDER

RANK	STATE	PERCENT
1	New York	5.0
2	Texas	4.2
3	Connecticut	3.9
4	Louisiana	3.8
4	Maine	3.8
6	Florida	3.7
7	Oklahoma	3.6
8	Delaware	3.5
8	Kentucky	3.5
10	North Carolina	3.4
11	Massachusetts	3.3
11	Mississippi	3.3
11	Vermont	3.3
14	Nevada	3.2
15	New Hampshire	3.1
16	Georgia	3.0
16	Rhode Island	3.0
16	South Carolina	3.0
19	Alabama	2.9
19	Arkansas	2.9
19	New Jersey	2.9
19	Ohio	2.9
23	Tennessee	2.8
24	Missouri	2.7
24	New Mexico	2.7
24	West Virginia	2.7
27	Colorado	2.4
27	Iowa	2.4
27	Michigan	2.4
30	Kansas	2.3
30	Utah	2.3
32	Arizona	2.2
32	Illinois	2.2
32	Pennsylvania	2.2
32	Virginia	2.2
36	Minnesota	2.1
37	Indiana	2.0
37	Maryland	2.0
37	Montana	2.0
37	Wisconsin	2.0
41	Washington	1.9
42	California	1.8
42	Idaho	1.8
44	Wyoming	1.7
45	Oregon	1.4
46	Hawaii	1.3
47	Nebraska	1.2
48	North Dakota	0.7
49	Alaska	0.4
49	South Dakota	0.4
	District of Columbia	1.3

Source: Morgan Quitno Press using data from U.S. Dept of Health & Human Services, Health Care Financing Admin. "State Health Care Expenditures" (http://www.hcfa.gov/stats/nhe-oact/stateestimates/)
*By state of provider. Includes spending for services and products by public and private freestanding home health agencies. Excludes home health care services provided by hospital-based agencies which are included in hospital expenditures.

Average Annual Change in Expenditures for Home Health Care: 1990 to 1998

National Percent Change = 10.5% Average Annual Increase*

ALPHA ORDER				RANK ORDER		
RANK	STATE	PERCENT CHANGE		RANK	STATE	PERCENT CHANGE
31	Alabama	10.8		1	Hawaii	25.1
4	Alaska	20.7		2	Louisiana	21.3
25	Arizona	12.3		3	Utah	20.8
14	Arkansas	15.0		4	Alaska	20.7
33	California	10.5		5	New Mexico	20.1
17	Colorado	14.3		6	Idaho	18.9
32	Connecticut	10.7		7	Nevada	18.6
10	Delaware	17.2		8	Oklahoma	18.1
30	Florida	11.3		9	Texas	17.6
28	Georgia	11.5		10	Delaware	17.2
1	Hawaii	25.1		11	Ohio	15.7
6	Idaho	18.9		12	North Carolina	15.3
34	Illinois	10.4		13	Kentucky	15.2
21	Indiana	13.8		14	Arkansas	15.0
20	Iowa	14.0		15	New Hampshire	14.5
21	Kansas	13.8		16	Maine	14.4
13	Kentucky	15.2		17	Colorado	14.3
2	Louisiana	21.3		17	South Carolina	14.3
16	Maine	14.4		17	West Virginia	14.3
39	Maryland	9.5		20	Iowa	14.0
43	Massachusetts	8.5		21	Indiana	13.8
50	Michigan	4.6		21	Kansas	13.8
42	Minnesota	9.2		23	Missouri	13.6
41	Mississippi	9.4		24	Oregon	13.2
23	Missouri	13.6		25	Arizona	12.3
46	Montana	7.7		26	Virginia	11.8
36	Nebraska	10.1		27	Wyoming	11.6
7	Nevada	18.6		28	Georgia	11.5
15	New Hampshire	14.5		28	Rhode Island	11.5
38	New Jersey	9.6		30	Florida	11.3
5	New Mexico	20.1		31	Alabama	10.8
49	New York	4.7		32	Connecticut	10.7
12	North Carolina	15.3		33	California	10.5
45	North Dakota	7.8		34	Illinois	10.4
11	Ohio	15.7		34	South Dakota	10.4
8	Oklahoma	18.1		36	Nebraska	10.1
24	Oregon	13.2		37	Pennsylvania	9.9
37	Pennsylvania	9.9		38	New Jersey	9.6
28	Rhode Island	11.5		39	Maryland	9.5
17	South Carolina	14.3		39	Vermont	9.5
34	South Dakota	10.4		41	Mississippi	9.4
48	Tennessee	6.0		42	Minnesota	9.2
9	Texas	17.6		43	Massachusetts	8.5
3	Utah	20.8		43	Washington	8.5
39	Vermont	9.5		45	North Dakota	7.8
26	Virginia	11.8		46	Montana	7.7
43	Washington	8.5		47	Wisconsin	6.8
17	West Virginia	14.3		48	Tennessee	6.0
47	Wisconsin	6.8		49	New York	4.7
27	Wyoming	11.6		50	Michigan	4.6
					District of Columbia	6.0

Source: U.S. Department of Health and Human Services, Health Care Financing Administration
  "State Health Care Expenditures" (http://www.hcfa.gov/stats/nhe-oact/stateestimates/)
By state of provider. Includes spending for services and products by public and private freestanding home health agencies. Excludes home health care services provided by hospital-based agencies which are included in hospital expenditures.

Per Capita Expenditures for Home Health Care in 1998

National Per Capita = $108*

ALPHA ORDER

RANK	STATE	PER CAPITA
18	Alabama	$108
49	Alaska	15
36	Arizona	71
25	Arkansas	95
42	California	60
31	Colorado	82
2	Connecticut	183
6	Delaware	148
5	Florida	149
19	Georgia	106
43	Hawaii	50
45	Idaho	49
33	Illinois	81
38	Indiana	70
28	Iowa	87
30	Kansas	83
10	Kentucky	129
8	Louisiana	144
4	Maine	151
34	Maryland	76
3	Massachusetts	163
29	Michigan	86
27	Minnesota	89
19	Mississippi	106
21	Missouri	104
40	Montana	64
47	Nebraska	43
22	Nevada	103
12	New Hampshire	122
14	New Jersey	116
31	New Mexico	82
1	New York	236
11	North Carolina	124
48	North Dakota	31
17	Ohio	109
13	Oklahoma	117
46	Oregon	46
26	Pennsylvania	92
9	Rhode Island	136
24	South Carolina	102
49	South Dakota	15
16	Tennessee	114
7	Texas	145
39	Utah	65
15	Vermont	115
36	Virginia	71
40	Washington	64
22	West Virginia	103
35	Wisconsin	75
43	Wyoming	50

RANK ORDER

RANK	STATE	PER CAPITA
1	New York	$236
2	Connecticut	183
3	Massachusetts	163
4	Maine	151
5	Florida	149
6	Delaware	148
7	Texas	145
8	Louisiana	144
9	Rhode Island	136
10	Kentucky	129
11	North Carolina	124
12	New Hampshire	122
13	Oklahoma	117
14	New Jersey	116
15	Vermont	115
16	Tennessee	114
17	Ohio	109
18	Alabama	108
19	Georgia	106
19	Mississippi	106
21	Missouri	104
22	Nevada	103
22	West Virginia	103
24	South Carolina	102
25	Arkansas	95
26	Pennsylvania	92
27	Minnesota	89
28	Iowa	87
29	Michigan	86
30	Kansas	83
31	Colorado	82
31	New Mexico	82
33	Illinois	81
34	Maryland	76
35	Wisconsin	75
36	Arizona	71
36	Virginia	71
38	Indiana	70
39	Utah	65
40	Montana	64
40	Washington	64
42	California	60
43	Hawaii	50
43	Wyoming	50
45	Idaho	49
46	Oregon	46
47	Nebraska	43
48	North Dakota	31
49	Alaska	15
49	South Dakota	15
	District of Columbia	104

Source: Morgan Quitno Press using data from U.S. Dept of Health & Human Services, Health Care Financing Admin. "State Health Care Expenditures" (http://www.hcfa.gov/stats/nhe-oact/stateestimates/)
*By state of provider. Includes spending for services and products by public and private freestanding home health agencies. Excludes home health care services provided by hospital-based agencies which are included in hospital expenditures.

Per Capita Medicare Expenditures for Home Health Care in 1998

National Per Capita = $38.27*

ALPHA ORDER				RANK ORDER		
RANK	STATE	PER CAPITA		RANK	STATE	PER CAPITA
12	Alabama	$44.82		1	Louisiana	$129.05
49	Alaska	6.50		2	Oklahoma	89.83
38	Arizona	19.07		3	Texas	85.02
32	Arkansas	23.24		4	Connecticut	75.78
29	California	26.37		5	Tennessee	73.63
39	Colorado	18.90		6	Rhode Island	72.90
4	Connecticut	75.78		7	Maine	72.14
20	Delaware	32.26		8	Mississippi	71.24
11	Florida	46.15		9	Vermont	71.12
21	Georgia	31.82		10	Massachusetts	66.73
45	Hawaii	8.40		11	Florida	46.15
37	Idaho	20.31		12	Alabama	44.82
31	Illinois	25.02		13	Michigan	39.00
27	Indiana	26.91		14	New Hampshire	38.79
43	Iowa	13.28		15	Pennsylvania	38.49
35	Kansas	22.74		16	West Virginia	34.77
18	Kentucky	32.53		17	North Carolina	33.26
1	Louisiana	129.05		18	Kentucky	32.53
7	Maine	72.14		19	South Carolina	32.30
24	Maryland	30.60		20	Delaware	32.26
10	Massachusetts	66.73		21	Georgia	31.82
13	Michigan	39.00		22	New York	31.44
42	Minnesota	13.96		23	New Jersey	31.38
8	Mississippi	71.24		24	Maryland	30.60
33	Missouri	23.17		25	New Mexico	29.42
41	Montana	18.19		26	Ohio	27.50
48	Nebraska	6.62		27	Indiana	26.91
28	Nevada	26.38		28	Nevada	26.38
14	New Hampshire	38.79		29	California	26.37
23	New Jersey	31.38		30	Utah	26.18
25	New Mexico	29.42		31	Illinois	25.02
22	New York	31.44		32	Arkansas	23.24
17	North Carolina	33.26		33	Missouri	23.17
50	North Dakota	6.27		34	Virginia	23.12
26	Ohio	27.50		35	Kansas	22.74
2	Oklahoma	89.83		36	Wisconsin	20.68
46	Oregon	8.23		37	Idaho	20.31
15	Pennsylvania	38.49		38	Arizona	19.07
6	Rhode Island	72.90		39	Colorado	18.90
19	South Carolina	32.30		40	Wyoming	18.75
47	South Dakota	8.21		41	Montana	18.19
5	Tennessee	73.63		42	Minnesota	13.96
3	Texas	85.02		43	Iowa	13.28
30	Utah	26.18		44	Washington	9.85
9	Vermont	71.12		45	Hawaii	8.40
34	Virginia	23.12		46	Oregon	8.23
44	Washington	9.85		47	South Dakota	8.21
16	West Virginia	34.77		48	Nebraska	6.62
36	Wisconsin	20.68		49	Alaska	6.50
40	Wyoming	18.75		50	North Dakota	6.27
					District of Columbia	51.78

Source: Morgan Quitno Press using data from U.S. Dept of Health & Human Services, Health Care Financing Admin.
"State Health Care Expenditures" (http://www.hcfa.gov/stats/nhe-oact/stateestimates/)
*By state of provider. Includes spending for services and products by public and private freestanding home health agencies. Excludes home health care services provided by hospital-based agencies which are included in hospital expenditures.

Per Capita Medicaid Expenditures for Home Health Care in 1998

National Per Capita = $18.48*

<table>
<tr><td colspan="3"><u>ALPHA ORDER</u></td><td colspan="3"><u>RANK ORDER</u></td></tr>
<tr><th>RANK</th><th>STATE</th><th>PER CAPITA</th><th>RANK</th><th>STATE</th><th>PER CAPITA</th></tr>
<tr><td>34</td><td>Alabama</td><td>$4.37</td><td>1</td><td>New York</td><td>$102.10</td></tr>
<tr><td>40</td><td>Alaska</td><td>3.25</td><td>2</td><td>Connecticut</td><td>58.98</td></tr>
<tr><td>44</td><td>Arizona</td><td>1.93</td><td>3</td><td>Massachusetts</td><td>45.08</td></tr>
<tr><td>17</td><td>Arkansas</td><td>12.61</td><td>4</td><td>Minnesota</td><td>30.68</td></tr>
<tr><td>18</td><td>California</td><td>11.60</td><td>5</td><td>New Jersey</td><td>27.55</td></tr>
<tr><td>19</td><td>Colorado</td><td>11.59</td><td>6</td><td>Wisconsin</td><td>25.47</td></tr>
<tr><td>2</td><td>Connecticut</td><td>58.98</td><td>7</td><td>Michigan</td><td>24.03</td></tr>
<tr><td>9</td><td>Delaware</td><td>21.50</td><td>8</td><td>Maryland</td><td>23.78</td></tr>
<tr><td>26</td><td>Florida</td><td>5.77</td><td>9</td><td>Delaware</td><td>21.50</td></tr>
<tr><td>37</td><td>Georgia</td><td>3.54</td><td>10</td><td>Texas</td><td>21.36</td></tr>
<tr><td>45</td><td>Hawaii</td><td>1.68</td><td>11</td><td>West Virginia</td><td>20.42</td></tr>
<tr><td>23</td><td>Idaho</td><td>8.94</td><td>12</td><td>North Carolina</td><td>18.02</td></tr>
<tr><td>49</td><td>Illinois</td><td>0.66</td><td>13</td><td>Vermont</td><td>16.93</td></tr>
<tr><td>29</td><td>Indiana</td><td>5.08</td><td>14</td><td>Kentucky</td><td>15.25</td></tr>
<tr><td>21</td><td>Iowa</td><td>10.14</td><td>15</td><td>Maine</td><td>15.23</td></tr>
<tr><td>27</td><td>Kansas</td><td>5.31</td><td>16</td><td>Washington</td><td>13.89</td></tr>
<tr><td>14</td><td>Kentucky</td><td>15.25</td><td>17</td><td>Arkansas</td><td>12.61</td></tr>
<tr><td>32</td><td>Louisiana</td><td>4.81</td><td>18</td><td>California</td><td>11.60</td></tr>
<tr><td>15</td><td>Maine</td><td>15.23</td><td>19</td><td>Colorado</td><td>11.59</td></tr>
<tr><td>8</td><td>Maryland</td><td>23.78</td><td>20</td><td>Missouri</td><td>10.30</td></tr>
<tr><td>3</td><td>Massachusetts</td><td>45.08</td><td>21</td><td>Iowa</td><td>10.14</td></tr>
<tr><td>7</td><td>Michigan</td><td>24.03</td><td>22</td><td>Montana</td><td>9.10</td></tr>
<tr><td>4</td><td>Minnesota</td><td>30.68</td><td>23</td><td>Idaho</td><td>8.94</td></tr>
<tr><td>39</td><td>Mississippi</td><td>3.27</td><td>24</td><td>Oklahoma</td><td>7.49</td></tr>
<tr><td>20</td><td>Missouri</td><td>10.30</td><td>25</td><td>Pennsylvania</td><td>6.42</td></tr>
<tr><td>22</td><td>Montana</td><td>9.10</td><td>26</td><td>Florida</td><td>5.77</td></tr>
<tr><td>42</td><td>Nebraska</td><td>3.01</td><td>27</td><td>Kansas</td><td>5.31</td></tr>
<tr><td>33</td><td>Nevada</td><td>4.59</td><td>28</td><td>Oregon</td><td>5.18</td></tr>
<tr><td>30</td><td>New Hampshire</td><td>5.06</td><td>29</td><td>Indiana</td><td>5.08</td></tr>
<tr><td>5</td><td>New Jersey</td><td>27.55</td><td>30</td><td>New Hampshire</td><td>5.06</td></tr>
<tr><td>38</td><td>New Mexico</td><td>3.46</td><td>30</td><td>Rhode Island</td><td>5.06</td></tr>
<tr><td>1</td><td>New York</td><td>102.10</td><td>32</td><td>Louisiana</td><td>4.81</td></tr>
<tr><td>12</td><td>North Carolina</td><td>18.02</td><td>33</td><td>Nevada</td><td>4.59</td></tr>
<tr><td>50</td><td>North Dakota</td><td>0.00</td><td>34</td><td>Alabama</td><td>4.37</td></tr>
<tr><td>41</td><td>Ohio</td><td>3.03</td><td>35</td><td>Wyoming</td><td>4.17</td></tr>
<tr><td>24</td><td>Oklahoma</td><td>7.49</td><td>36</td><td>Tennessee</td><td>3.87</td></tr>
<tr><td>28</td><td>Oregon</td><td>5.18</td><td>37</td><td>Georgia</td><td>3.54</td></tr>
<tr><td>25</td><td>Pennsylvania</td><td>6.42</td><td>38</td><td>New Mexico</td><td>3.46</td></tr>
<tr><td>30</td><td>Rhode Island</td><td>5.06</td><td>39</td><td>Mississippi</td><td>3.27</td></tr>
<tr><td>43</td><td>South Carolina</td><td>2.86</td><td>40</td><td>Alaska</td><td>3.25</td></tr>
<tr><td>47</td><td>South Dakota</td><td>1.37</td><td>41</td><td>Ohio</td><td>3.03</td></tr>
<tr><td>36</td><td>Tennessee</td><td>3.87</td><td>42</td><td>Nebraska</td><td>3.01</td></tr>
<tr><td>10</td><td>Texas</td><td>21.36</td><td>43</td><td>South Carolina</td><td>2.86</td></tr>
<tr><td>46</td><td>Utah</td><td>1.43</td><td>44</td><td>Arizona</td><td>1.93</td></tr>
<tr><td>13</td><td>Vermont</td><td>16.93</td><td>45</td><td>Hawaii</td><td>1.68</td></tr>
<tr><td>48</td><td>Virginia</td><td>0.74</td><td>46</td><td>Utah</td><td>1.43</td></tr>
<tr><td>16</td><td>Washington</td><td>13.89</td><td>47</td><td>South Dakota</td><td>1.37</td></tr>
<tr><td>11</td><td>West Virginia</td><td>20.42</td><td>48</td><td>Virginia</td><td>0.74</td></tr>
<tr><td>6</td><td>Wisconsin</td><td>25.47</td><td>49</td><td>Illinois</td><td>0.66</td></tr>
<tr><td>35</td><td>Wyoming</td><td>4.17</td><td>50</td><td>North Dakota</td><td>0.00</td></tr>
<tr><td></td><td></td><td></td><td></td><td>District of Columbia</td><td>30.69</td></tr>
</table>

Source: Morgan Quitno Press using data from U.S. Dept of Health & Human Services, Health Care Financing Admin.
"State Health Care Expenditures" (http://www.hcfa.gov/stats/nhe-oact/stateestimates/)
*By state of provider. Includes spending for services and products by public and private freestanding home health agencies. Excludes home health care services provided by hospital-based agencies which are included in hospital expenditures.

Expenditures for Over-the-Counter Drugs and Other Medical Non-Durables in 1998
National Total = $121,906,000,000*

ALPHA ORDER

RANK	STATE	EXPENDITURES	% of USA
21	Alabama	$2,049,000,000	1.7%
49	Alaska	221,000,000	0.2%
20	Arizona	2,066,000,000	1.7%
32	Arkansas	1,177,000,000	1.0%
1	California	11,604,000,000	9.5%
27	Colorado	1,546,000,000	1.3%
26	Connecticut	1,705,000,000	1.4%
44	Delaware	390,000,000	0.3%
4	Florida	8,226,000,000	6.7%
11	Georgia	3,367,000,000	2.8%
41	Hawaii	514,000,000	0.4%
43	Idaho	474,000,000	0.4%
6	Illinois	5,174,000,000	4.2%
15	Indiana	2,649,000,000	2.2%
31	Iowa	1,219,000,000	1.0%
33	Kansas	1,087,000,000	0.9%
24	Kentucky	1,966,000,000	1.6%
23	Louisiana	1,992,000,000	1.6%
39	Maine	559,000,000	0.5%
18	Maryland	2,304,000,000	1.9%
13	Massachusetts	2,882,000,000	2.4%
8	Michigan	4,884,000,000	4.0%
22	Minnesota	2,004,000,000	1.6%
30	Mississippi	1,222,000,000	1.0%
16	Missouri	2,403,000,000	2.0%
45	Montana	349,000,000	0.3%
37	Nebraska	791,000,000	0.6%
36	Nevada	825,000,000	0.7%
40	New Hampshire	539,000,000	0.4%
9	New Jersey	4,564,000,000	3.7%
38	New Mexico	630,000,000	0.5%
2	New York	8,940,000,000	7.3%
10	North Carolina	3,411,000,000	2.8%
47	North Dakota	250,000,000	0.2%
7	Ohio	5,027,000,000	4.1%
28	Oklahoma	1,418,000,000	1.2%
29	Oregon	1,386,000,000	1.1%
5	Pennsylvania	6,162,000,000	5.1%
42	Rhode Island	505,000,000	0.4%
25	South Carolina	1,721,000,000	1.4%
46	South Dakota	268,000,000	0.2%
14	Tennessee	2,751,000,000	2.3%
3	Texas	8,672,000,000	7.1%
35	Utah	828,000,000	0.7%
48	Vermont	237,000,000	0.2%
12	Virginia	2,947,000,000	2.4%
17	Washington	2,365,000,000	1.9%
34	West Virginia	949,000,000	0.8%
19	Wisconsin	2,269,000,000	1.9%
50	Wyoming	178,000,000	0.1%

RANK ORDER

RANK	STATE	EXPENDITURES	% of USA
1	California	$11,604,000,000	9.5%
2	New York	8,940,000,000	7.3%
3	Texas	8,672,000,000	7.1%
4	Florida	8,226,000,000	6.7%
5	Pennsylvania	6,162,000,000	5.1%
6	Illinois	5,174,000,000	4.2%
7	Ohio	5,027,000,000	4.1%
8	Michigan	4,884,000,000	4.0%
9	New Jersey	4,564,000,000	3.7%
10	North Carolina	3,411,000,000	2.8%
11	Georgia	3,367,000,000	2.8%
12	Virginia	2,947,000,000	2.4%
13	Massachusetts	2,882,000,000	2.4%
14	Tennessee	2,751,000,000	2.3%
15	Indiana	2,649,000,000	2.2%
16	Missouri	2,403,000,000	2.0%
17	Washington	2,365,000,000	1.9%
18	Maryland	2,304,000,000	1.9%
19	Wisconsin	2,269,000,000	1.9%
20	Arizona	2,066,000,000	1.7%
21	Alabama	2,049,000,000	1.7%
22	Minnesota	2,004,000,000	1.6%
23	Louisiana	1,992,000,000	1.6%
24	Kentucky	1,966,000,000	1.6%
25	South Carolina	1,721,000,000	1.4%
26	Connecticut	1,705,000,000	1.4%
27	Colorado	1,546,000,000	1.3%
28	Oklahoma	1,418,000,000	1.2%
29	Oregon	1,386,000,000	1.1%
30	Mississippi	1,222,000,000	1.0%
31	Iowa	1,219,000,000	1.0%
32	Arkansas	1,177,000,000	1.0%
33	Kansas	1,087,000,000	0.9%
34	West Virginia	949,000,000	0.8%
35	Utah	828,000,000	0.7%
36	Nevada	825,000,000	0.7%
37	Nebraska	791,000,000	0.6%
38	New Mexico	630,000,000	0.5%
39	Maine	559,000,000	0.5%
40	New Hampshire	539,000,000	0.4%
41	Hawaii	514,000,000	0.4%
42	Rhode Island	505,000,000	0.4%
43	Idaho	474,000,000	0.4%
44	Delaware	390,000,000	0.3%
45	Montana	349,000,000	0.3%
46	South Dakota	268,000,000	0.2%
47	North Dakota	250,000,000	0.2%
48	Vermont	237,000,000	0.2%
49	Alaska	221,000,000	0.2%
50	Wyoming	178,000,000	0.1%
	District of Columbia	239,000,000	0.2%

Source: U.S. Department of Health and Human Services, Health Care Financing Administration
"State Health Care Expenditures" (http://www.hcfa.gov/stats/nhe-oact/stateestimates/)
*Purchases in retail outlets. By state of outlet. Includes over-the-counter drugs and sundries.

Percent of Total Personal Health Care Expenditures
Spent on Over-the-Counter Drugs and Other Medical Non-Durables in 1998
National Percent = 12.0%*

ALPHA ORDER

RANK ORDER

RANK	STATE	PERCENT		RANK	STATE	PERCENT
16	Alabama	12.8		1	Nevada	14.7
47	Alaska	9.6		2	Arizona	14.0
2	Arizona	14.0		2	Idaho	14.0
5	Arkansas	13.9		2	New Jersey	14.0
44	California	10.5		5	Arkansas	13.9
40	Colorado	11.3		5	Utah	13.9
41	Connecticut	11.2		7	Florida	13.8
20	Delaware	12.6		7	Mississippi	13.8
7	Florida	13.8		9	Michigan	13.7
24	Georgia	12.4		10	Kentucky	13.6
43	Hawaii	11.0		11	West Virginia	13.5
2	Idaho	14.0		12	Virginia	13.2
32	Illinois	11.7		13	Nebraska	13.0
21	Indiana	12.5		13	South Carolina	13.0
28	Iowa	12.0		15	Oklahoma	12.9
34	Kansas	11.6		16	Alabama	12.8
10	Kentucky	13.6		16	Oregon	12.8
27	Louisiana	12.1		16	Texas	12.8
38	Maine	11.4		19	Wyoming	12.7
32	Maryland	11.7		20	Delaware	12.6
47	Massachusetts	9.6		21	Indiana	12.5
9	Michigan	13.7		21	North Carolina	12.5
46	Minnesota	9.9		21	Tennessee	12.5
7	Mississippi	13.8		24	Georgia	12.4
36	Missouri	11.5		25	Montana	12.3
25	Montana	12.3		25	Washington	12.3
13	Nebraska	13.0		27	Louisiana	12.1
1	Nevada	14.7		28	Iowa	12.0
34	New Hampshire	11.6		28	Pennsylvania	12.0
2	New Jersey	14.0		30	New Mexico	11.8
30	New Mexico	11.8		30	Ohio	11.8
45	New York	10.4		32	Illinois	11.7
21	North Carolina	12.5		32	Maryland	11.7
50	North Dakota	9.3		34	Kansas	11.6
30	Ohio	11.8		34	New Hampshire	11.6
15	Oklahoma	12.9		36	Missouri	11.5
16	Oregon	12.8		36	Vermont	11.5
28	Pennsylvania	12.0		38	Maine	11.4
41	Rhode Island	11.2		38	Wisconsin	11.4
13	South Carolina	13.0		40	Colorado	11.3
49	South Dakota	9.4		41	Connecticut	11.2
21	Tennessee	12.5		41	Rhode Island	11.2
16	Texas	12.8		43	Hawaii	11.0
5	Utah	13.9		44	California	10.5
36	Vermont	11.5		45	New York	10.4
12	Virginia	13.2		46	Minnesota	9.9
25	Washington	12.3		47	Alaska	9.6
11	West Virginia	13.5		47	Massachusetts	9.6
38	Wisconsin	11.4		49	South Dakota	9.4
19	Wyoming	12.7		50	North Dakota	9.3
					District of Columbia	5.6

Source: Morgan Quitno Press using data from U.S. Dept of Health & Human Services, Health Care Financing Admin.
"State Health Care Expenditures" (http://www.hcfa.gov/stats/nhe-oact/stateestimates/)
*Purchases in retail outlets. By state of outlet. Includes over-the-counter drugs and sundries.

Average Annual Change in Expenditures for Over-the-Counter Drugs and Other Medical Non-Durables: 1990 to 1998
National Percent Change = 9.3% Average Annual Increase*

ALPHA ORDER

RANK	STATE	PERCENT CHANGE
23	Alabama	9.3
47	Alaska	8.0
3	Arizona	11.4
20	Arkansas	9.5
49	California	7.1
8	Colorado	10.4
29	Connecticut	9.1
3	Delaware	11.4
2	Florida	11.6
12	Georgia	10.2
50	Hawaii	5.6
5	Idaho	10.6
40	Illinois	8.5
31	Indiana	8.9
31	Iowa	8.9
39	Kansas	8.6
17	Kentucky	9.6
44	Louisiana	8.2
8	Maine	10.4
44	Maryland	8.2
37	Massachusetts	8.8
23	Michigan	9.3
14	Minnesota	10.0
23	Mississippi	9.3
37	Missouri	8.8
27	Montana	9.2
13	Nebraska	10.1
1	Nevada	14.3
27	New Hampshire	9.2
16	New Jersey	9.9
31	New Mexico	8.9
22	New York	9.4
8	North Carolina	10.4
48	North Dakota	7.6
40	Ohio	8.5
31	Oklahoma	8.9
5	Oregon	10.6
20	Pennsylvania	9.5
40	Rhode Island	8.5
5	South Carolina	10.6
40	South Dakota	8.5
14	Tennessee	10.0
17	Texas	9.6
11	Utah	10.3
31	Vermont	8.9
31	Virginia	8.9
23	Washington	9.3
30	West Virginia	9.0
17	Wisconsin	9.6
44	Wyoming	8.2

RANK ORDER

RANK	STATE	PERCENT CHANGE
1	Nevada	14.3
2	Florida	11.6
3	Arizona	11.4
3	Delaware	11.4
5	Idaho	10.6
5	Oregon	10.6
5	South Carolina	10.6
8	Colorado	10.4
8	Maine	10.4
8	North Carolina	10.4
11	Utah	10.3
12	Georgia	10.2
13	Nebraska	10.1
14	Minnesota	10.0
14	Tennessee	10.0
16	New Jersey	9.9
17	Kentucky	9.6
17	Texas	9.6
17	Wisconsin	9.6
20	Arkansas	9.5
20	Pennsylvania	9.5
22	New York	9.4
23	Alabama	9.3
23	Michigan	9.3
23	Mississippi	9.3
23	Washington	9.3
27	Montana	9.2
27	New Hampshire	9.2
29	Connecticut	9.1
30	West Virginia	9.0
31	Indiana	8.9
31	Iowa	8.9
31	New Mexico	8.9
31	Oklahoma	8.9
31	Vermont	8.9
31	Virginia	8.9
37	Massachusetts	8.8
37	Missouri	8.8
39	Kansas	8.6
40	Illinois	8.5
40	Ohio	8.5
40	Rhode Island	8.5
40	South Dakota	8.5
44	Louisiana	8.2
44	Maryland	8.2
44	Wyoming	8.2
47	Alaska	8.0
48	North Dakota	7.6
49	California	7.1
50	Hawaii	5.6
	District of Columbia	6.5

Source: U.S. Department of Health and Human Services, Health Care Financing Administration
"State Health Care Expenditures" (http://www.hcfa.gov/stats/nhe-oact/stateestimates/)
*Purchases in retail outlets. By state of outlet. Includes over-the-counter drugs and sundries.

Per Capita Expenditures for Over-the-Counter Drugs and Other Medical Non-Durables in 1998
National Per Capita = $451*

ALPHA ORDER

RANK	STATE	PER CAPITA
14	Alabama	$471
49	Alaska	359
26	Arizona	443
16	Arkansas	464
50	California	355
44	Colorado	390
5	Connecticut	521
3	Delaware	524
2	Florida	552
28	Georgia	441
32	Hawaii	432
45	Idaho	385
33	Illinois	429
21	Indiana	448
34	Iowa	426
39	Kansas	412
9	Kentucky	500
17	Louisiana	457
21	Maine	448
20	Maryland	449
15	Massachusetts	469
10	Michigan	497
36	Minnesota	424
25	Mississippi	444
27	Missouri	442
41	Montana	397
12	Nebraska	476
13	Nevada	473
18	New Hampshire	455
1	New Jersey	564
48	New Mexico	363
11	New York	492
19	North Carolina	452
43	North Dakota	392
24	Ohio	447
35	Oklahoma	425
37	Oregon	422
6	Pennsylvania	513
7	Rhode Island	511
21	South Carolina	448
47	South Dakota	367
8	Tennessee	506
29	Texas	440
42	Utah	394
40	Vermont	401
30	Virginia	434
38	Washington	416
3	West Virginia	524
30	Wisconsin	434
46	Wyoming	371

RANK ORDER

RANK	STATE	PER CAPITA
1	New Jersey	$564
2	Florida	552
3	Delaware	524
3	West Virginia	524
5	Connecticut	521
6	Pennsylvania	513
7	Rhode Island	511
8	Tennessee	506
9	Kentucky	500
10	Michigan	497
11	New York	492
12	Nebraska	476
13	Nevada	473
14	Alabama	471
15	Massachusetts	469
16	Arkansas	464
17	Louisiana	457
18	New Hampshire	455
19	North Carolina	452
20	Maryland	449
21	Indiana	448
21	Maine	448
21	South Carolina	448
24	Ohio	447
25	Mississippi	444
26	Arizona	443
27	Missouri	442
28	Georgia	441
29	Texas	440
30	Virginia	434
30	Wisconsin	434
32	Hawaii	432
33	Illinois	429
34	Iowa	426
35	Oklahoma	425
36	Minnesota	424
37	Oregon	422
38	Washington	416
39	Kansas	412
40	Vermont	401
41	Montana	397
42	Utah	394
43	North Dakota	392
44	Colorado	390
45	Idaho	385
46	Wyoming	371
47	South Dakota	367
48	New Mexico	363
49	Alaska	359
50	California	355

District of Columbia 458

Source: Morgan Quitno Press using data from U.S. Dept of Health & Human Services, Health Care Financing Admin. "State Health Care Expenditures" (http://www.hcfa.gov/stats/nhe-oact/stateestimates/)
*Purchases in retail outlets. By state of outlet. Includes over-the-counter drugs and sundries. Per capita calculated using resident population. These figures may be skewed due to residents crossing state borders to make purchases.

Expenditures for Vision Products and Other Medical Durables in 1998

National Total = $15,499,000,000*

ALPHA ORDER

ALPHA ORDER

RANK	STATE	EXPENDITURES	% of USA
25	Alabama	$186,000,000	1.2%
46	Alaska	38,000,000	0.2%
22	Arizona	267,000,000	1.7%
36	Arkansas	87,000,000	0.6%
1	California	1,656,000,000	10.7%
18	Colorado	323,000,000	2.1%
23	Connecticut	231,000,000	1.5%
43	Delaware	49,000,000	0.3%
2	Florida	1,184,000,000	7.6%
10	Georgia	432,000,000	2.8%
38	Hawaii	78,000,000	0.5%
41	Idaho	59,000,000	0.4%
6	Illinois	662,000,000	4.3%
17	Indiana	328,000,000	2.1%
27	Iowa	177,000,000	1.1%
31	Kansas	128,000,000	0.8%
26	Kentucky	185,000,000	1.2%
24	Louisiana	198,000,000	1.3%
42	Maine	58,000,000	0.4%
19	Maryland	322,000,000	2.1%
12	Massachusetts	347,000,000	2.2%
8	Michigan	626,000,000	4.0%
14	Minnesota	343,000,000	2.2%
35	Mississippi	93,000,000	0.6%
20	Missouri	280,000,000	1.8%
44	Montana	41,000,000	0.3%
34	Nebraska	119,000,000	0.8%
32	Nevada	123,000,000	0.8%
40	New Hampshire	68,000,000	0.4%
9	New Jersey	552,000,000	3.6%
39	New Mexico	77,000,000	0.5%
4	New York	1,099,000,000	7.1%
15	North Carolina	338,000,000	2.2%
47	North Dakota	35,000,000	0.2%
7	Ohio	647,000,000	4.2%
30	Oklahoma	142,000,000	0.9%
28	Oregon	169,000,000	1.1%
5	Pennsylvania	688,000,000	4.4%
47	Rhode Island	35,000,000	0.2%
29	South Carolina	168,000,000	1.1%
45	South Dakota	40,000,000	0.3%
21	Tennessee	271,000,000	1.7%
3	Texas	1,176,000,000	7.6%
33	Utah	121,000,000	0.8%
49	Vermont	29,000,000	0.2%
11	Virginia	392,000,000	2.5%
13	Washington	346,000,000	2.2%
36	West Virginia	87,000,000	0.6%
16	Wisconsin	333,000,000	2.1%
50	Wyoming	22,000,000	0.1%

RANK ORDER

RANK	STATE	EXPENDITURES	% of USA
1	California	$1,656,000,000	10.7%
2	Florida	1,184,000,000	7.6%
3	Texas	1,176,000,000	7.6%
4	New York	1,099,000,000	7.1%
5	Pennsylvania	688,000,000	4.4%
6	Illinois	662,000,000	4.3%
7	Ohio	647,000,000	4.2%
8	Michigan	626,000,000	4.0%
9	New Jersey	552,000,000	3.6%
10	Georgia	432,000,000	2.8%
11	Virginia	392,000,000	2.5%
12	Massachusetts	347,000,000	2.2%
13	Washington	346,000,000	2.2%
14	Minnesota	343,000,000	2.2%
15	North Carolina	338,000,000	2.2%
16	Wisconsin	333,000,000	2.1%
17	Indiana	328,000,000	2.1%
18	Colorado	323,000,000	2.1%
19	Maryland	322,000,000	2.1%
20	Missouri	280,000,000	1.8%
21	Tennessee	271,000,000	1.7%
22	Arizona	267,000,000	1.7%
23	Connecticut	231,000,000	1.5%
24	Louisiana	198,000,000	1.3%
25	Alabama	186,000,000	1.2%
26	Kentucky	185,000,000	1.2%
27	Iowa	177,000,000	1.1%
28	Oregon	169,000,000	1.1%
29	South Carolina	168,000,000	1.1%
30	Oklahoma	142,000,000	0.9%
31	Kansas	128,000,000	0.8%
32	Nevada	123,000,000	0.8%
33	Utah	121,000,000	0.8%
34	Nebraska	119,000,000	0.8%
35	Mississippi	93,000,000	0.6%
36	Arkansas	87,000,000	0.6%
36	West Virginia	87,000,000	0.6%
38	Hawaii	78,000,000	0.5%
39	New Mexico	77,000,000	0.5%
40	New Hampshire	68,000,000	0.4%
41	Idaho	59,000,000	0.4%
42	Maine	58,000,000	0.4%
43	Delaware	49,000,000	0.3%
44	Montana	41,000,000	0.3%
45	South Dakota	40,000,000	0.3%
46	Alaska	38,000,000	0.2%
47	North Dakota	35,000,000	0.2%
47	Rhode Island	35,000,000	0.2%
49	Vermont	29,000,000	0.2%
50	Wyoming	22,000,000	0.1%
	District of Columbia	42,000,000	0.3%

Source: U.S. Department of Health and Human Services, Health Care Financing Administration
"State Health Care Expenditures" (http://www.hcfa.gov/stats/nhe-oact/stateestimates/)
*By state of provider. Includes eyeglasses, hearing aids, surgical appliances and supplies, bulk and cylinder oxygen and medical equipment rentals.

Percent of Total Personal Health Care Expenditures
Spent on Vision Products and Other Medical Durables in 1998
National Percent = 1.5%*

ALPHA ORDER				RANK ORDER		
RANK	**STATE**	**PERCENT**		**RANK**	**STATE**	**PERCENT**
41	Alabama	1.2		1	Colorado	2.4
10	Alaska	1.7		2	Nevada	2.2
6	Arizona	1.8		3	Florida	2.0
48	Arkansas	1.0		3	Nebraska	2.0
23	California	1.5		3	Utah	2.0
1	Colorado	2.4		6	Arizona	1.8
23	Connecticut	1.5		6	Michigan	1.8
18	Delaware	1.6		6	Virginia	1.8
3	Florida	2.0		6	Washington	1.8
18	Georgia	1.6		10	Alaska	1.7
10	Hawaii	1.7		10	Hawaii	1.7
10	Idaho	1.7		10	Idaho	1.7
23	Illinois	1.5		10	Iowa	1.7
23	Indiana	1.5		10	Minnesota	1.7
10	Iowa	1.7		10	New Jersey	1.7
29	Kansas	1.4		10	Texas	1.7
34	Kentucky	1.3		10	Wisconsin	1.7
41	Louisiana	1.2		18	Delaware	1.6
41	Maine	1.2		18	Georgia	1.6
18	Maryland	1.6		18	Maryland	1.6
41	Massachusetts	1.2		18	Oregon	1.6
6	Michigan	1.8		18	Wyoming	1.6
10	Minnesota	1.7		23	California	1.5
48	Mississippi	1.0		23	Connecticut	1.5
34	Missouri	1.3		23	Illinois	1.5
29	Montana	1.4		23	Indiana	1.5
3	Nebraska	2.0		23	New Hampshire	1.5
2	Nevada	2.2		23	Ohio	1.5
23	New Hampshire	1.5		29	Kansas	1.4
10	New Jersey	1.7		29	Montana	1.4
29	New Mexico	1.4		29	New Mexico	1.4
34	New York	1.3		29	South Dakota	1.4
41	North Carolina	1.2		29	Vermont	1.4
34	North Dakota	1.3		34	Kentucky	1.3
23	Ohio	1.5		34	Missouri	1.3
34	Oklahoma	1.3		34	New York	1.3
18	Oregon	1.6		34	North Dakota	1.3
34	Pennsylvania	1.3		34	Oklahoma	1.3
50	Rhode Island	0.8		34	Pennsylvania	1.3
34	South Carolina	1.3		34	South Carolina	1.3
29	South Dakota	1.4		41	Alabama	1.2
41	Tennessee	1.2		41	Louisiana	1.2
10	Texas	1.7		41	Maine	1.2
3	Utah	2.0		41	Massachusetts	1.2
29	Vermont	1.4		41	North Carolina	1.2
6	Virginia	1.8		41	Tennessee	1.2
6	Washington	1.8		41	West Virginia	1.2
41	West Virginia	1.2		48	Arkansas	1.0
10	Wisconsin	1.7		48	Mississippi	1.0
18	Wyoming	1.6		50	Rhode Island	0.8
					District of Columbia	1.0

Source: Morgan Quitno Press using data from U.S. Dept of Health & Human Services, Health Care Financing Admin. "State Health Care Expenditures" (http://www.hcfa.gov/stats/nhe-oact/stateestimates/)
*By state of provider. Includes eyeglasses, hearing aids, surgical appliances and supplies, bulk and cylinder oxygen and medical equipment rentals.

Average Annual Change in Expenditures for Vision Products and Other Medical Durables: 1990 to 1998
National Percent Change = 5.0% Average Annual Increase*

ALPHA ORDER			RANK ORDER		
RANK	STATE	PERCENT CHANGE	RANK	STATE	PERCENT CHANGE
22	Alabama	5.2	1	Nevada	8.9
19	Alaska	5.4	2	Colorado	7.5
8	Arizona	6.4	2	Idaho	7.5
16	Arkansas	5.9	4	Oregon	7.0
45	California	4.0	5	Washington	6.6
2	Colorado	7.5	6	Mississippi	6.5
38	Connecticut	4.3	6	Utah	6.5
10	Delaware	6.3	8	Arizona	6.4
10	Florida	6.3	8	Georgia	6.4
8	Georgia	6.4	10	Delaware	6.3
41	Hawaii	4.2	10	Florida	6.3
2	Idaho	7.5	10	Texas	6.3
41	Illinois	4.2	13	New Hampshire	6.2
31	Indiana	4.7	13	South Carolina	6.2
38	Iowa	4.3	15	North Carolina	6.0
33	Kansas	4.5	16	Arkansas	5.9
17	Kentucky	5.6	17	Kentucky	5.6
27	Louisiana	4.9	17	Virginia	5.6
43	Maine	4.1	19	Alaska	5.4
32	Maryland	4.6	19	Wisconsin	5.4
29	Massachusetts	4.8	21	Tennessee	5.3
22	Michigan	5.2	22	Alabama	5.2
22	Minnesota	5.2	22	Michigan	5.2
6	Mississippi	6.5	22	Minnesota	5.2
35	Missouri	4.4	25	New Mexico	5.0
45	Montana	4.0	25	South Dakota	5.0
27	Nebraska	4.9	27	Louisiana	4.9
1	Nevada	8.9	27	Nebraska	4.9
13	New Hampshire	6.2	29	Massachusetts	4.8
33	New Jersey	4.5	29	Vermont	4.8
25	New Mexico	5.0	31	Indiana	4.7
49	New York	3.4	32	Maryland	4.6
15	North Carolina	6.0	33	Kansas	4.5
38	North Dakota	4.3	33	New Jersey	4.5
35	Ohio	4.4	35	Missouri	4.4
35	Oklahoma	4.4	35	Ohio	4.4
4	Oregon	7.0	35	Oklahoma	4.4
47	Pennsylvania	3.9	38	Connecticut	4.3
50	Rhode Island	3.3	38	Iowa	4.3
13	South Carolina	6.2	38	North Dakota	4.3
25	South Dakota	5.0	41	Hawaii	4.2
21	Tennessee	5.3	41	Illinois	4.2
10	Texas	6.3	43	Maine	4.1
6	Utah	6.5	43	Wyoming	4.1
29	Vermont	4.8	45	California	4.0
17	Virginia	5.6	45	Montana	4.0
5	Washington	6.6	47	Pennsylvania	3.9
48	West Virginia	3.7	48	West Virginia	3.7
19	Wisconsin	5.4	49	New York	3.4
43	Wyoming	4.1	50	Rhode Island	3.3
				District of Columbia	3.5

Source: U.S. Department of Health and Human Services, Health Care Financing Administration
    "State Health Care Expenditures" (http://www.hcfa.gov/stats/nhe-oact/stateestimates/)
*By state of provider. Includes eyeglasses, hearing aids, surgical appliances and supplies, bulk and cylinder oxygen and medical equipment rentals.

Per Capita Expenditures for Vision Products and Other Medical Durables in 1998

National Per Capita = $57*

ALPHA ORDER			RANK ORDER		
RANK	STATE	PER CAPITA	RANK	STATE	PER CAPITA
46	Alabama	$43	1	Colorado	$81
13	Alaska	62	2	Florida	79
21	Arizona	57	3	Minnesota	73
49	Arkansas	34	4	Nebraska	72
30	California	51	5	Connecticut	71
1	Colorado	81	5	Nevada	71
5	Connecticut	71	7	New Jersey	68
8	Delaware	66	8	Delaware	66
2	Florida	79	8	Hawaii	66
21	Georgia	57	10	Michigan	64
8	Hawaii	66	10	Wisconsin	64
36	Idaho	48	12	Maryland	63
27	Illinois	55	13	Alaska	62
25	Indiana	56	13	Iowa	62
13	Iowa	62	15	New York	61
34	Kansas	49	15	Washington	61
38	Kentucky	47	17	Texas	60
42	Louisiana	45	18	Ohio	58
40	Maine	46	18	Utah	58
12	Maryland	63	18	Virginia	58
25	Massachusetts	56	21	Arizona	57
10	Michigan	64	21	Georgia	57
3	Minnesota	73	21	New Hampshire	57
49	Mississippi	34	21	Pennsylvania	57
30	Missouri	51	25	Indiana	56
38	Montana	47	25	Massachusetts	56
4	Nebraska	72	27	Illinois	55
5	Nevada	71	27	North Dakota	55
21	New Hampshire	57	27	South Dakota	55
7	New Jersey	68	30	California	51
44	New Mexico	44	30	Missouri	51
15	New York	61	30	Oregon	51
42	North Carolina	45	33	Tennessee	50
27	North Dakota	55	34	Kansas	49
18	Ohio	58	34	Vermont	49
46	Oklahoma	43	36	Idaho	48
30	Oregon	51	36	West Virginia	48
21	Pennsylvania	57	38	Kentucky	47
48	Rhode Island	35	38	Montana	47
44	South Carolina	44	40	Maine	46
27	South Dakota	55	40	Wyoming	46
33	Tennessee	50	42	Louisiana	45
17	Texas	60	42	North Carolina	45
18	Utah	58	44	New Mexico	44
34	Vermont	49	44	South Carolina	44
18	Virginia	58	46	Alabama	43
15	Washington	61	46	Oklahoma	43
36	West Virginia	48	48	Rhode Island	35
10	Wisconsin	64	49	Arkansas	34
40	Wyoming	46	49	Mississippi	34
				District of Columbia	81

Source: Morgan Quitno Press using data from U.S. Dept of Health & Human Services, Health Care Financing Admin. "State Health Care Expenditures" (http://www.hcfa.gov/stats/nhe-oact/stateestimates/)
*By state of provider. Includes eyeglasses, hearing aids, surgical appliances and supplies, bulk and cylinder oxygen and medical equipment rentals.

Expenditures for Nursing Home Care in 1998

National Total = $87,826,000,000*

ALPHA ORDER				RANK ORDER			
RANK	STATE	EXPENDITURES	% of USA	RANK	STATE	EXPENDITURES	% of USA
25	Alabama	$1,064,000,000	1.2%	1	New York	$10,586,000,000	12.1%
50	Alaska	42,000,000	0.0%	2	Pennsylvania	5,883,000,000	6.7%
30	Arizona	839,000,000	1.0%	3	California	5,626,000,000	6.4%
32	Arkansas	776,000,000	0.9%	4	Ohio	4,978,000,000	5.7%
3	California	5,626,000,000	6.4%	5	Florida	4,880,000,000	5.6%
29	Colorado	904,000,000	1.0%	6	Texas	4,346,000,000	4.9%
13	Connecticut	2,264,000,000	2.6%	7	Illinois	3,924,000,000	4.5%
40	Delaware	290,000,000	0.3%	8	Massachusetts	3,568,000,000	4.1%
5	Florida	4,880,000,000	5.6%	9	New Jersey	3,233,000,000	3.7%
20	Georgia	1,545,000,000	1.8%	10	Michigan	2,459,000,000	2.8%
46	Hawaii	204,000,000	0.2%	11	North Carolina	2,347,000,000	2.7%
43	Idaho	264,000,000	0.3%	12	Indiana	2,337,000,000	2.7%
7	Illinois	3,924,000,000	4.5%	13	Connecticut	2,264,000,000	2.6%
12	Indiana	2,337,000,000	2.7%	14	Wisconsin	2,110,000,000	2.4%
24	Iowa	1,186,000,000	1.4%	15	Missouri	2,002,000,000	2.3%
27	Kansas	920,000,000	1.0%	16	Tennessee	2,001,000,000	2.3%
22	Kentucky	1,283,000,000	1.5%	17	Minnesota	1,964,000,000	2.2%
23	Louisiana	1,248,000,000	1.4%	18	Maryland	1,695,000,000	1.9%
36	Maine	476,000,000	0.5%	19	Virginia	1,546,000,000	1.8%
18	Maryland	1,695,000,000	1.9%	20	Georgia	1,545,000,000	1.8%
8	Massachusetts	3,568,000,000	4.1%	21	Washington	1,492,000,000	1.7%
10	Michigan	2,459,000,000	2.8%	22	Kentucky	1,283,000,000	1.5%
17	Minnesota	1,964,000,000	2.2%	23	Louisiana	1,248,000,000	1.4%
34	Mississippi	687,000,000	0.8%	24	Iowa	1,186,000,000	1.4%
15	Missouri	2,002,000,000	2.3%	25	Alabama	1,064,000,000	1.2%
45	Montana	222,000,000	0.3%	26	Oklahoma	954,000,000	1.1%
33	Nebraska	697,000,000	0.8%	27	Kansas	920,000,000	1.0%
48	Nevada	164,000,000	0.2%	28	South Carolina	907,000,000	1.0%
38	New Hampshire	425,000,000	0.5%	29	Colorado	904,000,000	1.0%
9	New Jersey	3,233,000,000	3.7%	30	Arizona	839,000,000	1.0%
44	New Mexico	257,000,000	0.3%	31	Oregon	838,000,000	1.0%
1	New York	10,586,000,000	12.1%	32	Arkansas	776,000,000	0.9%
11	North Carolina	2,347,000,000	2.7%	33	Nebraska	697,000,000	0.8%
41	North Dakota	287,000,000	0.3%	34	Mississippi	687,000,000	0.8%
4	Ohio	4,978,000,000	5.7%	35	West Virginia	515,000,000	0.6%
26	Oklahoma	954,000,000	1.1%	36	Maine	476,000,000	0.5%
31	Oregon	838,000,000	1.0%	37	Rhode Island	468,000,000	0.5%
2	Pennsylvania	5,883,000,000	6.7%	38	New Hampshire	425,000,000	0.5%
37	Rhode Island	468,000,000	0.5%	39	Utah	300,000,000	0.3%
28	South Carolina	907,000,000	1.0%	40	Delaware	290,000,000	0.3%
42	South Dakota	286,000,000	0.3%	41	North Dakota	287,000,000	0.3%
16	Tennessee	2,001,000,000	2.3%	42	South Dakota	286,000,000	0.3%
6	Texas	4,346,000,000	4.9%	43	Idaho	264,000,000	0.3%
39	Utah	300,000,000	0.3%	44	New Mexico	257,000,000	0.3%
47	Vermont	177,000,000	0.2%	45	Montana	222,000,000	0.3%
19	Virginia	1,546,000,000	1.8%	46	Hawaii	204,000,000	0.2%
21	Washington	1,492,000,000	1.7%	47	Vermont	177,000,000	0.2%
35	West Virginia	515,000,000	0.6%	48	Nevada	164,000,000	0.2%
14	Wisconsin	2,110,000,000	2.4%	49	Wyoming	113,000,000	0.1%
49	Wyoming	113,000,000	0.1%	50	Alaska	42,000,000	0.0%
					District of Columbia	245,000,000	0.3%

Source: U.S. Department of Health and Human Services, Health Care Financing Administration
"State Health Care Expenditures" (http://www.hcfa.gov/stats/nhe-oact/stateestimates/)
By state of provider. Includes freestanding nursing and personal-care facilities. Includes Medicare- and Medicaid-certified skilled nursing and intermediate care facilities as well as facilities that are not certified. Excludes hospital-based facilities as they are counted in hospital care expenditures.

Percent of Total Personal Health Care Expenditures
Spent on Nursing Home Care in 1998
National Percent = 8.6%*

ALPHA ORDER

RANK ORDER

RANK	STATE	PERCENT		RANK	STATE	PERCENT
40	Alabama	6.6		1	Connecticut	14.9
50	Alaska	1.8		2	New York	12.3
43	Arizona	5.7		3	Massachusetts	11.9
19	Arkansas	9.2		4	Ohio	11.7
45	California	5.1		5	Iowa	11.6
40	Colorado	6.6		6	Pennsylvania	11.5
1	Connecticut	14.9		7	Nebraska	11.4
18	Delaware	9.3		8	Indiana	11.0
28	Florida	8.2		9	North Dakota	10.7
43	Georgia	5.7		10	Wisconsin	10.6
48	Hawaii	4.4		11	Rhode Island	10.4
30	Idaho	7.8		12	South Dakota	10.1
22	Illinois	8.9		13	New Jersey	9.9
8	Indiana	11.0		14	Kansas	9.8
5	Iowa	11.6		15	Maine	9.7
14	Kansas	9.8		15	Minnesota	9.7
22	Kentucky	8.9		17	Missouri	9.6
35	Louisiana	7.6		18	Delaware	9.3
15	Maine	9.7		19	Arkansas	9.2
25	Maryland	8.6		20	New Hampshire	9.1
3	Massachusetts	11.9		20	Tennessee	9.1
37	Michigan	6.9		22	Illinois	8.9
15	Minnesota	9.7		22	Kentucky	8.9
32	Mississippi	7.7		24	Oklahoma	8.7
17	Missouri	9.6		25	Maryland	8.6
30	Montana	7.8		25	North Carolina	8.6
7	Nebraska	11.4		25	Vermont	8.6
49	Nevada	2.9		28	Florida	8.2
20	New Hampshire	9.1		29	Wyoming	8.0
13	New Jersey	9.9		30	Idaho	7.8
47	New Mexico	4.8		30	Montana	7.8
2	New York	12.3		32	Mississippi	7.7
25	North Carolina	8.6		32	Oregon	7.7
9	North Dakota	10.7		32	Washington	7.7
4	Ohio	11.7		35	Louisiana	7.6
24	Oklahoma	8.7		36	West Virginia	7.3
32	Oregon	7.7		37	Michigan	6.9
6	Pennsylvania	11.5		37	South Carolina	6.9
11	Rhode Island	10.4		37	Virginia	6.9
37	South Carolina	6.9		40	Alabama	6.6
12	South Dakota	10.1		40	Colorado	6.6
20	Tennessee	9.1		42	Texas	6.4
42	Texas	6.4		43	Arizona	5.7
46	Utah	5.0		43	Georgia	5.7
25	Vermont	8.6		45	California	5.1
37	Virginia	6.9		46	Utah	5.0
32	Washington	7.7		47	New Mexico	4.8
36	West Virginia	7.3		48	Hawaii	4.4
10	Wisconsin	10.6		49	Nevada	2.9
29	Wyoming	8.0		50	Alaska	1.8

District of Columbia   5.8

Source: Morgan Quitno Press using data from U.S. Dept of Health & Human Services, Health Care Financing Admin.
"State Health Care Expenditures" (http://www.hcfa.gov/stats/nhe-oact/stateestimates/)
*By state of provider. Includes freestanding nursing and personal-care facilities. Includes Medicare- and Medicaid-certified skilled nursing and intermediate care facilities as well as facilities that are not certified. Excludes hospital-based facilities as they are counted in hospital care expenditures.

Average Annual Change in Expenditures for Nursing Home Care: 1990 to 1998

National Percent Change = 7.1% Average Annual Increase*

ALPHA ORDER

RANK	STATE	PERCENT CHANGE
5	Alabama	10.1
50	Alaska	(0.9)
14	Arizona	8.2
20	Arkansas	7.7
24	California	6.8
22	Colorado	7.3
32	Connecticut	6.1
27	Delaware	6.7
3	Florida	10.2
10	Georgia	9.0
41	Hawaii	4.9
9	Idaho	9.2
24	Illinois	6.8
36	Indiana	5.9
29	Iowa	6.2
32	Kansas	6.1
8	Kentucky	9.5
36	Louisiana	5.9
47	Maine	3.6
16	Maryland	7.9
42	Massachusetts	4.8
28	Michigan	6.4
47	Minnesota	3.6
2	Mississippi	10.5
19	Missouri	7.8
42	Montana	4.8
16	Nebraska	7.9
40	Nevada	5.0
11	New Hampshire	8.8
15	New Jersey	8.1
34	New Mexico	6.0
39	New York	5.3
3	North Carolina	10.2
45	North Dakota	4.6
22	Ohio	7.3
29	Oklahoma	6.2
34	Oregon	6.0
21	Pennsylvania	7.6
49	Rhode Island	2.8
16	South Carolina	7.9
24	South Dakota	6.8
1	Tennessee	12.7
13	Texas	8.4
44	Utah	4.7
46	Vermont	3.9
6	Virginia	9.7
29	Washington	6.2
12	West Virginia	8.7
38	Wisconsin	5.4
6	Wyoming	9.7

RANK ORDER

RANK	STATE	PERCENT CHANGE
1	Tennessee	12.7
2	Mississippi	10.5
3	Florida	10.2
3	North Carolina	10.2
5	Alabama	10.1
6	Virginia	9.7
6	Wyoming	9.7
8	Kentucky	9.5
9	Idaho	9.2
10	Georgia	9.0
11	New Hampshire	8.8
12	West Virginia	8.7
13	Texas	8.4
14	Arizona	8.2
15	New Jersey	8.1
16	Maryland	7.9
16	Nebraska	7.9
16	South Carolina	7.9
19	Missouri	7.8
20	Arkansas	7.7
21	Pennsylvania	7.6
22	Colorado	7.3
22	Ohio	7.3
24	California	6.8
24	Illinois	6.8
24	South Dakota	6.8
27	Delaware	6.7
28	Michigan	6.4
29	Iowa	6.2
29	Oklahoma	6.2
29	Washington	6.2
32	Connecticut	6.1
32	Kansas	6.1
34	New Mexico	6.0
34	Oregon	6.0
36	Indiana	5.9
36	Louisiana	5.9
38	Wisconsin	5.4
39	New York	5.3
40	Nevada	5.0
41	Hawaii	4.9
42	Massachusetts	4.8
42	Montana	4.8
44	Utah	4.7
45	North Dakota	4.6
46	Vermont	3.9
47	Maine	3.6
47	Minnesota	3.6
49	Rhode Island	2.8
50	Alaska	(0.9)

	District of Columbia	7.2

Source: U.S. Department of Health and Human Services, Health Care Financing Administration
"State Health Care Expenditures" (http://www.hcfa.gov/stats/nhe-oact/stateestimates/)
*By state of provider. Includes freestanding nursing and personal-care facilities. Includes Medicare- and Medicaid-certified skilled nursing and intermediate care facilities as well as facilities that are not certified. Excludes hospital-based facilities as they are counted in hospital care expenditures.

Per Capita Expenditures for Nursing Home Care in 1998

National Per Capita = $325*

ALPHA ORDER

RANK	STATE	PER CAPITA
36	Alabama	$245
50	Alaska	68
44	Arizona	180
26	Arkansas	306
45	California	172
39	Colorado	228
1	Connecticut	692
15	Delaware	390
22	Florida	327
43	Georgia	202
46	Hawaii	171
42	Idaho	214
24	Illinois	325
13	Indiana	396
10	Iowa	415
20	Kansas	349
23	Kentucky	326
28	Louisiana	286
16	Maine	382
21	Maryland	330
3	Massachusetts	581
34	Michigan	250
9	Minnesota	416
34	Mississippi	250
17	Missouri	368
33	Montana	252
8	Nebraska	420
49	Nevada	94
19	New Hampshire	358
12	New Jersey	399
47	New Mexico	148
2	New York	583
25	North Carolina	311
6	North Dakota	450
7	Ohio	443
28	Oklahoma	286
32	Oregon	255
4	Pennsylvania	490
5	Rhode Island	474
37	South Carolina	236
14	South Dakota	391
17	Tennessee	368
41	Texas	220
48	Utah	143
27	Vermont	300
39	Virginia	228
31	Washington	262
30	West Virginia	284
11	Wisconsin	404
38	Wyoming	235

RANK ORDER

RANK	STATE	PER CAPITA
1	Connecticut	$692
2	New York	583
3	Massachusetts	581
4	Pennsylvania	490
5	Rhode Island	474
6	North Dakota	450
7	Ohio	443
8	Nebraska	420
9	Minnesota	416
10	Iowa	415
11	Wisconsin	404
12	New Jersey	399
13	Indiana	396
14	South Dakota	391
15	Delaware	390
16	Maine	382
17	Missouri	368
17	Tennessee	368
19	New Hampshire	358
20	Kansas	349
21	Maryland	330
22	Florida	327
23	Kentucky	326
24	Illinois	325
25	North Carolina	311
26	Arkansas	306
27	Vermont	300
28	Louisiana	286
28	Oklahoma	286
30	West Virginia	284
31	Washington	262
32	Oregon	255
33	Montana	252
34	Michigan	250
34	Mississippi	250
36	Alabama	245
37	South Carolina	236
38	Wyoming	235
39	Colorado	228
39	Virginia	228
41	Texas	220
42	Idaho	214
43	Georgia	202
44	Arizona	180
45	California	172
46	Hawaii	171
47	New Mexico	148
48	Utah	143
49	Nevada	94
50	Alaska	68
	District of Columbia	470

Source: Morgan Quitno Press using data from U.S. Dept of Health & Human Services, Health Care Financing Admin.
"State Health Care Expenditures" (http://www.hcfa.gov/stats/nhe-oact/stateestimates/)
*By state of provider. Includes freestanding nursing and personal-care facilities. Includes Medicare- and Medicaid-certified skilled nursing and intermediate care facilities as well as facilities that are not certified.
Excludes hospital-based facilities as they are counted in hospital care expenditures.

Per Capita Medicare Expenditures for Nursing Home Care in 1998

National Per Capita = $38.62*

RANK	STATE	PER CAPITA
14	Alabama	$39.07
50	Alaska	3.25
26	Arizona	31.71
30	Arkansas	29.15
27	California	30.66
17	Colorado	37.04
1	Connecticut	89.84
23	Delaware	33.60
4	Florida	67.81
35	Georgia	27.63
49	Hawaii	10.92
21	Idaho	34.12
33	Illinois	28.50
6	Indiana	49.43
44	Iowa	22.02
37	Kansas	26.91
34	Kentucky	28.47
46	Louisiana	20.86
11	Maine	44.89
20	Maryland	34.50
2	Massachusetts	71.12
16	Michigan	37.37
24	Minnesota	33.01
40	Mississippi	25.08
19	Missouri	35.13
42	Montana	22.74
39	Nebraska	25.89
47	Nevada	20.64
12	New Hampshire	43.01
9	New Jersey	47.43
45	New Mexico	21.92
10	New York	47.41
22	North Carolina	33.66
48	North Dakota	15.68
8	Ohio	47.70
43	Oklahoma	22.46
36	Oregon	27.42
7	Pennsylvania	48.16
3	Rhode Island	70.87
28	South Carolina	29.69
18	South Dakota	35.58
15	Tennessee	38.84
25	Texas	32.01
41	Utah	23.33
31	Vermont	28.79
38	Virginia	26.81
13	Washington	41.84
32	West Virginia	28.70
5	Wisconsin	54.00
29	Wyoming	29.16

RANK	STATE	PER CAPITA
1	Connecticut	$89.84
2	Massachusetts	71.12
3	Rhode Island	70.87
4	Florida	67.81
5	Wisconsin	54.00
6	Indiana	49.43
7	Pennsylvania	48.16
8	Ohio	47.70
9	New Jersey	47.43
10	New York	47.41
11	Maine	44.89
12	New Hampshire	43.01
13	Washington	41.84
14	Alabama	39.07
15	Tennessee	38.84
16	Michigan	37.37
17	Colorado	37.04
18	South Dakota	35.58
19	Missouri	35.13
20	Maryland	34.50
21	Idaho	34.12
22	North Carolina	33.66
23	Delaware	33.60
24	Minnesota	33.01
25	Texas	32.01
26	Arizona	31.71
27	California	30.66
28	South Carolina	29.69
29	Wyoming	29.16
30	Arkansas	29.15
31	Vermont	28.79
32	West Virginia	28.70
33	Illinois	28.50
34	Kentucky	28.47
35	Georgia	27.63
36	Oregon	27.42
37	Kansas	26.91
38	Virginia	26.81
39	Nebraska	25.89
40	Mississippi	25.08
41	Utah	23.33
42	Montana	22.74
43	Oklahoma	22.46
44	Iowa	22.02
45	New Mexico	21.92
46	Louisiana	20.86
47	Nevada	20.64
48	North Dakota	15.68
49	Hawaii	10.92
50	Alaska	3.25
	District of Columbia	23.01

Source: Morgan Quitno Press using data from U.S. Dept of Health & Human Services, Health Care Financing Admin.
"State Health Care Expenditures" (http://www.hcfa.gov/stats/nhe-oact/stateestimates/)
By state of provider. Includes freestanding nursing and personal-care facilities. Includes Medicare-certified skilled nursing and intermediate care facilities as well as facilities that are not certified. Excludes hospital-based facilities as they are counted in hospital care expenditures.

Per Capita Medicaid Expenditures for Nursing Home Care in 1998

National Per Capita = $150*

ALPHA ORDER

RANK ORDER

RANK	STATE	PER CAPITA		RANK	STATE	PER CAPITA
31	Alabama	$128		1	New York	$417
47	Alaska	60		2	Connecticut	317
50	Arizona	3		3	Pennsylvania	275
24	Arkansas	136		4	Massachusetts	239
49	California	46		5	Rhode Island	227
44	Colorado	73		6	North Dakota	198
2	Connecticut	317		7	Ohio	194
20	Delaware	155		8	Minnesota	189
38	Florida	104		8	Wisconsin	189
41	Georgia	86		10	Louisiana	188
28	Hawaii	131		10	Nebraska	188
36	Idaho	107		12	New Jersey	185
22	Illinois	146		13	Maine	180
19	Indiana	159		14	New Hampshire	175
15	Iowa	174		15	Iowa	174
36	Kansas	107		16	Tennessee	172
27	Kentucky	133		17	South Dakota	170
10	Louisiana	188		18	West Virginia	166
13	Maine	180		19	Indiana	159
33	Maryland	116		20	Delaware	155
4	Massachusetts	239		21	Missouri	153
25	Michigan	135		22	Illinois	146
8	Minnesota	189		23	North Carolina	137
25	Mississippi	135		24	Arkansas	136
21	Missouri	153		25	Michigan	135
42	Montana	80		25	Mississippi	135
10	Nebraska	188		27	Kentucky	133
48	Nevada	53		28	Hawaii	131
14	New Hampshire	175		28	Wyoming	131
12	New Jersey	185		30	Vermont	129
40	New Mexico	88		31	Alabama	128
1	New York	417		31	Oklahoma	128
23	North Carolina	137		33	Maryland	116
6	North Dakota	198		34	South Carolina	115
7	Ohio	194		35	Washington	111
31	Oklahoma	128		36	Idaho	107
43	Oregon	79		36	Kansas	107
3	Pennsylvania	275		38	Florida	104
5	Rhode Island	227		39	Texas	97
34	South Carolina	115		40	New Mexico	88
17	South Dakota	170		41	Georgia	86
16	Tennessee	172		42	Montana	80
39	Texas	97		43	Oregon	79
46	Utah	62		44	Colorado	73
30	Vermont	129		45	Virginia	68
45	Virginia	68		46	Utah	62
35	Washington	111		47	Alaska	60
18	West Virginia	166		48	Nevada	53
8	Wisconsin	189		49	California	46
28	Wyoming	131		50	Arizona	3

District of Columbia   407

Source: Morgan Quitno Press using data from U.S. Dept of Health & Human Services, Health Care Financing Admin.
"State Health Care Expenditures" (http://www.hcfa.gov/stats/nhe-oact/stateestimates/)
*By state of provider. Includes freestanding nursing and personal-care facilities. Includes Medicaid-certified skilled nursing and intermediate care facilities as well as facilities that are not certified. Excludes hospital-based facilities as they are counted in hospital care expenditures.

Persons Not Covered by Health Insurance in 1999

National Total = 42,267,000 Uninsured

RANK	STATE	UNINSURED	% of USA
21	Alabama	625,000	1.5%
44	Alaska	118,000	0.3%
12	Arizona	1,013,000	2.4%
31	Arkansas	375,000	0.9%
1	California	6,728,000	15.9%
17	Colorado	681,000	1.6%
33	Connecticut	322,000	0.8%
46	Delaware	86,000	0.2%
4	Florida	2,901,000	6.9%
6	Georgia	1,254,000	3.0%
42	Hawaii	132,000	0.3%
37	Idaho	239,000	0.6%
5	Illinois	1,710,000	4.0%
19	Indiana	642,000	1.5%
38	Iowa	238,000	0.6%
34	Kansas	321,000	0.8%
25	Kentucky	574,000	1.4%
13	Louisiana	984,000	2.3%
41	Maine	149,000	0.4%
22	Maryland	610,000	1.4%
18	Massachusetts	648,000	1.5%
10	Michigan	1,105,000	2.6%
30	Minnesota	382,000	0.9%
28	Mississippi	460,000	1.1%
27	Missouri	470,000	1.1%
40	Montana	164,000	0.4%
39	Nebraska	180,000	0.4%
31	Nevada	375,000	0.9%
43	New Hampshire	123,000	0.3%
11	New Jersey	1,091,000	2.6%
29	New Mexico	449,000	1.1%
3	New York	2,984,000	7.1%
8	North Carolina	1,178,000	2.8%
48	North Dakota	75,000	0.2%
7	Ohio	1,238,000	2.9%
23	Oklahoma	588,000	1.4%
26	Oregon	484,000	1.1%
9	Pennsylvania	1,127,000	2.7%
50	Rhode Island	68,000	0.2%
16	South Carolina	684,000	1.6%
45	South Dakota	87,000	0.2%
20	Tennessee	631,000	1.5%
2	Texas	4,670,000	11.0%
36	Utah	302,000	0.7%
49	Vermont	73,000	0.2%
14	Virginia	969,000	2.3%
15	Washington	910,000	2.2%
35	West Virginia	309,000	0.7%
24	Wisconsin	578,000	1.4%
47	Wyoming	77,000	0.2%

RANK	STATE	UNINSURED	% of USA
1	California	6,728,000	15.9%
2	Texas	4,670,000	11.0%
3	New York	2,984,000	7.1%
4	Florida	2,901,000	6.9%
5	Illinois	1,710,000	4.0%
6	Georgia	1,254,000	3.0%
7	Ohio	1,238,000	2.9%
8	North Carolina	1,178,000	2.8%
9	Pennsylvania	1,127,000	2.7%
10	Michigan	1,105,000	2.6%
11	New Jersey	1,091,000	2.6%
12	Arizona	1,013,000	2.4%
13	Louisiana	984,000	2.3%
14	Virginia	969,000	2.3%
15	Washington	910,000	2.2%
16	South Carolina	684,000	1.6%
17	Colorado	681,000	1.6%
18	Massachusetts	648,000	1.5%
19	Indiana	642,000	1.5%
20	Tennessee	631,000	1.5%
21	Alabama	625,000	1.5%
22	Maryland	610,000	1.4%
23	Oklahoma	588,000	1.4%
24	Wisconsin	578,000	1.4%
25	Kentucky	574,000	1.4%
26	Oregon	484,000	1.1%
27	Missouri	470,000	1.1%
28	Mississippi	460,000	1.1%
29	New Mexico	449,000	1.1%
30	Minnesota	382,000	0.9%
31	Arkansas	375,000	0.9%
31	Nevada	375,000	0.9%
33	Connecticut	322,000	0.8%
34	Kansas	321,000	0.8%
35	West Virginia	309,000	0.7%
36	Utah	302,000	0.7%
37	Idaho	239,000	0.6%
38	Iowa	238,000	0.6%
39	Nebraska	180,000	0.4%
40	Montana	164,000	0.4%
41	Maine	149,000	0.4%
42	Hawaii	132,000	0.3%
43	New Hampshire	123,000	0.3%
44	Alaska	118,000	0.3%
45	South Dakota	87,000	0.2%
46	Delaware	86,000	0.2%
47	Wyoming	77,000	0.2%
48	North Dakota	75,000	0.2%
49	Vermont	73,000	0.2%
50	Rhode Island	68,000	0.2%
	District of Columbia	80,000	0.2%

Source: Morgan Quitno Press using data from U.S. Bureau of the Census
"Health Insurance Historical Table 4" (http://www.census.gov/hhes/hlthins/historic/hihistt4.html)

Percent of Population Not Covered by Health Insurance in 1999

National Percent = 15.5% of Population*

ALPHA ORDER

RANK	STATE	PERCENT
24	Alabama	14.3
8	Alaska	19.1
4	Arizona	21.2
21	Arkansas	14.7
6	California	20.3
14	Colorado	16.8
45	Connecticut	9.8
36	Delaware	11.4
7	Florida	19.2
17	Georgia	16.1
38	Hawaii	11.1
8	Idaho	19.1
26	Illinois	14.1
41	Indiana	10.8
48	Iowa	8.3
30	Kansas	12.1
23	Kentucky	14.5
3	Louisiana	22.5
31	Maine	11.9
32	Maryland	11.8
43	Massachusetts	10.5
37	Michigan	11.2
49	Minnesota	8.0
15	Mississippi	16.6
47	Missouri	8.6
10	Montana	18.6
41	Nebraska	10.8
5	Nevada	20.7
44	New Hampshire	10.2
28	New Jersey	13.4
1	New Mexico	25.8
16	New York	16.4
20	North Carolina	15.4
32	North Dakota	11.8
39	Ohio	11.0
12	Oklahoma	17.5
22	Oregon	14.6
46	Pennsylvania	9.4
50	Rhode Island	6.9
11	South Carolina	17.6
32	South Dakota	11.8
35	Tennessee	11.5
2	Texas	23.3
25	Utah	14.2
29	Vermont	12.3
26	Virginia	14.1
19	Washington	15.8
13	West Virginia	17.1
39	Wisconsin	11.0
17	Wyoming	16.1

RANK ORDER

RANK	STATE	PERCENT
1	New Mexico	25.8
2	Texas	23.3
3	Louisiana	22.5
4	Arizona	21.2
5	Nevada	20.7
6	California	20.3
7	Florida	19.2
8	Alaska	19.1
8	Idaho	19.1
10	Montana	18.6
11	South Carolina	17.6
12	Oklahoma	17.5
13	West Virginia	17.1
14	Colorado	16.8
15	Mississippi	16.6
16	New York	16.4
17	Georgia	16.1
17	Wyoming	16.1
19	Washington	15.8
20	North Carolina	15.4
21	Arkansas	14.7
22	Oregon	14.6
23	Kentucky	14.5
24	Alabama	14.3
25	Utah	14.2
26	Illinois	14.1
26	Virginia	14.1
28	New Jersey	13.4
29	Vermont	12.3
30	Kansas	12.1
31	Maine	11.9
32	Maryland	11.8
32	North Dakota	11.8
32	South Dakota	11.8
35	Tennessee	11.5
36	Delaware	11.4
37	Michigan	11.2
38	Hawaii	11.1
39	Ohio	11.0
39	Wisconsin	11.0
41	Indiana	10.8
41	Nebraska	10.8
43	Massachusetts	10.5
44	New Hampshire	10.2
45	Connecticut	9.8
46	Pennsylvania	9.4
47	Missouri	8.6
48	Iowa	8.3
49	Minnesota	8.0
50	Rhode Island	6.9

District of Columbia 15.4

Source: U.S. Bureau of the Census
"Health Insurance Coverage: 1999" (http://www.census.gov/hhes/hlthins/hlthin99/hi99te.html)

Persons Covered by Health Insurance in 1999

National Total = 231,533,000 Insured

<table>
<tr><td colspan="4"><u>ALPHA ORDER</u></td><td colspan="4"><u>RANK ORDER</u></td></tr>
<tr><td>RANK</td><td>STATE</td><td>INSURED</td><td>% of USA</td><td>RANK</td><td>STATE</td><td>INSURED</td><td>% of USA</td></tr>
<tr><td>22</td><td>Alabama</td><td>3,801,000</td><td>1.6%</td><td>1</td><td>California</td><td>27,057,000</td><td>11.7%</td></tr>
<tr><td>49</td><td>Alaska</td><td>509,000</td><td>0.2%</td><td>2</td><td>New York</td><td>15,464,000</td><td>6.7%</td></tr>
<tr><td>21</td><td>Arizona</td><td>3,838,000</td><td>1.7%</td><td>3</td><td>Texas</td><td>15,380,000</td><td>6.6%</td></tr>
<tr><td>33</td><td>Arkansas</td><td>2,183,000</td><td>0.9%</td><td>4</td><td>Florida</td><td>12,159,000</td><td>5.3%</td></tr>
<tr><td>1</td><td>California</td><td>27,057,000</td><td>11.7%</td><td>5</td><td>Pennsylvania</td><td>10,674,000</td><td>4.6%</td></tr>
<tr><td>23</td><td>Colorado</td><td>3,516,000</td><td>1.5%</td><td>6</td><td>Illinois</td><td>10,448,000</td><td>4.5%</td></tr>
<tr><td>27</td><td>Connecticut</td><td>3,005,000</td><td>1.3%</td><td>7</td><td>Ohio</td><td>10,046,000</td><td>4.3%</td></tr>
<tr><td>45</td><td>Delaware</td><td>679,000</td><td>0.3%</td><td>8</td><td>Michigan</td><td>8,996,000</td><td>3.9%</td></tr>
<tr><td>4</td><td>Florida</td><td>12,159,000</td><td>5.3%</td><td>9</td><td>New Jersey</td><td>7,015,000</td><td>3.0%</td></tr>
<tr><td>10</td><td>Georgia</td><td>6,550,000</td><td>2.8%</td><td>10</td><td>Georgia</td><td>6,550,000</td><td>2.8%</td></tr>
<tr><td>41</td><td>Hawaii</td><td>1,080,000</td><td>0.5%</td><td>11</td><td>North Carolina</td><td>6,355,000</td><td>2.7%</td></tr>
<tr><td>42</td><td>Idaho</td><td>1,014,000</td><td>0.4%</td><td>12</td><td>Virginia</td><td>5,875,000</td><td>2.5%</td></tr>
<tr><td>6</td><td>Illinois</td><td>10,448,000</td><td>4.5%</td><td>13</td><td>Massachusetts</td><td>5,546,000</td><td>2.4%</td></tr>
<tr><td>14</td><td>Indiana</td><td>5,261,000</td><td>2.3%</td><td>14</td><td>Indiana</td><td>5,261,000</td><td>2.3%</td></tr>
<tr><td>30</td><td>Iowa</td><td>2,599,000</td><td>1.1%</td><td>15</td><td>Missouri</td><td>5,003,000</td><td>2.2%</td></tr>
<tr><td>32</td><td>Kansas</td><td>2,300,000</td><td>1.0%</td><td>16</td><td>Tennessee</td><td>4,900,000</td><td>2.1%</td></tr>
<tr><td>24</td><td>Kentucky</td><td>3,332,000</td><td>1.4%</td><td>17</td><td>Wisconsin</td><td>4,806,000</td><td>2.1%</td></tr>
<tr><td>25</td><td>Louisiana</td><td>3,328,000</td><td>1.4%</td><td>18</td><td>Washington</td><td>4,799,000</td><td>2.1%</td></tr>
<tr><td>40</td><td>Maine</td><td>1,120,000</td><td>0.5%</td><td>19</td><td>Maryland</td><td>4,457,000</td><td>1.9%</td></tr>
<tr><td>19</td><td>Maryland</td><td>4,457,000</td><td>1.9%</td><td>20</td><td>Minnesota</td><td>4,417,000</td><td>1.9%</td></tr>
<tr><td>13</td><td>Massachusetts</td><td>5,546,000</td><td>2.4%</td><td>21</td><td>Arizona</td><td>3,838,000</td><td>1.7%</td></tr>
<tr><td>8</td><td>Michigan</td><td>8,996,000</td><td>3.9%</td><td>22</td><td>Alabama</td><td>3,801,000</td><td>1.6%</td></tr>
<tr><td>20</td><td>Minnesota</td><td>4,417,000</td><td>1.9%</td><td>23</td><td>Colorado</td><td>3,516,000</td><td>1.5%</td></tr>
<tr><td>31</td><td>Mississippi</td><td>2,304,000</td><td>1.0%</td><td>24</td><td>Kentucky</td><td>3,332,000</td><td>1.4%</td></tr>
<tr><td>15</td><td>Missouri</td><td>5,003,000</td><td>2.2%</td><td>25</td><td>Louisiana</td><td>3,328,000</td><td>1.4%</td></tr>
<tr><td>44</td><td>Montana</td><td>732,000</td><td>0.3%</td><td>26</td><td>South Carolina</td><td>3,145,000</td><td>1.4%</td></tr>
<tr><td>36</td><td>Nebraska</td><td>1,480,000</td><td>0.6%</td><td>27</td><td>Connecticut</td><td>3,005,000</td><td>1.3%</td></tr>
<tr><td>35</td><td>Nevada</td><td>1,532,000</td><td>0.7%</td><td>28</td><td>Oregon</td><td>2,912,000</td><td>1.3%</td></tr>
<tr><td>39</td><td>New Hampshire</td><td>1,127,000</td><td>0.5%</td><td>29</td><td>Oklahoma</td><td>2,698,000</td><td>1.2%</td></tr>
<tr><td>9</td><td>New Jersey</td><td>7,015,000</td><td>3.0%</td><td>30</td><td>Iowa</td><td>2,599,000</td><td>1.1%</td></tr>
<tr><td>38</td><td>New Mexico</td><td>1,335,000</td><td>0.6%</td><td>31</td><td>Mississippi</td><td>2,304,000</td><td>1.0%</td></tr>
<tr><td>2</td><td>New York</td><td>15,464,000</td><td>6.7%</td><td>32</td><td>Kansas</td><td>2,300,000</td><td>1.0%</td></tr>
<tr><td>11</td><td>North Carolina</td><td>6,355,000</td><td>2.7%</td><td>33</td><td>Arkansas</td><td>2,183,000</td><td>0.9%</td></tr>
<tr><td>47</td><td>North Dakota</td><td>543,000</td><td>0.2%</td><td>34</td><td>Utah</td><td>1,846,000</td><td>0.8%</td></tr>
<tr><td>7</td><td>Ohio</td><td>10,046,000</td><td>4.3%</td><td>35</td><td>Nevada</td><td>1,532,000</td><td>0.7%</td></tr>
<tr><td>29</td><td>Oklahoma</td><td>2,698,000</td><td>1.2%</td><td>36</td><td>Nebraska</td><td>1,480,000</td><td>0.6%</td></tr>
<tr><td>28</td><td>Oregon</td><td>2,912,000</td><td>1.3%</td><td>37</td><td>West Virginia</td><td>1,456,000</td><td>0.6%</td></tr>
<tr><td>5</td><td>Pennsylvania</td><td>10,674,000</td><td>4.6%</td><td>38</td><td>New Mexico</td><td>1,335,000</td><td>0.6%</td></tr>
<tr><td>43</td><td>Rhode Island</td><td>915,000</td><td>0.4%</td><td>39</td><td>New Hampshire</td><td>1,127,000</td><td>0.5%</td></tr>
<tr><td>26</td><td>South Carolina</td><td>3,145,000</td><td>1.4%</td><td>40</td><td>Maine</td><td>1,120,000</td><td>0.5%</td></tr>
<tr><td>46</td><td>South Dakota</td><td>621,000</td><td>0.3%</td><td>41</td><td>Hawaii</td><td>1,080,000</td><td>0.5%</td></tr>
<tr><td>16</td><td>Tennessee</td><td>4,900,000</td><td>2.1%</td><td>42</td><td>Idaho</td><td>1,014,000</td><td>0.4%</td></tr>
<tr><td>3</td><td>Texas</td><td>15,380,000</td><td>6.6%</td><td>43</td><td>Rhode Island</td><td>915,000</td><td>0.4%</td></tr>
<tr><td>34</td><td>Utah</td><td>1,846,000</td><td>0.8%</td><td>44</td><td>Montana</td><td>732,000</td><td>0.3%</td></tr>
<tr><td>48</td><td>Vermont</td><td>531,000</td><td>0.2%</td><td>45</td><td>Delaware</td><td>679,000</td><td>0.3%</td></tr>
<tr><td>12</td><td>Virginia</td><td>5,875,000</td><td>2.5%</td><td>46</td><td>South Dakota</td><td>621,000</td><td>0.3%</td></tr>
<tr><td>18</td><td>Washington</td><td>4,799,000</td><td>2.1%</td><td>47</td><td>North Dakota</td><td>543,000</td><td>0.2%</td></tr>
<tr><td>37</td><td>West Virginia</td><td>1,456,000</td><td>0.6%</td><td>48</td><td>Vermont</td><td>531,000</td><td>0.2%</td></tr>
<tr><td>17</td><td>Wisconsin</td><td>4,806,000</td><td>2.1%</td><td>49</td><td>Alaska</td><td>509,000</td><td>0.2%</td></tr>
<tr><td>50</td><td>Wyoming</td><td>405,000</td><td>0.2%</td><td>50</td><td>Wyoming</td><td>405,000</td><td>0.2%</td></tr>
<tr><td></td><td></td><td></td><td></td><td></td><td>District of Columbia</td><td>437,000</td><td>0.2%</td></tr>
</table>

Source: U.S. Bureau of the Census
"Health Insurance Historical Table 4" (http://www.census.gov/hhes/hlthins/historic/hihistt4.html)

Percent of Population Covered by Health Insurance in 1999

National Percent = 84.5% of Population

RANK	STATE	PERCENT
27	Alabama	85.7
42	Alaska	80.9
47	Arizona	78.8
30	Arkansas	85.3
45	California	79.7
37	Colorado	83.2
6	Connecticut	90.2
15	Delaware	88.6
44	Florida	80.8
33	Georgia	83.9
13	Hawaii	88.9
42	Idaho	80.9
24	Illinois	85.9
9	Indiana	89.2
3	Iowa	91.7
21	Kansas	87.9
28	Kentucky	85.5
48	Louisiana	77.5
20	Maine	88.1
17	Maryland	88.2
8	Massachusetts	89.5
14	Michigan	88.8
2	Minnesota	92.0
36	Mississippi	83.4
4	Missouri	91.4
41	Montana	81.4
9	Nebraska	89.2
46	Nevada	79.2
7	New Hampshire	89.8
23	New Jersey	86.6
50	New Mexico	74.2
35	New York	83.6
31	North Carolina	84.6
17	North Dakota	88.2
11	Ohio	89.0
39	Oklahoma	82.5
29	Oregon	85.4
5	Pennsylvania	90.6
1	Rhode Island	93.1
40	South Carolina	82.4
17	South Dakota	88.2
16	Tennessee	88.5
49	Texas	76.7
26	Utah	85.8
22	Vermont	87.7
24	Virginia	85.9
32	Washington	84.2
38	West Virginia	82.9
11	Wisconsin	89.0
33	Wyoming	83.9

RANK	STATE	PERCENT
1	Rhode Island	93.1
2	Minnesota	92.0
3	Iowa	91.7
4	Missouri	91.4
5	Pennsylvania	90.6
6	Connecticut	90.2
7	New Hampshire	89.8
8	Massachusetts	89.5
9	Indiana	89.2
9	Nebraska	89.2
11	Ohio	89.0
11	Wisconsin	89.0
13	Hawaii	88.9
14	Michigan	88.8
15	Delaware	88.6
16	Tennessee	88.5
17	Maryland	88.2
17	North Dakota	88.2
17	South Dakota	88.2
20	Maine	88.1
21	Kansas	87.9
22	Vermont	87.7
23	New Jersey	86.6
24	Illinois	85.9
24	Virginia	85.9
26	Utah	85.8
27	Alabama	85.7
28	Kentucky	85.5
29	Oregon	85.4
30	Arkansas	85.3
31	North Carolina	84.6
32	Washington	84.2
33	Georgia	83.9
33	Wyoming	83.9
35	New York	83.6
36	Mississippi	83.4
37	Colorado	83.2
38	West Virginia	82.9
39	Oklahoma	82.5
40	South Carolina	82.4
41	Montana	81.4
42	Alaska	80.9
42	Idaho	80.9
44	Florida	80.8
45	California	79.7
46	Nevada	79.2
47	Arizona	78.8
48	Louisiana	77.5
49	Texas	76.7
50	New Mexico	74.2
	District of Columbia	84.6

Source: U.S. Bureau of the Census
"Health Insurance Historical Table 4" (http://www.census.gov/hhes/hlthins/historic/hihistt4.html)

Persons Not Covered by Health Insurance in 1995

National Total = 39,070,000 Uninsured

<u>ALPHA ORDER</u>

RANK	STATE	UNINSURED	% of USA
26	Alabama	459,000	1.2%
50	Alaska	49,000	0.1%
15	Arizona	846,000	2.2%
27	Arkansas	401,000	1.0%
1	California	5,977,000	15.3%
25	Colorado	490,000	1.3%
34	Connecticut	267,000	0.7%
43	Delaware	116,000	0.3%
4	Florida	2,461,000	6.3%
8	Georgia	1,223,000	3.1%
45	Hawaii	98,000	0.3%
39	Idaho	172,000	0.4%
5	Illinois	1,381,000	3.5%
16	Indiana	820,000	2.1%
33	Iowa	272,000	0.7%
28	Kansas	364,000	0.9%
23	Kentucky	528,000	1.4%
14	Louisiana	900,000	2.3%
38	Maine	177,000	0.5%
18	Maryland	674,000	1.7%
20	Massachusetts	662,000	1.7%
12	Michigan	954,000	2.4%
29	Minnesota	345,000	0.9%
22	Mississippi	532,000	1.4%
13	Missouri	909,000	2.3%
44	Montana	107,000	0.3%
41	Nebraska	131,000	0.3%
35	Nevada	255,000	0.7%
42	New Hampshire	119,000	0.3%
10	New Jersey	1,184,000	3.0%
30	New Mexico	338,000	0.9%
3	New York	2,629,000	6.7%
7	North Carolina	1,234,000	3.2%
49	North Dakota	57,000	0.1%
6	Ohio	1,261,000	3.2%
17	Oklahoma	675,000	1.7%
31	Oregon	324,000	0.8%
9	Pennsylvania	1,196,000	3.1%
40	Rhode Island	150,000	0.4%
24	South Carolina	495,000	1.3%
47	South Dakota	69,000	0.2%
21	Tennessee	572,000	1.5%
2	Texas	4,490,000	11.5%
36	Utah	210,000	0.5%
48	Vermont	64,000	0.2%
11	Virginia	1,080,000	2.8%
19	Washington	672,000	1.7%
32	West Virginia	298,000	0.8%
37	Wisconsin	207,000	0.5%
46	Wyoming	72,000	0.2%

<u>RANK ORDER</u>

RANK	STATE	UNINSURED	% of USA
1	California	5,977,000	15.3%
2	Texas	4,490,000	11.5%
3	New York	2,629,000	6.7%
4	Florida	2,461,000	6.3%
5	Illinois	1,381,000	3.5%
6	Ohio	1,261,000	3.2%
7	North Carolina	1,234,000	3.2%
8	Georgia	1,223,000	3.1%
9	Pennsylvania	1,196,000	3.1%
10	New Jersey	1,184,000	3.0%
11	Virginia	1,080,000	2.8%
12	Michigan	954,000	2.4%
13	Missouri	909,000	2.3%
14	Louisiana	900,000	2.3%
15	Arizona	846,000	2.2%
16	Indiana	820,000	2.1%
17	Oklahoma	675,000	1.7%
18	Maryland	674,000	1.7%
19	Washington	672,000	1.7%
20	Massachusetts	662,000	1.7%
21	Tennessee	572,000	1.5%
22	Mississippi	532,000	1.4%
23	Kentucky	528,000	1.4%
24	South Carolina	495,000	1.3%
25	Colorado	490,000	1.3%
26	Alabama	459,000	1.2%
27	Arkansas	401,000	1.0%
28	Kansas	364,000	0.9%
29	Minnesota	345,000	0.9%
30	New Mexico	338,000	0.9%
31	Oregon	324,000	0.8%
32	West Virginia	298,000	0.8%
33	Iowa	272,000	0.7%
34	Connecticut	267,000	0.7%
35	Nevada	255,000	0.7%
36	Utah	210,000	0.5%
37	Wisconsin	207,000	0.5%
38	Maine	177,000	0.5%
39	Idaho	172,000	0.4%
40	Rhode Island	150,000	0.4%
41	Nebraska	131,000	0.3%
42	New Hampshire	119,000	0.3%
43	Delaware	116,000	0.3%
44	Montana	107,000	0.3%
45	Hawaii	98,000	0.3%
46	Wyoming	72,000	0.2%
47	South Dakota	69,000	0.2%
48	Vermont	64,000	0.2%
49	North Dakota	57,000	0.1%
50	Alaska	49,000	0.1%
	District of Columbia	92,000	0.2%

Source: Morgan Quitno Press using data from U.S. Bureau of the Census
"Health Insurance Historical Table 4" (http://www.census.gov/hhes/hlthins/historic/hihistt4.html)

Percent of Population Not Covered by Health Insurance in 1995

National Percent = 15.4% of Population

ALPHA ORDER

RANK	STATE	PERCENT
25	Alabama	13.5
32	Alaska	12.5
5	Arizona	20.4
10	Arkansas	17.9
3	California	20.6
17	Colorado	14.8
46	Connecticut	8.8
13	Delaware	15.7
9	Florida	18.3
10	Georgia	17.9
45	Hawaii	8.9
24	Idaho	14.0
40	Illinois	11.0
31	Indiana	12.6
38	Iowa	11.3
34	Kansas	12.4
19	Kentucky	14.6
4	Louisiana	20.5
25	Maine	13.5
14	Maryland	15.3
39	Massachusetts	11.1
42	Michigan	9.7
48	Minnesota	8.0
6	Mississippi	19.7
19	Missouri	14.6
30	Montana	12.7
44	Nebraska	9.0
8	Nevada	18.7
41	New Hampshire	10.0
23	New Jersey	14.2
1	New Mexico	25.6
16	New York	15.2
22	North Carolina	14.3
47	North Dakota	8.3
36	Ohio	11.9
7	Oklahoma	19.2
32	Oregon	12.5
43	Pennsylvania	9.6
29	Rhode Island	12.9
19	South Carolina	14.6
48	South Dakota	8.0
17	Tennessee	14.8
2	Texas	24.5
37	Utah	11.7
28	Vermont	13.2
25	Virginia	13.5
34	Washington	12.4
14	West Virginia	15.3
50	Wisconsin	7.3
12	Wyoming	15.9

RANK ORDER

RANK	STATE	PERCENT
1	New Mexico	25.6
2	Texas	24.5
3	California	20.6
4	Louisiana	20.5
5	Arizona	20.4
6	Mississippi	19.7
7	Oklahoma	19.2
8	Nevada	18.7
9	Florida	18.3
10	Arkansas	17.9
10	Georgia	17.9
12	Wyoming	15.9
13	Delaware	15.7
14	Maryland	15.3
14	West Virginia	15.3
16	New York	15.2
17	Colorado	14.8
17	Tennessee	14.8
19	Kentucky	14.6
19	Missouri	14.6
19	South Carolina	14.6
22	North Carolina	14.3
23	New Jersey	14.2
24	Idaho	14.0
25	Alabama	13.5
25	Maine	13.5
25	Virginia	13.5
28	Vermont	13.2
29	Rhode Island	12.9
30	Montana	12.7
31	Indiana	12.6
32	Alaska	12.5
32	Oregon	12.5
34	Kansas	12.4
34	Washington	12.4
36	Ohio	11.9
37	Utah	11.7
38	Iowa	11.3
39	Massachusetts	11.1
40	Illinois	11.0
41	New Hampshire	10.0
42	Michigan	9.7
43	Pennsylvania	9.6
44	Nebraska	9.0
45	Hawaii	8.9
46	Connecticut	8.8
47	North Dakota	8.3
48	Minnesota	8.0
48	South Dakota	8.0
50	Wisconsin	7.3
	District of Columbia	17.3

Source: Morgan Quitno Press using data from U.S. Bureau of the Census
"Health Insurance Historical Table 4" (http://www.census.gov/hhes/hlthins/historic/hihistt4.html)

Change in Number of Persons Uninsured: 1995 to 1999

National Change = 3,197,000 Increase

ALPHA ORDER

RANK	STATE	CHANGE
11	Alabama	166,000
18	Alaska	69,000
10	Arizona	167,000
36	Arkansas	(26,000)
1	California	751,000
7	Colorado	191,000
22	Connecticut	55,000
38	Delaware	(30,000)
2	Florida	440,000
27	Georgia	31,000
26	Hawaii	34,000
19	Idaho	67,000
5	Illinois	329,000
49	Indiana	(178,000)
39	Iowa	(34,000)
40	Kansas	(43,000)
24	Kentucky	46,000
17	Louisiana	84,000
37	Maine	(28,000)
42	Maryland	(64,000)
34	Massachusetts	(14,000)
13	Michigan	151,000
25	Minnesota	37,000
44	Mississippi	(72,000)
50	Missouri	(439,000)
21	Montana	57,000
23	Nebraska	49,000
14	Nevada	120,000
33	New Hampshire	4,000
47	New Jersey	(93,000)
15	New Mexico	111,000
4	New York	355,000
41	North Carolina	(56,000)
28	North Dakota	18,000
35	Ohio	(23,000)
46	Oklahoma	(87,000)
12	Oregon	160,000
43	Pennsylvania	(69,000)
45	Rhode Island	(82,000)
8	South Carolina	189,000
28	South Dakota	18,000
20	Tennessee	59,000
9	Texas	180,000
16	Utah	92,000
31	Vermont	9,000
48	Virginia	(111,000)
6	Washington	238,000
30	West Virginia	11,000
3	Wisconsin	371,000
32	Wyoming	5,000

RANK ORDER

RANK	STATE	CHANGE
1	California	751,000
2	Florida	440,000
3	Wisconsin	371,000
4	New York	355,000
5	Illinois	329,000
6	Washington	238,000
7	Colorado	191,000
8	South Carolina	189,000
9	Texas	180,000
10	Arizona	167,000
11	Alabama	166,000
12	Oregon	160,000
13	Michigan	151,000
14	Nevada	120,000
15	New Mexico	111,000
16	Utah	92,000
17	Louisiana	84,000
18	Alaska	69,000
19	Idaho	67,000
20	Tennessee	59,000
21	Montana	57,000
22	Connecticut	55,000
23	Nebraska	49,000
24	Kentucky	46,000
25	Minnesota	37,000
26	Hawaii	34,000
27	Georgia	31,000
28	North Dakota	18,000
28	South Dakota	18,000
30	West Virginia	11,000
31	Vermont	9,000
32	Wyoming	5,000
33	New Hampshire	4,000
34	Massachusetts	(14,000)
35	Ohio	(23,000)
36	Arkansas	(26,000)
37	Maine	(28,000)
38	Delaware	(30,000)
39	Iowa	(34,000)
40	Kansas	(43,000)
41	North Carolina	(56,000)
42	Maryland	(64,000)
43	Pennsylvania	(69,000)
44	Mississippi	(72,000)
45	Rhode Island	(82,000)
46	Oklahoma	(87,000)
47	New Jersey	(93,000)
48	Virginia	(111,000)
49	Indiana	(178,000)
50	Missouri	(439,000)
	District of Columbia	(12,000)

Source: Morgan Quitno Press using data from U.S. Bureau of the Census
"Health Insurance Historical Table 4" (http://www.census.gov/hhes/hlthins/historic/hihistt4.html)
Table HI-4: "Health Insurance Coverage Status and Type of Coverage by State - 1987 to 1997"

Percent Change in Number of Uninsured: 1995 to 1999

National Percent Change = 8.2% Increase

ALPHA ORDER

RANK	STATE	PERCENT CHANGE
11	Alabama	36.2
2	Alaska	140.8
19	Arizona	19.7
38	Arkansas	(6.5)
24	California	12.6
7	Colorado	39.0
18	Connecticut	20.6
48	Delaware	(25.9)
20	Florida	17.9
33	Georgia	2.5
13	Hawaii	34.7
7	Idaho	39.0
17	Illinois	23.8
47	Indiana	(21.7)
43	Iowa	(12.5)
42	Kansas	(11.8)
28	Kentucky	8.7
27	Louisiana	9.3
46	Maine	(15.8)
40	Maryland	(9.5)
35	Massachusetts	(2.1)
21	Michigan	15.8
25	Minnesota	10.7
45	Mississippi	(13.5)
49	Missouri	(48.3)
3	Montana	53.3
10	Nebraska	37.4
5	Nevada	47.1
32	New Hampshire	3.4
39	New Jersey	(7.9)
14	New Mexico	32.8
23	New York	13.5
36	North Carolina	(4.5)
15	North Dakota	31.6
34	Ohio	(1.8)
44	Oklahoma	(12.9)
4	Oregon	49.4
37	Pennsylvania	(5.8)
50	Rhode Island	(54.7)
9	South Carolina	38.2
16	South Dakota	26.1
26	Tennessee	10.3
30	Texas	4.0
6	Utah	43.8
22	Vermont	14.1
41	Virginia	(10.3)
12	Washington	35.4
31	West Virginia	3.7
1	Wisconsin	179.2
29	Wyoming	6.9

RANK ORDER

RANK	STATE	PERCENT CHANGE
1	Wisconsin	179.2
2	Alaska	140.8
3	Montana	53.3
4	Oregon	49.4
5	Nevada	47.1
6	Utah	43.8
7	Colorado	39.0
7	Idaho	39.0
9	South Carolina	38.2
10	Nebraska	37.4
11	Alabama	36.2
12	Washington	35.4
13	Hawaii	34.7
14	New Mexico	32.8
15	North Dakota	31.6
16	South Dakota	26.1
17	Illinois	23.8
18	Connecticut	20.6
19	Arizona	19.7
20	Florida	17.9
21	Michigan	15.8
22	Vermont	14.1
23	New York	13.5
24	California	12.6
25	Minnesota	10.7
26	Tennessee	10.3
27	Louisiana	9.3
28	Kentucky	8.7
29	Wyoming	6.9
30	Texas	4.0
31	West Virginia	3.7
32	New Hampshire	3.4
33	Georgia	2.5
34	Ohio	(1.8)
35	Massachusetts	(2.1)
36	North Carolina	(4.5)
37	Pennsylvania	(5.8)
38	Arkansas	(6.5)
39	New Jersey	(7.9)
40	Maryland	(9.5)
41	Virginia	(10.3)
42	Kansas	(11.8)
43	Iowa	(12.5)
44	Oklahoma	(12.9)
45	Mississippi	(13.5)
46	Maine	(15.8)
47	Indiana	(21.7)
48	Delaware	(25.9)
49	Missouri	(48.3)
50	Rhode Island	(54.7)
	District of Columbia	(13.0)

Source: Morgan Quitno Press using data from U.S. Bureau of the Census
"Health Insurance Historical Table 4" (http://www.census.gov/hhes/hlthins/historic/hihistt4.html)
Table HI-4: "Health Insurance Coverage Status and Type of Coverage by State - 1987 to 1997"

Change in Percent of Population Uninsured: 1995 to 1999

National Percent Change = 0.6% Increase

<table>
<tr><td colspan="3">ALPHA ORDER</td><td colspan="3">RANK ORDER</td></tr>
<tr><td>RANK</td><td>STATE</td><td>PERCENT CHANGE</td><td>RANK</td><td>STATE</td><td>PERCENT CHANGE</td></tr>
<tr><td>22</td><td>Alabama</td><td>5.9</td><td>1</td><td>Alaska</td><td>52.8</td></tr>
<tr><td>1</td><td>Alaska</td><td>52.8</td><td>2</td><td>Wisconsin</td><td>50.7</td></tr>
<tr><td>25</td><td>Arizona</td><td>3.9</td><td>3</td><td>South Dakota</td><td>47.5</td></tr>
<tr><td>44</td><td>Arkansas</td><td>(17.9)</td><td>4</td><td>Montana</td><td>46.5</td></tr>
<tr><td>31</td><td>California</td><td>(1.5)</td><td>5</td><td>North Dakota</td><td>42.2</td></tr>
<tr><td>15</td><td>Colorado</td><td>13.5</td><td>6</td><td>Idaho</td><td>36.4</td></tr>
<tr><td>17</td><td>Connecticut</td><td>11.4</td><td>7</td><td>Illinois</td><td>28.2</td></tr>
<tr><td>48</td><td>Delaware</td><td>(27.4)</td><td>8</td><td>Washington</td><td>27.4</td></tr>
<tr><td>23</td><td>Florida</td><td>4.9</td><td>9</td><td>Hawaii</td><td>24.7</td></tr>
<tr><td>40</td><td>Georgia</td><td>(10.1)</td><td>10</td><td>Utah</td><td>21.4</td></tr>
<tr><td>9</td><td>Hawaii</td><td>24.7</td><td>11</td><td>South Carolina</td><td>20.5</td></tr>
<tr><td>6</td><td>Idaho</td><td>36.4</td><td>12</td><td>Nebraska</td><td>20.0</td></tr>
<tr><td>7</td><td>Illinois</td><td>28.2</td><td>13</td><td>Oregon</td><td>16.8</td></tr>
<tr><td>42</td><td>Indiana</td><td>(14.3)</td><td>14</td><td>Michigan</td><td>15.5</td></tr>
<tr><td>47</td><td>Iowa</td><td>(26.5)</td><td>15</td><td>Colorado</td><td>13.5</td></tr>
<tr><td>33</td><td>Kansas</td><td>(2.4)</td><td>16</td><td>West Virginia</td><td>11.8</td></tr>
<tr><td>30</td><td>Kentucky</td><td>(0.7)</td><td>17</td><td>Connecticut</td><td>11.4</td></tr>
<tr><td>19</td><td>Louisiana</td><td>9.8</td><td>18</td><td>Nevada</td><td>10.7</td></tr>
<tr><td>41</td><td>Maine</td><td>(11.9)</td><td>19</td><td>Louisiana</td><td>9.8</td></tr>
<tr><td>46</td><td>Maryland</td><td>(22.9)</td><td>20</td><td>New York</td><td>7.9</td></tr>
<tr><td>35</td><td>Massachusetts</td><td>(5.4)</td><td>21</td><td>North Carolina</td><td>7.7</td></tr>
<tr><td>14</td><td>Michigan</td><td>15.5</td><td>22</td><td>Alabama</td><td>5.9</td></tr>
<tr><td>29</td><td>Minnesota</td><td>0.0</td><td>23</td><td>Florida</td><td>4.9</td></tr>
<tr><td>43</td><td>Mississippi</td><td>(15.7)</td><td>24</td><td>Virginia</td><td>4.4</td></tr>
<tr><td>49</td><td>Missouri</td><td>(41.1)</td><td>25</td><td>Arizona</td><td>3.9</td></tr>
<tr><td>4</td><td>Montana</td><td>46.5</td><td>26</td><td>New Hampshire</td><td>2.0</td></tr>
<tr><td>12</td><td>Nebraska</td><td>20.0</td><td>27</td><td>Wyoming</td><td>1.3</td></tr>
<tr><td>18</td><td>Nevada</td><td>10.7</td><td>28</td><td>New Mexico</td><td>0.8</td></tr>
<tr><td>26</td><td>New Hampshire</td><td>2.0</td><td>29</td><td>Minnesota</td><td>0.0</td></tr>
<tr><td>36</td><td>New Jersey</td><td>(5.6)</td><td>30</td><td>Kentucky</td><td>(0.7)</td></tr>
<tr><td>28</td><td>New Mexico</td><td>0.8</td><td>31</td><td>California</td><td>(1.5)</td></tr>
<tr><td>20</td><td>New York</td><td>7.9</td><td>32</td><td>Pennsylvania</td><td>(2.1)</td></tr>
<tr><td>21</td><td>North Carolina</td><td>7.7</td><td>33</td><td>Kansas</td><td>(2.4)</td></tr>
<tr><td>5</td><td>North Dakota</td><td>42.2</td><td>34</td><td>Texas</td><td>(4.9)</td></tr>
<tr><td>38</td><td>Ohio</td><td>(7.6)</td><td>35</td><td>Massachusetts</td><td>(5.4)</td></tr>
<tr><td>39</td><td>Oklahoma</td><td>(8.9)</td><td>36</td><td>New Jersey</td><td>(5.6)</td></tr>
<tr><td>13</td><td>Oregon</td><td>16.8</td><td>37</td><td>Vermont</td><td>(6.8)</td></tr>
<tr><td>32</td><td>Pennsylvania</td><td>(2.1)</td><td>38</td><td>Ohio</td><td>(7.6)</td></tr>
<tr><td>50</td><td>Rhode Island</td><td>(46.5)</td><td>39</td><td>Oklahoma</td><td>(8.9)</td></tr>
<tr><td>11</td><td>South Carolina</td><td>20.5</td><td>40</td><td>Georgia</td><td>(10.1)</td></tr>
<tr><td>3</td><td>South Dakota</td><td>47.5</td><td>41</td><td>Maine</td><td>(11.9)</td></tr>
<tr><td>45</td><td>Tennessee</td><td>(22.3)</td><td>42</td><td>Indiana</td><td>(14.3)</td></tr>
<tr><td>34</td><td>Texas</td><td>(4.9)</td><td>43</td><td>Mississippi</td><td>(15.7)</td></tr>
<tr><td>10</td><td>Utah</td><td>21.4</td><td>44</td><td>Arkansas</td><td>(17.9)</td></tr>
<tr><td>37</td><td>Vermont</td><td>(6.8)</td><td>45</td><td>Tennessee</td><td>(22.3)</td></tr>
<tr><td>24</td><td>Virginia</td><td>4.4</td><td>46</td><td>Maryland</td><td>(22.9)</td></tr>
<tr><td>8</td><td>Washington</td><td>27.4</td><td>47</td><td>Iowa</td><td>(26.5)</td></tr>
<tr><td>16</td><td>West Virginia</td><td>11.8</td><td>48</td><td>Delaware</td><td>(27.4)</td></tr>
<tr><td>2</td><td>Wisconsin</td><td>50.7</td><td>49</td><td>Missouri</td><td>(41.1)</td></tr>
<tr><td>27</td><td>Wyoming</td><td>1.3</td><td>50</td><td>Rhode Island</td><td>(46.5)</td></tr>
<tr><td></td><td></td><td></td><td></td><td>District of Columbia</td><td>(11.0)</td></tr>
</table>

Source: Morgan Quitno Press using data from U.S. Bureau of the Census
"Health Insurance Historical Table 4" (http://www.census.gov/hhes/hlthins/historic/hihistt4.html)

Percent of Population Covered by Private Health Insurance in 1999

National Percent = 71.0% of Population

ALPHA ORDER   RANK ORDER

RANK	STATE	PERCENT
31	Alabama	70.8
41	Alaska	66.8
46	Arizona	63.8
38	Arkansas	68.8
47	California	63.7
26	Colorado	72.1
3	Connecticut	80.9
24	Delaware	73.5
45	Florida	64.8
40	Georgia	68.3
18	Hawaii	76.2
25	Idaho	72.5
20	Illinois	75.3
6	Indiana	80.1
1	Iowa	82.8
14	Kansas	77.8
34	Kentucky	69.9
49	Louisiana	61.4
21	Maine	75.1
8	Maryland	79.6
28	Massachusetts	71.8
15	Michigan	77.6
1	Minnesota	82.8
42	Mississippi	66.5
5	Missouri	80.2
35	Montana	69.4
12	Nebraska	78.3
39	Nevada	68.7
9	New Hampshire	79.3
19	New Jersey	76.1
50	New Mexico	56.6
43	New York	65.9
30	North Carolina	71.0
17	North Dakota	76.3
16	Ohio	77.4
35	Oklahoma	69.4
23	Oregon	73.6
12	Pennsylvania	78.3
4	Rhode Island	80.6
35	South Carolina	69.4
11	South Dakota	78.6
33	Tennessee	70.3
48	Texas	63.3
10	Utah	79.1
32	Vermont	70.4
22	Virginia	73.9
29	Washington	71.7
44	West Virginia	65.5
7	Wisconsin	79.8
26	Wyoming	72.1

RANK	STATE	PERCENT
1	Iowa	82.8
1	Minnesota	82.8
3	Connecticut	80.9
4	Rhode Island	80.6
5	Missouri	80.2
6	Indiana	80.1
7	Wisconsin	79.8
8	Maryland	79.6
9	New Hampshire	79.3
10	Utah	79.1
11	South Dakota	78.6
12	Nebraska	78.3
12	Pennsylvania	78.3
14	Kansas	77.8
15	Michigan	77.6
16	Ohio	77.4
17	North Dakota	76.3
18	Hawaii	76.2
19	New Jersey	76.1
20	Illinois	75.3
21	Maine	75.1
22	Virginia	73.9
23	Oregon	73.6
24	Delaware	73.5
25	Idaho	72.5
26	Colorado	72.1
26	Wyoming	72.1
28	Massachusetts	71.8
29	Washington	71.7
30	North Carolina	71.0
31	Alabama	70.8
32	Vermont	70.4
33	Tennessee	70.3
34	Kentucky	69.9
35	Montana	69.4
35	Oklahoma	69.4
35	South Carolina	69.4
38	Arkansas	68.8
39	Nevada	68.7
40	Georgia	68.3
41	Alaska	66.8
42	Mississippi	66.5
43	New York	65.9
44	West Virginia	65.5
45	Florida	64.8
46	Arizona	63.8
47	California	63.7
48	Texas	63.3
49	Louisiana	61.4
50	New Mexico	56.6
	District of Columbia	64.1

Source: U.S. Bureau of the Census
   "Health Insurance Historical Table 4" (http://www.census.gov/hhes/hlthins/historic/hihistt4.html)

Percent of Population Covered by Government Health Insurance in 1999

National Percent = 26.5% of Population*

ALPHA ORDER

RANK	STATE	PERCENT
19	Alabama	28.5
14	Alaska	29.1
23	Arizona	27.6
2	Arkansas	34.3
27	California	26.8
43	Colorado	22.3
41	Connecticut	23.5
13	Delaware	29.2
7	Florida	30.9
33	Georgia	25.8
22	Hawaii	27.9
42	Idaho	22.9
48	Illinois	21.1
37	Indiana	24.2
36	Iowa	24.5
16	Kansas	28.9
8	Kentucky	30.6
12	Louisiana	29.5
21	Maine	28.0
38	Maryland	24.0
10	Massachusetts	30.2
40	Michigan	23.6
44	Minnesota	22.2
3	Mississippi	34.1
34	Missouri	24.9
20	Montana	28.2
29	Nebraska	26.3
48	Nevada	21.1
47	New Hampshire	21.2
46	New Jersey	21.7
5	New Mexico	31.8
9	New York	30.3
24	North Carolina	27.3
6	North Dakota	31.0
34	Ohio	24.9
15	Oklahoma	29.0
31	Oregon	26.0
24	Pennsylvania	27.3
18	Rhode Island	28.6
16	South Carolina	28.9
26	South Dakota	27.0
11	Tennessee	29.8
39	Texas	23.7
50	Utah	16.9
4	Vermont	34.0
27	Virginia	26.8
31	Washington	26.0
1	West Virginia	35.3
45	Wisconsin	22.0
30	Wyoming	26.1

RANK ORDER

RANK	STATE	PERCENT
1	West Virginia	35.3
2	Arkansas	34.3
3	Mississippi	34.1
4	Vermont	34.0
5	New Mexico	31.8
6	North Dakota	31.0
7	Florida	30.9
8	Kentucky	30.6
9	New York	30.3
10	Massachusetts	30.2
11	Tennessee	29.8
12	Louisiana	29.5
13	Delaware	29.2
14	Alaska	29.1
15	Oklahoma	29.0
16	Kansas	28.9
16	South Carolina	28.9
18	Rhode Island	28.6
19	Alabama	28.5
20	Montana	28.2
21	Maine	28.0
22	Hawaii	27.9
23	Arizona	27.6
24	North Carolina	27.3
24	Pennsylvania	27.3
26	South Dakota	27.0
27	California	26.8
27	Virginia	26.8
29	Nebraska	26.3
30	Wyoming	26.1
31	Oregon	26.0
31	Washington	26.0
33	Georgia	25.8
34	Missouri	24.9
34	Ohio	24.9
36	Iowa	24.5
37	Indiana	24.2
38	Maryland	24.0
39	Texas	23.7
40	Michigan	23.6
41	Connecticut	23.5
42	Idaho	22.9
43	Colorado	22.3
44	Minnesota	22.2
45	Wisconsin	22.0
46	New Jersey	21.7
47	New Hampshire	21.2
48	Illinois	21.1
48	Nevada	21.1
50	Utah	16.9
	District of Columbia	34.1

Source: Morgan Quitno Press using data from U.S. Bureau of the Census
   "Health Insurance Historical Table 4" (http://www.census.gov/hhes/hlthins/historic/hihistt4.html)
*Includes Medicaid, Medicare and Military health care.

Percent of Population Covered by Military Health Insurance in 1999

National Percent = 3.1% of Population*

ALPHA ORDER				RANK ORDER		
RANK	STATE	PERCENT		RANK	STATE	PERCENT
30	Alabama	2.8		1	Alaska	12.1
1	Alaska	12.1		2	Virginia	8.7
10	Arizona	5.9		3	Kansas	7.7
6	Arkansas	6.8		4	Colorado	6.9
30	California	2.8		4	Kentucky	6.9
4	Colorado	6.9		6	Arkansas	6.8
39	Connecticut	2.0		6	North Dakota	6.8
28	Delaware	3.0		8	Hawaii	6.5
24	Florida	3.6		9	Nebraska	6.0
20	Georgia	4.0		10	Arizona	5.9
8	Hawaii	6.5		11	Wyoming	5.7
33	Idaho	2.7		12	Mississippi	5.5
47	Illinois	1.4		13	Washington	5.3
34	Indiana	2.6		14	Maine	4.9
30	Iowa	2.8		15	Montana	4.7
3	Kansas	7.7		15	Oklahoma	4.7
4	Kentucky	6.9		17	Louisiana	4.6
17	Louisiana	4.6		17	South Dakota	4.6
14	Maine	4.9		19	North Carolina	4.2
22	Maryland	3.8		20	Georgia	4.0
37	Massachusetts	2.3		21	New Mexico	3.9
49	Michigan	1.0		22	Maryland	3.8
40	Minnesota	1.8		23	South Carolina	3.7
12	Mississippi	5.5		24	Florida	3.6
37	Missouri	2.3		24	Utah	3.6
15	Montana	4.7		26	Nevada	3.4
9	Nebraska	6.0		27	Vermont	3.2
26	Nevada	3.4		28	Delaware	3.0
34	New Hampshire	2.6		29	Texas	2.9
50	New Jersey	0.8		30	Alabama	2.8
21	New Mexico	3.9		30	California	2.8
43	New York	1.6		30	Iowa	2.8
19	North Carolina	4.2		33	Idaho	2.7
6	North Dakota	6.8		34	Indiana	2.6
43	Ohio	1.6		34	New Hampshire	2.6
15	Oklahoma	4.7		36	Tennessee	2.5
42	Oregon	1.7		37	Massachusetts	2.3
47	Pennsylvania	1.4		37	Missouri	2.3
43	Rhode Island	1.6		39	Connecticut	2.0
23	South Carolina	3.7		40	Minnesota	1.8
17	South Dakota	4.6		40	West Virginia	1.8
36	Tennessee	2.5		42	Oregon	1.7
29	Texas	2.9		43	New York	1.6
24	Utah	3.6		43	Ohio	1.6
27	Vermont	3.2		43	Rhode Island	1.6
2	Virginia	8.7		46	Wisconsin	1.5
13	Washington	5.3		47	Illinois	1.4
40	West Virginia	1.8		47	Pennsylvania	1.4
46	Wisconsin	1.5		49	Michigan	1.0
11	Wyoming	5.7		50	New Jersey	0.8
					District of Columbia	2.0

Source: Morgan Quitno Press using data from U.S. Bureau of the Census
   "Health Insurance Historical Table 4" (http://www.census.gov/hhes/hlthins/historic/hihistt4.html)
*Includes CHAMPUS (Comprehensive Health and Medical Plan for Uniformed Services)/Tricare, Veterans
and military health care.

Percent of Children Not Covered by Health Insurance in 1999

National Percent = 13.9% of Children*

ALPHA ORDER			RANK ORDER		
RANK	STATE	PERCENT	RANK	STATE	PERCENT
29	Alabama	10.6	1	New Mexico	27.7
12	Alaska	16.2	2	Louisiana	24.6
5	Arizona	22.0	3	Texas	24.1
25	Arkansas	11.8	4	Nevada	22.1
9	California	18.3	5	Arizona	22.0
13	Colorado	16.0	6	Idaho	20.5
36	Connecticut	9.2	7	South Carolina	19.4
46	Delaware	6.7	8	Montana	18.9
11	Florida	16.5	9	California	18.3
21	Georgia	12.6	10	Oklahoma	17.0
29	Hawaii	10.6	11	Florida	16.5
6	Idaho	20.5	12	Alaska	16.2
24	Illinois	12.1	13	Colorado	16.0
39	Indiana	8.9	14	Mississippi	15.5
48	Iowa	6.2	15	Wyoming	14.5
22	Kansas	12.5	16	Virginia	14.1
18	Kentucky	13.7	17	West Virginia	13.8
2	Louisiana	24.6	18	Kentucky	13.7
46	Maine	6.7	19	Washington	13.3
34	Maryland	9.5	20	Oregon	13.2
37	Massachusetts	9.1	21	Georgia	12.6
33	Michigan	9.7	22	Kansas	12.5
44	Minnesota	7.4	23	North Carolina	12.4
14	Mississippi	15.5	24	Illinois	12.1
50	Missouri	5.4	25	Arkansas	11.8
8	Montana	18.9	26	New York	11.5
39	Nebraska	8.9	27	Utah	11.4
4	Nevada	22.1	28	Wisconsin	10.7
49	New Hampshire	5.9	29	Alabama	10.6
32	New Jersey	9.8	29	Hawaii	10.6
1	New Mexico	27.7	31	North Dakota	10.4
26	New York	11.5	32	New Jersey	9.8
23	North Carolina	12.4	33	Michigan	9.7
31	North Dakota	10.4	34	Maryland	9.5
39	Ohio	8.9	35	Tennessee	9.4
10	Oklahoma	17.0	36	Connecticut	9.2
20	Oregon	13.2	37	Massachusetts	9.1
43	Pennsylvania	7.6	37	South Dakota	9.1
45	Rhode Island	6.9	39	Indiana	8.9
7	South Carolina	19.4	39	Nebraska	8.9
37	South Dakota	9.1	39	Ohio	8.9
35	Tennessee	9.4	42	Vermont	8.0
3	Texas	24.1	43	Pennsylvania	7.6
27	Utah	11.4	44	Minnesota	7.4
42	Vermont	8.0	45	Rhode Island	6.9
16	Virginia	14.1	46	Delaware	6.7
19	Washington	13.3	46	Maine	6.7
17	West Virginia	13.8	48	Iowa	6.2
28	Wisconsin	10.7	49	New Hampshire	5.9
15	Wyoming	14.5	50	Missouri	5.4
				District of Columbia	17.2

Source: Morgan Quitno Press using data from U.S. Bureau of the Census
   "Health Insurance Historical Table 5" (http://www.census.gov/hhes/hlthins/historic/hihistt5.html)
*Children under 18 years old.

State Children's Health Insurance Program Enrollment in 2000

National Total = 3,333,879 Children*

RANK	STATE	CHILDREN	% of USA
22	Alabama	37,587	1.1%
35	Alaska	13,413	0.4%
14	Arizona	60,803	1.8%
49	Arkansas	1,892	0.1%
2	California	477,615	14.3%
25	Colorado	34,889	1.0%
32	Connecticut	18,804	0.6%
42	Delaware	4,474	0.1%
3	Florida	227,463	6.8%
5	Georgia	120,626	3.6%
48	Hawaii	2,256	0.1%
36	Idaho	12,449	0.4%
13	Illinois	62,507	1.9%
20	Indiana	44,373	1.3%
31	Iowa	19,958	0.6%
26	Kansas	26,306	0.8%
17	Kentucky	55,593	1.7%
18	Louisiana	49,995	1.5%
28	Maine	22,742	0.7%
10	Maryland	93,081	2.8%
7	Massachusetts	113,034	3.4%
23	Michigan	37,148	1.1%
50	Minnesota	24	0.0%
30	Mississippi	20,451	0.6%
12	Missouri	73,825	2.2%
39	Montana	8,317	0.2%
38	Nebraska	11,400	0.3%
33	Nevada	15,946	0.5%
43	New Hampshire	4,272	0.1%
11	New Jersey	89,034	2.7%
40	New Mexico	6,106	0.2%
1	New York	769,457	23.1%
9	North Carolina	103,567	3.1%
46	North Dakota	2,573	0.1%
8	Ohio	111,436	3.3%
16	Oklahoma	57,719	1.7%
24	Oregon	37,092	1.1%
6	Pennsylvania	119,710	3.6%
37	Rhode Island	11,539	0.3%
15	South Carolina	59,853	1.8%
41	South Dakota	5,888	0.2%
34	Tennessee	14,861	0.4%
4	Texas	130,519	3.9%
27	Utah	25,294	0.8%
44	Vermont	4,081	0.1%
21	Virginia	37,681	1.1%
45	Washington	2,616	0.1%
29	West Virginia	21,659	0.6%
19	Wisconsin	47,140	1.4%
47	Wyoming	2,547	0.1%

RANK	STATE	CHILDREN	% of USA
1	New York	769,457	23.1%
2	California	477,615	14.3%
3	Florida	227,463	6.8%
4	Texas	130,519	3.9%
5	Georgia	120,626	3.6%
6	Pennsylvania	119,710	3.6%
7	Massachusetts	113,034	3.4%
8	Ohio	111,436	3.3%
9	North Carolina	103,567	3.1%
10	Maryland	93,081	2.8%
11	New Jersey	89,034	2.7%
12	Missouri	73,825	2.2%
13	Illinois	62,507	1.9%
14	Arizona	60,803	1.8%
15	South Carolina	59,853	1.8%
16	Oklahoma	57,719	1.7%
17	Kentucky	55,593	1.7%
18	Louisiana	49,995	1.5%
19	Wisconsin	47,140	1.4%
20	Indiana	44,373	1.3%
21	Virginia	37,681	1.1%
22	Alabama	37,587	1.1%
23	Michigan	37,148	1.1%
24	Oregon	37,092	1.1%
25	Colorado	34,889	1.0%
26	Kansas	26,306	0.8%
27	Utah	25,294	0.8%
28	Maine	22,742	0.7%
29	West Virginia	21,659	0.6%
30	Mississippi	20,451	0.6%
31	Iowa	19,958	0.6%
32	Connecticut	18,804	0.6%
33	Nevada	15,946	0.5%
34	Tennessee	14,861	0.4%
35	Alaska	13,413	0.4%
36	Idaho	12,449	0.4%
37	Rhode Island	11,539	0.3%
38	Nebraska	11,400	0.3%
39	Montana	8,317	0.2%
40	New Mexico	6,106	0.2%
41	South Dakota	5,888	0.2%
42	Delaware	4,474	0.1%
43	New Hampshire	4,272	0.1%
44	Vermont	4,081	0.1%
45	Washington	2,616	0.1%
46	North Dakota	2,573	0.1%
47	Wyoming	2,547	0.1%
48	Hawaii	2,256	0.1%
49	Arkansas	1,892	0.1%
50	Minnesota	24	0.0%
	District of Columbia	2,264	0.1%

Source: U.S. Department of Health and Human Services, Health Care Financing Administration
    "Children's Health Insurance Program" (http://www.hcfa.gov/init/children.htm)
*For fiscal year 2000. The State Children's Health Insurance Program (SCHIP) was created in 1997 to help states expand health insurance to children whose families earn too much to qualify for Medicaid, yet not enough to afford private health insurance.

Health Maintenance Organizations (HMOs) in 2000

National Total = 563 HMOs*

<table>
<tr><th colspan="4">ALPHA ORDER</th><th colspan="4">RANK ORDER</th></tr>
<tr><th>RANK</th><th>STATE</th><th>HMOs</th><th>% of USA</th><th>RANK</th><th>STATE</th><th>HMOs</th><th>% of USA</th></tr>
<tr><td>25</td><td>Alabama</td><td>7</td><td>1.2%</td><td>1</td><td>Texas</td><td>37</td><td>6.6%</td></tr>
<tr><td>50</td><td>Alaska</td><td>0</td><td>0.0%</td><td>2</td><td>California</td><td>35</td><td>6.2%</td></tr>
<tr><td>18</td><td>Arizona</td><td>11</td><td>2.0%</td><td>3</td><td>Florida</td><td>34</td><td>6.0%</td></tr>
<tr><td>37</td><td>Arkansas</td><td>4</td><td>0.7%</td><td>4</td><td>Ohio</td><td>33</td><td>5.9%</td></tr>
<tr><td>2</td><td>California</td><td>35</td><td>6.2%</td><td>5</td><td>New York</td><td>31</td><td>5.5%</td></tr>
<tr><td>13</td><td>Colorado</td><td>16</td><td>2.8%</td><td>6</td><td>Michigan</td><td>22</td><td>3.9%</td></tr>
<tr><td>20</td><td>Connecticut</td><td>10</td><td>1.8%</td><td>6</td><td>Pennsylvania</td><td>22</td><td>3.9%</td></tr>
<tr><td>33</td><td>Delaware</td><td>5</td><td>0.9%</td><td>8</td><td>Illinois</td><td>21</td><td>3.7%</td></tr>
<tr><td>3</td><td>Florida</td><td>34</td><td>6.0%</td><td>9</td><td>Missouri</td><td>20</td><td>3.6%</td></tr>
<tr><td>18</td><td>Georgia</td><td>11</td><td>2.0%</td><td>9</td><td>Wisconsin</td><td>20</td><td>3.6%</td></tr>
<tr><td>31</td><td>Hawaii</td><td>6</td><td>1.1%</td><td>11</td><td>North Carolina</td><td>18</td><td>3.2%</td></tr>
<tr><td>41</td><td>Idaho</td><td>3</td><td>0.5%</td><td>12</td><td>Tennessee</td><td>17</td><td>3.0%</td></tr>
<tr><td>8</td><td>Illinois</td><td>21</td><td>3.7%</td><td>13</td><td>Colorado</td><td>16</td><td>2.8%</td></tr>
<tr><td>14</td><td>Indiana</td><td>15</td><td>2.7%</td><td>14</td><td>Indiana</td><td>15</td><td>2.7%</td></tr>
<tr><td>41</td><td>Iowa</td><td>3</td><td>0.5%</td><td>15</td><td>New Jersey</td><td>13</td><td>2.3%</td></tr>
<tr><td>25</td><td>Kansas</td><td>7</td><td>1.2%</td><td>15</td><td>Virginia</td><td>13</td><td>2.3%</td></tr>
<tr><td>25</td><td>Kentucky</td><td>7</td><td>1.2%</td><td>17</td><td>Louisiana</td><td>12</td><td>2.1%</td></tr>
<tr><td>17</td><td>Louisiana</td><td>12</td><td>2.1%</td><td>18</td><td>Arizona</td><td>11</td><td>2.0%</td></tr>
<tr><td>33</td><td>Maine</td><td>5</td><td>0.9%</td><td>18</td><td>Georgia</td><td>11</td><td>2.0%</td></tr>
<tr><td>20</td><td>Maryland</td><td>10</td><td>1.8%</td><td>20</td><td>Connecticut</td><td>10</td><td>1.8%</td></tr>
<tr><td>20</td><td>Massachusetts</td><td>10</td><td>1.8%</td><td>20</td><td>Maryland</td><td>10</td><td>1.8%</td></tr>
<tr><td>6</td><td>Michigan</td><td>22</td><td>3.9%</td><td>20</td><td>Massachusetts</td><td>10</td><td>1.8%</td></tr>
<tr><td>23</td><td>Minnesota</td><td>8</td><td>1.4%</td><td>23</td><td>Minnesota</td><td>8</td><td>1.4%</td></tr>
<tr><td>41</td><td>Mississippi</td><td>3</td><td>0.5%</td><td>23</td><td>Oklahoma</td><td>8</td><td>1.4%</td></tr>
<tr><td>9</td><td>Missouri</td><td>20</td><td>3.6%</td><td>25</td><td>Alabama</td><td>7</td><td>1.2%</td></tr>
<tr><td>41</td><td>Montana</td><td>3</td><td>0.5%</td><td>25</td><td>Kansas</td><td>7</td><td>1.2%</td></tr>
<tr><td>25</td><td>Nebraska</td><td>7</td><td>1.2%</td><td>25</td><td>Kentucky</td><td>7</td><td>1.2%</td></tr>
<tr><td>25</td><td>Nevada</td><td>7</td><td>1.2%</td><td>25</td><td>Nebraska</td><td>7</td><td>1.2%</td></tr>
<tr><td>37</td><td>New Hampshire</td><td>4</td><td>0.7%</td><td>25</td><td>Nevada</td><td>7</td><td>1.2%</td></tr>
<tr><td>15</td><td>New Jersey</td><td>13</td><td>2.3%</td><td>25</td><td>Utah</td><td>7</td><td>1.2%</td></tr>
<tr><td>37</td><td>New Mexico</td><td>4</td><td>0.7%</td><td>31</td><td>Hawaii</td><td>6</td><td>1.1%</td></tr>
<tr><td>5</td><td>New York</td><td>31</td><td>5.5%</td><td>31</td><td>Oregon</td><td>6</td><td>1.1%</td></tr>
<tr><td>11</td><td>North Carolina</td><td>18</td><td>3.2%</td><td>33</td><td>Delaware</td><td>5</td><td>0.9%</td></tr>
<tr><td>46</td><td>North Dakota</td><td>2</td><td>0.4%</td><td>33</td><td>Maine</td><td>5</td><td>0.9%</td></tr>
<tr><td>4</td><td>Ohio</td><td>33</td><td>5.9%</td><td>33</td><td>South Carolina</td><td>5</td><td>0.9%</td></tr>
<tr><td>23</td><td>Oklahoma</td><td>8</td><td>1.4%</td><td>33</td><td>Washington</td><td>5</td><td>0.9%</td></tr>
<tr><td>31</td><td>Oregon</td><td>6</td><td>1.1%</td><td>37</td><td>Arkansas</td><td>4</td><td>0.7%</td></tr>
<tr><td>6</td><td>Pennsylvania</td><td>22</td><td>3.9%</td><td>37</td><td>New Hampshire</td><td>4</td><td>0.7%</td></tr>
<tr><td>46</td><td>Rhode Island</td><td>2</td><td>0.4%</td><td>37</td><td>New Mexico</td><td>4</td><td>0.7%</td></tr>
<tr><td>33</td><td>South Carolina</td><td>5</td><td>0.9%</td><td>37</td><td>West Virginia</td><td>4</td><td>0.7%</td></tr>
<tr><td>41</td><td>South Dakota</td><td>3</td><td>0.5%</td><td>41</td><td>Idaho</td><td>3</td><td>0.5%</td></tr>
<tr><td>12</td><td>Tennessee</td><td>17</td><td>3.0%</td><td>41</td><td>Iowa</td><td>3</td><td>0.5%</td></tr>
<tr><td>1</td><td>Texas</td><td>37</td><td>6.6%</td><td>41</td><td>Mississippi</td><td>3</td><td>0.5%</td></tr>
<tr><td>25</td><td>Utah</td><td>7</td><td>1.2%</td><td>41</td><td>Montana</td><td>3</td><td>0.5%</td></tr>
<tr><td>48</td><td>Vermont</td><td>1</td><td>0.2%</td><td>41</td><td>South Dakota</td><td>3</td><td>0.5%</td></tr>
<tr><td>15</td><td>Virginia</td><td>13</td><td>2.3%</td><td>46</td><td>North Dakota</td><td>2</td><td>0.4%</td></tr>
<tr><td>33</td><td>Washington</td><td>5</td><td>0.9%</td><td>46</td><td>Rhode Island</td><td>2</td><td>0.4%</td></tr>
<tr><td>37</td><td>West Virginia</td><td>4</td><td>0.7%</td><td>48</td><td>Vermont</td><td>1</td><td>0.2%</td></tr>
<tr><td>9</td><td>Wisconsin</td><td>20</td><td>3.6%</td><td>48</td><td>Wyoming</td><td>1</td><td>0.2%</td></tr>
<tr><td>48</td><td>Wyoming</td><td>1</td><td>0.2%</td><td>50</td><td>Alaska</td><td>0</td><td>0.0%</td></tr>
<tr><td></td><td></td><td></td><td></td><td></td><td>District of Columbia</td><td>5</td><td>0.9%</td></tr>
</table>

Source: InterStudy Publications (Minneapolis, MN)
   "HMO Industry Report 10.2" (Press Release, October 30, 2000)
*As of January 1, 2000. Total does not include two HMOs in Guam and three in Puerto Rico. Health plans are allocated to states based upon their primary service areas. This means each plan is counted once. However, many plans serve more than one state.

Enrollees in Health Maintenance Organizations (HMOs) in 2000

National Total = 79,537,787 Enrollees*

ALPHA ORDER

RANK	STATE	ENROLLEES	% of USA
36	Alabama	314,977	0.4%
50	Alaska	0	0.0%
16	Arizona	1,475,853	1.9%
38	Arkansas	265,009	0.3%
1	California	17,740,759	22.3%
14	Colorado	1,603,307	2.0%
17	Connecticut	1,464,687	1.8%
42	Delaware	165,474	0.2%
3	Florida	4,748,377	6.0%
21	Georgia	1,352,683	1.7%
35	Hawaii	355,432	0.4%
43	Idaho	98,681	0.1%
9	Illinois	2,550,863	3.2%
27	Indiana	736,172	0.9%
39	Iowa	212,456	0.3%
30	Kansas	476,189	0.6%
23	Kentucky	1,247,228	1.6%
26	Louisiana	744,002	0.9%
37	Maine	279,222	0.4%
11	Maryland**	2,270,181	2.9%
6	Massachusetts	3,271,525	4.1%
8	Michigan	2,670,190	3.4%
18	Minnesota	1,427,393	1.8%
46	Mississippi	30,468	0.0%
12	Missouri	1,927,393	2.4%
44	Montana	61,498	0.1%
40	Nebraska	187,226	0.2%
31	Nevada	424,994	0.5%
32	New Hampshire	405,219	0.5%
10	New Jersey	2,519,850	3.2%
28	New Mexico	656,425	0.8%
2	New York	6,511,040	8.2%
19	North Carolina	1,364,668	1.7%
48	North Dakota	15,827	0.0%
7	Ohio	2,830,995	3.6%
29	Oklahoma	491,955	0.6%
20	Oregon	1,362,335	1.7%
4	Pennsylvania	4,064,919	5.1%
34	Rhode Island	377,286	0.5%
33	South Carolina	385,512	0.5%
45	South Dakota	49,395	0.1%
13	Tennessee	1,807,330	2.3%
5	Texas	3,704,612	4.7%
25	Utah	751,948	0.9%
47	Vermont	27,349	0.0%
22	Virginia**	1,269,280	1.6%
24	Washington	876,290	1.1%
41	West Virginia**	186,508	0.2%
15	Wisconsin	1,587,643	2.0%
49	Wyoming	6,625	0.0%

RANK ORDER

RANK	STATE	ENROLLEES	% of USA
1	California	17,740,759	22.3%
2	New York	6,511,040	8.2%
3	Florida	4,748,377	6.0%
4	Pennsylvania	4,064,919	5.1%
5	Texas	3,704,612	4.7%
6	Massachusetts	3,271,525	4.1%
7	Ohio	2,830,995	3.6%
8	Michigan	2,670,190	3.4%
9	Illinois	2,550,863	3.2%
10	New Jersey	2,519,850	3.2%
11	Maryland**	2,270,181	2.9%
12	Missouri	1,927,393	2.4%
13	Tennessee	1,807,330	2.3%
14	Colorado	1,603,307	2.0%
15	Wisconsin	1,587,643	2.0%
16	Arizona	1,475,853	1.9%
17	Connecticut	1,464,687	1.8%
18	Minnesota	1,427,393	1.8%
19	North Carolina	1,364,668	1.7%
20	Oregon	1,362,335	1.7%
21	Georgia	1,352,683	1.7%
22	Virginia**	1,269,280	1.6%
23	Kentucky	1,247,228	1.6%
24	Washington	876,290	1.1%
25	Utah	751,948	0.9%
26	Louisiana	744,002	0.9%
27	Indiana	736,172	0.9%
28	New Mexico	656,425	0.8%
29	Oklahoma	491,955	0.6%
30	Kansas	476,189	0.6%
31	Nevada	424,994	0.5%
32	New Hampshire	405,219	0.5%
33	South Carolina	385,512	0.5%
34	Rhode Island	377,286	0.5%
35	Hawaii	355,432	0.4%
36	Alabama	314,977	0.4%
37	Maine	279,222	0.4%
38	Arkansas	265,009	0.3%
39	Iowa	212,456	0.3%
40	Nebraska	187,226	0.2%
41	West Virginia**	186,508	0.2%
42	Delaware	165,474	0.2%
43	Idaho	98,681	0.1%
44	Montana	61,498	0.1%
45	South Dakota	49,395	0.1%
46	Mississippi	30,468	0.0%
47	Vermont	27,349	0.0%
48	North Dakota	15,827	0.0%
49	Wyoming	6,625	0.0%
50	Alaska	0	0.0%
	District of Columbia	182,537	0.2%

Source: InterStudy Publications (Minneapolis, MN)
   "HMO Industry Report 10.2" (Press Release, October 30, 2000)
*As of January 1, 2000. Total does not include 1,361,318 enrollees in U.S. territories.
**Maryland, Virginia and West Virginia include partial enrollment from five HMOs serving the Washington, DC metropolitan area.

Percent Change in Enrollees in Health Maintenance Organizations (HMOs): 1999 to 2000
National Percent Change = 0.4% Increase*

ALPHA ORDER

RANK ORDER

RANK	STATE	PERCENT CHANGE	RANK	STATE	PERCENT CHANGE
47	Alabama	(28.0)	1	Iowa	52.8
24	Alaska	0.0	2	Idaho	25.3
28	Arizona	(1.4)	3	Vermont	16.8
46	Arkansas	(15.1)	4	Connecticut	15.2
12	California	4.2	5	Wyoming	15.0
16	Colorado	2.6	6	Maine	11.2
4	Connecticut	15.2	7	Georgia	9.1
49	Delaware	(51.3)	7	South Dakota	9.1
34	Florida	(3.1)	9	Kansas	7.8
7	Georgia	9.1	10	Montana	5.6
44	Hawaii	(11.6)	11	New Jersey	5.4
2	Idaho	25.3	12	California	4.2
17	Illinois	1.8	13	Nevada	3.7
40	Indiana	(5.3)	14	Missouri	3.6
1	Iowa	52.8	15	Oklahoma	3.3
9	Kansas	7.8	16	Colorado	2.6
33	Kentucky	(2.7)	17	Illinois	1.8
37	Louisiana	(4.0)	17	Utah	1.8
6	Maine	11.2	19	Michigan	0.8
36	Maryland	(3.9)	19	Texas	0.8
23	Massachusetts	0.6	21	Pennsylvania	0.7
19	Michigan	0.8	21	South Carolina	0.7
26	Minnesota	(0.6)	23	Massachusetts	0.6
50	Mississippi	(65.9)	24	Alaska	0.0
14	Missouri	3.6	25	Ohio	(0.4)
10	Montana	5.6	26	Minnesota	(0.6)
48	Nebraska	(38.7)	27	New Mexico	(0.7)
13	Nevada	3.7	28	Arizona	(1.4)
31	New Hampshire	(1.9)	29	West Virginia	(1.5)
11	New Jersey	5.4	30	Wisconsin	(1.6)
27	New Mexico	(0.7)	31	New Hampshire	(1.9)
42	New York	(6.2)	32	North Dakota	(2.0)
35	North Carolina	(3.6)	33	Kentucky	(2.7)
32	North Dakota	(2.0)	34	Florida	(3.1)
25	Ohio	(0.4)	35	North Carolina	(3.6)
15	Oklahoma	3.3	36	Maryland	(3.9)
38	Oregon	(4.2)	37	Louisiana	(4.0)
21	Pennsylvania	0.7	38	Oregon	(4.2)
41	Rhode Island	(5.8)	39	Virginia	(4.7)
21	South Carolina	0.7	40	Indiana	(5.3)
7	South Dakota	9.1	41	Rhode Island	(5.8)
44	Tennessee	(11.6)	42	New York	(6.2)
19	Texas	0.8	43	Washington	(11.0)
17	Utah	1.8	44	Hawaii	(11.6)
3	Vermont	16.8	44	Tennessee	(11.6)
39	Virginia	(4.7)	46	Arkansas	(15.1)
43	Washington	(11.0)	47	Alabama	(28.0)
29	West Virginia	(1.5)	48	Nebraska	(38.7)
30	Wisconsin	(1.6)	49	Delaware	(51.3)
5	Wyoming	15.0	50	Mississippi	(65.9)

District of Columbia   3.6

Source: InterStudy Publications (Minneapolis, MN)
    "HMO Industry Report 10.2" (Press Release, October 30, 2000)
As of January 1, 2000. National rate does not include enrollees in U.S. territories.
**Not applicable.*

Percent of Population Enrolled in Health Maintenance Organizations (HMOs) in 2000
National Percent = 28.3% Enrolled in HMOs*

ALPHA ORDER

RANK	STATE	PERCENT
43	Alabama	7.2
50	Alaska	0.0
17	Arizona	30.9
38	Arkansas	10.4
1	California	53.5
6	Colorado	39.5
3	Connecticut	44.6
26	Delaware	22.0
16	Florida	31.4
32	Georgia	17.4
20	Hawaii	30.0
41	Idaho	7.9
27	Illinois	21.0
36	Indiana	12.4
42	Iowa	7.4
30	Kansas	17.9
15	Kentucky	31.5
33	Louisiana	17.0
25	Maine	22.3
4	Maryland	43.9
2	Massachusetts	53.0
22	Michigan	27.1
21	Minnesota	29.9
49	Mississippi	1.1
11	Missouri	35.2
44	Montana	7.0
37	Nebraska	11.2
24	Nevada	23.5
13	New Hampshire	33.7
17	New Jersey	30.9
8	New Mexico	37.7
9	New York	35.8
31	North Carolina	17.8
47	North Dakota	2.5
23	Ohio	25.1
35	Oklahoma	14.7
5	Oregon	41.1
12	Pennsylvania	33.9
7	Rhode Island	38.1
40	South Carolina	9.9
45	South Dakota	6.7
14	Tennessee	33.0
28	Texas	18.5
10	Utah	35.3
46	Vermont	4.6
28	Virginia	18.5
34	Washington	15.2
39	West Virginia	10.3
19	Wisconsin	30.2
48	Wyoming	1.4

RANK ORDER

RANK	STATE	PERCENT
1	California	53.5
2	Massachusetts	53.0
3	Connecticut	44.6
4	Maryland	43.9
5	Oregon	41.1
6	Colorado	39.5
7	Rhode Island	38.1
8	New Mexico	37.7
9	New York	35.8
10	Utah	35.3
11	Missouri	35.2
12	Pennsylvania	33.9
13	New Hampshire	33.7
14	Tennessee	33.0
15	Kentucky	31.5
16	Florida	31.4
17	Arizona	30.9
17	New Jersey	30.9
19	Wisconsin	30.2
20	Hawaii	30.0
21	Minnesota	29.9
22	Michigan	27.1
23	Ohio	25.1
24	Nevada	23.5
25	Maine	22.3
26	Delaware	22.0
27	Illinois	21.0
28	Texas	18.5
28	Virginia	18.5
30	Kansas	17.9
31	North Carolina	17.8
32	Georgia	17.4
33	Louisiana	17.0
34	Washington	15.2
35	Oklahoma	14.7
36	Indiana	12.4
37	Nebraska	11.2
38	Arkansas	10.4
39	West Virginia	10.3
40	South Carolina	9.9
41	Idaho	7.9
42	Iowa	7.4
43	Alabama	7.2
44	Montana	7.0
45	South Dakota	6.7
46	Vermont	4.6
47	North Dakota	2.5
48	Wyoming	1.4
49	Mississippi	1.1
50	Alaska	0.0
	District of Columbia	35.2

Source: InterStudy Publications (Minneapolis, MN)
    "HMO Industry Report 10.2" (Press Release, October 30, 2000)
*As of January 1, 2000. National percent does not include enrollees or population in U.S. territories.

Percent of Insured Population Enrolled in
Health Maintenance Organizations (HMOs) in 2000
National Percent = 34.4% of Insured are Enrolled in HMOs*

ALPHA ORDER

RANK	STATE	PERCENT
43	Alabama	8.3
50	Alaska	0.0
12	Arizona	38.5
40	Arkansas	12.1
1	California	65.6
7	Colorado	45.6
5	Connecticut	48.7
26	Delaware	24.4
11	Florida	39.1
32	Georgia	20.7
20	Hawaii	32.9
41	Idaho	9.7
26	Illinois	24.4
36	Indiana	14.0
44	Iowa	8.2
32	Kansas	20.7
15	Kentucky	37.4
29	Louisiana	22.4
25	Maine	24.9
3	Maryland	50.9
2	Massachusetts	59.0
22	Michigan	29.7
21	Minnesota	32.3
49	Mississippi	1.3
12	Missouri	38.5
42	Montana	8.4
38	Nebraska	12.7
24	Nevada	27.7
17	New Hampshire	36.0
18	New Jersey	35.9
4	New Mexico	49.2
8	New York	42.1
31	North Carolina	21.5
47	North Dakota	2.9
23	Ohio	28.2
35	Oklahoma	18.2
6	Oregon	46.8
14	Pennsylvania	38.1
9	Rhode Island	41.2
39	South Carolina	12.3
45	South Dakota	8.0
16	Tennessee	36.9
28	Texas	24.1
10	Utah	40.7
46	Vermont	5.2
30	Virginia	21.6
34	Washington	18.3
37	West Virginia	12.8
19	Wisconsin	33.0
48	Wyoming	1.6

RANK ORDER

RANK	STATE	PERCENT
1	California	65.6
2	Massachusetts	59.0
3	Maryland	50.9
4	New Mexico	49.2
5	Connecticut	48.7
6	Oregon	46.8
7	Colorado	45.6
8	New York	42.1
9	Rhode Island	41.2
10	Utah	40.7
11	Florida	39.1
12	Arizona	38.5
12	Missouri	38.5
14	Pennsylvania	38.1
15	Kentucky	37.4
16	Tennessee	36.9
17	New Hampshire	36.0
18	New Jersey	35.9
19	Wisconsin	33.0
20	Hawaii	32.9
21	Minnesota	32.3
22	Michigan	29.7
23	Ohio	28.2
24	Nevada	27.7
25	Maine	24.9
26	Delaware	24.4
26	Illinois	24.4
28	Texas	24.1
29	Louisiana	22.4
30	Virginia	21.6
31	North Carolina	21.5
32	Georgia	20.7
32	Kansas	20.7
34	Washington	18.3
35	Oklahoma	18.2
36	Indiana	14.0
37	West Virginia	12.8
38	Nebraska	12.7
39	South Carolina	12.3
40	Arkansas	12.1
41	Idaho	9.7
42	Montana	8.4
43	Alabama	8.3
44	Iowa	8.2
45	South Dakota	8.0
46	Vermont	5.2
47	North Dakota	2.9
48	Wyoming	1.6
49	Mississippi	1.3
50	Alaska	0.0
	District of Columbia	41.8

Source: Morgan Quitno Press using data from InterStudy Publications (Minneapolis, MN)
    "HMO Industry Report 10.2" (Press Release, October 30, 2000)
*As of January 1, 2000. Calculated using estimated number of insured as of 1999 from the U.S. Census Bureau.

Medicare Enrollees in 1999

National Total = 39,027,270 Enrollees*

ALPHA ORDER

RANK	STATE	ENROLLEES	% of USA
19	Alabama	675,013	1.7%
50	Alaska	40,096	0.1%
20	Arizona	658,751	1.7%
31	Arkansas	434,684	1.1%
1	California	3,822,301	9.8%
30	Colorado	457,787	1.2%
26	Connecticut	509,627	1.3%
46	Delaware	109,661	0.3%
2	Florida	2,763,922	7.1%
12	Georgia	896,553	2.3%
43	Hawaii	161,436	0.4%
42	Idaho	161,575	0.4%
7	Illinois	1,620,900	4.2%
15	Indiana	842,865	2.2%
29	Iowa	474,586	1.2%
33	Kansas	387,940	1.0%
23	Kentucky	614,087	1.6%
24	Louisiana	595,653	1.5%
38	Maine	212,942	0.5%
22	Maryland	632,471	1.6%
11	Massachusetts	949,735	2.4%
8	Michigan	1,384,283	3.5%
21	Minnesota	646,683	1.7%
32	Mississippi	413,041	1.1%
14	Missouri	852,418	2.2%
44	Montana	135,239	0.3%
35	Nebraska	251,564	0.6%
36	Nevada	229,367	0.6%
41	New Hampshire	166,683	0.4%
9	New Jersey	1,187,988	3.0%
37	New Mexico	229,029	0.6%
3	New York	2,677,201	6.9%
10	North Carolina	1,111,998	2.8%
47	North Dakota	102,740	0.3%
6	Ohio	1,686,485	4.3%
27	Oklahoma	501,844	1.3%
28	Oregon	482,560	1.2%
5	Pennsylvania	2,080,610	5.3%
40	Rhode Island	169,569	0.4%
25	South Carolina	555,881	1.4%
45	South Dakota	118,706	0.3%
16	Tennessee	814,298	2.1%
4	Texas	2,218,856	5.7%
39	Utah	200,996	0.5%
48	Vermont	87,573	0.2%
13	Virginia	874,965	2.2%
18	Washington	722,836	1.9%
34	West Virginia	334,490	0.9%
17	Wisconsin	775,484	2.0%
49	Wyoming	64,317	0.2%

RANK ORDER

RANK	STATE	ENROLLEES	% of USA
1	California	3,822,301	9.8%
2	Florida	2,763,922	7.1%
3	New York	2,677,201	6.9%
4	Texas	2,218,856	5.7%
5	Pennsylvania	2,080,610	5.3%
6	Ohio	1,686,485	4.3%
7	Illinois	1,620,900	4.2%
8	Michigan	1,384,283	3.5%
9	New Jersey	1,187,988	3.0%
10	North Carolina	1,111,998	2.8%
11	Massachusetts	949,735	2.4%
12	Georgia	896,553	2.3%
13	Virginia	874,965	2.2%
14	Missouri	852,418	2.2%
15	Indiana	842,865	2.2%
16	Tennessee	814,298	2.1%
17	Wisconsin	775,484	2.0%
18	Washington	722,836	1.9%
19	Alabama	675,013	1.7%
20	Arizona	658,751	1.7%
21	Minnesota	646,683	1.7%
22	Maryland	632,471	1.6%
23	Kentucky	614,087	1.6%
24	Louisiana	595,653	1.5%
25	South Carolina	555,881	1.4%
26	Connecticut	509,627	1.3%
27	Oklahoma	501,844	1.3%
28	Oregon	482,560	1.2%
29	Iowa	474,586	1.2%
30	Colorado	457,787	1.2%
31	Arkansas	434,684	1.1%
32	Mississippi	413,041	1.1%
33	Kansas	387,940	1.0%
34	West Virginia	334,490	0.9%
35	Nebraska	251,564	0.6%
36	Nevada	229,367	0.6%
37	New Mexico	229,029	0.6%
38	Maine	212,942	0.5%
39	Utah	200,996	0.5%
40	Rhode Island	169,569	0.4%
41	New Hampshire	166,683	0.4%
42	Idaho	161,575	0.4%
43	Hawaii	161,436	0.4%
44	Montana	135,239	0.3%
45	South Dakota	118,706	0.3%
46	Delaware	109,661	0.3%
47	North Dakota	102,740	0.3%
48	Vermont	87,573	0.2%
49	Wyoming	64,317	0.2%
50	Alaska	40,096	0.1%
	District of Columbia	75,041	0.2%

Source: U.S. Department of Health and Human Services, Health Care Financing Administration
"Medicare Estimated Benefit Payments by State" (http://www.hcfa.gov/stats/BENEPAY/bnpay99i.htm)
For fiscal year 1999. Includes aged and disabled enrollees. Total includes 523,963 enrollees in Puerto Rico and 327,977 enrollees in "other outlying areas."

Medicare Benefit Payments in 1999

National Total = $208,623,563,538*

ALPHA ORDER

RANK	STATE	BENEFITS	% of USA
19	Alabama	$3,817,396,530	1.8%
50	Alaska	133,480,125	0.1%
24	Arizona	2,827,734,758	1.4%
30	Arkansas	2,044,027,481	1.0%
1	California	23,305,723,494	11.2%
27	Colorado	2,327,582,779	1.1%
23	Connecticut	2,985,509,581	1.4%
47	Delaware	386,467,560	0.2%
2	Florida	18,389,206,288	8.8%
18	Georgia	3,895,108,054	1.9%
41	Hawaii	600,476,783	0.3%
42	Idaho	580,302,396	0.3%
7	Illinois	7,605,610,448	3.6%
13	Indiana	4,730,109,977	2.3%
34	Iowa	1,416,873,428	0.7%
31	Kansas	1,739,329,004	0.8%
21	Kentucky	3,120,201,506	1.5%
14	Louisiana	4,257,731,541	2.0%
40	Maine	659,651,613	0.3%
15	Maryland	4,095,719,519	2.0%
12	Massachusetts	4,832,685,785	2.3%
9	Michigan	6,716,357,961	3.2%
22	Minnesota	2,991,679,494	1.4%
28	Mississippi	2,231,394,305	1.1%
16	Missouri	4,061,920,145	1.9%
44	Montana	508,924,248	0.2%
35	Nebraska	1,055,877,294	0.5%
36	Nevada	1,047,877,402	0.5%
43	New Hampshire	557,216,453	0.3%
8	New Jersey	7,474,563,686	3.6%
39	New Mexico	794,664,887	0.4%
3	New York	16,838,053,507	8.1%
10	North Carolina	5,808,687,639	2.8%
46	North Dakota	459,480,874	0.2%
6	Ohio	9,304,893,988	4.5%
29	Oklahoma	2,065,542,544	1.0%
33	Oregon	1,648,723,895	0.8%
5	Pennsylvania	12,953,469,729	6.2%
37	Rhode Island	973,152,273	0.5%
25	South Carolina	2,801,284,695	1.3%
45	South Dakota	486,673,168	0.2%
11	Tennessee	4,855,360,413	2.3%
4	Texas	14,227,830,241	6.8%
38	Utah	836,291,181	0.4%
48	Vermont	253,949,833	0.1%
17	Virginia	4,049,543,351	1.9%
26	Washington	2,504,808,594	1.2%
32	West Virginia	1,652,563,616	0.8%
20	Wisconsin	3,355,504,649	1.6%
49	Wyoming	210,883,286	0.1%

RANK ORDER

RANK	STATE	BENEFITS	% of USA
1	California	$23,305,723,494	11.2%
2	Florida	18,389,206,288	8.8%
3	New York	16,838,053,507	8.1%
4	Texas	14,227,830,241	6.8%
5	Pennsylvania	12,953,469,729	6.2%
6	Ohio	9,304,893,988	4.5%
7	Illinois	7,605,610,448	3.6%
8	New Jersey	7,474,563,686	3.6%
9	Michigan	6,716,357,961	3.2%
10	North Carolina	5,808,687,639	2.8%
11	Tennessee	4,855,360,413	2.3%
12	Massachusetts	4,832,685,785	2.3%
13	Indiana	4,730,109,977	2.3%
14	Louisiana	4,257,731,541	2.0%
15	Maryland	4,095,719,519	2.0%
16	Missouri	4,061,920,145	1.9%
17	Virginia	4,049,543,351	1.9%
18	Georgia	3,895,108,054	1.9%
19	Alabama	3,817,396,530	1.8%
20	Wisconsin	3,355,504,649	1.6%
21	Kentucky	3,120,201,506	1.5%
22	Minnesota	2,991,679,494	1.4%
23	Connecticut	2,985,509,581	1.4%
24	Arizona	2,827,734,758	1.4%
25	South Carolina	2,801,284,695	1.3%
26	Washington	2,504,808,594	1.2%
27	Colorado	2,327,582,779	1.1%
28	Mississippi	2,231,394,305	1.1%
29	Oklahoma	2,065,542,544	1.0%
30	Arkansas	2,044,027,481	1.0%
31	Kansas	1,739,329,004	0.8%
32	West Virginia	1,652,563,616	0.8%
33	Oregon	1,648,723,895	0.8%
34	Iowa	1,416,873,428	0.7%
35	Nebraska	1,055,877,294	0.5%
36	Nevada	1,047,877,402	0.5%
37	Rhode Island	973,152,273	0.5%
38	Utah	836,291,181	0.4%
39	New Mexico	794,664,887	0.4%
40	Maine	659,651,613	0.3%
41	Hawaii	600,476,783	0.3%
42	Idaho	580,302,396	0.3%
43	New Hampshire	557,216,453	0.3%
44	Montana	508,924,248	0.2%
45	South Dakota	486,673,168	0.2%
46	North Dakota	459,480,874	0.2%
47	Delaware	386,467,560	0.2%
48	Vermont	253,949,833	0.1%
49	Wyoming	210,883,286	0.1%
50	Alaska	133,480,125	0.1%
	District of Columbia	825,298,033	0.4%

Source: U.S. Department of Health and Human Services, Health Care Financing Administration
"Medicare Estimated Benefit Payments by State" (http://www.hcfa.gov/stats/BENEPAY/bnpay99i.htm)
For fiscal year 1999. Includes payments to aged and disabled enrollees. Total includes $1,264,153,750 in payments to enrollees in Puerto Rico and $56,009,752 to enrollees in "other outlying areas."

Medicare Payments per Enrollee in 1999

National Rate = $5,346*

ALPHA ORDER

RANK	STATE	PER ENROLLEE
12	Alabama	$5,655
46	Alaska	3,329
33	Arizona	4,293
24	Arkansas	4,702
8	California	6,097
18	Colorado	5,084
10	Connecticut	5,858
41	Delaware	3,524
2	Florida	6,653
31	Georgia	4,345
39	Hawaii	3,720
40	Idaho	3,592
25	Illinois	4,692
13	Indiana	5,612
49	Iowa	2,985
29	Kansas	4,484
19	Kentucky	5,081
1	Louisiana	7,148
48	Maine	3,098
3	Maryland	6,476
17	Massachusetts	5,088
22	Michigan	4,852
27	Minnesota	4,626
15	Mississippi	5,402
23	Missouri	4,765
38	Montana	3,763
34	Nebraska	4,197
28	Nevada	4,569
45	New Hampshire	3,343
5	New Jersey	6,292
42	New Mexico	3,470
6	New York	6,289
16	North Carolina	5,224
30	North Dakota	4,472
14	Ohio	5,517
36	Oklahoma	4,116
44	Oregon	3,417
7	Pennsylvania	6,226
11	Rhode Island	5,739
20	South Carolina	5,039
37	South Dakota	4,100
9	Tennessee	5,963
4	Texas	6,412
35	Utah	4,161
50	Vermont	2,900
26	Virginia	4,628
43	Washington	3,465
21	West Virginia	4,941
32	Wisconsin	4,327
47	Wyoming	3,279

RANK ORDER

RANK	STATE	PER ENROLLEE
1	Louisiana	$7,148
2	Florida	6,653
3	Maryland	6,476
4	Texas	6,412
5	New Jersey	6,292
6	New York	6,289
7	Pennsylvania	6,226
8	California	6,097
9	Tennessee	5,963
10	Connecticut	5,858
11	Rhode Island	5,739
12	Alabama	5,655
13	Indiana	5,612
14	Ohio	5,517
15	Mississippi	5,402
16	North Carolina	5,224
17	Massachusetts	5,088
18	Colorado	5,084
19	Kentucky	5,081
20	South Carolina	5,039
21	West Virginia	4,941
22	Michigan	4,852
23	Missouri	4,765
24	Arkansas	4,702
25	Illinois	4,692
26	Virginia	4,628
27	Minnesota	4,626
28	Nevada	4,569
29	Kansas	4,484
30	North Dakota	4,472
31	Georgia	4,345
32	Wisconsin	4,327
33	Arizona	4,293
34	Nebraska	4,197
35	Utah	4,161
36	Oklahoma	4,116
37	South Dakota	4,100
38	Montana	3,763
39	Hawaii	3,720
40	Idaho	3,592
41	Delaware	3,524
42	New Mexico	3,470
43	Washington	3,465
44	Oregon	3,417
45	New Hampshire	3,343
46	Alaska	3,329
47	Wyoming	3,279
48	Maine	3,098
49	Iowa	2,985
50	Vermont	2,900

District of Columbia 10,998

Source: U.S. Department of Health and Human Services, Health Care Financing Administration
"Medicare Estimated Benefit Payments by State" (http://www.hcfa.gov/stats/BENEPAY/bnpay99i.htm)
*For fiscal year 1999. Includes aged and disabled enrollees. National rate includes payments to enrollees in Puerto Rico and in "other outlying areas."

Percent of Population Enrolled in Medicare in 1999

National Percent = 14.1% of Population*

ALPHA ORDER

RANK	STATE	PERCENT
13	Alabama	15.4
50	Alaska	6.5
33	Arizona	13.8
5	Arkansas	17.0
45	California	11.5
47	Colorado	11.3
11	Connecticut	15.5
24	Delaware	14.6
2	Florida	18.3
45	Georgia	11.5
34	Hawaii	13.6
40	Idaho	12.9
37	Illinois	13.4
30	Indiana	14.2
7	Iowa	16.5
24	Kansas	14.6
11	Kentucky	15.5
34	Louisiana	13.6
5	Maine	17.0
44	Maryland	12.2
13	Massachusetts	15.4
31	Michigan	14.0
36	Minnesota	13.5
18	Mississippi	14.9
10	Missouri	15.6
15	Montana	15.3
16	Nebraska	15.1
41	Nevada	12.7
32	New Hampshire	13.9
24	New Jersey	14.6
39	New Mexico	13.2
22	New York	14.7
28	North Carolina	14.5
8	North Dakota	16.2
17	Ohio	15.0
18	Oklahoma	14.9
24	Oregon	14.6
3	Pennsylvania	17.3
4	Rhode Island	17.1
29	South Carolina	14.3
8	South Dakota	16.2
20	Tennessee	14.8
48	Texas	11.1
49	Utah	9.4
22	Vermont	14.7
41	Virginia	12.7
43	Washington	12.6
1	West Virginia	18.5
20	Wisconsin	14.8
37	Wyoming	13.4

RANK ORDER

RANK	STATE	PERCENT
1	West Virginia	18.5
2	Florida	18.3
3	Pennsylvania	17.3
4	Rhode Island	17.1
5	Arkansas	17.0
5	Maine	17.0
7	Iowa	16.5
8	North Dakota	16.2
8	South Dakota	16.2
10	Missouri	15.6
11	Connecticut	15.5
11	Kentucky	15.5
13	Alabama	15.4
13	Massachusetts	15.4
15	Montana	15.3
16	Nebraska	15.1
17	Ohio	15.0
18	Mississippi	14.9
18	Oklahoma	14.9
20	Tennessee	14.8
20	Wisconsin	14.8
22	New York	14.7
22	Vermont	14.7
24	Delaware	14.6
24	Kansas	14.6
24	New Jersey	14.6
24	Oregon	14.6
28	North Carolina	14.5
29	South Carolina	14.3
30	Indiana	14.2
31	Michigan	14.0
32	New Hampshire	13.9
33	Arizona	13.8
34	Hawaii	13.6
34	Louisiana	13.6
36	Minnesota	13.5
37	Illinois	13.4
37	Wyoming	13.4
39	New Mexico	13.2
40	Idaho	12.9
41	Nevada	12.7
41	Virginia	12.7
43	Washington	12.6
44	Maryland	12.2
45	California	11.5
45	Georgia	11.5
47	Colorado	11.3
48	Texas	11.1
49	Utah	9.4
50	Alaska	6.5
	District of Columbia	14.5

*Source: Morgan Quitno Press using data from U.S. Dept. of Health and Human Services, Health Care Financing Admn
"Medicare Estimated Benefit Payments by State" (http://www.hcfa.gov/stats/BENEPAY/bnpay99i.htm)*
For fiscal year 1999. Includes aged and disabled enrollees. National rate includes only residents of the 50 states and the District of Columbia.

Medicare Managed Care Enrollees in 2001

National Total = 6,199,297 Enrollees*

RANK	STATE	ENROLLEES	% of USA
22	Alabama	53,748	0.9%
45	Alaska	0	0.0%
7	Arizona	240,511	3.9%
32	Arkansas	17,462	0.3%
1	California	1,561,809	25.2%
12	Colorado	153,093	2.5%
19	Connecticut	73,778	1.2%
42	Delaware	890	0.0%
2	Florida	693,752	11.2%
26	Georgia	40,859	0.7%
21	Hawaii	54,979	0.9%
34	Idaho	13,479	0.2%
11	Illinois	159,032	2.6%
30	Indiana	19,976	0.3%
38	Iowa	7,056	0.1%
35	Kansas	10,285	0.2%
33	Kentucky	15,555	0.3%
15	Louisiana	97,257	1.6%
45	Maine	0	0.0%
27	Maryland	34,764	0.6%
8	Massachusetts	225,239	3.6%
18	Michigan	77,788	1.3%
16	Minnesota	82,132	1.3%
39	Mississippi	4,359	0.1%
10	Missouri	162,836	2.6%
45	Montana	0	0.0%
36	Nebraska	10,269	0.2%
17	Nevada	81,044	1.3%
41	New Hampshire	1,021	0.0%
13	New Jersey	151,329	2.4%
29	New Mexico	28,281	0.5%
4	New York	455,495	7.3%
24	North Carolina	45,142	0.7%
43	North Dakota	685	0.0%
6	Ohio	248,402	4.0%
23	Oklahoma	47,370	0.8%
9	Oregon	191,457	3.1%
3	Pennsylvania	515,246	8.3%
20	Rhode Island	57,240	0.9%
45	South Carolina	0	0.0%
44	South Dakota	633	0.0%
28	Tennessee	34,241	0.6%
5	Texas	249,117	4.0%
31	Utah	18,323	0.3%
45	Vermont	0	0.0%
40	Virginia	3,207	0.1%
14	Washington	150,033	2.4%
37	West Virginia	9,023	0.1%
25	Wisconsin	41,842	0.7%
45	Wyoming	0	0.0%

RANK	STATE	ENROLLEES	% of USA
1	California	1,561,809	25.2%
2	Florida	693,752	11.2%
3	Pennsylvania	515,246	8.3%
4	New York	455,495	7.3%
5	Texas	249,117	4.0%
6	Ohio	248,402	4.0%
7	Arizona	240,511	3.9%
8	Massachusetts	225,239	3.6%
9	Oregon	191,457	3.1%
10	Missouri	162,836	2.6%
11	Illinois	159,032	2.6%
12	Colorado	153,093	2.5%
13	New Jersey	151,329	2.4%
14	Washington	150,033	2.4%
15	Louisiana	97,257	1.6%
16	Minnesota	82,132	1.3%
17	Nevada	81,044	1.3%
18	Michigan	77,788	1.3%
19	Connecticut	73,778	1.2%
20	Rhode Island	57,240	0.9%
21	Hawaii	54,979	0.9%
22	Alabama	53,748	0.9%
23	Oklahoma	47,370	0.8%
24	North Carolina	45,142	0.7%
25	Wisconsin	41,842	0.7%
26	Georgia	40,859	0.7%
27	Maryland	34,764	0.6%
28	Tennessee	34,241	0.6%
29	New Mexico	28,281	0.5%
30	Indiana	19,976	0.3%
31	Utah	18,323	0.3%
32	Arkansas	17,462	0.3%
33	Kentucky	15,555	0.3%
34	Idaho	13,479	0.2%
35	Kansas	10,285	0.2%
36	Nebraska	10,269	0.2%
37	West Virginia	9,023	0.1%
38	Iowa	7,056	0.1%
39	Mississippi	4,359	0.1%
40	Virginia	3,207	0.1%
41	New Hampshire	1,021	0.0%
42	Delaware	890	0.0%
43	North Dakota	685	0.0%
44	South Dakota	633	0.0%
45	Alaska	0	0.0%
45	Maine	0	0.0%
45	Montana	0	0.0%
45	South Carolina	0	0.0%
45	Vermont	0	0.0%
45	Wyoming	0	0.0%
	District of Columbia	1,093	0.0%

Source: U.S. Department of Health and Human Services, Health Care Financing Administration
"Medicare Managed Care Contract Report" (February 1, 2001, http://www.hcfa.gov/stats/mmCC0201.txt)
*As of February 1st. Includes TEFRA, Cost, and Health Care Prepayment Plans (HCPP) and other demo plans.
National total includes 58,165 enrollees in the United Mine Workers' plan not shown separately by state.

Percent of Medicare Enrollees in Managed Care Programs in 2001

National Percent = 16.3% of Medicare Enrollees*

RANK	STATE	PERCENT
25	Alabama	8.0
45	Alaska	0.0
3	Arizona	36.9
33	Arkansas	4.0
1	California	41.3
6	Colorado	33.9
16	Connecticut	14.5
40	Delaware	0.8
8	Florida	25.1
29	Georgia	4.6
5	Hawaii	34.6
24	Idaho	8.5
21	Illinois	9.8
37	Indiana	2.4
38	Iowa	1.5
35	Kansas	2.6
35	Kentucky	2.6
14	Louisiana	16.3
45	Maine	0.0
27	Maryland	5.5
10	Massachusetts	23.7
26	Michigan	5.6
17	Minnesota	12.8
39	Mississippi	1.1
12	Missouri	19.1
45	Montana	0.0
31	Nebraska	4.1
4	Nevada	36.3
42	New Hampshire	0.6
18	New Jersey	12.7
19	New Mexico	12.6
13	New York	17.1
31	North Carolina	4.1
41	North Dakota	0.7
15	Ohio	14.7
22	Oklahoma	9.5
2	Oregon	39.8
9	Pennsylvania	24.7
7	Rhode Island	33.7
45	South Carolina	0.0
43	South Dakota	0.5
30	Tennessee	4.2
20	Texas	11.3
23	Utah	9.3
45	Vermont	0.0
44	Virginia	0.4
11	Washington	20.9
34	West Virginia	2.7
28	Wisconsin	5.4
45	Wyoming	0.0

RANK	STATE	PERCENT
1	California	41.3
2	Oregon	39.8
3	Arizona	36.9
4	Nevada	36.3
5	Hawaii	34.6
6	Colorado	33.9
7	Rhode Island	33.7
8	Florida	25.1
9	Pennsylvania	24.7
10	Massachusetts	23.7
11	Washington	20.9
12	Missouri	19.1
13	New York	17.1
14	Louisiana	16.3
15	Ohio	14.7
16	Connecticut	14.5
17	Minnesota	12.8
18	New Jersey	12.7
19	New Mexico	12.6
20	Texas	11.3
21	Illinois	9.8
22	Oklahoma	9.5
23	Utah	9.3
24	Idaho	8.5
25	Alabama	8.0
26	Michigan	5.6
27	Maryland	5.5
28	Wisconsin	5.4
29	Georgia	4.6
30	Tennessee	4.2
31	Nebraska	4.1
31	North Carolina	4.1
33	Arkansas	4.0
34	West Virginia	2.7
35	Kansas	2.6
35	Kentucky	2.6
37	Indiana	2.4
38	Iowa	1.5
39	Mississippi	1.1
40	Delaware	0.8
41	North Dakota	0.7
42	New Hampshire	0.6
43	South Dakota	0.5
44	Virginia	0.4
45	Alaska	0.0
45	Maine	0.0
45	Montana	0.0
45	South Carolina	0.0
45	Vermont	0.0
45	Wyoming	0.0

District of Columbia 1.4

Source: Morgan Quitno Press using data from U.S. Dept. of Health and Human Services, Health Care Financing Admin.
"Medicare Managed Care Contract Report" (February 1, 2001, http://www.hcfa.gov/stats/mmCC0201.txt)
*As of February 1st. Based on December 1999 Medicare enrollees. Includes aged and disabled enrollees.
National percent does not include enrollees in Puerto Rico and other outlying areas.

Medicare Physicians in 1999

National Total = 830,372 Physicians*

<u>ALPHA ORDER</u>

RANK	STATE	PHYSICIANS	% of USA
26	Alabama	9,629	1.2%
49	Alaska	1,481	0.2%
24	Arizona	11,587	1.4%
31	Arkansas	6,972	0.8%
1	California	98,515	11.9%
22	Colorado	13,131	1.6%
23	Connecticut	12,279	1.5%
45	Delaware	2,440	0.3%
5	Florida	43,006	5.2%
12	Georgia	19,217	2.3%
40	Hawaii**	4,011	0.5%
27	Idaho	8,769	1.1%
44	Illinois	2,549	0.3%
7	Indiana	32,663	3.9%
18	Iowa	15,726	1.9%
32	Kansas	6,591	0.8%
29	Kentucky	8,620	1.0%
21	Louisiana	13,533	1.6%
9	Maine	28,566	3.4%
11	Maryland	19,364	2.3%
36	Massachusetts	4,646	0.6%
8	Michigan	29,112	3.5%
19	Minnesota	15,552	1.9%
17	Mississippi	16,560	2.0%
33	Missouri	5,414	0.7%
43	Montana	2,611	0.3%
13	Nebraska	18,405	2.2%
46	Nevada	2,311	0.3%
38	New Hampshire	4,234	0.5%
37	New Jersey	4,355	0.5%
10	New Mexico	28,374	3.4%
39	New York	4,197	0.5%
41	North Carolina	3,575	0.4%
2	North Dakota	73,216	8.8%
6	Ohio	32,841	4.0%
30	Oklahoma	7,570	0.9%
25	Oregon	9,934	1.2%
3	Pennsylvania	52,530	6.3%
42	Rhode Island	3,485	0.4%
28	South Carolina	8,682	1.0%
47	South Dakota	2,227	0.3%
20	Tennessee	15,149	1.8%
4	Texas	51,304	6.2%
34	Utah	5,001	0.6%
14	Vermont	17,312	2.1%
48	Virginia	2,226	0.3%
15	Washington	17,218	2.1%
16	West Virginia	16,627	2.0%
35	Wisconsin	4,948	0.6%
50	Wyoming	1,277	0.2%

<u>RANK ORDER</u>

RANK	STATE	PHYSICIANS	% of USA
1	California	98,515	11.9%
2	North Dakota	73,216	8.8%
3	Pennsylvania	52,530	6.3%
4	Texas	51,304	6.2%
5	Florida	43,006	5.2%
6	Ohio	32,841	4.0%
7	Indiana	32,663	3.9%
8	Michigan	29,112	3.5%
9	Maine	28,566	3.4%
10	New Mexico	28,374	3.4%
11	Maryland	19,364	2.3%
12	Georgia	19,217	2.3%
13	Nebraska	18,405	2.2%
14	Vermont	17,312	2.1%
15	Washington	17,218	2.1%
16	West Virginia	16,627	2.0%
17	Mississippi	16,560	2.0%
18	Iowa	15,726	1.9%
19	Minnesota	15,552	1.9%
20	Tennessee	15,149	1.8%
21	Louisiana	13,533	1.6%
22	Colorado	13,131	1.6%
23	Connecticut	12,279	1.5%
24	Arizona	11,587	1.4%
25	Oregon	9,934	1.2%
26	Alabama	9,629	1.2%
27	Idaho	8,769	1.1%
28	South Carolina	8,682	1.0%
29	Kentucky	8,620	1.0%
30	Oklahoma	7,570	0.9%
31	Arkansas	6,972	0.8%
32	Kansas	6,591	0.8%
33	Missouri	5,414	0.7%
34	Utah	5,001	0.6%
35	Wisconsin	4,948	0.6%
36	Massachusetts	4,646	0.6%
37	New Jersey	4,355	0.5%
38	New Hampshire	4,234	0.5%
39	New York	4,197	0.5%
40	Hawaii**	4,011	0.5%
41	North Carolina	3,575	0.4%
42	Rhode Island	3,485	0.4%
43	Montana	2,611	0.3%
44	Illinois	2,549	0.3%
45	Delaware	2,440	0.3%
46	Nevada	2,311	0.3%
47	South Dakota	2,227	0.3%
48	Virginia	2,226	0.3%
49	Alaska	1,481	0.2%
50	Wyoming	1,277	0.2%
	District of Columbia	4,449	0.5%

*Source: U.S. Department of Health and Human Services, Health Care Financing Administration
"Medicare Physician Registry" (July 1999)*
*Medicare Part B. "Physicians" include MD, DO, DDM, DDS, DPM, OD and CH. National total includes 6,376
physicians in Puerto Rico and the Virgin Islands.
**Physicians for Guam are included in Hawaii's total.*

Percent of Physicians Participating in Medicare in 1999

National Percent = 84.6% of Physicians Participate in Medicare*

ALPHA ORDER

RANK	STATE	PERCENT
2	Alabama	94.5
41	Alaska	81.4
21	Arizona	89.7
39	Arkansas	83.1
42	California	81.0
33	Colorado	84.6
25	Connecticut	88.7
35	Delaware	84.1
46	Florida	77.6
37	Georgia	83.3
31	Hawaii	85.6
47	Idaho	75.6
34	Illinois	84.2
44	Indiana	79.0
16	Iowa	91.1
1	Kansas	94.7
10	Kentucky	92.3
49	Louisiana	73.5
6	Maine	93.8
14	Maryland	91.7
5	Massachusetts	94.0
27	Michigan	87.7
45	Minnesota	78.1
40	Mississippi	82.6
24	Missouri	89.2
32	Montana	84.7
9	Nebraska	92.4
7	Nevada	93.3
11	New Hampshire	92.2
43	New Jersey	80.1
23	New Mexico	89.3
48	New York	75.3
26	North Carolina	88.3
3	North Dakota	94.3
8	Ohio	93.2
19	Oklahoma	89.9
20	Oregon	89.8
36	Pennsylvania	83.5
50	Rhode Island	71.7
18	South Carolina	90.0
30	South Dakota	85.7
17	Tennessee	90.9
37	Texas	83.3
4	Utah	94.1
13	Vermont	91.8
28	Virginia	87.2
14	Washington	91.7
12	West Virginia	92.1
22	Wisconsin	89.4
29	Wyoming	86.4

RANK ORDER

RANK	STATE	PERCENT
1	Kansas	94.7
2	Alabama	94.5
3	North Dakota	94.3
4	Utah	94.1
5	Massachusetts	94.0
6	Maine	93.8
7	Nevada	93.3
8	Ohio	93.2
9	Nebraska	92.4
10	Kentucky	92.3
11	New Hampshire	92.2
12	West Virginia	92.1
13	Vermont	91.8
14	Maryland	91.7
14	Washington	91.7
16	Iowa	91.1
17	Tennessee	90.9
18	South Carolina	90.0
19	Oklahoma	89.9
20	Oregon	89.8
21	Arizona	89.7
22	Wisconsin	89.4
23	New Mexico	89.3
24	Missouri	89.2
25	Connecticut	88.7
26	North Carolina	88.3
27	Michigan	87.7
28	Virginia	87.2
29	Wyoming	86.4
30	South Dakota	85.7
31	Hawaii	85.6
32	Montana	84.7
33	Colorado	84.6
34	Illinois	84.2
35	Delaware	84.1
36	Pennsylvania	83.5
37	Georgia	83.3
37	Texas	83.3
39	Arkansas	83.1
40	Mississippi	82.6
41	Alaska	81.4
42	California	81.0
43	New Jersey	80.1
44	Indiana	79.0
45	Minnesota	78.1
46	Florida	77.6
47	Idaho	75.6
48	New York	75.3
49	Louisiana	73.5
50	Rhode Island	71.7
	District of Columbia	81.0

Source: U.S. Department of Health and Human Services, Health Care Financing Administration
"1999 Data Compendium" (July 1999)
*Medicare Part B. Physicians include MD's, DO's, limited license practitioners and non-physician practitioners.

Medicaid Recipients in 1998

National Total = 40,649,482 Recipients*

ALPHA ORDER

RANK	STATE	RECIPIENTS	% of USA
23	Alabama	527,078	1.3%
48	Alaska	74,508	0.2%
26	Arizona	507,668	1.2%
28	Arkansas	424,727	1.0%
1	California	7,082,175	17.4%
30	Colorado	344,916	0.8%
29	Connecticut	381,208	0.9%
44	Delaware	101,436	0.2%
4	Florida	1,904,591	4.7%
11	Georgia	1,221,978	3.0%
38	Hawaii	184,614	0.5%
43	Idaho	123,176	0.3%
8	Illinois	1,363,856	3.4%
19	Indiana	607,293	1.5%
34	Iowa	314,936	0.8%
35	Kansas	241,933	0.6%
18	Kentucky	644,482	1.6%
16	Louisiana	720,615	1.8%
39	Maine	170,456	0.4%
21	Maryland	561,085	1.4%
13	Massachusetts	908,238	2.2%
9	Michigan	1,362,890	3.4%
22	Minnesota	538,413	1.3%
27	Mississippi	485,767	1.2%
15	Missouri	734,015	1.8%
45	Montana	100,760	0.2%
37	Nebraska	211,188	0.5%
41	Nevada	128,144	0.3%
46	New Hampshire	93,970	0.2%
14	New Jersey	813,251	2.0%
33	New Mexico	329,418	0.8%
2	New York	3,073,241	7.6%
12	North Carolina	1,167,988	2.9%
49	North Dakota	62,280	0.2%
10	Ohio	1,290,776	3.2%
32	Oklahoma	342,475	0.8%
25	Oregon	511,171	1.3%
6	Pennsylvania	1,523,120	3.7%
40	Rhode Island	153,130	0.4%
20	South Carolina	594,962	1.5%
47	South Dakota	89,537	0.2%
5	Tennessee	1,843,661	4.5%
3	Texas	2,324,810	5.7%
36	Utah	215,801	0.5%
42	Vermont	123,992	0.3%
17	Virginia	653,236	1.6%
7	Washington	1,413,208	3.5%
31	West Virginia	342,668	0.8%
24	Wisconsin	518,595	1.3%
50	Wyoming	46,121	0.1%

RANK ORDER

RANK	STATE	RECIPIENTS	% of USA
1	California	7,082,175	17.4%
2	New York	3,073,241	7.6%
3	Texas	2,324,810	5.7%
4	Florida	1,904,591	4.7%
5	Tennessee	1,843,661	4.5%
6	Pennsylvania	1,523,120	3.7%
7	Washington	1,413,208	3.5%
8	Illinois	1,363,856	3.4%
9	Michigan	1,362,890	3.4%
10	Ohio	1,290,776	3.2%
11	Georgia	1,221,978	3.0%
12	North Carolina	1,167,988	2.9%
13	Massachusetts	908,238	2.2%
14	New Jersey	813,251	2.0%
15	Missouri	734,015	1.8%
16	Louisiana	720,615	1.8%
17	Virginia	653,236	1.6%
18	Kentucky	644,482	1.6%
19	Indiana	607,293	1.5%
20	South Carolina	594,962	1.5%
21	Maryland	561,085	1.4%
22	Minnesota	538,413	1.3%
23	Alabama	527,078	1.3%
24	Wisconsin	518,595	1.3%
25	Oregon	511,171	1.3%
26	Arizona	507,668	1.2%
27	Mississippi	485,767	1.2%
28	Arkansas	424,727	1.0%
29	Connecticut	381,208	0.9%
30	Colorado	344,916	0.8%
31	West Virginia	342,668	0.8%
32	Oklahoma	342,475	0.8%
33	New Mexico	329,418	0.8%
34	Iowa	314,936	0.8%
35	Kansas	241,933	0.6%
36	Utah	215,801	0.5%
37	Nebraska	211,188	0.5%
38	Hawaii	184,614	0.5%
39	Maine	170,456	0.4%
40	Rhode Island	153,130	0.4%
41	Nevada	128,144	0.3%
42	Vermont	123,992	0.3%
43	Idaho	123,176	0.3%
44	Delaware	101,436	0.2%
45	Montana	100,760	0.2%
46	New Hampshire	93,970	0.2%
47	South Dakota	89,537	0.2%
48	Alaska	74,508	0.2%
49	North Dakota	62,280	0.2%
50	Wyoming	46,121	0.1%
	District of Columbia	166,146	0.4%

Source: U.S. Department of Health and Human Services, Health Care Financing Administration
"Medicaid Recipients by Basis of Eligibility and by State: FY 1998" (HCFA-2082)
For fiscal year 1998. National total includes recipients for U.S. territories.

Medicaid Recipients in 1997

National Total = 34,872,275 Recipients*

ALPHA ORDER

RANK ORDER

RANK	STATE	RECIPIENTS	% of USA
17	Alabama	546,140	1.6%
48	Alaska	73,050	0.2%
18	Arizona	540,785	1.6%
28	Arkansas	370,386	1.1%
1	California	4,854,546	13.9%
33	Colorado	251,423	0.7%
37	Connecticut	201,779	0.6%
46	Delaware	83,956	0.2%
4	Florida	1,597,461	4.6%
8	Georgia	1,208,445	3.5%
35	Hawaii	206,081	0.6%
41	Idaho	115,087	0.3%
6	Illinois	1,399,960	4.0%
23	Indiana	514,683	1.5%
32	Iowa	293,596	0.8%
34	Kansas	232,888	0.7%
14	Kentucky	664,454	1.9%
12	Louisiana	746,461	2.1%
38	Maine	167,221	0.5%
25	Maryland	402,002	1.2%
13	Massachusetts	723,472	2.1%
9	Michigan	1,132,783	3.2%
27	Minnesota	371,483	1.1%
24	Mississippi	504,017	1.4%
19	Missouri	540,487	1.5%
44	Montana	95,562	0.3%
36	Nebraska	203,340	0.6%
43	Nevada	105,588	0.3%
45	New Hampshire	95,215	0.3%
20	New Jersey	537,890	1.5%
30	New Mexico	320,223	0.9%
2	New York	3,151,837	9.0%
10	North Carolina	1,112,931	3.2%
49	North Dakota	61,117	0.2%
7	Ohio	1,395,540	4.0%
31	Oklahoma	315,801	0.9%
21	Oregon	531,242	1.5%
11	Pennsylvania	1,024,993	2.9%
40	Rhode Island	116,766	0.3%
22	South Carolina	519,875	1.5%
47	South Dakota	75,444	0.2%
5	Tennessee	1,415,612	4.1%
3	Texas	2,538,655	7.3%
39	Utah	144,749	0.4%
42	Vermont	109,283	0.3%
16	Virginia	595,234	1.7%
15	Washington	630,165	1.8%
29	West Virginia	359,091	1.0%
26	Wisconsin	392,223	1.1%
50	Wyoming	48,865	0.1%

RANK	STATE	RECIPIENTS	% of USA
1	California	4,854,546	13.9%
2	New York	3,151,837	9.0%
3	Texas	2,538,655	7.3%
4	Florida	1,597,461	4.6%
5	Tennessee	1,415,612	4.1%
6	Illinois	1,399,960	4.0%
7	Ohio	1,395,540	4.0%
8	Georgia	1,208,445	3.5%
9	Michigan	1,132,783	3.2%
10	North Carolina	1,112,931	3.2%
11	Pennsylvania	1,024,993	2.9%
12	Louisiana	746,461	2.1%
13	Massachusetts	723,472	2.1%
14	Kentucky	664,454	1.9%
15	Washington	630,165	1.8%
16	Virginia	595,234	1.7%
17	Alabama	546,140	1.6%
18	Arizona	540,785	1.6%
19	Missouri	540,487	1.5%
20	New Jersey	537,890	1.5%
21	Oregon	531,242	1.5%
22	South Carolina	519,875	1.5%
23	Indiana	514,683	1.5%
24	Mississippi	504,017	1.4%
25	Maryland	402,002	1.2%
26	Wisconsin	392,223	1.1%
27	Minnesota	371,483	1.1%
28	Arkansas	370,386	1.1%
29	West Virginia	359,091	1.0%
30	New Mexico	320,223	0.9%
31	Oklahoma	315,801	0.9%
32	Iowa	293,596	0.8%
33	Colorado	251,423	0.7%
34	Kansas	232,888	0.7%
35	Hawaii	206,081	0.6%
36	Nebraska	203,340	0.6%
37	Connecticut	201,779	0.6%
38	Maine	167,221	0.5%
39	Utah	144,749	0.4%
40	Rhode Island	116,766	0.3%
41	Idaho	115,087	0.3%
42	Vermont	109,283	0.3%
43	Nevada	105,588	0.3%
44	Montana	95,562	0.3%
45	New Hampshire	95,215	0.3%
46	Delaware	83,956	0.2%
47	South Dakota	75,444	0.2%
48	Alaska	73,050	0.2%
49	North Dakota	61,117	0.2%
50	Wyoming	48,865	0.1%
	District of Columbia	128,008	0.4%

Source: U.S. Department of Health and Human Services, Health Care Financing Administration
"Medicaid Recipients by Basis of Eligibility and by State: FY 1997" (HCFA-2082)
*For fiscal year 1997. National total includes recipients for U.S. territories.

Percent Change in Number of Medicaid Recipients: 1994 to 1997

National Percent Change = 0.5% Decrease*

ALPHA ORDER

ALPHA ORDER

RANK	STATE	PERCENT CHANGE	RANK	STATE	PERCENT CHANGE
23	Alabama	0.5	1	Hawaii	70.6
15	Alaska	6.1	2	Tennessee	50.8
15	Arizona	6.1	3	Oregon	29.2
12	Arkansas	9.0	4	Nebraska	23.7
29	California	(3.1)	5	New Mexico	19.4
43	Colorado	(13.1)	6	Vermont	16.1
50	Connecticut	(43.1)	7	North Carolina	13.0
8	Delaware	12.2	8	Delaware	12.2
38	Florida	(7.5)	9	Georgia	11.4
9	Georgia	11.4	10	New Hampshire	11.3
1	Hawaii	70.6	11	Nevada	10.7
17	Idaho	4.6	12	Arkansas	9.0
27	Illinois	(2.9)	13	New York	8.4
44	Indiana	(14.9)	14	South Carolina	6.9
28	Iowa	(3.0)	15	Alaska	6.1
38	Kansas	(7.5)	15	Arizona	6.1
19	Kentucky	4.2	17	Idaho	4.6
32	Louisiana	(4.1)	17	South Dakota	4.6
34	Maine	(5.5)	19	Kentucky	4.2
30	Maryland	(3.2)	20	Massachusetts	1.8
20	Massachusetts	1.8	21	Rhode Island	1.7
33	Michigan	(4.5)	22	Texas	1.0
42	Minnesota	(12.7)	23	Alabama	0.5
36	Mississippi	(6.1)	24	Montana	(0.7)
47	Missouri	(19.2)	25	West Virginia	(2.1)
24	Montana	(0.7)	26	North Dakota	(2.6)
4	Nebraska	23.7	27	Illinois	(2.9)
11	Nevada	10.7	28	Iowa	(3.0)
10	New Hampshire	11.3	29	California	(3.1)
49	New Jersey	(31.9)	30	Maryland	(3.2)
5	New Mexico	19.4	31	Wyoming	(3.3)
13	New York	8.4	32	Louisiana	(4.1)
7	North Carolina	13.0	33	Michigan	(4.5)
26	North Dakota	(2.6)	34	Maine	(5.5)
41	Ohio	(8.4)	35	Washington	(5.7)
47	Oklahoma	(19.2)	36	Mississippi	(6.1)
3	Oregon	29.2	37	Virginia	(7.4)
46	Pennsylvania	(18.4)	38	Florida	(7.5)
21	Rhode Island	1.7	38	Kansas	(7.5)
14	South Carolina	6.9	40	Utah	(7.9)
17	South Dakota	4.6	41	Ohio	(8.4)
2	Tennessee	50.8	42	Minnesota	(12.7)
22	Texas	1.0	43	Colorado	(13.1)
40	Utah	(7.9)	44	Indiana	(14.9)
6	Vermont	16.1	45	Wisconsin	(17.2)
37	Virginia	(7.4)	46	Pennsylvania	(18.4)
35	Washington	(5.7)	47	Missouri	(19.2)
25	West Virginia	(2.1)	47	Oklahoma	(19.2)
45	Wisconsin	(17.2)	49	New Jersey	(31.9)
31	Wyoming	(3.3)	50	Connecticut	(43.1)
				District of Columbia	0.6

Source: Morgan Quitno Press using data from U.S. Dept. of Health & Human Services, Health Care Financing Admin.
"Medicaid Recipients by Basis of Eligibility and by State: FY 1994 and 1997" (HCFA-2082)
*For fiscal years 1994 and 1997. National figure includes recipients for U.S. territories.

Medicaid Expenditures in 1997

National Total = $160,528,502,653*

ALPHA ORDER

RANK	STATE	PAYMENTS	% of USA
24	Alabama	$2,201,307,097	1.4%
46	Alaska	364,110,087	0.2%
26	Arizona	1,740,017,249	1.1%
30	Arkansas	1,313,630,245	0.8%
2	California	16,240,099,854	10.1%
29	Colorado	1,523,356,381	0.9%
17	Connecticut	2,932,104,706	1.8%
44	Delaware	409,213,692	0.3%
6	Florida	6,447,889,401	4.0%
12	Georgia	3,584,015,676	2.2%
40	Hawaii	628,742,323	0.4%
43	Idaho	423,261,391	0.3%
5	Illinois	6,503,829,004	4.1%
22	Indiana	2,493,114,385	1.6%
31	Iowa	1,262,327,643	0.8%
35	Kansas	1,028,739,139	0.6%
21	Kentucky	2,571,547,988	1.6%
16	Louisiana	3,055,407,383	1.9%
34	Maine	1,090,325,858	0.7%
19	Maryland	2,706,411,626	1.7%
9	Massachusetts	5,509,187,324	3.4%
8	Michigan	5,560,326,710	3.5%
18	Minnesota	2,746,987,575	1.7%
27	Mississippi	1,702,265,458	1.1%
15	Missouri	3,142,586,502	2.0%
45	Montana	392,064,609	0.2%
39	Nebraska	731,656,067	0.5%
42	Nevada	489,276,626	0.3%
38	New Hampshire	731,879,670	0.5%
10	New Jersey	5,478,127,337	3.4%
36	New Mexico	945,547,063	0.6%
1	New York	24,525,116,698	15.3%
11	North Carolina	4,529,992,284	2.8%
48	North Dakota	331,970,747	0.2%
7	Ohio	6,443,156,403	4.0%
32	Oklahoma	1,195,881,195	0.7%
28	Oregon	1,544,061,944	1.0%
4	Pennsylvania	8,075,706,681	5.0%
37	Rhode Island	917,489,179	0.6%
25	South Carolina	2,152,056,132	1.3%
49	South Dakota	331,629,892	0.2%
13	Tennessee	3,434,971,957	2.1%
3	Texas	9,600,126,934	6.0%
41	Utah	626,662,383	0.4%
47	Vermont	358,490,340	0.2%
23	Virginia	2,274,509,097	1.4%
14	Washington	3,197,051,126	2.0%
33	West Virginia	1,193,977,808	0.7%
20	Wisconsin	2,573,586,437	1.6%
50	Wyoming	194,261,299	0.1%

RANK ORDER

RANK	STATE	PAYMENTS	% of USA
1	New York	$24,525,116,698	15.3%
2	California	16,240,099,854	10.1%
3	Texas	9,600,126,934	6.0%
4	Pennsylvania	8,075,706,681	5.0%
5	Illinois	6,503,829,004	4.1%
6	Florida	6,447,889,401	4.0%
7	Ohio	6,443,156,403	4.0%
8	Michigan	5,560,326,710	3.5%
9	Massachusetts	5,509,187,324	3.4%
10	New Jersey	5,478,127,337	3.4%
11	North Carolina	4,529,992,284	2.8%
12	Georgia	3,584,015,676	2.2%
13	Tennessee	3,434,971,957	2.1%
14	Washington	3,197,051,126	2.0%
15	Missouri	3,142,586,502	2.0%
16	Louisiana	3,055,407,383	1.9%
17	Connecticut	2,932,104,706	1.8%
18	Minnesota	2,746,987,575	1.7%
19	Maryland	2,706,411,626	1.7%
20	Wisconsin	2,573,586,437	1.6%
21	Kentucky	2,571,547,988	1.6%
22	Indiana	2,493,114,385	1.6%
23	Virginia	2,274,509,097	1.4%
24	Alabama	2,201,307,097	1.4%
25	South Carolina	2,152,056,132	1.3%
26	Arizona	1,740,017,249	1.1%
27	Mississippi	1,702,265,458	1.1%
28	Oregon	1,544,061,944	1.0%
29	Colorado	1,523,356,381	0.9%
30	Arkansas	1,313,630,245	0.8%
31	Iowa	1,262,327,643	0.8%
32	Oklahoma	1,195,881,195	0.7%
33	West Virginia	1,193,977,808	0.7%
34	Maine	1,090,325,858	0.7%
35	Kansas	1,028,739,139	0.6%
36	New Mexico	945,547,063	0.6%
37	Rhode Island	917,489,179	0.6%
38	New Hampshire	731,879,670	0.5%
39	Nebraska	731,656,067	0.5%
40	Hawaii	628,742,323	0.4%
41	Utah	626,662,383	0.4%
42	Nevada	489,276,626	0.3%
43	Idaho	423,261,391	0.3%
44	Delaware	409,213,692	0.3%
45	Montana	392,064,609	0.2%
46	Alaska	364,110,087	0.2%
47	Vermont	358,490,340	0.2%
48	North Dakota	331,970,747	0.2%
49	South Dakota	331,629,892	0.2%
50	Wyoming	194,261,299	0.1%
	District of Columbia	796,084,288	0.5%

Source: U.S. Department of Health and Human Services, Health Care Financing Administration
"Medicaid Financial Statistics Tables (HCFA-64 Report)"
For fiscal year 1997. National total includes payments for U.S. territories. These figures differ from those previously listed in this book. In the past, we had used HCFA-2082 report. In response to reader requests, we have switched to HCFA-64 report which includes additional expenditures.

Percent Change in Medicaid Expenditures: 1994 to 1997

National Percent Change = 16.7% Increase*

ALPHA ORDER

RANK	STATE	PERCENT CHANGE
21	Alabama	23.9
14	Alaska	26.9
46	Arizona	2.2
23	Arkansas	23.2
42	California	11.3
7	Colorado	37.1
13	Connecticut	27.3
1	Delaware	46.9
20	Florida	24.1
42	Georgia	11.3
6	Hawaii	37.4
8	Idaho	36.9
15	Illinois	26.3
47	Indiana	1.2
26	Iowa	20.9
45	Kansas	5.6
3	Kentucky	40.1
50	Louisiana	(27.2)
28	Maine	19.9
27	Maryland	20.8
15	Massachusetts	26.3
41	Michigan	11.8
42	Minnesota	11.3
9	Mississippi	29.9
17	Missouri	24.7
29	Montana	19.4
29	Nebraska	19.4
11	Nevada	28.4
49	New Hampshire	(23.2)
37	New Jersey	14.7
5	New Mexico	38.8
38	New York	14.2
2	North Carolina	45.6
25	North Dakota	22.1
33	Ohio	16.7
39	Oklahoma	13.6
4	Oregon	39.3
33	Pennsylvania	16.7
32	Rhode Island	17.0
35	South Carolina	16.0
36	South Dakota	15.1
10	Tennessee	28.6
31	Texas	17.9
22	Utah	23.7
18	Vermont	24.6
24	Virginia	23.0
19	Washington	24.3
48	West Virginia	(3.9)
40	Wisconsin	11.9
12	Wyoming	27.4

RANK ORDER

RANK	STATE	PERCENT CHANGE
1	Delaware	46.9
2	North Carolina	45.6
3	Kentucky	40.1
4	Oregon	39.3
5	New Mexico	38.8
6	Hawaii	37.4
7	Colorado	37.1
8	Idaho	36.9
9	Mississippi	29.9
10	Tennessee	28.6
11	Nevada	28.4
12	Wyoming	27.4
13	Connecticut	27.3
14	Alaska	26.9
15	Illinois	26.3
15	Massachusetts	26.3
17	Missouri	24.7
18	Vermont	24.6
19	Washington	24.3
20	Florida	24.1
21	Alabama	23.9
22	Utah	23.7
23	Arkansas	23.2
24	Virginia	23.0
25	North Dakota	22.1
26	Iowa	20.9
27	Maryland	20.8
28	Maine	19.9
29	Montana	19.4
29	Nebraska	19.4
31	Texas	17.9
32	Rhode Island	17.0
33	Ohio	16.7
33	Pennsylvania	16.7
35	South Carolina	16.0
36	South Dakota	15.1
37	New Jersey	14.7
38	New York	14.2
39	Oklahoma	13.6
40	Wisconsin	11.9
41	Michigan	11.8
42	California	11.3
42	Georgia	11.3
42	Minnesota	11.3
45	Kansas	5.6
46	Arizona	2.2
47	Indiana	1.2
48	West Virginia	(3.9)
49	New Hampshire	(23.2)
50	Louisiana	(27.2)

District of Columbia 1.3

Source: Morgan Quitno Press using data from U.S. Dept. of Health & Human Services, Health Care Financing Admin. "Medicaid Financial Statistics Tables (HCFA-64 Report)"
For fiscal years 1994 and 1997. National figure includes payments for U.S. territories. These figures differ from those previously listed in this book. In the past, we had used HCFA-2082 report. In response to reader requests, we have switched to HCFA-64 report which includes additional expenditures.

Medicaid Expenditures per Recipient in 1997

National Rate = $4,603 per Recipient*

ALPHA ORDER				RANK ORDER		
RANK	STATE	PER RECIPIENT		RANK	STATE	PER RECIPIENT
31	Alabama	$4,031		1	New Jersey	$10,184
15	Alaska	4,984		2	Pennsylvania	7,879
44	Arizona	3,218		3	Rhode Island	7,858
39	Arkansas	3,547		4	New York	7,781
41	California	3,345		5	New Hampshire	7,687
11	Colorado	6,059		6	Massachusetts	7,615
NA	Connecticut**	NA		7	Minnesota	7,395
17	Delaware	4,874		8	Maryland	6,732
30	Florida	4,036		9	Wisconsin	6,562
46	Georgia	2,966		10	Maine	6,520
45	Hawaii	3,051		11	Colorado	6,059
37	Idaho	3,678		12	Missouri	5,814
19	Illinois	4,646		13	North Dakota	5,432
18	Indiana	4,844		14	Washington	5,073
25	Iowa	4,300		15	Alaska	4,984
22	Kansas	4,417		16	Michigan	4,909
33	Kentucky	3,870		17	Delaware	4,874
28	Louisiana	4,093		18	Indiana	4,844
10	Maine	6,520		19	Illinois	4,646
8	Maryland	6,732		20	Nevada	4,634
6	Massachusetts	7,615		21	Ohio	4,617
16	Michigan	4,909		22	Kansas	4,417
7	Minnesota	7,395		23	South Dakota	4,396
40	Mississippi	3,377		24	Utah	4,329
12	Missouri	5,814		25	Iowa	4,300
27	Montana	4,103		26	South Carolina	4,140
38	Nebraska	3,598		27	Montana	4,103
20	Nevada	4,634		28	Louisiana	4,093
5	New Hampshire	7,687		29	North Carolina	4,070
1	New Jersey	10,184		30	Florida	4,036
47	New Mexico	2,953		31	Alabama	4,031
4	New York	7,781		32	Wyoming	3,975
29	North Carolina	4,070		33	Kentucky	3,870
13	North Dakota	5,432		34	Virginia	3,821
21	Ohio	4,617		35	Oklahoma	3,787
35	Oklahoma	3,787		36	Texas	3,782
48	Oregon	2,907		37	Idaho	3,678
2	Pennsylvania	7,879		38	Nebraska	3,598
3	Rhode Island	7,858		39	Arkansas	3,547
26	South Carolina	4,140		40	Mississippi	3,377
23	South Dakota	4,396		41	California	3,345
49	Tennessee	2,426		42	West Virginia	3,325
36	Texas	3,782		43	Vermont	3,280
24	Utah	4,329		44	Arizona	3,218
43	Vermont	3,280		45	Hawaii	3,051
34	Virginia	3,821		46	Georgia	2,966
14	Washington	5,073		47	New Mexico	2,953
42	West Virginia	3,325		48	Oregon	2,907
9	Wisconsin	6,562		49	Tennessee	2,426
32	Wyoming	3,975		NA	Connecticut**	NA
					District of Columbia	6,219

Source: Morgan Quitno Press using data from U.S. Dept. of Health & Human Services, Health Care Financing Admin.
    "Medicaid Financial Statistics Tables (HCFA-64 Report)"
*For fiscal years 1994 and 1997. National figure includes payments and recipients in U.S. territories. These
figures differ from those previously listed in this book. In the past, we had used HCFA-2082 report for expenditures
and recipients. In response to reader requests, we have switched to HCFA-64 report for expenditures which
includes additional payments. **Not available.

Percent Change in Expenditures per Medicaid Recipient: 1994 to 1997

National Percent Change = 17.2% Increase*

RANK	STATE	PERCENT CHANGE
25	Alabama	23.3
27	Alaska	19.6
45	Arizona	(3.6)
36	Arkansas	13.1
34	California	14.8
2	Colorado	57.8
NA	Connecticut**	NA
14	Delaware	30.9
9	Florida	34.2
42	Georgia	0.0
47	Hawaii	(19.4)
14	Idaho	30.9
16	Illinois	30.1
28	Indiana	18.9
23	Iowa	24.6
35	Kansas	14.1
8	Kentucky	34.5
48	Louisiana	(24.1)
20	Maine	26.9
22	Maryland	24.7
24	Massachusetts	24.0
29	Michigan	17.1
18	Minnesota	27.5
6	Mississippi	38.4
3	Missouri	54.3
26	Montana	20.3
44	Nebraska	(3.5)
32	Nevada	16.1
49	New Hampshire	(31.0)
1	New Jersey	68.4
31	New Mexico	16.3
41	New York	5.4
17	North Carolina	28.9
21	North Dakota	25.5
19	Ohio	27.4
5	Oklahoma	40.6
39	Oregon	7.9
4	Pennsylvania	43.0
33	Rhode Island	15.1
38	South Carolina	8.5
37	South Dakota	10.1
46	Tennessee	(14.8)
30	Texas	16.8
9	Utah	34.2
40	Vermont	7.3
11	Virginia	32.9
12	Washington	31.8
43	West Virginia	(1.9)
7	Wisconsin	35.2
12	Wyoming	31.8

RANK	STATE	PERCENT CHANGE
1	New Jersey	68.4
2	Colorado	57.8
3	Missouri	54.3
4	Pennsylvania	43.0
5	Oklahoma	40.6
6	Mississippi	38.4
7	Wisconsin	35.2
8	Kentucky	34.5
9	Florida	34.2
9	Utah	34.2
11	Virginia	32.9
12	Washington	31.8
12	Wyoming	31.8
14	Delaware	30.9
14	Idaho	30.9
16	Illinois	30.1
17	North Carolina	28.9
18	Minnesota	27.5
19	Ohio	27.4
20	Maine	26.9
21	North Dakota	25.5
22	Maryland	24.7
23	Iowa	24.6
24	Massachusetts	24.0
25	Alabama	23.3
26	Montana	20.3
27	Alaska	19.6
28	Indiana	18.9
29	Michigan	17.1
30	Texas	16.8
31	New Mexico	16.3
32	Nevada	16.1
33	Rhode Island	15.1
34	California	14.8
35	Kansas	14.1
36	Arkansas	13.1
37	South Dakota	10.1
38	South Carolina	8.5
39	Oregon	7.9
40	Vermont	7.3
41	New York	5.4
42	Georgia	0.0
43	West Virginia	(1.9)
44	Nebraska	(3.5)
45	Arizona	(3.6)
46	Tennessee	(14.8)
47	Hawaii	(19.4)
48	Louisiana	(24.1)
49	New Hampshire	(31.0)
NA	Connecticut**	NA

| | District of Columbia | 0.7 |

Source: Morgan Quitno Press using data from U.S. Dept. of Health & Human Services, Health Care Financing Admin. "Medicaid Financial Statistics Tables (HCFA-64 Report)"

*For fiscal years 1994 and 1997. National figure includes payments and recipients in U.S. territories. These figures differ from those previously listed in this book. In the past, we had used HCFA-2082 report for expenditures and recipients. In response to reader requests, we have switched to HCFA-64 report for expenditures which includes additional payments. **Not available.

Percent of Population Receiving Medicaid in 1998

National Percent = 14.7% of Population*

ALPHA ORDER

RANK ORDER

RANK	STATE	PERCENT	RANK	STATE	PERCENT
27	Alabama	12.1	1	Tennessee	33.9
27	Alaska	12.1	2	Washington	24.8
36	Arizona	10.9	3	California	21.7
9	Arkansas	16.7	4	Vermont	21.0
3	California	21.7	5	New Mexico	19.0
48	Colorado	8.7	6	West Virginia	18.9
30	Connecticut	11.6	7	Mississippi	17.7
21	Delaware	13.6	8	New York	16.9
23	Florida	12.8	9	Arkansas	16.7
12	Georgia	16.0	10	Louisiana	16.5
14	Hawaii	15.5	11	Kentucky	16.4
41	Idaho	10.0	12	Georgia	16.0
34	Illinois	11.3	13	Oregon	15.6
38	Indiana	10.3	14	Hawaii	15.5
35	Iowa	11.0	14	North Carolina	15.5
47	Kansas	9.2	14	Rhode Island	15.5
11	Kentucky	16.4	14	South Carolina	15.5
10	Louisiana	16.5	18	Massachusetts	14.8
20	Maine	13.7	19	Michigan	13.9
36	Maryland	10.9	20	Maine	13.7
18	Massachusetts	14.8	21	Delaware	13.6
19	Michigan	13.9	22	Missouri	13.5
33	Minnesota	11.4	23	Florida	12.8
7	Mississippi	17.7	24	Nebraska	12.7
22	Missouri	13.5	24	Pennsylvania	12.7
31	Montana	11.5	26	South Dakota	12.3
24	Nebraska	12.7	27	Alabama	12.1
50	Nevada	7.3	27	Alaska	12.1
49	New Hampshire	7.9	29	Texas	11.8
41	New Jersey	10.0	30	Connecticut	11.6
5	New Mexico	19.0	31	Montana	11.5
8	New York	16.9	31	Ohio	11.5
14	North Carolina	15.5	33	Minnesota	11.4
44	North Dakota	9.8	34	Illinois	11.3
31	Ohio	11.5	35	Iowa	11.0
38	Oklahoma	10.3	36	Arizona	10.9
13	Oregon	15.6	36	Maryland	10.9
24	Pennsylvania	12.7	38	Indiana	10.3
14	Rhode Island	15.5	38	Oklahoma	10.3
14	South Carolina	15.5	38	Utah	10.3
26	South Dakota	12.3	41	Idaho	10.0
1	Tennessee	33.9	41	New Jersey	10.0
29	Texas	11.8	43	Wisconsin	9.9
38	Utah	10.3	44	North Dakota	9.8
4	Vermont	21.0	45	Virginia	9.6
45	Virginia	9.6	45	Wyoming	9.6
2	Washington	24.8	47	Kansas	9.2
6	West Virginia	18.9	48	Colorado	8.7
43	Wisconsin	9.9	49	New Hampshire	7.9
45	Wyoming	9.6	50	Nevada	7.3

District of Columbia   31.9

Source: Morgan Quitno Press using data from U.S. Dept. of Health & Human Services, Health Care Financing Admin.
"Medicaid Recipients by Basis of Eligibility and by State: FY 1998" (HCFA-2082)
*For fiscal year 1998. National percent does not include recipients or population in U.S. territories.

Medicaid Managed Care Enrollment in 1999

National Total = 17,756,603 Enrollees*

ALPHA ORDER

RANK	STATE	ENROLLEES	% of USA
11	Alabama	377,952	2.1%
49	Alaska	0	0.0%
12	Arizona	363,662	2.0%
23	Arkansas	232,123	1.3%
1	California	2,540,902	14.3%
25	Colorado	216,357	1.2%
24	Connecticut	230,217	1.3%
39	Delaware	68,869	0.4%
5	Florida	912,045	5.1%
9	Georgia	638,082	3.6%
33	Hawaii	120,246	0.7%
44	Idaho	31,184	0.2%
31	Illinois	158,888	0.9%
16	Indiana	331,363	1.9%
30	Iowa	176,487	1.0%
36	Kansas	95,868	0.5%
17	Kentucky	324,447	1.8%
42	Louisiana	44,741	0.3%
46	Maine	23,720	0.1%
15	Maryland	347,937	2.0%
10	Massachusetts	575,186	3.2%
3	Michigan	1,130,608	6.4%
21	Minnesota	268,360	1.5%
27	Mississippi	200,347	1.1%
20	Missouri	276,628	1.6%
38	Montana	69,738	0.4%
32	Nebraska	122,006	0.7%
43	Nevada	36,945	0.2%
48	New Hampshire	5,812	0.0%
13	New Jersey	356,956	2.0%
26	New Mexico	208,528	1.2%
8	New York	659,569	3.7%
7	North Carolina	689,104	3.9%
45	North Dakota	23,886	0.1%
22	Ohio	244,888	1.4%
28	Oklahoma	193,902	1.1%
18	Oregon	308,798	1.7%
4	Pennsylvania	1,004,601	5.7%
37	Rhode Island	85,900	0.5%
47	South Carolina	23,149	0.1%
41	South Dakota	50,220	0.3%
2	Tennessee	1,312,969	7.4%
14	Texas	352,062	2.0%
34	Utah	118,601	0.7%
40	Vermont	65,692	0.4%
19	Virginia	292,214	1.6%
6	Washington	706,202	4.0%
35	West Virginia	111,532	0.6%
29	Wisconsin	187,543	1.1%
49	Wyoming	0	0.0%

RANK ORDER

RANK	STATE	ENROLLEES	% of USA
1	California	2,540,902	14.3%
2	Tennessee	1,312,969	7.4%
3	Michigan	1,130,608	6.4%
4	Pennsylvania	1,004,601	5.7%
5	Florida	912,045	5.1%
6	Washington	706,202	4.0%
7	North Carolina	689,104	3.9%
8	New York	659,569	3.7%
9	Georgia	638,082	3.6%
10	Massachusetts	575,186	3.2%
11	Alabama	377,952	2.1%
12	Arizona	363,662	2.0%
13	New Jersey	356,956	2.0%
14	Texas	352,062	2.0%
15	Maryland	347,937	2.0%
16	Indiana	331,363	1.9%
17	Kentucky	324,447	1.8%
18	Oregon	308,798	1.7%
19	Virginia	292,214	1.6%
20	Missouri	276,628	1.6%
21	Minnesota	268,360	1.5%
22	Ohio	244,888	1.4%
23	Arkansas	232,123	1.3%
24	Connecticut	230,217	1.3%
25	Colorado	216,357	1.2%
26	New Mexico	208,528	1.2%
27	Mississippi	200,347	1.1%
28	Oklahoma	193,902	1.1%
29	Wisconsin	187,543	1.1%
30	Iowa	176,487	1.0%
31	Illinois	158,888	0.9%
32	Nebraska	122,006	0.7%
33	Hawaii	120,246	0.7%
34	Utah	118,601	0.7%
35	West Virginia	111,532	0.6%
36	Kansas	95,868	0.5%
37	Rhode Island	85,900	0.5%
38	Montana	69,738	0.4%
39	Delaware	68,869	0.4%
40	Vermont	65,692	0.4%
41	South Dakota	50,220	0.3%
42	Louisiana	44,741	0.3%
43	Nevada	36,945	0.2%
44	Idaho	31,184	0.2%
45	North Dakota	23,886	0.1%
46	Maine	23,720	0.1%
47	South Carolina	23,149	0.1%
48	New Hampshire	5,812	0.0%
49	Alaska	0	0.0%
49	Wyoming	0	0.0%
	District of Columbia	75,499	0.4%

Source: U.S. Department of Health and Human Services, Health Care Financing Administration
"Medicaid Managed Care State Enrollment" (http://www.hcfa.gov/medicaid/mcsten99.htm)
*As of June 30, 1999. Enrollment in state health care reform programs that expand eligibility beyond traditional Medicaid standards. National total includes 764,068 Medicaid managed care enrollees in Puerto Rico.

Percent of Medicaid Enrollees in Managed Care in 1999

National Percent = 55.6% of Medicaid Enrollees*

ALPHA ORDER				RANK ORDER		
RANK	STATE	PERCENT		RANK	STATE	PERCENT
15	Alabama	73.6		1	Michigan	100.0
49	Alaska	0.0		1	Montana	100.0
6	Arizona	90.7		1	Tennessee	100.0
28	Arkansas	59.8		4	Washington	99.9
34	California	51.1		5	Colorado	92.2
5	Colorado	92.2		6	Arizona	90.7
18	Connecticut	71.5		7	Utah	89.5
12	Delaware	78.1		8	Iowa	85.3
26	Florida	60.3		9	North Carolina	82.9
14	Georgia	75.2		10	Oregon	81.5
11	Hawaii	78.7		11	Hawaii	78.7
40	Idaho	35.8		12	Delaware	78.1
45	Illinois	12.1		13	Pennsylvania	77.0
21	Indiana	66.2		14	Georgia	75.2
8	Iowa	85.3		15	Alabama	73.6
32	Kansas	53.1		15	South Dakota	73.6
27	Kentucky	60.1		17	New Mexico	73.2
47	Louisiana	5.8		18	Connecticut	71.5
44	Maine	14.1		19	Nebraska	71.1
20	Maryland	69.5		20	Maryland	69.5
22	Massachusetts	64.5		21	Indiana	66.2
1	Michigan	100.0		22	Massachusetts	64.5
25	Minnesota	61.3		23	Rhode Island	64.1
37	Mississippi	41.3		24	Virginia	63.5
39	Missouri	38.7		25	Minnesota	61.3
1	Montana	100.0		26	Florida	60.3
19	Nebraska	71.1		27	Kentucky	60.1
38	Nevada	39.7		28	Arkansas	59.8
46	New Hampshire	8.1		29	New Jersey	58.4
29	New Jersey	58.4		30	Vermont	57.7
17	New Mexico	73.2		31	North Dakota	55.1
41	New York	29.2		32	Kansas	53.1
9	North Carolina	82.9		33	Oklahoma	52.1
31	North Dakota	55.1		34	California	51.1
42	Ohio	25.1		35	Wisconsin	47.4
33	Oklahoma	52.1		36	West Virginia	43.4
10	Oregon	81.5		37	Mississippi	41.3
13	Pennsylvania	77.0		38	Nevada	39.7
23	Rhode Island	64.1		39	Missouri	38.7
48	South Carolina	4.7		40	Idaho	35.8
15	South Dakota	73.6		41	New York	29.2
1	Tennessee	100.0		42	Ohio	25.1
43	Texas	19.7		43	Texas	19.7
7	Utah	89.5		44	Maine	14.1
30	Vermont	57.7		45	Illinois	12.1
24	Virginia	63.5		46	New Hampshire	8.1
4	Washington	99.9		47	Louisiana	5.8
36	West Virginia	43.4		48	South Carolina	4.7
35	Wisconsin	47.4		49	Alaska	0.0
49	Wyoming	0.0		49	Wyoming	0.0
				District of Columbia		61.4

Source: U.S. Department of Health and Human Services, Health Care Financing Administration
"Medicaid Managed Care State Enrollment" (http://www.hcfa.gov/medicaid/mcsten99.htm)
As of June 30, 1999. Enrollment in state health care reform programs that expand eligibility beyond traditional
Medicaid standards. National percent includes Medicaid enrollees in Puerto Rico and the Virgin Islands.

Federal Medicaid Matching Fund Rate for 2001

National Average = 72.55% of States' Funds Matched by Federal Government*

ALPHA ORDER

RANK ORDER

RANK	STATE	RATE		RANK	STATE	RATE
12	Alabama	78.99		1	Mississippi	83.77
33	Alaska	69.23		2	West Virginia	82.74
16	Arizona	76.04		3	New Mexico	81.66
5	Arkansas	81.11		4	Montana	81.13
38	California	65.88		5	Arkansas	81.11
42	Colorado	65.00		6	Utah	80.01
42	Connecticut	65.00		7	Oklahoma	79.87
42	Delaware	65.00		8	Idaho	79.53
31	Florida	69.63		9	Louisiana	79.37
28	Georgia	71.77		10	South Carolina	79.31
34	Hawaii	67.70		11	Kentucky	79.27
8	Idaho	79.53		12	Alabama	78.99
42	Illinois	65.00		12	North Dakota	78.99
22	Indiana	73.43		14	South Dakota	77.82
19	Iowa	73.87		15	Maine	76.28
27	Kansas	71.90		16	Arizona	76.04
11	Kentucky	79.27		17	Wyoming	75.22
9	Louisiana	79.37		18	Tennessee	74.65
15	Maine	76.28		19	Iowa	73.87
42	Maryland	65.00		20	North Carolina	73.73
42	Massachusetts	65.00		21	Vermont	73.68
32	Michigan	69.33		22	Indiana	73.43
39	Minnesota	65.78		23	Missouri	72.72
1	Mississippi	83.77		24	Texas	72.40
23	Missouri	72.72		25	Nebraska	72.27
4	Montana	81.13		26	Oregon	72.00
25	Nebraska	72.27		27	Kansas	71.90
41	Nevada	65.25		28	Georgia	71.77
42	New Hampshire	65.00		29	Wisconsin	71.50
42	New Jersey	65.00		30	Ohio	71.32
3	New Mexico	81.66		31	Florida	69.63
42	New York	65.00		32	Michigan	69.33
20	North Carolina	73.73		33	Alaska	69.23
12	North Dakota	78.99		34	Hawaii	67.70
30	Ohio	71.32		35	Rhode Island	67.65
7	Oklahoma	79.87		36	Pennsylvania	67.53
26	Oregon	72.00		37	Virginia	66.30
36	Pennsylvania	67.53		38	California	65.88
35	Rhode Island	67.65		39	Minnesota	65.78
10	South Carolina	79.31		40	Washington	65.49
14	South Dakota	77.82		41	Nevada	65.25
18	Tennessee	74.65		42	Colorado	65.00
24	Texas	72.40		42	Connecticut	65.00
6	Utah	80.01		42	Delaware	65.00
21	Vermont	73.68		42	Illinois	65.00
37	Virginia	66.30		42	Maryland	65.00
40	Washington	65.49		42	Massachusetts	65.00
2	West Virginia	82.74		42	New Hampshire	65.00
29	Wisconsin	71.50		42	New Jersey	65.00
17	Wyoming	75.22		42	New York	65.00
					District of Columbia	79.00

Source: U.S. Department of Health and Human Services, Health Care Financing Administration
"Enhanced Federal Medical Assistance Percentages" (Federal Register, 2/23/00)
*For fiscal year 2001. These are "enhanced" matching rates established by the Children's Health Insurance
Program, signed into law in August 1997. Sixty-five percent is the minimum. National average is a simple average of
the 51 individual rates and is not weighted for population or funds.

Estimated State Funds from the Tobacco Settlement Through 2025

National Total = $195,918,675,920*

ALPHA ORDER

RANK	STATE	FUNDS	% of USA
21	Alabama	$3,166,302,119	1.6%
45	Alaska	668,903,057	0.3%
22	Arizona	2,887,614,909	1.5%
30	Arkansas	1,622,336,126	0.8%
1	California	25,006,972,511	12.8%
23	Colorado	2,685,773,549	1.4%
19	Connecticut	3,637,303,382	1.9%
41	Delaware	774,798,677	0.4%
NA	Florida**	NA	NA
9	Georgia	4,808,740,669	2.5%
35	Hawaii	1,179,165,923	0.6%
43	Idaho	711,700,479	0.4%
5	Illinois	9,118,539,559	4.7%
18	Indiana	3,996,355,551	2.0%
28	Iowa	1,703,839,986	0.9%
29	Kansas	1,633,317,646	0.8%
20	Kentucky	3,450,438,586	1.8%
14	Louisiana	4,418,657,915	2.3%
31	Maine	1,507,301,276	0.8%
13	Maryland	4,428,657,384	2.3%
7	Massachusetts	7,913,114,213	4.0%
6	Michigan	8,526,278,034	4.4%
NA	Minnesota**	NA	NA
NA	Mississippi**	NA	NA
12	Missouri	4,456,368,286	2.3%
39	Montana	832,182,431	0.4%
37	Nebraska	1,165,683,457	0.6%
34	Nevada	1,194,976,855	0.6%
33	New Hampshire	1,304,689,150	0.7%
8	New Jersey	7,576,167,918	3.9%
36	New Mexico	1,168,438,809	0.6%
2	New York	25,003,202,243	12.8%
11	North Carolina	4,569,381,898	2.3%
42	North Dakota	717,089,369	0.4%
4	Ohio	9,869,422,449	5.0%
26	Oklahoma	2,029,985,862	1.0%
25	Oregon	2,248,476,833	1.1%
3	Pennsylvania	11,259,169,603	5.7%
32	Rhode Island	1,408,469,747	0.7%
24	South Carolina	2,304,693,120	1.2%
44	South Dakota	683,650,009	0.3%
10	Tennessee	4,782,168,127	2.4%
NA	Texas**	NA	NA
38	Utah	871,616,513	0.4%
40	Vermont	805,588,329	0.4%
17	Virginia	4,006,037,550	2.0%
16	Washington	4,022,716,267	2.1%
27	West Virginia	1,736,741,427	0.9%
15	Wisconsin	4,059,511,421	2.1%
46	Wyoming	486,553,976	0.2%

RANK ORDER

RANK	STATE	FUNDS	% of USA
1	California	$25,006,972,511	12.8%
2	New York	25,003,202,243	12.8%
3	Pennsylvania	11,259,169,603	5.7%
4	Ohio	9,869,422,449	5.0%
5	Illinois	9,118,539,559	4.7%
6	Michigan	8,526,278,034	4.4%
7	Massachusetts	7,913,114,213	4.0%
8	New Jersey	7,576,167,918	3.9%
9	Georgia	4,808,740,669	2.5%
10	Tennessee	4,782,168,127	2.4%
11	North Carolina	4,569,381,898	2.3%
12	Missouri	4,456,368,286	2.3%
13	Maryland	4,428,657,384	2.3%
14	Louisiana	4,418,657,915	2.3%
15	Wisconsin	4,059,511,421	2.1%
16	Washington	4,022,716,267	2.1%
17	Virginia	4,006,037,550	2.0%
18	Indiana	3,996,355,551	2.0%
19	Connecticut	3,637,303,382	1.9%
20	Kentucky	3,450,438,586	1.8%
21	Alabama	3,166,302,119	1.6%
22	Arizona	2,887,614,909	1.5%
23	Colorado	2,685,773,549	1.4%
24	South Carolina	2,304,693,120	1.2%
25	Oregon	2,248,476,833	1.1%
26	Oklahoma	2,029,985,862	1.0%
27	West Virginia	1,736,741,427	0.9%
28	Iowa	1,703,839,986	0.9%
29	Kansas	1,633,317,646	0.8%
30	Arkansas	1,622,336,126	0.8%
31	Maine	1,507,301,276	0.8%
32	Rhode Island	1,408,469,747	0.7%
33	New Hampshire	1,304,689,150	0.7%
34	Nevada	1,194,976,855	0.6%
35	Hawaii	1,179,165,923	0.6%
36	New Mexico	1,168,438,809	0.6%
37	Nebraska	1,165,683,457	0.6%
38	Utah	871,616,513	0.4%
39	Montana	832,182,431	0.4%
40	Vermont	805,588,329	0.4%
41	Delaware	774,798,677	0.4%
42	North Dakota	717,089,369	0.4%
43	Idaho	711,700,479	0.4%
44	South Dakota	683,650,009	0.3%
45	Alaska	668,903,057	0.3%
46	Wyoming	486,553,976	0.2%
NA	Florida**	NA	NA
NA	Minnesota**	NA	NA
NA	Mississippi**	NA	NA
NA	Texas**	NA	NA
	District of Columbia	1,189,458,106	0.6%

Source: National Association of Attorneys General
"Attorneys General Announce Tobacco Settlement Proposal" (News release, http://www.naag.org/tob2.htm)
This settlement was reached in November 1998. National total includes $4,640,249,229 for U.S. territories.
***Total does not include $40 billion in previous settlements with Florida, Minnesota, Mississippi and Texas.*

State Government Expenditures for Health Programs in 1998

National Total = $35,066,884,000*

ALPHA ORDER

RANK	STATE	EXPENDITURES	% of USA
18	Alabama	$554,980,000	1.6%
41	Alaska	161,108,000	0.5%
15	Arizona	656,826,000	1.9%
31	Arkansas	271,451,000	0.8%
1	California	6,388,493,000	18.2%
30	Colorado	282,136,000	0.8%
24	Connecticut	402,252,000	1.1%
39	Delaware	184,013,000	0.5%
4	Florida	1,840,385,000	5.2%
14	Georgia	681,884,000	1.9%
32	Hawaii	269,974,000	0.8%
45	Idaho	93,361,000	0.3%
5	Illinois	1,733,954,000	4.9%
23	Indiana	421,808,000	1.2%
37	Iowa	194,559,000	0.6%
29	Kansas	293,522,000	0.8%
28	Kentucky	318,865,000	0.9%
25	Louisiana	380,552,000	1.1%
34	Maine	251,644,000	0.7%
13	Maryland	773,271,000	2.2%
8	Massachusetts	1,396,566,000	4.0%
3	Michigan	2,200,499,000	6.3%
22	Minnesota	467,222,000	1.3%
35	Mississippi	248,810,000	0.7%
17	Missouri	603,186,000	1.7%
38	Montana	188,941,000	0.5%
36	Nebraska	217,079,000	0.6%
46	Nevada	92,485,000	0.3%
44	New Hampshire	122,456,000	0.3%
12	New Jersey	813,249,000	2.3%
33	New Mexico	267,416,000	0.8%
2	New York	2,351,440,000	6.7%
11	North Carolina	961,591,000	2.7%
50	North Dakota	45,534,000	0.1%
6	Ohio	1,480,747,000	4.2%
27	Oklahoma	340,508,000	1.0%
26	Oregon	371,130,000	1.1%
9	Pennsylvania	1,360,888,000	3.9%
43	Rhode Island	129,777,000	0.4%
16	South Carolina	627,252,000	1.8%
48	South Dakota	59,841,000	0.2%
21	Tennessee	522,405,000	1.5%
7	Texas	1,450,106,000	4.1%
40	Utah	183,665,000	0.5%
49	Vermont	58,618,000	0.2%
19	Virginia	535,124,000	1.5%
10	Washington	1,081,493,000	3.1%
42	West Virginia	131,488,000	0.4%
20	Wisconsin	524,385,000	1.5%
47	Wyoming	77,945,000	0.2%

RANK ORDER

RANK	STATE	EXPENDITURES	% of USA
1	California	$6,388,493,000	18.2%
2	New York	2,351,440,000	6.7%
3	Michigan	2,200,499,000	6.3%
4	Florida	1,840,385,000	5.2%
5	Illinois	1,733,954,000	4.9%
6	Ohio	1,480,747,000	4.2%
7	Texas	1,450,106,000	4.1%
8	Massachusetts	1,396,566,000	4.0%
9	Pennsylvania	1,360,888,000	3.9%
10	Washington	1,081,493,000	3.1%
11	North Carolina	961,591,000	2.7%
12	New Jersey	813,249,000	2.3%
13	Maryland	773,271,000	2.2%
14	Georgia	681,884,000	1.9%
15	Arizona	656,826,000	1.9%
16	South Carolina	627,252,000	1.8%
17	Missouri	603,186,000	1.7%
18	Alabama	554,980,000	1.6%
19	Virginia	535,124,000	1.5%
20	Wisconsin	524,385,000	1.5%
21	Tennessee	522,405,000	1.5%
22	Minnesota	467,222,000	1.3%
23	Indiana	421,808,000	1.2%
24	Connecticut	402,252,000	1.1%
25	Louisiana	380,552,000	1.1%
26	Oregon	371,130,000	1.1%
27	Oklahoma	340,508,000	1.0%
28	Kentucky	318,865,000	0.9%
29	Kansas	293,522,000	0.8%
30	Colorado	282,136,000	0.8%
31	Arkansas	271,451,000	0.8%
32	Hawaii	269,974,000	0.8%
33	New Mexico	267,416,000	0.8%
34	Maine	251,644,000	0.7%
35	Mississippi	248,810,000	0.7%
36	Nebraska	217,079,000	0.6%
37	Iowa	194,559,000	0.6%
38	Montana	188,941,000	0.5%
39	Delaware	184,013,000	0.5%
40	Utah	183,665,000	0.5%
41	Alaska	161,108,000	0.5%
42	West Virginia	131,488,000	0.4%
43	Rhode Island	129,777,000	0.4%
44	New Hampshire	122,456,000	0.3%
45	Idaho	93,361,000	0.3%
46	Nevada	92,485,000	0.3%
47	Wyoming	77,945,000	0.2%
48	South Dakota	59,841,000	0.2%
49	Vermont	58,618,000	0.2%
50	North Dakota	45,534,000	0.1%
	District of Columbia**	NA	NA

Source: U.S. Bureau of the Census, Governments Division
   "1998 State Government Finance Data" (http://www.census.gov/govs/www/state98.html)
*Includes outpatient health services other than hospital care, research and education, categorical health programs, treatment and immunization clinics, nursing and environmental health activities. Includes capital expenditures.
**Not applicable.

Per Capita State Government Expenditures for Health Programs in 1998

National Per Capita = $130*

RANK	STATE	PER CAPITA
20	Alabama	$128
1	Alaska	262
15	Arizona	141
28	Arkansas	107
8	California	195
46	Colorado	71
22	Connecticut	123
2	Delaware	247
22	Florida	123
37	Georgia	89
3	Hawaii	227
43	Idaho	76
14	Illinois	144
46	Indiana	71
49	Iowa	68
26	Kansas	111
41	Kentucky	81
38	Louisiana	87
7	Maine	202
13	Maryland	151
3	Massachusetts	227
5	Michigan	224
33	Minnesota	99
36	Mississippi	90
26	Missouri	111
6	Montana	215
17	Nebraska	131
50	Nevada	53
29	New Hampshire	103
31	New Jersey	100
12	New Mexico	154
19	New York	129
21	North Carolina	127
46	North Dakota	71
16	Ohio	132
30	Oklahoma	102
24	Oregon	113
24	Pennsylvania	113
17	Rhode Island	131
10	South Carolina	163
40	South Dakota	82
35	Tennessee	96
44	Texas	74
38	Utah	87
33	Vermont	99
42	Virginia	79
9	Washington	190
45	West Virginia	73
31	Wisconsin	100
11	Wyoming	162

RANK	STATE	PER CAPITA
1	Alaska	$262
2	Delaware	247
3	Hawaii	227
3	Massachusetts	227
5	Michigan	224
6	Montana	215
7	Maine	202
8	California	195
9	Washington	190
10	South Carolina	163
11	Wyoming	162
12	New Mexico	154
13	Maryland	151
14	Illinois	144
15	Arizona	141
16	Ohio	132
17	Nebraska	131
17	Rhode Island	131
19	New York	129
20	Alabama	128
21	North Carolina	127
22	Connecticut	123
22	Florida	123
24	Oregon	113
24	Pennsylvania	113
26	Kansas	111
26	Missouri	111
28	Arkansas	107
29	New Hampshire	103
30	Oklahoma	102
31	New Jersey	100
31	Wisconsin	100
33	Minnesota	99
33	Vermont	99
35	Tennessee	96
36	Mississippi	90
37	Georgia	89
38	Louisiana	87
38	Utah	87
40	South Dakota	82
41	Kentucky	81
42	Virginia	79
43	Idaho	76
44	Texas	74
45	West Virginia	73
46	Colorado	71
46	Indiana	71
46	North Dakota	71
49	Iowa	68
50	Nevada	53
	District of Columbia**	NA

Source: Morgan Quitno Press using data from U.S. Bureau of the Census, Governments Division
"1998 State Government Finance Data" (http://www.census.gov/govs/www/state98.html)
Includes outpatient health services other than hospital care, research and education, categorical health programs, treatment and immunization clinics, nursing and environmental health activities. Includes capital expenditures.
**Not applicable.*

State Government Expenditures for Hospitals in 1998

National Total = $28,928,103,000*

ALPHA ORDER

RANK	STATE	EXPENDITURES	% of USA
11	Alabama	$948,312,000	3.3%
49	Alaska	26,311,000	0.1%
40	Arizona	62,466,000	0.2%
26	Arkansas	371,271,000	1.3%
2	California	2,431,517,000	8.4%
35	Colorado	150,831,000	0.5%
8	Connecticut	1,054,818,000	3.6%
41	Delaware	56,801,000	0.2%
20	Florida	502,081,000	1.7%
15	Georgia	700,255,000	2.4%
33	Hawaii	231,668,000	0.8%
44	Idaho	45,164,000	0.2%
13	Illinois	806,842,000	2.8%
34	Indiana	216,860,000	0.7%
18	Iowa	537,465,000	1.9%
30	Kansas	285,042,000	1.0%
25	Kentucky	444,045,000	1.5%
6	Louisiana	1,212,424,000	4.2%
42	Maine	49,431,000	0.2%
28	Maryland	336,751,000	1.2%
19	Massachusetts	524,659,000	1.8%
7	Michigan	1,118,566,000	3.9%
32	Minnesota	231,861,000	0.8%
23	Mississippi	466,143,000	1.6%
24	Missouri	460,591,000	1.6%
47	Montana	39,852,000	0.1%
36	Nebraska	140,758,000	0.5%
37	Nevada	82,491,000	0.3%
43	New Hampshire	46,904,000	0.2%
9	New Jersey	1,022,082,000	3.5%
29	New Mexico	319,694,000	1.1%
1	New York	3,346,194,000	11.6%
12	North Carolina	829,645,000	2.9%
45	North Dakota	45,006,000	0.2%
10	Ohio	1,014,384,000	3.5%
31	Oklahoma	257,278,000	0.9%
22	Oregon	467,787,000	1.6%
4	Pennsylvania	1,538,005,000	5.3%
39	Rhode Island	77,953,000	0.3%
14	South Carolina	707,356,000	2.4%
46	South Dakota	40,654,000	0.1%
17	Tennessee	555,729,000	1.9%
3	Texas	2,305,130,000	8.0%
27	Utah	353,279,000	1.2%
50	Vermont	8,672,000	0.0%
5	Virginia	1,274,442,000	4.4%
16	Washington	587,524,000	2.0%
38	West Virginia	78,360,000	0.3%
21	Wisconsin	487,563,000	1.7%
48	Wyoming	29,186,000	0.1%

RANK ORDER

RANK	STATE	EXPENDITURES	% of USA
1	New York	$3,346,194,000	11.6%
2	California	2,431,517,000	8.4%
3	Texas	2,305,130,000	8.0%
4	Pennsylvania	1,538,005,000	5.3%
5	Virginia	1,274,442,000	4.4%
6	Louisiana	1,212,424,000	4.2%
7	Michigan	1,118,566,000	3.9%
8	Connecticut	1,054,818,000	3.6%
9	New Jersey	1,022,082,000	3.5%
10	Ohio	1,014,384,000	3.5%
11	Alabama	948,312,000	3.3%
12	North Carolina	829,645,000	2.9%
13	Illinois	806,842,000	2.8%
14	South Carolina	707,356,000	2.4%
15	Georgia	700,255,000	2.4%
16	Washington	587,524,000	2.0%
17	Tennessee	555,729,000	1.9%
18	Iowa	537,465,000	1.9%
19	Massachusetts	524,659,000	1.8%
20	Florida	502,081,000	1.7%
21	Wisconsin	487,563,000	1.7%
22	Oregon	467,787,000	1.6%
23	Mississippi	466,143,000	1.6%
24	Missouri	460,591,000	1.6%
25	Kentucky	444,045,000	1.5%
26	Arkansas	371,271,000	1.3%
27	Utah	353,279,000	1.2%
28	Maryland	336,751,000	1.2%
29	New Mexico	319,694,000	1.1%
30	Kansas	285,042,000	1.0%
31	Oklahoma	257,278,000	0.9%
32	Minnesota	231,861,000	0.8%
33	Hawaii	231,668,000	0.8%
34	Indiana	216,860,000	0.7%
35	Colorado	150,831,000	0.5%
36	Nebraska	140,758,000	0.5%
37	Nevada	82,491,000	0.3%
38	West Virginia	78,360,000	0.3%
39	Rhode Island	77,953,000	0.3%
40	Arizona	62,466,000	0.2%
41	Delaware	56,801,000	0.2%
42	Maine	49,431,000	0.2%
43	New Hampshire	46,904,000	0.2%
44	Idaho	45,164,000	0.2%
45	North Dakota	45,006,000	0.2%
46	South Dakota	40,654,000	0.1%
47	Montana	39,852,000	0.1%
48	Wyoming	29,186,000	0.1%
49	Alaska	26,311,000	0.1%
50	Vermont	8,672,000	0.0%
	District of Columbia**	NA	NA

Source: U.S. Bureau of the Census, Governments Division
"1998 State Government Finance Data" (http://www.census.gov/govs/www/state98.html)
*Financing, construction, acquisition, maintenance or operation of hospital facilities, provision of hospital care and support of public or private hospitals.
**Not applicable.

Per Capita State Government Expenditures for Hospitals in 1998

National Per Capita = $107*

<u>ALPHA ORDER</u>

RANK	STATE	PER CAPITA
3	Alabama	$218
41	Alaska	43
50	Arizona	13
12	Arkansas	146
32	California	74
45	Colorado	38
1	Connecticut	322
31	Delaware	76
48	Florida	34
24	Georgia	92
4	Hawaii	195
46	Idaho	37
34	Illinois	67
46	Indiana	37
5	Iowa	188
20	Kansas	108
18	Kentucky	113
2	Louisiana	278
43	Maine	40
35	Maryland	66
26	Massachusetts	85
17	Michigan	114
38	Minnesota	49
10	Mississippi	169
26	Missouri	85
40	Montana	45
26	Nebraska	85
39	Nevada	47
43	New Hampshire	40
15	New Jersey	126
7	New Mexico	184
7	New York	184
19	North Carolina	110
33	North Dakota	71
25	Ohio	90
30	Oklahoma	77
13	Oregon	143
14	Pennsylvania	128
29	Rhode Island	79
7	South Carolina	184
37	South Dakota	56
22	Tennessee	102
16	Texas	117
11	Utah	168
49	Vermont	15
5	Virginia	188
21	Washington	103
41	West Virginia	43
23	Wisconsin	93
36	Wyoming	61

<u>RANK ORDER</u>

RANK	STATE	PER CAPITA
1	Connecticut	$322
2	Louisiana	278
3	Alabama	218
4	Hawaii	195
5	Iowa	188
5	Virginia	188
7	New Mexico	184
7	New York	184
7	South Carolina	184
10	Mississippi	169
11	Utah	168
12	Arkansas	146
13	Oregon	143
14	Pennsylvania	128
15	New Jersey	126
16	Texas	117
17	Michigan	114
18	Kentucky	113
19	North Carolina	110
20	Kansas	108
21	Washington	103
22	Tennessee	102
23	Wisconsin	93
24	Georgia	92
25	Ohio	90
26	Massachusetts	85
26	Missouri	85
26	Nebraska	85
29	Rhode Island	79
30	Oklahoma	77
31	Delaware	76
32	California	74
33	North Dakota	71
34	Illinois	67
35	Maryland	66
36	Wyoming	61
37	South Dakota	56
38	Minnesota	49
39	Nevada	47
40	Montana	45
41	Alaska	43
41	West Virginia	43
43	Maine	40
43	New Hampshire	40
45	Colorado	38
46	Idaho	37
46	Indiana	37
48	Florida	34
49	Vermont	15
50	Arizona	13
	District of Columbia**	NA

Source: Morgan Quitno Press using data from U.S. Bureau of the Census, Governments Division
    "1998 State Government Finance Data" (http://www.census.gov/govs/www/state98.html)
*Financing, construction, acquisition, maintenance or operation of hospital facilities, provision of hospital care and support of public or private hospitals.
**Not applicable.

Payroll of Health Care Establishments in 1998

National Total = $369,790,601,000*

ALPHA ORDER

RANK	STATE	PAYROLL	% of USA
23	Alabama	$5,521,348,000	1.5%
48	Alaska	941,317,000	0.3%
24	Arizona	5,206,664,000	1.4%
33	Arkansas	2,984,552,000	0.8%
1	California	37,148,398,000	10.0%
25	Colorado	4,896,457,000	1.3%
21	Connecticut	6,156,674,000	1.7%
43	Delaware	1,279,822,000	0.3%
4	Florida	20,723,891,000	5.6%
12	Georgia	9,206,579,000	2.5%
42	Hawaii	1,545,432,000	0.4%
44	Idaho	1,210,752,000	0.3%
6	Illinois	16,597,261,000	4.5%
15	Indiana	7,923,784,000	2.1%
30	Iowa	3,852,386,000	1.0%
31	Kansas	3,541,538,000	1.0%
26	Kentucky	4,756,652,000	1.3%
22	Louisiana	5,597,165,000	1.5%
39	Maine	1,829,124,000	0.5%
20	Maryland	7,032,205,000	1.9%
9	Massachusetts	12,454,933,000	3.4%
8	Michigan	13,513,127,000	3.7%
17	Minnesota	7,672,589,000	2.1%
32	Mississippi	3,171,648,000	0.9%
13	Missouri	8,035,157,000	2.2%
47	Montana	984,457,000	0.3%
35	Nebraska	2,342,276,000	0.6%
38	Nevada	1,835,682,000	0.5%
41	New Hampshire	1,686,826,000	0.5%
10	New Jersey	12,437,156,000	3.4%
37	New Mexico	1,843,067,000	0.5%
2	New York	32,881,306,000	8.9%
11	North Carolina	9,924,165,000	2.7%
46	North Dakota	1,089,193,000	0.3%
7	Ohio	16,350,171,000	4.4%
28	Oklahoma	3,917,220,000	1.1%
29	Oregon	3,888,155,000	1.1%
5	Pennsylvania	19,622,962,000	5.3%
40	Rhode Island	1,773,152,000	0.5%
27	South Carolina	4,379,008,000	1.2%
45	South Dakota	1,200,868,000	0.3%
14	Tennessee	7,957,223,000	2.2%
3	Texas	23,315,869,000	6.3%
36	Utah	2,154,573,000	0.6%
49	Vermont	819,150,000	0.2%
16	Virginia	7,759,393,000	2.1%
19	Washington	7,139,187,000	1.9%
34	West Virginia	2,373,420,000	0.6%
18	Wisconsin	7,349,343,000	2.0%
50	Wyoming	556,515,000	0.2%

RANK ORDER

RANK	STATE	PAYROLL	% of USA
1	California	$37,148,398,000	10.0%
2	New York	32,881,306,000	8.9%
3	Texas	23,315,869,000	6.3%
4	Florida	20,723,891,000	5.6%
5	Pennsylvania	19,622,962,000	5.3%
6	Illinois	16,597,261,000	4.5%
7	Ohio	16,350,171,000	4.4%
8	Michigan	13,513,127,000	3.7%
9	Massachusetts	12,454,933,000	3.4%
10	New Jersey	12,437,156,000	3.4%
11	North Carolina	9,924,165,000	2.7%
12	Georgia	9,206,579,000	2.5%
13	Missouri	8,035,157,000	2.2%
14	Tennessee	7,957,223,000	2.2%
15	Indiana	7,923,784,000	2.1%
16	Virginia	7,759,393,000	2.1%
17	Minnesota	7,672,589,000	2.1%
18	Wisconsin	7,349,343,000	2.0%
19	Washington	7,139,187,000	1.9%
20	Maryland	7,032,205,000	1.9%
21	Connecticut	6,156,674,000	1.7%
22	Louisiana	5,597,165,000	1.5%
23	Alabama	5,521,348,000	1.5%
24	Arizona	5,206,664,000	1.4%
25	Colorado	4,896,457,000	1.3%
26	Kentucky	4,756,652,000	1.3%
27	South Carolina	4,379,008,000	1.2%
28	Oklahoma	3,917,220,000	1.1%
29	Oregon	3,888,155,000	1.1%
30	Iowa	3,852,386,000	1.0%
31	Kansas	3,541,538,000	1.0%
32	Mississippi	3,171,648,000	0.9%
33	Arkansas	2,984,552,000	0.8%
34	West Virginia	2,373,420,000	0.6%
35	Nebraska	2,342,276,000	0.6%
36	Utah	2,154,573,000	0.6%
37	New Mexico	1,843,067,000	0.5%
38	Nevada	1,835,682,000	0.5%
39	Maine	1,829,124,000	0.5%
40	Rhode Island	1,773,152,000	0.5%
41	New Hampshire	1,686,826,000	0.5%
42	Hawaii	1,545,432,000	0.4%
43	Delaware	1,279,822,000	0.3%
44	Idaho	1,210,752,000	0.3%
45	South Dakota	1,200,868,000	0.3%
46	North Dakota	1,089,193,000	0.3%
47	Montana	984,457,000	0.3%
48	Alaska	941,317,000	0.3%
49	Vermont	819,150,000	0.2%
50	Wyoming	556,515,000	0.2%
	District of Columbia	1,789,594,000	0.5%

Source: U.S. Bureau of the Census
"County Business Patterns 1998 (NACIS)" (http://tier2.census.gov/cbp_naics/index.html)
*Includes establishments exempt from as well as subject to the federal income tax. Includes those establishments within the North American Industry Classification System (NACIS) classifications 621 (ambulatory health care services), 622 (hospitals) and 623 (nursing and residential care facilities). See Facilities Chapter for establishments.

Average Pay per Health Care Establishment Employee in 1998

National Average = $30,804 per Employee*

ALPHA ORDER

RANK	STATE	AVERAGE PAY	% of USA
22	Alabama	30,246	0.0%
1	Alaska	41,181	0.0%
10	Arizona	31,742	0.0%
42	Arkansas	26,598	0.0%
6	California	33,720	0.0%
13	Colorado	31,420	0.0%
7	Connecticut	33,657	0.0%
18	Delaware	31,062	0.0%
17	Florida	31,211	0.0%
8	Georgia	32,032	0.0%
2	Hawaii	38,430	0.0%
40	Idaho	27,194	0.0%
13	Illinois	31,420	0.0%
33	Indiana	28,532	0.0%
46	Iowa	25,599	0.0%
43	Kansas	26,450	0.0%
36	Kentucky	27,840	0.0%
41	Louisiana	26,902	0.0%
38	Maine	27,324	0.0%
11	Maryland	31,549	0.0%
9	Massachusetts	31,829	0.0%
15	Michigan	31,371	0.0%
27	Minnesota	29,673	0.0%
37	Mississippi	27,734	0.0%
32	Missouri	28,625	0.0%
45	Montana	25,872	0.0%
35	Nebraska	28,033	0.0%
3	Nevada	34,868	0.0%
24	New Hampshire	30,011	0.0%
4	New Jersey	34,856	0.0%
34	New Mexico	28,274	0.0%
5	New York	33,735	0.0%
25	North Carolina	29,898	0.0%
49	North Dakota	23,733	0.0%
29	Ohio	29,551	0.0%
44	Oklahoma	26,003	0.0%
21	Oregon	30,314	0.0%
23	Pennsylvania	30,166	0.0%
26	Rhode Island	29,889	0.0%
19	South Carolina	30,697	0.0%
48	South Dakota	24,895	0.0%
12	Tennessee	31,423	0.0%
31	Texas	28,704	0.0%
30	Utah	29,067	0.0%
47	Vermont	24,986	0.0%
20	Virginia	30,480	0.0%
16	Washington	31,298	0.0%
39	West Virginia	27,314	0.0%
28	Wisconsin	29,576	0.0%
50	Wyoming	23,488	0.0%

RANK ORDER

RANK	STATE	AVERAGE PAY	% of USA
1	Alaska	41,181	0.0%
2	Hawaii	38,430	0.0%
3	Nevada	34,868	0.0%
4	New Jersey	34,856	0.0%
5	New York	33,735	0.0%
6	California	33,720	0.0%
7	Connecticut	33,657	0.0%
8	Georgia	32,032	0.0%
9	Massachusetts	31,829	0.0%
10	Arizona	31,742	0.0%
11	Maryland	31,549	0.0%
12	Tennessee	31,423	0.0%
13	Colorado	31,420	0.0%
13	Illinois	31,420	0.0%
15	Michigan	31,371	0.0%
16	Washington	31,298	0.0%
17	Florida	31,211	0.0%
18	Delaware	31,062	0.0%
19	South Carolina	30,697	0.0%
20	Virginia	30,480	0.0%
21	Oregon	30,314	0.0%
22	Alabama	30,246	0.0%
23	Pennsylvania	30,166	0.0%
24	New Hampshire	30,011	0.0%
25	North Carolina	29,898	0.0%
26	Rhode Island	29,889	0.0%
27	Minnesota	29,673	0.0%
28	Wisconsin	29,576	0.0%
29	Ohio	29,551	0.0%
30	Utah	29,067	0.0%
31	Texas	28,704	0.0%
32	Missouri	28,625	0.0%
33	Indiana	28,532	0.0%
34	New Mexico	28,274	0.0%
35	Nebraska	28,033	0.0%
36	Kentucky	27,840	0.0%
37	Mississippi	27,734	0.0%
38	Maine	27,324	0.0%
39	West Virginia	27,314	0.0%
40	Idaho	27,194	0.0%
41	Louisiana	26,902	0.0%
42	Arkansas	26,598	0.0%
43	Kansas	26,450	0.0%
44	Oklahoma	26,003	0.0%
45	Montana	25,872	0.0%
46	Iowa	25,599	0.0%
47	Vermont	24,986	0.0%
48	South Dakota	24,895	0.0%
49	North Dakota	23,733	0.0%
50	Wyoming	23,488	0.0%
	District of Columbia	37,136	0.0%

Source: Morgan Quitno Press using data from U.S. Bureau of the Census
   "County Business Patterns 1998 (NACIS)" (http://tier2.census.gov/cbp_naics/index.html)
*Includes establishments exempt from as well as subject to the federal income tax. Includes those establishments
within the North American Industry Classification System (NACIS) classifications 621 (ambulatory health care
services), 622 (hospitals) and 623 (nursing and residential care facilities). See Facilities Chapter for establishments.

Receipts of Health Services Establishments in 1997

National Total = $885,054,001,000*

<table>
<tr><td colspan="4">ALPHA ORDER</td><td colspan="4">RANK ORDER</td></tr>
<tr><th>RANK</th><th>STATE</th><th>RECEIPTS</th><th>% of USA</th><th>RANK</th><th>STATE</th><th>RECEIPTS</th><th>% of USA</th></tr>
<tr><td>23</td><td>Alabama</td><td>$13,192,253,000</td><td>1.5%</td><td>1</td><td>California</td><td>$100,746,815,000</td><td>11.4%</td></tr>
<tr><td>48</td><td>Alaska</td><td>2,041,248,000</td><td>0.2%</td><td>2</td><td>New York</td><td>74,767,808,000</td><td>8.4%</td></tr>
<tr><td>24</td><td>Arizona</td><td>12,841,177,000</td><td>1.5%</td><td>3</td><td>Texas</td><td>56,758,770,000</td><td>6.4%</td></tr>
<tr><td>33</td><td>Arkansas</td><td>7,297,065,000</td><td>0.8%</td><td>4</td><td>Florida</td><td>51,974,200,000</td><td>5.9%</td></tr>
<tr><td>1</td><td>California</td><td>100,746,815,000</td><td>11.4%</td><td>5</td><td>Pennsylvania</td><td>45,253,553,000</td><td>5.1%</td></tr>
<tr><td>26</td><td>Colorado</td><td>11,657,625,000</td><td>1.3%</td><td>6</td><td>Illinois</td><td>39,775,490,000</td><td>4.5%</td></tr>
<tr><td>22</td><td>Connecticut</td><td>13,907,989,000</td><td>1.6%</td><td>7</td><td>Ohio</td><td>36,863,598,000</td><td>4.2%</td></tr>
<tr><td>44</td><td>Delaware</td><td>2,631,828,000</td><td>0.3%</td><td>8</td><td>Michigan</td><td>31,270,014,000</td><td>3.5%</td></tr>
<tr><td>4</td><td>Florida</td><td>51,974,200,000</td><td>5.9%</td><td>9</td><td>New Jersey</td><td>28,531,121,000</td><td>3.2%</td></tr>
<tr><td>11</td><td>Georgia</td><td>23,711,573,000</td><td>2.7%</td><td>10</td><td>Massachusetts</td><td>27,452,916,000</td><td>3.1%</td></tr>
<tr><td>41</td><td>Hawaii</td><td>3,975,313,000</td><td>0.4%</td><td>11</td><td>Georgia</td><td>23,711,573,000</td><td>2.7%</td></tr>
<tr><td>43</td><td>Idaho</td><td>2,835,543,000</td><td>0.3%</td><td>12</td><td>North Carolina</td><td>23,109,073,000</td><td>2.6%</td></tr>
<tr><td>6</td><td>Illinois</td><td>39,775,490,000</td><td>4.5%</td><td>13</td><td>Tennessee</td><td>19,212,914,000</td><td>2.2%</td></tr>
<tr><td>16</td><td>Indiana</td><td>18,042,945,000</td><td>2.0%</td><td>14</td><td>Virginia</td><td>18,835,208,000</td><td>2.1%</td></tr>
<tr><td>30</td><td>Iowa</td><td>8,765,614,000</td><td>1.0%</td><td>15</td><td>Missouri</td><td>18,421,088,000</td><td>2.1%</td></tr>
<tr><td>31</td><td>Kansas</td><td>8,198,279,000</td><td>0.9%</td><td>16</td><td>Indiana</td><td>18,042,945,000</td><td>2.0%</td></tr>
<tr><td>25</td><td>Kentucky</td><td>11,962,976,000</td><td>1.4%</td><td>17</td><td>Maryland</td><td>17,465,676,000</td><td>2.0%</td></tr>
<tr><td>21</td><td>Louisiana</td><td>14,444,944,000</td><td>1.6%</td><td>18</td><td>Minnesota</td><td>16,829,464,000</td><td>1.9%</td></tr>
<tr><td>39</td><td>Maine</td><td>4,249,374,000</td><td>0.5%</td><td>19</td><td>Washington</td><td>16,779,905,000</td><td>1.9%</td></tr>
<tr><td>17</td><td>Maryland</td><td>17,465,676,000</td><td>2.0%</td><td>20</td><td>Wisconsin</td><td>16,572,139,000</td><td>1.9%</td></tr>
<tr><td>10</td><td>Massachusetts</td><td>27,452,916,000</td><td>3.1%</td><td>21</td><td>Louisiana</td><td>14,444,944,000</td><td>1.6%</td></tr>
<tr><td>8</td><td>Michigan</td><td>31,270,014,000</td><td>3.5%</td><td>22</td><td>Connecticut</td><td>13,907,989,000</td><td>1.6%</td></tr>
<tr><td>18</td><td>Minnesota</td><td>16,829,464,000</td><td>1.9%</td><td>23</td><td>Alabama</td><td>13,192,253,000</td><td>1.5%</td></tr>
<tr><td>32</td><td>Mississippi</td><td>7,881,283,000</td><td>0.9%</td><td>24</td><td>Arizona</td><td>12,841,177,000</td><td>1.5%</td></tr>
<tr><td>15</td><td>Missouri</td><td>18,421,088,000</td><td>2.1%</td><td>25</td><td>Kentucky</td><td>11,962,976,000</td><td>1.4%</td></tr>
<tr><td>46</td><td>Montana</td><td>2,368,999,000</td><td>0.3%</td><td>26</td><td>Colorado</td><td>11,657,625,000</td><td>1.3%</td></tr>
<tr><td>35</td><td>Nebraska</td><td>5,102,506,000</td><td>0.6%</td><td>27</td><td>South Carolina</td><td>10,048,402,000</td><td>1.1%</td></tr>
<tr><td>37</td><td>Nevada</td><td>4,668,075,000</td><td>0.5%</td><td>28</td><td>Oklahoma</td><td>9,344,954,000</td><td>1.1%</td></tr>
<tr><td>40</td><td>New Hampshire</td><td>3,980,324,000</td><td>0.4%</td><td>29</td><td>Oregon</td><td>9,300,512,000</td><td>1.1%</td></tr>
<tr><td>9</td><td>New Jersey</td><td>28,531,121,000</td><td>3.2%</td><td>30</td><td>Iowa</td><td>8,765,614,000</td><td>1.0%</td></tr>
<tr><td>38</td><td>New Mexico</td><td>4,469,602,000</td><td>0.5%</td><td>31</td><td>Kansas</td><td>8,198,279,000</td><td>0.9%</td></tr>
<tr><td>2</td><td>New York</td><td>74,767,808,000</td><td>8.4%</td><td>32</td><td>Mississippi</td><td>7,881,283,000</td><td>0.9%</td></tr>
<tr><td>12</td><td>North Carolina</td><td>23,109,073,000</td><td>2.6%</td><td>33</td><td>Arkansas</td><td>7,297,065,000</td><td>0.8%</td></tr>
<tr><td>47</td><td>North Dakota</td><td>2,367,774,000</td><td>0.3%</td><td>34</td><td>West Virginia</td><td>5,825,082,000</td><td>0.7%</td></tr>
<tr><td>7</td><td>Ohio</td><td>36,863,598,000</td><td>4.2%</td><td>35</td><td>Nebraska</td><td>5,102,506,000</td><td>0.6%</td></tr>
<tr><td>28</td><td>Oklahoma</td><td>9,344,954,000</td><td>1.1%</td><td>36</td><td>Utah</td><td>5,059,071,000</td><td>0.6%</td></tr>
<tr><td>29</td><td>Oregon</td><td>9,300,512,000</td><td>1.1%</td><td>37</td><td>Nevada</td><td>4,668,075,000</td><td>0.5%</td></tr>
<tr><td>5</td><td>Pennsylvania</td><td>45,253,553,000</td><td>5.1%</td><td>38</td><td>New Mexico</td><td>4,469,602,000</td><td>0.5%</td></tr>
<tr><td>42</td><td>Rhode Island</td><td>3,902,244,000</td><td>0.4%</td><td>39</td><td>Maine</td><td>4,249,374,000</td><td>0.5%</td></tr>
<tr><td>27</td><td>South Carolina</td><td>10,048,402,000</td><td>1.1%</td><td>40</td><td>New Hampshire</td><td>3,980,324,000</td><td>0.4%</td></tr>
<tr><td>45</td><td>South Dakota</td><td>2,528,389,000</td><td>0.3%</td><td>41</td><td>Hawaii</td><td>3,975,313,000</td><td>0.4%</td></tr>
<tr><td>13</td><td>Tennessee</td><td>19,212,914,000</td><td>2.2%</td><td>42</td><td>Rhode Island</td><td>3,902,244,000</td><td>0.4%</td></tr>
<tr><td>3</td><td>Texas</td><td>56,758,770,000</td><td>6.4%</td><td>43</td><td>Idaho</td><td>2,835,543,000</td><td>0.3%</td></tr>
<tr><td>36</td><td>Utah</td><td>5,059,071,000</td><td>0.6%</td><td>44</td><td>Delaware</td><td>2,631,828,000</td><td>0.3%</td></tr>
<tr><td>49</td><td>Vermont</td><td>1,760,664,000</td><td>0.2%</td><td>45</td><td>South Dakota</td><td>2,528,389,000</td><td>0.3%</td></tr>
<tr><td>14</td><td>Virginia</td><td>18,835,208,000</td><td>2.1%</td><td>46</td><td>Montana</td><td>2,368,999,000</td><td>0.3%</td></tr>
<tr><td>19</td><td>Washington</td><td>16,779,905,000</td><td>1.9%</td><td>47</td><td>North Dakota</td><td>2,367,774,000</td><td>0.3%</td></tr>
<tr><td>34</td><td>West Virginia</td><td>5,825,082,000</td><td>0.7%</td><td>48</td><td>Alaska</td><td>2,041,248,000</td><td>0.2%</td></tr>
<tr><td>20</td><td>Wisconsin</td><td>16,572,139,000</td><td>1.9%</td><td>49</td><td>Vermont</td><td>1,760,664,000</td><td>0.2%</td></tr>
<tr><td>50</td><td>Wyoming</td><td>1,189,498,000</td><td>0.1%</td><td>50</td><td>Wyoming</td><td>1,189,498,000</td><td>0.1%</td></tr>
<tr><td></td><td></td><td></td><td></td><td></td><td>District of Columbia</td><td>4,881,124,000</td><td>0.6%</td></tr>
</table>

Source: Morgan Quitno Press using data from U.S. Bureau of the Census
   "1997 Economic Census, Health Care and Social Assistance" (EC97562A, October 1999)
*Includes establishments exempt from as well as subject to the federal income tax. These include those primarily engaged in furnishing medical, surgical and other health services to persons. See Facilities Chapter for establishments.

Receipts per Health Service Establishment in 1997

National Rate = $1,370,364 per Establishment*

<table>
<tr><td colspan="3">ALPHA ORDER</td><td colspan="3">RANK ORDER</td></tr>
<tr><td>RANK</td><td>STATE</td><td>PER ESTABLISHMENT</td><td>RANK</td><td>STATE</td><td>PER ESTABLISHMENT</td></tr>
<tr><td>5</td><td>Alabama</td><td>$1,552,760</td><td>1</td><td>Massachusetts</td><td>$1,671,512</td></tr>
<tr><td>32</td><td>Alaska</td><td>1,300,158</td><td>2</td><td>New York</td><td>1,627,723</td></tr>
<tr><td>38</td><td>Arizona</td><td>1,220,528</td><td>3</td><td>Mississippi</td><td>1,580,683</td></tr>
<tr><td>35</td><td>Arkansas</td><td>1,263,342</td><td>4</td><td>Tennessee</td><td>1,562,915</td></tr>
<tr><td>36</td><td>California</td><td>1,250,395</td><td>5</td><td>Alabama</td><td>1,552,760</td></tr>
<tr><td>42</td><td>Colorado</td><td>1,129,615</td><td>6</td><td>Minnesota</td><td>1,535,255</td></tr>
<tr><td>10</td><td>Connecticut</td><td>1,488,600</td><td>7</td><td>Illinois</td><td>1,527,359</td></tr>
<tr><td>15</td><td>Delaware</td><td>1,438,157</td><td>8</td><td>North Dakota</td><td>1,525,628</td></tr>
<tr><td>28</td><td>Florida</td><td>1,307,922</td><td>9</td><td>North Carolina</td><td>1,502,931</td></tr>
<tr><td>11</td><td>Georgia</td><td>1,483,086</td><td>10</td><td>Connecticut</td><td>1,488,600</td></tr>
<tr><td>22</td><td>Hawaii</td><td>1,351,688</td><td>11</td><td>Georgia</td><td>1,483,086</td></tr>
<tr><td>48</td><td>Idaho</td><td>923,630</td><td>12</td><td>Ohio</td><td>1,464,119</td></tr>
<tr><td>7</td><td>Illinois</td><td>1,527,359</td><td>13</td><td>Rhode Island</td><td>1,456,061</td></tr>
<tr><td>19</td><td>Indiana</td><td>1,409,495</td><td>14</td><td>Missouri</td><td>1,439,935</td></tr>
<tr><td>39</td><td>Iowa</td><td>1,218,292</td><td>15</td><td>Delaware</td><td>1,438,157</td></tr>
<tr><td>34</td><td>Kansas</td><td>1,278,185</td><td>16</td><td>Pennsylvania</td><td>1,436,074</td></tr>
<tr><td>18</td><td>Kentucky</td><td>1,426,882</td><td>17</td><td>Louisiana</td><td>1,432,178</td></tr>
<tr><td>17</td><td>Louisiana</td><td>1,432,178</td><td>18</td><td>Kentucky</td><td>1,426,882</td></tr>
<tr><td>44</td><td>Maine</td><td>1,117,962</td><td>19</td><td>Indiana</td><td>1,409,495</td></tr>
<tr><td>23</td><td>Maryland</td><td>1,341,244</td><td>20</td><td>West Virginia</td><td>1,374,164</td></tr>
<tr><td>1</td><td>Massachusetts</td><td>1,671,512</td><td>21</td><td>Wisconsin</td><td>1,353,159</td></tr>
<tr><td>26</td><td>Michigan</td><td>1,323,486</td><td>22</td><td>Hawaii</td><td>1,351,688</td></tr>
<tr><td>6</td><td>Minnesota</td><td>1,535,255</td><td>23</td><td>Maryland</td><td>1,341,244</td></tr>
<tr><td>3</td><td>Mississippi</td><td>1,580,683</td><td>24</td><td>South Carolina</td><td>1,334,095</td></tr>
<tr><td>14</td><td>Missouri</td><td>1,439,935</td><td>25</td><td>Virginia</td><td>1,330,452</td></tr>
<tr><td>50</td><td>Montana</td><td>869,357</td><td>26</td><td>Michigan</td><td>1,323,486</td></tr>
<tr><td>33</td><td>Nebraska</td><td>1,284,942</td><td>27</td><td>New Jersey</td><td>1,318,017</td></tr>
<tr><td>31</td><td>Nevada</td><td>1,301,387</td><td>28</td><td>Florida</td><td>1,307,922</td></tr>
<tr><td>37</td><td>New Hampshire</td><td>1,241,136</td><td>29</td><td>South Dakota</td><td>1,305,312</td></tr>
<tr><td>27</td><td>New Jersey</td><td>1,318,017</td><td>30</td><td>Texas</td><td>1,304,200</td></tr>
<tr><td>40</td><td>New Mexico</td><td>1,207,674</td><td>31</td><td>Nevada</td><td>1,301,387</td></tr>
<tr><td>2</td><td>New York</td><td>1,627,723</td><td>32</td><td>Alaska</td><td>1,300,158</td></tr>
<tr><td>9</td><td>North Carolina</td><td>1,502,931</td><td>33</td><td>Nebraska</td><td>1,284,942</td></tr>
<tr><td>8</td><td>North Dakota</td><td>1,525,628</td><td>34</td><td>Kansas</td><td>1,278,185</td></tr>
<tr><td>12</td><td>Ohio</td><td>1,464,119</td><td>35</td><td>Arkansas</td><td>1,263,342</td></tr>
<tr><td>45</td><td>Oklahoma</td><td>1,105,388</td><td>36</td><td>California</td><td>1,250,395</td></tr>
<tr><td>46</td><td>Oregon</td><td>1,020,240</td><td>37</td><td>New Hampshire</td><td>1,241,136</td></tr>
<tr><td>16</td><td>Pennsylvania</td><td>1,436,074</td><td>38</td><td>Arizona</td><td>1,220,528</td></tr>
<tr><td>13</td><td>Rhode Island</td><td>1,456,061</td><td>39</td><td>Iowa</td><td>1,218,292</td></tr>
<tr><td>24</td><td>South Carolina</td><td>1,334,095</td><td>40</td><td>New Mexico</td><td>1,207,674</td></tr>
<tr><td>29</td><td>South Dakota</td><td>1,305,312</td><td>41</td><td>Utah</td><td>1,157,153</td></tr>
<tr><td>4</td><td>Tennessee</td><td>1,562,915</td><td>42</td><td>Colorado</td><td>1,129,615</td></tr>
<tr><td>30</td><td>Texas</td><td>1,304,200</td><td>43</td><td>Washington</td><td>1,127,303</td></tr>
<tr><td>41</td><td>Utah</td><td>1,157,153</td><td>44</td><td>Maine</td><td>1,117,962</td></tr>
<tr><td>47</td><td>Vermont</td><td>949,657</td><td>45</td><td>Oklahoma</td><td>1,105,388</td></tr>
<tr><td>25</td><td>Virginia</td><td>1,330,452</td><td>46</td><td>Oregon</td><td>1,020,240</td></tr>
<tr><td>43</td><td>Washington</td><td>1,127,303</td><td>47</td><td>Vermont</td><td>949,657</td></tr>
<tr><td>20</td><td>West Virginia</td><td>1,374,164</td><td>48</td><td>Idaho</td><td>923,630</td></tr>
<tr><td>21</td><td>Wisconsin</td><td>1,353,159</td><td>49</td><td>Wyoming</td><td>877,211</td></tr>
<tr><td>49</td><td>Wyoming</td><td>877,211</td><td>50</td><td>Montana</td><td>869,357</td></tr>
<tr><td></td><td></td><td></td><td></td><td>District of Columbia</td><td>2,303,504</td></tr>
</table>

*Source: Morgan Quitno Press using data from U.S. Bureau of the Census
"1997 Economic Census, Health Care and Social Assistance" (EC97562A, October 1999)*
Includes establishments exempt from as well as subject to the federal income tax. These include those primarily engaged in furnishing medical, surgical and other health services to persons. See Facilities Chapter for establishments.

Receipts of Hospitals in 1997

National Total = $379,178,312,000*

ALPHA ORDER

RANK	STATE	RECEIPTS	% of USA
20	Alabama	$6,354,027,000	1.7%
48	Alaska	1,005,475,000	0.3%
26	Arizona	4,787,752,000	1.3%
31	Arkansas	3,531,991,000	0.9%
1	California	35,729,221,000	9.4%
27	Colorado	4,442,729,000	1.2%
25	Connecticut**	4,797,486,000	1.3%
45	Delaware**	1,157,237,000	0.3%
4	Florida	21,117,137,000	5.6%
12	Georgia	10,623,885,000	2.8%
41	Hawaii**	1,527,862,000	0.4%
44	Idaho	1,245,683,000	0.3%
6	Illinois	18,515,836,000	4.9%
16	Indiana	8,157,243,000	2.2%
30	Iowa**	4,052,045,000	1.1%
33	Kansas**	2,999,713,000	0.8%
23	Kentucky	5,603,713,000	1.5%
17	Louisiana	7,244,276,000	1.9%
40	Maine**	1,702,483,000	0.4%
18	Maryland	6,801,682,000	1.8%
10	Massachusetts	10,966,399,000	2.9%
8	Michigan	14,580,184,000	3.8%
22	Minnesota**	5,814,780,000	1.5%
28	Mississippi	4,292,837,000	1.1%
13	Missouri	9,013,034,000	2.4%
46	Montana**	1,100,902,000	0.3%
35	Nebraska**	2,346,897,000	0.6%
38	Nevada	1,882,577,000	0.5%
42	New Hampshire	1,527,161,000	0.4%
9	New Jersey	11,677,458,000	3.1%
37	New Mexico	2,030,749,000	0.5%
2	New York	33,493,372,000	8.8%
11	North Carolina	10,729,994,000	2.8%
47	North Dakota**	1,051,689,000	0.3%
7	Ohio	16,408,126,000	4.3%
29	Oklahoma	4,143,476,000	1.1%
32	Oregon	3,464,752,000	0.9%
5	Pennsylvania	20,306,035,000	5.4%
39	Rhode Island**	1,727,436,000	0.5%
24	South Carolina	5,057,641,000	1.3%
43	South Dakota	1,272,118,000	0.3%
14	Tennessee	8,623,439,000	2.3%
3	Texas	24,502,981,000	6.5%
36	Utah	2,211,878,000	0.6%
49	Vermont	689,929,000	0.2%
15	Virginia	8,373,942,000	2.2%
21	Washington	6,197,449,000	1.6%
34	West Virginia	2,961,078,000	0.8%
19	Wisconsin	6,623,633,000	1.7%
50	Wyoming	565,835,000	0.1%

RANK ORDER

RANK	STATE	RECEIPTS	% of USA
1	California	$35,729,221,000	9.4%
2	New York	33,493,372,000	8.8%
3	Texas	24,502,981,000	6.5%
4	Florida	21,117,137,000	5.6%
5	Pennsylvania	20,306,035,000	5.4%
6	Illinois	18,515,836,000	4.9%
7	Ohio	16,408,126,000	4.3%
8	Michigan	14,580,184,000	3.8%
9	New Jersey	11,677,458,000	3.1%
10	Massachusetts	10,966,399,000	2.9%
11	North Carolina	10,729,994,000	2.8%
12	Georgia	10,623,885,000	2.8%
13	Missouri	9,013,034,000	2.4%
14	Tennessee	8,623,439,000	2.3%
15	Virginia	8,373,942,000	2.2%
16	Indiana	8,157,243,000	2.2%
17	Louisiana	7,244,276,000	1.9%
18	Maryland	6,801,682,000	1.8%
19	Wisconsin	6,623,633,000	1.7%
20	Alabama	6,354,027,000	1.7%
21	Washington	6,197,449,000	1.6%
22	Minnesota**	5,814,780,000	1.5%
23	Kentucky	5,603,713,000	1.5%
24	South Carolina	5,057,641,000	1.3%
25	Connecticut**	4,797,486,000	1.3%
26	Arizona	4,787,752,000	1.3%
27	Colorado	4,442,729,000	1.2%
28	Mississippi	4,292,837,000	1.1%
29	Oklahoma	4,143,476,000	1.1%
30	Iowa**	4,052,045,000	1.1%
31	Arkansas	3,531,991,000	0.9%
32	Oregon	3,464,752,000	0.9%
33	Kansas**	2,999,713,000	0.8%
34	West Virginia	2,961,078,000	0.8%
35	Nebraska**	2,346,897,000	0.6%
36	Utah	2,211,878,000	0.6%
37	New Mexico	2,030,749,000	0.5%
38	Nevada	1,882,577,000	0.5%
39	Rhode Island**	1,727,436,000	0.5%
40	Maine**	1,702,483,000	0.4%
41	Hawaii**	1,527,862,000	0.4%
42	New Hampshire	1,527,161,000	0.4%
43	South Dakota	1,272,118,000	0.3%
44	Idaho	1,245,683,000	0.3%
45	Delaware**	1,157,237,000	0.3%
46	Montana**	1,100,902,000	0.3%
47	North Dakota**	1,051,689,000	0.3%
48	Alaska	1,005,475,000	0.3%
49	Vermont	689,929,000	0.2%
50	Wyoming	565,835,000	0.1%
	District of Columbia	2,978,620,000	0.8%

Source: Morgan Quitno Press using data from U.S. Bureau of the Census
 "1997 Economic Census, Health Care and Social Assistance" (EC97562A, October 1999)
*Includes establishments exempt from as well as subject to the federal income tax. Includes general medical and surgical hospitals, psychiatric hospitals and other specialty hospitals. Includes government owned hospitals.
**Amounts shown for these states are only for establishments exempt from federal income tax.

Receipts per Hospital in 1997

National Rate = $56,720,765 per Hospital*

ALPHA ORDER

RANK ORDER

RANK	STATE	PER HOSPITAL		RANK	STATE	PER HOSPITAL
27	Alabama	$46,379,759		1	New York	$108,392,790
39	Alaska	37,239,815		2	Delaware**	96,436,417
22	Arizona	52,040,783		3	Connecticut**	95,949,720
40	Arkansas	36,040,724		4	New Jersey	91,948,488
13	California	66,287,980		5	Rhode Island**	90,917,684
23	Colorado	51,659,640		6	Maryland	79,089,326
3	Connecticut**	95,949,720		7	Massachusetts	76,688,105
2	Delaware**	96,436,417		8	Illinois	75,884,574
11	Florida	69,236,515		9	Ohio	73,910,477
24	Georgia	51,572,257		10	Michigan	71,471,490
20	Hawaii**	54,566,500		11	Florida	69,236,515
44	Idaho	23,503,453		12	Pennsylvania	68,141,057
8	Illinois	75,884,574		13	California	66,287,980
26	Indiana	49,140,018		14	North Carolina	65,828,184
42	Iowa**	31,905,866		15	Virginia	61,573,103
46	Kansas**	21,895,715		16	South Carolina	58,809,779
30	Kentucky	43,779,008		17	Missouri	56,331,463
36	Louisiana	38,533,383		18	Nevada	55,369,912
35	Maine**	40,535,310		19	Washington	54,844,681
6	Maryland	79,089,326		20	Hawaii**	54,566,500
7	Massachusetts	76,688,105		21	Tennessee	52,581,945
10	Michigan	71,471,490		22	Arizona	52,040,783
37	Minnesota**	37,758,312		23	Colorado	51,659,640
38	Mississippi	37,329,017		24	Georgia	51,572,257
17	Missouri	56,331,463		25	Oregon	50,952,235
49	Montana**	19,658,964		26	Indiana	49,140,018
45	Nebraska**	23,468,970		27	Alabama	46,379,759
18	Nevada	55,369,912		28	Wisconsin	46,319,112
31	New Hampshire	42,421,139		29	Texas	45,460,076
4	New Jersey	91,948,488		30	Kentucky	43,779,008
41	New Mexico	32,234,111		31	New Hampshire	42,421,139
1	New York	108,392,790		32	Utah	41,733,547
14	North Carolina	65,828,184		33	West Virginia	41,705,324
47	North Dakota**	21,463,041		34	Vermont	40,584,059
9	Ohio	73,910,477		35	Maine**	40,535,310
43	Oklahoma	28,186,912		36	Louisiana	38,533,383
25	Oregon	50,952,235		37	Minnesota**	37,758,312
12	Pennsylvania	68,141,057		38	Mississippi	37,329,017
5	Rhode Island**	90,917,684		39	Alaska	37,239,815
16	South Carolina	58,809,779		40	Arkansas	36,040,724
48	South Dakota	20,518,032		41	New Mexico	32,234,111
21	Tennessee	52,581,945		42	Iowa**	31,905,866
29	Texas	45,460,076		43	Oklahoma	28,186,912
32	Utah	41,733,547		44	Idaho	23,503,453
34	Vermont	40,584,059		45	Nebraska**	23,468,970
15	Virginia	61,573,103		46	Kansas**	21,895,715
19	Washington	54,844,681		47	North Dakota**	21,463,041
33	West Virginia	41,705,324		48	South Dakota	20,518,032
28	Wisconsin	46,319,112		49	Montana**	19,658,964
50	Wyoming	18,252,742		50	Wyoming	18,252,742
					District of Columbia	165,478,889

Source: Morgan Quitno Press using data from U.S. Bureau of the Census
"1997 Economic Census, Health Care and Social Assistance" (EC97562A, October 1999)

Includes establishments exempt from as well as subject to the federal income tax. Includes general medical and surgical hospitals, psychiatric hospitals and other specialty hospitals. Includes government owned hospitals.
**Amounts shown for these states are only for establishments exempt from federal income tax.*

Receipts of Offices and Clinics of Doctors of Medicine in 1997

National Total = $168,251,883,000*

RANK	STATE	RECEIPTS	% of USA		RANK	STATE	RECEIPTS	% of USA
20	Alabama	$2,780,846,000	1.7%		1	California	$22,317,451,000	13.3%
48	Alaska	316,616,000	0.2%		2	Texas	12,439,354,000	7.4%
22	Arizona	2,684,355,000	1.6%		3	New York	11,965,964,000	7.1%
32	Arkansas	1,402,756,000	0.8%		4	Florida	11,676,140,000	6.9%
1	California	22,317,451,000	13.3%		5	Pennsylvania	7,594,668,000	4.5%
26	Colorado	2,286,435,000	1.4%		6	Illinois	7,233,092,000	4.3%
23	Connecticut	2,616,269,000	1.6%		7	Ohio	6,785,438,000	4.0%
44	Delaware	500,577,000	0.3%		8	New Jersey	6,087,711,000	3.6%
4	Florida	11,676,140,000	6.9%		9	Michigan	5,137,607,000	3.1%
10	Georgia	4,785,337,000	2.8%		10	Georgia	4,785,337,000	2.8%
38	Hawaii	720,675,000	0.4%		11	North Carolina	4,271,873,000	2.5%
42	Idaho	600,721,000	0.4%		12	Tennessee	4,137,600,000	2.5%
6	Illinois	7,233,092,000	4.3%		13	Virginia	3,983,290,000	2.4%
15	Indiana	3,475,948,000	2.1%		14	Massachusetts	3,574,465,000	2.1%
31	Iowa	1,465,067,000	0.9%		15	Indiana	3,475,948,000	2.1%
30	Kansas	1,566,643,000	0.9%		16	Maryland	3,354,135,000	2.0%
25	Kentucky	2,342,075,000	1.4%		17	Missouri	3,134,275,000	1.9%
21	Louisiana	2,741,786,000	1.6%		18	Wisconsin	3,049,648,000	1.8%
39	Maine	635,181,000	0.4%		19	Washington	2,818,141,000	1.7%
16	Maryland	3,354,135,000	2.0%		20	Alabama	2,780,846,000	1.7%
14	Massachusetts	3,574,465,000	2.1%		21	Louisiana	2,741,786,000	1.6%
9	Michigan	5,137,607,000	3.1%		22	Arizona	2,684,355,000	1.6%
24	Minnesota	2,367,336,000	1.4%		23	Connecticut	2,616,269,000	1.6%
33	Mississippi	1,392,642,000	0.8%		24	Minnesota	2,367,336,000	1.4%
17	Missouri	3,134,275,000	1.9%		25	Kentucky	2,342,075,000	1.4%
45	Montana	438,816,000	0.3%		26	Colorado	2,286,435,000	1.4%
37	Nebraska	882,168,000	0.5%		27	South Carolina	2,055,054,000	1.2%
34	Nevada	1,220,665,000	0.7%		28	Oregon	1,862,397,000	1.1%
41	New Hampshire	613,805,000	0.4%		29	Oklahoma	1,812,514,000	1.1%
8	New Jersey	6,087,711,000	3.6%		30	Kansas	1,566,643,000	0.9%
40	New Mexico	626,170,000	0.4%		31	Iowa	1,465,067,000	0.9%
3	New York	11,965,964,000	7.1%		32	Arkansas	1,402,756,000	0.8%
11	North Carolina	4,271,873,000	2.5%		33	Mississippi	1,392,642,000	0.8%
46	North Dakota	427,765,000	0.3%		34	Nevada	1,220,665,000	0.7%
7	Ohio	6,785,438,000	4.0%		35	West Virginia	1,124,036,000	0.7%
29	Oklahoma	1,812,514,000	1.1%		36	Utah	1,039,815,000	0.6%
28	Oregon	1,862,397,000	1.1%		37	Nebraska	882,168,000	0.5%
5	Pennsylvania	7,594,668,000	4.5%		38	Hawaii	720,675,000	0.4%
43	Rhode Island	525,592,000	0.3%		39	Maine	635,181,000	0.4%
27	South Carolina	2,055,054,000	1.2%		40	New Mexico	626,170,000	0.4%
47	South Dakota	424,223,000	0.3%		41	New Hampshire	613,805,000	0.4%
12	Tennessee	4,137,600,000	2.5%		42	Idaho	600,721,000	0.4%
2	Texas	12,439,354,000	7.4%		43	Rhode Island	525,592,000	0.3%
36	Utah	1,039,815,000	0.6%		44	Delaware	500,577,000	0.3%
49	Vermont	278,755,000	0.2%		45	Montana	438,816,000	0.3%
13	Virginia	3,983,290,000	2.4%		46	North Dakota	427,765,000	0.3%
19	Washington	2,818,141,000	1.7%		47	South Dakota	424,223,000	0.3%
35	West Virginia	1,124,036,000	0.7%		48	Alaska	316,616,000	0.2%
18	Wisconsin	3,049,648,000	1.8%		49	Vermont	278,755,000	0.2%
50	Wyoming	215,604,000	0.1%		50	Wyoming	215,604,000	0.1%
						District of Columbia	462,387,000	0.3%

Source: U.S. Bureau of the Census
"1997 Economic Census, Health Care and Social Assistance" (EC97562A, October 1999)
*Includes only establishments subject to the federal income tax. See Facilities Chapter for establishments.

Receipts per Office or Clinic of Doctors of Medicine in 1997

National Rate = $909,008 per Establishment*

ALPHA ORDER

RANK	STATE	PER ESTABLISHMENT
10	Alabama	$1,032,237
28	Alaska	889,371
38	Arizona	821,155
33	Arkansas	852,739
21	California	926,843
30	Colorado	884,159
13	Connecticut	983,190
31	Delaware	875,135
34	Florida	847,079
16	Georgia	941,810
47	Hawaii	705,161
39	Idaho	798,831
14	Illinois	972,190
11	Indiana	1,026,262
7	Iowa	1,141,907
5	Kansas	1,145,207
15	Kentucky	946,675
26	Louisiana	898,652
45	Maine	757,973
44	Maryland	772,308
19	Massachusetts	929,882
37	Michigan	824,127
2	Minnesota	1,945,223
23	Mississippi	916,212
12	Missouri	991,859
46	Montana	748,833
8	Nebraska	1,139,752
24	Nevada	914,356
17	New Hampshire	935,678
40	New Jersey	796,404
49	New Mexico	665,430
42	New York	790,511
9	North Carolina	1,107,277
1	North Dakota	2,239,607
27	Ohio	896,004
36	Oklahoma	828,010
25	Oregon	912,940
35	Pennsylvania	836,601
48	Rhode Island	687,948
20	South Carolina	927,371
4	South Dakota	1,277,780
6	Tennessee	1,142,983
29	Texas	885,931
32	Utah	853,007
43	Vermont	774,319
18	Virginia	931,328
22	Washington	921,563
41	West Virginia	794,372
3	Wisconsin	1,387,465
50	Wyoming	624,939

RANK ORDER

RANK	STATE	PER ESTABLISHMENT
1	North Dakota	$2,239,607
2	Minnesota	1,945,223
3	Wisconsin	1,387,465
4	South Dakota	1,277,780
5	Kansas	1,145,207
6	Tennessee	1,142,983
7	Iowa	1,141,907
8	Nebraska	1,139,752
9	North Carolina	1,107,277
10	Alabama	1,032,237
11	Indiana	1,026,262
12	Missouri	991,859
13	Connecticut	983,190
14	Illinois	972,190
15	Kentucky	946,675
16	Georgia	941,810
17	New Hampshire	935,678
18	Virginia	931,328
19	Massachusetts	929,882
20	South Carolina	927,371
21	California	926,843
22	Washington	921,563
23	Mississippi	916,212
24	Nevada	914,356
25	Oregon	912,940
26	Louisiana	898,652
27	Ohio	896,004
28	Alaska	889,371
29	Texas	885,931
30	Colorado	884,159
31	Delaware	875,135
32	Utah	853,007
33	Arkansas	852,739
34	Florida	847,079
35	Pennsylvania	836,601
36	Oklahoma	828,010
37	Michigan	824,127
38	Arizona	821,155
39	Idaho	798,831
40	New Jersey	796,404
41	West Virginia	794,372
42	New York	790,511
43	Vermont	774,319
44	Maryland	772,308
45	Maine	757,973
46	Montana	748,833
47	Hawaii	705,161
48	Rhode Island	687,948
49	New Mexico	665,430
50	Wyoming	624,939
	District of Columbia	787,712

Source: Morgan Quitno Press using data from U.S. Bureau of the Census
"1997 Economic Census, Health Care and Social Assistance" (EC97562A, October 1999)
*Includes only establishments subject to the federal income tax. See Facilities Chapter for establishments.

Receipts of Offices and Clinics of Dentists in 1997

National Total = $48,482,037,000*

ALPHA ORDER				RANK ORDER			
RANK	STATE	RECEIPTS	% of USA	RANK	STATE	RECEIPTS	% of USA
26	Alabama	$585,733,000	1.2%	1	California	$7,262,097,000	15.0%
44	Alaska	158,519,000	0.3%	2	New York	3,365,098,000	6.9%
24	Arizona	758,561,000	1.6%	3	Texas	2,811,112,000	5.8%
33	Arkansas	348,004,000	0.7%	4	Florida	2,677,391,000	5.5%
1	California	7,262,097,000	15.0%	5	Pennsylvania	2,040,175,000	4.2%
19	Colorado	833,314,000	1.7%	6	Illinois	2,032,882,000	4.2%
20	Connecticut	826,385,000	1.7%	7	Michigan	1,960,298,000	4.0%
45	Delaware	142,256,000	0.3%	8	New Jersey	1,803,107,000	3.7%
4	Florida	2,677,391,000	5.5%	9	Ohio	1,778,689,000	3.7%
12	Georgia	1,228,077,000	2.5%	10	Washington	1,554,248,000	3.2%
36	Hawaii	267,597,000	0.6%	11	Massachusetts	1,343,014,000	2.8%
40	Idaho	226,822,000	0.5%	12	Georgia	1,228,077,000	2.5%
6	Illinois	2,032,882,000	4.2%	13	North Carolina	1,171,773,000	2.4%
18	Indiana	902,891,000	1.9%	14	Virginia	1,135,960,000	2.3%
30	Iowa	430,789,000	0.9%	15	Wisconsin	979,157,000	2.0%
31	Kansas	428,608,000	0.9%	16	Maryland	952,528,000	2.0%
28	Kentucky	479,806,000	1.0%	17	Minnesota	942,837,000	1.9%
25	Louisiana	642,671,000	1.3%	18	Indiana	902,891,000	1.9%
41	Maine	205,278,000	0.4%	19	Colorado	833,314,000	1.7%
16	Maryland	952,528,000	2.0%	20	Connecticut	826,385,000	1.7%
11	Massachusetts	1,343,014,000	2.8%	21	Tennessee	813,990,000	1.7%
7	Michigan	1,960,298,000	4.0%	22	Oregon	810,438,000	1.7%
17	Minnesota	942,837,000	1.9%	23	Missouri	783,697,000	1.6%
35	Mississippi	290,042,000	0.6%	24	Arizona	758,561,000	1.6%
23	Missouri	783,697,000	1.6%	25	Louisiana	642,671,000	1.3%
46	Montana	138,694,000	0.3%	26	Alabama	585,733,000	1.2%
37	Nebraska	252,505,000	0.5%	27	South Carolina	531,705,000	1.1%
34	Nevada	328,676,000	0.7%	28	Kentucky	479,806,000	1.0%
38	New Hampshire	248,132,000	0.5%	29	Oklahoma	455,446,000	0.9%
8	New Jersey	1,803,107,000	3.7%	30	Iowa	430,789,000	0.9%
39	New Mexico	232,855,000	0.5%	31	Kansas	428,608,000	0.9%
2	New York	3,365,098,000	6.9%	32	Utah	402,171,000	0.8%
13	North Carolina	1,171,773,000	2.4%	33	Arkansas	348,004,000	0.7%
49	North Dakota	98,802,000	0.2%	34	Nevada	328,676,000	0.7%
9	Ohio	1,778,689,000	3.7%	35	Mississippi	290,042,000	0.6%
29	Oklahoma	455,446,000	0.9%	36	Hawaii	267,597,000	0.6%
22	Oregon	810,438,000	1.7%	37	Nebraska	252,505,000	0.5%
5	Pennsylvania	2,040,175,000	4.2%	38	New Hampshire	248,132,000	0.5%
43	Rhode Island	193,380,000	0.4%	39	New Mexico	232,855,000	0.5%
27	South Carolina	531,705,000	1.1%	40	Idaho	226,822,000	0.5%
48	South Dakota	109,481,000	0.2%	41	Maine	205,278,000	0.4%
21	Tennessee	813,990,000	1.7%	42	West Virginia	200,351,000	0.4%
3	Texas	2,811,112,000	5.8%	43	Rhode Island	193,380,000	0.4%
32	Utah	402,171,000	0.8%	44	Alaska	158,519,000	0.3%
47	Vermont	110,917,000	0.2%	45	Delaware	142,256,000	0.3%
14	Virginia	1,135,960,000	2.3%	46	Montana	138,694,000	0.3%
10	Washington	1,554,248,000	3.2%	47	Vermont	110,917,000	0.2%
42	West Virginia	200,351,000	0.4%	48	South Dakota	109,481,000	0.2%
15	Wisconsin	979,157,000	2.0%	49	North Dakota	98,802,000	0.2%
50	Wyoming	69,332,000	0.1%	50	Wyoming	69,332,000	0.1%
					District of Columbia	135,746,000	0.3%

Source: U.S. Bureau of the Census
   "1997 Economic Census, Health Care and Social Assistance" (EC97562A, October 1999)
*Includes only establishments subject to the federal income tax. See Facilities Chapter for establishments.

Receipts per Office or Clinic of Dentists in 1997

National Rate = $424,618 per Establishment*

ALPHA ORDER

RANK	STATE	PER ESTABLISHMENT
22	Alabama	$431,956
4	Alaska	542,873
12	Arizona	462,255
37	Arkansas	387,532
16	California	446,376
31	Colorado	408,087
10	Connecticut	465,831
1	Delaware	652,550
21	Florida	433,095
7	Georgia	477,108
32	Hawaii	407,301
14	Idaho	451,837
41	Illinois	377,649
30	Indiana	408,918
39	Iowa	387,052
24	Kansas	423,526
50	Kentucky	316,495
28	Louisiana	417,048
18	Maine	444,325
33	Maryland	401,741
13	Massachusetts	458,523
15	Michigan	450,436
9	Minnesota	470,948
43	Mississippi	371,849
40	Missouri	381,919
49	Montana	331,012
47	Nebraska	334,887
2	Nevada	571,610
11	New Hampshire	465,538
25	New Jersey	422,076
27	New Mexico	418,052
38	New York	387,060
5	North Carolina	504,422
34	North Dakota	401,634
36	Ohio	393,602
45	Oklahoma	359,185
6	Oregon	482,404
42	Pennsylvania	375,515
8	Rhode Island	471,659
19	South Carolina	437,257
29	South Dakota	410,041
35	Tennessee	397,068
26	Texas	420,133
44	Utah	369,642
20	Vermont	433,270
23	Virginia	429,474
3	Washington	549,787
46	West Virginia	340,733
17	Wisconsin	444,465
48	Wyoming	331,732

RANK ORDER

RANK	STATE	PER ESTABLISHMENT
1	Delaware	$652,550
2	Nevada	571,610
3	Washington	549,787
4	Alaska	542,873
5	North Carolina	504,422
6	Oregon	482,404
7	Georgia	477,108
8	Rhode Island	471,659
9	Minnesota	470,948
10	Connecticut	465,831
11	New Hampshire	465,538
12	Arizona	462,255
13	Massachusetts	458,523
14	Idaho	451,837
15	Michigan	450,436
16	California	446,376
17	Wisconsin	444,465
18	Maine	444,325
19	South Carolina	437,257
20	Vermont	433,270
21	Florida	433,095
22	Alabama	431,956
23	Virginia	429,474
24	Kansas	423,526
25	New Jersey	422,076
26	Texas	420,133
27	New Mexico	418,052
28	Louisiana	417,048
29	South Dakota	410,041
30	Indiana	408,918
31	Colorado	408,087
32	Hawaii	407,301
33	Maryland	401,741
34	North Dakota	401,634
35	Tennessee	397,068
36	Ohio	393,602
37	Arkansas	387,532
38	New York	387,060
39	Iowa	387,052
40	Missouri	381,919
41	Illinois	377,649
42	Pennsylvania	375,515
43	Mississippi	371,849
44	Utah	369,642
45	Oklahoma	359,185
46	West Virginia	340,733
47	Nebraska	334,887
48	Wyoming	331,732
49	Montana	331,012
50	Kentucky	316,495
	District of Columbia	412,602

Source: Morgan Quitno Press using data from U.S. Bureau of the Census
"1997 Economic Census, Health Care and Social Assistance" (EC97562A, October 1999)
*Includes only establishments subject to the federal income tax. See Facilities Chapter for establishments.

V. INCIDENCE OF DISEASE

V. INCIDENCE OF DISEASE (Continued)

Estimated New Cancer Cases in 2001

National Estimated Total = 1,268,000 New Cases*

ALPHA ORDER

RANK ORDER

RANK	STATE	CASES	% of USA	RANK	STATE	CASES	% of USA
20	Alabama	22,600	1.8%	1	California	117,400	9.3%
50	Alaska	1,600	0.1%	2	Florida	91,600	7.2%
22	Arizona	21,300	1.7%	3	New York	83,200	6.6%
31	Arkansas	14,100	1.1%	4	Texas	78,900	6.2%
1	California	117,400	9.3%	5	Pennsylvania	68,400	5.4%
30	Colorado	14,300	1.1%	6	Ohio	58,200	4.6%
28	Connecticut	16,000	1.3%	7	Illinois	56,800	4.5%
45	Delaware	4,000	0.3%	8	Michigan	45,300	3.6%
2	Florida	91,600	7.2%	9	New Jersey	41,200	3.2%
12	Georgia	31,100	2.5%	10	North Carolina	37,300	2.9%
43	Hawaii	4,700	0.4%	11	Massachusetts	31,300	2.5%
42	Idaho	5,000	0.4%	12	Georgia	31,100	2.5%
7	Illinois	56,800	4.5%	13	Virginia	30,500	2.4%
14	Indiana	29,300	2.3%	14	Indiana	29,300	2.3%
29	Iowa	14,800	1.2%	15	Tennessee	28,800	2.3%
33	Kansas	12,100	1.0%	16	Missouri	28,400	2.2%
23	Kentucky	21,100	1.7%	17	Wisconsin	25,000	2.0%
21	Louisiana	21,700	1.7%	18	Washington	24,800	2.0%
37	Maine	6,900	0.5%	19	Maryland	23,500	1.9%
19	Maryland	23,500	1.9%	20	Alabama	22,600	1.8%
11	Massachusetts	31,300	2.5%	21	Louisiana	21,700	1.7%
8	Michigan	45,300	3.6%	22	Arizona	21,300	1.7%
24	Minnesota	20,600	1.6%	23	Kentucky	21,100	1.7%
32	Mississippi	13,900	1.1%	24	Minnesota	20,600	1.6%
16	Missouri	28,400	2.2%	25	South Carolina	18,800	1.5%
44	Montana	4,300	0.3%	26	Oregon	16,700	1.3%
36	Nebraska	7,500	0.6%	27	Oklahoma	16,600	1.3%
35	Nevada	9,200	0.7%	28	Connecticut	16,000	1.3%
39	New Hampshire	5,800	0.5%	29	Iowa	14,800	1.2%
9	New Jersey	41,200	3.2%	30	Colorado	14,300	1.1%
37	New Mexico	6,900	0.5%	31	Arkansas	14,100	1.1%
3	New York	83,200	6.6%	32	Mississippi	13,900	1.1%
10	North Carolina	37,300	2.9%	33	Kansas	12,100	1.0%
47	North Dakota	3,100	0.2%	34	West Virginia	10,900	0.9%
6	Ohio	58,200	4.6%	35	Nevada	9,200	0.7%
27	Oklahoma	16,600	1.3%	36	Nebraska	7,500	0.6%
26	Oregon	16,700	1.3%	37	Maine	6,900	0.5%
5	Pennsylvania	68,400	5.4%	37	New Mexico	6,900	0.5%
40	Rhode Island	5,600	0.4%	39	New Hampshire	5,800	0.5%
25	South Carolina	18,800	1.5%	40	Rhode Island	5,600	0.4%
46	South Dakota	3,600	0.3%	40	Utah	5,600	0.4%
15	Tennessee	28,800	2.3%	42	Idaho	5,000	0.4%
4	Texas	78,900	6.2%	43	Hawaii	4,700	0.4%
40	Utah	5,600	0.4%	44	Montana	4,300	0.3%
48	Vermont	2,900	0.2%	45	Delaware	4,000	0.3%
13	Virginia	30,500	2.4%	46	South Dakota	3,600	0.3%
18	Washington	24,800	2.0%	47	North Dakota	3,100	0.2%
34	West Virginia	10,900	0.9%	48	Vermont	2,900	0.2%
17	Wisconsin	25,000	2.0%	49	Wyoming	2,200	0.2%
49	Wyoming	2,200	0.2%	50	Alaska	1,600	0.1%
					District of Columbia	2,800	0.2%

Source: American Cancer Society
   "Cancer Facts & Figures 2001" (Copyright 2001, Reprinted with permission from the American Cancer Society)
*These estimates are offered as a rough guide and should not be regarded as definitive. They are calculated according to the distribution of estimated 2001 cancer deaths by state. Totals do not include basal and squamous cell skin cancers or in situ carcinomas except urinary bladder.

Estimated Rate of New Cancer Cases in 2001

National Estimated Rate = 450.6 New Cases per 100,000 Population*

ALPHA ORDER

RANK	STATE	RATE
10	Alabama	508.2
49	Alaska	255.2
41	Arizona	415.2
6	Arkansas	527.4
47	California	346.6
48	Colorado	332.5
25	Connecticut	469.8
9	Delaware	510.5
2	Florida	573.1
44	Georgia	379.9
42	Hawaii	387.9
43	Idaho	386.4
31	Illinois	457.4
20	Indiana	481.9
13	Iowa	505.8
33	Kansas	450.1
7	Kentucky	522.0
18	Louisiana	485.6
4	Maine	541.2
35	Maryland	443.7
14	Massachusetts	493.0
32	Michigan	455.8
40	Minnesota	418.7
16	Mississippi	488.6
11	Missouri	507.6
23	Montana	476.6
37	Nebraska	438.3
30	Nevada	460.4
26	New Hampshire	469.3
15	New Jersey	489.6
45	New Mexico	379.3
36	New York	438.4
29	North Carolina	463.4
19	North Dakota	482.7
8	Ohio	512.6
21	Oklahoma	481.1
17	Oregon	488.1
3	Pennsylvania	557.0
5	Rhode Island	534.2
27	South Carolina	468.6
22	South Dakota	476.9
12	Tennessee	506.2
46	Texas	378.4
50	Utah	250.8
24	Vermont	476.3
38	Virginia	430.9
39	Washington	420.8
1	West Virginia	602.8
28	Wisconsin	466.1
34	Wyoming	445.5

RANK ORDER

RANK	STATE	RATE
1	West Virginia	602.8
2	Florida	573.1
3	Pennsylvania	557.0
4	Maine	541.2
5	Rhode Island	534.2
6	Arkansas	527.4
7	Kentucky	522.0
8	Ohio	512.6
9	Delaware	510.5
10	Alabama	508.2
11	Missouri	507.6
12	Tennessee	506.2
13	Iowa	505.8
14	Massachusetts	493.0
15	New Jersey	489.6
16	Mississippi	488.6
17	Oregon	488.1
18	Louisiana	485.6
19	North Dakota	482.7
20	Indiana	481.9
21	Oklahoma	481.1
22	South Dakota	476.9
23	Montana	476.6
24	Vermont	476.3
25	Connecticut	469.8
26	New Hampshire	469.3
27	South Carolina	468.6
28	Wisconsin	466.1
29	North Carolina	463.4
30	Nevada	460.4
31	Illinois	457.4
32	Michigan	455.8
33	Kansas	450.1
34	Wyoming	445.5
35	Maryland	443.7
36	New York	438.4
37	Nebraska	438.3
38	Virginia	430.9
39	Washington	420.8
40	Minnesota	418.7
41	Arizona	415.2
42	Hawaii	387.9
43	Idaho	386.4
44	Georgia	379.9
45	New Mexico	379.3
46	Texas	378.4
47	California	346.6
48	Colorado	332.5
49	Alaska	255.2
50	Utah	250.8
	District of Columbia	489.5

Source: Morgan Quitno Press using data from American Cancer Society
"Cancer Facts & Figures 2001" (Copyright 2001, Reprinted with permission from the American Cancer Society)
These estimates are offered as a rough guide and should not be regarded as definitive. They are calculated according to the distribution of estimated 2001 cancer deaths by state. Totals do not include basal and squamous cell skin cancers or in situ carcinomas except urinary bladder. Rates calculated using 2000 Census resident population figures

Estimated New Cases of Bladder Cancer in 2001

National Estimated Total = 54,300 New Cases*

RANK	STATE	CASES	% of USA
21	Alabama	800	1.5%
45	Alaska	100	0.2%
19	Arizona	900	1.7%
31	Arkansas	500	0.9%
1	California	5,300	9.8%
29	Colorado	600	1.1%
21	Connecticut	800	1.5%
37	Delaware	300	0.6%
2	Florida	4,400	8.1%
13	Georgia	1,100	2.0%
45	Hawaii	100	0.2%
37	Idaho	300	0.6%
7	Illinois	2,400	4.4%
12	Indiana	1,200	2.2%
25	Iowa	700	1.3%
31	Kansas	500	0.9%
25	Kentucky	700	1.3%
21	Louisiana	800	1.5%
34	Maine	400	0.7%
18	Maryland	1,000	1.8%
10	Massachusetts	1,600	2.9%
8	Michigan	2,000	3.7%
19	Minnesota	900	1.7%
34	Mississippi	400	0.7%
13	Missouri	1,100	2.0%
42	Montana	200	0.4%
37	Nebraska	300	0.6%
34	Nevada	400	0.7%
37	New Hampshire	300	0.6%
8	New Jersey	2,000	3.7%
42	New Mexico	200	0.4%
3	New York	4,200	7.7%
11	North Carolina	1,300	2.4%
45	North Dakota	100	0.2%
6	Ohio	2,500	4.6%
29	Oklahoma	600	1.1%
25	Oregon	700	1.3%
4	Pennsylvania	3,200	5.9%
42	Rhode Island	200	0.4%
25	South Carolina	700	1.3%
45	South Dakota	100	0.2%
21	Tennessee	800	1.5%
5	Texas	2,900	5.3%
37	Utah	300	0.6%
45	Vermont	100	0.2%
13	Virginia	1,100	2.0%
13	Washington	1,100	2.0%
31	West Virginia	500	0.9%
13	Wisconsin	1,100	2.0%
45	Wyoming	100	0.2%

RANK	STATE	CASES	% of USA
1	California	5,300	9.8%
2	Florida	4,400	8.1%
3	New York	4,200	7.7%
4	Pennsylvania	3,200	5.9%
5	Texas	2,900	5.3%
6	Ohio	2,500	4.6%
7	Illinois	2,400	4.4%
8	Michigan	2,000	3.7%
8	New Jersey	2,000	3.7%
10	Massachusetts	1,600	2.9%
11	North Carolina	1,300	2.4%
12	Indiana	1,200	2.2%
13	Georgia	1,100	2.0%
13	Missouri	1,100	2.0%
13	Virginia	1,100	2.0%
13	Washington	1,100	2.0%
13	Wisconsin	1,100	2.0%
18	Maryland	1,000	1.8%
19	Arizona	900	1.7%
19	Minnesota	900	1.7%
21	Alabama	800	1.5%
21	Connecticut	800	1.5%
21	Louisiana	800	1.5%
21	Tennessee	800	1.5%
25	Iowa	700	1.3%
25	Kentucky	700	1.3%
25	Oregon	700	1.3%
25	South Carolina	700	1.3%
29	Colorado	600	1.1%
29	Oklahoma	600	1.1%
31	Arkansas	500	0.9%
31	Kansas	500	0.9%
31	West Virginia	500	0.9%
34	Maine	400	0.7%
34	Mississippi	400	0.7%
34	Nevada	400	0.7%
37	Delaware	300	0.6%
37	Idaho	300	0.6%
37	Nebraska	300	0.6%
37	New Hampshire	300	0.6%
37	Utah	300	0.6%
42	Montana	200	0.4%
42	New Mexico	200	0.4%
42	Rhode Island	200	0.4%
45	Alaska	100	0.2%
45	Hawaii	100	0.2%
45	North Dakota	100	0.2%
45	South Dakota	100	0.2%
45	Vermont	100	0.2%
45	Wyoming	100	0.2%
	District of Columbia	100	0.2%

Source: American Cancer Society

"Cancer Facts & Figures 2001" (Copyright 2001, Reprinted with permission from the American Cancer Society)
*These estimates are offered as a rough guide and should be interpreted with caution. They are calculated according to the distribution of estimated 2001 cancer deaths by state.

Estimated Rate of New Cases of Bladder Cancer in 2001

National Estimated Rate = 19.3 New Cases per 100,000 Population*

ALPHA ORDER

RANK	STATE	RATE
29	Alabama	18.0
38	Alaska	16.0
31	Arizona	17.5
25	Arkansas	18.7
39	California	15.6
44	Colorado	13.9
10	Connecticut	23.5
1	Delaware	38.3
4	Florida	27.5
46	Georgia	13.4
50	Hawaii	8.3
11	Idaho	23.2
22	Illinois	19.3
20	Indiana	19.7
8	Iowa	23.9
27	Kansas	18.6
35	Kentucky	17.3
30	Louisiana	17.9
2	Maine	31.4
24	Maryland	18.9
6	Massachusetts	25.2
18	Michigan	20.1
28	Minnesota	18.3
42	Mississippi	14.1
20	Missouri	19.7
12	Montana	22.2
31	Nebraska	17.5
19	Nevada	20.0
7	New Hampshire	24.3
9	New Jersey	23.8
49	New Mexico	11.0
13	New York	22.1
37	North Carolina	16.2
39	North Dakota	15.6
14	Ohio	22.0
33	Oklahoma	17.4
15	Oregon	20.5
5	Pennsylvania	26.1
23	Rhode Island	19.1
33	South Carolina	17.4
48	South Dakota	13.2
42	Tennessee	14.1
44	Texas	13.9
46	Utah	13.4
36	Vermont	16.4
41	Virginia	15.5
25	Washington	18.7
3	West Virginia	27.6
15	Wisconsin	20.5
17	Wyoming	20.3

RANK ORDER

RANK	STATE	RATE
1	Delaware	38.3
2	Maine	31.4
3	West Virginia	27.6
4	Florida	27.5
5	Pennsylvania	26.1
6	Massachusetts	25.2
7	New Hampshire	24.3
8	Iowa	23.9
9	New Jersey	23.8
10	Connecticut	23.5
11	Idaho	23.2
12	Montana	22.2
13	New York	22.1
14	Ohio	22.0
15	Oregon	20.5
15	Wisconsin	20.5
17	Wyoming	20.3
18	Michigan	20.1
19	Nevada	20.0
20	Indiana	19.7
20	Missouri	19.7
22	Illinois	19.3
23	Rhode Island	19.1
24	Maryland	18.9
25	Arkansas	18.7
25	Washington	18.7
27	Kansas	18.6
28	Minnesota	18.3
29	Alabama	18.0
30	Louisiana	17.9
31	Arizona	17.5
31	Nebraska	17.5
33	Oklahoma	17.4
33	South Carolina	17.4
35	Kentucky	17.3
36	Vermont	16.4
37	North Carolina	16.2
38	Alaska	16.0
39	California	15.6
39	North Dakota	15.6
41	Virginia	15.5
42	Mississippi	14.1
42	Tennessee	14.1
44	Colorado	13.9
44	Texas	13.9
46	Georgia	13.4
46	Utah	13.4
48	South Dakota	13.2
49	New Mexico	11.0
50	Hawaii	8.3
	District of Columbia	17.5

Source: Morgan Quitno Press using data from American Cancer Society
"Cancer Facts & Figures 2001" (Copyright 2001, Reprinted with permission from the American Cancer Society)
These estimates are offered as a rough guide and should be interpreted with caution. They are calculated according to the distribution of estimated 2001 cancer deaths by state. Rates calculated using 2000 Census resident population figures

358

Estimated New Female Breast Cancer Cases in 2001

National Estimated Total = 192,200 New Cases*

ALPHA ORDER

RANK	STATE	CASES	% of USA
23	Alabama	2,900	1.5%
50	Alaska	200	0.1%
21	Arizona	3,200	1.7%
32	Arkansas	1,900	1.0%
1	California	18,800	9.8%
30	Colorado	2,100	1.1%
26	Connecticut	2,500	1.3%
43	Delaware	600	0.3%
3	Florida	12,500	6.5%
11	Georgia	5,000	2.6%
43	Hawaii	600	0.3%
40	Idaho	800	0.4%
6	Illinois	9,100	4.7%
14	Indiana	4,400	2.3%
29	Iowa	2,300	1.2%
33	Kansas	1,700	0.9%
23	Kentucky	2,900	1.5%
20	Louisiana	3,300	1.7%
38	Maine	1,000	0.5%
16	Maryland	4,000	2.1%
12	Massachusetts	4,600	2.4%
8	Michigan	6,800	3.5%
21	Minnesota	3,200	1.7%
31	Mississippi	2,000	1.0%
17	Missouri	3,800	2.0%
43	Montana	600	0.3%
35	Nebraska	1,200	0.6%
35	Nevada	1,200	0.6%
40	New Hampshire	800	0.4%
9	New Jersey	6,700	3.5%
37	New Mexico	1,100	0.6%
2	New York	14,200	7.4%
10	North Carolina	5,500	2.9%
46	North Dakota	500	0.3%
7	Ohio	8,900	4.6%
26	Oklahoma	2,500	1.3%
28	Oregon	2,400	1.2%
5	Pennsylvania	10,300	5.4%
40	Rhode Island	800	0.4%
25	South Carolina	2,800	1.5%
46	South Dakota	500	0.3%
15	Tennessee	4,200	2.2%
4	Texas	12,300	6.4%
38	Utah	1,000	0.5%
48	Vermont	400	0.2%
12	Virginia	4,600	2.4%
18	Washington	3,600	1.9%
34	West Virginia	1,500	0.8%
18	Wisconsin	3,600	1.9%
49	Wyoming	300	0.2%

RANK ORDER

RANK	STATE	CASES	% of USA
1	California	18,800	9.8%
2	New York	14,200	7.4%
3	Florida	12,500	6.5%
4	Texas	12,300	6.4%
5	Pennsylvania	10,300	5.4%
6	Illinois	9,100	4.7%
7	Ohio	8,900	4.6%
8	Michigan	6,800	3.5%
9	New Jersey	6,700	3.5%
10	North Carolina	5,500	2.9%
11	Georgia	5,000	2.6%
12	Massachusetts	4,600	2.4%
12	Virginia	4,600	2.4%
14	Indiana	4,400	2.3%
15	Tennessee	4,200	2.2%
16	Maryland	4,000	2.1%
17	Missouri	3,800	2.0%
18	Washington	3,600	1.9%
18	Wisconsin	3,600	1.9%
20	Louisiana	3,300	1.7%
21	Arizona	3,200	1.7%
21	Minnesota	3,200	1.7%
23	Alabama	2,900	1.5%
23	Kentucky	2,900	1.5%
25	South Carolina	2,800	1.5%
26	Connecticut	2,500	1.3%
26	Oklahoma	2,500	1.3%
28	Oregon	2,400	1.2%
29	Iowa	2,300	1.2%
30	Colorado	2,100	1.1%
31	Mississippi	2,000	1.0%
32	Arkansas	1,900	1.0%
33	Kansas	1,700	0.9%
34	West Virginia	1,500	0.8%
35	Nebraska	1,200	0.6%
35	Nevada	1,200	0.6%
37	New Mexico	1,100	0.6%
38	Maine	1,000	0.5%
38	Utah	1,000	0.5%
40	Idaho	800	0.4%
40	New Hampshire	800	0.4%
40	Rhode Island	800	0.4%
43	Delaware	600	0.3%
43	Hawaii	600	0.3%
43	Montana	600	0.3%
46	North Dakota	500	0.3%
46	South Dakota	500	0.3%
48	Vermont	400	0.2%
49	Wyoming	300	0.2%
50	Alaska	200	0.1%
	District of Columbia	600	0.3%

Source: American Cancer Society
   "Cancer Facts & Figures 2001" (Copyright 2001, Reprinted with permission from the American Cancer Society)
*These estimates are offered as a rough guide and should be interpreted with caution. They are calculated
according to the distribution of estimated 2001 cancer deaths by state.

Estimated Rate of New Female Breast Cancer in 2001

National Estimated Rate = 137.9 New Cases per 100,000 Female Population*

ALPHA ORDER

RANK	STATE	RATE
38	Alabama	127.6
50	Alaska	67.9
33	Arizona	132.6
19	Arkansas	144.1
46	California	113.5
47	Colorado	102.7
14	Connecticut	148.0
9	Delaware	154.9
2	Florida	160.6
42	Georgia	125.1
48	Hawaii	101.1
38	Idaho	127.6
15	Illinois	146.5
18	Indiana	144.2
6	Iowa	156.2
40	Kansas	126.1
22	Kentucky	142.4
16	Louisiana	145.5
7	Maine	155.9
12	Maryland	150.5
20	Massachusetts	143.9
31	Michigan	134.3
35	Minnesota	132.1
26	Mississippi	138.7
29	Missouri	134.8
27	Montana	135.1
23	Nebraska	141.0
27	Nevada	135.1
36	New Hampshire	131.1
4	New Jersey	159.6
43	New Mexico	124.5
11	New York	150.7
24	North Carolina	139.6
5	North Dakota	157.0
10	Ohio	153.0
16	Oklahoma	145.5
21	Oregon	143.0
1	Pennsylvania	165.4
8	Rhode Island	155.5
25	South Carolina	139.3
32	South Dakota	134.2
13	Tennessee	148.1
45	Texas	121.1
49	Utah	93.4
33	Vermont	132.6
37	Virginia	130.9
44	Washington	124.4
3	West Virginia	160.2
29	Wisconsin	134.8
41	Wyoming	125.7

RANK ORDER

RANK	STATE	RATE
1	Pennsylvania	165.4
2	Florida	160.6
3	West Virginia	160.2
4	New Jersey	159.6
5	North Dakota	157.0
6	Iowa	156.2
7	Maine	155.9
8	Rhode Island	155.5
9	Delaware	154.9
10	Ohio	153.0
11	New York	150.7
12	Maryland	150.5
13	Tennessee	148.1
14	Connecticut	148.0
15	Illinois	146.5
16	Louisiana	145.5
16	Oklahoma	145.5
18	Indiana	144.2
19	Arkansas	144.1
20	Massachusetts	143.9
21	Oregon	143.0
22	Kentucky	142.4
23	Nebraska	141.0
24	North Carolina	139.6
25	South Carolina	139.3
26	Mississippi	138.7
27	Montana	135.1
27	Nevada	135.1
29	Missouri	134.8
29	Wisconsin	134.8
31	Michigan	134.3
32	South Dakota	134.2
33	Arizona	132.6
33	Vermont	132.6
35	Minnesota	132.1
36	New Hampshire	131.1
37	Virginia	130.9
38	Alabama	127.6
38	Idaho	127.6
40	Kansas	126.1
41	Wyoming	125.7
42	Georgia	125.1
43	New Mexico	124.5
44	Washington	124.4
45	Texas	121.1
46	California	113.5
47	Colorado	102.7
48	Hawaii	101.1
49	Utah	93.4
50	Alaska	67.9
	District of Columbia	217.4

Source: Morgan Quitno Press using data from American Cancer Society
    "Cancer Facts & Figures 2001" (Copyright 2001, Reprinted with permission from the American Cancer Society)
*These estimates are offered as a rough guide and should be interpreted with caution. They are calculated according to the distribution of estimated 2001 cancer deaths by state. Rates calculated using 1999 Census female resident population estimates.

Percent of Women 40 and Older
Who Have Ever Had a Mammogram: 1999
National Median = 86.2% of Women 40 and Older

ALPHA ORDER

RANK	STATE	PERCENT
28	Alabama	86.0
45	Alaska	82.6
17	Arizona	88.0
48	Arkansas	81.1
NA	California*	NA
36	Colorado	84.4
1	Connecticut	91.9
3	Delaware	91.2
6	Florida	90.5
33	Georgia	85.5
13	Hawaii	88.5
39	Idaho	84.0
21	Illinois	86.6
34	Indiana	85.4
26	Iowa	86.1
29	Kansas	85.9
32	Kentucky	85.6
47	Louisiana	82.1
5	Maine	90.9
10	Maryland	89.3
7	Massachusetts	90.2
9	Michigan	89.5
39	Minnesota	84.0
49	Mississippi	80.6
43	Missouri	83.1
30	Montana	85.8
37	Nebraska	84.3
11	Nevada	88.9
15	New Hampshire	88.2
35	New Jersey	84.6
41	New Mexico	83.6
30	New York	85.8
20	North Carolina	86.7
21	North Dakota	86.6
14	Ohio	88.4
43	Oklahoma	83.1
2	Oregon	91.5
15	Pennsylvania	88.2
4	Rhode Island	91.0
19	South Carolina	87.4
23	South Dakota	86.3
37	Tennessee	84.3
25	Texas	86.2
26	Utah	86.1
18	Vermont	87.8
23	Virginia	86.3
8	Washington	90.0
45	West Virginia	82.6
12	Wisconsin	88.8
42	Wyoming	83.3

RANK ORDER

RANK	STATE	PERCENT
1	Connecticut	91.9
2	Oregon	91.5
3	Delaware	91.2
4	Rhode Island	91.0
5	Maine	90.9
6	Florida	90.5
7	Massachusetts	90.2
8	Washington	90.0
9	Michigan	89.5
10	Maryland	89.3
11	Nevada	88.9
12	Wisconsin	88.8
13	Hawaii	88.5
14	Ohio	88.4
15	New Hampshire	88.2
15	Pennsylvania	88.2
17	Arizona	88.0
18	Vermont	87.8
19	South Carolina	87.4
20	North Carolina	86.7
21	Illinois	86.6
21	North Dakota	86.6
23	South Dakota	86.3
23	Virginia	86.3
25	Texas	86.2
26	Iowa	86.1
26	Utah	86.1
28	Alabama	86.0
29	Kansas	85.9
30	Montana	85.8
30	New York	85.8
32	Kentucky	85.6
33	Georgia	85.5
34	Indiana	85.4
35	New Jersey	84.6
36	Colorado	84.4
37	Nebraska	84.3
37	Tennessee	84.3
39	Idaho	84.0
39	Minnesota	84.0
41	New Mexico	83.6
42	Wyoming	83.3
43	Missouri	83.1
43	Oklahoma	83.1
45	Alaska	82.6
45	West Virginia	82.6
47	Louisiana	82.1
48	Arkansas	81.1
49	Mississippi	80.6
NA	California*	NA

District of Columbia   89.5

Source: U.S. Department of Health and Human Services, Centers for Disease Control and Prevention
"1999 Behavioral Risk Factor Surveillance Summary Prevalence Report" (June 23, 2000)
*Not available.

Estimated New Colon and Rectum Cancer Cases in 2001

National Estimated Total = 135,400 New Cases*

ALPHA ORDER

RANK	STATE	CASES	% of USA
24	Alabama	2,000	1.5%
50	Alaska	100	0.1%
21	Arizona	2,200	1.6%
31	Arkansas	1,300	1.0%
1	California	11,700	8.6%
30	Colorado	1,500	1.1%
28	Connecticut	1,600	1.2%
44	Delaware	400	0.3%
3	Florida	9,400	6.9%
15	Georgia	2,900	2.1%
42	Hawaii	500	0.4%
42	Idaho	500	0.4%
7	Illinois	6,200	4.6%
12	Indiana	3,200	2.4%
26	Iowa	1,900	1.4%
33	Kansas	1,200	0.9%
21	Kentucky	2,200	1.6%
19	Louisiana	2,400	1.8%
37	Maine	700	0.5%
17	Maryland	2,700	2.0%
11	Massachusetts	3,600	2.7%
8	Michigan	4,900	3.6%
23	Minnesota	2,100	1.6%
31	Mississippi	1,300	1.0%
14	Missouri	3,100	2.3%
44	Montana	400	0.3%
35	Nebraska	1,000	0.7%
35	Nevada	1,000	0.7%
40	New Hampshire	600	0.4%
9	New Jersey	4,500	3.3%
37	New Mexico	700	0.5%
2	New York	9,700	7.2%
10	North Carolina	4,000	3.0%
48	North Dakota	300	0.2%
6	Ohio	6,400	4.7%
27	Oklahoma	1,800	1.3%
28	Oregon	1,600	1.2%
5	Pennsylvania	8,000	5.9%
40	Rhode Island	600	0.4%
24	South Carolina	2,000	1.5%
44	South Dakota	400	0.3%
15	Tennessee	2,900	2.1%
4	Texas	8,700	6.4%
37	Utah	700	0.5%
44	Vermont	400	0.3%
12	Virginia	3,200	2.4%
19	Washington	2,400	1.8%
34	West Virginia	1,100	0.8%
18	Wisconsin	2,600	1.9%
48	Wyoming	300	0.2%

RANK ORDER

RANK	STATE	CASES	% of USA
1	California	11,700	8.6%
2	New York	9,700	7.2%
3	Florida	9,400	6.9%
4	Texas	8,700	6.4%
5	Pennsylvania	8,000	5.9%
6	Ohio	6,400	4.7%
7	Illinois	6,200	4.6%
8	Michigan	4,900	3.6%
9	New Jersey	4,500	3.3%
10	North Carolina	4,000	3.0%
11	Massachusetts	3,600	2.7%
12	Indiana	3,200	2.4%
12	Virginia	3,200	2.4%
14	Missouri	3,100	2.3%
15	Georgia	2,900	2.1%
15	Tennessee	2,900	2.1%
17	Maryland	2,700	2.0%
18	Wisconsin	2,600	1.9%
19	Louisiana	2,400	1.8%
19	Washington	2,400	1.8%
21	Arizona	2,200	1.6%
21	Kentucky	2,200	1.6%
23	Minnesota	2,100	1.6%
24	Alabama	2,000	1.5%
24	South Carolina	2,000	1.5%
26	Iowa	1,900	1.4%
27	Oklahoma	1,800	1.3%
28	Connecticut	1,600	1.2%
28	Oregon	1,600	1.2%
30	Colorado	1,500	1.1%
31	Arkansas	1,300	1.0%
31	Mississippi	1,300	1.0%
33	Kansas	1,200	0.9%
34	West Virginia	1,100	0.8%
35	Nebraska	1,000	0.7%
35	Nevada	1,000	0.7%
37	Maine	700	0.5%
37	New Mexico	700	0.5%
37	Utah	700	0.5%
40	New Hampshire	600	0.4%
40	Rhode Island	600	0.4%
42	Hawaii	500	0.4%
42	Idaho	500	0.4%
44	Delaware	400	0.3%
44	Montana	400	0.3%
44	South Dakota	400	0.3%
44	Vermont	400	0.3%
48	North Dakota	300	0.2%
48	Wyoming	300	0.2%
50	Alaska	100	0.1%
	District of Columbia	300	0.2%

Source: American Cancer Society

"Cancer Facts & Figures 2001" (Copyright 2001, Reprinted with permission from the American Cancer Society)
*These estimates are offered as a rough guide and should be interpreted with caution. They are calculated according to the distribution of estimated 2001 cancer deaths by state.

Estimated Rate of New Colon and Rectum Cancer Cases in 2001

National Estimated Rate = 48.1 New Cases per 100,000 Population*

ALPHA ORDER

RANK	STATE	RATE
36	Alabama	45.0
50	Alaska	16.0
39	Arizona	42.9
28	Arkansas	48.6
48	California	34.5
47	Colorado	34.9
31	Connecticut	47.0
20	Delaware	51.0
6	Florida	58.8
46	Georgia	35.4
42	Hawaii	41.3
44	Idaho	38.6
24	Illinois	49.9
17	Indiana	52.6
3	Iowa	64.9
37	Kansas	44.6
13	Kentucky	54.4
14	Louisiana	53.7
12	Maine	54.9
20	Maryland	51.0
9	Massachusetts	56.7
27	Michigan	49.3
40	Minnesota	42.7
34	Mississippi	45.7
11	Missouri	55.4
38	Montana	44.3
7	Nebraska	58.4
23	Nevada	50.0
28	New Hampshire	48.6
15	New Jersey	53.5
45	New Mexico	38.5
19	New York	51.1
26	North Carolina	49.7
33	North Dakota	46.7
10	Ohio	56.4
18	Oklahoma	52.2
32	Oregon	46.8
2	Pennsylvania	65.1
8	Rhode Island	57.2
24	South Carolina	49.9
16	South Dakota	53.0
20	Tennessee	51.0
41	Texas	41.7
49	Utah	31.3
1	Vermont	65.7
35	Virginia	45.2
43	Washington	40.7
4	West Virginia	60.8
30	Wisconsin	48.5
4	Wyoming	60.8

RANK ORDER

RANK	STATE	RATE
1	Vermont	65.7
2	Pennsylvania	65.1
3	Iowa	64.9
4	West Virginia	60.8
4	Wyoming	60.8
6	Florida	58.8
7	Nebraska	58.4
8	Rhode Island	57.2
9	Massachusetts	56.7
10	Ohio	56.4
11	Missouri	55.4
12	Maine	54.9
13	Kentucky	54.4
14	Louisiana	53.7
15	New Jersey	53.5
16	South Dakota	53.0
17	Indiana	52.6
18	Oklahoma	52.2
19	New York	51.1
20	Delaware	51.0
20	Maryland	51.0
20	Tennessee	51.0
23	Nevada	50.0
24	Illinois	49.9
24	South Carolina	49.9
26	North Carolina	49.7
27	Michigan	49.3
28	Arkansas	48.6
28	New Hampshire	48.6
30	Wisconsin	48.5
31	Connecticut	47.0
32	Oregon	46.8
33	North Dakota	46.7
34	Mississippi	45.7
35	Virginia	45.2
36	Alabama	45.0
37	Kansas	44.6
38	Montana	44.3
39	Arizona	42.9
40	Minnesota	42.7
41	Texas	41.7
42	Hawaii	41.3
43	Washington	40.7
44	Idaho	38.6
45	New Mexico	38.5
46	Georgia	35.4
47	Colorado	34.9
48	California	34.5
49	Utah	31.3
50	Alaska	16.0
	District of Columbia	52.4

Source: Morgan Quitno Press using data from American Cancer Society
"Cancer Facts & Figures 2001" (Copyright 2001, Reprinted with permission from the American Cancer Society)
These estimates are offered as a rough guide and should be interpreted with caution. They are calculated according to the distribution of estimated 2001 cancer deaths by state. Rates calculated using 2000 Census resident population figures

Estimated New Leukemia Cases in 2001

National Estimated Total = 31,500 New Cases*

ALPHA ORDER					RANK ORDER			

RANK	STATE	CASES	% of USA
20	Alabama	500	1.6%
NA	Alaska**	NA	NA
20	Arizona	500	1.6%
27	Arkansas	400	1.3%
1	California	3,000	9.5%
27	Colorado	400	1.3%
27	Connecticut	400	1.3%
39	Delaware	100	0.3%
2	Florida	2,300	7.3%
11	Georgia	700	2.2%
39	Hawaii	100	0.3%
39	Idaho	100	0.3%
6	Illinois	1,500	4.8%
11	Indiana	700	2.2%
20	Iowa	500	1.6%
32	Kansas	300	1.0%
20	Kentucky	500	1.6%
20	Louisiana	500	1.6%
39	Maine	100	0.3%
20	Maryland	500	1.6%
11	Massachusetts	700	2.2%
8	Michigan	1,100	3.5%
19	Minnesota	600	1.9%
32	Mississippi	300	1.0%
11	Missouri	700	2.2%
39	Montana	100	0.3%
35	Nebraska	200	0.6%
35	Nevada	200	0.6%
39	New Hampshire	100	0.3%
8	New Jersey	1,100	3.5%
35	New Mexico	200	0.6%
3	New York	2,000	6.3%
10	North Carolina	900	2.9%
39	North Dakota	100	0.3%
7	Ohio	1,400	4.4%
27	Oklahoma	400	1.3%
27	Oregon	400	1.3%
5	Pennsylvania	1,700	5.4%
39	Rhode Island	100	0.3%
20	South Carolina	500	1.6%
39	South Dakota	100	0.3%
11	Tennessee	700	2.2%
3	Texas	2,000	6.3%
35	Utah	200	0.6%
39	Vermont	100	0.3%
11	Virginia	700	2.2%
11	Washington	700	2.2%
32	West Virginia	300	1.0%
11	Wisconsin	700	2.2%
39	Wyoming	100	0.3%

RANK	STATE	CASES	% of USA
1	California	3,000	9.5%
2	Florida	2,300	7.3%
3	New York	2,000	6.3%
3	Texas	2,000	6.3%
5	Pennsylvania	1,700	5.4%
6	Illinois	1,500	4.8%
7	Ohio	1,400	4.4%
8	Michigan	1,100	3.5%
8	New Jersey	1,100	3.5%
10	North Carolina	900	2.9%
11	Georgia	700	2.2%
11	Indiana	700	2.2%
11	Massachusetts	700	2.2%
11	Missouri	700	2.2%
11	Tennessee	700	2.2%
11	Virginia	700	2.2%
11	Washington	700	2.2%
11	Wisconsin	700	2.2%
19	Minnesota	600	1.9%
20	Alabama	500	1.6%
20	Arizona	500	1.6%
20	Iowa	500	1.6%
20	Kentucky	500	1.6%
20	Louisiana	500	1.6%
20	Maryland	500	1.6%
20	South Carolina	500	1.6%
27	Arkansas	400	1.3%
27	Colorado	400	1.3%
27	Connecticut	400	1.3%
27	Oklahoma	400	1.3%
27	Oregon	400	1.3%
32	Kansas	300	1.0%
32	Mississippi	300	1.0%
32	West Virginia	300	1.0%
35	Nebraska	200	0.6%
35	Nevada	200	0.6%
35	New Mexico	200	0.6%
35	Utah	200	0.6%
39	Delaware	100	0.3%
39	Hawaii	100	0.3%
39	Idaho	100	0.3%
39	Maine	100	0.3%
39	Montana	100	0.3%
39	New Hampshire	100	0.3%
39	North Dakota	100	0.3%
39	Rhode Island	100	0.3%
39	South Dakota	100	0.3%
39	Vermont	100	0.3%
39	Wyoming	100	0.3%
NA	Alaska**	NA	NA
	District of Columbia**	NA	NA

Source: American Cancer Society
"Cancer Facts & Figures 2001" (Copyright 2001, Reprinted with permission from the American Cancer Society)
These estimates are offered as a rough guide and should be interpreted with caution. They are calculated according to the distribution of estimated 2001 cancer deaths by state.

Estimated Rate of New Leukemia Cases in 2001

National Estimated Rate = 11.2 New Cases per 100,000 Population*

ALPHA ORDER

RANK	STATE	RATE
26	Alabama	11.2
NA	Alaska**	NA
38	Arizona	9.7
6	Arkansas	15.0
44	California	8.9
42	Colorado	9.3
21	Connecticut	11.7
12	Delaware	12.8
7	Florida	14.4
45	Georgia	8.6
46	Hawaii	8.3
49	Idaho	7.7
19	Illinois	12.1
25	Indiana	11.5
2	Iowa	17.1
26	Kansas	11.2
15	Kentucky	12.4
26	Louisiana	11.2
48	Maine	7.8
41	Maryland	9.4
32	Massachusetts	11.0
30	Michigan	11.1
18	Minnesota	12.2
34	Mississippi	10.5
13	Missouri	12.5
30	Montana	11.1
21	Nebraska	11.7
36	Nevada	10.0
47	New Hampshire	8.1
10	New Jersey	13.1
32	New Mexico	11.0
34	New York	10.5
26	North Carolina	11.2
5	North Dakota	15.6
16	Ohio	12.3
24	Oklahoma	11.6
21	Oregon	11.7
8	Pennsylvania	13.8
40	Rhode Island	9.5
13	South Carolina	12.5
9	South Dakota	13.2
16	Tennessee	12.3
39	Texas	9.6
43	Utah	9.0
4	Vermont	16.4
37	Virginia	9.9
20	Washington	11.9
3	West Virginia	16.6
10	Wisconsin	13.1
1	Wyoming	20.3

RANK ORDER

RANK	STATE	RATE
1	Wyoming	20.3
2	Iowa	17.1
3	West Virginia	16.6
4	Vermont	16.4
5	North Dakota	15.6
6	Arkansas	15.0
7	Florida	14.4
8	Pennsylvania	13.8
9	South Dakota	13.2
10	New Jersey	13.1
10	Wisconsin	13.1
12	Delaware	12.8
13	Missouri	12.5
13	South Carolina	12.5
15	Kentucky	12.4
16	Ohio	12.3
16	Tennessee	12.3
18	Minnesota	12.2
19	Illinois	12.1
20	Washington	11.9
21	Connecticut	11.7
21	Nebraska	11.7
21	Oregon	11.7
24	Oklahoma	11.6
25	Indiana	11.5
26	Alabama	11.2
26	Kansas	11.2
26	Louisiana	11.2
26	North Carolina	11.2
30	Michigan	11.1
30	Montana	11.1
32	Massachusetts	11.0
32	New Mexico	11.0
34	Mississippi	10.5
34	New York	10.5
36	Nevada	10.0
37	Virginia	9.9
38	Arizona	9.7
39	Texas	9.6
40	Rhode Island	9.5
41	Maryland	9.4
42	Colorado	9.3
43	Utah	9.0
44	California	8.9
45	Georgia	8.6
46	Hawaii	8.3
47	New Hampshire	8.1
48	Maine	7.8
49	Idaho	7.7
NA	Alaska**	NA
	District of Columbia**	NA

Source: Morgan Quitno Press using data from American Cancer Society
"Cancer Facts & Figures 2001" (Copyright 2001, Reprinted with permission from the American Cancer Society)
*These estimates are offered as a rough guide and should be interpreted with caution. They are calculated according to the distribution of estimated 2001 cancer deaths by state. Rates calculated using 2000 Census resident population figures

Estimated New Lung Cancer Cases in 2001

National Estimated Total = 169,500 New Cases*

ALPHA ORDER					RANK ORDER			
RANK	STATE		CASES	% of USA	RANK	STATE	CASES	% of USA
20	Alabama		3,100	1.8%	1	California	14,200	8.4%
50	Alaska		200	0.1%	2	Florida	12,900	7.6%
23	Arizona		2,800	1.7%	3	Texas	11,000	6.5%
28	Arkansas		2,200	1.3%	4	New York	10,000	5.9%
1	California		14,200	8.4%	5	Pennsylvania	8,900	5.3%
33	Colorado		1,600	0.9%	6	Ohio	8,100	4.8%
29	Connecticut		2,000	1.2%	7	Illinois	7,400	4.4%
41	Delaware		600	0.4%	8	Michigan	6,200	3.7%
2	Florida		12,900	7.6%	9	North Carolina	5,400	3.2%
11	Georgia		4,400	2.6%	10	New Jersey	5,000	2.9%
41	Hawaii		600	0.4%	11	Georgia	4,400	2.6%
41	Idaho		600	0.4%	12	Missouri	4,300	2.5%
7	Illinois		7,400	4.4%	12	Tennessee	4,300	2.5%
14	Indiana		4,200	2.5%	14	Indiana	4,200	2.5%
31	Iowa		1,900	1.1%	14	Virginia	4,200	2.5%
33	Kansas		1,600	0.9%	16	Massachusetts	4,000	2.4%
17	Kentucky		3,400	2.0%	17	Kentucky	3,400	2.0%
22	Louisiana		2,900	1.7%	18	Washington	3,300	1.9%
36	Maine		1,000	0.6%	19	Maryland	3,200	1.9%
19	Maryland		3,200	1.9%	20	Alabama	3,100	1.8%
16	Massachusetts		4,000	2.4%	21	Wisconsin	3,000	1.8%
8	Michigan		6,200	3.7%	22	Louisiana	2,900	1.7%
26	Minnesota		2,400	1.4%	23	Arizona	2,800	1.7%
29	Mississippi		2,000	1.2%	24	Oklahoma	2,600	1.5%
12	Missouri		4,300	2.5%	24	South Carolina	2,600	1.5%
41	Montana		600	0.4%	26	Minnesota	2,400	1.4%
37	Nebraska		900	0.5%	27	Oregon	2,300	1.4%
35	Nevada		1,300	0.8%	28	Arkansas	2,200	1.3%
38	New Hampshire		800	0.5%	29	Connecticut	2,000	1.2%
10	New Jersey		5,000	2.9%	29	Mississippi	2,000	1.2%
38	New Mexico		800	0.5%	31	Iowa	1,900	1.1%
4	New York		10,000	5.9%	32	West Virginia	1,700	1.0%
9	North Carolina		5,400	3.2%	33	Colorado	1,600	0.9%
45	North Dakota		400	0.2%	33	Kansas	1,600	0.9%
6	Ohio		8,100	4.8%	35	Nevada	1,300	0.8%
24	Oklahoma		2,600	1.5%	36	Maine	1,000	0.6%
27	Oregon		2,300	1.4%	37	Nebraska	900	0.5%
5	Pennsylvania		8,900	5.3%	38	New Hampshire	800	0.5%
38	Rhode Island		800	0.5%	38	New Mexico	800	0.5%
24	South Carolina		2,600	1.5%	38	Rhode Island	800	0.5%
45	South Dakota		400	0.2%	41	Delaware	600	0.4%
12	Tennessee		4,300	2.5%	41	Hawaii	600	0.4%
3	Texas		11,000	6.5%	41	Idaho	600	0.4%
45	Utah		400	0.2%	41	Montana	600	0.4%
45	Vermont		400	0.2%	45	North Dakota	400	0.2%
14	Virginia		4,200	2.5%	45	South Dakota	400	0.2%
18	Washington		3,300	1.9%	45	Utah	400	0.2%
32	West Virginia		1,700	1.0%	45	Vermont	400	0.2%
21	Wisconsin		3,000	1.8%	49	Wyoming	300	0.2%
49	Wyoming		300	0.2%	50	Alaska	200	0.1%
						District of Columbia	300	0.2%

Source: American Cancer Society
   "Cancer Facts & Figures 2001" (Copyright 2001, Reprinted with permission from the American Cancer Society)
These estimates are offered as a rough guide and should be interpreted with caution. They are calculated according to the distribution of estimated 2001 cancer deaths by state.

Estimated Rate of New Lung Cancer Cases in 2001

National Estimated Rate = 60.2 New Cases per 100,000 Population*

ALPHA ORDER

RANK	STATE	RATE
14	Alabama	69.7
49	Alaska	31.9
37	Arizona	54.6
3	Arkansas	82.3
47	California	41.9
48	Colorado	37.2
34	Connecticut	58.7
7	Delaware	76.6
4	Florida	80.7
38	Georgia	53.7
43	Hawaii	49.5
45	Idaho	46.4
30	Illinois	59.6
15	Indiana	69.1
21	Iowa	64.9
31	Kansas	59.5
2	Kentucky	84.1
21	Louisiana	64.9
5	Maine	78.4
29	Maryland	60.4
25	Massachusetts	63.0
26	Michigan	62.4
44	Minnesota	48.8
13	Mississippi	70.3
6	Missouri	76.9
18	Montana	66.5
42	Nebraska	52.6
20	Nevada	65.1
24	New Hampshire	64.7
32	New Jersey	59.4
46	New Mexico	44.0
41	New York	52.7
17	North Carolina	67.1
27	North Dakota	62.3
12	Ohio	71.3
10	Oklahoma	75.3
16	Oregon	67.2
11	Pennsylvania	72.5
8	Rhode Island	76.3
23	South Carolina	64.8
39	South Dakota	53.0
9	Tennessee	75.6
40	Texas	52.8
50	Utah	17.9
19	Vermont	65.7
33	Virginia	59.3
35	Washington	56.0
1	West Virginia	94.0
36	Wisconsin	55.9
28	Wyoming	60.8

RANK ORDER

RANK	STATE	RATE
1	West Virginia	94.0
2	Kentucky	84.1
3	Arkansas	82.3
4	Florida	80.7
5	Maine	78.4
6	Missouri	76.9
7	Delaware	76.6
8	Rhode Island	76.3
9	Tennessee	75.6
10	Oklahoma	75.3
11	Pennsylvania	72.5
12	Ohio	71.3
13	Mississippi	70.3
14	Alabama	69.7
15	Indiana	69.1
16	Oregon	67.2
17	North Carolina	67.1
18	Montana	66.5
19	Vermont	65.7
20	Nevada	65.1
21	Iowa	64.9
21	Louisiana	64.9
23	South Carolina	64.8
24	New Hampshire	64.7
25	Massachusetts	63.0
26	Michigan	62.4
27	North Dakota	62.3
28	Wyoming	60.8
29	Maryland	60.4
30	Illinois	59.6
31	Kansas	59.5
32	New Jersey	59.4
33	Virginia	59.3
34	Connecticut	58.7
35	Washington	56.0
36	Wisconsin	55.9
37	Arizona	54.6
38	Georgia	53.7
39	South Dakota	53.0
40	Texas	52.8
41	New York	52.7
42	Nebraska	52.6
43	Hawaii	49.5
44	Minnesota	48.8
45	Idaho	46.4
46	New Mexico	44.0
47	California	41.9
48	Colorado	37.2
49	Alaska	31.9
50	Utah	17.9

District of Columbia	52.4

*Source: Morgan Quitno Press using data from American Cancer Society
"Cancer Facts & Figures 2001" (Copyright 2001, Reprinted with permission from the American Cancer Society)*
*These estimates are offered as a rough guide and should be interpreted with caution. They are calculated according to the distribution of estimated 2001 cancer deaths by state. Rates calculated using 2000 Census resident population figures

Estimated New Non-Hodgkin's Lymphoma Cases in 2001

National Estimated Total = 56,200 New Cases*

RANK	STATE	CASES	% of USA
24	Alabama	800	1.4%
47	Alaska	100	0.2%
20	Arizona	1,000	1.8%
31	Arkansas	600	1.1%
1	California	5,300	9.4%
27	Colorado	700	1.2%
24	Connecticut	800	1.4%
43	Delaware	200	0.4%
2	Florida	4,200	7.5%
18	Georgia	1,100	2.0%
36	Hawaii	300	0.5%
43	Idaho	200	0.4%
7	Illinois	2,500	4.4%
12	Indiana	1,300	2.3%
27	Iowa	700	1.2%
32	Kansas	500	0.9%
21	Kentucky	900	1.6%
21	Louisiana	900	1.6%
36	Maine	300	0.5%
21	Maryland	900	1.6%
10	Massachusetts	1,400	2.5%
8	Michigan	2,200	3.9%
14	Minnesota	1,200	2.1%
32	Mississippi	500	0.9%
14	Missouri	1,200	2.1%
43	Montana	200	0.4%
36	Nebraska	300	0.5%
35	Nevada	400	0.7%
36	New Hampshire	300	0.5%
9	New Jersey	2,000	3.6%
36	New Mexico	300	0.5%
3	New York	3,700	6.6%
10	North Carolina	1,400	2.5%
47	North Dakota	100	0.2%
6	Ohio	2,700	4.8%
27	Oklahoma	700	1.2%
24	Oregon	800	1.4%
5	Pennsylvania	3,000	5.3%
36	Rhode Island	300	0.5%
27	South Carolina	700	1.2%
43	South Dakota	200	0.4%
14	Tennessee	1,200	2.1%
4	Texas	3,600	6.4%
36	Utah	300	0.5%
47	Vermont	100	0.2%
14	Virginia	1,200	2.1%
18	Washington	1,100	2.0%
32	West Virginia	500	0.9%
12	Wisconsin	1,300	2.3%
47	Wyoming	100	0.2%

RANK	STATE	CASES	% of USA
1	California	5,300	9.4%
2	Florida	4,200	7.5%
3	New York	3,700	6.6%
4	Texas	3,600	6.4%
5	Pennsylvania	3,000	5.3%
6	Ohio	2,700	4.8%
7	Illinois	2,500	4.4%
8	Michigan	2,200	3.9%
9	New Jersey	2,000	3.6%
10	Massachusetts	1,400	2.5%
10	North Carolina	1,400	2.5%
12	Indiana	1,300	2.3%
12	Wisconsin	1,300	2.3%
14	Minnesota	1,200	2.1%
14	Missouri	1,200	2.1%
14	Tennessee	1,200	2.1%
14	Virginia	1,200	2.1%
18	Georgia	1,100	2.0%
18	Washington	1,100	2.0%
20	Arizona	1,000	1.8%
21	Kentucky	900	1.6%
21	Louisiana	900	1.6%
21	Maryland	900	1.6%
24	Alabama	800	1.4%
24	Connecticut	800	1.4%
24	Oregon	800	1.4%
27	Colorado	700	1.2%
27	Iowa	700	1.2%
27	Oklahoma	700	1.2%
27	South Carolina	700	1.2%
31	Arkansas	600	1.1%
32	Kansas	500	0.9%
32	Mississippi	500	0.9%
32	West Virginia	500	0.9%
35	Nevada	400	0.7%
36	Hawaii	300	0.5%
36	Maine	300	0.5%
36	Nebraska	300	0.5%
36	New Hampshire	300	0.5%
36	New Mexico	300	0.5%
36	Rhode Island	300	0.5%
36	Utah	300	0.5%
43	Delaware	200	0.4%
43	Idaho	200	0.4%
43	Montana	200	0.4%
43	South Dakota	200	0.4%
47	Alaska	100	0.2%
47	North Dakota	100	0.2%
47	Vermont	100	0.2%
47	Wyoming	100	0.2%
	District of Columbia	100	0.2%

Source: American Cancer Society

"Cancer Facts & Figures 2001" (Copyright 2001, Reprinted with permission from the American Cancer Society)
These estimates are offered as a rough guide and should be interpreted with caution. They are calculated according to the distribution of estimated 2001 cancer deaths by state.

Estimated Rate of New Non-Hodgkin's Lymphoma Cases in 2001

National Estimated Rate = 20.0 New Cases per 100,000 Population*

ALPHA ORDER

RANK	STATE	RATE
34	Alabama	18.0
45	Alaska	16.0
30	Arizona	19.5
17	Arkansas	22.4
46	California	15.6
44	Colorado	16.3
14	Connecticut	23.5
5	Delaware	25.5
4	Florida	26.3
49	Georgia	13.4
6	Hawaii	24.8
48	Idaho	15.5
27	Illinois	20.1
22	Indiana	21.4
11	Iowa	23.9
33	Kansas	18.6
18	Kentucky	22.3
27	Louisiana	20.1
14	Maine	23.5
40	Maryland	17.0
20	Massachusetts	22.1
20	Michigan	22.1
7	Minnesota	24.4
35	Mississippi	17.6
22	Missouri	21.4
19	Montana	22.2
36	Nebraska	17.5
29	Nevada	20.0
9	New Hampshire	24.3
12	New Jersey	23.8
42	New Mexico	16.5
30	New York	19.5
37	North Carolina	17.4
46	North Dakota	15.6
12	Ohio	23.8
25	Oklahoma	20.3
16	Oregon	23.4
7	Pennsylvania	24.4
1	Rhode Island	28.6
37	South Carolina	17.4
3	South Dakota	26.5
24	Tennessee	21.1
39	Texas	17.3
49	Utah	13.4
43	Vermont	16.4
40	Virginia	17.0
32	Washington	18.7
2	West Virginia	27.6
10	Wisconsin	24.2
25	Wyoming	20.3

RANK ORDER

RANK	STATE	RATE
1	Rhode Island	28.6
2	West Virginia	27.6
3	South Dakota	26.5
4	Florida	26.3
5	Delaware	25.5
6	Hawaii	24.8
7	Minnesota	24.4
7	Pennsylvania	24.4
9	New Hampshire	24.3
10	Wisconsin	24.2
11	Iowa	23.9
12	New Jersey	23.8
12	Ohio	23.8
14	Connecticut	23.5
14	Maine	23.5
16	Oregon	23.4
17	Arkansas	22.4
18	Kentucky	22.3
19	Montana	22.2
20	Massachusetts	22.1
20	Michigan	22.1
22	Indiana	21.4
22	Missouri	21.4
24	Tennessee	21.1
25	Oklahoma	20.3
25	Wyoming	20.3
27	Illinois	20.1
27	Louisiana	20.1
29	Nevada	20.0
30	Arizona	19.5
30	New York	19.5
32	Washington	18.7
33	Kansas	18.6
34	Alabama	18.0
35	Mississippi	17.6
36	Nebraska	17.5
37	North Carolina	17.4
37	South Carolina	17.4
39	Texas	17.3
40	Maryland	17.0
40	Virginia	17.0
42	New Mexico	16.5
43	Vermont	16.4
44	Colorado	16.3
45	Alaska	16.0
46	California	15.6
46	North Dakota	15.6
48	Idaho	15.5
49	Georgia	13.4
49	Utah	13.4
	District of Columbia	17.5

Source: Morgan Quitno Press using data from American Cancer Society
  "Cancer Facts & Figures 2001" (Copyright 2001, Reprinted with permission from the American Cancer Society)
*These estimates are offered as a rough guide and should be interpreted with caution. They are calculated
according to the distribution of estimated 2001 cancer deaths by state. Rates calculated using 2000 Census
resident population figures

Estimated New Prostate Cancer Cases in 2001

National Estimated Total = 198,100 New Cases*

RANK	STATE	CASES	% of USA
16	Alabama	4,100	2.1%
50	Alaska	200	0.1%
20	Arizona	3,600	1.8%
30	Arkansas	2,400	1.2%
1	California	17,500	8.8%
32	Colorado	2,100	1.1%
27	Connecticut	2,500	1.3%
45	Delaware	600	0.3%
2	Florida	15,000	7.6%
11	Georgia	4,900	2.5%
44	Hawaii	700	0.4%
39	Idaho	900	0.5%
6	Illinois	9,000	4.5%
14	Indiana	4,400	2.2%
27	Iowa	2,500	1.3%
33	Kansas	2,000	1.0%
26	Kentucky	2,800	1.4%
22	Louisiana	3,500	1.8%
39	Maine	900	0.5%
19	Maryland	3,700	1.9%
13	Massachusetts	4,600	2.3%
8	Michigan	7,100	3.6%
20	Minnesota	3,600	1.8%
27	Mississippi	2,500	1.3%
17	Missouri	4,000	2.0%
41	Montana	800	0.4%
38	Nebraska	1,200	0.6%
36	Nevada	1,300	0.7%
41	New Hampshire	800	0.4%
9	New Jersey	6,200	3.1%
36	New Mexico	1,300	0.7%
3	New York	12,700	6.4%
10	North Carolina	6,000	3.0%
47	North Dakota	500	0.3%
7	Ohio	8,700	4.4%
31	Oklahoma	2,200	1.1%
25	Oregon	3,000	1.5%
5	Pennsylvania	10,900	5.5%
41	Rhode Island	800	0.4%
24	South Carolina	3,200	1.6%
45	South Dakota	600	0.3%
18	Tennessee	3,900	2.0%
4	Texas	12,500	6.3%
34	Utah	1,400	0.7%
49	Vermont	300	0.2%
11	Virginia	4,900	2.5%
23	Washington	3,400	1.7%
34	West Virginia	1,400	0.7%
15	Wisconsin	4,300	2.2%
48	Wyoming	400	0.2%

RANK	STATE	CASES	% of USA
1	California	17,500	8.8%
2	Florida	15,000	7.6%
3	New York	12,700	6.4%
4	Texas	12,500	6.3%
5	Pennsylvania	10,900	5.5%
6	Illinois	9,000	4.5%
7	Ohio	8,700	4.4%
8	Michigan	7,100	3.6%
9	New Jersey	6,200	3.1%
10	North Carolina	6,000	3.0%
11	Georgia	4,900	2.5%
11	Virginia	4,900	2.5%
13	Massachusetts	4,600	2.3%
14	Indiana	4,400	2.2%
15	Wisconsin	4,300	2.2%
16	Alabama	4,100	2.1%
17	Missouri	4,000	2.0%
18	Tennessee	3,900	2.0%
19	Maryland	3,700	1.9%
20	Arizona	3,600	1.8%
20	Minnesota	3,600	1.8%
22	Louisiana	3,500	1.8%
23	Washington	3,400	1.7%
24	South Carolina	3,200	1.6%
25	Oregon	3,000	1.5%
26	Kentucky	2,800	1.4%
27	Connecticut	2,500	1.3%
27	Iowa	2,500	1.3%
27	Mississippi	2,500	1.3%
30	Arkansas	2,400	1.2%
31	Oklahoma	2,200	1.1%
32	Colorado	2,100	1.1%
33	Kansas	2,000	1.0%
34	Utah	1,400	0.7%
34	West Virginia	1,400	0.7%
36	Nevada	1,300	0.7%
36	New Mexico	1,300	0.7%
38	Nebraska	1,200	0.6%
39	Idaho	900	0.5%
39	Maine	900	0.5%
41	Montana	800	0.4%
41	New Hampshire	800	0.4%
41	Rhode Island	800	0.4%
44	Hawaii	700	0.4%
45	Delaware	600	0.3%
45	South Dakota	600	0.3%
47	North Dakota	500	0.3%
48	Wyoming	400	0.2%
49	Vermont	300	0.2%
50	Alaska	200	0.1%
	District of Columbia	500	0.3%

Source: American Cancer Society
"Cancer Facts & Figures 2001" (Copyright 2001, Reprinted with permission from the American Cancer Society)
*These estimates are offered as a rough guide and should be interpreted with caution. They are calculated according to the distribution of estimated 2001 cancer deaths by state.

Estimated Rate of New Prostate Cancer Cases in 2001

National Estimated Rate = 148.6 New Cases per 100,000 Male Population*

ALPHA ORDER

RANK	STATE	RATE
2	Alabama	195.5
50	Alaska	61.5
25	Arizona	152.3
3	Arkansas	194.7
47	California	105.6
48	Colorado	104.4
21	Connecticut	157.0
15	Delaware	163.8
1	Florida	204.6
43	Georgia	129.2
46	Hawaii	118.2
38	Idaho	144.1
27	Illinois	152.1
26	Indiana	152.2
8	Iowa	178.9
23	Kansas	153.2
36	Kentucky	145.6
12	Louisiana	166.4
33	Maine	147.2
33	Maryland	147.2
22	Massachusetts	154.5
30	Michigan	147.9
24	Minnesota	153.0
5	Mississippi	188.4
29	Missouri	151.0
7	Montana	182.3
32	Nebraska	147.3
39	Nevada	141.1
40	New Hampshire	135.4
20	New Jersey	157.1
28	New Mexico	151.9
37	New York	144.8
16	North Carolina	161.7
19	North Dakota	158.6
18	Ohio	159.9
41	Oklahoma	134.2
6	Oregon	183.2
4	Pennsylvania	189.1
10	Rhode Island	168.0
9	South Carolina	170.7
12	South Dakota	166.4
31	Tennessee	147.4
44	Texas	126.4
42	Utah	132.2
49	Vermont	102.7
35	Virginia	145.9
45	Washington	118.8
17	West Virginia	160.9
11	Wisconsin	166.7
14	Wyoming	166.0

RANK ORDER

RANK	STATE	RATE
1	Florida	204.6
2	Alabama	195.5
3	Arkansas	194.7
4	Pennsylvania	189.1
5	Mississippi	188.4
6	Oregon	183.2
7	Montana	182.3
8	Iowa	178.9
9	South Carolina	170.7
10	Rhode Island	168.0
11	Wisconsin	166.7
12	Louisiana	166.4
12	South Dakota	166.4
14	Wyoming	166.0
15	Delaware	163.8
16	North Carolina	161.7
17	West Virginia	160.9
18	Ohio	159.9
19	North Dakota	158.6
20	New Jersey	157.1
21	Connecticut	157.0
22	Massachusetts	154.5
23	Kansas	153.2
24	Minnesota	153.0
25	Arizona	152.3
26	Indiana	152.2
27	Illinois	152.1
28	New Mexico	151.9
29	Missouri	151.0
30	Michigan	147.9
31	Tennessee	147.4
32	Nebraska	147.3
33	Maine	147.2
33	Maryland	147.2
35	Virginia	145.9
36	Kentucky	145.6
37	New York	144.8
38	Idaho	144.1
39	Nevada	141.1
40	New Hampshire	135.4
41	Oklahoma	134.2
42	Utah	132.2
43	Georgia	129.2
44	Texas	126.4
45	Washington	118.8
46	Hawaii	118.2
47	California	105.6
48	Colorado	104.4
49	Vermont	102.7
50	Alaska	61.5
	District of Columbia	205.7

Source: Morgan Quitno Press using data from American Cancer Society
"Cancer Facts & Figures 2001" (Copyright 2001, Reprinted with permission from the American Cancer Society)
*These estimates are offered as a rough guide and should be interpreted with caution. They are calculated according to the distribution of estimated 2001 cancer deaths by state. Rates calculated using 1999 Census male resident population estimates.

Estimated New Skin Melanoma Cases in 2001

National Estimated Total = 51,400 New Cases*

ALPHA ORDER

RANK	STATE	CASES	% of USA
20	Alabama	900	1.8%
47	Alaska	100	0.2%
17	Arizona	1,100	2.1%
31	Arkansas	500	1.0%
1	California	5,300	10.3%
22	Colorado	800	1.6%
27	Connecticut	700	1.4%
41	Delaware	200	0.4%
2	Florida	3,800	7.4%
14	Georgia	1,200	2.3%
47	Hawaii	100	0.2%
37	Idaho	300	0.6%
6	Illinois	2,100	4.1%
17	Indiana	1,100	2.1%
31	Iowa	500	1.0%
29	Kansas	600	1.2%
20	Kentucky	900	1.8%
27	Louisiana	700	1.4%
37	Maine	300	0.6%
22	Maryland	800	1.6%
10	Massachusetts	1,400	2.7%
9	Michigan	1,600	3.1%
22	Minnesota	800	1.6%
31	Mississippi	500	1.0%
14	Missouri	1,200	2.3%
41	Montana	200	0.4%
37	Nebraska	300	0.6%
34	Nevada	400	0.8%
41	New Hampshire	200	0.4%
8	New Jersey	1,800	3.5%
37	New Mexico	300	0.6%
4	New York	2,800	5.4%
10	North Carolina	1,400	2.7%
47	North Dakota	100	0.2%
6	Ohio	2,100	4.1%
22	Oklahoma	800	1.6%
22	Oregon	800	1.6%
5	Pennsylvania	2,700	5.3%
41	Rhode Island	200	0.4%
29	South Carolina	600	1.2%
41	South Dakota	200	0.4%
10	Tennessee	1,400	2.7%
3	Texas	3,400	6.6%
34	Utah	400	0.8%
41	Vermont	200	0.4%
13	Virginia	1,300	2.5%
14	Washington	1,200	2.3%
34	West Virginia	400	0.8%
17	Wisconsin	1,100	2.1%
47	Wyoming	100	0.2%

RANK ORDER

RANK	STATE	CASES	% of USA
1	California	5,300	10.3%
2	Florida	3,800	7.4%
3	Texas	3,400	6.6%
4	New York	2,800	5.4%
5	Pennsylvania	2,700	5.3%
6	Illinois	2,100	4.1%
6	Ohio	2,100	4.1%
8	New Jersey	1,800	3.5%
9	Michigan	1,600	3.1%
10	Massachusetts	1,400	2.7%
10	North Carolina	1,400	2.7%
10	Tennessee	1,400	2.7%
13	Virginia	1,300	2.5%
14	Georgia	1,200	2.3%
14	Missouri	1,200	2.3%
14	Washington	1,200	2.3%
17	Arizona	1,100	2.1%
17	Indiana	1,100	2.1%
17	Wisconsin	1,100	2.1%
20	Alabama	900	1.8%
20	Kentucky	900	1.8%
22	Colorado	800	1.6%
22	Maryland	800	1.6%
22	Minnesota	800	1.6%
22	Oklahoma	800	1.6%
22	Oregon	800	1.6%
27	Connecticut	700	1.4%
27	Louisiana	700	1.4%
29	Kansas	600	1.2%
29	South Carolina	600	1.2%
31	Arkansas	500	1.0%
31	Iowa	500	1.0%
31	Mississippi	500	1.0%
34	Nevada	400	0.8%
34	Utah	400	0.8%
34	West Virginia	400	0.8%
37	Idaho	300	0.6%
37	Maine	300	0.6%
37	Nebraska	300	0.6%
37	New Mexico	300	0.6%
41	Delaware	200	0.4%
41	Montana	200	0.4%
41	New Hampshire	200	0.4%
41	Rhode Island	200	0.4%
41	South Dakota	200	0.4%
41	Vermont	200	0.4%
47	Alaska	100	0.2%
47	Hawaii	100	0.2%
47	North Dakota	100	0.2%
47	Wyoming	100	0.2%
	District of Columbia**	NA	NA

Source: American Cancer Society
 "Cancer Facts & Figures 2001" (Copyright 2001, Reprinted with permission from the American Cancer Society)
*These estimates are offered as a rough guide and should be interpreted with caution. They are calculated according to the distribution of estimated 2001 cancer deaths by state.

Estimated Rate of New Skin Melanoma Cases in 2001

National Estimated Rate = 18.3 New Cases per 100,000 Population*

ALPHA ORDER

RANK	STATE	RATE
23	Alabama	20.2
42	Alaska	16.0
16	Arizona	21.4
26	Arkansas	18.7
44	California	15.6
27	Colorado	18.6
19	Connecticut	20.6
3	Delaware	25.5
5	Florida	23.8
49	Georgia	14.7
50	Hawaii	8.3
8	Idaho	23.2
36	Illinois	16.9
30	Indiana	18.1
35	Iowa	17.1
10	Kansas	22.3
10	Kentucky	22.3
43	Louisiana	15.7
6	Maine	23.5
46	Maryland	15.1
13	Massachusetts	22.1
41	Michigan	16.1
38	Minnesota	16.3
32	Mississippi	17.6
16	Missouri	21.4
12	Montana	22.2
33	Nebraska	17.5
24	Nevada	20.0
40	New Hampshire	16.2
16	New Jersey	21.4
37	New Mexico	16.5
48	New York	14.8
34	North Carolina	17.4
44	North Dakota	15.6
28	Ohio	18.5
8	Oklahoma	23.2
7	Oregon	23.4
15	Pennsylvania	22.0
25	Rhode Island	19.1
47	South Carolina	15.0
2	South Dakota	26.5
4	Tennessee	24.6
38	Texas	16.3
31	Utah	17.9
1	Vermont	32.9
29	Virginia	18.4
21	Washington	20.4
13	West Virginia	22.1
20	Wisconsin	20.5
22	Wyoming	20.3

RANK ORDER

RANK	STATE	RATE
1	Vermont	32.9
2	South Dakota	26.5
3	Delaware	25.5
4	Tennessee	24.6
5	Florida	23.8
6	Maine	23.5
7	Oregon	23.4
8	Idaho	23.2
8	Oklahoma	23.2
10	Kansas	22.3
10	Kentucky	22.3
12	Montana	22.2
13	Massachusetts	22.1
13	West Virginia	22.1
15	Pennsylvania	22.0
16	Arizona	21.4
16	Missouri	21.4
16	New Jersey	21.4
19	Connecticut	20.6
20	Wisconsin	20.5
21	Washington	20.4
22	Wyoming	20.3
23	Alabama	20.2
24	Nevada	20.0
25	Rhode Island	19.1
26	Arkansas	18.7
27	Colorado	18.6
28	Ohio	18.5
29	Virginia	18.4
30	Indiana	18.1
31	Utah	17.9
32	Mississippi	17.6
33	Nebraska	17.5
34	North Carolina	17.4
35	Iowa	17.1
36	Illinois	16.9
37	New Mexico	16.5
38	Minnesota	16.3
38	Texas	16.3
40	New Hampshire	16.2
41	Michigan	16.1
42	Alaska	16.0
43	Louisiana	15.7
44	California	15.6
44	North Dakota	15.6
46	Maryland	15.1
47	South Carolina	15.0
48	New York	14.8
49	Georgia	14.7
50	Hawaii	8.3

District of Columbia**   NA

Source: Morgan Quitno Press using data from American Cancer Society
    "Cancer Facts & Figures 2001" (Copyright 2001, Reprinted with permission from the American Cancer Society)
*These estimates are offered as a rough guide and should be interpreted with caution. They are calculated
according to the distribution of estimated 2001 cancer deaths by state. Rates calculated using 2000 Census
resident population figures

Estimated New Cancer of the Uterus (Cervix) Cases in 2001

National Estimated Total = 12,900 New Cases*

ALPHA ORDER

RANK	STATE	CASES	% of USA
19	Alabama	200	1.6%
NA	Alaska**	NA	NA
19	Arizona	200	1.6%
19	Arkansas	200	1.6%
1	California	1,400	10.9%
28	Colorado	100	0.8%
28	Connecticut	100	0.8%
28	Delaware	100	0.8%
3	Florida	900	7.0%
8	Georgia	400	3.1%
NA	Hawaii**	NA	NA
NA	Idaho**	NA	NA
5	Illinois	600	4.7%
12	Indiana	300	2.3%
28	Iowa	100	0.8%
28	Kansas	100	0.8%
19	Kentucky	200	1.6%
12	Louisiana	300	2.3%
28	Maine	100	0.8%
12	Maryland	300	2.3%
12	Massachusetts	300	2.3%
8	Michigan	400	3.1%
28	Minnesota	100	0.8%
19	Mississippi	200	1.6%
12	Missouri	300	2.3%
NA	Montana**	NA	NA
28	Nebraska	100	0.8%
28	Nevada	100	0.8%
NA	New Hampshire**	NA	NA
8	New Jersey	400	3.1%
28	New Mexico	100	0.8%
3	New York	900	7.0%
8	North Carolina	400	3.1%
NA	North Dakota**	NA	NA
5	Ohio	600	4.7%
19	Oklahoma	200	1.6%
28	Oregon	100	0.8%
5	Pennsylvania	600	4.7%
28	Rhode Island	100	0.8%
19	South Carolina	200	1.6%
NA	South Dakota**	NA	NA
12	Tennessee	300	2.3%
2	Texas	1,000	7.8%
NA	Utah**	NA	NA
NA	Vermont**	NA	NA
12	Virginia	300	2.3%
19	Washington	200	1.6%
28	West Virginia	100	0.8%
19	Wisconsin	200	1.6%
NA	Wyoming**	NA	NA

RANK ORDER

RANK	STATE	CASES	% of USA
1	California	1,400	10.9%
2	Texas	1,000	7.8%
3	Florida	900	7.0%
3	New York	900	7.0%
5	Illinois	600	4.7%
5	Ohio	600	4.7%
5	Pennsylvania	600	4.7%
8	Georgia	400	3.1%
8	Michigan	400	3.1%
8	New Jersey	400	3.1%
8	North Carolina	400	3.1%
12	Indiana	300	2.3%
12	Louisiana	300	2.3%
12	Maryland	300	2.3%
12	Massachusetts	300	2.3%
12	Missouri	300	2.3%
12	Tennessee	300	2.3%
12	Virginia	300	2.3%
19	Alabama	200	1.6%
19	Arizona	200	1.6%
19	Arkansas	200	1.6%
19	Kentucky	200	1.6%
19	Mississippi	200	1.6%
19	Oklahoma	200	1.6%
19	South Carolina	200	1.6%
19	Washington	200	1.6%
19	Wisconsin	200	1.6%
28	Colorado	100	0.8%
28	Connecticut	100	0.8%
28	Delaware	100	0.8%
28	Iowa	100	0.8%
28	Kansas	100	0.8%
28	Maine	100	0.8%
28	Minnesota	100	0.8%
28	Nebraska	100	0.8%
28	Nevada	100	0.8%
28	New Mexico	100	0.8%
28	Oregon	100	0.8%
28	Rhode Island	100	0.8%
28	West Virginia	100	0.8%
NA	Alaska**	NA	NA
NA	Hawaii**	NA	NA
NA	Idaho**	NA	NA
NA	Montana**	NA	NA
NA	New Hampshire**	NA	NA
NA	North Dakota**	NA	NA
NA	South Dakota**	NA	NA
NA	Utah**	NA	NA
NA	Vermont**	NA	NA
NA	Wyoming**	NA	NA
	District of Columbia**	NA	NA

Source: American Cancer Society
"Cancer Facts & Figures 2001" (Copyright 2001, Reprinted with permission from the American Cancer Society)
*These estimates are offered as a rough guide and should be interpreted with caution. They are calculated according to the distribution of estimated 2001 cancer deaths by state.

Estimated Rate of New Cancer of the Uterus (Cervix) Cases in 2001

National Estimated Rate = 9.3 New Cases per 100,000 Female Population*

ALPHA ORDER

RANK	STATE	RATE
28	Alabama	8.8
NA	Alaska**	NA
31	Arizona	8.3
4	Arkansas	15.2
29	California	8.5
39	Colorado	4.9
38	Connecticut	5.9
1	Delaware	25.8
8	Florida	11.6
18	Georgia	10.0
NA	Hawaii**	NA
NA	Idaho**	NA
23	Illinois	9.7
20	Indiana	9.8
36	Iowa	6.8
34	Kansas	7.4
20	Kentucky	9.8
6	Louisiana	13.2
3	Maine	15.6
10	Maryland	11.3
27	Massachusetts	9.4
32	Michigan	7.9
40	Minnesota	4.1
5	Mississippi	13.9
14	Missouri	10.6
NA	Montana**	NA
7	Nebraska	11.7
10	Nevada	11.3
NA	New Hampshire**	NA
25	New Jersey	9.5
10	New Mexico	11.3
25	New York	9.5
17	North Carolina	10.2
NA	North Dakota**	NA
16	Ohio	10.3
8	Oklahoma	11.6
37	Oregon	6.0
24	Pennsylvania	9.6
2	Rhode Island	19.4
19	South Carolina	9.9
NA	South Dakota**	NA
14	Tennessee	10.6
20	Texas	9.8
NA	Utah**	NA
NA	Vermont**	NA
29	Virginia	8.5
35	Washington	6.9
13	West Virginia	10.7
33	Wisconsin	7.5
NA	Wyoming**	NA

RANK ORDER

RANK	STATE	RATE
1	Delaware	25.8
2	Rhode Island	19.4
3	Maine	15.6
4	Arkansas	15.2
5	Mississippi	13.9
6	Louisiana	13.2
7	Nebraska	11.7
8	Florida	11.6
8	Oklahoma	11.6
10	Maryland	11.3
10	Nevada	11.3
10	New Mexico	11.3
13	West Virginia	10.7
14	Missouri	10.6
14	Tennessee	10.6
16	Ohio	10.3
17	North Carolina	10.2
18	Georgia	10.0
19	South Carolina	9.9
20	Indiana	9.8
20	Kentucky	9.8
20	Texas	9.8
23	Illinois	9.7
24	Pennsylvania	9.6
25	New Jersey	9.5
25	New York	9.5
27	Massachusetts	9.4
28	Alabama	8.8
29	California	8.5
29	Virginia	8.5
31	Arizona	8.3
32	Michigan	7.9
33	Wisconsin	7.5
34	Kansas	7.4
35	Washington	6.9
36	Iowa	6.8
37	Oregon	6.0
38	Connecticut	5.9
39	Colorado	4.9
40	Minnesota	4.1
NA	Alaska**	NA
NA	Hawaii**	NA
NA	Idaho**	NA
NA	Montana**	NA
NA	New Hampshire**	NA
NA	North Dakota**	NA
NA	South Dakota**	NA
NA	Utah**	NA
NA	Vermont**	NA
NA	Wyoming**	NA
	District of Columbia**	NA

Source: Morgan Quitno Press using data from American Cancer Society
"Cancer Facts & Figures 2001" (Copyright 2001, Reprinted with permission from the American Cancer Society)
*These estimates are offered as a rough guide and should be interpreted with caution. They are calculated according to the distribution of estimated 2001 cancer deaths by state. Rates calculated using 1999 Census female resident population estimates.

Percent of Women 18 Years and Older
Who Had a Pap Smear Within the Past Three Years: 1999
National Median = 85.4% of Women 18 Years and Older*

ALPHA ORDER				RANK ORDER		
RANK	STATE	PERCENT		RANK	STATE	PERCENT
16	Alabama	86.6		1	Alaska	90.9
1	Alaska	90.9		1	North Carolina	90.9
19	Arizona	86.1		3	Maine	89.5
44	Arkansas	82.6		4	Maryland	89.2
NA	California**	NA		5	New Hampshire	88.4
12	Colorado	87.4		5	Vermont	88.4
7	Connecticut	88.3		7	Connecticut	88.3
9	Delaware	87.7		8	Georgia	88.0
27	Florida	85.3		9	Delaware	87.7
8	Georgia	88.0		10	Oregon	87.6
14	Hawaii	87.1		11	Minnesota	87.5
48	Idaho	79.3		12	Colorado	87.4
31	Illinois	84.9		12	Kansas	87.4
45	Indiana	82.4		14	Hawaii	87.1
27	Iowa	85.3		15	South Carolina	87.0
12	Kansas	87.4		16	Alabama	86.6
42	Kentucky	83.4		16	North Dakota	86.6
25	Louisiana	85.4		18	Massachusetts	86.2
3	Maine	89.5		19	Arizona	86.1
4	Maryland	89.2		20	Rhode Island	86.0
18	Massachusetts	86.2		21	Washington	85.9
22	Michigan	85.8		22	Michigan	85.8
11	Minnesota	87.5		23	Ohio	85.5
37	Mississippi	84.1		23	Virginia	85.5
34	Missouri	84.6		25	Louisiana	85.4
29	Montana	85.2		25	South Dakota	85.4
32	Nebraska	84.8		27	Florida	85.3
49	Nevada	78.5		27	Iowa	85.3
5	New Hampshire	88.4		29	Montana	85.2
35	New Jersey	84.3		30	Tennessee	85.1
40	New Mexico	83.7		31	Illinois	84.9
36	New York	84.2		32	Nebraska	84.8
1	North Carolina	90.9		33	Wisconsin	84.7
16	North Dakota	86.6		34	Missouri	84.6
23	Ohio	85.5		35	New Jersey	84.3
38	Oklahoma	83.8		36	New York	84.2
10	Oregon	87.6		37	Mississippi	84.1
41	Pennsylvania	83.6		38	Oklahoma	83.8
20	Rhode Island	86.0		38	Wyoming	83.8
15	South Carolina	87.0		40	New Mexico	83.7
25	South Dakota	85.4		41	Pennsylvania	83.6
30	Tennessee	85.1		42	Kentucky	83.4
43	Texas	82.7		43	Texas	82.7
46	Utah	80.8		44	Arkansas	82.6
5	Vermont	88.4		45	Indiana	82.4
23	Virginia	85.5		46	Utah	80.8
21	Washington	85.9		47	West Virginia	80.7
47	West Virginia	80.7		48	Idaho	79.3
33	Wisconsin	84.7		49	Nevada	78.5
38	Wyoming	83.8		NA	California**	NA
					District of Columbia	90.8

Source: U.S. Department of Health and Human Services, Centers for Disease Control and Prevention
   "1999 Behavioral Risk Factor Surveillance Summary Prevalence Report" (June 23, 2000)
*Of women with intact cervix. Pap smear is a test for cancer, especially of the female genital tract. Named after George Papanicolaou (1883-1962), American anatomist.
**Not available.

376

AIDS Cases Reported in 2000

National Total = 36,091 New AIDS Cases*

RANK	STATE	CASES	% of USA
20	Alabama	457	1.3%
45	Alaska	22	0.1%
21	Arizona	427	1.2%
31	Arkansas	172	0.5%
3	California	4,479	12.4%
26	Colorado	300	0.8%
17	Connecticut	546	1.5%
28	Delaware	199	0.6%
2	Florida	4,613	12.8%
10	Georgia	1,117	3.1%
37	Hawaii	99	0.3%
46	Idaho	20	0.1%
5	Illinois	1,693	4.7%
24	Indiana	352	1.0%
39	Iowa	86	0.2%
36	Kansas	121	0.3%
30	Kentucky	186	0.5%
16	Louisiana	649	1.8%
42	Maine	38	0.1%
8	Maryland	1,197	3.3%
9	Massachusetts	1,137	3.2%
15	Michigan	652	1.8%
33	Minnesota	160	0.4%
22	Mississippi	395	1.1%
23	Missouri	368	1.0%
47	Montana	14	0.0%
40	Nebraska	68	0.2%
27	Nevada	275	0.8%
44	New Hampshire	31	0.1%
6	New Jersey	1,592	4.4%
34	New Mexico	140	0.4%
1	New York	4,634	12.8%
14	North Carolina	667	1.8%
50	North Dakota	3	0.0%
17	Ohio	546	1.5%
25	Oklahoma	320	0.9%
32	Oregon	171	0.5%
7	Pennsylvania	1,479	4.1%
38	Rhode Island	95	0.3%
13	South Carolina	755	2.1%
49	South Dakota	7	0.0%
11	Tennessee	771	2.1%
4	Texas	2,567	7.1%
35	Utah	137	0.4%
43	Vermont	37	0.1%
12	Virginia	764	2.1%
19	Washington	480	1.3%
41	West Virginia	60	0.2%
28	Wisconsin	199	0.6%
48	Wyoming	9	0.0%

RANK	STATE	CASES	% of USA
1	New York	4,634	12.8%
2	Florida	4,613	12.8%
3	California	4,479	12.4%
4	Texas	2,567	7.1%
5	Illinois	1,693	4.7%
6	New Jersey	1,592	4.4%
7	Pennsylvania	1,479	4.1%
8	Maryland	1,197	3.3%
9	Massachusetts	1,137	3.2%
10	Georgia	1,117	3.1%
11	Tennessee	771	2.1%
12	Virginia	764	2.1%
13	South Carolina	755	2.1%
14	North Carolina	667	1.8%
15	Michigan	652	1.8%
16	Louisiana	649	1.8%
17	Connecticut	546	1.5%
17	Ohio	546	1.5%
19	Washington	480	1.3%
20	Alabama	457	1.3%
21	Arizona	427	1.2%
22	Mississippi	395	1.1%
23	Missouri	368	1.0%
24	Indiana	352	1.0%
25	Oklahoma	320	0.9%
26	Colorado	300	0.8%
27	Nevada	275	0.8%
28	Delaware	199	0.6%
28	Wisconsin	199	0.6%
30	Kentucky	186	0.5%
31	Arkansas	172	0.5%
32	Oregon	171	0.5%
33	Minnesota	160	0.4%
34	New Mexico	140	0.4%
35	Utah	137	0.4%
36	Kansas	121	0.3%
37	Hawaii	99	0.3%
38	Rhode Island	95	0.3%
39	Iowa	86	0.2%
40	Nebraska	68	0.2%
41	West Virginia	60	0.2%
42	Maine	38	0.1%
43	Vermont	37	0.1%
44	New Hampshire	31	0.1%
45	Alaska	22	0.1%
46	Idaho	20	0.1%
47	Montana	14	0.0%
48	Wyoming	9	0.0%
49	South Dakota	7	0.0%
50	North Dakota	3	0.0%
	District of Columbia	785	2.2%

Source: U.S. Department of Health and Human Services, National Center for Health Statistics
"Morbidity and Mortality Weekly Report" (January 5, 2001, Vol. 49, No. 51)
*Provisional data. AIDS is Acquired Immunodeficiency Syndrome. It is a specific group of diseases or conditions which are indicative of severe immunosuppression related to infection with the Human Immunodeficiency Virus (HIV). National total does not include 589 cases in Puerto Rico.

AIDS Rate in 2000

National Rate = 12.8 New AIDS Cases Reported per 100,000 Population*

ALPHA ORDER

RANK	STATE	RATE
19	Alabama	10.3
40	Alaska	3.5
22	Arizona	8.3
30	Arkansas	6.4
15	California	13.2
27	Colorado	7.0
8	Connecticut	16.0
2	Delaware	25.4
1	Florida	28.9
12	Georgia	13.6
24	Hawaii	8.2
48	Idaho	1.5
12	Illinois	13.6
33	Indiana	5.8
44	Iowa	2.9
37	Kansas	4.5
36	Kentucky	4.6
9	Louisiana	14.5
43	Maine	3.0
4	Maryland	22.6
7	Massachusetts	17.9
28	Michigan	6.6
41	Minnesota	3.3
10	Mississippi	13.9
28	Missouri	6.6
47	Montana	1.6
38	Nebraska	4.0
11	Nevada	13.8
45	New Hampshire	2.5
5	New Jersey	18.9
26	New Mexico	7.7
3	New York	24.4
22	North Carolina	8.3
50	North Dakota	0.5
35	Ohio	4.8
20	Oklahoma	9.3
34	Oregon	5.0
17	Pennsylvania	12.0
21	Rhode Island	9.1
6	South Carolina	18.8
49	South Dakota	0.9
12	Tennessee	13.6
16	Texas	12.3
31	Utah	6.1
31	Vermont	6.1
18	Virginia	10.8
25	Washington	8.1
41	West Virginia	3.3
39	Wisconsin	3.7
46	Wyoming	1.8

RANK ORDER

RANK	STATE	RATE
1	Florida	28.9
2	Delaware	25.4
3	New York	24.4
4	Maryland	22.6
5	New Jersey	18.9
6	South Carolina	18.8
7	Massachusetts	17.9
8	Connecticut	16.0
9	Louisiana	14.5
10	Mississippi	13.9
11	Nevada	13.8
12	Georgia	13.6
12	Illinois	13.6
12	Tennessee	13.6
15	California	13.2
16	Texas	12.3
17	Pennsylvania	12.0
18	Virginia	10.8
19	Alabama	10.3
20	Oklahoma	9.3
21	Rhode Island	9.1
22	Arizona	8.3
22	North Carolina	8.3
24	Hawaii	8.2
25	Washington	8.1
26	New Mexico	7.7
27	Colorado	7.0
28	Michigan	6.6
28	Missouri	6.6
30	Arkansas	6.4
31	Utah	6.1
31	Vermont	6.1
33	Indiana	5.8
34	Oregon	5.0
35	Ohio	4.8
36	Kentucky	4.6
37	Kansas	4.5
38	Nebraska	4.0
39	Wisconsin	3.7
40	Alaska	3.5
41	Minnesota	3.3
41	West Virginia	3.3
43	Maine	3.0
44	Iowa	2.9
45	New Hampshire	2.5
46	Wyoming	1.8
47	Montana	1.6
48	Idaho	1.5
49	South Dakota	0.9
50	North Dakota	0.5

District of Columbia 137.2

Source: Morgan Quitno Press using data from U.S. Dept. of Health & Human Serv's, National Center for Health Statistics "Morbidity and Mortality Weekly Report" (January 5, 2001, Vol. 49, No. 51)
*Provisional data. AIDS is Acquired Immunodeficiency Syndrome. It is a specific group of diseases or conditions which are indicative of severe immunosuppression related to infection with the Human Immunodeficiency Virus (HIV). National rate does not include cases or population.

AIDS Cases Reported Through June 2000

National Total = 720,299 Reported AIDS Cases*

ALPHA ORDER

RANK	STATE	CASES	% of USA
23	Alabama	5,979	0.8%
45	Alaska	459	0.1%
21	Arizona	7,196	1.0%
32	Arkansas	2,848	0.4%
2	California	116,925	16.2%
22	Colorado	6,888	1.0%
13	Connecticut	11,139	1.5%
33	Delaware	2,436	0.3%
3	Florida	76,656	10.6%
8	Georgia	21,995	3.1%
34	Hawaii	2,410	0.3%
44	Idaho	486	0.1%
6	Illinois	24,158	3.4%
24	Indiana	5,910	0.8%
39	Iowa	1,267	0.2%
35	Kansas	2,322	0.3%
31	Kentucky	3,221	0.4%
12	Louisiana	12,185	1.7%
42	Maine	923	0.1%
9	Maryland	20,534	2.9%
10	Massachusetts	15,701	2.2%
15	Michigan	10,714	1.5%
28	Minnesota	3,643	0.5%
27	Mississippi	4,201	0.6%
19	Missouri	8,863	1.2%
47	Montana	316	0.0%
40	Nebraska	1,038	0.1%
26	Nevada	4,265	0.6%
43	New Hampshire	860	0.1%
5	New Jersey	40,501	5.6%
36	New Mexico	1,987	0.3%
1	New York	137,015	19.0%
16	North Carolina	9,962	1.4%
50	North Dakota	104	0.0%
14	Ohio	10,980	1.5%
29	Oklahoma	3,567	0.5%
25	Oregon	4,662	0.6%
7	Pennsylvania	23,365	3.2%
37	Rhode Island	1,981	0.3%
18	South Carolina	9,075	1.3%
49	South Dakota	158	0.0%
20	Tennessee	8,082	1.1%
4	Texas	52,292	7.3%
38	Utah	1,872	0.3%
46	Vermont	374	0.1%
11	Virginia	12,422	1.7%
17	Washington	9,246	1.3%
40	West Virginia	1,038	0.1%
30	Wisconsin	3,453	0.5%
48	Wyoming	178	0.0%

RANK ORDER

RANK	STATE	CASES	% of USA
1	New York	137,015	19.0%
2	California	116,925	16.2%
3	Florida	76,656	10.6%
4	Texas	52,292	7.3%
5	New Jersey	40,501	5.6%
6	Illinois	24,158	3.4%
7	Pennsylvania	23,365	3.2%
8	Georgia	21,995	3.1%
9	Maryland	20,534	2.9%
10	Massachusetts	15,701	2.2%
11	Virginia	12,422	1.7%
12	Louisiana	12,185	1.7%
13	Connecticut	11,139	1.5%
14	Ohio	10,980	1.5%
15	Michigan	10,714	1.5%
16	North Carolina	9,962	1.4%
17	Washington	9,246	1.3%
18	South Carolina	9,075	1.3%
19	Missouri	8,863	1.2%
20	Tennessee	8,082	1.1%
21	Arizona	7,196	1.0%
22	Colorado	6,888	1.0%
23	Alabama	5,979	0.8%
24	Indiana	5,910	0.8%
25	Oregon	4,662	0.6%
26	Nevada	4,265	0.6%
27	Mississippi	4,201	0.6%
28	Minnesota	3,643	0.5%
29	Oklahoma	3,567	0.5%
30	Wisconsin	3,453	0.5%
31	Kentucky	3,221	0.4%
32	Arkansas	2,848	0.4%
33	Delaware	2,436	0.3%
34	Hawaii	2,410	0.3%
35	Kansas	2,322	0.3%
36	New Mexico	1,987	0.3%
37	Rhode Island	1,981	0.3%
38	Utah	1,872	0.3%
39	Iowa	1,267	0.2%
40	Nebraska	1,038	0.1%
40	West Virginia	1,038	0.1%
42	Maine	923	0.1%
43	New Hampshire	860	0.1%
44	Idaho	486	0.1%
45	Alaska	459	0.1%
46	Vermont	374	0.1%
47	Montana	316	0.0%
48	Wyoming	178	0.0%
49	South Dakota	158	0.0%
50	North Dakota	104	0.0%
	District of Columbia	12,447	1.7%

Source: U.S. Department of Health and Human Services, Centers for Disease Control and Prevention
   "HIV/AIDS Surveillance Report, 2000" (Mid-year Edition, Vol. 12, No. 1)

Cumulative through June 2000. AIDS is Acquired Immunodeficiency Syndrome. It is a specific group of diseases or conditions which are indicative of severe immunosuppression related to infection with the Human Immunodeficiency Virus (HIV). National total does not include 23,675 cases in Puerto Rico, 453 cases in the Virgin Islands and 50 cases in other U.S. territories.

AIDS Cases in Children 12 Years and Younger Through June 2000

National Total = 8,395 Juvenile AIDS Cases*

ALPHA ORDER

RANK	STATE	CASES	% of USA
18	Alabama	70	0.8%
44	Alaska	5	0.1%
23	Arizona	38	0.5%
23	Arkansas	38	0.5%
4	California	596	7.1%
26	Colorado	29	0.3%
11	Connecticut	175	2.1%
32	Delaware	22	0.3%
2	Florida	1,387	16.5%
10	Georgia	202	2.4%
36	Hawaii	15	0.2%
48	Idaho	2	0.0%
8	Illinois	267	3.2%
22	Indiana	40	0.5%
39	Iowa	9	0.1%
37	Kansas	13	0.2%
28	Kentucky	26	0.3%
13	Louisiana	121	1.4%
39	Maine	9	0.1%
7	Maryland	299	3.6%
9	Massachusetts	206	2.5%
16	Michigan	106	1.3%
31	Minnesota	23	0.3%
20	Mississippi	55	0.7%
19	Missouri	56	0.7%
47	Montana	3	0.0%
38	Nebraska	10	0.1%
28	Nevada	26	0.3%
39	New Hampshire	9	0.1%
3	New Jersey	744	8.9%
43	New Mexico	8	0.1%
1	New York	2,233	26.6%
15	North Carolina	113	1.3%
50	North Dakota	1	0.0%
13	Ohio	121	1.4%
28	Oklahoma	26	0.3%
35	Oregon	17	0.2%
6	Pennsylvania	313	3.7%
33	Rhode Island	21	0.3%
17	South Carolina	79	0.9%
46	South Dakota	4	0.0%
21	Tennessee	52	0.6%
5	Texas	375	4.5%
33	Utah	21	0.3%
44	Vermont	5	0.1%
12	Virginia	164	2.0%
25	Washington	34	0.4%
39	West Virginia	9	0.1%
27	Wisconsin	27	0.3%
48	Wyoming	2	0.0%

RANK ORDER

RANK	STATE	CASES	% of USA
1	New York	2,233	26.6%
2	Florida	1,387	16.5%
3	New Jersey	744	8.9%
4	California	596	7.1%
5	Texas	375	4.5%
6	Pennsylvania	313	3.7%
7	Maryland	299	3.6%
8	Illinois	267	3.2%
9	Massachusetts	206	2.5%
10	Georgia	202	2.4%
11	Connecticut	175	2.1%
12	Virginia	164	2.0%
13	Louisiana	121	1.4%
13	Ohio	121	1.4%
15	North Carolina	113	1.3%
16	Michigan	106	1.3%
17	South Carolina	79	0.9%
18	Alabama	70	0.8%
19	Missouri	56	0.7%
20	Mississippi	55	0.7%
21	Tennessee	52	0.6%
22	Indiana	40	0.5%
23	Arizona	38	0.5%
23	Arkansas	38	0.5%
25	Washington	34	0.4%
26	Colorado	29	0.3%
27	Wisconsin	27	0.3%
28	Kentucky	26	0.3%
28	Nevada	26	0.3%
28	Oklahoma	26	0.3%
31	Minnesota	23	0.3%
32	Delaware	22	0.3%
33	Rhode Island	21	0.3%
33	Utah	21	0.3%
35	Oregon	17	0.2%
36	Hawaii	15	0.2%
37	Kansas	13	0.2%
38	Nebraska	10	0.1%
39	Iowa	9	0.1%
39	Maine	9	0.1%
39	New Hampshire	9	0.1%
39	West Virginia	9	0.1%
43	New Mexico	8	0.1%
44	Alaska	5	0.1%
44	Vermont	5	0.1%
46	South Dakota	4	0.0%
47	Montana	3	0.0%
48	Idaho	2	0.0%
48	Wyoming	2	0.0%
50	North Dakota	1	0.0%
	District of Columbia	169	2.0%

Source: U.S. Department of Health and Human Services, Centers for Disease Control and Prevention
"HIV/AIDS Surveillance Report, 2000" (Mid-year Edition, Vol. 12, No. 1)
*Cumulative through June 2000. AIDS is Acquired Immunodeficiency Syndrome. It is a specific group of diseases or conditions which are indicative of severe immunosuppression related to infection with the Human Immunodeficiency Virus (HIV). National total does not include 386 cases in Puerto Rico AND 17 cases in the Virgin Islands.

E-Coli Cases Reported in 2000

National Total = 7,679 Cases*

ALPHA ORDER					RANK ORDER			
RANK	STATE		CASES	% of USA	RANK	STATE	CASES	% of USA
48	Alabama		20	0.3%	1	Ohio	500	6.5%
43	Alaska		31	0.4%	2	Minnesota	494	6.4%
26	Arizona		100	1.3%	3	California	453	5.9%
27	Arkansas		95	1.2%	4	Wisconsin	440	5.7%
3	California		453	5.9%	5	Washington	428	5.6%
9	Colorado		273	3.6%	6	New York	401	5.2%
17	Connecticut		180	2.3%	7	Massachusetts	332	4.3%
50	Delaware		2	0.0%	8	Iowa	329	4.3%
18	Florida		170	2.2%	9	Colorado	273	3.6%
29	Georgia		79	1.0%	10	Oregon	271	3.5%
47	Hawaii		26	0.3%	11	Michigan	243	3.2%
25	Idaho		109	1.4%	12	Indiana	225	2.9%
14	Illinois		214	2.8%	13	Texas	222	2.9%
12	Indiana		225	2.9%	14	Illinois	214	2.8%
8	Iowa		329	4.3%	15	Missouri	208	2.7%
36	Kansas		46	0.6%	16	New Jersey	207	2.7%
32	Kentucky		72	0.9%	17	Connecticut	180	2.3%
33	Louisiana		63	0.8%	18	Florida	170	2.2%
34	Maine		59	0.8%	19	North Carolina	158	2.1%
42	Maryland		34	0.4%	20	Virginia	142	1.8%
7	Massachusetts		332	4.3%	21	Utah	122	1.6%
11	Michigan		243	3.2%	22	Nebraska	115	1.5%
2	Minnesota		494	6.4%	22	Tennessee	115	1.5%
35	Mississippi		57	0.7%	24	South Dakota	114	1.5%
15	Missouri		208	2.7%	25	Idaho	109	1.4%
43	Montana		31	0.4%	26	Arizona	100	1.3%
22	Nebraska		115	1.5%	27	Arkansas	95	1.2%
49	Nevada		15	0.2%	28	Pennsylvania	87	1.1%
30	New Hampshire		76	1.0%	29	Georgia	79	1.0%
16	New Jersey		207	2.7%	30	New Hampshire	76	1.0%
38	New Mexico		39	0.5%	31	Vermont	73	1.0%
6	New York		401	5.2%	32	Kentucky	72	0.9%
19	North Carolina		158	2.1%	33	Louisiana	63	0.8%
37	North Dakota		41	0.5%	34	Maine	59	0.8%
1	Ohio		500	6.5%	35	Mississippi	57	0.7%
40	Oklahoma		36	0.5%	36	Kansas	46	0.6%
10	Oregon		271	3.5%	37	North Dakota	41	0.5%
28	Pennsylvania		87	1.1%	38	New Mexico	39	0.5%
39	Rhode Island		37	0.5%	39	Rhode Island	37	0.5%
41	South Carolina		35	0.5%	40	Oklahoma	36	0.5%
24	South Dakota		114	1.5%	41	South Carolina	35	0.5%
22	Tennessee		115	1.5%	42	Maryland	34	0.4%
13	Texas		222	2.9%	43	Alaska	31	0.4%
21	Utah		122	1.6%	43	Montana	31	0.4%
31	Vermont		73	1.0%	43	Wyoming	31	0.4%
20	Virginia		142	1.8%	46	West Virginia	28	0.4%
5	Washington		428	5.6%	47	Hawaii	26	0.3%
46	West Virginia		28	0.4%	48	Alabama	20	0.3%
4	Wisconsin		440	5.7%	49	Nevada	15	0.2%
43	Wyoming		31	0.4%	50	Delaware	2	0.0%
						District of Columbia	1	0.0%

Source: U.S. Department of Health and Human Services, National Center for Health Statistics
   "Morbidity and Mortality Weekly Report" (January 5, 2001, Vol. 49, No. 51)

*Individual cases may be reported through both the Public Health Laboratory Information System and the National Electronic Telecommunications System for Surveillance. Escherichia Coli is a common bacterium that normally inhabits the intestinal tracts of humans and animals but can cause infection in other parts of the body, especially the urinary tract. One strain, sometimes transmitted in hamburger meat, can cause serious infection resulting in sickness and death.

E-Coli Rate in 2000

National Rate = 2.7 Cases per 100,000 Population*

ALPHA ORDER

RANK	STATE	RATE
49	Alabama	0.4
17	Alaska	4.9
34	Arizona	1.9
22	Arkansas	3.6
40	California	1.3
11	Colorado	6.3
15	Connecticut	5.3
50	Delaware	0.3
41	Florida	1.1
43	Georgia	1.0
27	Hawaii	2.1
5	Idaho	8.4
36	Illinois	1.7
20	Indiana	3.7
3	Iowa	11.2
36	Kansas	1.7
35	Kentucky	1.8
39	Louisiana	1.4
18	Maine	4.6
48	Maryland	0.6
16	Massachusetts	5.2
26	Michigan	2.4
4	Minnesota	10.0
30	Mississippi	2.0
20	Missouri	3.7
24	Montana	3.4
9	Nebraska	6.7
46	Nevada	0.8
13	New Hampshire	6.1
25	New Jersey	2.5
27	New Mexico	2.1
27	New York	2.1
30	North Carolina	2.0
10	North Dakota	6.4
19	Ohio	4.4
43	Oklahoma	1.0
7	Oregon	7.9
47	Pennsylvania	0.7
23	Rhode Island	3.5
45	South Carolina	0.9
1	South Dakota	15.1
30	Tennessee	2.0
41	Texas	1.1
14	Utah	5.5
2	Vermont	12.0
30	Virginia	2.0
8	Washington	7.3
38	West Virginia	1.5
6	Wisconsin	8.2
11	Wyoming	6.3

RANK ORDER

RANK	STATE	RATE
1	South Dakota	15.1
2	Vermont	12.0
3	Iowa	11.2
4	Minnesota	10.0
5	Idaho	8.4
6	Wisconsin	8.2
7	Oregon	7.9
8	Washington	7.3
9	Nebraska	6.7
10	North Dakota	6.4
11	Colorado	6.3
11	Wyoming	6.3
13	New Hampshire	6.1
14	Utah	5.5
15	Connecticut	5.3
16	Massachusetts	5.2
17	Alaska	4.9
18	Maine	4.6
19	Ohio	4.4
20	Indiana	3.7
20	Missouri	3.7
22	Arkansas	3.6
23	Rhode Island	3.5
24	Montana	3.4
25	New Jersey	2.5
26	Michigan	2.4
27	Hawaii	2.1
27	New Mexico	2.1
27	New York	2.1
30	Mississippi	2.0
30	North Carolina	2.0
30	Tennessee	2.0
30	Virginia	2.0
34	Arizona	1.9
35	Kentucky	1.8
36	Illinois	1.7
36	Kansas	1.7
38	West Virginia	1.5
39	Louisiana	1.4
40	California	1.3
41	Florida	1.1
41	Texas	1.1
43	Georgia	1.0
43	Oklahoma	1.0
45	South Carolina	0.9
46	Nevada	0.8
47	Pennsylvania	0.7
48	Maryland	0.6
49	Alabama	0.4
50	Delaware	0.3

District of Columbia 0.2

Source: Morgan Quitno Press using data from U.S. Dept. of Health & Human Serv's, National Center for Health Statistics
"Morbidity and Mortality Weekly Report" (January 5, 2001, Vol. 49, No. 51)
*Individual cases may be reported through both the Public Health Laboratory Information System and the National Electronic Telecommunications System for Surveillance. Escherichia Coli is a common bacterium that normally inhabits the intestinal tracts of humans and animals but can cause infection in other parts of the body, especially the urinary tract. One strain, sometimes transmitted in hamburger meat, can cause serious infection resulting in sickness and death.

German Measles (Rubella) Cases Reported in 2000

National Total = 152 Cases*

ALPHA ORDER

RANK	STATE	CASES	% of USA
8	Alabama	3	2.0%
23	Alaska	0	0.0%
11	Arizona	1	0.7%
23	Arkansas	0	0.0%
2	California	10	6.6%
11	Colorado	1	0.7%
11	Connecticut	1	0.7%
11	Delaware	1	0.7%
9	Florida	2	1.3%
23	Georgia	0	0.0%
23	Hawaii	0	0.0%
23	Idaho	0	0.0%
11	Illinois	1	0.7%
23	Indiana	0	0.0%
23	Iowa	0	0.0%
23	Kansas	0	0.0%
11	Kentucky	1	0.7%
11	Louisiana	1	0.7%
23	Maine	0	0.0%
23	Maryland	0	0.0%
5	Massachusetts	9	5.9%
23	Michigan	0	0.0%
11	Minnesota	1	0.7%
23	Mississippi	0	0.0%
11	Missouri	1	0.7%
23	Montana	0	0.0%
11	Nebraska	1	0.7%
23	Nevada	0	0.0%
9	New Hampshire	2	1.3%
23	New Jersey	0	0.0%
23	New Mexico	0	0.0%
2	New York	10	6.6%
1	North Carolina	82	53.9%
23	North Dakota	0	0.0%
23	Ohio	0	0.0%
23	Oklahoma	0	0.0%
23	Oregon	0	0.0%
23	Pennsylvania	0	0.0%
11	Rhode Island	1	0.7%
2	South Carolina	10	6.6%
23	South Dakota	0	0.0%
11	Tennessee	1	0.7%
7	Texas	5	3.3%
23	Utah	0	0.0%
23	Vermont	0	0.0%
23	Virginia	0	0.0%
6	Washington	7	4.6%
23	West Virginia	0	0.0%
23	Wisconsin	0	0.0%
23	Wyoming	0	0.0%

RANK ORDER

RANK	STATE	CASES	% of USA
1	North Carolina	82	53.9%
2	California	10	6.6%
2	New York	10	6.6%
2	South Carolina	10	6.6%
5	Massachusetts	9	5.9%
6	Washington	7	4.6%
7	Texas	5	3.3%
8	Alabama	3	2.0%
9	Florida	2	1.3%
9	New Hampshire	2	1.3%
11	Arizona	1	0.7%
11	Colorado	1	0.7%
11	Connecticut	1	0.7%
11	Delaware	1	0.7%
11	Illinois	1	0.7%
11	Kentucky	1	0.7%
11	Louisiana	1	0.7%
11	Minnesota	1	0.7%
11	Missouri	1	0.7%
11	Nebraska	1	0.7%
11	Rhode Island	1	0.7%
11	Tennessee	1	0.7%
23	Alaska	0	0.0%
23	Arkansas	0	0.0%
23	Georgia	0	0.0%
23	Hawaii	0	0.0%
23	Idaho	0	0.0%
23	Indiana	0	0.0%
23	Iowa	0	0.0%
23	Kansas	0	0.0%
23	Maine	0	0.0%
23	Maryland	0	0.0%
23	Michigan	0	0.0%
23	Mississippi	0	0.0%
23	Montana	0	0.0%
23	Nevada	0	0.0%
23	New Jersey	0	0.0%
23	New Mexico	0	0.0%
23	North Dakota	0	0.0%
23	Ohio	0	0.0%
23	Oklahoma	0	0.0%
23	Oregon	0	0.0%
23	Pennsylvania	0	0.0%
23	South Dakota	0	0.0%
23	Utah	0	0.0%
23	Vermont	0	0.0%
23	Virginia	0	0.0%
23	West Virginia	0	0.0%
23	Wisconsin	0	0.0%
23	Wyoming	0	0.0%
	District of Columbia	0	0.0%

Source: U.S. Department of Health and Human Services, National Center for Health Statistics
   "Morbidity and Mortality Weekly Report" (January 5, 2001, Vol. 49, No. 51)
*Provisional data. A mild, contagious, eruptive disease caused by a virus and capable of producing congenital defects in infants born to mothers infected during the first three months of pregnancy.

German Measles (Rubella) Rate in 2000

National Rate = 0.05 Cases per 100,000 Population*

ALPHA ORDER

RANK	STATE	RATE
8	Alabama	0.07
23	Alaska	0.00
13	Arizona	0.02
23	Arkansas	0.00
11	California	0.03
13	Colorado	0.02
11	Connecticut	0.03
5	Delaware	0.13
21	Florida	0.01
23	Georgia	0.00
23	Hawaii	0.00
23	Idaho	0.00
21	Illinois	0.01
23	Indiana	0.00
23	Iowa	0.00
23	Kansas	0.00
13	Kentucky	0.02
13	Louisiana	0.02
23	Maine	0.00
23	Maryland	0.00
4	Massachusetts	0.14
23	Michigan	0.00
13	Minnesota	0.02
23	Mississippi	0.00
13	Missouri	0.02
23	Montana	0.00
9	Nebraska	0.06
23	Nevada	0.00
3	New Hampshire	0.16
23	New Jersey	0.00
23	New Mexico	0.00
10	New York	0.05
1	North Carolina	1.02
23	North Dakota	0.00
23	Ohio	0.00
23	Oklahoma	0.00
23	Oregon	0.00
23	Pennsylvania	0.00
7	Rhode Island	0.10
2	South Carolina	0.25
23	South Dakota	0.00
13	Tennessee	0.02
13	Texas	0.02
23	Utah	0.00
23	Vermont	0.00
23	Virginia	0.00
6	Washington	0.12
23	West Virginia	0.00
23	Wisconsin	0.00
23	Wyoming	0.00

RANK ORDER

RANK	STATE	RATE
1	North Carolina	1.02
2	South Carolina	0.25
3	New Hampshire	0.16
4	Massachusetts	0.14
5	Delaware	0.13
6	Washington	0.12
7	Rhode Island	0.10
8	Alabama	0.07
9	Nebraska	0.06
10	New York	0.05
11	California	0.03
11	Connecticut	0.03
13	Arizona	0.02
13	Colorado	0.02
13	Kentucky	0.02
13	Louisiana	0.02
13	Minnesota	0.02
13	Missouri	0.02
13	Tennessee	0.02
13	Texas	0.02
21	Florida	0.01
21	Illinois	0.01
23	Alaska	0.00
23	Arkansas	0.00
23	Georgia	0.00
23	Hawaii	0.00
23	Idaho	0.00
23	Indiana	0.00
23	Iowa	0.00
23	Kansas	0.00
23	Maine	0.00
23	Maryland	0.00
23	Michigan	0.00
23	Mississippi	0.00
23	Montana	0.00
23	Nevada	0.00
23	New Jersey	0.00
23	New Mexico	0.00
23	North Dakota	0.00
23	Ohio	0.00
23	Oklahoma	0.00
23	Oregon	0.00
23	Pennsylvania	0.00
23	South Dakota	0.00
23	Utah	0.00
23	Vermont	0.00
23	Virginia	0.00
23	West Virginia	0.00
23	Wisconsin	0.00
23	Wyoming	0.00

District of Columbia 0.00

Source: Morgan Quitno Press using data from U.S. Dept. of Health & Human Serv's, National Center for Health Statistics "Morbidity and Mortality Weekly Report" (January 5, 2001, Vol. 49, No. 51)
*Provisional data. A mild, contagious, eruptive disease caused by a virus and capable of producing congenital defects in infants born to mothers infected during the first three months of pregnancy.

Hepatitis A and B Cases Reported in 2000

National Total = 18,921 Cases*

ALPHA ORDER

RANK	STATE	CASES	% of USA
32	Alabama	132	0.7%
44	Alaska	23	0.1%
7	Arizona	712	3.8%
23	Arkansas	190	1.0%
1	California	3,841	20.3%
18	Colorado	318	1.7%
22	Connecticut	194	1.0%
50	Delaware	0	0.0%
4	Florida	1,059	5.6%
10	Georgia	511	2.7%
43	Hawaii	24	0.1%
39	Idaho	56	0.3%
6	Illinois	762	4.0%
25	Indiana	172	0.9%
34	Iowa	101	0.5%
31	Kansas	134	0.7%
30	Kentucky	139	0.7%
26	Louisiana	164	0.9%
42	Maine	26	0.1%
16	Maryland	355	1.9%
28	Massachusetts	142	0.8%
5	Michigan	936	4.9%
21	Minnesota	230	1.2%
20	Mississippi	248	1.3%
8	Missouri	701	3.7%
46	Montana	14	0.1%
37	Nebraska	85	0.4%
29	Nevada	140	0.7%
41	New Hampshire	38	0.2%
27	New Jersey	157	0.8%
24	New Mexico	186	1.0%
3	New York	1,198	6.3%
12	North Carolina	410	2.2%
48	North Dakota	7	0.0%
14	Ohio	378	2.0%
11	Oklahoma	412	2.2%
19	Oregon	316	1.7%
9	Pennsylvania	592	3.1%
40	Rhode Island	48	0.3%
33	South Carolina	109	0.6%
49	South Dakota	5	0.0%
15	Tennessee	365	1.9%
2	Texas	2,196	11.6%
34	Utah	101	0.5%
45	Vermont	16	0.1%
17	Virginia	320	1.7%
13	Washington	400	2.1%
38	West Virginia	81	0.4%
46	Wisconsin	14	0.1%
36	Wyoming	88	0.5%

RANK ORDER

RANK	STATE	CASES	% of USA
1	California	3,841	20.3%
2	Texas	2,196	11.6%
3	New York	1,198	6.3%
4	Florida	1,059	5.6%
5	Michigan	936	4.9%
6	Illinois	762	4.0%
7	Arizona	712	3.8%
8	Missouri	701	3.7%
9	Pennsylvania	592	3.1%
10	Georgia	511	2.7%
11	Oklahoma	412	2.2%
12	North Carolina	410	2.2%
13	Washington	400	2.1%
14	Ohio	378	2.0%
15	Tennessee	365	1.9%
16	Maryland	355	1.9%
17	Virginia	320	1.7%
18	Colorado	318	1.7%
19	Oregon	316	1.7%
20	Mississippi	248	1.3%
21	Minnesota	230	1.2%
22	Connecticut	194	1.0%
23	Arkansas	190	1.0%
24	New Mexico	186	1.0%
25	Indiana	172	0.9%
26	Louisiana	164	0.9%
27	New Jersey	157	0.8%
28	Massachusetts	142	0.8%
29	Nevada	140	0.7%
30	Kentucky	139	0.7%
31	Kansas	134	0.7%
32	Alabama	132	0.7%
33	South Carolina	109	0.6%
34	Iowa	101	0.5%
34	Utah	101	0.5%
36	Wyoming	88	0.5%
37	Nebraska	85	0.4%
38	West Virginia	81	0.4%
39	Idaho	56	0.3%
40	Rhode Island	48	0.3%
41	New Hampshire	38	0.2%
42	Maine	26	0.1%
43	Hawaii	24	0.1%
44	Alaska	23	0.1%
45	Vermont	16	0.1%
46	Montana	14	0.1%
46	Wisconsin	14	0.1%
48	North Dakota	7	0.0%
49	South Dakota	5	0.0%
50	Delaware	0	0.0%
	District of Columbia	75	0.4%

Source: U.S. Department of Health and Human Services, National Center for Health Statistics "Morbidity and Mortality Weekly Report" (January 5, 2001, Vol. 49, No. 51)
*Provisional data. An inflammation of the liver.

Hepatitis A and B Rate in 2000

National Rate = 6.7 Cases per 100,000 Population*

ALPHA ORDER				RANK ORDER		
RANK	STATE	RATE		RANK	STATE	RATE
38	Alabama	3.0		1	Wyoming	17.8
32	Alaska	3.7		2	Arizona	13.9
2	Arizona	13.9		3	Missouri	12.5
12	Arkansas	7.1		4	Oklahoma	11.9
5	California	11.3		5	California	11.3
11	Colorado	7.4		6	Texas	10.5
21	Connecticut	5.7		7	New Mexico	10.2
50	Delaware	0.0		8	Michigan	9.4
16	Florida	6.6		9	Oregon	9.2
19	Georgia	6.2		10	Mississippi	8.7
43	Hawaii	2.0		11	Colorado	7.4
31	Idaho	4.3		12	Arkansas	7.1
20	Illinois	6.1		13	Nevada	7.0
39	Indiana	2.8		14	Washington	6.8
34	Iowa	3.5		15	Maryland	6.7
23	Kansas	5.0		16	Florida	6.6
35	Kentucky	3.4		17	Tennessee	6.4
32	Louisiana	3.7		18	New York	6.3
43	Maine	2.0		19	Georgia	6.2
15	Maryland	6.7		20	Illinois	6.1
42	Massachusetts	2.2		21	Connecticut	5.7
8	Michigan	9.4		22	North Carolina	5.1
26	Minnesota	4.7		23	Kansas	5.0
10	Mississippi	8.7		23	Nebraska	5.0
3	Missouri	12.5		25	Pennsylvania	4.8
46	Montana	1.6		26	Minnesota	4.7
23	Nebraska	5.0		27	Rhode Island	4.6
13	Nevada	7.0		28	Utah	4.5
37	New Hampshire	3.1		28	Virginia	4.5
45	New Jersey	1.9		28	West Virginia	4.5
7	New Mexico	10.2		31	Idaho	4.3
18	New York	6.3		32	Alaska	3.7
22	North Carolina	5.1		32	Louisiana	3.7
47	North Dakota	1.1		34	Iowa	3.5
36	Ohio	3.3		35	Kentucky	3.4
4	Oklahoma	11.9		36	Ohio	3.3
9	Oregon	9.2		37	New Hampshire	3.1
25	Pennsylvania	4.8		38	Alabama	3.0
27	Rhode Island	4.6		39	Indiana	2.8
40	South Carolina	2.7		40	South Carolina	2.7
48	South Dakota	0.7		41	Vermont	2.6
17	Tennessee	6.4		42	Massachusetts	2.2
6	Texas	10.5		43	Hawaii	2.0
28	Utah	4.5		43	Maine	2.0
41	Vermont	2.6		45	New Jersey	1.9
28	Virginia	4.5		46	Montana	1.6
14	Washington	6.8		47	North Dakota	1.1
28	West Virginia	4.5		48	South Dakota	0.7
49	Wisconsin	0.3		49	Wisconsin	0.3
1	Wyoming	17.8		50	Delaware	0.0

District of Columbia   13.1

Source: Morgan Quitno Press using data from U.S. Dept. of Health & Human Serv's, National Center for Health Statistics "Morbidity and Mortality Weekly Report" (January 5, 2001, Vol. 49, No. 51)
Provisional data. An inflammation of the liver.

Hepatitis C Cases Reported in 2000

National Total = 2,895 Cases*

ALPHA ORDER

RANK	STATE	CASES	% of USA
28	Alabama	8	0.3%
45	Alaska	0	0.0%
17	Arizona	21	0.7%
27	Arkansas	9	0.3%
7	California	115	4.0%
15	Colorado	31	1.1%
45	Connecticut	0	0.0%
45	Delaware	0	0.0%
11	Florida	58	2.0%
35	Georgia	3	0.1%
39	Hawaii	2	0.1%
35	Idaho	3	0.1%
21	Illinois	19	0.7%
43	Indiana	1	0.0%
39	Iowa	2	0.1%
25	Kansas	10	0.3%
12	Kentucky	37	1.3%
4	Louisiana	308	10.6%
39	Maine	2	0.1%
18	Maryland	20	0.7%
33	Massachusetts	4	0.1%
6	Michigan	191	6.6%
29	Minnesota	7	0.2%
5	Mississippi	287	9.9%
2	Missouri	414	14.3%
32	Montana	5	0.2%
29	Nebraska	7	0.2%
22	Nevada	18	0.6%
45	New Hampshire	0	0.0%
1	New Jersey	510	17.6%
23	New Mexico	16	0.6%
10	New York	71	2.5%
18	North Carolina	20	0.7%
43	North Dakota	1	0.0%
24	Ohio	12	0.4%
25	Oklahoma	10	0.3%
16	Oregon	29	1.0%
13	Pennsylvania	36	1.2%
31	Rhode Island	6	0.2%
35	South Carolina	3	0.1%
45	South Dakota	0	0.0%
9	Tennessee	100	3.5%
7	Texas	115	4.0%
39	Utah	2	0.1%
33	Vermont	4	0.1%
35	Virginia	3	0.1%
14	Washington	34	1.2%
18	West Virginia	20	0.7%
45	Wisconsin	0	0.0%
3	Wyoming	318	11.0%

RANK ORDER

RANK	STATE	CASES	% of USA
1	New Jersey	510	17.6%
2	Missouri	414	14.3%
3	Wyoming	318	11.0%
4	Louisiana	308	10.6%
5	Mississippi	287	9.9%
6	Michigan	191	6.6%
7	California	115	4.0%
7	Texas	115	4.0%
9	Tennessee	100	3.5%
10	New York	71	2.5%
11	Florida	58	2.0%
12	Kentucky	37	1.3%
13	Pennsylvania	36	1.2%
14	Washington	34	1.2%
15	Colorado	31	1.1%
16	Oregon	29	1.0%
17	Arizona	21	0.7%
18	Maryland	20	0.7%
18	North Carolina	20	0.7%
18	West Virginia	20	0.7%
21	Illinois	19	0.7%
22	Nevada	18	0.6%
23	New Mexico	16	0.6%
24	Ohio	12	0.4%
25	Kansas	10	0.3%
25	Oklahoma	10	0.3%
27	Arkansas	9	0.3%
28	Alabama	8	0.3%
29	Minnesota	7	0.2%
29	Nebraska	7	0.2%
31	Rhode Island	6	0.2%
32	Montana	5	0.2%
33	Massachusetts	4	0.1%
33	Vermont	4	0.1%
35	Georgia	3	0.1%
35	Idaho	3	0.1%
35	South Carolina	3	0.1%
35	Virginia	3	0.1%
39	Hawaii	2	0.1%
39	Iowa	2	0.1%
39	Maine	2	0.1%
39	Utah	2	0.1%
43	Indiana	1	0.0%
43	North Dakota	1	0.0%
45	Alaska	0	0.0%
45	Connecticut	0	0.0%
45	Delaware	0	0.0%
45	New Hampshire	0	0.0%
45	South Dakota	0	0.0%
45	Wisconsin	0	0.0%
	District of Columbia	3	0.1%

Source: U.S. Department of Health and Human Services, National Center for Health Statistics
    "Morbidity and Mortality Weekly Report" (January 5, 2001, Vol. 49, No. 51)
*Provisional data. An inflammation of the liver. It is the leading cause for liver transplantation and is transmitted by blood-to-blood contact. Most new cases of C are caused by high-risk drug behaviors.

Hepatitis C Rate in 2000

National Rate = 1.0 Cases per 100,000 Population*

ALPHA ORDER

RANK	STATE	RATE
30	Alabama	0.2
42	Alaska	0.0
19	Arizona	0.4
25	Arkansas	0.3
25	California	0.3
13	Colorado	0.7
42	Connecticut	0.0
42	Delaware	0.0
19	Florida	0.4
42	Georgia	0.0
30	Hawaii	0.2
30	Idaho	0.2
30	Illinois	0.2
42	Indiana	0.0
36	Iowa	0.1
19	Kansas	0.4
9	Kentucky	0.9
4	Louisiana	6.9
30	Maine	0.2
19	Maryland	0.4
36	Massachusetts	0.1
6	Michigan	1.9
36	Minnesota	0.1
2	Mississippi	10.1
3	Missouri	7.4
15	Montana	0.6
19	Nebraska	0.4
9	Nevada	0.9
42	New Hampshire	0.0
5	New Jersey	6.1
9	New Mexico	0.9
19	New York	0.4
25	North Carolina	0.3
30	North Dakota	0.2
36	Ohio	0.1
25	Oklahoma	0.3
9	Oregon	0.9
25	Pennsylvania	0.3
15	Rhode Island	0.6
36	South Carolina	0.1
42	South Dakota	0.0
7	Tennessee	1.8
15	Texas	0.6
36	Utah	0.1
13	Vermont	0.7
42	Virginia	0.0
15	Washington	0.6
8	West Virginia	1.1
42	Wisconsin	0.0
1	Wyoming	64.4

RANK ORDER

RANK	STATE	RATE
1	Wyoming	64.4
2	Mississippi	10.1
3	Missouri	7.4
4	Louisiana	6.9
5	New Jersey	6.1
6	Michigan	1.9
7	Tennessee	1.8
8	West Virginia	1.1
9	Kentucky	0.9
9	Nevada	0.9
9	New Mexico	0.9
9	Oregon	0.9
13	Colorado	0.7
13	Vermont	0.7
15	Montana	0.6
15	Rhode Island	0.6
15	Texas	0.6
15	Washington	0.6
19	Arizona	0.4
19	Florida	0.4
19	Kansas	0.4
19	Maryland	0.4
19	Nebraska	0.4
19	New York	0.4
25	Arkansas	0.3
25	California	0.3
25	North Carolina	0.3
25	Oklahoma	0.3
25	Pennsylvania	0.3
30	Alabama	0.2
30	Hawaii	0.2
30	Idaho	0.2
30	Illinois	0.2
30	Maine	0.2
30	North Dakota	0.2
36	Iowa	0.1
36	Massachusetts	0.1
36	Minnesota	0.1
36	Ohio	0.1
36	South Carolina	0.1
36	Utah	0.1
42	Alaska	0.0
42	Connecticut	0.0
42	Delaware	0.0
42	Georgia	0.0
42	Indiana	0.0
42	New Hampshire	0.0
42	South Dakota	0.0
42	Virginia	0.0
42	Wisconsin	0.0
	District of Columbia	0.5

Source: Morgan Quitno Press using data from U.S. Dept. of Health & Human Serv's, National Center for Health Statistics "Morbidity and Mortality Weekly Report" (January 5, 2001, Vol. 49, No. 51)
Provisional data. An inflammation of the liver. It is the leading cause for liver transplantation and is transmitted by blood-to-blood contact. Most new cases of C are caused by high-risk drug behaviors.

Legionellosis Cases Reported in 2000

National Total = 969 Cases*

ALPHA ORDER

RANK	STATE	CASES	% of USA
34	Alabama	4	0.4%
46	Alaska	0	0.0%
26	Arizona	8	0.8%
46	Arkansas	0	0.0%
5	California	56	5.8%
16	Colorado	16	1.7%
14	Connecticut	18	1.9%
24	Delaware	10	1.0%
7	Florida	48	5.0%
25	Georgia	9	0.9%
46	Hawaii	0	0.0%
31	Idaho	5	0.5%
14	Illinois	18	1.9%
8	Indiana	41	4.2%
19	Iowa	15	1.5%
34	Kansas	4	0.4%
12	Kentucky	21	2.2%
29	Louisiana	6	0.6%
38	Maine	2	0.2%
4	Maryland	68	7.0%
16	Massachusetts	16	1.7%
6	Michigan	50	5.2%
21	Minnesota	13	1.3%
42	Mississippi	1	0.1%
11	Missouri	25	2.6%
38	Montana	2	0.2%
34	Nebraska	4	0.4%
42	Nevada	1	0.1%
34	New Hampshire	4	0.4%
19	New Jersey	15	1.5%
42	New Mexico	1	0.1%
2	New York	99	10.2%
16	North Carolina	16	1.7%
42	North Dakota	1	0.1%
1	Ohio	122	12.6%
31	Oklahoma	5	0.5%
NA	Oregon**	NA	NA
3	Pennsylvania	98	10.1%
26	Rhode Island	8	0.8%
29	South Carolina	6	0.6%
38	South Dakota	2	0.2%
22	Tennessee	12	1.2%
28	Texas	7	0.7%
22	Utah	12	1.2%
31	Vermont	5	0.5%
9	Virginia	33	3.4%
13	Washington	20	2.1%
NA	West Virginia**	NA	NA
9	Wisconsin	33	3.4%
38	Wyoming	2	0.2%

RANK ORDER

RANK	STATE	CASES	% of USA
1	Ohio	122	12.6%
2	New York	99	10.2%
3	Pennsylvania	98	10.1%
4	Maryland	68	7.0%
5	California	56	5.8%
6	Michigan	50	5.2%
7	Florida	48	5.0%
8	Indiana	41	4.2%
9	Virginia	33	3.4%
9	Wisconsin	33	3.4%
11	Missouri	25	2.6%
12	Kentucky	21	2.2%
13	Washington	20	2.1%
14	Connecticut	18	1.9%
14	Illinois	18	1.9%
16	Colorado	16	1.7%
16	Massachusetts	16	1.7%
16	North Carolina	16	1.7%
19	Iowa	15	1.5%
19	New Jersey	15	1.5%
21	Minnesota	13	1.3%
22	Tennessee	12	1.2%
22	Utah	12	1.2%
24	Delaware	10	1.0%
25	Georgia	9	0.9%
26	Arizona	8	0.8%
26	Rhode Island	8	0.8%
28	Texas	7	0.7%
29	Louisiana	6	0.6%
29	South Carolina	6	0.6%
31	Idaho	5	0.5%
31	Oklahoma	5	0.5%
31	Vermont	5	0.5%
34	Alabama	4	0.4%
34	Kansas	4	0.4%
34	Nebraska	4	0.4%
34	New Hampshire	4	0.4%
38	Maine	2	0.2%
38	Montana	2	0.2%
38	South Dakota	2	0.2%
38	Wyoming	2	0.2%
42	Mississippi	1	0.1%
42	Nevada	1	0.1%
42	New Mexico	1	0.1%
42	North Dakota	1	0.1%
46	Alaska	0	0.0%
46	Arkansas	0	0.0%
46	Hawaii	0	0.0%
NA	Oregon**	NA	NA
NA	West Virginia**	NA	NA
	District of Columbia	7	0.7%

Source: U.S. Department of Health and Human Services, National Center for Health Statistics
    "Morbidity and Mortality Weekly Report" (January 5, 2001, Vol. 49, No. 51)
*Provisional data. A pneumonia-like disease (Legionnaire's Disease).
**Not notifiable.

Legionellosis Rate in 2000

National Rate = 0.3 Cases per 100,000 Population*

ALPHA ORDER

RANK	STATE	RATE
37	Alabama	0.1
44	Alaska	0.0
26	Arizona	0.2
44	Arkansas	0.0
26	California	0.2
17	Colorado	0.4
9	Connecticut	0.5
1	Delaware	1.3
20	Florida	0.3
37	Georgia	0.1
44	Hawaii	0.0
17	Idaho	0.4
37	Illinois	0.1
7	Indiana	0.7
9	Iowa	0.5
26	Kansas	0.2
9	Kentucky	0.5
37	Louisiana	0.1
26	Maine	0.2
1	Maryland	1.3
20	Massachusetts	0.3
9	Michigan	0.5
20	Minnesota	0.3
44	Mississippi	0.0
9	Missouri	0.5
26	Montana	0.2
26	Nebraska	0.2
37	Nevada	0.1
20	New Hampshire	0.3
26	New Jersey	0.2
37	New Mexico	0.1
9	New York	0.5
26	North Carolina	0.2
26	North Dakota	0.2
3	Ohio	1.1
37	Oklahoma	0.1
NA	Oregon**	NA
4	Pennsylvania	0.8
4	Rhode Island	0.8
26	South Carolina	0.2
20	South Dakota	0.3
26	Tennessee	0.2
44	Texas	0.0
9	Utah	0.5
4	Vermont	0.8
9	Virginia	0.5
20	Washington	0.3
NA	West Virginia**	NA
8	Wisconsin	0.6
17	Wyoming	0.4

RANK ORDER

RANK	STATE	RATE
1	Delaware	1.3
1	Maryland	1.3
3	Ohio	1.1
4	Pennsylvania	0.8
4	Rhode Island	0.8
4	Vermont	0.8
7	Indiana	0.7
8	Wisconsin	0.6
9	Connecticut	0.5
9	Iowa	0.5
9	Kentucky	0.5
9	Michigan	0.5
9	Missouri	0.5
9	New York	0.5
9	Utah	0.5
9	Virginia	0.5
17	Colorado	0.4
17	Idaho	0.4
17	Wyoming	0.4
20	Florida	0.3
20	Massachusetts	0.3
20	Minnesota	0.3
20	New Hampshire	0.3
20	South Dakota	0.3
20	Washington	0.3
26	Arizona	0.2
26	California	0.2
26	Kansas	0.2
26	Maine	0.2
26	Montana	0.2
26	Nebraska	0.2
26	New Jersey	0.2
26	North Carolina	0.2
26	North Dakota	0.2
26	South Carolina	0.2
26	Tennessee	0.2
37	Alabama	0.1
37	Georgia	0.1
37	Illinois	0.1
37	Louisiana	0.1
37	Nevada	0.1
37	New Mexico	0.1
37	Oklahoma	0.1
44	Alaska	0.0
44	Arkansas	0.0
44	Hawaii	0.0
44	Mississippi	0.0
44	Texas	0.0
NA	Oregon**	NA
NA	West Virginia**	NA

District of Columbia 1.2

Source: Morgan Quitno Press using data from U.S. Dept. of Health & Human Serv's, National Center for Health Statistics "Morbidity and Mortality Weekly Report" (January 5, 2001, Vol. 49, No. 51)
Provisional data. A pneumonia-like disease (Legionnaire's Disease).
***Not notifiable.*

Lyme Disease Cases in 2000

National Total = 13,309 Cases*

ALPHA ORDER

RANK	STATE	CASES	% of USA
32	Alabama	7	0.1%
39	Alaska	2	0.0%
43	Arizona	0	0.0%
33	Arkansas	4	0.0%
12	California	104	0.8%
28	Colorado	11	0.1%
2	Connecticut	2,550	19.2%
11	Delaware	142	1.1%
15	Florida	50	0.4%
43	Georgia	0	0.0%
NA	Hawaii**	NA	NA
33	Idaho	4	0.0%
28	Illinois	11	0.1%
22	Indiana	32	0.2%
20	Iowa	34	0.3%
24	Kansas	17	0.1%
27	Kentucky	13	0.1%
33	Louisiana	4	0.0%
43	Maine	0	0.0%
7	Maryland	559	4.2%
5	Massachusetts	1,098	8.3%
43	Michigan	0	0.0%
8	Minnesota	393	3.0%
41	Mississippi	1	0.0%
17	Missouri	45	0.3%
43	Montana	0	0.0%
33	Nebraska	4	0.0%
33	Nevada	4	0.0%
14	New Hampshire	84	0.6%
3	New Jersey	1,467	11.0%
43	New Mexico	0	0.0%
1	New York	4,027	30.3%
16	North Carolina	46	0.3%
39	North Dakota	2	0.0%
13	Ohio	89	0.7%
41	Oklahoma	1	0.0%
26	Oregon	15	0.1%
4	Pennsylvania	1,276	9.6%
6	Rhode Island	590	4.4%
24	South Carolina	17	0.1%
43	South Dakota	0	0.0%
23	Tennessee	28	0.2%
19	Texas	36	0.3%
38	Utah	3	0.0%
18	Vermont	39	0.3%
10	Virginia	146	1.1%
30	Washington	9	0.1%
20	West Virginia	34	0.3%
9	Wisconsin	291	2.2%
30	Wyoming	9	0.1%

RANK ORDER

RANK	STATE	CASES	% of USA
1	New York	4,027	30.3%
2	Connecticut	2,550	19.2%
3	New Jersey	1,467	11.0%
4	Pennsylvania	1,276	9.6%
5	Massachusetts	1,098	8.3%
6	Rhode Island	590	4.4%
7	Maryland	559	4.2%
8	Minnesota	393	3.0%
9	Wisconsin	291	2.2%
10	Virginia	146	1.1%
11	Delaware	142	1.1%
12	California	104	0.8%
13	Ohio	89	0.7%
14	New Hampshire	84	0.6%
15	Florida	50	0.4%
16	North Carolina	46	0.3%
17	Missouri	45	0.3%
18	Vermont	39	0.3%
19	Texas	36	0.3%
20	Iowa	34	0.3%
20	West Virginia	34	0.3%
22	Indiana	32	0.2%
23	Tennessee	28	0.2%
24	Kansas	17	0.1%
24	South Carolina	17	0.1%
26	Oregon	15	0.1%
27	Kentucky	13	0.1%
28	Colorado	11	0.1%
28	Illinois	11	0.1%
30	Washington	9	0.1%
30	Wyoming	9	0.1%
32	Alabama	7	0.1%
33	Arkansas	4	0.0%
33	Idaho	4	0.0%
33	Louisiana	4	0.0%
33	Nebraska	4	0.0%
33	Nevada	4	0.0%
38	Utah	3	0.0%
39	Alaska	2	0.0%
39	North Dakota	2	0.0%
41	Mississippi	1	0.0%
41	Oklahoma	1	0.0%
43	Arizona	0	0.0%
43	Georgia	0	0.0%
43	Maine	0	0.0%
43	Michigan	0	0.0%
43	Montana	0	0.0%
43	New Mexico	0	0.0%
43	South Dakota	0	0.0%
NA	Hawaii**	NA	NA
	District of Columbia	11	0.1%

Source: U.S. Department of Health and Human Services, National Center for Health Statistics
   "Morbidity and Mortality Weekly Report" (January 5, 2001, Vol. 49, No. 51)
Provisional data. Caused by ticks-lesions, followed by arthritis of large joints, myalgia, malaise and neurologic and cardiac manifestations. Named after Old Lyme, CT, where the disease was first reported.
**Not notifiable.*

Lyme Disease Rate in 2000

National Rate = 4.7 Cases per 100,000 Population*

ALPHA ORDER

RANK	STATE	RATE
32	Alabama	0.2
25	Alaska	0.3
41	Arizona	0.0
37	Arkansas	0.1
25	California	0.3
25	Colorado	0.3
1	Connecticut	74.9
4	Delaware	18.1
25	Florida	0.3
41	Georgia	0.0
NA	Hawaii**	NA
25	Idaho	0.3
37	Illinois	0.1
21	Indiana	0.5
16	Iowa	1.2
19	Kansas	0.6
25	Kentucky	0.3
37	Louisiana	0.1
41	Maine	0.0
7	Maryland	10.6
6	Massachusetts	17.3
41	Michigan	0.0
9	Minnesota	8.0
41	Mississippi	0.0
17	Missouri	0.8
41	Montana	0.0
32	Nebraska	0.2
32	Nevada	0.2
10	New Hampshire	6.8
5	New Jersey	17.4
41	New Mexico	0.0
3	New York	21.2
19	North Carolina	0.6
25	North Dakota	0.3
17	Ohio	0.8
41	Oklahoma	0.0
23	Oregon	0.4
8	Pennsylvania	10.4
2	Rhode Island	56.3
23	South Carolina	0.4
41	South Dakota	0.0
21	Tennessee	0.5
32	Texas	0.2
37	Utah	0.1
11	Vermont	6.4
13	Virginia	2.1
32	Washington	0.2
14	West Virginia	1.9
12	Wisconsin	5.4
15	Wyoming	1.8

RANK ORDER

RANK	STATE	RATE
1	Connecticut	74.9
2	Rhode Island	56.3
3	New York	21.2
4	Delaware	18.1
5	New Jersey	17.4
6	Massachusetts	17.3
7	Maryland	10.6
8	Pennsylvania	10.4
9	Minnesota	8.0
10	New Hampshire	6.8
11	Vermont	6.4
12	Wisconsin	5.4
13	Virginia	2.1
14	West Virginia	1.9
15	Wyoming	1.8
16	Iowa	1.2
17	Missouri	0.8
17	Ohio	0.8
19	Kansas	0.6
19	North Carolina	0.6
21	Indiana	0.5
21	Tennessee	0.5
23	Oregon	0.4
23	South Carolina	0.4
25	Alaska	0.3
25	California	0.3
25	Colorado	0.3
25	Florida	0.3
25	Idaho	0.3
25	Kentucky	0.3
25	North Dakota	0.3
32	Alabama	0.2
32	Nebraska	0.2
32	Nevada	0.2
32	Texas	0.2
32	Washington	0.2
37	Arkansas	0.1
37	Illinois	0.1
37	Louisiana	0.1
37	Utah	0.1
41	Arizona	0.0
41	Georgia	0.0
41	Maine	0.0
41	Michigan	0.0
41	Mississippi	0.0
41	Montana	0.0
41	New Mexico	0.0
41	Oklahoma	0.0
41	South Dakota	0.0
NA	Hawaii**	NA

District of Columbia   1.9

Source: Morgan Quitno Press using data from U.S. Dept. of Health & Human Serv's, National Center for Health Statistics "Morbidity and Mortality Weekly Report" (January 5, 2001, Vol. 49, No. 51)
*Provisional data. Caused by ticks-lesions, followed by arthritis of large joints, myalgia, malaise and neurologic and cardiac manifestations. Named after Old Lyme, CT, where the disease was first reported.
**Not notifiable.

Malaria Cases Reported in 2000

National Total = 1,288 Cases*

ALPHA ORDER

RANK	STATE	CASES	% of USA
21	Alabama	16	1.2%
47	Alaska	0	0.0%
25	Arizona	9	0.7%
39	Arkansas	3	0.2%
2	California	186	14.4%
16	Colorado	25	1.9%
19	Connecticut	20	1.6%
35	Delaware	5	0.4%
4	Florida	74	5.7%
14	Georgia	30	2.3%
24	Hawaii	11	0.9%
35	Idaho	5	0.4%
5	Illinois	54	4.2%
32	Indiana	6	0.5%
41	Iowa	2	0.2%
29	Kansas	7	0.5%
20	Kentucky	18	1.4%
27	Louisiana	8	0.6%
32	Maine	6	0.5%
3	Maryland	128	9.9%
15	Massachusetts	27	2.1%
11	Michigan	33	2.6%
8	Minnesota	40	3.1%
43	Mississippi	1	0.1%
18	Missouri	21	1.6%
43	Montana	1	0.1%
29	Nebraska	7	0.5%
29	Nevada	7	0.5%
43	New Hampshire	1	0.1%
9	New Jersey	39	3.0%
47	New Mexico	0	0.0%
1	New York	202	15.7%
10	North Carolina	36	2.8%
39	North Dakota	3	0.2%
17	Ohio	23	1.8%
25	Oklahoma	9	0.7%
7	Oregon	42	3.3%
13	Pennsylvania	31	2.4%
27	Rhode Island	8	0.6%
41	South Carolina	2	0.2%
43	South Dakota	1	0.1%
23	Tennessee	12	0.9%
47	Texas	0	0.0%
32	Utah	6	0.5%
37	Vermont	4	0.3%
6	Virginia	50	3.9%
11	Washington	33	2.6%
37	West Virginia	4	0.3%
22	Wisconsin	15	1.2%
47	Wyoming	0	0.0%

RANK ORDER

RANK	STATE	CASES	% of USA
1	New York	202	15.7%
2	California	186	14.4%
3	Maryland	128	9.9%
4	Florida	74	5.7%
5	Illinois	54	4.2%
6	Virginia	50	3.9%
7	Oregon	42	3.3%
8	Minnesota	40	3.1%
9	New Jersey	39	3.0%
10	North Carolina	36	2.8%
11	Michigan	33	2.6%
11	Washington	33	2.6%
13	Pennsylvania	31	2.4%
14	Georgia	30	2.3%
15	Massachusetts	27	2.1%
16	Colorado	25	1.9%
17	Ohio	23	1.8%
18	Missouri	21	1.6%
19	Connecticut	20	1.6%
20	Kentucky	18	1.4%
21	Alabama	16	1.2%
22	Wisconsin	15	1.2%
23	Tennessee	12	0.9%
24	Hawaii	11	0.9%
25	Arizona	9	0.7%
25	Oklahoma	9	0.7%
27	Louisiana	8	0.6%
27	Rhode Island	8	0.6%
29	Kansas	7	0.5%
29	Nebraska	7	0.5%
29	Nevada	7	0.5%
32	Indiana	6	0.5%
32	Maine	6	0.5%
32	Utah	6	0.5%
35	Delaware	5	0.4%
35	Idaho	5	0.4%
37	Vermont	4	0.3%
37	West Virginia	4	0.3%
39	Arkansas	3	0.2%
39	North Dakota	3	0.2%
41	Iowa	2	0.2%
41	South Carolina	2	0.2%
43	Mississippi	1	0.1%
43	Montana	1	0.1%
43	New Hampshire	1	0.1%
43	South Dakota	1	0.1%
47	Alaska	0	0.0%
47	New Mexico	0	0.0%
47	Texas	0	0.0%
47	Wyoming	0	0.0%
	District of Columbia	17	1.3%

Source: U.S. Department of Health and Human Services, National Center for Health Statistics
    "Morbidity and Mortality Weekly Report" (January 5, 2001, Vol. 49, No. 51)
*Provisional data. Infectious disease usually transmitted by bites of infected mosquitoes. Symptoms include high fever, shaking chills, sweating and anemia.

Malaria Rate in 2000

National Rate = 0.5 Cases per 100,000 Population*

ALPHA ORDER

RANK	STATE	RATE
20	Alabama	0.4
46	Alaska	0.0
34	Arizona	0.2
39	Arkansas	0.1
9	California	0.6
9	Colorado	0.6
9	Connecticut	0.6
9	Delaware	0.6
14	Florida	0.5
20	Georgia	0.4
4	Hawaii	0.9
20	Idaho	0.4
20	Illinois	0.4
39	Indiana	0.1
39	Iowa	0.1
28	Kansas	0.3
14	Kentucky	0.5
34	Louisiana	0.2
14	Maine	0.5
1	Maryland	2.4
20	Massachusetts	0.4
28	Michigan	0.3
5	Minnesota	0.8
46	Mississippi	0.0
20	Missouri	0.4
39	Montana	0.1
20	Nebraska	0.4
20	Nevada	0.4
39	New Hampshire	0.1
14	New Jersey	0.5
46	New Mexico	0.0
3	New York	1.1
14	North Carolina	0.5
14	North Dakota	0.5
34	Ohio	0.2
28	Oklahoma	0.3
2	Oregon	1.2
28	Pennsylvania	0.3
5	Rhode Island	0.8
39	South Carolina	0.1
39	South Dakota	0.1
34	Tennessee	0.2
46	Texas	0.0
28	Utah	0.3
7	Vermont	0.7
7	Virginia	0.7
9	Washington	0.6
34	West Virginia	0.2
28	Wisconsin	0.3
46	Wyoming	0.0

RANK ORDER

RANK	STATE	RATE
1	Maryland	2.4
2	Oregon	1.2
3	New York	1.1
4	Hawaii	0.9
5	Minnesota	0.8
5	Rhode Island	0.8
7	Vermont	0.7
7	Virginia	0.7
9	California	0.6
9	Colorado	0.6
9	Connecticut	0.6
9	Delaware	0.6
9	Washington	0.6
14	Florida	0.5
14	Kentucky	0.5
14	Maine	0.5
14	New Jersey	0.5
14	North Carolina	0.5
14	North Dakota	0.5
20	Alabama	0.4
20	Georgia	0.4
20	Idaho	0.4
20	Illinois	0.4
20	Massachusetts	0.4
20	Missouri	0.4
20	Nebraska	0.4
20	Nevada	0.4
28	Kansas	0.3
28	Michigan	0.3
28	Oklahoma	0.3
28	Pennsylvania	0.3
28	Utah	0.3
28	Wisconsin	0.3
34	Arizona	0.2
34	Louisiana	0.2
34	Ohio	0.2
34	Tennessee	0.2
34	West Virginia	0.2
39	Arkansas	0.1
39	Indiana	0.1
39	Iowa	0.1
39	Montana	0.1
39	New Hampshire	0.1
39	South Carolina	0.1
39	South Dakota	0.1
46	Alaska	0.0
46	Mississippi	0.0
46	New Mexico	0.0
46	Texas	0.0
46	Wyoming	0.0

District of Columbia 3.0

*Source: Morgan Quitno Press using data from U.S. Dept. of Health & Human Serv's, National Center for Health Statistics
"Morbidity and Mortality Weekly Report" (January 5, 2001, Vol. 49, No. 51)*
*Provisional data. Infectious disease usually transmitted by bites of infected mosquitoes. Symptoms include high
fever, shaking chills, sweating and anemia.*

Measles (Rubeola) Cases Reported in 2000

National Total = 81 Cases*

ALPHA ORDER

RANK	STATE	CASES	% of USA
21	Alabama	0	0.0%
17	Alaska	1	1.2%
21	Arizona	0	0.0%
21	Arkansas	0	0.0%
2	California	15	18.5%
5	Colorado	3	3.7%
21	Connecticut	0	0.0%
21	Delaware	0	0.0%
13	Florida	2	2.5%
21	Georgia	0	0.0%
5	Hawaii	3	3.7%
21	Idaho	0	0.0%
4	Illinois	4	4.9%
21	Indiana	0	0.0%
13	Iowa	2	2.5%
13	Kansas	2	2.5%
21	Kentucky	0	0.0%
21	Louisiana	0	0.0%
21	Maine	0	0.0%
21	Maryland	0	0.0%
17	Massachusetts	1	1.2%
5	Michigan	3	3.7%
17	Minnesota	1	1.2%
21	Mississippi	0	0.0%
21	Missouri	0	0.0%
21	Montana	0	0.0%
21	Nebraska	0	0.0%
3	Nevada	7	8.6%
5	New Hampshire	3	3.7%
21	New Jersey	0	0.0%
21	New Mexico	0	0.0%
1	New York	19	23.5%
21	North Carolina	0	0.0%
21	North Dakota	0	0.0%
5	Ohio	3	3.7%
21	Oklahoma	0	0.0%
21	Oregon	0	0.0%
17	Pennsylvania	1	1.2%
21	Rhode Island	0	0.0%
21	South Carolina	0	0.0%
21	South Dakota	0	0.0%
21	Tennessee	0	0.0%
21	Texas	0	0.0%
5	Utah	3	3.7%
5	Vermont	3	3.7%
13	Virginia	2	2.5%
5	Washington	3	3.7%
21	West Virginia	0	0.0%
21	Wisconsin	0	0.0%
21	Wyoming	0	0.0%

RANK ORDER

RANK	STATE	CASES	% of USA
1	New York	19	23.5%
2	California	15	18.5%
3	Nevada	7	8.6%
4	Illinois	4	4.9%
5	Colorado	3	3.7%
5	Hawaii	3	3.7%
5	Michigan	3	3.7%
5	New Hampshire	3	3.7%
5	Ohio	3	3.7%
5	Utah	3	3.7%
5	Vermont	3	3.7%
5	Washington	3	3.7%
13	Florida	2	2.5%
13	Iowa	2	2.5%
13	Kansas	2	2.5%
13	Virginia	2	2.5%
17	Alaska	1	1.2%
17	Massachusetts	1	1.2%
17	Minnesota	1	1.2%
17	Pennsylvania	1	1.2%
21	Alabama	0	0.0%
21	Arizona	0	0.0%
21	Arkansas	0	0.0%
21	Connecticut	0	0.0%
21	Delaware	0	0.0%
21	Georgia	0	0.0%
21	Idaho	0	0.0%
21	Indiana	0	0.0%
21	Kentucky	0	0.0%
21	Louisiana	0	0.0%
21	Maine	0	0.0%
21	Maryland	0	0.0%
21	Mississippi	0	0.0%
21	Missouri	0	0.0%
21	Montana	0	0.0%
21	Nebraska	0	0.0%
21	New Jersey	0	0.0%
21	New Mexico	0	0.0%
21	North Carolina	0	0.0%
21	North Dakota	0	0.0%
21	Oklahoma	0	0.0%
21	Oregon	0	0.0%
21	Rhode Island	0	0.0%
21	South Carolina	0	0.0%
21	South Dakota	0	0.0%
21	Tennessee	0	0.0%
21	Texas	0	0.0%
21	West Virginia	0	0.0%
21	Wisconsin	0	0.0%
21	Wyoming	0	0.0%
	District of Columbia	0	0.0%

Source: U.S. Department of Health and Human Services, National Center for Health Statistics
    "Morbidity and Mortality Weekly Report" (January 5, 2001, Vol. 49, No. 51)
*Provisional data. Includes indigenous and imported cases.

Measles (Rubeola) Rate in 2000

National Rate = 0.03 Cases per 100,000 Population*

ALPHA ORDER			RANK ORDER		
RANK	STATE	RATE	RANK	STATE	RATE
21	Alabama	0.00	1	Vermont	0.49
5	Alaska	0.16	2	Nevada	0.35
21	Arizona	0.00	3	Hawaii	0.25
21	Arkansas	0.00	4	New Hampshire	0.24
12	California	0.04	5	Alaska	0.16
8	Colorado	0.07	6	Utah	0.13
21	Connecticut	0.00	7	New York	0.10
21	Delaware	0.00	8	Colorado	0.07
19	Florida	0.01	8	Iowa	0.07
21	Georgia	0.00	8	Kansas	0.07
3	Hawaii	0.25	11	Washington	0.05
21	Idaho	0.00	12	California	0.04
13	Illinois	0.03	13	Illinois	0.03
21	Indiana	0.00	13	Michigan	0.03
8	Iowa	0.07	13	Ohio	0.03
8	Kansas	0.07	13	Virginia	0.03
21	Kentucky	0.00	17	Massachusetts	0.02
21	Louisiana	0.00	17	Minnesota	0.02
21	Maine	0.00	19	Florida	0.01
21	Maryland	0.00	19	Pennsylvania	0.01
17	Massachusetts	0.02	21	Alabama	0.00
13	Michigan	0.03	21	Arizona	0.00
17	Minnesota	0.02	21	Arkansas	0.00
21	Mississippi	0.00	21	Connecticut	0.00
21	Missouri	0.00	21	Delaware	0.00
21	Montana	0.00	21	Georgia	0.00
21	Nebraska	0.00	21	Idaho	0.00
2	Nevada	0.35	21	Indiana	0.00
4	New Hampshire	0.24	21	Kentucky	0.00
21	New Jersey	0.00	21	Louisiana	0.00
21	New Mexico	0.00	21	Maine	0.00
7	New York	0.10	21	Maryland	0.00
21	North Carolina	0.00	21	Mississippi	0.00
21	North Dakota	0.00	21	Missouri	0.00
13	Ohio	0.03	21	Montana	0.00
21	Oklahoma	0.00	21	Nebraska	0.00
21	Oregon	0.00	21	New Jersey	0.00
19	Pennsylvania	0.01	21	New Mexico	0.00
21	Rhode Island	0.00	21	North Carolina	0.00
21	South Carolina	0.00	21	North Dakota	0.00
21	South Dakota	0.00	21	Oklahoma	0.00
21	Tennessee	0.00	21	Oregon	0.00
21	Texas	0.00	21	Rhode Island	0.00
6	Utah	0.13	21	South Carolina	0.00
1	Vermont	0.49	21	South Dakota	0.00
13	Virginia	0.03	21	Tennessee	0.00
11	Washington	0.05	21	Texas	0.00
21	West Virginia	0.00	21	West Virginia	0.00
21	Wisconsin	0.00	21	Wisconsin	0.00
21	Wyoming	0.00	21	Wyoming	0.00
				District of Columbia	0.00

Source: Morgan Quitno Press using data from U.S. Dept. of Health & Human Serv's, National Center for Health Statistics "Morbidity and Mortality Weekly Report" (January 5, 2001, Vol. 49, No. 51)
Provisional data. Includes indigenous and imported cases.

Meningococcal Infections Reported in 2000

National Total = 2,035 Cases*

RANK	STATE	CASES	% of USA
22	Alabama	35	1.7%
37	Alaska	9	0.4%
5	Arizona	97	4.8%
31	Arkansas	15	0.7%
1	California	274	13.5%
24	Colorado	34	1.7%
30	Connecticut	19	0.9%
50	Delaware	1	0.0%
2	Florida	123	6.0%
14	Georgia	48	2.4%
39	Hawaii	8	0.4%
43	Idaho	7	0.3%
7	Illinois	79	3.9%
14	Indiana	48	2.4%
20	Iowa	37	1.8%
36	Kansas	11	0.5%
27	Kentucky	26	1.3%
22	Louisiana	35	1.7%
39	Maine	8	0.4%
26	Maryland	27	1.3%
9	Massachusetts	72	3.5%
3	Michigan	106	5.2%
29	Minnesota	22	1.1%
32	Mississippi	14	0.7%
10	Missouri	70	3.4%
44	Montana	6	0.3%
39	Nebraska	8	0.4%
46	Nevada	5	0.2%
34	New Hampshire	12	0.6%
16	New Jersey	46	2.3%
34	New Mexico	12	0.6%
4	New York	103	5.1%
19	North Carolina	39	1.9%
49	North Dakota	3	0.1%
6	Ohio	96	4.7%
25	Oklahoma	28	1.4%
8	Oregon	77	3.8%
17	Pennsylvania	45	2.2%
37	Rhode Island	9	0.4%
27	South Carolina	26	1.3%
44	South Dakota	6	0.3%
12	Tennessee	56	2.8%
12	Texas	56	2.8%
39	Utah	8	0.4%
47	Vermont	4	0.2%
18	Virginia	42	2.1%
11	Washington	69	3.4%
33	West Virginia	13	0.6%
20	Wisconsin	37	1.8%
47	Wyoming	4	0.2%

RANK	STATE	CASES	% of USA
1	California	274	13.5%
2	Florida	123	6.0%
3	Michigan	106	5.2%
4	New York	103	5.1%
5	Arizona	97	4.8%
6	Ohio	96	4.7%
7	Illinois	79	3.9%
8	Oregon	77	3.8%
9	Massachusetts	72	3.5%
10	Missouri	70	3.4%
11	Washington	69	3.4%
12	Tennessee	56	2.8%
12	Texas	56	2.8%
14	Georgia	48	2.4%
14	Indiana	48	2.4%
16	New Jersey	46	2.3%
17	Pennsylvania	45	2.2%
18	Virginia	42	2.1%
19	North Carolina	39	1.9%
20	Iowa	37	1.8%
20	Wisconsin	37	1.8%
22	Alabama	35	1.7%
22	Louisiana	35	1.7%
24	Colorado	34	1.7%
25	Oklahoma	28	1.4%
26	Maryland	27	1.3%
27	Kentucky	26	1.3%
27	South Carolina	26	1.3%
29	Minnesota	22	1.1%
30	Connecticut	19	0.9%
31	Arkansas	15	0.7%
32	Mississippi	14	0.7%
33	West Virginia	13	0.6%
34	New Hampshire	12	0.6%
34	New Mexico	12	0.6%
36	Kansas	11	0.5%
37	Alaska	9	0.4%
37	Rhode Island	9	0.4%
39	Hawaii	8	0.4%
39	Maine	8	0.4%
39	Nebraska	8	0.4%
39	Utah	8	0.4%
43	Idaho	7	0.3%
44	Montana	6	0.3%
44	South Dakota	6	0.3%
46	Nevada	5	0.2%
47	Vermont	4	0.2%
47	Wyoming	4	0.2%
49	North Dakota	3	0.1%
50	Delaware	1	0.0%
	District of Columbia	0	0.0%

Source: U.S. Department of Health and Human Services, National Center for Health Statistics "Morbidity and Mortality Weekly Report" (January 5, 2001, Vol. 49, No. 51)
Provisional data. A bacterium (Neisseria meningitidis) that causes cerebrospinal meningitis.

Meningococcal Infection Rate in 2000

National Rate = 0.7 Cases per 100,000 Population*

ALPHA ORDER			RANK ORDER		
RANK	STATE	RATE	RANK	STATE	RATE
12	Alabama	0.8	1	Oregon	2.3
3	Alaska	1.4	2	Arizona	1.9
2	Arizona	1.9	3	Alaska	1.4
28	Arkansas	0.6	4	Iowa	1.3
12	California	0.8	4	Missouri	1.3
12	Colorado	0.8	6	Washington	1.2
28	Connecticut	0.6	7	Massachusetts	1.1
50	Delaware	0.1	7	Michigan	1.1
12	Florida	0.8	9	New Hampshire	1.0
28	Georgia	0.6	9	Tennessee	1.0
22	Hawaii	0.7	11	Rhode Island	0.9
36	Idaho	0.5	12	Alabama	0.8
28	Illinois	0.6	12	California	0.8
12	Indiana	0.8	12	Colorado	0.8
4	Iowa	1.3	12	Florida	0.8
44	Kansas	0.4	12	Indiana	0.8
28	Kentucky	0.6	12	Louisiana	0.8
12	Louisiana	0.8	12	Ohio	0.8
28	Maine	0.6	12	Oklahoma	0.8
36	Maryland	0.5	12	South Dakota	0.8
7	Massachusetts	1.1	12	Wyoming	0.8
7	Michigan	1.1	22	Hawaii	0.7
44	Minnesota	0.4	22	Montana	0.7
36	Mississippi	0.5	22	New Mexico	0.7
4	Missouri	1.3	22	Vermont	0.7
22	Montana	0.7	22	West Virginia	0.7
36	Nebraska	0.5	22	Wisconsin	0.7
48	Nevada	0.3	28	Arkansas	0.6
9	New Hampshire	1.0	28	Connecticut	0.6
36	New Jersey	0.5	28	Georgia	0.6
22	New Mexico	0.7	28	Illinois	0.6
36	New York	0.5	28	Kentucky	0.6
36	North Carolina	0.5	28	Maine	0.6
36	North Dakota	0.5	28	South Carolina	0.6
12	Ohio	0.8	28	Virginia	0.6
12	Oklahoma	0.8	36	Idaho	0.5
1	Oregon	2.3	36	Maryland	0.5
44	Pennsylvania	0.4	36	Mississippi	0.5
11	Rhode Island	0.9	36	Nebraska	0.5
28	South Carolina	0.6	36	New Jersey	0.5
12	South Dakota	0.8	36	New York	0.5
9	Tennessee	1.0	36	North Carolina	0.5
48	Texas	0.3	36	North Dakota	0.5
44	Utah	0.4	44	Kansas	0.4
22	Vermont	0.7	44	Minnesota	0.4
28	Virginia	0.6	44	Pennsylvania	0.4
6	Washington	1.2	44	Utah	0.4
22	West Virginia	0.7	48	Nevada	0.3
22	Wisconsin	0.7	48	Texas	0.3
12	Wyoming	0.8	50	Delaware	0.1
				District of Columbia	0.0

Source: Morgan Quitno Press using data from U.S. Dept. of Health & Human Serv's, National Center for Health Statistics "Morbidity and Mortality Weekly Report" (January 5, 2001, Vol. 49, No. 51)
*Provisional data. A bacterium (Neisseria meningitidis) that causes cerebrospinal meningitis.

Mumps Cases Reported in 2000

National Total = 323 Cases*

ALPHA ORDER

RANK	STATE	CASES	% of USA
21	Alabama	4	1.2%
13	Alaska	7	2.2%
16	Arizona	6	1.9%
20	Arkansas	5	1.5%
1	California	87	26.9%
28	Colorado	3	0.9%
28	Connecticut	3	0.9%
40	Delaware	0	0.0%
13	Florida	7	2.2%
30	Georgia	2	0.6%
5	Hawaii	14	4.3%
33	Idaho	1	0.3%
16	Illinois	6	1.9%
33	Indiana	1	0.3%
11	Iowa	8	2.5%
21	Kansas	4	1.2%
33	Kentucky	1	0.3%
21	Louisiana	4	1.2%
40	Maine	0	0.0%
9	Maryland	10	3.1%
33	Massachusetts	1	0.3%
4	Michigan	17	5.3%
40	Minnesota	0	0.0%
30	Mississippi	2	0.6%
21	Missouri	4	1.2%
33	Montana	1	0.3%
21	Nebraska	4	1.2%
16	Nevada	6	1.9%
40	New Hampshire	0	0.0%
21	New Jersey	4	1.2%
33	New Mexico	1	0.3%
3	New York	18	5.6%
11	North Carolina	8	2.5%
40	North Dakota	0	0.0%
10	Ohio	9	2.8%
40	Oklahoma	0	0.0%
NA	Oregon**	NA	NA
16	Pennsylvania	6	1.9%
33	Rhode Island	1	0.3%
6	South Carolina	11	3.4%
40	South Dakota	0	0.0%
30	Tennessee	2	0.6%
2	Texas	22	6.8%
13	Utah	7	2.2%
40	Vermont	0	0.0%
6	Virginia	11	3.4%
6	Washington	11	3.4%
40	West Virginia	0	0.0%
40	Wisconsin	0	0.0%
21	Wyoming	4	1.2%

RANK ORDER

RANK	STATE	CASES	% of USA
1	California	87	26.9%
2	Texas	22	6.8%
3	New York	18	5.6%
4	Michigan	17	5.3%
5	Hawaii	14	4.3%
6	South Carolina	11	3.4%
6	Virginia	11	3.4%
6	Washington	11	3.4%
9	Maryland	10	3.1%
10	Ohio	9	2.8%
11	Iowa	8	2.5%
11	North Carolina	8	2.5%
13	Alaska	7	2.2%
13	Florida	7	2.2%
13	Utah	7	2.2%
16	Arizona	6	1.9%
16	Illinois	6	1.9%
16	Nevada	6	1.9%
16	Pennsylvania	6	1.9%
20	Arkansas	5	1.5%
21	Alabama	4	1.2%
21	Kansas	4	1.2%
21	Louisiana	4	1.2%
21	Missouri	4	1.2%
21	Nebraska	4	1.2%
21	New Jersey	4	1.2%
21	Wyoming	4	1.2%
28	Colorado	3	0.9%
28	Connecticut	3	0.9%
30	Georgia	2	0.6%
30	Mississippi	2	0.6%
30	Tennessee	2	0.6%
33	Idaho	1	0.3%
33	Indiana	1	0.3%
33	Kentucky	1	0.3%
33	Massachusetts	1	0.3%
33	Montana	1	0.3%
33	New Mexico	1	0.3%
33	Rhode Island	1	0.3%
40	Delaware	0	0.0%
40	Maine	0	0.0%
40	Minnesota	0	0.0%
40	New Hampshire	0	0.0%
40	North Dakota	0	0.0%
40	Oklahoma	0	0.0%
40	South Dakota	0	0.0%
40	Vermont	0	0.0%
40	West Virginia	0	0.0%
40	Wisconsin	0	0.0%
NA	Oregon**	NA	NA
	District of Columbia	0	0.0%

Source: U.S. Department of Health and Human Services, National Center for Health Statistics
"Morbidity and Mortality Weekly Report" (January 5, 2001, Vol. 49, No. 51)
*Provisional data. An acute, inflammatory, contagious disease caused by a paramyxovirus and characterized by swelling of the salivary glands, especially the parotids, and sometimes of the pancreas, ovaries, or testes. This disease, mainly affecting children, can be prevented by vaccination.
**Mumps is not a notifiable disease in Oregon.

Mumps Rate in 2000

National Rate = 0.11 Cases per 100,000 Population*

ALPHA ORDER

RANK	STATE	RATE
21	Alabama	0.09
2	Alaska	1.12
16	Arizona	0.12
10	Arkansas	0.19
8	California	0.26
27	Colorado	0.07
21	Connecticut	0.09
40	Delaware	0.00
34	Florida	0.04
36	Georgia	0.02
1	Hawaii	1.16
25	Idaho	0.08
30	Illinois	0.05
36	Indiana	0.02
6	Iowa	0.27
15	Kansas	0.15
36	Kentucky	0.02
21	Louisiana	0.09
40	Maine	0.00
10	Maryland	0.19
36	Massachusetts	0.02
13	Michigan	0.17
40	Minnesota	0.00
27	Mississippi	0.07
27	Missouri	0.07
17	Montana	0.11
9	Nebraska	0.23
5	Nevada	0.30
40	New Hampshire	0.00
30	New Jersey	0.05
30	New Mexico	0.05
21	New York	0.09
19	North Carolina	0.10
40	North Dakota	0.00
25	Ohio	0.08
40	Oklahoma	0.00
NA	Oregon**	NA
30	Pennsylvania	0.05
19	Rhode Island	0.10
6	South Carolina	0.27
40	South Dakota	0.00
34	Tennessee	0.04
17	Texas	0.11
4	Utah	0.31
40	Vermont	0.00
14	Virginia	0.16
10	Washington	0.19
40	West Virginia	0.00
40	Wisconsin	0.00
3	Wyoming	0.81

RANK ORDER

RANK	STATE	RATE
1	Hawaii	1.16
2	Alaska	1.12
3	Wyoming	0.81
4	Utah	0.31
5	Nevada	0.30
6	Iowa	0.27
6	South Carolina	0.27
8	California	0.26
9	Nebraska	0.23
10	Arkansas	0.19
10	Maryland	0.19
10	Washington	0.19
13	Michigan	0.17
14	Virginia	0.16
15	Kansas	0.15
16	Arizona	0.12
17	Montana	0.11
17	Texas	0.11
19	North Carolina	0.10
19	Rhode Island	0.10
21	Alabama	0.09
21	Connecticut	0.09
21	Louisiana	0.09
21	New York	0.09
25	Idaho	0.08
25	Ohio	0.08
27	Colorado	0.07
27	Mississippi	0.07
27	Missouri	0.07
30	Illinois	0.05
30	New Jersey	0.05
30	New Mexico	0.05
30	Pennsylvania	0.05
34	Florida	0.04
34	Tennessee	0.04
36	Georgia	0.02
36	Indiana	0.02
36	Kentucky	0.02
36	Massachusetts	0.02
40	Delaware	0.00
40	Maine	0.00
40	Minnesota	0.00
40	New Hampshire	0.00
40	North Dakota	0.00
40	Oklahoma	0.00
40	South Dakota	0.00
40	Vermont	0.00
40	West Virginia	0.00
40	Wisconsin	0.00
NA	Oregon**	NA

District of Columbia   0.00

Source: Morgan Quitno Press using data from U.S. Dept. of Health & Human Serv's, National Center for Health Statistics
"Morbidity and Mortality Weekly Report" (January 5, 2001, Vol. 49, No. 51)
Provisional data. An acute, inflammatory, contagious disease caused by a paramyxovirus and characterized by swelling of the salivary glands, especially the parotids, and sometimes of the pancreas, ovaries, or testes. This disease, mainly affecting children, can be prevented by vaccination.
**Mumps is not a notifiable disease in Oregon.*

Rabies (Animal) Cases Reported in 2000

National Total = 5,834 Cases*

RANK	STATE	CASES	% of USA
20	Alabama	81	1.4%
32	Alaska	24	0.4%
22	Arizona	79	1.4%
37	Arkansas	20	0.3%
8	California	258	4.4%
46	Colorado	0	0.0%
7	Connecticut	271	4.6%
31	Delaware	49	0.8%
10	Florida	162	2.8%
5	Georgia	344	5.9%
46	Hawaii	0	0.0%
40	Idaho	9	0.2%
33	Illinois	22	0.4%
38	Indiana	15	0.3%
21	Iowa	80	1.4%
17	Kansas	100	1.7%
34	Kentucky	21	0.4%
46	Louisiana	0	0.0%
12	Maine	132	2.3%
4	Maryland	407	7.0%
6	Massachusetts	276	4.7%
24	Michigan	68	1.2%
18	Minnesota	96	1.6%
45	Mississippi	1	0.0%
30	Missouri	50	0.9%
25	Montana	65	1.1%
44	Nebraska	2	0.0%
40	Nevada	9	0.2%
34	New Hampshire	21	0.4%
9	New Jersey	195	3.3%
34	New Mexico	21	0.4%
1	New York	812	13.9%
3	North Carolina	551	9.4%
14	North Dakota	116	2.0%
29	Ohio	52	0.9%
27	Oklahoma	57	1.0%
43	Oregon	7	0.1%
13	Pennsylvania	127	2.2%
26	Rhode Island	61	1.0%
11	South Carolina	155	2.7%
19	South Dakota	90	1.5%
16	Tennessee	103	1.8%
46	Texas	0	0.0%
39	Utah	10	0.2%
27	Vermont	57	1.0%
2	Virginia	559	9.6%
46	Washington	0	0.0%
15	West Virginia	113	1.9%
40	Wisconsin	9	0.2%
23	Wyoming	77	1.3%

RANK	STATE	CASES	% of USA
1	New York	812	13.9%
2	Virginia	559	9.6%
3	North Carolina	551	9.4%
4	Maryland	407	7.0%
5	Georgia	344	5.9%
6	Massachusetts	276	4.7%
7	Connecticut	271	4.6%
8	California	258	4.4%
9	New Jersey	195	3.3%
10	Florida	162	2.8%
11	South Carolina	155	2.7%
12	Maine	132	2.3%
13	Pennsylvania	127	2.2%
14	North Dakota	116	2.0%
15	West Virginia	113	1.9%
16	Tennessee	103	1.8%
17	Kansas	100	1.7%
18	Minnesota	96	1.6%
19	South Dakota	90	1.5%
20	Alabama	81	1.4%
21	Iowa	80	1.4%
22	Arizona	79	1.4%
23	Wyoming	77	1.3%
24	Michigan	68	1.2%
25	Montana	65	1.1%
26	Rhode Island	61	1.0%
27	Oklahoma	57	1.0%
27	Vermont	57	1.0%
29	Ohio	52	0.9%
30	Missouri	50	0.9%
31	Delaware	49	0.8%
32	Alaska	24	0.4%
33	Illinois	22	0.4%
34	Kentucky	21	0.4%
34	New Hampshire	21	0.4%
34	New Mexico	21	0.4%
37	Arkansas	20	0.3%
38	Indiana	15	0.3%
39	Utah	10	0.2%
40	Idaho	9	0.2%
40	Nevada	9	0.2%
40	Wisconsin	9	0.2%
43	Oregon	7	0.1%
44	Nebraska	2	0.0%
45	Mississippi	1	0.0%
46	Colorado	0	0.0%
46	Hawaii	0	0.0%
46	Louisiana	0	0.0%
46	Texas	0	0.0%
46	Washington	0	0.0%
	District of Columbia	0	0.0%

Source: U.S. Department of Health and Human Services, National Center for Health Statistics
"Morbidity and Mortality Weekly Report" (January 5, 2001, Vol. 49, No. 51)
*Provisional data. An acute, infectious, often fatal viral disease of most warm-blooded animals, especially wolves, cats, and dogs, that attacks the central nervous system and is transmitted by the bite of infected animals.

Rabies (Animal) Rate in 2000

National Rate = 2.1 Cases per 100,000 Human Population*

ALPHA ORDER			RANK ORDER		
RANK	STATE	RATE	RANK	STATE	RATE
23	Alabama	1.8	1	North Dakota	18.1
18	Alaska	3.8	2	Wyoming	15.6
27	Arizona	1.5	3	South Dakota	11.9
33	Arkansas	0.7	4	Maine	10.4
32	California	0.8	5	Vermont	9.4
45	Colorado	0.0	6	Connecticut	8.0
6	Connecticut	8.0	7	Virginia	7.9
11	Delaware	6.3	8	Maryland	7.7
29	Florida	1.0	9	Montana	7.2
16	Georgia	4.2	10	North Carolina	6.8
45	Hawaii	0.0	11	Delaware	6.3
33	Idaho	0.7	12	West Virginia	6.2
40	Illinois	0.2	13	Rhode Island	5.8
40	Indiana	0.2	14	Massachusetts	4.3
20	Iowa	2.7	14	New York	4.3
19	Kansas	3.7	16	Georgia	4.2
36	Kentucky	0.5	17	South Carolina	3.9
45	Louisiana	0.0	18	Alaska	3.8
4	Maine	10.4	19	Kansas	3.7
8	Maryland	7.7	20	Iowa	2.7
14	Massachusetts	4.3	21	New Jersey	2.3
33	Michigan	0.7	22	Minnesota	2.0
22	Minnesota	2.0	23	Alabama	1.8
45	Mississippi	0.0	23	Tennessee	1.8
31	Missouri	0.9	25	New Hampshire	1.7
9	Montana	7.2	25	Oklahoma	1.7
44	Nebraska	0.1	27	Arizona	1.5
36	Nevada	0.5	28	New Mexico	1.2
25	New Hampshire	1.7	29	Florida	1.0
21	New Jersey	2.3	29	Pennsylvania	1.0
28	New Mexico	1.2	31	Missouri	0.9
14	New York	4.3	32	California	0.8
10	North Carolina	6.8	33	Arkansas	0.7
1	North Dakota	18.1	33	Idaho	0.7
36	Ohio	0.5	33	Michigan	0.7
25	Oklahoma	1.7	36	Kentucky	0.5
40	Oregon	0.2	36	Nevada	0.5
29	Pennsylvania	1.0	36	Ohio	0.5
13	Rhode Island	5.8	39	Utah	0.4
17	South Carolina	3.9	40	Illinois	0.2
3	South Dakota	11.9	40	Indiana	0.2
23	Tennessee	1.8	40	Oregon	0.2
45	Texas	0.0	40	Wisconsin	0.2
39	Utah	0.4	44	Nebraska	0.1
5	Vermont	9.4	45	Colorado	0.0
7	Virginia	7.9	45	Hawaii	0.0
45	Washington	0.0	45	Louisiana	0.0
12	West Virginia	6.2	45	Mississippi	0.0
40	Wisconsin	0.2	45	Texas	0.0
2	Wyoming	15.6	45	Washington	0.0
				District of Columbia	0.0

Source: Morgan Quitno Press using data from U.S. Dept. of Health & Human Serv's, National Center for Health Statistics "Morbidity and Mortality Weekly Report" (January 5, 2001, Vol. 49, No. 51)
*Provisional data. An acute, infectious, often fatal viral disease of most warm-blooded animals, especially wolves, cats, and dogs, that attacks the central nervous system and is transmitted by the bite of infected animals.

Salmonellosis Cases Reported in 2000

National Total = 67,231 Cases*

ALPHA ORDER

RANK ORDER

RANK	STATE	CASES	% of USA
23	Alabama	1,203	1.8%
50	Alaska	85	0.1%
16	Arizona	1,524	2.3%
19	Arkansas	1,347	2.0%
1	California	7,636	11.4%
18	Colorado	1,356	2.0%
28	Connecticut	881	1.3%
42	Delaware	254	0.4%
6	Florida	2,884	4.3%
4	Georgia	3,079	4.6%
35	Hawaii	462	0.7%
44	Idaho	229	0.3%
13	Illinois	1,617	2.4%
24	Indiana	1,200	1.8%
30	Iowa	684	1.0%
33	Kansas	660	1.0%
34	Kentucky	647	1.0%
25	Louisiana	1,041	1.5%
45	Maine	223	0.3%
14	Maryland	1,612	2.4%
8	Massachusetts	2,401	3.6%
11	Michigan	1,815	2.7%
22	Minnesota	1,240	1.8%
29	Mississippi	804	1.2%
15	Missouri	1,600	2.4%
49	Montana	97	0.1%
37	Nebraska	362	0.5%
41	Nevada	258	0.4%
40	New Hampshire	288	0.4%
12	New Jersey	1,693	2.5%
36	New Mexico	423	0.6%
3	New York	4,369	6.5%
9	North Carolina	2,245	3.3%
47	North Dakota	142	0.2%
5	Ohio	2,978	4.4%
31	Oklahoma	682	1.0%
32	Oregon	661	1.0%
7	Pennsylvania	2,424	3.6%
39	Rhode Island	299	0.4%
20	South Carolina	1,280	1.9%
46	South Dakota	206	0.3%
17	Tennessee	1,426	2.1%
2	Texas	5,072	7.5%
27	Utah	970	1.4%
43	Vermont	230	0.3%
10	Virginia	1,837	2.7%
21	Washington	1,260	1.9%
38	West Virginia	320	0.5%
26	Wisconsin	1,038	1.5%
48	Wyoming	123	0.2%

RANK	STATE	CASES	% of USA
1	California	7,636	11.4%
2	Texas	5,072	7.5%
3	New York	4,369	6.5%
4	Georgia	3,079	4.6%
5	Ohio	2,978	4.4%
6	Florida	2,884	4.3%
7	Pennsylvania	2,424	3.6%
8	Massachusetts	2,401	3.6%
9	North Carolina	2,245	3.3%
10	Virginia	1,837	2.7%
11	Michigan	1,815	2.7%
12	New Jersey	1,693	2.5%
13	Illinois	1,617	2.4%
14	Maryland	1,612	2.4%
15	Missouri	1,600	2.4%
16	Arizona	1,524	2.3%
17	Tennessee	1,426	2.1%
18	Colorado	1,356	2.0%
19	Arkansas	1,347	2.0%
20	South Carolina	1,280	1.9%
21	Washington	1,260	1.9%
22	Minnesota	1,240	1.8%
23	Alabama	1,203	1.8%
24	Indiana	1,200	1.8%
25	Louisiana	1,041	1.5%
26	Wisconsin	1,038	1.5%
27	Utah	970	1.4%
28	Connecticut	881	1.3%
29	Mississippi	804	1.2%
30	Iowa	684	1.0%
31	Oklahoma	682	1.0%
32	Oregon	661	1.0%
33	Kansas	660	1.0%
34	Kentucky	647	1.0%
35	Hawaii	462	0.7%
36	New Mexico	423	0.6%
37	Nebraska	362	0.5%
38	West Virginia	320	0.5%
39	Rhode Island	299	0.4%
40	New Hampshire	288	0.4%
41	Nevada	258	0.4%
42	Delaware	254	0.4%
43	Vermont	230	0.3%
44	Idaho	229	0.3%
45	Maine	223	0.3%
46	South Dakota	206	0.3%
47	North Dakota	142	0.2%
48	Wyoming	123	0.2%
49	Montana	97	0.1%
50	Alaska	85	0.1%
	District of Columbia	64	0.1%

Source: U.S. Department of Health and Human Services, National Center for Health Statistics
"Morbidity and Mortality Weekly Report" (January 5, 2001, Vol. 49, No. 51)
*Provisional data. Any disease caused by a salmonella infection, which may be manifested as food poisoning with acute gastroenteritis, vomiting and diarrhea. Reported through Public Health Laboratory Information System and the National Electronic Telecommunications System for Surveillance.

Salmonellosis Rate in 2000

National Rate = 23.9 Cases per 100,000 Population*

ALPHA ORDER

RANK	STATE	RATE
17	Alabama	27.1
47	Alaska	13.6
11	Arizona	29.7
1	Arkansas	50.4
31	California	22.5
9	Colorado	31.5
20	Connecticut	25.9
7	Delaware	32.4
42	Florida	18.0
6	Georgia	37.6
3	Hawaii	38.1
43	Idaho	17.7
48	Illinois	13.0
37	Indiana	19.7
26	Iowa	23.4
24	Kansas	24.5
46	Kentucky	16.0
27	Louisiana	23.3
45	Maine	17.5
10	Maryland	30.4
4	Massachusetts	37.8
41	Michigan	18.3
21	Minnesota	25.2
14	Mississippi	28.3
12	Missouri	28.6
50	Montana	10.8
34	Nebraska	21.2
49	Nevada	12.9
27	New Hampshire	23.3
35	New Jersey	20.1
27	New Mexico	23.3
30	New York	23.0
15	North Carolina	27.9
32	North Dakota	22.1
18	Ohio	26.2
36	Oklahoma	19.8
40	Oregon	19.3
37	Pennsylvania	19.7
13	Rhode Island	28.5
8	South Carolina	31.9
16	South Dakota	27.3
22	Tennessee	25.1
25	Texas	24.3
2	Utah	43.4
4	Vermont	37.8
19	Virginia	26.0
33	Washington	21.4
43	West Virginia	17.7
39	Wisconsin	19.4
23	Wyoming	24.9

RANK ORDER

RANK	STATE	RATE
1	Arkansas	50.4
2	Utah	43.4
3	Hawaii	38.1
4	Massachusetts	37.8
4	Vermont	37.8
6	Georgia	37.6
7	Delaware	32.4
8	South Carolina	31.9
9	Colorado	31.5
10	Maryland	30.4
11	Arizona	29.7
12	Missouri	28.6
13	Rhode Island	28.5
14	Mississippi	28.3
15	North Carolina	27.9
16	South Dakota	27.3
17	Alabama	27.1
18	Ohio	26.2
19	Virginia	26.0
20	Connecticut	25.9
21	Minnesota	25.2
22	Tennessee	25.1
23	Wyoming	24.9
24	Kansas	24.5
25	Texas	24.3
26	Iowa	23.4
27	Louisiana	23.3
27	New Hampshire	23.3
27	New Mexico	23.3
30	New York	23.0
31	California	22.5
32	North Dakota	22.1
33	Washington	21.4
34	Nebraska	21.2
35	New Jersey	20.1
36	Oklahoma	19.8
37	Indiana	19.7
37	Pennsylvania	19.7
39	Wisconsin	19.4
40	Oregon	19.3
41	Michigan	18.3
42	Florida	18.0
43	Idaho	17.7
43	West Virginia	17.7
45	Maine	17.5
46	Kentucky	16.0
47	Alaska	13.6
48	Illinois	13.0
49	Nevada	12.9
50	Montana	10.8

District of Columbia   11.2

Source: Morgan Quitno Press using data from U.S. Dept. of Health & Human Serv's, National Center for Health Statistics "Morbidity and Mortality Weekly Report" (January 5, 2001, Vol. 49, No. 51)
*Provisional data. Any disease caused by a salmonella infection, which may be manifested as food poisoning with acute gastroenteritis, vomiting and diarrhea. Reported through Public Health Laboratory Information System and the National Electronic Telecommunications System for Surveillance.

Shigellosis Cases Reported in 2000

National Total = 31,274 Cases*

ALPHA ORDER

RANK	STATE	CASES	% of USA
33	Alabama	177	0.6%
47	Alaska	11	0.0%
10	Arizona	952	3.0%
30	Arkansas	269	0.9%
2	California	2,689	8.6%
20	Colorado	475	1.5%
36	Connecticut	135	0.4%
42	Delaware	47	0.2%
6	Florida	1,544	4.9%
22	Georgia	441	1.4%
39	Hawaii	74	0.2%
40	Idaho	70	0.2%
9	Illinois	1,098	3.5%
5	Indiana	1,660	5.3%
11	Iowa	887	2.8%
23	Kansas	393	1.3%
18	Kentucky	631	2.0%
24	Louisiana	334	1.1%
44	Maine	23	0.1%
25	Maryland	327	1.0%
19	Massachusetts	520	1.7%
7	Michigan	1,257	4.0%
4	Minnesota	1,728	5.5%
32	Mississippi	209	0.7%
8	Missouri	1,130	3.6%
48	Montana	8	0.0%
29	Nebraska	271	0.9%
37	Nevada	122	0.4%
45	New Hampshire	15	0.0%
14	New Jersey	773	2.5%
27	New Mexico	285	0.9%
3	New York	2,228	7.1%
17	North Carolina	665	2.1%
38	North Dakota	109	0.3%
15	Ohio	754	2.4%
34	Oklahoma	170	0.5%
28	Oregon	272	0.9%
21	Pennsylvania	454	1.5%
41	Rhode Island	67	0.2%
31	South Carolina	228	0.7%
46	South Dakota	12	0.0%
16	Tennessee	704	2.3%
1	Texas	4,810	15.4%
35	Utah	164	0.5%
50	Vermont	5	0.0%
13	Virginia	794	2.5%
12	Washington	863	2.8%
43	West Virginia	39	0.1%
26	Wisconsin	293	0.9%
48	Wyoming	8	0.0%

RANK ORDER

RANK	STATE	CASES	% of USA
1	Texas	4,810	15.4%
2	California	2,689	8.6%
3	New York	2,228	7.1%
4	Minnesota	1,728	5.5%
5	Indiana	1,660	5.3%
6	Florida	1,544	4.9%
7	Michigan	1,257	4.0%
8	Missouri	1,130	3.6%
9	Illinois	1,098	3.5%
10	Arizona	952	3.0%
11	Iowa	887	2.8%
12	Washington	863	2.8%
13	Virginia	794	2.5%
14	New Jersey	773	2.5%
15	Ohio	754	2.4%
16	Tennessee	704	2.3%
17	North Carolina	665	2.1%
18	Kentucky	631	2.0%
19	Massachusetts	520	1.7%
20	Colorado	475	1.5%
21	Pennsylvania	454	1.5%
22	Georgia	441	1.4%
23	Kansas	393	1.3%
24	Louisiana	334	1.1%
25	Maryland	327	1.0%
26	Wisconsin	293	0.9%
27	New Mexico	285	0.9%
28	Oregon	272	0.9%
29	Nebraska	271	0.9%
30	Arkansas	269	0.9%
31	South Carolina	228	0.7%
32	Mississippi	209	0.7%
33	Alabama	177	0.6%
34	Oklahoma	170	0.5%
35	Utah	164	0.5%
36	Connecticut	135	0.4%
37	Nevada	122	0.4%
38	North Dakota	109	0.3%
39	Hawaii	74	0.2%
40	Idaho	70	0.2%
41	Rhode Island	67	0.2%
42	Delaware	47	0.2%
43	West Virginia	39	0.1%
44	Maine	23	0.1%
45	New Hampshire	15	0.0%
46	South Dakota	12	0.0%
47	Alaska	11	0.0%
48	Montana	8	0.0%
48	Wyoming	8	0.0%
50	Vermont	5	0.0%
	District of Columbia	80	0.3%

Source: U.S. Department of Health and Human Services, National Center for Health Statistics
"Morbidity and Mortality Weekly Report" (January 5, 2001, Vol. 49, No. 51)
*Provisional data. Dysentery caused by any of various species of shigellae, occurring most frequently in areas where poor sanitation and malnutrition are prevalent and commonly affecting children and infants. Reported through Public Health Laboratory Information System and the National Electronic Telecommunications System for Surveillance.

Shigellosis Rate in 2000

National Rate = 11.1 Cases per 100,000 Population*

ALPHA ORDER			RANK ORDER		
RANK	STATE	RATE	RANK	STATE	RATE
40	Alabama	4.0	1	Minnesota	35.1
44	Alaska	1.8	2	Iowa	30.3
6	Arizona	18.6	3	Indiana	27.3
18	Arkansas	10.1	4	Texas	23.1
24	California	7.9	5	Missouri	20.2
17	Colorado	11.0	6	Arizona	18.6
40	Connecticut	4.0	7	North Dakota	17.0
34	Delaware	6.0	8	Nebraska	15.8
19	Florida	9.7	9	New Mexico	15.7
37	Georgia	5.4	10	Kentucky	15.6
32	Hawaii	6.1	11	Kansas	14.6
37	Idaho	5.4	11	Washington	14.6
21	Illinois	8.8	13	Michigan	12.6
3	Indiana	27.3	14	Tennessee	12.4
2	Iowa	30.3	15	New York	11.7
11	Kansas	14.6	16	Virginia	11.2
10	Kentucky	15.6	17	Colorado	11.0
26	Louisiana	7.5	18	Arkansas	10.1
44	Maine	1.8	19	Florida	9.7
31	Maryland	6.2	20	New Jersey	9.2
23	Massachusetts	8.2	21	Illinois	8.8
13	Michigan	12.6	22	North Carolina	8.3
1	Minnesota	35.1	23	Massachusetts	8.2
27	Mississippi	7.3	24	California	7.9
5	Missouri	20.2	24	Oregon	7.9
49	Montana	0.9	26	Louisiana	7.5
8	Nebraska	15.8	27	Mississippi	7.3
32	Nevada	6.1	27	Utah	7.3
48	New Hampshire	1.2	29	Ohio	6.6
20	New Jersey	9.2	30	Rhode Island	6.4
9	New Mexico	15.7	31	Maryland	6.2
15	New York	11.7	32	Hawaii	6.1
22	North Carolina	8.3	32	Nevada	6.1
7	North Dakota	17.0	34	Delaware	6.0
29	Ohio	6.6	35	South Carolina	5.7
39	Oklahoma	4.9	36	Wisconsin	5.5
24	Oregon	7.9	37	Georgia	5.4
42	Pennsylvania	3.7	37	Idaho	5.4
30	Rhode Island	6.4	39	Oklahoma	4.9
35	South Carolina	5.7	40	Alabama	4.0
46	South Dakota	1.6	40	Connecticut	4.0
14	Tennessee	12.4	42	Pennsylvania	3.7
4	Texas	23.1	43	West Virginia	2.2
27	Utah	7.3	44	Alaska	1.8
50	Vermont	0.8	44	Maine	1.8
16	Virginia	11.2	46	South Dakota	1.6
11	Washington	14.6	46	Wyoming	1.6
43	West Virginia	2.2	48	New Hampshire	1.2
36	Wisconsin	5.5	49	Montana	0.9
46	Wyoming	1.6	50	Vermont	0.8
				District of Columbia	14.0

Source: Morgan Quitno Press using data from U.S. Dept. of Health & Human Serv's, National Center for Health Statistics "Morbidity and Mortality Weekly Report" (January 5, 2001, Vol. 49, No. 51)
*Provisional data. Dysentery caused by any of various species of shigellae, occurring most frequently in areas where poor sanitation and malnutrition are prevalent and commonly affecting children and infants. Reported through Public Health Laboratory Information System and the National Electronic Telecommunications System for Surveillance.

Tuberculosis Cases Reported in 2000

National Total = 12,942 Cases*

ALPHA ORDER

RANK	STATE	CASES	% of USA
10	Alabama	310	2.4%
28	Alaska	96	0.7%
16	Arizona	237	1.8%
21	Arkansas	159	1.2%
1	California	2,652	20.5%
33	Colorado	70	0.5%
29	Connecticut	91	0.7%
46	Delaware	14	0.1%
3	Florida	922	7.1%
6	Georgia	576	4.5%
24	Hawaii	132	1.0%
42	Idaho	19	0.1%
4	Illinois	670	5.2%
27	Indiana	110	0.8%
35	Iowa	39	0.3%
36	Kansas	37	0.3%
26	Kentucky	114	0.9%
32	Louisiana	74	0.6%
47	Maine	12	0.1%
15	Maryland	247	1.9%
12	Massachusetts	302	2.3%
17	Michigan	229	1.8%
20	Minnesota	165	1.3%
22	Mississippi	137	1.1%
19	Missouri	196	1.5%
44	Montana	17	0.1%
41	Nebraska	23	0.2%
30	Nevada	89	0.7%
42	New Hampshire	19	0.1%
7	New Jersey	551	4.3%
36	New Mexico	37	0.3%
2	New York	1,572	12.1%
8	North Carolina	447	3.5%
48	North Dakota	5	0.0%
9	Ohio	314	2.4%
25	Oklahoma	130	1.0%
40	Oregon	25	0.2%
18	Pennsylvania	208	1.6%
39	Rhode Island	32	0.2%
23	South Carolina	135	1.0%
45	South Dakota	16	0.1%
11	Tennessee	305	2.4%
5	Texas	659	5.1%
34	Utah	49	0.4%
49	Vermont	4	0.0%
13	Virginia	289	2.2%
14	Washington	250	1.9%
38	West Virginia	33	0.3%
31	Wisconsin	81	0.6%
49	Wyoming	4	0.0%

RANK ORDER

RANK	STATE	CASES	% of USA
1	California	2,652	20.5%
2	New York	1,572	12.1%
3	Florida	922	7.1%
4	Illinois	670	5.2%
5	Texas	659	5.1%
6	Georgia	576	4.5%
7	New Jersey	551	4.3%
8	North Carolina	447	3.5%
9	Ohio	314	2.4%
10	Alabama	310	2.4%
11	Tennessee	305	2.4%
12	Massachusetts	302	2.3%
13	Virginia	289	2.2%
14	Washington	250	1.9%
15	Maryland	247	1.9%
16	Arizona	237	1.8%
17	Michigan	229	1.8%
18	Pennsylvania	208	1.6%
19	Missouri	196	1.5%
20	Minnesota	165	1.3%
21	Arkansas	159	1.2%
22	Mississippi	137	1.1%
23	South Carolina	135	1.0%
24	Hawaii	132	1.0%
25	Oklahoma	130	1.0%
26	Kentucky	114	0.9%
27	Indiana	110	0.8%
28	Alaska	96	0.7%
29	Connecticut	91	0.7%
30	Nevada	89	0.7%
31	Wisconsin	81	0.6%
32	Louisiana	74	0.6%
33	Colorado	70	0.5%
34	Utah	49	0.4%
35	Iowa	39	0.3%
36	Kansas	37	0.3%
36	New Mexico	37	0.3%
38	West Virginia	33	0.3%
39	Rhode Island	32	0.2%
40	Oregon	25	0.2%
41	Nebraska	23	0.2%
42	Idaho	19	0.1%
42	New Hampshire	19	0.1%
44	Montana	17	0.1%
45	South Dakota	16	0.1%
46	Delaware	14	0.1%
47	Maine	12	0.1%
48	North Dakota	5	0.0%
49	Vermont	4	0.0%
49	Wyoming	4	0.0%
	District of Columbia	38	0.3%

Source: U.S. Department of Health and Human Services, National Center for Health Statistics
   "Morbidity and Mortality Weekly Report" (January 5, 2001, Vol. 49, No. 51)
*Provisional data. An infectious disease caused by the tubercle bacillus and causing the formation of tubercles on
the lungs and other tissues of the body, often developing long after the initial infection. Characterized by the
coughing up of mucus and sputum, fever, weight loss, and chest pain.

Tuberculosis Rate in 2000

National Rate = 4.6 Cases per 100,000 Population*

<table>
<tr><td colspan="3">ALPHA ORDER</td><td colspan="3">RANK ORDER</td></tr>
<tr><td>RANK</td><td>STATE</td><td>RATE</td><td>RANK</td><td>STATE</td><td>RATE</td></tr>
<tr><td>5</td><td>Alabama</td><td>7.0</td><td>1</td><td>Alaska</td><td>15.3</td></tr>
<tr><td>1</td><td>Alaska</td><td>15.3</td><td>2</td><td>Hawaii</td><td>10.9</td></tr>
<tr><td>16</td><td>Arizona</td><td>4.6</td><td>3</td><td>New York</td><td>8.3</td></tr>
<tr><td>8</td><td>Arkansas</td><td>5.9</td><td>4</td><td>California</td><td>7.8</td></tr>
<tr><td>4</td><td>California</td><td>7.8</td><td>5</td><td>Alabama</td><td>7.0</td></tr>
<tr><td>39</td><td>Colorado</td><td>1.6</td><td>5</td><td>Georgia</td><td>7.0</td></tr>
<tr><td>28</td><td>Connecticut</td><td>2.7</td><td>7</td><td>New Jersey</td><td>6.5</td></tr>
<tr><td>34</td><td>Delaware</td><td>1.8</td><td>8</td><td>Arkansas</td><td>5.9</td></tr>
<tr><td>9</td><td>Florida</td><td>5.8</td><td>9</td><td>Florida</td><td>5.8</td></tr>
<tr><td>5</td><td>Georgia</td><td>7.0</td><td>10</td><td>North Carolina</td><td>5.6</td></tr>
<tr><td>2</td><td>Hawaii</td><td>10.9</td><td>11</td><td>Illinois</td><td>5.4</td></tr>
<tr><td>40</td><td>Idaho</td><td>1.5</td><td>11</td><td>Tennessee</td><td>5.4</td></tr>
<tr><td>11</td><td>Illinois</td><td>5.4</td><td>13</td><td>Massachusetts</td><td>4.8</td></tr>
<tr><td>34</td><td>Indiana</td><td>1.8</td><td>13</td><td>Mississippi</td><td>4.8</td></tr>
<tr><td>44</td><td>Iowa</td><td>1.3</td><td>15</td><td>Maryland</td><td>4.7</td></tr>
<tr><td>43</td><td>Kansas</td><td>1.4</td><td>16</td><td>Arizona</td><td>4.6</td></tr>
<tr><td>26</td><td>Kentucky</td><td>2.8</td><td>17</td><td>Nevada</td><td>4.5</td></tr>
<tr><td>37</td><td>Louisiana</td><td>1.7</td><td>18</td><td>Washington</td><td>4.2</td></tr>
<tr><td>46</td><td>Maine</td><td>0.9</td><td>19</td><td>Virginia</td><td>4.1</td></tr>
<tr><td>15</td><td>Maryland</td><td>4.7</td><td>20</td><td>Oklahoma</td><td>3.8</td></tr>
<tr><td>13</td><td>Massachusetts</td><td>4.8</td><td>21</td><td>Missouri</td><td>3.5</td></tr>
<tr><td>29</td><td>Michigan</td><td>2.3</td><td>22</td><td>Minnesota</td><td>3.4</td></tr>
<tr><td>22</td><td>Minnesota</td><td>3.4</td><td>22</td><td>South Carolina</td><td>3.4</td></tr>
<tr><td>13</td><td>Mississippi</td><td>4.8</td><td>24</td><td>Texas</td><td>3.2</td></tr>
<tr><td>21</td><td>Missouri</td><td>3.5</td><td>25</td><td>Rhode Island</td><td>3.1</td></tr>
<tr><td>33</td><td>Montana</td><td>1.9</td><td>26</td><td>Kentucky</td><td>2.8</td></tr>
<tr><td>44</td><td>Nebraska</td><td>1.3</td><td>26</td><td>Ohio</td><td>2.8</td></tr>
<tr><td>17</td><td>Nevada</td><td>4.5</td><td>28</td><td>Connecticut</td><td>2.7</td></tr>
<tr><td>40</td><td>New Hampshire</td><td>1.5</td><td>29</td><td>Michigan</td><td>2.3</td></tr>
<tr><td>7</td><td>New Jersey</td><td>6.5</td><td>30</td><td>Utah</td><td>2.2</td></tr>
<tr><td>32</td><td>New Mexico</td><td>2.0</td><td>31</td><td>South Dakota</td><td>2.1</td></tr>
<tr><td>3</td><td>New York</td><td>8.3</td><td>32</td><td>New Mexico</td><td>2.0</td></tr>
<tr><td>10</td><td>North Carolina</td><td>5.6</td><td>33</td><td>Montana</td><td>1.9</td></tr>
<tr><td>47</td><td>North Dakota</td><td>0.8</td><td>34</td><td>Delaware</td><td>1.8</td></tr>
<tr><td>26</td><td>Ohio</td><td>2.8</td><td>34</td><td>Indiana</td><td>1.8</td></tr>
<tr><td>20</td><td>Oklahoma</td><td>3.8</td><td>34</td><td>West Virginia</td><td>1.8</td></tr>
<tr><td>49</td><td>Oregon</td><td>0.7</td><td>37</td><td>Louisiana</td><td>1.7</td></tr>
<tr><td>37</td><td>Pennsylvania</td><td>1.7</td><td>37</td><td>Pennsylvania</td><td>1.7</td></tr>
<tr><td>25</td><td>Rhode Island</td><td>3.1</td><td>39</td><td>Colorado</td><td>1.6</td></tr>
<tr><td>22</td><td>South Carolina</td><td>3.4</td><td>40</td><td>Idaho</td><td>1.5</td></tr>
<tr><td>31</td><td>South Dakota</td><td>2.1</td><td>40</td><td>New Hampshire</td><td>1.5</td></tr>
<tr><td>11</td><td>Tennessee</td><td>5.4</td><td>40</td><td>Wisconsin</td><td>1.5</td></tr>
<tr><td>24</td><td>Texas</td><td>3.2</td><td>43</td><td>Kansas</td><td>1.4</td></tr>
<tr><td>30</td><td>Utah</td><td>2.2</td><td>44</td><td>Iowa</td><td>1.3</td></tr>
<tr><td>49</td><td>Vermont</td><td>0.7</td><td>44</td><td>Nebraska</td><td>1.3</td></tr>
<tr><td>19</td><td>Virginia</td><td>4.1</td><td>46</td><td>Maine</td><td>0.9</td></tr>
<tr><td>18</td><td>Washington</td><td>4.2</td><td>47</td><td>North Dakota</td><td>0.8</td></tr>
<tr><td>34</td><td>West Virginia</td><td>1.8</td><td>47</td><td>Wyoming</td><td>0.8</td></tr>
<tr><td>40</td><td>Wisconsin</td><td>1.5</td><td>49</td><td>Oregon</td><td>0.7</td></tr>
<tr><td>47</td><td>Wyoming</td><td>0.8</td><td>49</td><td>Vermont</td><td>0.7</td></tr>
<tr><td></td><td></td><td></td><td></td><td>District of Columbia</td><td>6.6</td></tr>
</table>

Source: Morgan Quitno Press using data from U.S. Dept. of Health & Human Serv's, National Center for Health Statistics
    "Morbidity and Mortality Weekly Report" (January 5, 2001, Vol. 49, No. 51)
*Provisional data. An infectious disease caused by the tubercle bacillus and causing the formation of tubercles on
the lungs and other tissues of the body, often developing long after the initial infection. Characterized by the
coughing up of mucus and sputum, fever, weight loss, and chest pain.

Whooping Cough (Pertussis) Cases Reported in 2000

National Total = 6,755 Cases*

ALPHA ORDER

RANK	STATE	CASES	% of USA
42	Alabama	21	0.3%
41	Alaska	22	0.3%
11	Arizona	143	2.1%
35	Arkansas	36	0.5%
2	California	550	8.1%
3	Colorado	457	6.8%
27	Connecticut	48	0.7%
46	Delaware	9	0.1%
23	Florida	65	1.0%
33	Georgia	40	0.6%
39	Hawaii	32	0.5%
24	Idaho	64	0.9%
21	Illinois	82	1.2%
14	Indiana	126	1.9%
25	Iowa	60	0.9%
33	Kansas	40	0.6%
26	Kentucky	56	0.8%
44	Louisiana	12	0.2%
28	Maine	45	0.7%
12	Maryland	136	2.0%
1	Massachusetts	1,151	17.0%
15	Michigan	125	1.9%
6	Minnesota	398	5.9%
49	Mississippi	1	0.0%
19	Missouri	110	1.6%
36	Montana	35	0.5%
38	Nebraska	33	0.5%
43	Nevada	15	0.2%
13	New Hampshire	128	1.9%
29	New Jersey	43	0.6%
20	New Mexico	91	1.3%
5	New York	411	6.1%
18	North Carolina	111	1.6%
47	North Dakota	7	0.1%
7	Ohio	392	5.8%
30	Oklahoma	41	0.6%
17	Oregon	114	1.7%
10	Pennsylvania	220	3.3%
40	Rhode Island	23	0.3%
30	South Carolina	41	0.6%
45	South Dakota	11	0.2%
37	Tennessee	34	0.5%
9	Texas	249	3.7%
30	Utah	41	0.6%
8	Vermont	252	3.7%
16	Virginia	115	1.7%
4	Washington	427	6.3%
49	West Virginia	1	0.0%
21	Wisconsin	82	1.2%
48	Wyoming	6	0.1%

RANK ORDER

RANK	STATE	CASES	% of USA
1	Massachusetts	1,151	17.0%
2	California	550	8.1%
3	Colorado	457	6.8%
4	Washington	427	6.3%
5	New York	411	6.1%
6	Minnesota	398	5.9%
7	Ohio	392	5.8%
8	Vermont	252	3.7%
9	Texas	249	3.7%
10	Pennsylvania	220	3.3%
11	Arizona	143	2.1%
12	Maryland	136	2.0%
13	New Hampshire	128	1.9%
14	Indiana	126	1.9%
15	Michigan	125	1.9%
16	Virginia	115	1.7%
17	Oregon	114	1.7%
18	North Carolina	111	1.6%
19	Missouri	110	1.6%
20	New Mexico	91	1.3%
21	Illinois	82	1.2%
21	Wisconsin	82	1.2%
23	Florida	65	1.0%
24	Idaho	64	0.9%
25	Iowa	60	0.9%
26	Kentucky	56	0.8%
27	Connecticut	48	0.7%
28	Maine	45	0.7%
29	New Jersey	43	0.6%
30	Oklahoma	41	0.6%
30	South Carolina	41	0.6%
30	Utah	41	0.6%
33	Georgia	40	0.6%
33	Kansas	40	0.6%
35	Arkansas	36	0.5%
36	Montana	35	0.5%
37	Tennessee	34	0.5%
38	Nebraska	33	0.5%
39	Hawaii	32	0.5%
40	Rhode Island	23	0.3%
41	Alaska	22	0.3%
42	Alabama	21	0.3%
43	Nevada	15	0.2%
44	Louisiana	12	0.2%
45	South Dakota	11	0.2%
46	Delaware	9	0.1%
47	North Dakota	7	0.1%
48	Wyoming	6	0.1%
49	Mississippi	1	0.0%
49	West Virginia	1	0.0%
	District of Columbia	3	0.0%

Source: U.S. Department of Health and Human Services, National Center for Health Statistics
"Morbidity and Mortality Weekly Report" (January 5, 2001, Vol. 49, No. 51)
*Provisional data. Acute, highly contagious infection of respiratory tract.

Whooping Cough (Pertussis) Rate in 2000

National Rate = 2.4 Cases per 100,000 Population*

<table>
<tr><td colspan="3">ALPHA ORDER</td><td colspan="3">RANK ORDER</td></tr>
<tr><th>RANK</th><th>STATE</th><th>RATE</th><th>RANK</th><th>STATE</th><th>RATE</th></tr>
<tr><td>44</td><td>Alabama</td><td>0.5</td><td>1</td><td>Vermont</td><td>41.4</td></tr>
<tr><td>10</td><td>Alaska</td><td>3.5</td><td>2</td><td>Massachusetts</td><td>18.1</td></tr>
<tr><td>14</td><td>Arizona</td><td>2.8</td><td>3</td><td>Colorado</td><td>10.6</td></tr>
<tr><td>33</td><td>Arkansas</td><td>1.3</td><td>4</td><td>New Hampshire</td><td>10.4</td></tr>
<tr><td>25</td><td>California</td><td>1.6</td><td>5</td><td>Minnesota</td><td>8.1</td></tr>
<tr><td>3</td><td>Colorado</td><td>10.6</td><td>6</td><td>Washington</td><td>7.2</td></tr>
<tr><td>30</td><td>Connecticut</td><td>1.4</td><td>7</td><td>New Mexico</td><td>5.0</td></tr>
<tr><td>38</td><td>Delaware</td><td>1.1</td><td>8</td><td>Idaho</td><td>4.9</td></tr>
<tr><td>47</td><td>Florida</td><td>0.4</td><td>9</td><td>Montana</td><td>3.9</td></tr>
<tr><td>44</td><td>Georgia</td><td>0.5</td><td>10</td><td>Alaska</td><td>3.5</td></tr>
<tr><td>15</td><td>Hawaii</td><td>2.6</td><td>10</td><td>Maine</td><td>3.5</td></tr>
<tr><td>8</td><td>Idaho</td><td>4.9</td><td>10</td><td>Ohio</td><td>3.5</td></tr>
<tr><td>42</td><td>Illinois</td><td>0.7</td><td>13</td><td>Oregon</td><td>3.3</td></tr>
<tr><td>19</td><td>Indiana</td><td>2.1</td><td>14</td><td>Arizona</td><td>2.8</td></tr>
<tr><td>19</td><td>Iowa</td><td>2.1</td><td>15</td><td>Hawaii</td><td>2.6</td></tr>
<tr><td>27</td><td>Kansas</td><td>1.5</td><td>15</td><td>Maryland</td><td>2.6</td></tr>
<tr><td>30</td><td>Kentucky</td><td>1.4</td><td>17</td><td>New York</td><td>2.2</td></tr>
<tr><td>48</td><td>Louisiana</td><td>0.3</td><td>17</td><td>Rhode Island</td><td>2.2</td></tr>
<tr><td>10</td><td>Maine</td><td>3.5</td><td>19</td><td>Indiana</td><td>2.1</td></tr>
<tr><td>15</td><td>Maryland</td><td>2.6</td><td>19</td><td>Iowa</td><td>2.1</td></tr>
<tr><td>2</td><td>Massachusetts</td><td>18.1</td><td>21</td><td>Missouri</td><td>2.0</td></tr>
<tr><td>33</td><td>Michigan</td><td>1.3</td><td>22</td><td>Nebraska</td><td>1.9</td></tr>
<tr><td>5</td><td>Minnesota</td><td>8.1</td><td>23</td><td>Pennsylvania</td><td>1.8</td></tr>
<tr><td>50</td><td>Mississippi</td><td>0.0</td><td>23</td><td>Utah</td><td>1.8</td></tr>
<tr><td>21</td><td>Missouri</td><td>2.0</td><td>25</td><td>California</td><td>1.6</td></tr>
<tr><td>9</td><td>Montana</td><td>3.9</td><td>25</td><td>Virginia</td><td>1.6</td></tr>
<tr><td>22</td><td>Nebraska</td><td>1.9</td><td>27</td><td>Kansas</td><td>1.5</td></tr>
<tr><td>41</td><td>Nevada</td><td>0.8</td><td>27</td><td>South Dakota</td><td>1.5</td></tr>
<tr><td>4</td><td>New Hampshire</td><td>10.4</td><td>27</td><td>Wisconsin</td><td>1.5</td></tr>
<tr><td>44</td><td>New Jersey</td><td>0.5</td><td>30</td><td>Connecticut</td><td>1.4</td></tr>
<tr><td>7</td><td>New Mexico</td><td>5.0</td><td>30</td><td>Kentucky</td><td>1.4</td></tr>
<tr><td>17</td><td>New York</td><td>2.2</td><td>30</td><td>North Carolina</td><td>1.4</td></tr>
<tr><td>30</td><td>North Carolina</td><td>1.4</td><td>33</td><td>Arkansas</td><td>1.3</td></tr>
<tr><td>38</td><td>North Dakota</td><td>1.1</td><td>33</td><td>Michigan</td><td>1.3</td></tr>
<tr><td>10</td><td>Ohio</td><td>3.5</td><td>35</td><td>Oklahoma</td><td>1.2</td></tr>
<tr><td>35</td><td>Oklahoma</td><td>1.2</td><td>35</td><td>Texas</td><td>1.2</td></tr>
<tr><td>13</td><td>Oregon</td><td>3.3</td><td>35</td><td>Wyoming</td><td>1.2</td></tr>
<tr><td>23</td><td>Pennsylvania</td><td>1.8</td><td>38</td><td>Delaware</td><td>1.1</td></tr>
<tr><td>17</td><td>Rhode Island</td><td>2.2</td><td>38</td><td>North Dakota</td><td>1.1</td></tr>
<tr><td>40</td><td>South Carolina</td><td>1.0</td><td>40</td><td>South Carolina</td><td>1.0</td></tr>
<tr><td>27</td><td>South Dakota</td><td>1.5</td><td>41</td><td>Nevada</td><td>0.8</td></tr>
<tr><td>43</td><td>Tennessee</td><td>0.6</td><td>42</td><td>Illinois</td><td>0.7</td></tr>
<tr><td>35</td><td>Texas</td><td>1.2</td><td>43</td><td>Tennessee</td><td>0.6</td></tr>
<tr><td>23</td><td>Utah</td><td>1.8</td><td>44</td><td>Alabama</td><td>0.5</td></tr>
<tr><td>1</td><td>Vermont</td><td>41.4</td><td>44</td><td>Georgia</td><td>0.5</td></tr>
<tr><td>25</td><td>Virginia</td><td>1.6</td><td>44</td><td>New Jersey</td><td>0.5</td></tr>
<tr><td>6</td><td>Washington</td><td>7.2</td><td>47</td><td>Florida</td><td>0.4</td></tr>
<tr><td>49</td><td>West Virginia</td><td>0.1</td><td>48</td><td>Louisiana</td><td>0.3</td></tr>
<tr><td>27</td><td>Wisconsin</td><td>1.5</td><td>49</td><td>West Virginia</td><td>0.1</td></tr>
<tr><td>35</td><td>Wyoming</td><td>1.2</td><td>50</td><td>Mississippi</td><td>0.0</td></tr>
<tr><td></td><td></td><td></td><td></td><td>District of Columbia</td><td>0.5</td></tr>
</table>

Source: Morgan Quitno Press using data from U.S. Dept. of Health & Human Serv's, National Center for Health Statistics
     "Morbidity and Mortality Weekly Report" (January 5, 2001, Vol. 49, No. 51)
*Provisional data. Acute, highly contagious infection of respiratory tract.

Percent of Children Aged 19 to 35 Months Fully Immunized in 1999

National Percent = 78.4%*

ALPHA ORDER

RANK	STATE	PERCENT
31	Alabama	78.4
28	Alaska	80.1
47	Arizona	72.4
36	Arkansas	77.1
39	California	75.3
38	Colorado	75.8
5	Connecticut	85.9
32	Delaware	78.2
25	Florida	80.3
14	Georgia	81.9
19	Hawaii	81.6
50	Idaho	69.4
35	Illinois	77.4
43	Indiana	74.3
10	Iowa	83.4
30	Kansas	78.9
2	Kentucky	87.6
37	Louisiana	76.8
11	Maine	82.9
29	Maryland	79.4
6	Massachusetts	85.2
42	Michigan	74.4
6	Minnesota	85.2
17	Mississippi	81.7
40	Missouri	75.0
13	Montana	82.5
15	Nebraska	81.8
44	Nevada	73.1
8	New Hampshire	84.5
22	New Jersey	80.8
45	New Mexico	73.0
20	New York	81.0
15	North Carolina	81.8
24	North Dakota	80.4
33	Ohio	78.1
46	Oklahoma	72.9
49	Oregon	72.3
4	Pennsylvania	86.0
3	Rhode Island	87.4
23	South Carolina	80.6
17	South Dakota	81.7
34	Tennessee	77.7
47	Texas	72.4
27	Utah	80.2
1	Vermont	90.5
25	Virginia	80.3
41	Washington	74.9
20	West Virginia	81.0
8	Wisconsin	84.5
12	Wyoming	82.8

RANK ORDER

RANK	STATE	PERCENT
1	Vermont	90.5
2	Kentucky	87.6
3	Rhode Island	87.4
4	Pennsylvania	86.0
5	Connecticut	85.9
6	Massachusetts	85.2
6	Minnesota	85.2
8	New Hampshire	84.5
8	Wisconsin	84.5
10	Iowa	83.4
11	Maine	82.9
12	Wyoming	82.8
13	Montana	82.5
14	Georgia	81.9
15	Nebraska	81.8
15	North Carolina	81.8
17	Mississippi	81.7
17	South Dakota	81.7
19	Hawaii	81.6
20	New York	81.0
20	West Virginia	81.0
22	New Jersey	80.8
23	South Carolina	80.6
24	North Dakota	80.4
25	Florida	80.3
25	Virginia	80.3
27	Utah	80.2
28	Alaska	80.1
29	Maryland	79.4
30	Kansas	78.9
31	Alabama	78.4
32	Delaware	78.2
33	Ohio	78.1
34	Tennessee	77.7
35	Illinois	77.4
36	Arkansas	77.1
37	Louisiana	76.8
38	Colorado	75.8
39	California	75.3
40	Missouri	75.0
41	Washington	74.9
42	Michigan	74.4
43	Indiana	74.3
44	Nevada	73.1
45	New Mexico	73.0
46	Oklahoma	72.9
47	Arizona	72.4
47	Texas	72.4
49	Oregon	72.3
50	Idaho	69.4
	District of Columbia	77.5

Source: U.S. Department of Health and Human Services, Centers for Disease Control and Prevention
    "State Vaccination Coverage Levels" (Morbidity and Mortality Weekly Report, Vol. 49, No. 26, July 7, 2000)
Fully immunized children received four doses of DTP/DT (Diphtheria, Tetanus, Pertussis (Whooping Cough)), three doses of OPV (Poliovirus), one dose of MCV (Measles Containing Vaccine) and three doses of Hib (Haemophilus influenzae type b).

Sexually Transmitted Diseases in 1999

National Total = 1,026,317 Cases*

ALPHA ORDER

ALPHA ORDER

RANK	STATE	CASES	% of USA
15	Alabama	23,466	2.3%
42	Alaska	2,189	0.2%
22	Arizona	16,616	1.6%
30	Arkansas	9,178	0.9%
1	California	104,118	10.1%
24	Colorado	13,382	1.3%
28	Connecticut	10,759	1.0%
36	Delaware	4,433	0.4%
4	Florida	55,068	5.4%
5	Georgia	52,043	5.1%
38	Hawaii	3,631	0.4%
43	Idaho	1,868	0.2%
3	Illinois	56,546	5.5%
21	Indiana	18,276	1.8%
33	Iowa	6,885	0.7%
31	Kansas	8,772	0.9%
27	Kentucky	10,828	1.1%
12	Louisiana	30,139	2.9%
46	Maine	1,303	0.1%
14	Maryland	24,341	2.4%
26	Massachusetts	11,267	1.1%
10	Michigan	39,263	3.8%
29	Minnesota	10,291	1.0%
17	Mississippi	22,150	2.2%
18	Missouri	21,638	2.1%
45	Montana	1,638	0.2%
35	Nebraska	5,093	0.5%
37	Nevada	4,394	0.4%
47	New Hampshire	1,092	0.1%
20	New Jersey	20,344	2.0%
34	New Mexico	6,003	0.6%
7	New York	46,781	4.6%
8	North Carolina	41,711	4.1%
48	North Dakota	1,030	0.1%
6	Ohio	47,631	4.6%
25	Oklahoma	12,403	1.2%
32	Oregon	7,039	0.7%
9	Pennsylvania	40,398	3.9%
39	Rhode Island	2,950	0.3%
11	South Carolina	33,853	3.3%
44	South Dakota	1,736	0.2%
13	Tennessee	26,223	2.6%
2	Texas	96,357	9.4%
40	Utah	2,475	0.2%
50	Vermont	540	0.1%
16	Virginia	23,293	2.3%
23	Washington	14,173	1.4%
41	West Virginia	2,409	0.2%
19	Wisconsin	21,169	2.1%
49	Wyoming	831	0.1%

RANK ORDER

RANK	STATE	CASES	% of USA
1	California	104,118	10.1%
2	Texas	96,357	9.4%
3	Illinois	56,546	5.5%
4	Florida	55,068	5.4%
5	Georgia	52,043	5.1%
6	Ohio	47,631	4.6%
7	New York	46,781	4.6%
8	North Carolina	41,711	4.1%
9	Pennsylvania	40,398	3.9%
10	Michigan	39,263	3.8%
11	South Carolina	33,853	3.3%
12	Louisiana	30,139	2.9%
13	Tennessee	26,223	2.6%
14	Maryland	24,341	2.4%
15	Alabama	23,466	2.3%
16	Virginia	23,293	2.3%
17	Mississippi	22,150	2.2%
18	Missouri	21,638	2.1%
19	Wisconsin	21,169	2.1%
20	New Jersey	20,344	2.0%
21	Indiana	18,276	1.8%
22	Arizona	16,616	1.6%
23	Washington	14,173	1.4%
24	Colorado	13,382	1.3%
25	Oklahoma	12,403	1.2%
26	Massachusetts	11,267	1.1%
27	Kentucky	10,828	1.1%
28	Connecticut	10,759	1.0%
29	Minnesota	10,291	1.0%
30	Arkansas	9,178	0.9%
31	Kansas	8,772	0.9%
32	Oregon	7,039	0.7%
33	Iowa	6,885	0.7%
34	New Mexico	6,003	0.6%
35	Nebraska	5,093	0.5%
36	Delaware	4,433	0.4%
37	Nevada	4,394	0.4%
38	Hawaii	3,631	0.4%
39	Rhode Island	2,950	0.3%
40	Utah	2,475	0.2%
41	West Virginia	2,409	0.2%
42	Alaska	2,189	0.2%
43	Idaho	1,868	0.2%
44	South Dakota	1,736	0.2%
45	Montana	1,638	0.2%
46	Maine	1,303	0.1%
47	New Hampshire	1,092	0.1%
48	North Dakota	1,030	0.1%
49	Wyoming	831	0.1%
50	Vermont	540	0.1%
	District of Columbia	6,301	0.6%

Source: Morgan Quitno Press using data from U.S. Dept. of Health and Human Services, Nat'l Center for Health Statistics "Sexually Transmitted Disease Surveillance 1999" (http://www.cdc.gov/nchstp/dstd/dstdp.html)
*Includes chancroid, chlamydia, gonorrhea and primary and secondary syphilis.

Sexually Transmitted Disease Rate in 1999

National Rate = 389.9 Cases per 100,000 Population*

ALPHA ORDER

RANK	STATE	RATE
7	Alabama	539.2
20	Alaska	356.6
21	Arizona	355.9
19	Arkansas	361.6
28	California	318.8
24	Colorado	337.0
27	Connecticut	328.6
5	Delaware	596.1
18	Florida	369.2
4	Georgia	681.0
31	Hawaii	304.4
45	Idaho	152.0
12	Illinois	469.5
29	Indiana	309.8
37	Iowa	240.5
26	Kansas	333.7
33	Kentucky	275.1
3	Louisiana	689.9
48	Maine	104.8
10	Maryland	474.0
42	Massachusetts	183.3
15	Michigan	399.9
39	Minnesota	217.8
2	Mississippi	804.8
16	Missouri	397.9
41	Montana	186.0
30	Nebraska	306.4
34	Nevada	251.6
49	New Hampshire	92.2
35	New Jersey	250.7
22	New Mexico	345.6
11	New York	470.8
6	North Carolina	552.6
44	North Dakota	161.4
13	Ohio	424.9
17	Oklahoma	370.6
40	Oregon	214.4
25	Pennsylvania	336.6
32	Rhode Island	298.4
1	South Carolina	882.6
38	South Dakota	235.2
9	Tennessee	482.9
8	Texas	487.7
47	Utah	117.9
50	Vermont	91.4
23	Virginia	342.9
36	Washington	249.2
46	West Virginia	133.0
14	Wisconsin	405.3
43	Wyoming	172.7

RANK ORDER

RANK	STATE	RATE
1	South Carolina	882.6
2	Mississippi	804.8
3	Louisiana	689.9
4	Georgia	681.0
5	Delaware	596.1
6	North Carolina	552.6
7	Alabama	539.2
8	Texas	487.7
9	Tennessee	482.9
10	Maryland	474.0
11	New York	470.8
12	Illinois	469.5
13	Ohio	424.9
14	Wisconsin	405.3
15	Michigan	399.9
16	Missouri	397.9
17	Oklahoma	370.6
18	Florida	369.2
19	Arkansas	361.6
20	Alaska	356.6
21	Arizona	355.9
22	New Mexico	345.6
23	Virginia	342.9
24	Colorado	337.0
25	Pennsylvania	336.6
26	Kansas	333.7
27	Connecticut	328.6
28	California	318.8
29	Indiana	309.8
30	Nebraska	306.4
31	Hawaii	304.4
32	Rhode Island	298.4
33	Kentucky	275.1
34	Nevada	251.6
35	New Jersey	250.7
36	Washington	249.2
37	Iowa	240.5
38	South Dakota	235.2
39	Minnesota	217.8
40	Oregon	214.4
41	Montana	186.0
42	Massachusetts	183.3
43	Wyoming	172.7
44	North Dakota	161.4
45	Idaho	152.0
46	West Virginia	133.0
47	Utah	117.9
48	Maine	104.8
49	New Hampshire	92.2
50	Vermont	91.4

District of Columbia 1,214.1

Source: Morgan Quitno Press using data from U.S. Dept. of Health and Human Services, Nat'l Center for Health Statistics
"Sexually Transmitted Disease Surveillance 1999" (http://www.cdc.gov/nchstp/dstd/dstdp.html)
*Includes chancroid, chlamydia, gonorrhea and primary and secondary syphilis.

Chancroid Cases Reported in 1999

National Total = 143 Cases*

ALPHA ORDER

RANK	STATE	CASES	% of USA
10	Alabama	1	0.7%
17	Alaska	0	0.0%
17	Arizona	0	0.0%
17	Arkansas	0	0.0%
5	California	7	4.9%
17	Colorado	0	0.0%
17	Connecticut	0	0.0%
17	Delaware	0	0.0%
8	Florida	3	2.1%
10	Georgia	1	0.7%
17	Hawaii	0	0.0%
17	Idaho	0	0.0%
17	Illinois	0	0.0%
17	Indiana	0	0.0%
17	Iowa	0	0.0%
17	Kansas	0	0.0%
17	Kentucky	0	0.0%
4	Louisiana	9	6.3%
17	Maine	0	0.0%
17	Maryland	0	0.0%
10	Massachusetts	1	0.7%
17	Michigan	0	0.0%
10	Minnesota	1	0.7%
17	Mississippi	0	0.0%
17	Missouri	0	0.0%
17	Montana	0	0.0%
17	Nebraska	0	0.0%
17	Nevada	0	0.0%
17	New Hampshire	0	0.0%
17	New Jersey	0	0.0%
17	New Mexico	0	0.0%
2	New York	39	27.3%
5	North Carolina	7	4.9%
17	North Dakota	0	0.0%
17	Ohio	0	0.0%
17	Oklahoma	0	0.0%
10	Oregon	1	0.7%
17	Pennsylvania	0	0.0%
10	Rhode Island	1	0.7%
1	South Carolina	48	33.6%
17	South Dakota	0	0.0%
17	Tennessee	0	0.0%
3	Texas	16	11.2%
17	Utah	0	0.0%
17	Vermont	0	0.0%
8	Virginia	3	2.1%
17	Washington	0	0.0%
17	West Virginia	0	0.0%
7	Wisconsin	4	2.8%
10	Wyoming	1	0.7%

RANK ORDER

RANK	STATE	CASES	% of USA
1	South Carolina	48	33.6%
2	New York	39	27.3%
3	Texas	16	11.2%
4	Louisiana	9	6.3%
5	California	7	4.9%
5	North Carolina	7	4.9%
7	Wisconsin	4	2.8%
8	Florida	3	2.1%
8	Virginia	3	2.1%
10	Alabama	1	0.7%
10	Georgia	1	0.7%
10	Massachusetts	1	0.7%
10	Minnesota	1	0.7%
10	Oregon	1	0.7%
10	Rhode Island	1	0.7%
10	Wyoming	1	0.7%
17	Alaska	0	0.0%
17	Arizona	0	0.0%
17	Arkansas	0	0.0%
17	Colorado	0	0.0%
17	Connecticut	0	0.0%
17	Delaware	0	0.0%
17	Hawaii	0	0.0%
17	Idaho	0	0.0%
17	Illinois	0	0.0%
17	Indiana	0	0.0%
17	Iowa	0	0.0%
17	Kansas	0	0.0%
17	Kentucky	0	0.0%
17	Maine	0	0.0%
17	Maryland	0	0.0%
17	Michigan	0	0.0%
17	Mississippi	0	0.0%
17	Missouri	0	0.0%
17	Montana	0	0.0%
17	Nebraska	0	0.0%
17	Nevada	0	0.0%
17	New Hampshire	0	0.0%
17	New Jersey	0	0.0%
17	New Mexico	0	0.0%
17	North Dakota	0	0.0%
17	Ohio	0	0.0%
17	Oklahoma	0	0.0%
17	Pennsylvania	0	0.0%
17	South Dakota	0	0.0%
17	Tennessee	0	0.0%
17	Utah	0	0.0%
17	Vermont	0	0.0%
17	Washington	0	0.0%
17	West Virginia	0	0.0%
	District of Columbia	0	0.0%

Source: U.S. Department of Health and Human Services, National Center for Health Statistics
"Sexually Transmitted Disease Surveillance 1999" (http://www.cdc.gov/nchstp/dstd/dstdp.html)
A soft, highly infectious, nonsyphilitic venereal ulcer of the genital region, caused by the bacillus Hemophilus ducreyi. Also called soft chancre.

Chancroid Rate in 1999

National Rate = 0.1 Cases per 100,000 Population*

<u>ALPHA ORDER</u>

<u>RANK ORDER</u>

RANK	STATE	RATE		RANK	STATE	RATE
9	Alabama	0.0		1	South Carolina	1.3
9	Alaska	0.0		2	Louisiana	0.2
9	Arizona	0.0		2	New York	0.2
9	Arkansas	0.0		2	Wyoming	0.2
9	California	0.0		5	North Carolina	0.1
9	Colorado	0.0		5	Rhode Island	0.1
9	Connecticut	0.0		5	Texas	0.1
9	Delaware	0.0		5	Wisconsin	0.1
9	Florida	0.0		9	Alabama	0.0
9	Georgia	0.0		9	Alaska	0.0
9	Hawaii	0.0		9	Arizona	0.0
9	Idaho	0.0		9	Arkansas	0.0
9	Illinois	0.0		9	California	0.0
9	Indiana	0.0		9	Colorado	0.0
9	Iowa	0.0		9	Connecticut	0.0
9	Kansas	0.0		9	Delaware	0.0
9	Kentucky	0.0		9	Florida	0.0
2	Louisiana	0.2		9	Georgia	0.0
9	Maine	0.0		9	Hawaii	0.0
9	Maryland	0.0		9	Idaho	0.0
9	Massachusetts	0.0		9	Illinois	0.0
9	Michigan	0.0		9	Indiana	0.0
9	Minnesota	0.0		9	Iowa	0.0
9	Mississippi	0.0		9	Kansas	0.0
9	Missouri	0.0		9	Kentucky	0.0
9	Montana	0.0		9	Maine	0.0
9	Nebraska	0.0		9	Maryland	0.0
9	Nevada	0.0		9	Massachusetts	0.0
9	New Hampshire	0.0		9	Michigan	0.0
9	New Jersey	0.0		9	Minnesota	0.0
9	New Mexico	0.0		9	Mississippi	0.0
2	New York	0.2		9	Missouri	0.0
5	North Carolina	0.1		9	Montana	0.0
9	North Dakota	0.0		9	Nebraska	0.0
9	Ohio	0.0		9	Nevada	0.0
9	Oklahoma	0.0		9	New Hampshire	0.0
9	Oregon	0.0		9	New Jersey	0.0
9	Pennsylvania	0.0		9	New Mexico	0.0
5	Rhode Island	0.1		9	North Dakota	0.0
1	South Carolina	1.3		9	Ohio	0.0
9	South Dakota	0.0		9	Oklahoma	0.0
9	Tennessee	0.0		9	Oregon	0.0
5	Texas	0.1		9	Pennsylvania	0.0
9	Utah	0.0		9	South Dakota	0.0
9	Vermont	0.0		9	Tennessee	0.0
9	Virginia	0.0		9	Utah	0.0
9	Washington	0.0		9	Vermont	0.0
9	West Virginia	0.0		9	Virginia	0.0
5	Wisconsin	0.1		9	Washington	0.0
2	Wyoming	0.2		9	West Virginia	0.0
					District of Columbia	0.0

Source: U.S. Department of Health and Human Services, National Center for Health Statistics
    "Sexually Transmitted Disease Surveillance 1999" (http://www.cdc.gov/nchstp/dstd/dstdp.html)
A soft, highly infectious, nonsyphilitic venereal ulcer of the genital region, caused by the bacillus Hemophilus ducreyi. Also called soft chancre.

Chlamydia Cases Reported in 1999

National Total = 659,441 Cases*

<u>ALPHA ORDER</u>

RANK	STATE	CASES	% of USA
19	Alabama	12,375	1.9%
41	Alaska	1,886	0.3%
20	Arizona	12,111	1.8%
32	Arkansas	5,865	0.9%
1	California	85,156	12.9%
24	Colorado	10,848	1.6%
28	Connecticut	7,422	1.1%
38	Delaware	2,761	0.4%
4	Florida	31,743	4.8%
5	Georgia	30,368	4.6%
36	Hawaii	3,165	0.5%
43	Idaho	1,778	0.3%
3	Illinois	32,870	5.0%
22	Indiana	11,734	1.8%
33	Iowa	5,511	0.8%
31	Kansas	6,093	0.9%
29	Kentucky	7,378	1.1%
12	Louisiana	16,635	2.5%
46	Maine	1,220	0.2%
16	Maryland	13,568	2.1%
25	Massachusetts	8,776	1.3%
9	Michigan	23,107	3.5%
27	Minnesota	7,450	1.1%
23	Mississippi	11,545	1.8%
17	Missouri	13,355	2.0%
44	Montana	1,584	0.2%
35	Nebraska	3,616	0.5%
37	Nevada	3,086	0.5%
47	New Hampshire	976	0.1%
18	New Jersey	12,424	1.9%
34	New Mexico	5,017	0.8%
8	New York	26,766	4.1%
10	North Carolina	21,812	3.3%
48	North Dakota	947	0.1%
6	Ohio	29,398	4.5%
26	Oklahoma	8,195	1.2%
30	Oregon	6,127	0.9%
7	Pennsylvania	27,019	4.1%
39	Rhode Island	2,345	0.4%
11	South Carolina	18,499	2.8%
45	South Dakota	1,544	0.2%
14	Tennessee	14,216	2.2%
2	Texas	62,958	9.5%
40	Utah	2,219	0.3%
50	Vermont	485	0.1%
15	Virginia	13,735	2.1%
21	Washington	11,964	1.8%
42	West Virginia	1,820	0.3%
13	Wisconsin	14,462	2.2%
49	Wyoming	787	0.1%

<u>RANK ORDER</u>

RANK	STATE	CASES	% of USA
1	California	85,156	12.9%
2	Texas	62,958	9.5%
3	Illinois	32,870	5.0%
4	Florida	31,743	4.8%
5	Georgia	30,368	4.6%
6	Ohio	29,398	4.5%
7	Pennsylvania	27,019	4.1%
8	New York	26,766	4.1%
9	Michigan	23,107	3.5%
10	North Carolina	21,812	3.3%
11	South Carolina	18,499	2.8%
12	Louisiana	16,635	2.5%
13	Wisconsin	14,462	2.2%
14	Tennessee	14,216	2.2%
15	Virginia	13,735	2.1%
16	Maryland	13,568	2.1%
17	Missouri	13,355	2.0%
18	New Jersey	12,424	1.9%
19	Alabama	12,375	1.9%
20	Arizona	12,111	1.8%
21	Washington	11,964	1.8%
22	Indiana	11,734	1.8%
23	Mississippi	11,545	1.8%
24	Colorado	10,848	1.6%
25	Massachusetts	8,776	1.3%
26	Oklahoma	8,195	1.2%
27	Minnesota	7,450	1.1%
28	Connecticut	7,422	1.1%
29	Kentucky	7,378	1.1%
30	Oregon	6,127	0.9%
31	Kansas	6,093	0.9%
32	Arkansas	5,865	0.9%
33	Iowa	5,511	0.8%
34	New Mexico	5,017	0.8%
35	Nebraska	3,616	0.5%
36	Hawaii	3,165	0.5%
37	Nevada	3,086	0.5%
38	Delaware	2,761	0.4%
39	Rhode Island	2,345	0.4%
40	Utah	2,219	0.3%
41	Alaska	1,886	0.3%
42	West Virginia	1,820	0.3%
43	Idaho	1,778	0.3%
44	Montana	1,584	0.2%
45	South Dakota	1,544	0.2%
46	Maine	1,220	0.2%
47	New Hampshire	976	0.1%
48	North Dakota	947	0.1%
49	Wyoming	787	0.1%
50	Vermont	485	0.1%
	District of Columbia	2,720	0.4%

*Source: U.S. Department of Health and Human Services, National Center for Health Statistics
"Sexually Transmitted Disease Surveillance 1999" (http://www.cdc.gov/nchstp/dstd/dstdp.html)*
Any of several common, often asymptomatic, sexually transmitted diseases caused by the microorganism Chlamydia trachomatis, including nonspecific urethritis in men.

Chlamydia Rate in 1999

National Rate = 254.1 Cases per 100,000 Population*

ALPHA ORDER

RANK	STATE	RATE
11	Alabama	284.4
8	Alaska	307.2
20	Arizona	259.4
26	Arkansas	231.1
19	California	260.7
13	Colorado	273.2
27	Connecticut	226.7
5	Delaware	371.3
30	Florida	212.8
3	Georgia	397.4
15	Hawaii	265.3
44	Idaho	144.7
14	Illinois	272.9
34	Indiana	198.9
35	Iowa	192.5
25	Kansas	231.8
36	Kentucky	187.4
4	Louisiana	380.8
48	Maine	98.1
16	Maryland	264.2
45	Massachusetts	142.8
24	Michigan	235.4
41	Minnesota	157.7
2	Mississippi	419.5
21	Missouri	245.6
38	Montana	179.9
29	Nebraska	217.5
39	Nevada	176.7
49	New Hampshire	82.4
42	New Jersey	153.1
10	New Mexico	288.8
6	New York	360.7
9	North Carolina	289.0
43	North Dakota	148.4
17	Ohio	262.3
22	Oklahoma	244.9
37	Oregon	186.7
28	Pennsylvania	225.1
23	Rhode Island	237.2
1	South Carolina	482.3
32	South Dakota	209.2
18	Tennessee	261.8
7	Texas	318.6
46	Utah	105.7
50	Vermont	82.1
33	Virginia	202.2
31	Washington	210.3
47	West Virginia	100.5
12	Wisconsin	276.9
40	Wyoming	163.6

RANK ORDER

RANK	STATE	RATE
1	South Carolina	482.3
2	Mississippi	419.5
3	Georgia	397.4
4	Louisiana	380.8
5	Delaware	371.3
6	New York	360.7
7	Texas	318.6
8	Alaska	307.2
9	North Carolina	289.0
10	New Mexico	288.8
11	Alabama	284.4
12	Wisconsin	276.9
13	Colorado	273.2
14	Illinois	272.9
15	Hawaii	265.3
16	Maryland	264.2
17	Ohio	262.3
18	Tennessee	261.8
19	California	260.7
20	Arizona	259.4
21	Missouri	245.6
22	Oklahoma	244.9
23	Rhode Island	237.2
24	Michigan	235.4
25	Kansas	231.8
26	Arkansas	231.1
27	Connecticut	226.7
28	Pennsylvania	225.1
29	Nebraska	217.5
30	Florida	212.8
31	Washington	210.3
32	South Dakota	209.2
33	Virginia	202.2
34	Indiana	198.9
35	Iowa	192.5
36	Kentucky	187.4
37	Oregon	186.7
38	Montana	179.9
39	Nevada	176.7
40	Wyoming	163.6
41	Minnesota	157.7
42	New Jersey	153.1
43	North Dakota	148.4
44	Idaho	144.7
45	Massachusetts	142.8
46	Utah	105.7
47	West Virginia	100.5
48	Maine	98.1
49	New Hampshire	82.4
50	Vermont	82.1
	District of Columbia	524.1

Source: U.S. Department of Health and Human Services, National Center for Health Statistics
    "Sexually Transmitted Disease Surveillance 1999" (http://www.cdc.gov/nchstp/dstd/dstdp.html)
*Any of several common, often asymptomatic, sexually transmitted diseases caused by the microorganism Chlamydia trachomatis, including nonspecific urethritis in men.

Gonorrhea Cases Reported in 1999

National Total = 360,076 Cases*

ALPHA ORDER

RANK	STATE	CASES	% of USA
14	Alabama	10,888	3.0%
41	Alaska	302	0.1%
22	Arizona	4,293	1.2%
26	Arkansas	3,226	0.9%
7	California	18,672	5.2%
29	Colorado	2,526	0.7%
25	Connecticut	3,321	0.9%
32	Delaware	1,662	0.5%
3	Florida	22,939	6.4%
4	Georgia	21,244	5.9%
40	Hawaii	463	0.1%
45	Idaho	89	0.0%
2	Illinois	23,254	6.5%
21	Indiana	6,092	1.7%
34	Iowa	1,365	0.4%
28	Kansas	2,665	0.7%
24	Kentucky	3,349	0.9%
12	Louisiana	13,189	3.7%
46	Maine	83	0.0%
15	Maryland	10,430	2.9%
30	Massachusetts	2,453	0.7%
9	Michigan	15,907	4.4%
27	Minnesota	2,830	0.8%
16	Mississippi	10,411	2.9%
18	Missouri	8,187	2.3%
48	Montana	53	0.0%
33	Nebraska	1,471	0.4%
35	Nevada	1,303	0.4%
44	New Hampshire	115	0.0%
19	New Jersey	7,852	2.2%
36	New Mexico	974	0.3%
5	New York	19,826	5.5%
6	North Carolina	19,428	5.4%
46	North Dakota	83	0.0%
8	Ohio	18,141	5.0%
23	Oklahoma	4,021	1.1%
37	Oregon	903	0.3%
11	Pennsylvania	13,295	3.7%
38	Rhode Island	601	0.2%
10	South Carolina	15,037	4.2%
43	South Dakota	192	0.1%
13	Tennessee	11,366	3.2%
1	Texas	32,910	9.1%
42	Utah	254	0.1%
49	Vermont	52	0.0%
17	Virginia	9,402	2.6%
31	Washington	2,132	0.6%
39	West Virginia	584	0.2%
20	Wisconsin	6,662	1.9%
50	Wyoming	43	0.0%

RANK ORDER

RANK	STATE	CASES	% of USA
1	Texas	32,910	9.1%
2	Illinois	23,254	6.5%
3	Florida	22,939	6.4%
4	Georgia	21,244	5.9%
5	New York	19,826	5.5%
6	North Carolina	19,428	5.4%
7	California	18,672	5.2%
8	Ohio	18,141	5.0%
9	Michigan	15,907	4.4%
10	South Carolina	15,037	4.2%
11	Pennsylvania	13,295	3.7%
12	Louisiana	13,189	3.7%
13	Tennessee	11,366	3.2%
14	Alabama	10,888	3.0%
15	Maryland	10,430	2.9%
16	Mississippi	10,411	2.9%
17	Virginia	9,402	2.6%
18	Missouri	8,187	2.3%
19	New Jersey	7,852	2.2%
20	Wisconsin	6,662	1.9%
21	Indiana	6,092	1.7%
22	Arizona	4,293	1.2%
23	Oklahoma	4,021	1.1%
24	Kentucky	3,349	0.9%
25	Connecticut	3,321	0.9%
26	Arkansas	3,226	0.9%
27	Minnesota	2,830	0.8%
28	Kansas	2,665	0.7%
29	Colorado	2,526	0.7%
30	Massachusetts	2,453	0.7%
31	Washington	2,132	0.6%
32	Delaware	1,662	0.5%
33	Nebraska	1,471	0.4%
34	Iowa	1,365	0.4%
35	Nevada	1,303	0.4%
36	New Mexico	974	0.3%
37	Oregon	903	0.3%
38	Rhode Island	601	0.2%
39	West Virginia	584	0.2%
40	Hawaii	463	0.1%
41	Alaska	302	0.1%
42	Utah	254	0.1%
43	South Dakota	192	0.1%
44	New Hampshire	115	0.0%
45	Idaho	89	0.0%
46	Maine	83	0.0%
46	North Dakota	83	0.0%
48	Montana	53	0.0%
49	Vermont	52	0.0%
50	Wyoming	43	0.0%
	District of Columbia	3,536	1.0%

*Source: U.S. Department of Health and Human Services, National Center for Health Statistics
"Sexually Transmitted Disease Surveillance 1999" (http://www.cdc.gov/nchstp/dstd/dstdp.html)*
Gonorrhea is a sexually transmitted disease caused by gonococcal bacteria that affects the mucous membrane chiefly of the genital and urinary tracts and is characterized by an acute purulent discharge and painful or difficult urination, though women often have no symptoms.

Gonorrhea Rate in 1999

National Rate = 133.2 Cases per 100,000 Population*

ALPHA ORDER

RANK ORDER

RANK	STATE	RATE		RANK	STATE	RATE
6	Alabama	250.2		1	South Carolina	392.0
35	Alaska	49.2		2	Mississippi	378.3
26	Arizona	92.0		3	Louisiana	301.9
18	Arkansas	127.1		4	Georgia	278.0
33	California	57.2		5	North Carolina	257.4
30	Colorado	63.6		6	Alabama	250.2
23	Connecticut	101.4		7	Delaware	223.5
7	Delaware	223.5		8	Tennessee	209.3
14	Florida	153.8		9	Maryland	203.1
4	Georgia	278.0		10	Illinois	193.1
38	Hawaii	38.8		11	Texas	166.6
48	Idaho	7.2		12	Michigan	162.0
10	Illinois	193.1		13	Ohio	161.8
22	Indiana	103.3		14	Florida	153.8
36	Iowa	47.7		15	Missouri	150.5
23	Kansas	101.4		16	Virginia	138.4
28	Kentucky	85.1		17	Wisconsin	127.5
3	Louisiana	301.9		18	Arkansas	127.1
49	Maine	6.7		19	Oklahoma	120.1
9	Maryland	203.1		20	Pennsylvania	110.8
37	Massachusetts	39.9		21	New York	109.1
12	Michigan	162.0		22	Indiana	103.3
32	Minnesota	59.9		23	Connecticut	101.4
2	Mississippi	378.3		23	Kansas	101.4
15	Missouri	150.5		25	New Jersey	96.8
50	Montana	6.0		26	Arizona	92.0
27	Nebraska	88.5		27	Nebraska	88.5
29	Nevada	74.6		28	Kentucky	85.1
45	New Hampshire	9.7		29	Nevada	74.6
25	New Jersey	96.8		30	Colorado	63.6
34	New Mexico	56.1		31	Rhode Island	60.8
21	New York	109.1		32	Minnesota	59.9
5	North Carolina	257.4		33	California	57.2
43	North Dakota	13.0		34	New Mexico	56.1
13	Ohio	161.8		35	Alaska	49.2
19	Oklahoma	120.1		36	Iowa	47.7
41	Oregon	27.5		37	Massachusetts	39.9
20	Pennsylvania	110.8		38	Hawaii	38.8
31	Rhode Island	60.8		39	Washington	37.5
1	South Carolina	392.0		40	West Virginia	32.2
42	South Dakota	26.0		41	Oregon	27.5
8	Tennessee	209.3		42	South Dakota	26.0
11	Texas	166.6		43	North Dakota	13.0
44	Utah	12.1		44	Utah	12.1
47	Vermont	8.8		45	New Hampshire	9.7
16	Virginia	138.4		46	Wyoming	8.9
39	Washington	37.5		47	Vermont	8.8
40	West Virginia	32.2		48	Idaho	7.2
17	Wisconsin	127.5		49	Maine	6.7
46	Wyoming	8.9		50	Montana	6.0

District of Columbia   681.3

Source: U.S. Department of Health and Human Services, National Center for Health Statistics
"Sexually Transmitted Disease Surveillance 1999" (http://www.cdc.gov/nchstp/dstd/dstdp.html)
*Gonorrhea is a sexually transmitted disease caused by gonococcal bacteria that affects the mucous membrane chiefly of the genital and urinary tracts and is characterized by an acute purulent discharge and painful or difficult urination, though women often have no symptoms.

Syphilis Cases Reported in 1999

National Total = 6,657 Cases*

ALPHA ORDER

RANK	STATE	CASES	% of USA
14	Alabama	202	3.0%
43	Alaska	1	0.0%
13	Arizona	212	3.2%
22	Arkansas	87	1.3%
10	California	283	4.3%
34	Colorado	8	0.1%
28	Connecticut	16	0.2%
31	Delaware	10	0.2%
7	Florida	383	5.8%
5	Georgia	430	6.5%
39	Hawaii	3	0.0%
43	Idaho	1	0.0%
6	Illinois	422	6.3%
4	Indiana	450	6.8%
33	Iowa	9	0.1%
29	Kansas	14	0.2%
19	Kentucky	101	1.5%
9	Louisiana	306	4.6%
47	Maine	0	0.0%
8	Maryland	343	5.2%
27	Massachusetts	37	0.6%
12	Michigan	249	3.7%
31	Minnesota	10	0.2%
15	Mississippi	194	2.9%
20	Missouri	96	1.4%
43	Montana	1	0.0%
36	Nebraska	6	0.1%
37	Nevada	5	0.1%
43	New Hampshire	1	0.0%
25	New Jersey	68	1.0%
30	New Mexico	12	0.2%
18	New York	150	2.3%
3	North Carolina	464	7.0%
47	North Dakota	0	0.0%
21	Ohio	92	1.4%
16	Oklahoma	187	2.8%
34	Oregon	8	0.1%
23	Pennsylvania	84	1.3%
39	Rhode Island	3	0.0%
11	South Carolina	269	4.0%
47	South Dakota	0	0.0%
1	Tennessee	641	9.6%
2	Texas	473	7.1%
42	Utah	2	0.0%
39	Vermont	3	0.0%
17	Virginia	153	2.3%
24	Washington	77	1.2%
37	West Virginia	5	0.1%
26	Wisconsin	41	0.6%
47	Wyoming	0	0.0%

RANK ORDER

RANK	STATE	CASES	% of USA
1	Tennessee	641	9.6%
2	Texas	473	7.1%
3	North Carolina	464	7.0%
4	Indiana	450	6.8%
5	Georgia	430	6.5%
6	Illinois	422	6.3%
7	Florida	383	5.8%
8	Maryland	343	5.2%
9	Louisiana	306	4.6%
10	California	283	4.3%
11	South Carolina	269	4.0%
12	Michigan	249	3.7%
13	Arizona	212	3.2%
14	Alabama	202	3.0%
15	Mississippi	194	2.9%
16	Oklahoma	187	2.8%
17	Virginia	153	2.3%
18	New York	150	2.3%
19	Kentucky	101	1.5%
20	Missouri	96	1.4%
21	Ohio	92	1.4%
22	Arkansas	87	1.3%
23	Pennsylvania	84	1.3%
24	Washington	77	1.2%
25	New Jersey	68	1.0%
26	Wisconsin	41	0.6%
27	Massachusetts	37	0.6%
28	Connecticut	16	0.2%
29	Kansas	14	0.2%
30	New Mexico	12	0.2%
31	Delaware	10	0.2%
31	Minnesota	10	0.2%
33	Iowa	9	0.1%
34	Colorado	8	0.1%
34	Oregon	8	0.1%
36	Nebraska	6	0.1%
37	Nevada	5	0.1%
37	West Virginia	5	0.1%
39	Hawaii	3	0.0%
39	Rhode Island	3	0.0%
39	Vermont	3	0.0%
42	Utah	2	0.0%
43	Alaska	1	0.0%
43	Idaho	1	0.0%
43	Montana	1	0.0%
43	New Hampshire	1	0.0%
47	Maine	0	0.0%
47	North Dakota	0	0.0%
47	South Dakota	0	0.0%
47	Wyoming	0	0.0%
	District of Columbia	45	0.7%

Source: U.S. Department of Health and Human Services, National Center for Health Statistics
"Sexually Transmitted Disease Surveillance 1999" (http://www.cdc.gov/nchstp/dstd/dstdp.html)
*Includes only primary and secondary cases. Does not include 28,971 cases in other stages. A chronic infectious disease caused by a spirochete (Treponema pallidum), either transmitted by direct contact, usually in sexual intercourse, or passed from mother to child in utero, and progressing through three stages characterized respectively by local formation of chancres, ulcerous skin eruptions, and systemic infection leading to general paresis.

Syphilis Rate in 1999

National Rate = 2.5 Cases per 100,000 Population*

ALPHA ORDER

RANK	STATE	RATE
10	Alabama	4.6
39	Alaska	0.2
11	Arizona	4.5
13	Arkansas	3.4
22	California	0.9
39	Colorado	0.2
30	Connecticut	0.5
21	Delaware	1.3
14	Florida	2.6
8	Georgia	5.6
34	Hawaii	0.3
43	Idaho	0.1
12	Illinois	3.5
2	Indiana	7.6
34	Iowa	0.3
30	Kansas	0.5
14	Kentucky	2.6
3	Louisiana	7.0
47	Maine	0.0
6	Maryland	6.7
29	Massachusetts	0.6
16	Michigan	2.5
39	Minnesota	0.2
3	Mississippi	7.0
19	Missouri	1.8
43	Montana	0.1
33	Nebraska	0.4
34	Nevada	0.3
43	New Hampshire	0.1
23	New Jersey	0.8
27	New Mexico	0.7
23	New York	0.8
7	North Carolina	6.1
47	North Dakota	0.0
23	Ohio	0.8
8	Oklahoma	5.6
39	Oregon	0.2
27	Pennsylvania	0.7
34	Rhode Island	0.3
3	South Carolina	7.0
47	South Dakota	0.0
1	Tennessee	11.8
17	Texas	2.4
43	Utah	0.1
30	Vermont	0.5
18	Virginia	2.3
20	Washington	1.4
34	West Virginia	0.3
23	Wisconsin	0.8
47	Wyoming	0.0

RANK ORDER

RANK	STATE	RATE
1	Tennessee	11.8
2	Indiana	7.6
3	Louisiana	7.0
3	Mississippi	7.0
3	South Carolina	7.0
6	Maryland	6.7
7	North Carolina	6.1
8	Georgia	5.6
8	Oklahoma	5.6
10	Alabama	4.6
11	Arizona	4.5
12	Illinois	3.5
13	Arkansas	3.4
14	Florida	2.6
14	Kentucky	2.6
16	Michigan	2.5
17	Texas	2.4
18	Virginia	2.3
19	Missouri	1.8
20	Washington	1.4
21	Delaware	1.3
22	California	0.9
23	New Jersey	0.8
23	New York	0.8
23	Ohio	0.8
23	Wisconsin	0.8
27	New Mexico	0.7
27	Pennsylvania	0.7
29	Massachusetts	0.6
30	Connecticut	0.5
30	Kansas	0.5
30	Vermont	0.5
33	Nebraska	0.4
34	Hawaii	0.3
34	Iowa	0.3
34	Nevada	0.3
34	Rhode Island	0.3
34	West Virginia	0.3
39	Alaska	0.2
39	Colorado	0.2
39	Minnesota	0.2
39	Oregon	0.2
43	Idaho	0.1
43	Montana	0.1
43	New Hampshire	0.1
43	Utah	0.1
47	Maine	0.0
47	North Dakota	0.0
47	South Dakota	0.0
47	Wyoming	0.0

District of Columbia	8.7

Source: U.S. Department of Health and Human Services, National Center for Health Statistics
"Sexually Transmitted Disease Surveillance 1999" (http://www.cdc.gov/nchstp/dstd/dstdp.html)
*Includes only primary and secondary cases. Does not include 28,971 cases in other stages. A chronic infectious disease caused by a spirochete (Treponema pallidum), either transmitted by direct contact, usually in sexual intercourse, or passed from mother to child in utero, and progressing through three stages characterized respectively by local formation of chancres, ulcerous skin eruptions, and systemic infection leading to general paresis.

VI. PROVIDERS

VI. PROVIDERS (continued)

Physicians in 1999

National Total = 785,899 Physicians*

ALPHA ORDER

RANK	STATE	PHYSICIANS	% of USA
25	Alabama	9,695	1.2%
49	Alaska	1,293	0.2%
23	Arizona	11,916	1.5%
32	Arkansas	5,607	0.7%
1	California	94,867	12.1%
24	Colorado	11,420	1.5%
20	Connecticut	13,185	1.7%
46	Delaware	2,034	0.3%
4	Florida	44,917	5.7%
14	Georgia	18,746	2.4%
38	Hawaii	3,840	0.5%
43	Idaho	2,313	0.3%
6	Illinois	35,395	4.5%
21	Indiana	13,148	1.7%
31	Iowa	5,826	0.7%
30	Kansas	6,356	0.8%
26	Kentucky	9,367	1.2%
22	Louisiana	12,027	1.5%
41	Maine	3,417	0.4%
11	Maryland	23,133	2.9%
8	Massachusetts	28,457	3.6%
10	Michigan	24,832	3.2%
18	Minnesota	13,718	1.7%
33	Mississippi	5,232	0.7%
17	Missouri	13,952	1.8%
45	Montana	2,065	0.3%
37	Nebraska	4,181	0.5%
40	Nevada	3,731	0.5%
42	New Hampshire	3,333	0.4%
9	New Jersey	26,891	3.4%
35	New Mexico	4,468	0.6%
2	New York	77,931	9.9%
12	North Carolina	20,509	2.6%
48	North Dakota	1,612	0.2%
7	Ohio	29,831	3.8%
29	Oklahoma	6,478	0.8%
28	Oregon	9,047	1.2%
5	Pennsylvania	39,024	5.0%
39	Rhode Island	3,747	0.5%
27	South Carolina	9,349	1.2%
47	South Dakota	1,647	0.2%
16	Tennessee	15,132	1.9%
3	Texas	45,876	5.8%
34	Utah	4,889	0.6%
44	Vermont	2,181	0.3%
13	Virginia	19,461	2.5%
15	Washington	16,229	2.1%
36	West Virginia	4,458	0.6%
19	Wisconsin	13,617	1.7%
50	Wyoming	988	0.1%

RANK ORDER

RANK	STATE	PHYSICIANS	% of USA
1	California	94,867	12.1%
2	New York	77,931	9.9%
3	Texas	45,876	5.8%
4	Florida	44,917	5.7%
5	Pennsylvania	39,024	5.0%
6	Illinois	35,395	4.5%
7	Ohio	29,831	3.8%
8	Massachusetts	28,457	3.6%
9	New Jersey	26,891	3.4%
10	Michigan	24,832	3.2%
11	Maryland	23,133	2.9%
12	North Carolina	20,509	2.6%
13	Virginia	19,461	2.5%
14	Georgia	18,746	2.4%
15	Washington	16,229	2.1%
16	Tennessee	15,132	1.9%
17	Missouri	13,952	1.8%
18	Minnesota	13,718	1.7%
19	Wisconsin	13,617	1.7%
20	Connecticut	13,185	1.7%
21	Indiana	13,148	1.7%
22	Louisiana	12,027	1.5%
23	Arizona	11,916	1.5%
24	Colorado	11,420	1.5%
25	Alabama	9,695	1.2%
26	Kentucky	9,367	1.2%
27	South Carolina	9,349	1.2%
28	Oregon	9,047	1.2%
29	Oklahoma	6,478	0.8%
30	Kansas	6,356	0.8%
31	Iowa	5,826	0.7%
32	Arkansas	5,607	0.7%
33	Mississippi	5,232	0.7%
34	Utah	4,889	0.6%
35	New Mexico	4,468	0.6%
36	West Virginia	4,458	0.6%
37	Nebraska	4,181	0.5%
38	Hawaii	3,840	0.5%
39	Rhode Island	3,747	0.5%
40	Nevada	3,731	0.5%
41	Maine	3,417	0.4%
42	New Hampshire	3,333	0.4%
43	Idaho	2,313	0.3%
44	Vermont	2,181	0.3%
45	Montana	2,065	0.3%
46	Delaware	2,034	0.3%
47	South Dakota	1,647	0.2%
48	North Dakota	1,612	0.2%
49	Alaska	1,293	0.2%
50	Wyoming	988	0.1%
	District of Columbia	4,531	0.6%

Source: American Medical Association (Chicago, Illinois)
"Physician Characteristics and Distribution in the U.S." (2001-2002 Edition)
As of December 31, 1999. Comprised of federal and nonfederal physicians. Total does not include 11,735 physicians in the U.S. territories and possessions, at APO's and FPO's and whose addresses are unknown.

Male Physicians in 1999

National Total = 602,400 Physicians*

ALPHA ORDER

RANK	STATE	PHYSICIANS	% of USA
25	Alabama	7,951	1.3%
49	Alaska	974	0.2%
23	Arizona	9,416	1.6%
32	Arkansas	4,606	0.8%
1	California	72,820	12.1%
24	Colorado	8,718	1.4%
21	Connecticut	9,965	1.7%
46	Delaware	1,545	0.3%
3	Florida	37,227	6.2%
14	Georgia	14,702	2.4%
39	Hawaii	2,961	0.5%
43	Idaho	1,993	0.3%
6	Illinois	25,683	4.3%
19	Indiana	10,494	1.7%
31	Iowa	4,722	0.8%
30	Kansas	5,019	0.8%
27	Kentucky	7,439	1.2%
22	Louisiana	9,500	1.6%
41	Maine	2,670	0.4%
11	Maryland	16,815	2.8%
8	Massachusetts	20,190	3.4%
10	Michigan	18,617	3.1%
20	Minnesota	10,466	1.7%
33	Mississippi	4,353	0.7%
17	Missouri	10,819	1.8%
44	Montana	1,745	0.3%
36	Nebraska	3,372	0.6%
38	Nevada	3,075	0.5%
42	New Hampshire	2,642	0.4%
9	New Jersey	19,654	3.3%
37	New Mexico	3,250	0.5%
2	New York	56,357	9.4%
12	North Carolina	15,983	2.7%
48	North Dakota	1,351	0.2%
7	Ohio	22,731	3.8%
29	Oklahoma	5,255	0.9%
28	Oregon	7,073	1.2%
5	Pennsylvania	29,567	4.9%
40	Rhode Island	2,763	0.5%
26	South Carolina	7,577	1.3%
47	South Dakota	1,375	0.2%
16	Tennessee	12,190	2.0%
4	Texas	35,733	5.9%
34	Utah	4,080	0.7%
45	Vermont	1,635	0.3%
13	Virginia	14,777	2.5%
15	Washington	12,451	2.1%
35	West Virginia	3,547	0.6%
18	Wisconsin	10,592	1.8%
50	Wyoming	843	0.1%

RANK ORDER

RANK	STATE	PHYSICIANS	% of USA
1	California	72,820	12.1%
2	New York	56,357	9.4%
3	Florida	37,227	6.2%
4	Texas	35,733	5.9%
5	Pennsylvania	29,567	4.9%
6	Illinois	25,683	4.3%
7	Ohio	22,731	3.8%
8	Massachusetts	20,190	3.4%
9	New Jersey	19,654	3.3%
10	Michigan	18,617	3.1%
11	Maryland	16,815	2.8%
12	North Carolina	15,983	2.7%
13	Virginia	14,777	2.5%
14	Georgia	14,702	2.4%
15	Washington	12,451	2.1%
16	Tennessee	12,190	2.0%
17	Missouri	10,819	1.8%
18	Wisconsin	10,592	1.8%
19	Indiana	10,494	1.7%
20	Minnesota	10,466	1.7%
21	Connecticut	9,965	1.7%
22	Louisiana	9,500	1.6%
23	Arizona	9,416	1.6%
24	Colorado	8,718	1.4%
25	Alabama	7,951	1.3%
26	South Carolina	7,577	1.3%
27	Kentucky	7,439	1.2%
28	Oregon	7,073	1.2%
29	Oklahoma	5,255	0.9%
30	Kansas	5,019	0.8%
31	Iowa	4,722	0.8%
32	Arkansas	4,606	0.8%
33	Mississippi	4,353	0.7%
34	Utah	4,080	0.7%
35	West Virginia	3,547	0.6%
36	Nebraska	3,372	0.6%
37	New Mexico	3,250	0.5%
38	Nevada	3,075	0.5%
39	Hawaii	2,961	0.5%
40	Rhode Island	2,763	0.5%
41	Maine	2,670	0.4%
42	New Hampshire	2,642	0.4%
43	Idaho	1,993	0.3%
44	Montana	1,745	0.3%
45	Vermont	1,635	0.3%
46	Delaware	1,545	0.3%
47	South Dakota	1,375	0.2%
48	North Dakota	1,351	0.2%
49	Alaska	974	0.2%
50	Wyoming	843	0.1%
	District of Columbia	3,117	0.5%

Source: American Medical Association (Chicago, Illinois)
    "Physician Characteristics and Distribution in the U.S." (2001-2002 Edition)
*As of December 31, 1999. Comprised of federal and nonfederal physicians. Total does not include 8,628 male physicians in the U.S. territories and possessions, at APO's and FPO's and whose addresses are unknown.

Female Physicians in 1999

National Total = 183,499 Physicians*

<table>
<tr><td colspan="4">ALPHA ORDER</td><td colspan="4">RANK ORDER</td></tr>
<tr><th>RANK</th><th>STATE</th><th>PHYSICIANS</th><th>% of USA</th><th>RANK</th><th>STATE</th><th>PHYSICIANS</th><th>% of USA</th></tr>
<tr><td>28</td><td>Alabama</td><td>1,744</td><td>1.0%</td><td>1</td><td>California</td><td>22,047</td><td>12.0%</td></tr>
<tr><td>47</td><td>Alaska</td><td>319</td><td>0.2%</td><td>2</td><td>New York</td><td>21,574</td><td>11.8%</td></tr>
<tr><td>24</td><td>Arizona</td><td>2,500</td><td>1.4%</td><td>3</td><td>Texas</td><td>10,143</td><td>5.5%</td></tr>
<tr><td>33</td><td>Arkansas</td><td>1,001</td><td>0.5%</td><td>4</td><td>Illinois</td><td>9,712</td><td>5.3%</td></tr>
<tr><td>1</td><td>California</td><td>22,047</td><td>12.0%</td><td>5</td><td>Pennsylvania</td><td>9,457</td><td>5.2%</td></tr>
<tr><td>21</td><td>Colorado</td><td>2,702</td><td>1.5%</td><td>6</td><td>Massachusetts</td><td>8,267</td><td>4.5%</td></tr>
<tr><td>17</td><td>Connecticut</td><td>3,220</td><td>1.8%</td><td>7</td><td>Florida</td><td>7,690</td><td>4.2%</td></tr>
<tr><td>44</td><td>Delaware</td><td>489</td><td>0.3%</td><td>8</td><td>New Jersey</td><td>7,237</td><td>3.9%</td></tr>
<tr><td>7</td><td>Florida</td><td>7,690</td><td>4.2%</td><td>9</td><td>Ohio</td><td>7,100</td><td>3.9%</td></tr>
<tr><td>14</td><td>Georgia</td><td>4,044</td><td>2.2%</td><td>10</td><td>Maryland</td><td>6,318</td><td>3.4%</td></tr>
<tr><td>36</td><td>Hawaii</td><td>879</td><td>0.5%</td><td>11</td><td>Michigan</td><td>6,215</td><td>3.4%</td></tr>
<tr><td>45</td><td>Idaho</td><td>320</td><td>0.2%</td><td>12</td><td>Virginia</td><td>4,684</td><td>2.6%</td></tr>
<tr><td>4</td><td>Illinois</td><td>9,712</td><td>5.3%</td><td>13</td><td>North Carolina</td><td>4,526</td><td>2.5%</td></tr>
<tr><td>22</td><td>Indiana</td><td>2,654</td><td>1.4%</td><td>14</td><td>Georgia</td><td>4,044</td><td>2.2%</td></tr>
<tr><td>32</td><td>Iowa</td><td>1,104</td><td>0.6%</td><td>15</td><td>Washington</td><td>3,778</td><td>2.1%</td></tr>
<tr><td>29</td><td>Kansas</td><td>1,337</td><td>0.7%</td><td>16</td><td>Minnesota</td><td>3,252</td><td>1.8%</td></tr>
<tr><td>26</td><td>Kentucky</td><td>1,928</td><td>1.1%</td><td>17</td><td>Connecticut</td><td>3,220</td><td>1.8%</td></tr>
<tr><td>23</td><td>Louisiana</td><td>2,527</td><td>1.4%</td><td>18</td><td>Missouri</td><td>3,133</td><td>1.7%</td></tr>
<tr><td>40</td><td>Maine</td><td>747</td><td>0.4%</td><td>19</td><td>Wisconsin</td><td>3,025</td><td>1.6%</td></tr>
<tr><td>10</td><td>Maryland</td><td>6,318</td><td>3.4%</td><td>20</td><td>Tennessee</td><td>2,942</td><td>1.6%</td></tr>
<tr><td>6</td><td>Massachusetts</td><td>8,267</td><td>4.5%</td><td>21</td><td>Colorado</td><td>2,702</td><td>1.5%</td></tr>
<tr><td>11</td><td>Michigan</td><td>6,215</td><td>3.4%</td><td>22</td><td>Indiana</td><td>2,654</td><td>1.4%</td></tr>
<tr><td>16</td><td>Minnesota</td><td>3,252</td><td>1.8%</td><td>23</td><td>Louisiana</td><td>2,527</td><td>1.4%</td></tr>
<tr><td>36</td><td>Mississippi</td><td>879</td><td>0.5%</td><td>24</td><td>Arizona</td><td>2,500</td><td>1.4%</td></tr>
<tr><td>18</td><td>Missouri</td><td>3,133</td><td>1.7%</td><td>25</td><td>Oregon</td><td>1,974</td><td>1.1%</td></tr>
<tr><td>45</td><td>Montana</td><td>320</td><td>0.2%</td><td>26</td><td>Kentucky</td><td>1,928</td><td>1.1%</td></tr>
<tr><td>38</td><td>Nebraska</td><td>809</td><td>0.4%</td><td>27</td><td>South Carolina</td><td>1,772</td><td>1.0%</td></tr>
<tr><td>42</td><td>Nevada</td><td>656</td><td>0.4%</td><td>28</td><td>Alabama</td><td>1,744</td><td>1.0%</td></tr>
<tr><td>41</td><td>New Hampshire</td><td>691</td><td>0.4%</td><td>29</td><td>Kansas</td><td>1,337</td><td>0.7%</td></tr>
<tr><td>8</td><td>New Jersey</td><td>7,237</td><td>3.9%</td><td>30</td><td>Oklahoma</td><td>1,223</td><td>0.7%</td></tr>
<tr><td>31</td><td>New Mexico</td><td>1,218</td><td>0.7%</td><td>31</td><td>New Mexico</td><td>1,218</td><td>0.7%</td></tr>
<tr><td>2</td><td>New York</td><td>21,574</td><td>11.8%</td><td>32</td><td>Iowa</td><td>1,104</td><td>0.6%</td></tr>
<tr><td>13</td><td>North Carolina</td><td>4,526</td><td>2.5%</td><td>33</td><td>Arkansas</td><td>1,001</td><td>0.5%</td></tr>
<tr><td>49</td><td>North Dakota</td><td>261</td><td>0.1%</td><td>34</td><td>Rhode Island</td><td>984</td><td>0.5%</td></tr>
<tr><td>9</td><td>Ohio</td><td>7,100</td><td>3.9%</td><td>35</td><td>West Virginia</td><td>911</td><td>0.5%</td></tr>
<tr><td>30</td><td>Oklahoma</td><td>1,223</td><td>0.7%</td><td>36</td><td>Hawaii</td><td>879</td><td>0.5%</td></tr>
<tr><td>25</td><td>Oregon</td><td>1,974</td><td>1.1%</td><td>36</td><td>Mississippi</td><td>879</td><td>0.5%</td></tr>
<tr><td>5</td><td>Pennsylvania</td><td>9,457</td><td>5.2%</td><td>38</td><td>Nebraska</td><td>809</td><td>0.4%</td></tr>
<tr><td>34</td><td>Rhode Island</td><td>984</td><td>0.5%</td><td>38</td><td>Utah</td><td>809</td><td>0.4%</td></tr>
<tr><td>27</td><td>South Carolina</td><td>1,772</td><td>1.0%</td><td>40</td><td>Maine</td><td>747</td><td>0.4%</td></tr>
<tr><td>48</td><td>South Dakota</td><td>272</td><td>0.1%</td><td>41</td><td>New Hampshire</td><td>691</td><td>0.4%</td></tr>
<tr><td>20</td><td>Tennessee</td><td>2,942</td><td>1.6%</td><td>42</td><td>Nevada</td><td>656</td><td>0.4%</td></tr>
<tr><td>3</td><td>Texas</td><td>10,143</td><td>5.5%</td><td>43</td><td>Vermont</td><td>546</td><td>0.3%</td></tr>
<tr><td>38</td><td>Utah</td><td>809</td><td>0.4%</td><td>44</td><td>Delaware</td><td>489</td><td>0.3%</td></tr>
<tr><td>43</td><td>Vermont</td><td>546</td><td>0.3%</td><td>45</td><td>Idaho</td><td>320</td><td>0.2%</td></tr>
<tr><td>12</td><td>Virginia</td><td>4,684</td><td>2.6%</td><td>45</td><td>Montana</td><td>320</td><td>0.2%</td></tr>
<tr><td>15</td><td>Washington</td><td>3,778</td><td>2.1%</td><td>47</td><td>Alaska</td><td>319</td><td>0.2%</td></tr>
<tr><td>35</td><td>West Virginia</td><td>911</td><td>0.5%</td><td>48</td><td>South Dakota</td><td>272</td><td>0.1%</td></tr>
<tr><td>19</td><td>Wisconsin</td><td>3,025</td><td>1.6%</td><td>49</td><td>North Dakota</td><td>261</td><td>0.1%</td></tr>
<tr><td>50</td><td>Wyoming</td><td>145</td><td>0.1%</td><td>50</td><td>Wyoming</td><td>145</td><td>0.1%</td></tr>
<tr><td></td><td></td><td></td><td></td><td></td><td>District of Columbia</td><td>1,414</td><td>0.8%</td></tr>
</table>

Source: American Medical Association (Chicago, Illinois)
  "Physician Characteristics and Distribution in the U.S." (2001-2002 Edition)
*As of December 31, 1999. Comprised of federal and nonfederal physicians. Total does not include 3,107 female physicians in the U.S. territories and possessions, at APO's and FPO's and whose addresses are unknown.

Percent of Physicians Who Are Female: 1999

National Percent = 23.3% of Physicians*

ALPHA ORDER				RANK ORDER		
RANK	STATE	PERCENT		RANK	STATE	PERCENT
40	Alabama	18.0		1	Massachusetts	29.1
10	Alaska	24.7		2	New York	27.7
28	Arizona	21.0		3	Illinois	27.4
41	Arkansas	17.9		4	Maryland	27.3
19	California	23.2		4	New Mexico	27.3
16	Colorado	23.7		6	New Jersey	26.9
11	Connecticut	24.4		7	Rhode Island	26.3
14	Delaware	24.0		8	Michigan	25.0
43	Florida	17.1		8	Vermont	25.0
27	Georgia	21.6		10	Alaska	24.7
20	Hawaii	22.9		11	Connecticut	24.4
50	Idaho	13.8		12	Pennsylvania	24.2
3	Illinois	27.4		13	Virginia	24.1
34	Indiana	20.2		14	Delaware	24.0
38	Iowa	18.9		15	Ohio	23.8
28	Kansas	21.0		16	Colorado	23.7
32	Kentucky	20.6		16	Minnesota	23.7
28	Louisiana	21.0		18	Washington	23.3
25	Maine	21.9		19	California	23.2
4	Maryland	27.3		20	Hawaii	22.9
1	Massachusetts	29.1		21	Missouri	22.5
8	Michigan	25.0		22	Wisconsin	22.2
16	Minnesota	23.7		23	North Carolina	22.1
44	Mississippi	16.8		23	Texas	22.1
21	Missouri	22.5		25	Maine	21.9
48	Montana	15.5		26	Oregon	21.8
36	Nebraska	19.3		27	Georgia	21.6
42	Nevada	17.6		28	Arizona	21.0
31	New Hampshire	20.7		28	Kansas	21.0
6	New Jersey	26.9		28	Louisiana	21.0
4	New Mexico	27.3		31	New Hampshire	20.7
2	New York	27.7		32	Kentucky	20.6
23	North Carolina	22.1		33	West Virginia	20.4
47	North Dakota	16.2		34	Indiana	20.2
15	Ohio	23.8		35	Tennessee	19.4
38	Oklahoma	18.9		36	Nebraska	19.3
26	Oregon	21.8		37	South Carolina	19.0
12	Pennsylvania	24.2		38	Iowa	18.9
7	Rhode Island	26.3		38	Oklahoma	18.9
37	South Carolina	19.0		40	Alabama	18.0
45	South Dakota	16.5		41	Arkansas	17.9
35	Tennessee	19.4		42	Nevada	17.6
23	Texas	22.1		43	Florida	17.1
45	Utah	16.5		44	Mississippi	16.8
8	Vermont	25.0		45	South Dakota	16.5
13	Virginia	24.1		45	Utah	16.5
18	Washington	23.3		47	North Dakota	16.2
33	West Virginia	20.4		48	Montana	15.5
22	Wisconsin	22.2		49	Wyoming	14.7
49	Wyoming	14.7		50	Idaho	13.8
					District of Columbia	31.2

Source: Morgan Quitno Press using data from American Medical Association (Chicago, Illinois)
    "Physician Characteristics and Distribution in the U.S." (2001-2002 Edition)
As of December 31, 1999. Comprised of federal and nonfederal physicians. National percent does not include physicians in the U.S. territories and possessions, at APO's and FPO's and whose addresses are unknown.

Physicians Under 35 Years Old in 1999

National Total = 134,479 Physicians*

ALPHA ORDER

RANK	STATE	PHYSICIANS	% of USA
25	Alabama	1,614	1.2%
48	Alaska	132	0.1%
26	Arizona	1,606	1.2%
32	Arkansas	884	0.7%
2	California	13,100	9.7%
24	Colorado	1,627	1.2%
19	Connecticut	2,258	1.7%
43	Delaware	338	0.3%
9	Florida	4,680	3.5%
14	Georgia	3,215	2.4%
39	Hawaii	511	0.4%
45	Idaho	224	0.2%
4	Illinois	7,862	5.8%
22	Indiana	2,080	1.5%
30	Iowa	997	0.7%
29	Kansas	1,030	0.8%
27	Kentucky	1,549	1.2%
17	Louisiana	2,530	1.9%
42	Maine	359	0.3%
10	Maryland	4,158	3.1%
7	Massachusetts	5,837	4.3%
8	Michigan	5,259	3.9%
18	Minnesota	2,462	1.8%
33	Mississippi	824	0.6%
15	Missouri	2,788	2.1%
49	Montana	123	0.1%
35	Nebraska	797	0.6%
41	Nevada	423	0.3%
40	New Hampshire	430	0.3%
11	New Jersey	4,049	3.0%
38	New Mexico	564	0.4%
1	New York	16,156	12.0%
12	North Carolina	3,928	2.9%
46	North Dakota	223	0.2%
6	Ohio	6,049	4.5%
31	Oklahoma	943	0.7%
28	Oregon	1,066	0.8%
5	Pennsylvania	7,339	5.5%
34	Rhode Island	809	0.6%
23	South Carolina	1,668	1.2%
47	South Dakota	179	0.1%
16	Tennessee	2,668	2.0%
3	Texas	8,530	6.3%
36	Utah	753	0.6%
44	Vermont	321	0.2%
13	Virginia	3,361	2.5%
21	Washington	2,091	1.6%
37	West Virginia	732	0.5%
20	Wisconsin	2,199	1.6%
50	Wyoming	107	0.1%

RANK ORDER

RANK	STATE	PHYSICIANS	% of USA
1	New York	16,156	12.0%
2	California	13,100	9.7%
3	Texas	8,530	6.3%
4	Illinois	7,862	5.8%
5	Pennsylvania	7,339	5.5%
6	Ohio	6,049	4.5%
7	Massachusetts	5,837	4.3%
8	Michigan	5,259	3.9%
9	Florida	4,680	3.5%
10	Maryland	4,158	3.1%
11	New Jersey	4,049	3.0%
12	North Carolina	3,928	2.9%
13	Virginia	3,361	2.5%
14	Georgia	3,215	2.4%
15	Missouri	2,788	2.1%
16	Tennessee	2,668	2.0%
17	Louisiana	2,530	1.9%
18	Minnesota	2,462	1.8%
19	Connecticut	2,258	1.7%
20	Wisconsin	2,199	1.6%
21	Washington	2,091	1.6%
22	Indiana	2,080	1.5%
23	South Carolina	1,668	1.2%
24	Colorado	1,627	1.2%
25	Alabama	1,614	1.2%
26	Arizona	1,606	1.2%
27	Kentucky	1,549	1.2%
28	Oregon	1,066	0.8%
29	Kansas	1,030	0.8%
30	Iowa	997	0.7%
31	Oklahoma	943	0.7%
32	Arkansas	884	0.7%
33	Mississippi	824	0.6%
34	Rhode Island	809	0.6%
35	Nebraska	797	0.6%
36	Utah	753	0.6%
37	West Virginia	732	0.5%
38	New Mexico	564	0.4%
39	Hawaii	511	0.4%
40	New Hampshire	430	0.3%
41	Nevada	423	0.3%
42	Maine	359	0.3%
43	Delaware	338	0.3%
44	Vermont	321	0.2%
45	Idaho	224	0.2%
46	North Dakota	223	0.2%
47	South Dakota	179	0.1%
48	Alaska	132	0.1%
49	Montana	123	0.1%
50	Wyoming	107	0.1%
	District of Columbia	1,047	0.8%

Source: American Medical Association (Chicago, Illinois)
"Physician Characteristics and Distribution in the U.S." (2001-2002 Edition)
As of December 31, 1999. Comprised of federal and nonfederal physicians. Total does not include 1,537 physicians in the U.S. territories and possessions, at APO's and FPO's and whose addresses are unknown.

Percent of Physicians Under 35 Years Old in 1999

National Percent = 17.1% of Physicians*

ALPHA ORDER			RANK ORDER		
RANK	STATE	PERCENT	RANK	STATE	PERCENT
21	Alabama	16.6	1	Illinois	22.2
48	Alaska	10.2	2	Rhode Island	21.6
37	Arizona	13.5	3	Michigan	21.2
27	Arkansas	15.8	4	Louisiana	21.0
35	California	13.8	5	New York	20.7
34	Colorado	14.2	6	Massachusetts	20.5
19	Connecticut	17.1	7	Ohio	20.3
21	Delaware	16.6	8	Missouri	20.0
47	Florida	10.4	9	North Carolina	19.2
18	Georgia	17.2	10	Nebraska	19.1
38	Hawaii	13.3	11	Pennsylvania	18.8
49	Idaho	9.7	12	Texas	18.6
1	Illinois	22.2	13	Maryland	18.0
27	Indiana	15.8	14	Minnesota	17.9
19	Iowa	17.1	15	South Carolina	17.8
25	Kansas	16.2	16	Tennessee	17.6
23	Kentucky	16.5	17	Virginia	17.3
4	Louisiana	21.0	18	Georgia	17.2
46	Maine	10.5	19	Connecticut	17.1
13	Maryland	18.0	19	Iowa	17.1
6	Massachusetts	20.5	21	Alabama	16.6
3	Michigan	21.2	21	Delaware	16.6
14	Minnesota	17.9	23	Kentucky	16.5
29	Mississippi	15.7	24	West Virginia	16.4
8	Missouri	20.0	25	Kansas	16.2
50	Montana	6.0	26	Wisconsin	16.1
10	Nebraska	19.1	27	Arkansas	15.8
43	Nevada	11.3	27	Indiana	15.8
39	New Hampshire	12.9	29	Mississippi	15.7
31	New Jersey	15.1	30	Utah	15.4
41	New Mexico	12.6	31	New Jersey	15.1
5	New York	20.7	32	Vermont	14.7
9	North Carolina	19.2	33	Oklahoma	14.6
35	North Dakota	13.8	34	Colorado	14.2
7	Ohio	20.3	35	California	13.8
33	Oklahoma	14.6	35	North Dakota	13.8
42	Oregon	11.8	37	Arizona	13.5
11	Pennsylvania	18.8	38	Hawaii	13.3
2	Rhode Island	21.6	39	New Hampshire	12.9
15	South Carolina	17.8	39	Washington	12.9
44	South Dakota	10.9	41	New Mexico	12.6
16	Tennessee	17.6	42	Oregon	11.8
12	Texas	18.6	43	Nevada	11.3
30	Utah	15.4	44	South Dakota	10.9
32	Vermont	14.7	45	Wyoming	10.8
17	Virginia	17.3	46	Maine	10.5
39	Washington	12.9	47	Florida	10.4
24	West Virginia	16.4	48	Alaska	10.2
26	Wisconsin	16.1	49	Idaho	9.7
45	Wyoming	10.8	50	Montana	6.0
				District of Columbia	23.1

Source: Morgan Quitno Press using data from American Medical Association (Chicago, Illinois)
"Physician Characteristics and Distribution in the U.S." (2001-2002 Edition)
*As of December 31, 1999. Comprised of federal and nonfederal physicians. National percent does not include physicians in the U.S. territories and possessions, at APO's and FPO's and whose addresses are unknown.

Physicians 35 to 44 Years Old in 1999

National Total = 210,133 Physicians*

RANK	STATE	PHYSICIANS	% of USA
25	Alabama	2,899	1.4%
49	Alaska	418	0.2%
24	Arizona	3,086	1.5%
31	Arkansas	1,604	0.8%
1	California	21,650	10.3%
23	Colorado	3,143	1.5%
21	Connecticut	3,524	1.7%
45	Delaware	550	0.3%
4	Florida	11,400	5.4%
13	Georgia	5,549	2.6%
40	Hawaii	993	0.5%
43	Idaho	635	0.3%
6	Illinois	9,357	4.5%
20	Indiana	3,741	1.8%
32	Iowa	1,594	0.8%
29	Kansas	1,713	0.8%
26	Kentucky	2,766	1.3%
22	Louisiana	3,222	1.5%
41	Maine	868	0.4%
11	Maryland	6,267	3.0%
8	Massachusetts	8,050	3.8%
10	Michigan	6,546	3.1%
18	Minnesota	3,969	1.9%
33	Mississippi	1,477	0.7%
18	Missouri	3,969	1.9%
46	Montana	542	0.3%
35	Nebraska	1,188	0.6%
37	Nevada	1,118	0.5%
42	New Hampshire	857	0.4%
9	New Jersey	7,324	3.5%
36	New Mexico	1,165	0.6%
2	New York	20,509	9.8%
12	North Carolina	6,121	2.9%
48	North Dakota	481	0.2%
7	Ohio	8,091	3.9%
30	Oklahoma	1,672	0.8%
28	Oregon	2,205	1.0%
5	Pennsylvania	10,420	5.0%
39	Rhode Island	998	0.5%
27	South Carolina	2,726	1.3%
47	South Dakota	494	0.2%
15	Tennessee	4,436	2.1%
3	Texas	13,070	6.2%
34	Utah	1,435	0.7%
44	Vermont	565	0.3%
14	Virginia	5,200	2.5%
16	Washington	4,155	2.0%
37	West Virginia	1,118	0.5%
17	Wisconsin	4,058	1.9%
50	Wyoming	228	0.1%

RANK	STATE	PHYSICIANS	% of USA
1	California	21,650	10.3%
2	New York	20,509	9.8%
3	Texas	13,070	6.2%
4	Florida	11,400	5.4%
5	Pennsylvania	10,420	5.0%
6	Illinois	9,357	4.5%
7	Ohio	8,091	3.9%
8	Massachusetts	8,050	3.8%
9	New Jersey	7,324	3.5%
10	Michigan	6,546	3.1%
11	Maryland	6,267	3.0%
12	North Carolina	6,121	2.9%
13	Georgia	5,549	2.6%
14	Virginia	5,200	2.5%
15	Tennessee	4,436	2.1%
16	Washington	4,155	2.0%
17	Wisconsin	4,058	1.9%
18	Minnesota	3,969	1.9%
18	Missouri	3,969	1.9%
20	Indiana	3,741	1.8%
21	Connecticut	3,524	1.7%
22	Louisiana	3,222	1.5%
23	Colorado	3,143	1.5%
24	Arizona	3,086	1.5%
25	Alabama	2,899	1.4%
26	Kentucky	2,766	1.3%
27	South Carolina	2,726	1.3%
28	Oregon	2,205	1.0%
29	Kansas	1,713	0.8%
30	Oklahoma	1,672	0.8%
31	Arkansas	1,604	0.8%
32	Iowa	1,594	0.8%
33	Mississippi	1,477	0.7%
34	Utah	1,435	0.7%
35	Nebraska	1,188	0.6%
36	New Mexico	1,165	0.6%
37	Nevada	1,118	0.5%
37	West Virginia	1,118	0.5%
39	Rhode Island	998	0.5%
40	Hawaii	993	0.5%
41	Maine	868	0.4%
42	New Hampshire	857	0.4%
43	Idaho	635	0.3%
44	Vermont	565	0.3%
45	Delaware	550	0.3%
46	Montana	542	0.3%
47	South Dakota	494	0.2%
48	North Dakota	481	0.2%
49	Alaska	418	0.2%
50	Wyoming	228	0.1%
	District of Columbia	967	0.5%

Source: American Medical Association (Chicago, Illinois)
"Physician Characteristics and Distribution in the U.S." (2001-2002 Edition)
*As of December 31, 1999. Comprised of federal and nonfederal physicians. Total does not include 3,275 physicians in the U.S. territories and possessions, at APO's and FPO's and whose addresses are unknown.

Physicians 45 to 54 Years Old in 1999

National Total = 190,661 Physicians*

<u>ALPHA ORDER</u>

RANK	STATE	PHYSICIANS	% of USA
26	Alabama	2,405	1.3%
49	Alaska	382	0.2%
24	Arizona	2,798	1.5%
32	Arkansas	1,410	0.7%
1	California	24,251	12.7%
22	Colorado	3,000	1.6%
21	Connecticut	3,219	1.7%
47	Delaware	452	0.2%
4	Florida	10,543	5.5%
14	Georgia	4,645	2.4%
38	Hawaii	1,003	0.5%
43	Idaho	620	0.3%
6	Illinois	8,065	4.2%
18	Indiana	3,373	1.8%
31	Iowa	1,430	0.8%
30	Kansas	1,532	0.8%
27	Kentucky	2,355	1.2%
23	Louisiana	2,870	1.5%
39	Maine	952	0.5%
11	Maryland	5,664	3.0%
9	Massachusetts	6,610	3.5%
10	Michigan	5,708	3.0%
17	Minnesota	3,444	1.8%
35	Mississippi	1,238	0.6%
20	Missouri	3,317	1.7%
44	Montana	588	0.3%
37	Nebraska	1,021	0.5%
40	Nevada	928	0.5%
41	New Hampshire	902	0.5%
7	New Jersey	6,807	3.6%
33	New Mexico	1,273	0.7%
2	New York	17,256	9.1%
13	North Carolina	4,747	2.5%
48	North Dakota	438	0.2%
8	Ohio	6,748	3.5%
29	Oklahoma	1,702	0.9%
25	Oregon	2,512	1.3%
5	Pennsylvania	9,311	4.9%
42	Rhode Island	779	0.4%
28	South Carolina	2,209	1.2%
46	South Dakota	480	0.3%
16	Tennessee	3,867	2.0%
3	Texas	10,999	5.8%
34	Utah	1,263	0.7%
45	Vermont	542	0.3%
12	Virginia	4,814	2.5%
15	Washington	4,557	2.4%
36	West Virginia	1,100	0.6%
19	Wisconsin	3,323	1.7%
50	Wyoming	286	0.2%

<u>RANK ORDER</u>

RANK	STATE	PHYSICIANS	% of USA
1	California	24,251	12.7%
2	New York	17,256	9.1%
3	Texas	10,999	5.8%
4	Florida	10,543	5.5%
5	Pennsylvania	9,311	4.9%
6	Illinois	8,065	4.2%
7	New Jersey	6,807	3.6%
8	Ohio	6,748	3.5%
9	Massachusetts	6,610	3.5%
10	Michigan	5,708	3.0%
11	Maryland	5,664	3.0%
12	Virginia	4,814	2.5%
13	North Carolina	4,747	2.5%
14	Georgia	4,645	2.4%
15	Washington	4,557	2.4%
16	Tennessee	3,867	2.0%
17	Minnesota	3,444	1.8%
18	Indiana	3,373	1.8%
19	Wisconsin	3,323	1.7%
20	Missouri	3,317	1.7%
21	Connecticut	3,219	1.7%
22	Colorado	3,000	1.6%
23	Louisiana	2,870	1.5%
24	Arizona	2,798	1.5%
25	Oregon	2,512	1.3%
26	Alabama	2,405	1.3%
27	Kentucky	2,355	1.2%
28	South Carolina	2,209	1.2%
29	Oklahoma	1,702	0.9%
30	Kansas	1,532	0.8%
31	Iowa	1,430	0.8%
32	Arkansas	1,410	0.7%
33	New Mexico	1,273	0.7%
34	Utah	1,263	0.7%
35	Mississippi	1,238	0.6%
36	West Virginia	1,100	0.6%
37	Nebraska	1,021	0.5%
38	Hawaii	1,003	0.5%
39	Maine	952	0.5%
40	Nevada	928	0.5%
41	New Hampshire	902	0.5%
42	Rhode Island	779	0.4%
43	Idaho	620	0.3%
44	Montana	588	0.3%
45	Vermont	542	0.3%
46	South Dakota	480	0.3%
47	Delaware	452	0.2%
48	North Dakota	438	0.2%
49	Alaska	382	0.2%
50	Wyoming	286	0.2%
	District of Columbia	923	0.5%

Source: American Medical Association (Chicago, Illinois)
   "Physician Characteristics and Distribution in the U.S." (2001-2002 Edition)
As of December 31, 1999. Comprised of federal and nonfederal physicians. Total does not include 2,663 physicians in the U.S. territories and possessions, at APO's and FPO's and whose addresses are unknown.

Physicians 55 to 64 Years Old in 1999

National Total = 112,242 Physicians*

ALPHA ORDER

RANK	STATE	PHYSICIANS	% of USA
26	Alabama	1,339	1.2%
49	Alaska	224	0.2%
20	Arizona	1,747	1.6%
31	Arkansas	796	0.7%
1	California	15,647	13.9%
23	Colorado	1,685	1.5%
19	Connecticut	1,816	1.6%
45	Delaware	311	0.3%
3	Florida	6,639	5.9%
13	Georgia	2,617	2.3%
37	Hawaii	575	0.5%
44	Idaho	364	0.3%
6	Illinois	5,094	4.5%
21	Indiana	1,741	1.6%
33	Iowa	783	0.7%
30	Kansas	904	0.8%
27	Kentucky	1,316	1.2%
24	Louisiana	1,600	1.4%
40	Maine	506	0.5%
11	Maryland	3,392	3.0%
9	Massachusetts	3,636	3.2%
10	Michigan	3,412	3.0%
22	Minnesota	1,712	1.5%
34	Mississippi	758	0.7%
17	Missouri	1,885	1.7%
43	Montana	384	0.3%
39	Nebraska	508	0.5%
38	Nevada	538	0.5%
42	New Hampshire	438	0.4%
7	New Jersey	4,211	3.8%
35	New Mexico	705	0.6%
2	New York	10,718	9.5%
14	North Carolina	2,482	2.2%
47	North Dakota	232	0.2%
8	Ohio	3,997	3.6%
29	Oklahoma	1,004	0.9%
25	Oregon	1,457	1.3%
5	Pennsylvania	5,123	4.6%
41	Rhode Island	495	0.4%
28	South Carolina	1,200	1.1%
48	South Dakota	229	0.2%
16	Tennessee	1,934	1.7%
4	Texas	6,316	5.6%
36	Utah	676	0.6%
46	Vermont	303	0.3%
12	Virginia	2,772	2.5%
15	Washington	2,414	2.2%
32	West Virginia	793	0.7%
18	Wisconsin	1,833	1.6%
50	Wyoming	159	0.1%

RANK ORDER

RANK	STATE	PHYSICIANS	% of USA
1	California	15,647	13.9%
2	New York	10,718	9.5%
3	Florida	6,639	5.9%
4	Texas	6,316	5.6%
5	Pennsylvania	5,123	4.6%
6	Illinois	5,094	4.5%
7	New Jersey	4,211	3.8%
8	Ohio	3,997	3.6%
9	Massachusetts	3,636	3.2%
10	Michigan	3,412	3.0%
11	Maryland	3,392	3.0%
12	Virginia	2,772	2.5%
13	Georgia	2,617	2.3%
14	North Carolina	2,482	2.2%
15	Washington	2,414	2.2%
16	Tennessee	1,934	1.7%
17	Missouri	1,885	1.7%
18	Wisconsin	1,833	1.6%
19	Connecticut	1,816	1.6%
20	Arizona	1,747	1.6%
21	Indiana	1,741	1.6%
22	Minnesota	1,712	1.5%
23	Colorado	1,685	1.5%
24	Louisiana	1,600	1.4%
25	Oregon	1,457	1.3%
26	Alabama	1,339	1.2%
27	Kentucky	1,316	1.2%
28	South Carolina	1,200	1.1%
29	Oklahoma	1,004	0.9%
30	Kansas	904	0.8%
31	Arkansas	796	0.7%
32	West Virginia	793	0.7%
33	Iowa	783	0.7%
34	Mississippi	758	0.7%
35	New Mexico	705	0.6%
36	Utah	676	0.6%
37	Hawaii	575	0.5%
38	Nevada	538	0.5%
39	Nebraska	508	0.5%
40	Maine	506	0.5%
41	Rhode Island	495	0.4%
42	New Hampshire	438	0.4%
43	Montana	384	0.3%
44	Idaho	364	0.3%
45	Delaware	311	0.3%
46	Vermont	303	0.3%
47	North Dakota	232	0.2%
48	South Dakota	229	0.2%
49	Alaska	224	0.2%
50	Wyoming	159	0.1%
	District of Columbia	822	0.7%

Source: American Medical Association (Chicago, Illinois)
   "Physician Characteristics and Distribution in the U.S." (2001-2002 Edition)
*As of December 31, 1999. Comprised of federal and nonfederal physicians. Total does not include 1,586 physicians in the U.S. territories and possessions, at APO's and FPO's and whose addresses are unknown.

Physicians 65 Years Old and Older in 1999

National Total = 138,384 Physicians*

ALPHA ORDER

RANK	STATE	PHYSICIANS	% of USA
27	Alabama	1,438	1.0%
50	Alaska	137	0.1%
16	Arizona	2,679	1.9%
33	Arkansas	913	0.7%
1	California	20,219	14.6%
23	Colorado	1,965	1.4%
17	Connecticut	2,368	1.7%
46	Delaware	383	0.3%
3	Florida	11,655	8.4%
15	Georgia	2,720	2.0%
36	Hawaii	758	0.5%
43	Idaho	470	0.3%
6	Illinois	5,017	3.6%
19	Indiana	2,213	1.6%
31	Iowa	1,022	0.7%
29	Kansas	1,177	0.9%
28	Kentucky	1,381	1.0%
25	Louisiana	1,805	1.3%
37	Maine	732	0.5%
11	Maryland	3,652	2.6%
9	Massachusetts	4,324	3.1%
10	Michigan	3,907	2.8%
21	Minnesota	2,131	1.5%
32	Mississippi	935	0.7%
22	Missouri	1,993	1.4%
45	Montana	428	0.3%
41	Nebraska	667	0.5%
38	Nevada	724	0.5%
40	New Hampshire	706	0.5%
8	New Jersey	4,500	3.3%
35	New Mexico	761	0.5%
2	New York	13,292	9.6%
13	North Carolina	3,231	2.3%
48	North Dakota	238	0.2%
7	Ohio	4,946	3.6%
30	Oklahoma	1,157	0.8%
24	Oregon	1,807	1.3%
5	Pennsylvania	6,831	4.9%
42	Rhode Island	666	0.5%
26	South Carolina	1,546	1.1%
47	South Dakota	265	0.2%
18	Tennessee	2,227	1.6%
4	Texas	6,961	5.0%
34	Utah	762	0.6%
44	Vermont	450	0.3%
12	Virginia	3,314	2.4%
14	Washington	3,012	2.2%
39	West Virginia	715	0.5%
20	Wisconsin	2,204	1.6%
49	Wyoming	208	0.2%

RANK ORDER

RANK	STATE	PHYSICIANS	% of USA
1	California	20,219	14.6%
2	New York	13,292	9.6%
3	Florida	11,655	8.4%
4	Texas	6,961	5.0%
5	Pennsylvania	6,831	4.9%
6	Illinois	5,017	3.6%
7	Ohio	4,946	3.6%
8	New Jersey	4,500	3.3%
9	Massachusetts	4,324	3.1%
10	Michigan	3,907	2.8%
11	Maryland	3,652	2.6%
12	Virginia	3,314	2.4%
13	North Carolina	3,231	2.3%
14	Washington	3,012	2.2%
15	Georgia	2,720	2.0%
16	Arizona	2,679	1.9%
17	Connecticut	2,368	1.7%
18	Tennessee	2,227	1.6%
19	Indiana	2,213	1.6%
20	Wisconsin	2,204	1.6%
21	Minnesota	2,131	1.5%
22	Missouri	1,993	1.4%
23	Colorado	1,965	1.4%
24	Oregon	1,807	1.3%
25	Louisiana	1,805	1.3%
26	South Carolina	1,546	1.1%
27	Alabama	1,438	1.0%
28	Kentucky	1,381	1.0%
29	Kansas	1,177	0.9%
30	Oklahoma	1,157	0.8%
31	Iowa	1,022	0.7%
32	Mississippi	935	0.7%
33	Arkansas	913	0.7%
34	Utah	762	0.6%
35	New Mexico	761	0.5%
36	Hawaii	758	0.5%
37	Maine	732	0.5%
38	Nevada	724	0.5%
39	West Virginia	715	0.5%
40	New Hampshire	706	0.5%
41	Nebraska	667	0.5%
42	Rhode Island	666	0.5%
43	Idaho	470	0.3%
44	Vermont	450	0.3%
45	Montana	428	0.3%
46	Delaware	383	0.3%
47	South Dakota	265	0.2%
48	North Dakota	238	0.2%
49	Wyoming	208	0.2%
50	Alaska	137	0.1%
	District of Columbia	772	0.6%

Source: American Medical Association (Chicago, Illinois)
"Physician Characteristics and Distribution in the U.S." (2001-2002 Edition)
*As of December 31, 1999. Comprised of federal and nonfederal physicians. Total does not include 2,674
physicians in the U.S. territories and possessions, at APO's and FPO's and whose addresses are unknown.

Percent of Physicians 65 Years Old and Older in 1999

National Percent = 17.7% of Physicians*

ALPHA ORDER

RANK	STATE	PERCENT
43	Alabama	14.8
50	Alaska	10.6
2	Arizona	22.5
30	Arkansas	16.3
4	California	21.3
22	Colorado	17.2
16	Connecticut	18.0
13	Delaware	18.8
1	Florida	25.9
47	Georgia	14.5
11	Hawaii	19.7
9	Idaho	20.3
49	Illinois	14.2
26	Indiana	16.8
20	Iowa	17.5
15	Kansas	18.5
45	Kentucky	14.7
42	Louisiana	15.0
3	Maine	21.4
35	Maryland	15.8
40	Massachusetts	15.2
37	Michigan	15.7
39	Minnesota	15.5
17	Mississippi	17.9
48	Missouri	14.3
7	Montana	20.7
33	Nebraska	16.0
12	Nevada	19.4
5	New Hampshire	21.2
27	New Jersey	16.7
24	New Mexico	17.0
23	New York	17.1
35	North Carolina	15.8
43	North Dakota	14.8
28	Ohio	16.6
17	Oklahoma	17.9
10	Oregon	20.0
20	Pennsylvania	17.5
19	Rhode Island	17.8
29	South Carolina	16.5
32	South Dakota	16.1
45	Tennessee	14.7
40	Texas	15.2
38	Utah	15.6
8	Vermont	20.6
24	Virginia	17.0
14	Washington	18.6
33	West Virginia	16.0
31	Wisconsin	16.2
6	Wyoming	21.1

RANK ORDER

RANK	STATE	PERCENT
1	Florida	25.9
2	Arizona	22.5
3	Maine	21.4
4	California	21.3
5	New Hampshire	21.2
6	Wyoming	21.1
7	Montana	20.7
8	Vermont	20.6
9	Idaho	20.3
10	Oregon	20.0
11	Hawaii	19.7
12	Nevada	19.4
13	Delaware	18.8
14	Washington	18.6
15	Kansas	18.5
16	Connecticut	18.0
17	Mississippi	17.9
17	Oklahoma	17.9
19	Rhode Island	17.8
20	Iowa	17.5
20	Pennsylvania	17.5
22	Colorado	17.2
23	New York	17.1
24	New Mexico	17.0
24	Virginia	17.0
26	Indiana	16.8
27	New Jersey	16.7
28	Ohio	16.6
29	South Carolina	16.5
30	Arkansas	16.3
31	Wisconsin	16.2
32	South Dakota	16.1
33	Nebraska	16.0
33	West Virginia	16.0
35	Maryland	15.8
35	North Carolina	15.8
37	Michigan	15.7
38	Utah	15.6
39	Minnesota	15.5
40	Massachusetts	15.2
40	Texas	15.2
42	Louisiana	15.0
43	Alabama	14.8
43	North Dakota	14.8
45	Kentucky	14.7
45	Tennessee	14.7
47	Georgia	14.5
48	Missouri	14.3
49	Illinois	14.2
50	Alaska	10.6

District of Columbia 17.0

Source: Morgan Quitno Press using data from American Medical Association (Chicago, Illinois)
"Physician Characteristics and Distribution in the U.S." (2001-2002 Edition)
*As of December 31, 1999. Comprised of federal and nonfederal physicians. National percent does not include physicians in the U.S. territories and possessions, at APO's and FPO's and whose addresses are unknown.

Federal Physicians in 1999

National Total = 18,307 Physicians*

ALPHA ORDER

RANK	STATE	PHYSICIANS	% of USA
26	Alabama	208	1.1%
35	Alaska	143	0.8%
13	Arizona	429	2.3%
33	Arkansas	149	0.8%
1	California	1,882	10.3%
16	Colorado	305	1.7%
31	Connecticut	165	0.9%
48	Delaware	49	0.3%
4	Florida	1,082	5.9%
7	Georgia	801	4.4%
26	Hawaii	208	1.1%
41	Idaho	73	0.4%
8	Illinois	555	3.0%
34	Indiana	148	0.8%
40	Iowa	92	0.5%
29	Kansas	185	1.0%
30	Kentucky	180	1.0%
25	Louisiana	221	1.2%
44	Maine	61	0.3%
2	Maryland	1,773	9.7%
14	Massachusetts	395	2.2%
18	Michigan	281	1.5%
23	Minnesota	233	1.3%
20	Mississippi	250	1.4%
19	Missouri	278	1.5%
46	Montana	55	0.3%
43	Nebraska	70	0.4%
37	Nevada	120	0.7%
45	New Hampshire	59	0.3%
17	New Jersey	285	1.6%
21	New Mexico	237	1.3%
6	New York	928	5.1%
11	North Carolina	473	2.6%
47	North Dakota	52	0.3%
11	Ohio	473	2.6%
28	Oklahoma	193	1.1%
24	Oregon	222	1.2%
10	Pennsylvania	500	2.7%
42	Rhode Island	71	0.4%
22	South Carolina	235	1.3%
39	South Dakota	96	0.5%
15	Tennessee	358	2.0%
3	Texas	1,443	7.9%
38	Utah	102	0.6%
50	Vermont	33	0.2%
5	Virginia	957	5.2%
9	Washington	541	3.0%
36	West Virginia	135	0.7%
31	Wisconsin	165	0.9%
49	Wyoming	38	0.2%

RANK ORDER

RANK	STATE	PHYSICIANS	% of USA
1	California	1,882	10.3%
2	Maryland	1,773	9.7%
3	Texas	1,443	7.9%
4	Florida	1,082	5.9%
5	Virginia	957	5.2%
6	New York	928	5.1%
7	Georgia	801	4.4%
8	Illinois	555	3.0%
9	Washington	541	3.0%
10	Pennsylvania	500	2.7%
11	North Carolina	473	2.6%
11	Ohio	473	2.6%
13	Arizona	429	2.3%
14	Massachusetts	395	2.2%
15	Tennessee	358	2.0%
16	Colorado	305	1.7%
17	New Jersey	285	1.6%
18	Michigan	281	1.5%
19	Missouri	278	1.5%
20	Mississippi	250	1.4%
21	New Mexico	237	1.3%
22	South Carolina	235	1.3%
23	Minnesota	233	1.3%
24	Oregon	222	1.2%
25	Louisiana	221	1.2%
26	Alabama	208	1.1%
26	Hawaii	208	1.1%
28	Oklahoma	193	1.1%
29	Kansas	185	1.0%
30	Kentucky	180	1.0%
31	Connecticut	165	0.9%
31	Wisconsin	165	0.9%
33	Arkansas	149	0.8%
34	Indiana	148	0.8%
35	Alaska	143	0.8%
36	West Virginia	135	0.7%
37	Nevada	120	0.7%
38	Utah	102	0.6%
39	South Dakota	96	0.5%
40	Iowa	92	0.5%
41	Idaho	73	0.4%
42	Rhode Island	71	0.4%
43	Nebraska	70	0.4%
44	Maine	61	0.3%
45	New Hampshire	59	0.3%
46	Montana	55	0.3%
47	North Dakota	52	0.3%
48	Delaware	49	0.3%
49	Wyoming	38	0.2%
50	Vermont	33	0.2%
	District of Columbia	320	1.7%

Source: American Medical Association (Chicago, Illinois)
"Physician Characteristics and Distribution in the U.S." (2001-2002 Edition)
*As of December 31, 1999. Total does not include 836 physicians in U.S. territories and possessions.

Rate of Federal Physicians in 1999

National Rate = 6.7 Physicians per 100,000 Population*

ALPHA ORDER

RANK	STATE	RATE
39	Alabama	4.8
2	Alaska	23.1
9	Arizona	9.0
27	Arkansas	5.8
29	California	5.7
13	Colorado	7.5
35	Connecticut	5.0
21	Delaware	6.5
15	Florida	7.2
7	Georgia	10.3
3	Hawaii	17.5
27	Idaho	5.8
41	Illinois	4.6
50	Indiana	2.5
47	Iowa	3.2
18	Kansas	7.0
42	Kentucky	4.5
32	Louisiana	5.1
36	Maine	4.9
1	Maryland	34.3
23	Massachusetts	6.4
49	Michigan	2.8
36	Minnesota	4.9
9	Mississippi	9.0
32	Missouri	5.1
24	Montana	6.2
43	Nebraska	4.2
20	Nevada	6.6
36	New Hampshire	4.9
46	New Jersey	3.5
5	New Mexico	13.6
32	New York	5.1
24	North Carolina	6.2
11	North Dakota	8.2
43	Ohio	4.2
29	Oklahoma	5.7
19	Oregon	6.7
43	Pennsylvania	4.2
15	Rhode Island	7.2
26	South Carolina	6.0
6	South Dakota	13.1
21	Tennessee	6.5
15	Texas	7.2
39	Utah	4.8
31	Vermont	5.6
4	Virginia	13.9
8	Washington	9.4
13	West Virginia	7.5
48	Wisconsin	3.1
12	Wyoming	7.9

RANK ORDER

RANK	STATE	RATE
1	Maryland	34.3
2	Alaska	23.1
3	Hawaii	17.5
4	Virginia	13.9
5	New Mexico	13.6
6	South Dakota	13.1
7	Georgia	10.3
8	Washington	9.4
9	Arizona	9.0
9	Mississippi	9.0
11	North Dakota	8.2
12	Wyoming	7.9
13	Colorado	7.5
13	West Virginia	7.5
15	Florida	7.2
15	Rhode Island	7.2
15	Texas	7.2
18	Kansas	7.0
19	Oregon	6.7
20	Nevada	6.6
21	Delaware	6.5
21	Tennessee	6.5
23	Massachusetts	6.4
24	Montana	6.2
24	North Carolina	6.2
26	South Carolina	6.0
27	Arkansas	5.8
27	Idaho	5.8
29	California	5.7
29	Oklahoma	5.7
31	Vermont	5.6
32	Louisiana	5.1
32	Missouri	5.1
32	New York	5.1
35	Connecticut	5.0
36	Maine	4.9
36	Minnesota	4.9
36	New Hampshire	4.9
39	Alabama	4.8
39	Utah	4.8
41	Illinois	4.6
42	Kentucky	4.5
43	Nebraska	4.2
43	Ohio	4.2
43	Pennsylvania	4.2
46	New Jersey	3.5
47	Iowa	3.2
48	Wisconsin	3.1
49	Michigan	2.8
50	Indiana	2.5

| | District of Columbia | 61.7 |

Source: Morgan Quitno Press using data from American Medical Association (Chicago, Illinois)
"Physician Characteristics and Distribution in the U.S." (2001-2002 Edition)
*As of December 31, 1999. National rate does not include physicians in U.S. territories and possessions.

Nonfederal Physicians in 1999

National Total = 767,592 Physicians*

ALPHA ORDER

RANK	STATE	PHYSICIANS	% of USA
25	Alabama	9,487	1.2%
49	Alaska	1,150	0.1%
23	Arizona	11,487	1.5%
32	Arkansas	5,458	0.7%
1	California	92,985	12.1%
24	Colorado	11,115	1.4%
20	Connecticut	13,020	1.7%
46	Delaware	1,985	0.3%
4	Florida	43,835	5.7%
14	Georgia	17,945	2.3%
39	Hawaii	3,632	0.5%
43	Idaho	2,240	0.3%
6	Illinois	34,840	4.5%
21	Indiana	13,000	1.7%
31	Iowa	5,734	0.7%
30	Kansas	6,171	0.8%
26	Kentucky	9,187	1.2%
22	Louisiana	11,806	1.5%
41	Maine	3,356	0.4%
11	Maryland	21,360	2.8%
8	Massachusetts	28,062	3.7%
10	Michigan	24,551	3.2%
18	Minnesota	13,485	1.8%
33	Mississippi	4,982	0.6%
17	Missouri	13,674	1.8%
45	Montana	2,010	0.3%
37	Nebraska	4,111	0.5%
40	Nevada	3,611	0.5%
42	New Hampshire	3,274	0.4%
9	New Jersey	26,606	3.5%
36	New Mexico	4,231	0.6%
2	New York	77,003	10.0%
12	North Carolina	20,036	2.6%
47	North Dakota	1,560	0.2%
7	Ohio	29,358	3.8%
29	Oklahoma	6,285	0.8%
28	Oregon	8,825	1.1%
5	Pennsylvania	38,524	5.0%
38	Rhode Island	3,676	0.5%
27	South Carolina	9,114	1.2%
48	South Dakota	1,551	0.2%
16	Tennessee	14,774	1.9%
3	Texas	44,433	5.8%
34	Utah	4,787	0.6%
44	Vermont	2,148	0.3%
13	Virginia	18,504	2.4%
15	Washington	15,688	2.0%
35	West Virginia	4,323	0.6%
19	Wisconsin	13,452	1.8%
50	Wyoming	950	0.1%

RANK ORDER

RANK	STATE	PHYSICIANS	% of USA
1	California	92,985	12.1%
2	New York	77,003	10.0%
3	Texas	44,433	5.8%
4	Florida	43,835	5.7%
5	Pennsylvania	38,524	5.0%
6	Illinois	34,840	4.5%
7	Ohio	29,358	3.8%
8	Massachusetts	28,062	3.7%
9	New Jersey	26,606	3.5%
10	Michigan	24,551	3.2%
11	Maryland	21,360	2.8%
12	North Carolina	20,036	2.6%
13	Virginia	18,504	2.4%
14	Georgia	17,945	2.3%
15	Washington	15,688	2.0%
16	Tennessee	14,774	1.9%
17	Missouri	13,674	1.8%
18	Minnesota	13,485	1.8%
19	Wisconsin	13,452	1.8%
20	Connecticut	13,020	1.7%
21	Indiana	13,000	1.7%
22	Louisiana	11,806	1.5%
23	Arizona	11,487	1.5%
24	Colorado	11,115	1.4%
25	Alabama	9,487	1.2%
26	Kentucky	9,187	1.2%
27	South Carolina	9,114	1.2%
28	Oregon	8,825	1.1%
29	Oklahoma	6,285	0.8%
30	Kansas	6,171	0.8%
31	Iowa	5,734	0.7%
32	Arkansas	5,458	0.7%
33	Mississippi	4,982	0.6%
34	Utah	4,787	0.6%
35	West Virginia	4,323	0.6%
36	New Mexico	4,231	0.6%
37	Nebraska	4,111	0.5%
38	Rhode Island	3,676	0.5%
39	Hawaii	3,632	0.5%
40	Nevada	3,611	0.5%
41	Maine	3,356	0.4%
42	New Hampshire	3,274	0.4%
43	Idaho	2,240	0.3%
44	Vermont	2,148	0.3%
45	Montana	2,010	0.3%
46	Delaware	1,985	0.3%
47	North Dakota	1,560	0.2%
48	South Dakota	1,551	0.2%
49	Alaska	1,150	0.1%
50	Wyoming	950	0.1%
	District of Columbia	4,211	0.5%

Source: American Medical Association (Chicago, Illinois)
    "Physician Characteristics and Distribution in the U.S." (2001-2002 Edition)
*As of December 31, 1999. Total does not include 10,899 nonfederal physicians in U.S. territories and possessions.

Rate of Nonfederal Physicians in 1999

National Rate = 281 Physicians per 100,000 Population*

ALPHA ORDER

RANK	STATE	RATE
41	Alabama	217
48	Alaska	186
31	Arizona	240
42	Arkansas	214
13	California	281
14	Colorado	274
4	Connecticut	397
22	Delaware	263
10	Florida	290
36	Georgia	230
9	Hawaii	306
50	Idaho	179
11	Illinois	287
40	Indiana	219
44	Iowa	200
34	Kansas	233
35	Kentucky	232
17	Louisiana	270
20	Maine	268
3	Maryland	413
1	Massachusetts	454
27	Michigan	249
12	Minnesota	282
49	Mississippi	180
26	Missouri	250
37	Montana	228
28	Nebraska	247
44	Nevada	200
15	New Hampshire	273
7	New Jersey	327
30	New Mexico	243
2	New York	423
23	North Carolina	262
29	North Dakota	246
24	Ohio	261
47	Oklahoma	187
21	Oregon	266
8	Pennsylvania	321
5	Rhode Island	371
33	South Carolina	235
43	South Dakota	212
18	Tennessee	269
39	Texas	222
38	Utah	225
6	Vermont	362
18	Virginia	269
15	Washington	273
32	West Virginia	239
25	Wisconsin	256
46	Wyoming	198

RANK ORDER

RANK	STATE	RATE
1	Massachusetts	454
2	New York	423
3	Maryland	413
4	Connecticut	397
5	Rhode Island	371
6	Vermont	362
7	New Jersey	327
8	Pennsylvania	321
9	Hawaii	306
10	Florida	290
11	Illinois	287
12	Minnesota	282
13	California	281
14	Colorado	274
15	New Hampshire	273
15	Washington	273
17	Louisiana	270
18	Tennessee	269
18	Virginia	269
20	Maine	268
21	Oregon	266
22	Delaware	263
23	North Carolina	262
24	Ohio	261
25	Wisconsin	256
26	Missouri	250
27	Michigan	249
28	Nebraska	247
29	North Dakota	246
30	New Mexico	243
31	Arizona	240
32	West Virginia	239
33	South Carolina	235
34	Kansas	233
35	Kentucky	232
36	Georgia	230
37	Montana	228
38	Utah	225
39	Texas	222
40	Indiana	219
41	Alabama	217
42	Arkansas	214
43	South Dakota	212
44	Iowa	200
44	Nevada	200
46	Wyoming	198
47	Oklahoma	187
48	Alaska	186
49	Mississippi	180
50	Idaho	179

| | District of Columbia | 811 |

Source: Morgan Quitno Press using data from American Medical Association (Chicago, Illinois)
"Physician Characteristics and Distribution in the U.S." (2001-2002 Edition)
*As of December 31, 1999.

Nonfederal Physicians in Patient Care in 1999

National Total = 602,639 Physicians*

ALPHA ORDER

RANK	STATE	PHYSICIANS	% of USA
25	Alabama	7,825	1.3%
49	Alaska	949	0.2%
24	Arizona	8,630	1.4%
31	Arkansas	4,468	0.7%
1	California	70,731	11.7%
23	Colorado	8,770	1.5%
21	Connecticut	10,087	1.7%
46	Delaware	1,565	0.3%
4	Florida	32,846	5.5%
14	Georgia	14,657	2.4%
40	Hawaii	2,842	0.5%
43	Idaho	1,802	0.3%
6	Illinois	27,779	4.6%
20	Indiana	10,523	1.7%
32	Iowa	4,411	0.7%
30	Kansas	4,877	0.8%
26	Kentucky	7,562	1.3%
22	Louisiana	9,690	1.6%
41	Maine	2,589	0.4%
11	Maryland	16,011	2.7%
9	Massachusetts	21,115	3.5%
10	Michigan	19,365	3.2%
19	Minnesota	10,701	1.8%
33	Mississippi	4,132	0.7%
17	Missouri	11,055	1.8%
45	Montana	1,568	0.3%
36	Nebraska	3,297	0.5%
38	Nevada	2,927	0.5%
42	New Hampshire	2,557	0.4%
8	New Jersey	21,262	3.5%
37	New Mexico	3,235	0.5%
2	New York	59,826	9.9%
12	North Carolina	15,849	2.6%
47	North Dakota	1,283	0.2%
7	Ohio	23,660	3.9%
29	Oklahoma	5,044	0.8%
28	Oregon	6,721	1.1%
5	Pennsylvania	30,371	5.0%
39	Rhode Island	2,905	0.5%
27	South Carolina	7,440	1.2%
48	South Dakota	1,272	0.2%
15	Tennessee	12,112	2.0%
3	Texas	36,061	6.0%
34	Utah	3,778	0.6%
44	Vermont	1,599	0.3%
13	Virginia	14,772	2.5%
16	Washington	11,888	2.0%
35	West Virginia	3,528	0.6%
18	Wisconsin	10,836	1.8%
50	Wyoming	745	0.1%

RANK ORDER

RANK	STATE	PHYSICIANS	% of USA
1	California	70,731	11.7%
2	New York	59,826	9.9%
3	Texas	36,061	6.0%
4	Florida	32,846	5.5%
5	Pennsylvania	30,371	5.0%
6	Illinois	27,779	4.6%
7	Ohio	23,660	3.9%
8	New Jersey	21,262	3.5%
9	Massachusetts	21,115	3.5%
10	Michigan	19,365	3.2%
11	Maryland	16,011	2.7%
12	North Carolina	15,849	2.6%
13	Virginia	14,772	2.5%
14	Georgia	14,657	2.4%
15	Tennessee	12,112	2.0%
16	Washington	11,888	2.0%
17	Missouri	11,055	1.8%
18	Wisconsin	10,836	1.8%
19	Minnesota	10,701	1.8%
20	Indiana	10,523	1.7%
21	Connecticut	10,087	1.7%
22	Louisiana	9,690	1.6%
23	Colorado	8,770	1.5%
24	Arizona	8,630	1.4%
25	Alabama	7,825	1.3%
26	Kentucky	7,562	1.3%
27	South Carolina	7,440	1.2%
28	Oregon	6,721	1.1%
29	Oklahoma	5,044	0.8%
30	Kansas	4,877	0.8%
31	Arkansas	4,468	0.7%
32	Iowa	4,411	0.7%
33	Mississippi	4,132	0.7%
34	Utah	3,778	0.6%
35	West Virginia	3,528	0.6%
36	Nebraska	3,297	0.5%
37	New Mexico	3,235	0.5%
38	Nevada	2,927	0.5%
39	Rhode Island	2,905	0.5%
40	Hawaii	2,842	0.5%
41	Maine	2,589	0.4%
42	New Hampshire	2,557	0.4%
43	Idaho	1,802	0.3%
44	Vermont	1,599	0.3%
45	Montana	1,568	0.3%
46	Delaware	1,565	0.3%
47	North Dakota	1,283	0.2%
48	South Dakota	1,272	0.2%
49	Alaska	949	0.2%
50	Wyoming	745	0.1%
	District of Columbia	3,121	0.5%

Source: American Medical Association (Chicago, Illinois)
"Physician Characteristics and Distribution in the U.S." (2001-2002 Edition)
*As of December 31, 1999. Total does not include 8,017 physicians in U.S. territories and possessions.

Rate of Nonfederal Physicians in Patient Care in 1999

National Rate = 221 Physicians per 100,000 Population*

ALPHA ORDER

RANK	STATE	RATE
38	Alabama	179
47	Alaska	153
36	Arizona	181
42	Arkansas	175
17	California	213
15	Colorado	216
4	Connecticut	307
20	Delaware	208
14	Florida	217
33	Georgia	188
9	Hawaii	240
50	Idaho	144
10	Illinois	229
40	Indiana	177
46	Iowa	154
35	Kansas	184
31	Kentucky	191
12	Louisiana	222
21	Maine	207
3	Maryland	310
1	Massachusetts	342
29	Michigan	196
11	Minnesota	224
49	Mississippi	149
26	Missouri	202
39	Montana	178
28	Nebraska	198
44	Nevada	162
17	New Hampshire	213
7	New Jersey	261
34	New Mexico	186
2	New York	329
21	North Carolina	207
26	North Dakota	202
19	Ohio	210
48	Oklahoma	150
25	Oregon	203
8	Pennsylvania	253
5	Rhode Island	293
31	South Carolina	191
43	South Dakota	174
13	Tennessee	221
37	Texas	180
40	Utah	177
6	Vermont	269
16	Virginia	215
21	Washington	207
30	West Virginia	195
24	Wisconsin	206
45	Wyoming	155

RANK ORDER

RANK	STATE	RATE
1	Massachusetts	342
2	New York	329
3	Maryland	310
4	Connecticut	307
5	Rhode Island	293
6	Vermont	269
7	New Jersey	261
8	Pennsylvania	253
9	Hawaii	240
10	Illinois	229
11	Minnesota	224
12	Louisiana	222
13	Tennessee	221
14	Florida	217
15	Colorado	216
16	Virginia	215
17	California	213
17	New Hampshire	213
19	Ohio	210
20	Delaware	208
21	Maine	207
21	North Carolina	207
21	Washington	207
24	Wisconsin	206
25	Oregon	203
26	Missouri	202
26	North Dakota	202
28	Nebraska	198
29	Michigan	196
30	West Virginia	195
31	Kentucky	191
31	South Carolina	191
33	Georgia	188
34	New Mexico	186
35	Kansas	184
36	Arizona	181
37	Texas	180
38	Alabama	179
39	Montana	178
40	Indiana	177
40	Utah	177
42	Arkansas	175
43	South Dakota	174
44	Nevada	162
45	Wyoming	155
46	Iowa	154
47	Alaska	153
48	Oklahoma	150
49	Mississippi	149
50	Idaho	144

	District of Columbia	601

Source: Morgan Quitno Press using data from American Medical Association (Chicago, Illinois)
   "Physician Characteristics and Distribution in the U.S." (2001-2002 Edition)
*As of December 31, 1999. National rate does not include physicians in U.S. territories and possessions.

438

Physicians in Primary Care in 1999

National Total = 262,004 Physicians*

ALPHA ORDER

ALPHA ORDER

RANK	STATE	PHYSICIANS	% of USA
25	Alabama	3,505	1.3%
49	Alaska	527	0.2%
24	Arizona	3,735	1.4%
31	Arkansas	2,063	0.8%
1	California	30,875	11.8%
23	Colorado	3,805	1.5%
21	Connecticut	4,175	1.6%
47	Delaware	656	0.3%
4	Florida	13,260	5.1%
14	Georgia	6,637	2.5%
38	Hawaii	1,366	0.5%
43	Idaho	822	0.3%
5	Illinois	12,855	4.9%
19	Indiana	4,634	1.8%
32	Iowa	1,996	0.8%
29	Kansas	2,285	0.9%
27	Kentucky	3,247	1.2%
22	Louisiana	3,972	1.5%
41	Maine	1,158	0.4%
11	Maryland	7,005	2.7%
10	Massachusetts	8,376	3.2%
9	Michigan	8,425	3.2%
17	Minnesota	4,989	1.9%
33	Mississippi	1,867	0.7%
20	Missouri	4,539	1.7%
45	Montana	690	0.3%
36	Nebraska	1,575	0.6%
39	Nevada	1,272	0.5%
42	New Hampshire	1,118	0.4%
8	New Jersey	9,348	3.6%
37	New Mexico	1,573	0.6%
2	New York	25,488	9.7%
12	North Carolina	6,944	2.7%
48	North Dakota	619	0.2%
7	Ohio	10,314	3.9%
30	Oklahoma	2,277	0.9%
28	Oregon	3,013	1.1%
6	Pennsylvania	12,429	4.7%
40	Rhode Island	1,267	0.5%
26	South Carolina	3,344	1.3%
46	South Dakota	660	0.3%
16	Tennessee	5,166	2.0%
3	Texas	15,390	5.9%
35	Utah	1,596	0.6%
44	Vermont	761	0.3%
13	Virginia	6,749	2.6%
15	Washington	5,466	2.1%
34	West Virginia	1,630	0.6%
18	Wisconsin	4,825	1.8%
50	Wyoming	396	0.2%

RANK ORDER

RANK	STATE	PHYSICIANS	% of USA
1	California	30,875	11.8%
2	New York	25,488	9.7%
3	Texas	15,390	5.9%
4	Florida	13,260	5.1%
5	Illinois	12,855	4.9%
6	Pennsylvania	12,429	4.7%
7	Ohio	10,314	3.9%
8	New Jersey	9,348	3.6%
9	Michigan	8,425	3.2%
10	Massachusetts	8,376	3.2%
11	Maryland	7,005	2.7%
12	North Carolina	6,944	2.7%
13	Virginia	6,749	2.6%
14	Georgia	6,637	2.5%
15	Washington	5,466	2.1%
16	Tennessee	5,166	2.0%
17	Minnesota	4,989	1.9%
18	Wisconsin	4,825	1.8%
19	Indiana	4,634	1.8%
20	Missouri	4,539	1.7%
21	Connecticut	4,175	1.6%
22	Louisiana	3,972	1.5%
23	Colorado	3,805	1.5%
24	Arizona	3,735	1.4%
25	Alabama	3,505	1.3%
26	South Carolina	3,344	1.3%
27	Kentucky	3,247	1.2%
28	Oregon	3,013	1.1%
29	Kansas	2,285	0.9%
30	Oklahoma	2,277	0.9%
31	Arkansas	2,063	0.8%
32	Iowa	1,996	0.8%
33	Mississippi	1,867	0.7%
34	West Virginia	1,630	0.6%
35	Utah	1,596	0.6%
36	Nebraska	1,575	0.6%
37	New Mexico	1,573	0.6%
38	Hawaii	1,366	0.5%
39	Nevada	1,272	0.5%
40	Rhode Island	1,267	0.5%
41	Maine	1,158	0.4%
42	New Hampshire	1,118	0.4%
43	Idaho	822	0.3%
44	Vermont	761	0.3%
45	Montana	690	0.3%
46	South Dakota	660	0.3%
47	Delaware	656	0.3%
48	North Dakota	619	0.2%
49	Alaska	527	0.2%
50	Wyoming	396	0.2%
	District of Columbia	1,320	0.5%

Source: American Medical Association (Chicago, Illinois)
   "Physician Characteristics and Distribution in the U.S." (2001-2002 Edition)
*Federal and nonfederal physicians as of December 31, 1999. National total does not include 4,776 physicians in U.S. territories and possessions. Primary Care Specialties include Family Practice, General Practice, Internal Medicine, Obstetrics/Gynecology and Pediatrics.

Rate of Physicians in Primary Care in 1999

National Rate = 96 Physicians per 100,000 Population*

ALPHA ORDER				RANK ORDER		
RANK	STATE			RANK	STATE	RATE
40	Alabama	80		1	New York	140
33	Alaska	85		2	Massachusetts	136
41	Arizona	78		3	Maryland	135
39	Arkansas	81		4	Rhode Island	128
18	California	93		4	Vermont	128
16	Colorado	94		6	Connecticut	127
6	Connecticut	127		7	Hawaii	115
30	Delaware	87		7	New Jersey	115
29	Florida	88		9	Illinois	106
33	Georgia	85		10	Minnesota	104
7	Hawaii	115		10	Pennsylvania	104
50	Idaho	66		12	North Dakota	98
9	Illinois	106		12	Virginia	98
41	Indiana	78		14	Nebraska	95
46	Iowa	70		14	Washington	95
31	Kansas	86		16	Colorado	94
38	Kentucky	82		16	Tennessee	94
23	Louisiana	91		18	California	93
20	Maine	92		18	New Hampshire	93
3	Maryland	135		20	Maine	92
2	Massachusetts	136		20	Ohio	92
33	Michigan	85		20	Wisconsin	92
10	Minnesota	104		23	Louisiana	91
49	Mississippi	67		23	North Carolina	91
36	Missouri	83		23	Oregon	91
41	Montana	78		26	New Mexico	90
14	Nebraska	95		26	South Dakota	90
46	Nevada	70		26	West Virginia	90
18	New Hampshire	93		29	Florida	88
7	New Jersey	115		30	Delaware	87
26	New Mexico	90		31	Kansas	86
1	New York	140		31	South Carolina	86
23	North Carolina	91		33	Alaska	85
12	North Dakota	98		33	Georgia	85
20	Ohio	92		33	Michigan	85
48	Oklahoma	68		36	Missouri	83
23	Oregon	91		36	Wyoming	83
10	Pennsylvania	104		38	Kentucky	82
4	Rhode Island	128		39	Arkansas	81
31	South Carolina	86		40	Alabama	80
26	South Dakota	90		41	Arizona	78
16	Tennessee	94		41	Indiana	78
44	Texas	77		41	Montana	78
45	Utah	75		44	Texas	77
4	Vermont	128		45	Utah	75
12	Virginia	98		46	Iowa	70
14	Washington	95		46	Nevada	70
26	West Virginia	90		48	Oklahoma	68
20	Wisconsin	92		49	Mississippi	67
36	Wyoming	83		50	Idaho	66
					District of Columbia	254

Source: Morgan Quitno Press using data from American Medical Association (Chicago, Illinois)
  "Physician Characteristics and Distribution in the U.S." (2001-2002 Edition)
Federal and nonfederal physicians as of January 1, 1999. National rate does not include physicians in U.S. territories and possessions. Primary Care Specialties include Family Practice, General Practice, Internal Medicine, Obstetrics/Gynecology and Pediatrics.

Percent of Physicians in Primary Care in 1999

National Percent = 33.3% of Physicians*

ALPHA ORDER

RANK	STATE	PERCENT
10	Alabama	36.2
1	Alaska	40.8
47	Arizona	31.3
6	Arkansas	36.8
42	California	32.5
37	Colorado	33.3
46	Connecticut	31.7
44	Delaware	32.3
49	Florida	29.5
16	Georgia	35.4
14	Hawaii	35.6
15	Idaho	35.5
9	Illinois	36.3
18	Indiana	35.2
26	Iowa	34.3
11	Kansas	36.0
23	Kentucky	34.7
39	Louisiana	33.0
29	Maine	33.9
48	Maryland	30.3
50	Massachusetts	29.4
29	Michigan	33.9
8	Minnesota	36.4
13	Mississippi	35.7
42	Missouri	32.5
36	Montana	33.4
5	Nebraska	37.7
27	Nevada	34.1
34	New Hampshire	33.5
22	New Jersey	34.8
18	New Mexico	35.2
40	New York	32.7
29	North Carolina	33.9
4	North Dakota	38.4
25	Ohio	34.6
20	Oklahoma	35.1
37	Oregon	33.3
45	Pennsylvania	31.8
32	Rhode Island	33.8
12	South Carolina	35.8
2	South Dakota	40.1
27	Tennessee	34.1
34	Texas	33.5
41	Utah	32.6
21	Vermont	34.9
23	Virginia	34.7
33	Washington	33.7
7	West Virginia	36.6
16	Wisconsin	35.4
2	Wyoming	40.1

RANK ORDER

RANK	STATE	PERCENT
1	Alaska	40.8
2	South Dakota	40.1
2	Wyoming	40.1
4	North Dakota	38.4
5	Nebraska	37.7
6	Arkansas	36.8
7	West Virginia	36.6
8	Minnesota	36.4
9	Illinois	36.3
10	Alabama	36.2
11	Kansas	36.0
12	South Carolina	35.8
13	Mississippi	35.7
14	Hawaii	35.6
15	Idaho	35.5
16	Georgia	35.4
16	Wisconsin	35.4
18	Indiana	35.2
18	New Mexico	35.2
20	Oklahoma	35.1
21	Vermont	34.9
22	New Jersey	34.8
23	Kentucky	34.7
23	Virginia	34.7
25	Ohio	34.6
26	Iowa	34.3
27	Nevada	34.1
27	Tennessee	34.1
29	Maine	33.9
29	Michigan	33.9
29	North Carolina	33.9
32	Rhode Island	33.8
33	Washington	33.7
34	New Hampshire	33.5
34	Texas	33.5
36	Montana	33.4
37	Colorado	33.3
37	Oregon	33.3
39	Louisiana	33.0
40	New York	32.7
41	Utah	32.6
42	California	32.5
42	Missouri	32.5
44	Delaware	32.3
45	Pennsylvania	31.8
46	Connecticut	31.7
47	Arizona	31.3
48	Maryland	30.3
49	Florida	29.5
50	Massachusetts	29.4
	District of Columbia	29.1

Source: Morgan Quitno Press using data from American Medical Association (Chicago, Illinois)
    "Physician Characteristics and Distribution in the U.S." (2001-2002 Edition)
*Federal and nonfederal physicians as of January 1, 1999. National rate does not include physicians in U.S. territories and possessions. Primary Care Specialties include Family Practice, General Practice, Internal Medicine, Obstetrics/Gynecology and Pediatrics.

Percent of Population Lacking Access to Primary Care in 2000

National Percent = 9.3% of Population*

ALPHA ORDER			RANK ORDER		
RANK	STATE	PERCENT	RANK	STATE	PERCENT
2	Alabama	22.7	1	Mississippi	26.9
13	Alaska	14.2	2	Alabama	22.7
33	Arizona	7.7	3	Utah	21.0
18	Arkansas	11.2	4	Idaho	20.3
44	California	4.9	5	South Dakota	19.2
34	Colorado	7.4	6	Louisiana	18.3
42	Connecticut	5.7	7	Wyoming	17.9
45	Delaware	4.5	8	Missouri	17.8
27	Florida	8.8	9	Georgia	16.3
9	Georgia	16.3	10	South Carolina	16.0
50	Hawaii	2.9	11	New Mexico	15.9
4	Idaho	20.3	12	North Dakota	15.5
38	Illinois	6.7	13	Alaska	14.2
27	Indiana	8.8	13	Kentucky	14.2
30	Iowa	8.4	15	Montana	13.5
41	Kansas	6.0	16	West Virginia	12.7
13	Kentucky	14.2	17	Texas	11.6
6	Louisiana	18.3	18	Arkansas	11.2
35	Maine	7.2	19	Minnesota	10.8
40	Maryland	6.2	20	Michigan	10.5
47	Massachusetts	4.0	21	Tennessee	10.1
20	Michigan	10.5	22	Nevada	9.8
19	Minnesota	10.8	23	North Carolina	9.5
1	Mississippi	26.9	24	Wisconsin	9.3
8	Missouri	17.8	25	New York	9.2
15	Montana	13.5	26	Washington	9.0
39	Nebraska	6.6	27	Florida	8.8
22	Nevada	9.8	27	Indiana	8.8
46	New Hampshire	4.3	29	Oregon	8.7
49	New Jersey	3.5	30	Iowa	8.4
11	New Mexico	15.9	31	Rhode Island	8.1
25	New York	9.2	32	Oklahoma	7.9
23	North Carolina	9.5	33	Arizona	7.7
12	North Dakota	15.5	34	Colorado	7.4
37	Ohio	7.0	35	Maine	7.2
32	Oklahoma	7.9	35	Virginia	7.2
29	Oregon	8.7	37	Ohio	7.0
43	Pennsylvania	5.5	38	Illinois	6.7
31	Rhode Island	8.1	39	Nebraska	6.6
10	South Carolina	16.0	40	Maryland	6.2
5	South Dakota	19.2	41	Kansas	6.0
21	Tennessee	10.1	42	Connecticut	5.7
17	Texas	11.6	43	Pennsylvania	5.5
3	Utah	21.0	44	California	4.9
48	Vermont	3.7	45	Delaware	4.5
35	Virginia	7.2	46	New Hampshire	4.3
26	Washington	9.0	47	Massachusetts	4.0
16	West Virginia	12.7	48	Vermont	3.7
24	Wisconsin	9.3	49	New Jersey	3.5
7	Wyoming	17.9	50	Hawaii	2.9
				District of Columbia	19.5

Source: Morgan Quitno Press using data from U.S. Dept. of Health and Human Services, Div. of Shortage Designation "Selected Statistics on Health Manpower Shortage Areas, As of December 31, 2000"

*Percent of population considered under-served by primary medical practitioners (Family & General Practice doctors, Internists, Ob/Gyns and Pediatricians). An under-served population does not have primary medical care within reasonable economic and geographic bounds.

Nonfederal Physicians in General/Family Practice in 1999

National Total = 81,154 Physicians*

<u>ALPHA ORDER</u>

RANK	STATE	PHYSICIANS	% of USA
23	Alabama	1,218	1.5%
47	Alaska	239	0.3%
20	Arizona	1,300	1.6%
28	Arkansas	1,089	1.3%
1	California	9,736	12.0%
18	Colorado	1,522	1.9%
36	Connecticut	595	0.7%
49	Delaware	208	0.3%
3	Florida	4,404	5.4%
15	Georgia	1,930	2.4%
45	Hawaii	317	0.4%
39	Idaho	463	0.6%
6	Illinois	3,622	4.5%
12	Indiana	2,234	2.8%
27	Iowa	1,121	1.4%
30	Kansas	1,052	1.3%
21	Kentucky	1,255	1.5%
24	Louisiana	1,217	1.5%
38	Maine	491	0.6%
21	Maryland	1,255	1.5%
26	Massachusetts	1,174	1.4%
8	Michigan	2,537	3.1%
10	Minnesota	2,409	3.0%
33	Mississippi	716	0.9%
25	Missouri	1,187	1.5%
43	Montana	345	0.4%
32	Nebraska	821	1.0%
40	Nevada	400	0.5%
41	New Hampshire	396	0.5%
17	New Jersey	1,582	1.9%
35	New Mexico	603	0.7%
5	New York	3,833	4.7%
11	North Carolina	2,398	3.0%
44	North Dakota	338	0.4%
7	Ohio	3,304	4.1%
31	Oklahoma	977	1.2%
29	Oregon	1,054	1.3%
4	Pennsylvania	3,877	4.8%
50	Rhode Island	207	0.3%
19	South Carolina	1,410	1.7%
42	South Dakota	350	0.4%
16	Tennessee	1,715	2.1%
2	Texas	5,556	6.8%
37	Utah	592	0.7%
46	Vermont	252	0.3%
12	Virginia	2,234	2.8%
9	Washington	2,478	3.1%
34	West Virginia	664	0.8%
14	Wisconsin	2,109	2.6%
48	Wyoming	216	0.3%

<u>RANK ORDER</u>

RANK	STATE	PHYSICIANS	% of USA
1	California	9,736	12.0%
2	Texas	5,556	6.8%
3	Florida	4,404	5.4%
4	Pennsylvania	3,877	4.8%
5	New York	3,833	4.7%
6	Illinois	3,622	4.5%
7	Ohio	3,304	4.1%
8	Michigan	2,537	3.1%
9	Washington	2,478	3.1%
10	Minnesota	2,409	3.0%
11	North Carolina	2,398	3.0%
12	Indiana	2,234	2.8%
12	Virginia	2,234	2.8%
14	Wisconsin	2,109	2.6%
15	Georgia	1,930	2.4%
16	Tennessee	1,715	2.1%
17	New Jersey	1,582	1.9%
18	Colorado	1,522	1.9%
19	South Carolina	1,410	1.7%
20	Arizona	1,300	1.6%
21	Kentucky	1,255	1.5%
21	Maryland	1,255	1.5%
23	Alabama	1,218	1.5%
24	Louisiana	1,217	1.5%
25	Missouri	1,187	1.5%
26	Massachusetts	1,174	1.4%
27	Iowa	1,121	1.4%
28	Arkansas	1,089	1.3%
29	Oregon	1,054	1.3%
30	Kansas	1,052	1.3%
31	Oklahoma	977	1.2%
32	Nebraska	821	1.0%
33	Mississippi	716	0.9%
34	West Virginia	664	0.8%
35	New Mexico	603	0.7%
36	Connecticut	595	0.7%
37	Utah	592	0.7%
38	Maine	491	0.6%
39	Idaho	463	0.6%
40	Nevada	400	0.5%
41	New Hampshire	396	0.5%
42	South Dakota	350	0.4%
43	Montana	345	0.4%
44	North Dakota	338	0.4%
45	Hawaii	317	0.4%
46	Vermont	252	0.3%
47	Alaska	239	0.3%
48	Wyoming	216	0.3%
49	Delaware	208	0.3%
50	Rhode Island	207	0.3%
	District of Columbia	152	0.2%

Source: American Medical Association (Chicago, Illinois)
   "Physician Characteristics and Distribution in the U.S." (2001-2002 Edition)
*As of December 31, 1999. Total does not include 2,031 physicians in U.S. territories and possessions.

Rate of Nonfederal Physicians in General/Family Practice in 1999

National Rate = 30 Physicians per 100,000 Population*

ALPHA ORDER

RANK	STATE	RATE
33	Alabama	28
11	Alaska	39
38	Arizona	27
6	Arkansas	43
29	California	29
15	Colorado	38
50	Connecticut	18
33	Delaware	28
29	Florida	29
42	Georgia	25
38	Hawaii	27
17	Idaho	37
28	Illinois	30
15	Indiana	38
11	Iowa	39
9	Kansas	40
23	Kentucky	32
33	Louisiana	28
11	Maine	39
43	Maryland	24
48	Massachusetts	19
40	Michigan	26
2	Minnesota	50
40	Mississippi	26
44	Missouri	22
11	Montana	39
3	Nebraska	49
44	Nevada	22
21	New Hampshire	33
48	New Jersey	19
20	New Mexico	35
46	New York	21
26	North Carolina	31
1	North Dakota	53
29	Ohio	29
29	Oklahoma	29
23	Oregon	32
23	Pennsylvania	32
46	Rhode Island	21
19	South Carolina	36
4	South Dakota	48
26	Tennessee	31
33	Texas	28
33	Utah	28
8	Vermont	42
21	Virginia	33
6	Washington	43
17	West Virginia	37
9	Wisconsin	40
5	Wyoming	45

RANK ORDER

RANK	STATE	RATE
1	North Dakota	53
2	Minnesota	50
3	Nebraska	49
4	South Dakota	48
5	Wyoming	45
6	Arkansas	43
6	Washington	43
8	Vermont	42
9	Kansas	40
9	Wisconsin	40
11	Alaska	39
11	Iowa	39
11	Maine	39
11	Montana	39
15	Colorado	38
15	Indiana	38
17	Idaho	37
17	West Virginia	37
19	South Carolina	36
20	New Mexico	35
21	New Hampshire	33
21	Virginia	33
23	Kentucky	32
23	Oregon	32
23	Pennsylvania	32
26	North Carolina	31
26	Tennessee	31
28	Illinois	30
29	California	29
29	Florida	29
29	Ohio	29
29	Oklahoma	29
33	Alabama	28
33	Delaware	28
33	Louisiana	28
33	Texas	28
33	Utah	28
38	Arizona	27
38	Hawaii	27
40	Michigan	26
40	Mississippi	26
42	Georgia	25
43	Maryland	24
44	Missouri	22
44	Nevada	22
46	New York	21
46	Rhode Island	21
48	Massachusetts	19
48	New Jersey	19
50	Connecticut	18
	District of Columbia	29

Source: Morgan Quitno Press using data from American Medical Association (Chicago, Illinois)
"Physician Characteristics and Distribution in the U.S." (2001-2002 Edition)
As of December 31, 1999. National rate does not include physicians in U.S. territories and possessions.

Percent of Nonfederal Physicians Who Are Specialists in 1999

National Percent = 73.3% of Physicians*

ALPHA ORDER

RANK	STATE	PERCENT
13	Alabama	74.2
43	Alaska	65.5
35	Arizona	68.3
41	Arkansas	65.7
25	California	70.9
26	Colorado	70.8
1	Connecticut	80.1
17	Delaware	73.4
33	Florida	68.7
9	Georgia	75.6
13	Hawaii	74.2
49	Idaho	61.7
12	Illinois	74.5
35	Indiana	68.3
47	Iowa	62.6
40	Kansas	66.2
21	Kentucky	72.5
8	Louisiana	76.1
38	Maine	67.4
7	Maryland	77.6
4	Massachusetts	78.9
16	Michigan	73.6
39	Minnesota	66.8
24	Mississippi	71.8
6	Missouri	77.7
46	Montana	63.6
44	Nebraska	64.6
19	Nevada	73.1
29	New Hampshire	70.2
2	New Jersey	79.3
37	New Mexico	68.0
4	New York	78.9
20	North Carolina	72.7
45	North Dakota	63.7
15	Ohio	74.0
32	Oklahoma	69.1
34	Oregon	68.6
10	Pennsylvania	75.1
2	Rhode Island	79.3
27	South Carolina	70.6
48	South Dakota	62.0
11	Tennessee	75.0
17	Texas	73.4
22	Utah	72.4
31	Vermont	69.3
22	Virginia	72.4
41	Washington	65.7
28	West Virginia	70.4
30	Wisconsin	69.9
50	Wyoming	59.9

RANK ORDER

RANK	STATE	PERCENT
1	Connecticut	80.1
2	New Jersey	79.3
2	Rhode Island	79.3
4	Massachusetts	78.9
4	New York	78.9
6	Missouri	77.7
7	Maryland	77.6
8	Louisiana	76.1
9	Georgia	75.6
10	Pennsylvania	75.1
11	Tennessee	75.0
12	Illinois	74.5
13	Alabama	74.2
13	Hawaii	74.2
15	Ohio	74.0
16	Michigan	73.6
17	Delaware	73.4
17	Texas	73.4
19	Nevada	73.1
20	North Carolina	72.7
21	Kentucky	72.5
22	Utah	72.4
22	Virginia	72.4
24	Mississippi	71.8
25	California	70.9
26	Colorado	70.8
27	South Carolina	70.6
28	West Virginia	70.4
29	New Hampshire	70.2
30	Wisconsin	69.9
31	Vermont	69.3
32	Oklahoma	69.1
33	Florida	68.7
34	Oregon	68.6
35	Arizona	68.3
35	Indiana	68.3
37	New Mexico	68.0
38	Maine	67.4
39	Minnesota	66.8
40	Kansas	66.2
41	Arkansas	65.7
41	Washington	65.7
43	Alaska	65.5
44	Nebraska	64.6
45	North Dakota	63.7
46	Montana	63.6
47	Iowa	62.6
48	South Dakota	62.0
49	Idaho	61.7
50	Wyoming	59.9
	District of Columbia	80.7

Source: Morgan Quitno Press using data from American Medical Association (Chicago, Illinois)
   "Physician Characteristics and Distribution in the U.S." (2001-2002 Edition)
*As of December 31, 1999. National rate does not include physicians in U.S. territories and possessions. Includes
physicians in medical, surgical and other specialties.

Nonfederal Physicians in Medical Specialties in 1999

National Total = 232,231 Physicians*

<u>ALPHA ORDER</u>

RANK	STATE	PHYSICIANS	% of USA
25	Alabama	2,863	1.2%
49	Alaska	240	0.1%
23	Arizona	2,976	1.3%
33	Arkansas	1,316	0.6%
2	California	26,741	11.5%
24	Colorado	2,955	1.3%
15	Connecticut	4,683	2.0%
44	Delaware	577	0.2%
4	Florida	12,406	5.3%
13	Georgia	5,346	2.3%
37	Hawaii	1,120	0.5%
45	Idaho	418	0.2%
6	Illinois	11,398	4.9%
22	Indiana	3,284	1.4%
35	Iowa	1,256	0.5%
30	Kansas	1,518	0.7%
26	Kentucky	2,542	1.1%
21	Louisiana	3,515	1.5%
42	Maine	835	0.4%
11	Maryland	7,229	3.1%
7	Massachusetts	10,098	4.3%
10	Michigan	7,507	3.2%
19	Minnesota	3,715	1.6%
32	Mississippi	1,318	0.6%
16	Missouri	4,510	1.9%
46	Montana	406	0.2%
40	Nebraska	986	0.4%
39	Nevada	1,044	0.4%
41	New Hampshire	857	0.4%
8	New Jersey	10,005	4.3%
38	New Mexico	1,113	0.5%
1	New York	28,114	12.1%
12	North Carolina	5,764	2.5%
48	North Dakota	351	0.2%
9	Ohio	8,989	3.9%
29	Oklahoma	1,635	0.7%
27	Oregon	2,323	1.0%
5	Pennsylvania	11,837	5.1%
31	Rhode Island	1,378	0.6%
28	South Carolina	2,319	1.0%
47	South Dakota	356	0.2%
17	Tennessee	4,504	1.9%
3	Texas	12,480	5.4%
34	Utah	1,285	0.6%
43	Vermont	593	0.3%
14	Virginia	5,327	2.3%
18	Washington	3,828	1.6%
36	West Virginia	1,174	0.5%
20	Wisconsin	3,571	1.5%
50	Wyoming	164	0.1%

<u>RANK ORDER</u>

RANK	STATE	PHYSICIANS	% of USA
1	New York	28,114	12.1%
2	California	26,741	11.5%
3	Texas	12,480	5.4%
4	Florida	12,406	5.3%
5	Pennsylvania	11,837	5.1%
6	Illinois	11,398	4.9%
7	Massachusetts	10,098	4.3%
8	New Jersey	10,005	4.3%
9	Ohio	8,989	3.9%
10	Michigan	7,507	3.2%
11	Maryland	7,229	3.1%
12	North Carolina	5,764	2.5%
13	Georgia	5,346	2.3%
14	Virginia	5,327	2.3%
15	Connecticut	4,683	2.0%
16	Missouri	4,510	1.9%
17	Tennessee	4,504	1.9%
18	Washington	3,828	1.6%
19	Minnesota	3,715	1.6%
20	Wisconsin	3,571	1.5%
21	Louisiana	3,515	1.5%
22	Indiana	3,284	1.4%
23	Arizona	2,976	1.3%
24	Colorado	2,955	1.3%
25	Alabama	2,863	1.2%
26	Kentucky	2,542	1.1%
27	Oregon	2,323	1.0%
28	South Carolina	2,319	1.0%
29	Oklahoma	1,635	0.7%
30	Kansas	1,518	0.7%
31	Rhode Island	1,378	0.6%
32	Mississippi	1,318	0.6%
33	Arkansas	1,316	0.6%
34	Utah	1,285	0.6%
35	Iowa	1,256	0.5%
36	West Virginia	1,174	0.5%
37	Hawaii	1,120	0.5%
38	New Mexico	1,113	0.5%
39	Nevada	1,044	0.4%
40	Nebraska	986	0.4%
41	New Hampshire	857	0.4%
42	Maine	835	0.4%
43	Vermont	593	0.3%
44	Delaware	577	0.2%
45	Idaho	418	0.2%
46	Montana	406	0.2%
47	South Dakota	356	0.2%
48	North Dakota	351	0.2%
49	Alaska	240	0.1%
50	Wyoming	164	0.1%
	District of Columbia	1,462	0.6%

Source: American Medical Association (Chicago, Illinois)
        "Physician Characteristics and Distribution in the U.S." (2001-2002 Edition)
As of December 31, 1999. Total does not include 2,740 physicians in U.S. territories and possessions. Medical Specialties are Allergy/Immunology, Cardiovascular Diseases, Dermatology, Gastroenterology, Internal Medicine, Pediatrics, Pediatric Cardiology and Pulmonary Diseases.

446

Rate of Nonfederal Physicians in Medical Specialties in 1999

National Rate = 85 Physicians per 100,000 Population*

ALPHA ORDER				RANK ORDER		
RANK	STATE	RATE		RANK	STATE	RATE
29	Alabama	66		1	Massachusetts	164
48	Alaska	39		2	New York	155
33	Arizona	62		3	Connecticut	143
42	Arkansas	52		4	Maryland	140
14	California	81		5	Rhode Island	139
22	Colorado	73		6	New Jersey	123
3	Connecticut	143		7	Vermont	100
19	Delaware	77		8	Pennsylvania	99
11	Florida	82		9	Hawaii	94
25	Georgia	69		9	Illinois	94
9	Hawaii	94		11	Florida	82
50	Idaho	33		11	Missouri	82
9	Illinois	94		11	Tennessee	82
40	Indiana	55		14	California	81
47	Iowa	44		15	Louisiana	80
39	Kansas	57		15	Ohio	80
31	Kentucky	64		17	Minnesota	78
15	Louisiana	80		17	Virginia	78
27	Maine	67		19	Delaware	77
4	Maryland	140		20	Michigan	76
1	Massachusetts	164		21	North Carolina	75
20	Michigan	76		22	Colorado	73
17	Minnesota	78		23	New Hampshire	71
45	Mississippi	48		24	Oregon	70
11	Missouri	82		25	Georgia	69
46	Montana	46		26	Wisconsin	68
37	Nebraska	59		27	Maine	67
38	Nevada	58		27	Washington	67
23	New Hampshire	71		29	Alabama	66
6	New Jersey	123		30	West Virginia	65
31	New Mexico	64		31	Kentucky	64
2	New York	155		31	New Mexico	64
21	North Carolina	75		33	Arizona	62
40	North Dakota	55		33	Texas	62
15	Ohio	80		35	South Carolina	60
43	Oklahoma	49		35	Utah	60
24	Oregon	70		37	Nebraska	59
8	Pennsylvania	99		38	Nevada	58
5	Rhode Island	139		39	Kansas	57
35	South Carolina	60		40	Indiana	55
43	South Dakota	49		40	North Dakota	55
11	Tennessee	82		42	Arkansas	52
33	Texas	62		43	Oklahoma	49
35	Utah	60		43	South Dakota	49
7	Vermont	100		45	Mississippi	48
17	Virginia	78		46	Montana	46
27	Washington	67		47	Iowa	44
30	West Virginia	65		48	Alaska	39
26	Wisconsin	68		49	Wyoming	34
49	Wyoming	34		50	Idaho	33
					District of Columbia	282

Source: Morgan Quitno Press using data from American Medical Association (Chicago, Illinois)
"Physician Characteristics and Distribution in the U.S." (2001-2002 Edition)
*As of December 31, 1999. National rate does not include physicians in U.S. territories and possessions. Medical Specialties are Allergy/Immunology, Cardiovascular Diseases, Dermatology, Gastroenterology, Internal Medicine, Pediatrics, Pediatric Cardiology and Pulmonary Diseases.

Nonfederal Physicians in Internal Medicine in 1999

National Total = 124,385 Physicians*

ALPHA ORDER

RANK	STATE	PHYSICIANS	% of USA
23	Alabama	1,541	1.2%
49	Alaska	114	0.1%
25	Arizona	1,453	1.2%
36	Arkansas	591	0.5%
2	California	13,961	11.2%
24	Colorado	1,521	1.2%
14	Connecticut	2,733	2.2%
44	Delaware	276	0.2%
6	Florida	6,045	4.9%
13	Georgia	2,812	2.3%
34	Hawaii	620	0.5%
46	Idaho	207	0.2%
4	Illinois	6,542	5.3%
22	Indiana	1,666	1.3%
35	Iowa	592	0.5%
30	Kansas	811	0.7%
27	Kentucky	1,270	1.0%
21	Louisiana	1,750	1.4%
41	Maine	466	0.4%
11	Maryland	4,054	3.3%
7	Massachusetts	5,956	4.8%
10	Michigan	4,204	3.4%
19	Minnesota	2,014	1.6%
32	Mississippi	669	0.5%
16	Missouri	2,406	1.9%
45	Montana	212	0.2%
40	Nebraska	490	0.4%
38	Nevada	576	0.5%
42	New Hampshire	439	0.4%
8	New Jersey	5,334	4.3%
37	New Mexico	577	0.5%
1	New York	16,156	13.0%
12	North Carolina	2,922	2.3%
47	North Dakota	201	0.2%
9	Ohio	4,728	3.8%
29	Oklahoma	824	0.7%
26	Oregon	1,393	1.1%
3	Pennsylvania	6,566	5.3%
31	Rhode Island	785	0.6%
28	South Carolina	1,120	0.9%
48	South Dakota	192	0.2%
17	Tennessee	2,335	1.9%
5	Texas	6,083	4.9%
39	Utah	569	0.5%
43	Vermont	343	0.3%
15	Virginia	2,731	2.2%
18	Washington	2,078	1.7%
33	West Virginia	646	0.5%
20	Wisconsin	1,925	1.5%
50	Wyoming	87	0.1%

RANK ORDER

RANK	STATE	PHYSICIANS	% of USA
1	New York	16,156	13.0%
2	California	13,961	11.2%
3	Pennsylvania	6,566	5.3%
4	Illinois	6,542	5.3%
5	Texas	6,083	4.9%
6	Florida	6,045	4.9%
7	Massachusetts	5,956	4.8%
8	New Jersey	5,334	4.3%
9	Ohio	4,728	3.8%
10	Michigan	4,204	3.4%
11	Maryland	4,054	3.3%
12	North Carolina	2,922	2.3%
13	Georgia	2,812	2.3%
14	Connecticut	2,733	2.2%
15	Virginia	2,731	2.2%
16	Missouri	2,406	1.9%
17	Tennessee	2,335	1.9%
18	Washington	2,078	1.7%
19	Minnesota	2,014	1.6%
20	Wisconsin	1,925	1.5%
21	Louisiana	1,750	1.4%
22	Indiana	1,666	1.3%
23	Alabama	1,541	1.2%
24	Colorado	1,521	1.2%
25	Arizona	1,453	1.2%
26	Oregon	1,393	1.1%
27	Kentucky	1,270	1.0%
28	South Carolina	1,120	0.9%
29	Oklahoma	824	0.7%
30	Kansas	811	0.7%
31	Rhode Island	785	0.6%
32	Mississippi	669	0.5%
33	West Virginia	646	0.5%
34	Hawaii	620	0.5%
35	Iowa	592	0.5%
36	Arkansas	591	0.5%
37	New Mexico	577	0.5%
38	Nevada	576	0.5%
39	Utah	569	0.5%
40	Nebraska	490	0.4%
41	Maine	466	0.4%
42	New Hampshire	439	0.4%
43	Vermont	343	0.3%
44	Delaware	276	0.2%
45	Montana	212	0.2%
46	Idaho	207	0.2%
47	North Dakota	201	0.2%
48	South Dakota	192	0.2%
49	Alaska	114	0.1%
50	Wyoming	87	0.1%
	District of Columbia	799	0.6%

Source: American Medical Association (Chicago, Illinois)
"Physician Characteristics and Distribution in the U.S." (2001-2002 Edition)

As of December 31, 1999. Total does not include 1,229 physicians in U.S. territories and possessions. Internal Medicine includes Diabetes, Endocrinology, Geriatrics, Hematology, Infectious Diseases, Nephrology, Nutrition, Medical Oncology and Rheumatology.

Rate of Nonfederal Physicians in Internal Medicine in 1999

National Rate = 46 Physicians per 100,000 Population*

ALPHA ORDER

RANK	STATE	RATE
30	Alabama	35
48	Alaska	18
36	Arizona	30
46	Arkansas	23
14	California	42
22	Colorado	37
3	Connecticut	83
22	Delaware	37
18	Florida	40
27	Georgia	36
10	Hawaii	52
50	Idaho	17
9	Illinois	54
40	Indiana	28
47	Iowa	21
35	Kansas	31
32	Kentucky	32
18	Louisiana	40
22	Maine	37
5	Maryland	78
1	Massachusetts	96
12	Michigan	43
14	Minnesota	42
44	Mississippi	24
11	Missouri	44
44	Montana	24
38	Nebraska	29
32	Nevada	32
22	New Hampshire	37
6	New Jersey	66
31	New Mexico	33
2	New York	89
21	North Carolina	38
32	North Dakota	32
14	Ohio	42
43	Oklahoma	25
14	Oregon	42
8	Pennsylvania	55
4	Rhode Island	79
38	South Carolina	29
42	South Dakota	26
12	Tennessee	43
36	Texas	30
41	Utah	27
7	Vermont	58
18	Virginia	40
27	Washington	36
27	West Virginia	36
22	Wisconsin	37
48	Wyoming	18

RANK ORDER

RANK	STATE	RATE
1	Massachusetts	96
2	New York	89
3	Connecticut	83
4	Rhode Island	79
5	Maryland	78
6	New Jersey	66
7	Vermont	58
8	Pennsylvania	55
9	Illinois	54
10	Hawaii	52
11	Missouri	44
12	Michigan	43
12	Tennessee	43
14	California	42
14	Minnesota	42
14	Ohio	42
14	Oregon	42
18	Florida	40
18	Louisiana	40
18	Virginia	40
21	North Carolina	38
22	Colorado	37
22	Delaware	37
22	Maine	37
22	New Hampshire	37
22	Wisconsin	37
27	Georgia	36
27	Washington	36
27	West Virginia	36
30	Alabama	35
31	New Mexico	33
32	Kentucky	32
32	Nevada	32
32	North Dakota	32
35	Kansas	31
36	Arizona	30
36	Texas	30
38	Nebraska	29
38	South Carolina	29
40	Indiana	28
41	Utah	27
42	South Dakota	26
43	Oklahoma	25
44	Mississippi	24
44	Montana	24
46	Arkansas	23
47	Iowa	21
48	Alaska	18
48	Wyoming	18
50	Idaho	17

District of Columbia   154

Source: Morgan Quitno Press using data from American Medical Association (Chicago, Illinois)
    "Physician Characteristics and Distribution in the U.S." (2001-2002 Edition)
*As of December 31, 1999. National rate does not include physicians in U.S. territories and possessions. Internal Medicine includes Diabetes, Endocrinology, Geriatrics, Hematology, Infectious Diseases, Nephrology, Nutrition, Medical Oncology and Rheumatology.

Nonfederal Physicians in Pediatrics in 1999

National Total = 57,738 Physicians*

ALPHA ORDER

RANK	STATE	PHYSICIANS	% of USA
25	Alabama	693	1.2%
47	Alaska	84	0.1%
23	Arizona	781	1.4%
31	Arkansas	390	0.7%
1	California	6,904	12.0%
24	Colorado	752	1.3%
17	Connecticut	1,021	1.8%
43	Delaware	187	0.3%
4	Florida	2,937	5.1%
14	Georgia	1,389	2.4%
36	Hawaii	314	0.5%
45	Idaho	89	0.2%
5	Illinois	2,728	4.7%
22	Indiana	808	1.4%
34	Iowa	325	0.6%
32	Kansas	377	0.7%
26	Kentucky	692	1.2%
18	Louisiana	953	1.7%
42	Maine	195	0.3%
11	Maryland	1,789	3.1%
9	Massachusetts	2,189	3.8%
10	Michigan	1,829	3.2%
21	Minnesota	845	1.5%
33	Mississippi	353	0.6%
16	Missouri	1,080	1.9%
46	Montana	86	0.1%
39	Nebraska	269	0.5%
41	Nevada	208	0.4%
40	New Hampshire	227	0.4%
6	New Jersey	2,547	4.4%
37	New Mexico	296	0.5%
2	New York	6,760	11.7%
12	North Carolina	1,543	2.7%
48	North Dakota	73	0.1%
8	Ohio	2,397	4.2%
29	Oklahoma	405	0.7%
28	Oregon	471	0.8%
7	Pennsylvania	2,500	4.3%
34	Rhode Island	325	0.6%
27	South Carolina	617	1.1%
48	South Dakota	73	0.1%
15	Tennessee	1,199	2.1%
3	Texas	3,472	6.0%
30	Utah	404	0.7%
44	Vermont	163	0.3%
13	Virginia	1,446	2.5%
19	Washington	938	1.6%
38	West Virginia	293	0.5%
20	Wisconsin	879	1.5%
50	Wyoming	44	0.1%

RANK ORDER

RANK	STATE	PHYSICIANS	% of USA
1	California	6,904	12.0%
2	New York	6,760	11.7%
3	Texas	3,472	6.0%
4	Florida	2,937	5.1%
5	Illinois	2,728	4.7%
6	New Jersey	2,547	4.4%
7	Pennsylvania	2,500	4.3%
8	Ohio	2,397	4.2%
9	Massachusetts	2,189	3.8%
10	Michigan	1,829	3.2%
11	Maryland	1,789	3.1%
12	North Carolina	1,543	2.7%
13	Virginia	1,446	2.5%
14	Georgia	1,389	2.4%
15	Tennessee	1,199	2.1%
16	Missouri	1,080	1.9%
17	Connecticut	1,021	1.8%
18	Louisiana	953	1.7%
19	Washington	938	1.6%
20	Wisconsin	879	1.5%
21	Minnesota	845	1.5%
22	Indiana	808	1.4%
23	Arizona	781	1.4%
24	Colorado	752	1.3%
25	Alabama	693	1.2%
26	Kentucky	692	1.2%
27	South Carolina	617	1.1%
28	Oregon	471	0.8%
29	Oklahoma	405	0.7%
30	Utah	404	0.7%
31	Arkansas	390	0.7%
32	Kansas	377	0.7%
33	Mississippi	353	0.6%
34	Iowa	325	0.6%
34	Rhode Island	325	0.6%
36	Hawaii	314	0.5%
37	New Mexico	296	0.5%
38	West Virginia	293	0.5%
39	Nebraska	269	0.5%
40	New Hampshire	227	0.4%
41	Nevada	208	0.4%
42	Maine	195	0.3%
43	Delaware	187	0.3%
44	Vermont	163	0.3%
45	Idaho	89	0.2%
46	Montana	86	0.1%
47	Alaska	84	0.1%
48	North Dakota	73	0.1%
48	South Dakota	73	0.1%
50	Wyoming	44	0.1%
	District of Columbia	399	0.7%

Source: American Medical Association (Chicago, Illinois)
    "Physician Characteristics and Distribution in the U.S." (2001-2002 Edition)
As of December 31, 1999. Total does not include 1,005 physicians in U.S. territories and possessions. Pediatrics includes Adolescent Medicine, Neonatal-Perinatal, Pediatric Allergy, Pediatric Endocrinology, Pediatric Pulmonology, Pediatric Hematology-Oncology and Pediatric Nephrology.

Rate of Nonfederal Physicians in Pediatrics in 1999

National Rate = 82 Physicians per 100,000 Population 17 Years and Younger*

ALPHA ORDER

RANK	STATE	RATE
28	Alabama	65
45	Alaska	43
35	Arizona	59
35	Arkansas	59
18	California	77
23	Colorado	71
6	Connecticut	123
9	Delaware	102
15	Florida	82
25	Georgia	68
8	Hawaii	109
50	Idaho	25
13	Illinois	86
40	Indiana	53
44	Iowa	45
39	Kansas	54
22	Kentucky	72
16	Louisiana	80
26	Maine	67
3	Maryland	137
2	Massachusetts	149
23	Michigan	71
27	Minnesota	66
41	Mississippi	47
18	Missouri	77
47	Montana	38
32	Nebraska	61
46	Nevada	42
20	New Hampshire	75
5	New Jersey	127
34	New Mexico	60
1	New York	152
17	North Carolina	79
42	North Dakota	46
14	Ohio	84
42	Oklahoma	46
37	Oregon	57
11	Pennsylvania	88
4	Rhode Island	135
28	South Carolina	65
48	South Dakota	37
10	Tennessee	89
32	Texas	61
37	Utah	57
7	Vermont	117
12	Virginia	87
31	Washington	63
21	West Virginia	73
28	Wisconsin	65
49	Wyoming	35

RANK ORDER

RANK	STATE	RATE
1	New York	152
2	Massachusetts	149
3	Maryland	137
4	Rhode Island	135
5	New Jersey	127
6	Connecticut	123
7	Vermont	117
8	Hawaii	109
9	Delaware	102
10	Tennessee	89
11	Pennsylvania	88
12	Virginia	87
13	Illinois	86
14	Ohio	84
15	Florida	82
16	Louisiana	80
17	North Carolina	79
18	California	77
18	Missouri	77
20	New Hampshire	75
21	West Virginia	73
22	Kentucky	72
23	Colorado	71
23	Michigan	71
25	Georgia	68
26	Maine	67
27	Minnesota	66
28	Alabama	65
28	South Carolina	65
28	Wisconsin	65
31	Washington	63
32	Nebraska	61
32	Texas	61
34	New Mexico	60
35	Arizona	59
35	Arkansas	59
37	Oregon	57
37	Utah	57
39	Kansas	54
40	Indiana	53
41	Mississippi	47
42	North Dakota	46
42	Oklahoma	46
44	Iowa	45
45	Alaska	43
46	Nevada	42
47	Montana	38
48	South Dakota	37
49	Wyoming	35
50	Idaho	25
	District of Columbia	419

Source: Morgan Quitno Press using data from American Medical Association (Chicago, Illinois)
"Physician Characteristics and Distribution in the U.S." (2001-2002 Edition)

As of December 31, 1999. National rate does not include physicians in U.S. territories and possessions. Pediatrics includes Adolescent Medicine, Neonatal-Perinatal, Pediatric Allergy, Pediatric Endocrinology, Pediatric Pulmonology, Pediatric Hematology-Oncology and Pediatric Nephrology.

Nonfederal Physicians in Surgical Specialties in 1999

National Total = 144,899 Physicians*

ALPHA ORDER

RANK	STATE	PHYSICIANS	% of USA
23	Alabama	2,111	1.5%
49	Alaska	228	0.2%
24	Arizona	2,108	1.5%
33	Arkansas	1,056	0.7%
1	California	16,621	11.5%
25	Colorado	2,075	1.4%
21	Connecticut	2,390	1.6%
45	Delaware	381	0.3%
4	Florida	8,219	5.7%
12	Georgia	3,894	2.7%
39	Hawaii	699	0.5%
43	Idaho	496	0.3%
6	Illinois	6,203	4.3%
20	Indiana	2,406	1.7%
32	Iowa	1,106	0.8%
31	Kansas	1,127	0.8%
27	Kentucky	1,865	1.3%
17	Louisiana	2,701	1.9%
42	Maine	594	0.4%
13	Maryland	3,801	2.6%
10	Massachusetts	4,379	3.0%
9	Michigan	4,579	3.2%
22	Minnesota	2,282	1.6%
30	Mississippi	1,160	0.8%
16	Missouri	2,840	2.0%
44	Montana	400	0.3%
36	Nebraska	804	0.6%
37	Nevada	734	0.5%
41	New Hampshire	626	0.4%
8	New Jersey	5,021	3.5%
38	New Mexico	715	0.5%
2	New York	13,497	9.3%
11	North Carolina	4,102	2.8%
48	North Dakota	295	0.2%
7	Ohio	5,796	4.0%
29	Oklahoma	1,249	0.9%
28	Oregon	1,618	1.1%
5	Pennsylvania	7,282	5.0%
40	Rhode Island	684	0.5%
26	South Carolina	1,944	1.3%
47	South Dakota	307	0.2%
15	Tennessee	3,183	2.2%
3	Texas	9,197	6.3%
34	Utah	994	0.7%
46	Vermont	360	0.2%
14	Virginia	3,717	2.6%
18	Washington	2,651	1.8%
35	West Virginia	896	0.6%
19	Wisconsin	2,483	1.7%
50	Wyoming	197	0.1%

RANK ORDER

RANK	STATE	PHYSICIANS	% of USA
1	California	16,621	11.5%
2	New York	13,497	9.3%
3	Texas	9,197	6.3%
4	Florida	8,219	5.7%
5	Pennsylvania	7,282	5.0%
6	Illinois	6,203	4.3%
7	Ohio	5,796	4.0%
8	New Jersey	5,021	3.5%
9	Michigan	4,579	3.2%
10	Massachusetts	4,379	3.0%
11	North Carolina	4,102	2.8%
12	Georgia	3,894	2.7%
13	Maryland	3,801	2.6%
14	Virginia	3,717	2.6%
15	Tennessee	3,183	2.2%
16	Missouri	2,840	2.0%
17	Louisiana	2,701	1.9%
18	Washington	2,651	1.8%
19	Wisconsin	2,483	1.7%
20	Indiana	2,406	1.7%
21	Connecticut	2,390	1.6%
22	Minnesota	2,282	1.6%
23	Alabama	2,111	1.5%
24	Arizona	2,108	1.5%
25	Colorado	2,075	1.4%
26	South Carolina	1,944	1.3%
27	Kentucky	1,865	1.3%
28	Oregon	1,618	1.1%
29	Oklahoma	1,249	0.9%
30	Mississippi	1,160	0.8%
31	Kansas	1,127	0.8%
32	Iowa	1,106	0.8%
33	Arkansas	1,056	0.7%
34	Utah	994	0.7%
35	West Virginia	896	0.6%
36	Nebraska	804	0.6%
37	Nevada	734	0.5%
38	New Mexico	715	0.5%
39	Hawaii	699	0.5%
40	Rhode Island	684	0.5%
41	New Hampshire	626	0.4%
42	Maine	594	0.4%
43	Idaho	496	0.3%
44	Montana	400	0.3%
45	Delaware	381	0.3%
46	Vermont	360	0.2%
47	South Dakota	307	0.2%
48	North Dakota	295	0.2%
49	Alaska	228	0.2%
50	Wyoming	197	0.1%
	District of Columbia	826	0.6%

Source: American Medical Association (Chicago, Illinois)
    "Physician Characteristics and Distribution in the U.S." (2001-2002 Edition)
*As of December 31, 1999. Total does not include 1,511 physicians in U.S. territories and possessions. Surgical Specialties include Colon and Rectal, General, Neurological, Obstetrics & Gynecology, Ophthalmology, Orthopedic, Otolaryngology, Plastic, Thoracic and Urological Surgeries.

Rate of Nonfederal Physicians in Surgical Specialties in 1999

National Rate = 53 Physicians per 100,000 Population*

ALPHA ORDER

RANK	STATE	RATE
26	Alabama	48
49	Alaska	37
38	Arizona	44
42	Arkansas	41
21	California	50
17	Colorado	51
2	Connecticut	73
17	Delaware	51
12	Florida	54
21	Georgia	50
10	Hawaii	59
46	Idaho	40
17	Illinois	51
46	Indiana	40
48	Iowa	39
39	Kansas	42
29	Kentucky	47
6	Louisiana	62
29	Maine	47
2	Maryland	73
4	Massachusetts	71
34	Michigan	46
26	Minnesota	48
39	Mississippi	42
15	Missouri	52
37	Montana	45
26	Nebraska	48
42	Nevada	41
15	New Hampshire	52
6	New Jersey	62
42	New Mexico	41
1	New York	74
12	North Carolina	54
29	North Dakota	47
17	Ohio	51
49	Oklahoma	37
25	Oregon	49
8	Pennsylvania	61
5	Rhode Island	69
21	South Carolina	50
39	South Dakota	42
11	Tennessee	58
34	Texas	46
29	Utah	47
8	Vermont	61
12	Virginia	54
34	Washington	46
21	West Virginia	50
29	Wisconsin	47
42	Wyoming	41

RANK ORDER

RANK	STATE	RATE
1	New York	74
2	Connecticut	73
2	Maryland	73
4	Massachusetts	71
5	Rhode Island	69
6	Louisiana	62
6	New Jersey	62
8	Pennsylvania	61
8	Vermont	61
10	Hawaii	59
11	Tennessee	58
12	Florida	54
12	North Carolina	54
12	Virginia	54
15	Missouri	52
15	New Hampshire	52
17	Colorado	51
17	Delaware	51
17	Illinois	51
17	Ohio	51
21	California	50
21	Georgia	50
21	South Carolina	50
21	West Virginia	50
25	Oregon	49
26	Alabama	48
26	Minnesota	48
26	Nebraska	48
29	Kentucky	47
29	Maine	47
29	North Dakota	47
29	Utah	47
29	Wisconsin	47
34	Michigan	46
34	Texas	46
34	Washington	46
37	Montana	45
38	Arizona	44
39	Kansas	42
39	Mississippi	42
39	South Dakota	42
42	Arkansas	41
42	Nevada	41
42	New Mexico	41
42	Wyoming	41
46	Idaho	40
46	Indiana	40
48	Iowa	39
49	Alaska	37
49	Oklahoma	37
	District of Columbia	159

Source: Morgan Quitno Press using data from American Medical Association (Chicago, Illinois)
"Physician Characteristics and Distribution in the U.S." (2001-2002 Edition)
*As of December 31, 1999. National rate does not include physicians in U.S. territories and possessions. Surgical Specialties include Colon and Rectal, General, Neurological, Obstetrics & Gynecology, Ophthalmology, Orthopedic, Otolaryngology, Plastic, Thoracic and Urological Surgeries.

453

Nonfederal Physicians in General Surgery in 1999

National Total = 37,902 Physicians*

ALPHA ORDER

RANK	STATE	PHYSICIANS	% of USA
22	Alabama	567	1.5%
49	Alaska	53	0.1%
25	Arizona	528	1.4%
34	Arkansas	284	0.7%
1	California	3,900	10.3%
27	Colorado	506	1.3%
21	Connecticut	613	1.6%
44	Delaware	112	0.3%
5	Florida	1,950	5.1%
13	Georgia	990	2.6%
41	Hawaii	172	0.5%
43	Idaho	120	0.3%
6	Illinois	1,663	4.4%
19	Indiana	617	1.6%
30	Iowa	312	0.8%
29	Kansas	322	0.8%
24	Kentucky	543	1.4%
17	Louisiana	695	1.8%
39	Maine	180	0.5%
12	Maryland	994	2.6%
10	Massachusetts	1,259	3.3%
9	Michigan	1,293	3.4%
22	Minnesota	567	1.5%
31	Mississippi	311	0.8%
16	Missouri	753	2.0%
46	Montana	103	0.3%
35	Nebraska	230	0.6%
38	Nevada	185	0.5%
42	New Hampshire	169	0.4%
8	New Jersey	1,301	3.4%
37	New Mexico	196	0.5%
2	New York	3,732	9.8%
11	North Carolina	1,031	2.7%
47	North Dakota	91	0.2%
7	Ohio	1,652	4.4%
31	Oklahoma	311	0.8%
28	Oregon	400	1.1%
4	Pennsylvania	2,147	5.7%
39	Rhode Island	180	0.5%
26	South Carolina	522	1.4%
48	South Dakota	84	0.2%
15	Tennessee	894	2.4%
3	Texas	2,311	6.1%
36	Utah	212	0.6%
45	Vermont	107	0.3%
14	Virginia	907	2.4%
20	Washington	614	1.6%
33	West Virginia	285	0.8%
18	Wisconsin	646	1.7%
50	Wyoming	46	0.1%

RANK ORDER

RANK	STATE	PHYSICIANS	% of USA
1	California	3,900	10.3%
2	New York	3,732	9.8%
3	Texas	2,311	6.1%
4	Pennsylvania	2,147	5.7%
5	Florida	1,950	5.1%
6	Illinois	1,663	4.4%
7	Ohio	1,652	4.4%
8	New Jersey	1,301	3.4%
9	Michigan	1,293	3.4%
10	Massachusetts	1,259	3.3%
11	North Carolina	1,031	2.7%
12	Maryland	994	2.6%
13	Georgia	990	2.6%
14	Virginia	907	2.4%
15	Tennessee	894	2.4%
16	Missouri	753	2.0%
17	Louisiana	695	1.8%
18	Wisconsin	646	1.7%
19	Indiana	617	1.6%
20	Washington	614	1.6%
21	Connecticut	613	1.6%
22	Alabama	567	1.5%
22	Minnesota	567	1.5%
24	Kentucky	543	1.4%
25	Arizona	528	1.4%
26	South Carolina	522	1.4%
27	Colorado	506	1.3%
28	Oregon	400	1.1%
29	Kansas	322	0.8%
30	Iowa	312	0.8%
31	Mississippi	311	0.8%
31	Oklahoma	311	0.8%
33	West Virginia	285	0.8%
34	Arkansas	284	0.7%
35	Nebraska	230	0.6%
36	Utah	212	0.6%
37	New Mexico	196	0.5%
38	Nevada	185	0.5%
39	Maine	180	0.5%
39	Rhode Island	180	0.5%
41	Hawaii	172	0.5%
42	New Hampshire	169	0.4%
43	Idaho	120	0.3%
44	Delaware	112	0.3%
45	Vermont	107	0.3%
46	Montana	103	0.3%
47	North Dakota	91	0.2%
48	South Dakota	84	0.2%
49	Alaska	53	0.1%
50	Wyoming	46	0.1%
	District of Columbia	242	0.6%

Source: American Medical Association (Chicago, Illinois)
   "Physician Characteristics and Distribution in the U.S." (2001-2002 Edition)
*As of December 31, 1999. Total does not include 410 physicians in U.S. territories and possessions. General Surgery includes Abdominal, Cardiovascular, Hand, Head and Neck, Pediatric, Traumatic and Vascular Surgeries.

Rate of Nonfederal Physicians in General Surgery in 1999

National Rate = 13.9 Physicians per 100,000 Population*

ALPHA ORDER

RANK	STATE	RATE
26	Alabama	13.0
50	Alaska	8.6
41	Arizona	11.0
40	Arkansas	11.1
34	California	11.8
29	Colorado	12.5
4	Connecticut	18.7
12	Delaware	14.9
27	Florida	12.9
28	Georgia	12.7
14	Hawaii	14.5
47	Idaho	9.6
20	Illinois	13.7
44	Indiana	10.4
42	Iowa	10.9
31	Kansas	12.1
20	Kentucky	13.7
10	Louisiana	15.9
15	Maine	14.4
3	Maryland	19.2
2	Massachusetts	20.4
25	Michigan	13.1
33	Minnesota	11.9
39	Mississippi	11.2
18	Missouri	13.8
35	Montana	11.7
18	Nebraska	13.8
45	Nevada	10.2
17	New Hampshire	14.1
9	New Jersey	16.0
38	New Mexico	11.3
1	New York	20.5
22	North Carolina	13.5
15	North Dakota	14.4
13	Ohio	14.7
49	Oklahoma	9.3
31	Oregon	12.1
7	Pennsylvania	17.9
5	Rhode Island	18.2
23	South Carolina	13.4
36	South Dakota	11.5
8	Tennessee	16.3
36	Texas	11.5
46	Utah	10.0
6	Vermont	18.0
24	Virginia	13.2
43	Washington	10.7
11	West Virginia	15.8
30	Wisconsin	12.3
47	Wyoming	9.6

RANK ORDER

RANK	STATE	RATE
1	New York	20.5
2	Massachusetts	20.4
3	Maryland	19.2
4	Connecticut	18.7
5	Rhode Island	18.2
6	Vermont	18.0
7	Pennsylvania	17.9
8	Tennessee	16.3
9	New Jersey	16.0
10	Louisiana	15.9
11	West Virginia	15.8
12	Delaware	14.9
13	Ohio	14.7
14	Hawaii	14.5
15	Maine	14.4
15	North Dakota	14.4
17	New Hampshire	14.1
18	Missouri	13.8
18	Nebraska	13.8
20	Illinois	13.7
20	Kentucky	13.7
22	North Carolina	13.5
23	South Carolina	13.4
24	Virginia	13.2
25	Michigan	13.1
26	Alabama	13.0
27	Florida	12.9
28	Georgia	12.7
29	Colorado	12.5
30	Wisconsin	12.3
31	Kansas	12.1
31	Oregon	12.1
33	Minnesota	11.9
34	California	11.8
35	Montana	11.7
36	South Dakota	11.5
36	Texas	11.5
38	New Mexico	11.3
39	Mississippi	11.2
40	Arkansas	11.1
41	Arizona	11.0
42	Iowa	10.9
43	Washington	10.7
44	Indiana	10.4
45	Nevada	10.2
46	Utah	10.0
47	Idaho	9.6
47	Wyoming	9.6
49	Oklahoma	9.3
50	Alaska	8.6

District of Columbia 46.6

Source: Morgan Quitno Press using data from American Medical Association (Chicago, Illinois)
     "Physician Characteristics and Distribution in the U.S." (2001-2002 Edition)
*As of December 31, 1999. National rate does not include physicians in U.S. territories and possessions. General Surgery includes Abdominal, Cardiovascular, Hand, Head and Neck, Pediatric, Traumatic and Vascular Surgeries.

Nonfederal Physicians in Obstetrics and Gynecology in 1999

National Total = 38,329 Physicians*

ALPHA ORDER

RANK	STATE	PHYSICIANS	% of USA
25	Alabama	524	1.4%
48	Alaska	58	0.2%
21	Arizona	583	1.5%
33	Arkansas	234	0.6%
1	California	4,477	11.7%
22	Colorado	550	1.4%
19	Connecticut	658	1.7%
44	Delaware	94	0.2%
4	Florida	2,019	5.3%
10	Georgia	1,197	3.1%
34	Hawaii	224	0.6%
43	Idaho	107	0.3%
5	Illinois	1,818	4.7%
20	Indiana	596	1.6%
36	Iowa	215	0.6%
31	Kansas	274	0.7%
27	Kentucky	463	1.2%
17	Louisiana	716	1.9%
42	Maine	132	0.3%
13	Maryland	1,091	2.8%
12	Massachusetts	1,109	2.9%
9	Michigan	1,308	3.4%
26	Minnesota	509	1.3%
30	Mississippi	299	0.8%
16	Missouri	724	1.9%
46	Montana	82	0.2%
40	Nebraska	169	0.4%
35	Nevada	216	0.6%
40	New Hampshire	169	0.4%
8	New Jersey	1,500	3.9%
38	New Mexico	187	0.5%
2	New York	3,618	9.4%
11	North Carolina	1,139	3.0%
49	North Dakota	54	0.1%
7	Ohio	1,520	4.0%
29	Oklahoma	304	0.8%
28	Oregon	391	1.0%
6	Pennsylvania	1,757	4.6%
39	Rhode Island	183	0.5%
24	South Carolina	529	1.4%
47	South Dakota	60	0.2%
15	Tennessee	810	2.1%
3	Texas	2,561	6.7%
32	Utah	254	0.7%
45	Vermont	86	0.2%
14	Virginia	1,063	2.8%
18	Washington	660	1.7%
37	West Virginia	210	0.5%
23	Wisconsin	548	1.4%
50	Wyoming	50	0.1%

RANK ORDER

RANK	STATE	PHYSICIANS	% of USA
1	California	4,477	11.7%
2	New York	3,618	9.4%
3	Texas	2,561	6.7%
4	Florida	2,019	5.3%
5	Illinois	1,818	4.7%
6	Pennsylvania	1,757	4.6%
7	Ohio	1,520	4.0%
8	New Jersey	1,500	3.9%
9	Michigan	1,308	3.4%
10	Georgia	1,197	3.1%
11	North Carolina	1,139	3.0%
12	Massachusetts	1,109	2.9%
13	Maryland	1,091	2.8%
14	Virginia	1,063	2.8%
15	Tennessee	810	2.1%
16	Missouri	724	1.9%
17	Louisiana	716	1.9%
18	Washington	660	1.7%
19	Connecticut	658	1.7%
20	Indiana	596	1.6%
21	Arizona	583	1.5%
22	Colorado	550	1.4%
23	Wisconsin	548	1.4%
24	South Carolina	529	1.4%
25	Alabama	524	1.4%
26	Minnesota	509	1.3%
27	Kentucky	463	1.2%
28	Oregon	391	1.0%
29	Oklahoma	304	0.8%
30	Mississippi	299	0.8%
31	Kansas	274	0.7%
32	Utah	254	0.7%
33	Arkansas	234	0.6%
34	Hawaii	224	0.6%
35	Nevada	216	0.6%
36	Iowa	215	0.6%
37	West Virginia	210	0.5%
38	New Mexico	187	0.5%
39	Rhode Island	183	0.5%
40	Nebraska	169	0.4%
40	New Hampshire	169	0.4%
42	Maine	132	0.3%
43	Idaho	107	0.3%
44	Delaware	94	0.2%
45	Vermont	86	0.2%
46	Montana	82	0.2%
47	South Dakota	60	0.2%
48	Alaska	58	0.2%
49	North Dakota	54	0.1%
50	Wyoming	50	0.1%
	District of Columbia	230	0.6%

Source: American Medical Association (Chicago, Illinois)
"Physician Characteristics and Distribution in the U.S." (2001-2002 Edition)
*As of December 31, 1999. Total does not include 543 physicians in U.S. territories and possessions. Obstetrics and Gynecology includes Gynecology and Oncology, Maternal and Fetal Medicine and Reproductive Endocrinology.

Rate of Nonfederal Physicians in Obstetrics and Gynecology in 1999

National Rate = 27 Physicians per 100,000 Female Population*

<u>ALPHA ORDER</u>

RANK	STATE	RATE
29	Alabama	23
40	Alaska	20
25	Arizona	24
44	Arkansas	18
17	California	27
17	Colorado	27
2	Connecticut	39
25	Delaware	24
19	Florida	26
9	Georgia	30
3	Hawaii	38
47	Idaho	17
11	Illinois	29
40	Indiana	20
50	Iowa	15
40	Kansas	20
29	Kentucky	23
8	Louisiana	32
34	Maine	21
1	Maryland	41
7	Massachusetts	35
19	Michigan	26
34	Minnesota	21
34	Mississippi	21
19	Missouri	26
44	Montana	18
40	Nebraska	20
25	Nevada	24
15	New Hampshire	28
5	New Jersey	36
34	New Mexico	21
3	New York	38
11	North Carolina	29
47	North Dakota	17
19	Ohio	26
44	Oklahoma	18
29	Oregon	23
15	Pennsylvania	28
5	Rhode Island	36
19	South Carolina	26
49	South Dakota	16
11	Tennessee	29
24	Texas	25
25	Utah	24
11	Vermont	29
9	Virginia	30
29	Washington	23
33	West Virginia	22
34	Wisconsin	21
34	Wyoming	21

<u>RANK ORDER</u>

RANK	STATE	RATE
1	Maryland	41
2	Connecticut	39
3	Hawaii	38
3	New York	38
5	New Jersey	36
5	Rhode Island	36
7	Massachusetts	35
8	Louisiana	32
9	Georgia	30
9	Virginia	30
11	Illinois	29
11	North Carolina	29
11	Tennessee	29
11	Vermont	29
15	New Hampshire	28
15	Pennsylvania	28
17	California	27
17	Colorado	27
19	Florida	26
19	Michigan	26
19	Missouri	26
19	Ohio	26
19	South Carolina	26
24	Texas	25
25	Arizona	24
25	Delaware	24
25	Nevada	24
25	Utah	24
29	Alabama	23
29	Kentucky	23
29	Oregon	23
29	Washington	23
33	West Virginia	22
34	Maine	21
34	Minnesota	21
34	Mississippi	21
34	New Mexico	21
34	Wisconsin	21
34	Wyoming	21
40	Alaska	20
40	Indiana	20
40	Kansas	20
40	Nebraska	20
44	Arkansas	18
44	Montana	18
44	Oklahoma	18
47	Idaho	17
47	North Dakota	17
49	South Dakota	16
50	Iowa	15

District of Columbia   83

Source: Morgan Quitno Press using data from American Medical Association (Chicago, Illinois)
   "Physician Characteristics and Distribution in the U.S." (2001-2002 Edition)
*As of December 31, 1999. National rate does not include physicians in U.S. territories and possessions. Obstetrics and Gynecology includes Gynecology and Oncology, Maternal and Fetal Medicine and Reproductive Endocrinology.

Nonfederal Physicians in Ophthalmology in 1999

National Total = 17,220 Physicians*

ALPHA ORDER

RANK	STATE	PHYSICIANS	% of USA
26	Alabama	211	1.2%
49	Alaska	30	0.2%
23	Arizona	262	1.5%
32	Arkansas	141	0.8%
1	California	2,083	12.1%
24	Colorado	252	1.5%
21	Connecticut	289	1.7%
44	Delaware	47	0.3%
3	Florida	1,090	6.3%
14	Georgia	369	2.1%
37	Hawaii	85	0.5%
42	Idaho	62	0.4%
6	Illinois	682	4.0%
22	Indiana	271	1.6%
30	Iowa	149	0.9%
29	Kansas	151	0.9%
28	Kentucky	191	1.1%
18	Louisiana	319	1.9%
39	Maine	75	0.4%
11	Maryland	476	2.8%
10	Massachusetts	532	3.1%
9	Michigan	538	3.1%
20	Minnesota	297	1.7%
33	Mississippi	138	0.8%
17	Missouri	334	1.9%
46	Montana	41	0.2%
35	Nebraska	96	0.6%
38	Nevada	82	0.5%
43	New Hampshire	61	0.4%
8	New Jersey	615	3.6%
39	New Mexico	75	0.4%
2	New York	1,743	10.1%
12	North Carolina	412	2.4%
47	North Dakota	38	0.2%
7	Ohio	637	3.7%
31	Oklahoma	145	0.8%
27	Oregon	203	1.2%
5	Pennsylvania	882	5.1%
41	Rhode Island	72	0.4%
25	South Carolina	229	1.3%
48	South Dakota	35	0.2%
15	Tennessee	339	2.0%
4	Texas	1,030	6.0%
34	Utah	114	0.7%
45	Vermont	43	0.2%
13	Virginia	409	2.4%
19	Washington	305	1.8%
36	West Virginia	94	0.5%
16	Wisconsin	336	2.0%
50	Wyoming	16	0.1%

RANK ORDER

RANK	STATE	PHYSICIANS	% of USA
1	California	2,083	12.1%
2	New York	1,743	10.1%
3	Florida	1,090	6.3%
4	Texas	1,030	6.0%
5	Pennsylvania	882	5.1%
6	Illinois	682	4.0%
7	Ohio	637	3.7%
8	New Jersey	615	3.6%
9	Michigan	538	3.1%
10	Massachusetts	532	3.1%
11	Maryland	476	2.8%
12	North Carolina	412	2.4%
13	Virginia	409	2.4%
14	Georgia	369	2.1%
15	Tennessee	339	2.0%
16	Wisconsin	336	2.0%
17	Missouri	334	1.9%
18	Louisiana	319	1.9%
19	Washington	305	1.8%
20	Minnesota	297	1.7%
21	Connecticut	289	1.7%
22	Indiana	271	1.6%
23	Arizona	262	1.5%
24	Colorado	252	1.5%
25	South Carolina	229	1.3%
26	Alabama	211	1.2%
27	Oregon	203	1.2%
28	Kentucky	191	1.1%
29	Kansas	151	0.9%
30	Iowa	149	0.9%
31	Oklahoma	145	0.8%
32	Arkansas	141	0.8%
33	Mississippi	138	0.8%
34	Utah	114	0.7%
35	Nebraska	96	0.6%
36	West Virginia	94	0.5%
37	Hawaii	85	0.5%
38	Nevada	82	0.5%
39	Maine	75	0.4%
39	New Mexico	75	0.4%
41	Rhode Island	72	0.4%
42	Idaho	62	0.4%
43	New Hampshire	61	0.4%
44	Delaware	47	0.3%
45	Vermont	43	0.2%
46	Montana	41	0.2%
47	North Dakota	38	0.2%
48	South Dakota	35	0.2%
49	Alaska	30	0.2%
50	Wyoming	16	0.1%
	District of Columbia	94	0.5%

Source: American Medical Association (Chicago, Illinois)
   "Physician Characteristics and Distribution in the U.S." (2001-2002 Edition)
As of December 31, 1999. Total does not include 180 physicians in U.S. territories and possessions.
Ophthalmology is the branch of medicine dealing with the anatomy, functions and diseases of the eye.

Rate of Nonfederal Physicians in Ophthalmology in 1999

National Rate = 6.3 Physicians per 100,000 Population*

ALPHA ORDER				RANK ORDER		
RANK	STATE	RATE		RANK	STATE	RATE
40	Alabama	4.8		1	New York	9.6
40	Alaska	4.8		2	Maryland	9.2
28	Arizona	5.5		3	Connecticut	8.8
28	Arkansas	5.5		4	Massachusetts	8.6
13	California	6.3		5	New Jersey	7.6
14	Colorado	6.2		6	Pennsylvania	7.4
3	Connecticut	8.8		7	Louisiana	7.3
14	Delaware	6.2		7	Rhode Island	7.3
9	Florida	7.2		9	Florida	7.2
44	Georgia	4.7		9	Hawaii	7.2
9	Hawaii	7.2		9	Vermont	7.2
38	Idaho	5.0		12	Wisconsin	6.4
27	Illinois	5.6		13	California	6.3
45	Indiana	4.6		14	Colorado	6.2
34	Iowa	5.2		14	Delaware	6.2
25	Kansas	5.7		14	Minnesota	6.2
40	Kentucky	4.8		14	Tennessee	6.2
7	Louisiana	7.3		18	Missouri	6.1
20	Maine	6.0		18	Oregon	6.1
2	Maryland	9.2		20	Maine	6.0
4	Massachusetts	8.6		20	North Dakota	6.0
28	Michigan	5.5		20	Virginia	6.0
14	Minnesota	6.2		23	South Carolina	5.9
38	Mississippi	5.0		24	Nebraska	5.8
18	Missouri	6.1		25	Kansas	5.7
45	Montana	4.6		25	Ohio	5.7
24	Nebraska	5.8		27	Illinois	5.6
47	Nevada	4.5		28	Arizona	5.5
36	New Hampshire	5.1		28	Arkansas	5.5
5	New Jersey	7.6		28	Michigan	5.5
48	New Mexico	4.3		31	North Carolina	5.4
1	New York	9.6		31	Utah	5.4
31	North Carolina	5.4		33	Washington	5.3
20	North Dakota	6.0		34	Iowa	5.2
25	Ohio	5.7		34	West Virginia	5.2
48	Oklahoma	4.3		36	New Hampshire	5.1
18	Oregon	6.1		36	Texas	5.1
6	Pennsylvania	7.4		38	Idaho	5.0
7	Rhode Island	7.3		38	Mississippi	5.0
23	South Carolina	5.9		40	Alabama	4.8
40	South Dakota	4.8		40	Alaska	4.8
14	Tennessee	6.2		40	Kentucky	4.8
36	Texas	5.1		40	South Dakota	4.8
31	Utah	5.4		44	Georgia	4.7
9	Vermont	7.2		45	Indiana	4.6
20	Virginia	6.0		45	Montana	4.6
33	Washington	5.3		47	Nevada	4.5
34	West Virginia	5.2		48	New Mexico	4.3
12	Wisconsin	6.4		48	Oklahoma	4.3
50	Wyoming	3.3		50	Wyoming	3.3
					District of Columbia	18.1

Source: Morgan Quitno Press using data from American Medical Association (Chicago, Illinois)
"Physician Characteristics and Distribution in the U.S." (2001-2002 Edition)
*As of December 31, 1999. National rate does not include physicians in U.S. territories and possessions.
Ophthalmology is the branch of medicine dealing with the anatomy, functions and diseases of the eye.

Nonfederal Physicians in Orthopedic Surgery in 1999

National Total = 21,055 Physicians*

ALPHA ORDER

RANK	STATE	PHYSICIANS	% of USA
25	Alabama	307	1.5%
48	Alaska	49	0.2%
24	Arizona	310	1.5%
31	Arkansas	168	0.8%
1	California	2,591	12.3%
23	Colorado	347	1.6%
22	Connecticut	353	1.7%
47	Delaware	51	0.2%
4	Florida	1,179	5.6%
12	Georgia	540	2.6%
43	Hawaii	93	0.4%
42	Idaho	98	0.5%
6	Illinois	831	3.9%
20	Indiana	391	1.9%
30	Iowa	176	0.8%
33	Kansas	165	0.8%
28	Kentucky	267	1.3%
21	Louisiana	382	1.8%
40	Maine	110	0.5%
14	Maryland	493	2.3%
8	Massachusetts	664	3.2%
11	Michigan	566	2.7%
19	Minnesota	402	1.9%
34	Mississippi	150	0.7%
18	Missouri	403	1.9%
44	Montana	83	0.4%
35	Nebraska	135	0.6%
41	Nevada	101	0.5%
38	New Hampshire	116	0.6%
9	New Jersey	656	3.1%
36	New Mexico	133	0.6%
2	New York	1,702	8.1%
10	North Carolina	591	2.8%
50	North Dakota	42	0.2%
7	Ohio	826	3.9%
29	Oklahoma	197	0.9%
27	Oregon	270	1.3%
5	Pennsylvania	1,019	4.8%
37	Rhode Island	117	0.6%
26	South Carolina	274	1.3%
46	South Dakota	56	0.3%
16	Tennessee	457	2.2%
3	Texas	1,280	6.1%
31	Utah	168	0.8%
45	Vermont	59	0.3%
13	Virginia	533	2.5%
15	Washington	463	2.2%
38	West Virginia	116	0.6%
17	Wisconsin	434	2.1%
49	Wyoming	47	0.2%

RANK ORDER

RANK	STATE	PHYSICIANS	% of USA
1	California	2,591	12.3%
2	New York	1,702	8.1%
3	Texas	1,280	6.1%
4	Florida	1,179	5.6%
5	Pennsylvania	1,019	4.8%
6	Illinois	831	3.9%
7	Ohio	826	3.9%
8	Massachusetts	664	3.2%
9	New Jersey	656	3.1%
10	North Carolina	591	2.8%
11	Michigan	566	2.7%
12	Georgia	540	2.6%
13	Virginia	533	2.5%
14	Maryland	493	2.3%
15	Washington	463	2.2%
16	Tennessee	457	2.2%
17	Wisconsin	434	2.1%
18	Missouri	403	1.9%
19	Minnesota	402	1.9%
20	Indiana	391	1.9%
21	Louisiana	382	1.8%
22	Connecticut	353	1.7%
23	Colorado	347	1.6%
24	Arizona	310	1.5%
25	Alabama	307	1.5%
26	South Carolina	274	1.3%
27	Oregon	270	1.3%
28	Kentucky	267	1.3%
29	Oklahoma	197	0.9%
30	Iowa	176	0.8%
31	Arkansas	168	0.8%
31	Utah	168	0.8%
33	Kansas	165	0.8%
34	Mississippi	150	0.7%
35	Nebraska	135	0.6%
36	New Mexico	133	0.6%
37	Rhode Island	117	0.6%
38	New Hampshire	116	0.6%
38	West Virginia	116	0.6%
40	Maine	110	0.5%
41	Nevada	101	0.5%
42	Idaho	98	0.5%
43	Hawaii	93	0.4%
44	Montana	83	0.4%
45	Vermont	59	0.3%
46	South Dakota	56	0.3%
47	Delaware	51	0.2%
48	Alaska	49	0.2%
49	Wyoming	47	0.2%
50	North Dakota	42	0.2%
	District of Columbia	94	0.4%

Source: American Medical Association (Chicago, Illinois)
"Physician Characteristics and Distribution in the U.S." (2001-2002 Edition)
*As of December 31, 1999. Total does not include 125 physicians in U.S. territories and possessions.
Orthopedics is the branch of medicine dealing with the skeletal system.

Rate of Nonfederal Physicians in Orthopedic Surgery in 1999

National Rate = 7.7 Physicians per 100,000 Population*

ALPHA ORDER

RANK ORDER

RANK	STATE	RATE		RANK	STATE	RATE
34	Alabama	7.0		1	Rhode Island	11.8
21	Alaska	7.9		2	Connecticut	10.8
42	Arizona	6.5		2	Massachusetts	10.8
39	Arkansas	6.6		4	Vermont	9.9
23	California	7.8		5	Wyoming	9.8
12	Colorado	8.6		6	New Hampshire	9.7
2	Connecticut	10.8		7	Maryland	9.5
37	Delaware	6.8		8	Montana	9.4
23	Florida	7.8		8	New York	9.4
35	Georgia	6.9		10	Maine	8.8
23	Hawaii	7.8		11	Louisiana	8.7
23	Idaho	7.8		12	Colorado	8.6
35	Illinois	6.9		13	Pennsylvania	8.5
39	Indiana	6.6		14	Minnesota	8.4
46	Iowa	6.1		15	Tennessee	8.3
45	Kansas	6.2		15	Wisconsin	8.3
38	Kentucky	6.7		17	Nebraska	8.1
11	Louisiana	8.7		17	New Jersey	8.1
10	Maine	8.8		17	Oregon	8.1
7	Maryland	9.5		20	Washington	8.0
2	Massachusetts	10.8		21	Alaska	7.9
48	Michigan	5.7		21	Utah	7.9
14	Minnesota	8.4		23	California	7.8
50	Mississippi	5.4		23	Florida	7.8
31	Missouri	7.4		23	Hawaii	7.8
8	Montana	9.4		23	Idaho	7.8
17	Nebraska	8.1		23	Virginia	7.8
49	Nevada	5.6		28	North Carolina	7.7
6	New Hampshire	9.7		29	New Mexico	7.6
17	New Jersey	8.1		29	South Dakota	7.6
29	New Mexico	7.6		31	Missouri	7.4
8	New York	9.4		32	Ohio	7.3
28	North Carolina	7.7		33	South Carolina	7.1
39	North Dakota	6.6		34	Alabama	7.0
32	Ohio	7.3		35	Georgia	6.9
47	Oklahoma	5.9		35	Illinois	6.9
17	Oregon	8.1		37	Delaware	6.8
13	Pennsylvania	8.5		38	Kentucky	6.7
1	Rhode Island	11.8		39	Arkansas	6.6
33	South Carolina	7.1		39	Indiana	6.6
29	South Dakota	7.6		39	North Dakota	6.6
15	Tennessee	8.3		42	Arizona	6.5
43	Texas	6.4		43	Texas	6.4
21	Utah	7.9		43	West Virginia	6.4
4	Vermont	9.9		45	Kansas	6.2
23	Virginia	7.8		46	Iowa	6.1
20	Washington	8.0		47	Oklahoma	5.9
43	West Virginia	6.4		48	Michigan	5.7
15	Wisconsin	8.3		49	Nevada	5.6
5	Wyoming	9.8		50	Mississippi	5.4

District of Columbia 18.1

Source: Morgan Quitno Press using data from American Medical Association (Chicago, Illinois)
"Physician Characteristics and Distribution in the U.S." (2001-2002 Edition)
*As of December 31, 1999. National rate does not include physicians in U.S. territories and possessions.
Orthopedics is the branch of medicine dealing with the skeletal system.

Nonfederal Physicians in Plastic Surgery in 1999

National Total = 5,829 Physicians*

ALPHA ORDER

RANK	STATE	PHYSICIANS	% of USA
23	Alabama	79	1.4%
49	Alaska	6	0.1%
17	Arizona	119	2.0%
35	Arkansas	30	0.5%
1	California	879	15.1%
19	Colorado	89	1.5%
20	Connecticut	87	1.5%
42	Delaware	18	0.3%
3	Florida	467	8.0%
14	Georgia	139	2.4%
34	Hawaii	31	0.5%
40	Idaho	19	0.3%
6	Illinois	208	3.6%
22	Indiana	80	1.4%
37	Iowa	24	0.4%
30	Kansas	48	0.8%
25	Kentucky	74	1.3%
21	Louisiana	81	1.4%
45	Maine	13	0.2%
13	Maryland	140	2.4%
11	Massachusetts	149	2.6%
9	Michigan	163	2.8%
26	Minnesota	71	1.2%
33	Mississippi	33	0.6%
16	Missouri	124	2.1%
43	Montana	17	0.3%
36	Nebraska	27	0.5%
32	Nevada	38	0.7%
44	New Hampshire	16	0.3%
8	New Jersey	185	3.2%
37	New Mexico	24	0.4%
2	New York	567	9.7%
10	North Carolina	152	2.6%
46	North Dakota	12	0.2%
7	Ohio	187	3.2%
31	Oklahoma	46	0.8%
29	Oregon	52	0.9%
5	Pennsylvania	229	3.9%
40	Rhode Island	19	0.3%
28	South Carolina	59	1.0%
48	South Dakota	8	0.1%
15	Tennessee	138	2.4%
4	Texas	420	7.2%
27	Utah	64	1.1%
47	Vermont	11	0.2%
12	Virginia	142	2.4%
18	Washington	107	1.8%
39	West Virginia	23	0.4%
23	Wisconsin	79	1.4%
50	Wyoming	3	0.1%

RANK ORDER

RANK	STATE	PHYSICIANS	% of USA
1	California	879	15.1%
2	New York	567	9.7%
3	Florida	467	8.0%
4	Texas	420	7.2%
5	Pennsylvania	229	3.9%
6	Illinois	208	3.6%
7	Ohio	187	3.2%
8	New Jersey	185	3.2%
9	Michigan	163	2.8%
10	North Carolina	152	2.6%
11	Massachusetts	149	2.6%
12	Virginia	142	2.4%
13	Maryland	140	2.4%
14	Georgia	139	2.4%
15	Tennessee	138	2.4%
16	Missouri	124	2.1%
17	Arizona	119	2.0%
18	Washington	107	1.8%
19	Colorado	89	1.5%
20	Connecticut	87	1.5%
21	Louisiana	81	1.4%
22	Indiana	80	1.4%
23	Alabama	79	1.4%
23	Wisconsin	79	1.4%
25	Kentucky	74	1.3%
26	Minnesota	71	1.2%
27	Utah	64	1.1%
28	South Carolina	59	1.0%
29	Oregon	52	0.9%
30	Kansas	48	0.8%
31	Oklahoma	46	0.8%
32	Nevada	38	0.7%
33	Mississippi	33	0.6%
34	Hawaii	31	0.5%
35	Arkansas	30	0.5%
36	Nebraska	27	0.5%
37	Iowa	24	0.4%
37	New Mexico	24	0.4%
39	West Virginia	23	0.4%
40	Idaho	19	0.3%
40	Rhode Island	19	0.3%
42	Delaware	18	0.3%
43	Montana	17	0.3%
44	New Hampshire	16	0.3%
45	Maine	13	0.2%
46	North Dakota	12	0.2%
47	Vermont	11	0.2%
48	South Dakota	8	0.1%
49	Alaska	6	0.1%
50	Wyoming	3	0.1%
	District of Columbia	33	0.6%

Source: American Medical Association (Chicago, Illinois)
    "Physician Characteristics and Distribution in the U.S." (2001-2002 Edition)
As of December 31, 1999. Total does not include 34 physicians in U.S. territories and possessions.

Rate of Nonfederal Physicians in Plastic Surgery in 1999

National Rate = 2.1 Physicians per 100,000 Population*

ALPHA ORDER

RANK	STATE	RATE
27	Alabama	1.8
47	Alaska	1.0
8	Arizona	2.5
44	Arkansas	1.2
4	California	2.7
14	Colorado	2.2
4	Connecticut	2.7
10	Delaware	2.4
1	Florida	3.1
27	Georgia	1.8
7	Hawaii	2.6
35	Idaho	1.5
30	Illinois	1.7
41	Indiana	1.3
49	Iowa	0.8
27	Kansas	1.8
19	Kentucky	1.9
19	Louisiana	1.9
47	Maine	1.0
4	Maryland	2.7
10	Massachusetts	2.4
30	Michigan	1.7
35	Minnesota	1.5
44	Mississippi	1.2
12	Missouri	2.3
19	Montana	1.9
33	Nebraska	1.6
15	Nevada	2.1
41	New Hampshire	1.3
12	New Jersey	2.3
39	New Mexico	1.4
1	New York	3.1
18	North Carolina	2.0
19	North Dakota	1.9
30	Ohio	1.7
39	Oklahoma	1.4
33	Oregon	1.6
19	Pennsylvania	1.9
19	Rhode Island	1.9
35	South Carolina	1.5
46	South Dakota	1.1
8	Tennessee	2.5
15	Texas	2.1
3	Utah	3.0
19	Vermont	1.9
15	Virginia	2.1
19	Washington	1.9
41	West Virginia	1.3
35	Wisconsin	1.5
50	Wyoming	0.6

RANK ORDER

RANK	STATE	RATE
1	Florida	3.1
1	New York	3.1
3	Utah	3.0
4	California	2.7
4	Connecticut	2.7
4	Maryland	2.7
7	Hawaii	2.6
8	Arizona	2.5
8	Tennessee	2.5
10	Delaware	2.4
10	Massachusetts	2.4
12	Missouri	2.3
12	New Jersey	2.3
14	Colorado	2.2
15	Nevada	2.1
15	Texas	2.1
15	Virginia	2.1
18	North Carolina	2.0
19	Kentucky	1.9
19	Louisiana	1.9
19	Montana	1.9
19	North Dakota	1.9
19	Pennsylvania	1.9
19	Rhode Island	1.9
19	Vermont	1.9
19	Washington	1.9
27	Alabama	1.8
27	Georgia	1.8
27	Kansas	1.8
30	Illinois	1.7
30	Michigan	1.7
30	Ohio	1.7
33	Nebraska	1.6
33	Oregon	1.6
35	Idaho	1.5
35	Minnesota	1.5
35	South Carolina	1.5
35	Wisconsin	1.5
39	New Mexico	1.4
39	Oklahoma	1.4
41	Indiana	1.3
41	New Hampshire	1.3
41	West Virginia	1.3
44	Arkansas	1.2
44	Mississippi	1.2
46	South Dakota	1.1
47	Alaska	1.0
47	Maine	1.0
49	Iowa	0.8
50	Wyoming	0.6

District of Columbia   6.4

*Source: Morgan Quitno Press using data from American Medical Association (Chicago, Illinois)
"Physician Characteristics and Distribution in the U.S." (2001-2002 Edition)*
As of December 31, 1999. National rate does not include physicians in U.S. territories and possessions.

Nonfederal Physicians in Other Specialties in 1999

National Total = 185,203 Physicians*

<u>ALPHA ORDER</u>

RANK	STATE	PHYSICIANS	% of USA
28	Alabama	2,062	1.1%
49	Alaska	285	0.2%
24	Arizona	2,756	1.5%
32	Arkansas	1,214	0.7%
1	California	22,564	12.2%
22	Colorado	2,840	1.5%
17	Connecticut	3,356	1.8%
44	Delaware	498	0.3%
5	Florida	9,472	5.1%
14	Georgia	4,327	2.3%
37	Hawaii	877	0.5%
46	Idaho	468	0.3%
6	Illinois	8,345	4.5%
20	Indiana	3,191	1.7%
31	Iowa	1,230	0.7%
30	Kansas	1,439	0.8%
25	Kentucky	2,252	1.2%
23	Louisiana	2,766	1.5%
41	Maine	832	0.4%
11	Maryland	5,542	3.0%
7	Massachusetts	7,673	4.1%
10	Michigan	5,988	3.2%
21	Minnesota	3,011	1.6%
34	Mississippi	1,100	0.6%
19	Missouri	3,278	1.8%
45	Montana	472	0.3%
38	Nebraska	865	0.5%
39	Nevada	863	0.5%
42	New Hampshire	815	0.4%
9	New Jersey	6,080	3.3%
35	New Mexico	1,048	0.6%
2	New York	19,129	10.3%
12	North Carolina	4,691	2.5%
47	North Dakota	348	0.2%
8	Ohio	6,949	3.8%
29	Oklahoma	1,458	0.8%
27	Oregon	2,117	1.1%
4	Pennsylvania	9,800	5.3%
40	Rhode Island	854	0.5%
26	South Carolina	2,176	1.2%
48	South Dakota	298	0.2%
16	Tennessee	3,395	1.8%
3	Texas	10,946	5.9%
33	Utah	1,185	0.6%
43	Vermont	535	0.3%
13	Virginia	4,351	2.3%
15	Washington	3,825	2.1%
36	West Virginia	975	0.5%
18	Wisconsin	3,343	1.8%
50	Wyoming	208	0.1%

<u>RANK ORDER</u>

RANK	STATE	PHYSICIANS	% of USA
1	California	22,564	12.2%
2	New York	19,129	10.3%
3	Texas	10,946	5.9%
4	Pennsylvania	9,800	5.3%
5	Florida	9,472	5.1%
6	Illinois	8,345	4.5%
7	Massachusetts	7,673	4.1%
8	Ohio	6,949	3.8%
9	New Jersey	6,080	3.3%
10	Michigan	5,988	3.2%
11	Maryland	5,542	3.0%
12	North Carolina	4,691	2.5%
13	Virginia	4,351	2.3%
14	Georgia	4,327	2.3%
15	Washington	3,825	2.1%
16	Tennessee	3,395	1.8%
17	Connecticut	3,356	1.8%
18	Wisconsin	3,343	1.8%
19	Missouri	3,278	1.8%
20	Indiana	3,191	1.7%
21	Minnesota	3,011	1.6%
22	Colorado	2,840	1.5%
23	Louisiana	2,766	1.5%
24	Arizona	2,756	1.5%
25	Kentucky	2,252	1.2%
26	South Carolina	2,176	1.2%
27	Oregon	2,117	1.1%
28	Alabama	2,062	1.1%
29	Oklahoma	1,458	0.8%
30	Kansas	1,439	0.8%
31	Iowa	1,230	0.7%
32	Arkansas	1,214	0.7%
33	Utah	1,185	0.6%
34	Mississippi	1,100	0.6%
35	New Mexico	1,048	0.6%
36	West Virginia	975	0.5%
37	Hawaii	877	0.5%
38	Nebraska	865	0.5%
39	Nevada	863	0.5%
40	Rhode Island	854	0.5%
41	Maine	832	0.4%
42	New Hampshire	815	0.4%
43	Vermont	535	0.3%
44	Delaware	498	0.3%
45	Montana	472	0.3%
46	Idaho	468	0.3%
47	North Dakota	348	0.2%
48	South Dakota	298	0.2%
49	Alaska	285	0.2%
50	Wyoming	208	0.1%
	District of Columbia	1,111	0.6%

Source: American Medical Association (Chicago, Illinois)
  "Physician Characteristics and Distribution in the U.S." (2001-2002 Edition)
As of December 31, 1999. Total does not include 2,130 physicians in U.S. territories and possessions. Other Specialties include Aerospace Medicine, Anesthesiology, Child Psychiatry, Diagnostic Radiology, Emergency Medicine, Forensic Pathology, Nuclear Medicine, Occupational Medicine, Neurology, Psychiatry, Public Health, Anatomic/Clinical Pathology, Radiology, Radiation Oncology and other specialties.

Rate of Nonfederal Physicians in Other Specialties in 1999

National Rate = 68 Physicians per 100,000 Population*

ALPHA ORDER				RANK ORDER		
RANK	STATE	RATE		RANK	STATE	RATE
43	Alabama	47		1	Massachusetts	124
44	Alaska	46		2	Maryland	107
29	Arizona	58		3	New York	105
41	Arkansas	48		4	Connecticut	102
12	California	68		5	Vermont	90
10	Colorado	70		6	Rhode Island	86
4	Connecticut	102		7	Pennsylvania	82
14	Delaware	66		8	New Jersey	75
19	Florida	63		9	Hawaii	74
31	Georgia	56		10	Colorado	70
9	Hawaii	74		11	Illinois	69
50	Idaho	37		12	California	68
11	Illinois	69		12	New Hampshire	68
36	Indiana	54		14	Delaware	66
45	Iowa	43		14	Maine	66
36	Kansas	54		14	Washington	66
30	Kentucky	57		17	Oregon	64
19	Louisiana	63		17	Wisconsin	64
14	Maine	66		19	Florida	63
2	Maryland	107		19	Louisiana	63
1	Massachusetts	124		19	Minnesota	63
25	Michigan	61		19	Virginia	63
19	Minnesota	63		23	Ohio	62
49	Mississippi	40		23	Tennessee	62
27	Missouri	60		25	Michigan	61
39	Montana	53		25	North Carolina	61
40	Nebraska	52		27	Missouri	60
41	Nevada	48		27	New Mexico	60
12	New Hampshire	68		29	Arizona	58
8	New Jersey	75		30	Kentucky	57
27	New Mexico	60		31	Georgia	56
3	New York	105		31	South Carolina	56
25	North Carolina	61		31	Utah	56
34	North Dakota	55		34	North Dakota	55
23	Ohio	62		34	Texas	55
45	Oklahoma	43		36	Indiana	54
17	Oregon	64		36	Kansas	54
7	Pennsylvania	82		36	West Virginia	54
6	Rhode Island	86		39	Montana	53
31	South Carolina	56		40	Nebraska	52
48	South Dakota	41		41	Arkansas	48
23	Tennessee	62		41	Nevada	48
34	Texas	55		43	Alabama	47
31	Utah	56		44	Alaska	46
5	Vermont	90		45	Iowa	43
19	Virginia	63		45	Oklahoma	43
14	Washington	66		45	Wyoming	43
36	West Virginia	54		48	South Dakota	41
17	Wisconsin	64		49	Mississippi	40
45	Wyoming	43		50	Idaho	37
					District of Columbia	214

Source: Morgan Quitno Press using data from American Medical Association (Chicago, Illinois)
    "Physician Characteristics and Distribution in the U.S." (2001-2002 Edition)
*As of December 31, 1999. National rate does not include physicians in U.S. territories and possessions. Other
Specialties include Aerospace Medicine, Anesthesiology, Child Psychiatry, Diagnostic Radiology, Emergency
Medicine, Forensic Pathology, Nuclear Medicine, Occupational Medicine, Neurology, Psychiatry, Public Health,
Anatomic/Clinical Pathology, Radiology, Radiation Oncology and other specialties.

465

Nonfederal Physicians in Anesthesiology in 1999

National Total = 33,929 Physicians*

ALPHA ORDER

RANK	STATE	PHYSICIANS	% of USA
27	Alabama	399	1.2%
47	Alaska	54	0.2%
19	Arizona	611	1.8%
32	Arkansas	258	0.8%
1	California	4,203	12.4%
22	Colorado	523	1.5%
21	Connecticut	524	1.5%
46	Delaware	60	0.2%
4	Florida	2,045	6.0%
13	Georgia	780	2.3%
41	Hawaii	129	0.4%
44	Idaho	82	0.2%
5	Illinois	1,647	4.9%
15	Indiana	745	2.2%
33	Iowa	254	0.7%
31	Kansas	267	0.8%
24	Kentucky	470	1.4%
25	Louisiana	454	1.3%
39	Maine	146	0.4%
10	Maryland	882	2.6%
9	Massachusetts	1,197	3.5%
11	Michigan	831	2.4%
23	Minnesota	478	1.4%
34	Mississippi	238	0.7%
20	Missouri	591	1.7%
42	Montana	105	0.3%
37	Nebraska	173	0.5%
35	Nevada	224	0.7%
40	New Hampshire	131	0.4%
8	New Jersey	1,212	3.6%
36	New Mexico	184	0.5%
2	New York	3,061	9.0%
14	North Carolina	770	2.3%
48	North Dakota	48	0.1%
7	Ohio	1,305	3.8%
29	Oklahoma	292	0.9%
26	Oregon	426	1.3%
6	Pennsylvania	1,567	4.6%
43	Rhode Island	99	0.3%
28	South Carolina	376	1.1%
49	South Dakota	46	0.1%
17	Tennessee	691	2.0%
3	Texas	2,482	7.3%
30	Utah	270	0.8%
45	Vermont	65	0.2%
16	Virginia	726	2.1%
12	Washington	828	2.4%
38	West Virginia	164	0.5%
18	Wisconsin	674	2.0%
50	Wyoming	43	0.1%

RANK ORDER

RANK	STATE	PHYSICIANS	% of USA
1	California	4,203	12.4%
2	New York	3,061	9.0%
3	Texas	2,482	7.3%
4	Florida	2,045	6.0%
5	Illinois	1,647	4.9%
6	Pennsylvania	1,567	4.6%
7	Ohio	1,305	3.8%
8	New Jersey	1,212	3.6%
9	Massachusetts	1,197	3.5%
10	Maryland	882	2.6%
11	Michigan	831	2.4%
12	Washington	828	2.4%
13	Georgia	780	2.3%
14	North Carolina	770	2.3%
15	Indiana	745	2.2%
16	Virginia	726	2.1%
17	Tennessee	691	2.0%
18	Wisconsin	674	2.0%
19	Arizona	611	1.8%
20	Missouri	591	1.7%
21	Connecticut	524	1.5%
22	Colorado	523	1.5%
23	Minnesota	478	1.4%
24	Kentucky	470	1.4%
25	Louisiana	454	1.3%
26	Oregon	426	1.3%
27	Alabama	399	1.2%
28	South Carolina	376	1.1%
29	Oklahoma	292	0.9%
30	Utah	270	0.8%
31	Kansas	267	0.8%
32	Arkansas	258	0.8%
33	Iowa	254	0.7%
34	Mississippi	238	0.7%
35	Nevada	224	0.7%
36	New Mexico	184	0.5%
37	Nebraska	173	0.5%
38	West Virginia	164	0.5%
39	Maine	146	0.4%
40	New Hampshire	131	0.4%
41	Hawaii	129	0.4%
42	Montana	105	0.3%
43	Rhode Island	99	0.3%
44	Idaho	82	0.2%
45	Vermont	65	0.2%
46	Delaware	60	0.2%
47	Alaska	54	0.2%
48	North Dakota	48	0.1%
49	South Dakota	46	0.1%
50	Wyoming	43	0.1%
	District of Columbia	99	0.3%

Source: American Medical Association (Chicago, Illinois)
"Physician Characteristics and Distribution in the U.S." (2001-2002 Edition)
*As of December 31, 1999. Total does not include 217 physicians in U.S. territories and possessions.

Rate of Nonfederal Physicians in Anesthesiology in 1999

National Rate = 12.4 Physicians per 100,000 Population*

RANK	STATE	RATE
39	Alabama	9.1
43	Alaska	8.7
11	Arizona	12.8
32	Arkansas	10.1
14	California	12.7
10	Colorado	12.9
4	Connecticut	16.0
47	Delaware	8.0
8	Florida	13.5
35	Georgia	10.0
24	Hawaii	10.9
49	Idaho	6.6
7	Illinois	13.6
17	Indiana	12.5
42	Iowa	8.9
32	Kansas	10.1
20	Kentucky	11.9
30	Louisiana	10.4
22	Maine	11.7
2	Maryland	17.1
1	Massachusetts	19.4
46	Michigan	8.4
35	Minnesota	10.0
45	Mississippi	8.6
27	Missouri	10.8
20	Montana	11.9
30	Nebraska	10.4
18	Nevada	12.4
24	New Hampshire	10.9
5	New Jersey	14.9
28	New Mexico	10.6
3	New York	16.8
32	North Carolina	10.1
48	North Dakota	7.6
23	Ohio	11.6
43	Oklahoma	8.7
11	Oregon	12.8
9	Pennsylvania	13.1
35	Rhode Island	10.0
38	South Carolina	9.7
50	South Dakota	6.3
16	Tennessee	12.6
18	Texas	12.4
14	Utah	12.7
24	Vermont	10.9
28	Virginia	10.6
6	Washington	14.4
39	West Virginia	9.1
11	Wisconsin	12.8
41	Wyoming	9.0

RANK	STATE	RATE
1	Massachusetts	19.4
2	Maryland	17.1
3	New York	16.8
4	Connecticut	16.0
5	New Jersey	14.9
6	Washington	14.4
7	Illinois	13.6
8	Florida	13.5
9	Pennsylvania	13.1
10	Colorado	12.9
11	Arizona	12.8
11	Oregon	12.8
11	Wisconsin	12.8
14	California	12.7
14	Utah	12.7
16	Tennessee	12.6
17	Indiana	12.5
18	Nevada	12.4
18	Texas	12.4
20	Kentucky	11.9
20	Montana	11.9
22	Maine	11.7
23	Ohio	11.6
24	Hawaii	10.9
24	New Hampshire	10.9
24	Vermont	10.9
27	Missouri	10.8
28	New Mexico	10.6
28	Virginia	10.6
30	Louisiana	10.4
30	Nebraska	10.4
32	Arkansas	10.1
32	Kansas	10.1
32	North Carolina	10.1
35	Georgia	10.0
35	Minnesota	10.0
35	Rhode Island	10.0
38	South Carolina	9.7
39	Alabama	9.1
39	West Virginia	9.1
41	Wyoming	9.0
42	Iowa	8.9
43	Alaska	8.7
43	Oklahoma	8.7
45	Mississippi	8.6
46	Michigan	8.4
47	Delaware	8.0
48	North Dakota	7.6
49	Idaho	6.6
50	South Dakota	6.3

	District of Columbia	19.1

Source: Morgan Quitno Press using data from American Medical Association (Chicago, Illinois)
   "Physician Characteristics and Distribution in the U.S." (2001-2002 Edition)
*As of December 31, 1999. National rate does not include physicians in U.S. territories and possessions.

Nonfederal Physicians in Psychiatry in 1999

National Total = 36,737 Physicians*

ALPHA ORDER

RANK	STATE	PHYSICIANS	% of USA
29	Alabama	290	0.8%
48	Alaska	58	0.2%
23	Arizona	463	1.3%
33	Arkansas	193	0.5%
2	California	4,964	13.5%
17	Colorado	557	1.5%
13	Connecticut	878	2.4%
44	Delaware	91	0.2%
6	Florida	1,556	4.2%
15	Georgia	802	2.2%
34	Hawaii	192	0.5%
47	Idaho	64	0.2%
7	Illinois	1,471	4.0%
24	Indiana	442	1.2%
37	Iowa	178	0.5%
28	Kansas	306	0.8%
27	Kentucky	350	1.0%
21	Louisiana	504	1.4%
35	Maine	190	0.5%
9	Maryland	1,224	3.3%
3	Massachusetts	1,939	5.3%
11	Michigan	1,067	2.9%
22	Minnesota	486	1.3%
40	Mississippi	154	0.4%
19	Missouri	516	1.4%
45	Montana	67	0.2%
42	Nebraska	143	0.4%
43	Nevada	124	0.3%
36	New Hampshire	186	0.5%
8	New Jersey	1,315	3.6%
31	New Mexico	216	0.6%
1	New York	5,374	14.6%
12	North Carolina	890	2.4%
46	North Dakota	65	0.2%
10	Ohio	1,105	3.0%
30	Oklahoma	254	0.7%
26	Oregon	377	1.0%
4	Pennsylvania	1,922	5.2%
32	Rhode Island	207	0.6%
25	South Carolina	432	1.2%
49	South Dakota	55	0.1%
20	Tennessee	509	1.4%
5	Texas	1,648	4.5%
38	Utah	161	0.4%
39	Vermont	155	0.4%
14	Virginia	873	2.4%
16	Washington	673	1.8%
41	West Virginia	150	0.4%
18	Wisconsin	540	1.5%
50	Wyoming	31	0.1%

RANK ORDER

RANK	STATE	PHYSICIANS	% of USA
1	New York	5,374	14.6%
2	California	4,964	13.5%
3	Massachusetts	1,939	5.3%
4	Pennsylvania	1,922	5.2%
5	Texas	1,648	4.5%
6	Florida	1,556	4.2%
7	Illinois	1,471	4.0%
8	New Jersey	1,315	3.6%
9	Maryland	1,224	3.3%
10	Ohio	1,105	3.0%
11	Michigan	1,067	2.9%
12	North Carolina	890	2.4%
13	Connecticut	878	2.4%
14	Virginia	873	2.4%
15	Georgia	802	2.2%
16	Washington	673	1.8%
17	Colorado	557	1.5%
18	Wisconsin	540	1.5%
19	Missouri	516	1.4%
20	Tennessee	509	1.4%
21	Louisiana	504	1.4%
22	Minnesota	486	1.3%
23	Arizona	463	1.3%
24	Indiana	442	1.2%
25	South Carolina	432	1.2%
26	Oregon	377	1.0%
27	Kentucky	350	1.0%
28	Kansas	306	0.8%
29	Alabama	290	0.8%
30	Oklahoma	254	0.7%
31	New Mexico	216	0.6%
32	Rhode Island	207	0.6%
33	Arkansas	193	0.5%
34	Hawaii	192	0.5%
35	Maine	190	0.5%
36	New Hampshire	186	0.5%
37	Iowa	178	0.5%
38	Utah	161	0.4%
39	Vermont	155	0.4%
40	Mississippi	154	0.4%
41	West Virginia	150	0.4%
42	Nebraska	143	0.4%
43	Nevada	124	0.3%
44	Delaware	91	0.2%
45	Montana	67	0.2%
46	North Dakota	65	0.2%
47	Idaho	64	0.2%
48	Alaska	58	0.2%
49	South Dakota	55	0.1%
50	Wyoming	31	0.1%
	District of Columbia	330	0.9%

Source: American Medical Association (Chicago, Illinois)
"Physician Characteristics and Distribution in the U.S." (2001-2002 Edition)
As of December 31, 1999. Total does not include 352 physicians in U.S. territories and possessions. Psychiatry includes psychoanalysis.

Rate of Nonfederal Physicians in Psychiatry in 1999

National Rate = 13.5 Physicians per 100,000 Population*

ALPHA ORDER

RANK	STATE	RATE
46	Alabama	6.6
32	Alaska	9.4
31	Arizona	9.7
39	Arkansas	7.6
12	California	15.0
13	Colorado	13.7
3	Connecticut	26.8
16	Delaware	12.1
25	Florida	10.3
25	Georgia	10.3
7	Hawaii	16.2
50	Idaho	5.1
16	Illinois	12.1
44	Indiana	7.4
48	Iowa	6.2
20	Kansas	11.5
35	Kentucky	8.8
20	Louisiana	11.5
11	Maine	15.2
5	Maryland	23.7
1	Massachusetts	31.4
24	Michigan	10.8
29	Minnesota	10.2
49	Mississippi	5.6
32	Missouri	9.4
39	Montana	7.6
36	Nebraska	8.6
45	Nevada	6.9
10	New Hampshire	15.5
8	New Jersey	16.1
15	New Mexico	12.4
2	New York	29.5
19	North Carolina	11.6
25	North Dakota	10.3
30	Ohio	9.8
39	Oklahoma	7.6
22	Oregon	11.4
9	Pennsylvania	16.0
6	Rhode Island	20.9
23	South Carolina	11.1
43	South Dakota	7.5
34	Tennessee	9.3
38	Texas	8.2
39	Utah	7.6
4	Vermont	26.1
14	Virginia	12.7
18	Washington	11.7
37	West Virginia	8.3
25	Wisconsin	10.3
47	Wyoming	6.5

RANK ORDER

RANK	STATE	RATE
1	Massachusetts	31.4
2	New York	29.5
3	Connecticut	26.8
4	Vermont	26.1
5	Maryland	23.7
6	Rhode Island	20.9
7	Hawaii	16.2
8	New Jersey	16.1
9	Pennsylvania	16.0
10	New Hampshire	15.5
11	Maine	15.2
12	California	15.0
13	Colorado	13.7
14	Virginia	12.7
15	New Mexico	12.4
16	Delaware	12.1
16	Illinois	12.1
18	Washington	11.7
19	North Carolina	11.6
20	Kansas	11.5
20	Louisiana	11.5
22	Oregon	11.4
23	South Carolina	11.1
24	Michigan	10.8
25	Florida	10.3
25	Georgia	10.3
25	North Dakota	10.3
25	Wisconsin	10.3
29	Minnesota	10.2
30	Ohio	9.8
31	Arizona	9.7
32	Alaska	9.4
32	Missouri	9.4
34	Tennessee	9.3
35	Kentucky	8.8
36	Nebraska	8.6
37	West Virginia	8.3
38	Texas	8.2
39	Arkansas	7.6
39	Montana	7.6
39	Oklahoma	7.6
39	Utah	7.6
43	South Dakota	7.5
44	Indiana	7.4
45	Nevada	6.9
46	Alabama	6.6
47	Wyoming	6.5
48	Iowa	6.2
49	Mississippi	5.6
50	Idaho	5.1

District of Columbia 63.6

Source: Morgan Quitno Press using data from American Medical Association (Chicago, Illinois)
"Physician Characteristics and Distribution in the U.S." (2001-2002 Edition)
*As of December 31, 1999. National rate does not include physicians in U.S. territories and possessions.
Psychiatry includes psychoanalysis.

Percent of Population Lacking Access to Mental Health Care in 2000

National Percent = 11.0% of Population*

<table>
<tr><td colspan="3">ALPHA ORDER</td><td colspan="3">RANK ORDER</td></tr>
<tr><td>RANK</td><td>STATE</td><td>PERCENT</td><td>RANK</td><td>STATE</td><td>PERCENT</td></tr>
<tr><td>1</td><td>Alabama</td><td>47.0</td><td>1</td><td>Alabama</td><td>47.0</td></tr>
<tr><td>22</td><td>Alaska</td><td>12.9</td><td>2</td><td>Montana</td><td>42.3</td></tr>
<tr><td>27</td><td>Arizona</td><td>10.8</td><td>3</td><td>Arkansas</td><td>41.9</td></tr>
<tr><td>3</td><td>Arkansas</td><td>41.9</td><td>4</td><td>New Mexico</td><td>37.3</td></tr>
<tr><td>40</td><td>California</td><td>2.8</td><td>5</td><td>Idaho</td><td>37.0</td></tr>
<tr><td>41</td><td>Colorado</td><td>2.0</td><td>6</td><td>North Dakota</td><td>34.8</td></tr>
<tr><td>47</td><td>Connecticut</td><td>0.5</td><td>7</td><td>Nebraska</td><td>33.5</td></tr>
<tr><td>48</td><td>Delaware</td><td>0.0</td><td>8</td><td>Iowa</td><td>33.3</td></tr>
<tr><td>38</td><td>Florida</td><td>3.3</td><td>9</td><td>South Carolina</td><td>31.0</td></tr>
<tr><td>24</td><td>Georgia</td><td>11.4</td><td>10</td><td>Kansas</td><td>29.6</td></tr>
<tr><td>39</td><td>Hawaii</td><td>3.1</td><td>11</td><td>Missouri</td><td>28.8</td></tr>
<tr><td>5</td><td>Idaho</td><td>37.0</td><td>12</td><td>Oklahoma</td><td>23.5</td></tr>
<tr><td>37</td><td>Illinois</td><td>3.9</td><td>13</td><td>Kentucky</td><td>22.2</td></tr>
<tr><td>36</td><td>Indiana</td><td>4.9</td><td>14</td><td>Wisconsin</td><td>21.5</td></tr>
<tr><td>8</td><td>Iowa</td><td>33.3</td><td>15</td><td>Texas</td><td>20.4</td></tr>
<tr><td>10</td><td>Kansas</td><td>29.6</td><td>16</td><td>Mississippi</td><td>19.2</td></tr>
<tr><td>13</td><td>Kentucky</td><td>22.2</td><td>17</td><td>Oregon</td><td>17.8</td></tr>
<tr><td>44</td><td>Louisiana</td><td>1.1</td><td>18</td><td>Tennessee</td><td>17.0</td></tr>
<tr><td>30</td><td>Maine</td><td>9.2</td><td>18</td><td>West Virginia</td><td>17.0</td></tr>
<tr><td>42</td><td>Maryland</td><td>1.3</td><td>20</td><td>Michigan</td><td>16.3</td></tr>
<tr><td>43</td><td>Massachusetts</td><td>1.2</td><td>21</td><td>Utah</td><td>15.7</td></tr>
<tr><td>20</td><td>Michigan</td><td>16.3</td><td>22</td><td>Alaska</td><td>12.9</td></tr>
<tr><td>23</td><td>Minnesota</td><td>12.5</td><td>23</td><td>Minnesota</td><td>12.5</td></tr>
<tr><td>16</td><td>Mississippi</td><td>19.2</td><td>24</td><td>Georgia</td><td>11.4</td></tr>
<tr><td>11</td><td>Missouri</td><td>28.8</td><td>24</td><td>Wyoming</td><td>11.4</td></tr>
<tr><td>2</td><td>Montana</td><td>42.3</td><td>26</td><td>Washington</td><td>11.1</td></tr>
<tr><td>7</td><td>Nebraska</td><td>33.5</td><td>27</td><td>Arizona</td><td>10.8</td></tr>
<tr><td>29</td><td>Nevada</td><td>9.5</td><td>28</td><td>North Carolina</td><td>10.0</td></tr>
<tr><td>33</td><td>New Hampshire</td><td>5.9</td><td>29</td><td>Nevada</td><td>9.5</td></tr>
<tr><td>46</td><td>New Jersey</td><td>0.6</td><td>30</td><td>Maine</td><td>9.2</td></tr>
<tr><td>4</td><td>New Mexico</td><td>37.3</td><td>31</td><td>Pennsylvania</td><td>6.6</td></tr>
<tr><td>35</td><td>New York</td><td>5.1</td><td>32</td><td>South Dakota</td><td>6.1</td></tr>
<tr><td>28</td><td>North Carolina</td><td>10.0</td><td>33</td><td>New Hampshire</td><td>5.9</td></tr>
<tr><td>6</td><td>North Dakota</td><td>34.8</td><td>34</td><td>Ohio</td><td>5.6</td></tr>
<tr><td>34</td><td>Ohio</td><td>5.6</td><td>35</td><td>New York</td><td>5.1</td></tr>
<tr><td>12</td><td>Oklahoma</td><td>23.5</td><td>36</td><td>Indiana</td><td>4.9</td></tr>
<tr><td>17</td><td>Oregon</td><td>17.8</td><td>37</td><td>Illinois</td><td>3.9</td></tr>
<tr><td>31</td><td>Pennsylvania</td><td>6.6</td><td>38</td><td>Florida</td><td>3.3</td></tr>
<tr><td>48</td><td>Rhode Island</td><td>0.0</td><td>39</td><td>Hawaii</td><td>3.1</td></tr>
<tr><td>9</td><td>South Carolina</td><td>31.0</td><td>40</td><td>California</td><td>2.8</td></tr>
<tr><td>32</td><td>South Dakota</td><td>6.1</td><td>41</td><td>Colorado</td><td>2.0</td></tr>
<tr><td>18</td><td>Tennessee</td><td>17.0</td><td>42</td><td>Maryland</td><td>1.3</td></tr>
<tr><td>15</td><td>Texas</td><td>20.4</td><td>43</td><td>Massachusetts</td><td>1.2</td></tr>
<tr><td>21</td><td>Utah</td><td>15.7</td><td>44</td><td>Louisiana</td><td>1.1</td></tr>
<tr><td>48</td><td>Vermont</td><td>0.0</td><td>44</td><td>Virginia</td><td>1.1</td></tr>
<tr><td>44</td><td>Virginia</td><td>1.1</td><td>46</td><td>New Jersey</td><td>0.6</td></tr>
<tr><td>26</td><td>Washington</td><td>11.1</td><td>47</td><td>Connecticut</td><td>0.5</td></tr>
<tr><td>18</td><td>West Virginia</td><td>17.0</td><td>48</td><td>Delaware</td><td>0.0</td></tr>
<tr><td>14</td><td>Wisconsin</td><td>21.5</td><td>48</td><td>Rhode Island</td><td>0.0</td></tr>
<tr><td>24</td><td>Wyoming</td><td>11.4</td><td>48</td><td>Vermont</td><td>0.0</td></tr>
<tr><td></td><td></td><td></td><td></td><td>District of Columbia</td><td>11.7</td></tr>
</table>

Source: Morgan Quitno Press using data from U.S. Dept. of Health and Human Services, Div. of Shortage Designation
"Selected Statistics on Health Manpower Shortage Areas, As of December 31, 2000"
*Percent of population considered under-served by mental health practitioners. An under-served population does not have primary medical care within reasonable economic and geographic bounds.

International Medical School Graduates Practicing in the U.S. in 1999

National Total = 181,781 Nonfederal Physicians*

ALPHA ORDER

RANK	STATE	PHYSICIANS	% of USA
26	Alabama	1,273	0.7%
48	Alaska	70	0.0%
20	Arizona	1,879	1.0%
34	Arkansas	601	0.3%
2	California	19,941	11.0%
33	Colorado	650	0.4%
13	Connecticut	3,517	1.9%
37	Delaware	546	0.3%
3	Florida	14,854	8.2%
14	Georgia	2,910	1.6%
36	Hawaii	551	0.3%
49	Idaho	55	0.0%
5	Illinois	11,764	6.5%
16	Indiana	2,316	1.3%
31	Iowa	879	0.5%
28	Kansas	1,023	0.6%
22	Kentucky	1,750	1.0%
21	Louisiana	1,821	1.0%
42	Maine	393	0.2%
10	Maryland	5,917	3.3%
11	Massachusetts	5,593	3.1%
9	Michigan	7,667	4.2%
23	Minnesota	1,652	0.9%
39	Mississippi	523	0.3%
15	Missouri	2,770	1.5%
47	Montana	79	0.0%
40	Nebraska	426	0.2%
32	Nevada	786	0.4%
41	New Hampshire	396	0.2%
4	New Jersey	11,880	6.5%
38	New Mexico	537	0.3%
1	New York	32,438	17.8%
18	North Carolina	2,088	1.1%
43	North Dakota	302	0.2%
8	Ohio	7,735	4.3%
27	Oklahoma	1,034	0.6%
35	Oregon	583	0.3%
7	Pennsylvania	8,848	4.9%
29	Rhode Island	981	0.5%
30	South Carolina	913	0.5%
46	South Dakota	164	0.1%
19	Tennessee	2,040	1.1%
6	Texas	9,688	5.3%
44	Utah	282	0.2%
45	Vermont	176	0.1%
12	Virginia	3,689	2.0%
25	Washington	1,460	0.8%
24	West Virginia	1,467	0.8%
17	Wisconsin	2,108	1.2%
50	Wyoming	50	0.0%

RANK ORDER

RANK	STATE	PHYSICIANS	% of USA
1	New York	32,438	17.8%
2	California	19,941	11.0%
3	Florida	14,854	8.2%
4	New Jersey	11,880	6.5%
5	Illinois	11,764	6.5%
6	Texas	9,688	5.3%
7	Pennsylvania	8,848	4.9%
8	Ohio	7,735	4.3%
9	Michigan	7,667	4.2%
10	Maryland	5,917	3.3%
11	Massachusetts	5,593	3.1%
12	Virginia	3,689	2.0%
13	Connecticut	3,517	1.9%
14	Georgia	2,910	1.6%
15	Missouri	2,770	1.5%
16	Indiana	2,316	1.3%
17	Wisconsin	2,108	1.2%
18	North Carolina	2,088	1.1%
19	Tennessee	2,040	1.1%
20	Arizona	1,879	1.0%
21	Louisiana	1,821	1.0%
22	Kentucky	1,750	1.0%
23	Minnesota	1,652	0.9%
24	West Virginia	1,467	0.8%
25	Washington	1,460	0.8%
26	Alabama	1,273	0.7%
27	Oklahoma	1,034	0.6%
28	Kansas	1,023	0.6%
29	Rhode Island	981	0.5%
30	South Carolina	913	0.5%
31	Iowa	879	0.5%
32	Nevada	786	0.4%
33	Colorado	650	0.4%
34	Arkansas	601	0.3%
35	Oregon	583	0.3%
36	Hawaii	551	0.3%
37	Delaware	546	0.3%
38	New Mexico	537	0.3%
39	Mississippi	523	0.3%
40	Nebraska	426	0.2%
41	New Hampshire	396	0.2%
42	Maine	393	0.2%
43	North Dakota	302	0.2%
44	Utah	282	0.2%
45	Vermont	176	0.1%
46	South Dakota	164	0.1%
47	Montana	79	0.0%
48	Alaska	70	0.0%
49	Idaho	55	0.0%
50	Wyoming	50	0.0%
	District of Columbia	766	0.4%

Source: American Medical Association (Chicago, Illinois)
    "Physician Characteristics and Distribution in the U.S." (2001-2002 Edition)
*Nonfederal physicians as of December 31, 1999. Total does not include 5,368 physicians in U.S. territories and possessions.

Rate of International Medical School Graduates Practicing in the U.S. in 1999

National Rate = 67 Nonfederal Physicians per 100,000 Population*

<table>
<tr><td colspan="3">ALPHA ORDER</td><td colspan="3">RANK ORDER</td></tr>
<tr><td>RANK</td><td>STATE</td><td>RATE</td><td>RANK</td><td>STATE</td><td>RATE</td></tr>
<tr><td>36</td><td>Alabama</td><td>29</td><td>1</td><td>New York</td><td>178</td></tr>
<tr><td>47</td><td>Alaska</td><td>11</td><td>2</td><td>New Jersey</td><td>146</td></tr>
<tr><td>24</td><td>Arizona</td><td>39</td><td>3</td><td>Maryland</td><td>114</td></tr>
<tr><td>40</td><td>Arkansas</td><td>24</td><td>4</td><td>Connecticut</td><td>107</td></tr>
<tr><td>14</td><td>California</td><td>60</td><td>5</td><td>Rhode Island</td><td>99</td></tr>
<tr><td>45</td><td>Colorado</td><td>16</td><td>6</td><td>Florida</td><td>98</td></tr>
<tr><td>4</td><td>Connecticut</td><td>107</td><td>7</td><td>Illinois</td><td>97</td></tr>
<tr><td>12</td><td>Delaware</td><td>72</td><td>8</td><td>Massachusetts</td><td>91</td></tr>
<tr><td>6</td><td>Florida</td><td>98</td><td>9</td><td>West Virginia</td><td>81</td></tr>
<tr><td>27</td><td>Georgia</td><td>37</td><td>10</td><td>Michigan</td><td>78</td></tr>
<tr><td>19</td><td>Hawaii</td><td>46</td><td>11</td><td>Pennsylvania</td><td>74</td></tr>
<tr><td>50</td><td>Idaho</td><td>4</td><td>12</td><td>Delaware</td><td>72</td></tr>
<tr><td>7</td><td>Illinois</td><td>97</td><td>13</td><td>Ohio</td><td>69</td></tr>
<tr><td>24</td><td>Indiana</td><td>39</td><td>14</td><td>California</td><td>60</td></tr>
<tr><td>31</td><td>Iowa</td><td>31</td><td>15</td><td>Virginia</td><td>54</td></tr>
<tr><td>24</td><td>Kansas</td><td>39</td><td>16</td><td>Missouri</td><td>51</td></tr>
<tr><td>20</td><td>Kentucky</td><td>44</td><td>17</td><td>North Dakota</td><td>48</td></tr>
<tr><td>22</td><td>Louisiana</td><td>42</td><td>17</td><td>Texas</td><td>48</td></tr>
<tr><td>31</td><td>Maine</td><td>31</td><td>19</td><td>Hawaii</td><td>46</td></tr>
<tr><td>3</td><td>Maryland</td><td>114</td><td>20</td><td>Kentucky</td><td>44</td></tr>
<tr><td>8</td><td>Massachusetts</td><td>91</td><td>21</td><td>Nevada</td><td>43</td></tr>
<tr><td>10</td><td>Michigan</td><td>78</td><td>22</td><td>Louisiana</td><td>42</td></tr>
<tr><td>29</td><td>Minnesota</td><td>35</td><td>23</td><td>Wisconsin</td><td>40</td></tr>
<tr><td>43</td><td>Mississippi</td><td>19</td><td>24</td><td>Arizona</td><td>39</td></tr>
<tr><td>16</td><td>Missouri</td><td>51</td><td>24</td><td>Indiana</td><td>39</td></tr>
<tr><td>49</td><td>Montana</td><td>9</td><td>24</td><td>Kansas</td><td>39</td></tr>
<tr><td>38</td><td>Nebraska</td><td>26</td><td>27</td><td>Georgia</td><td>37</td></tr>
<tr><td>21</td><td>Nevada</td><td>43</td><td>27</td><td>Tennessee</td><td>37</td></tr>
<tr><td>30</td><td>New Hampshire</td><td>33</td><td>29</td><td>Minnesota</td><td>35</td></tr>
<tr><td>2</td><td>New Jersey</td><td>146</td><td>30</td><td>New Hampshire</td><td>33</td></tr>
<tr><td>31</td><td>New Mexico</td><td>31</td><td>31</td><td>Iowa</td><td>31</td></tr>
<tr><td>1</td><td>New York</td><td>178</td><td>31</td><td>Maine</td><td>31</td></tr>
<tr><td>37</td><td>North Carolina</td><td>27</td><td>31</td><td>New Mexico</td><td>31</td></tr>
<tr><td>17</td><td>North Dakota</td><td>48</td><td>31</td><td>Oklahoma</td><td>31</td></tr>
<tr><td>13</td><td>Ohio</td><td>69</td><td>35</td><td>Vermont</td><td>30</td></tr>
<tr><td>31</td><td>Oklahoma</td><td>31</td><td>36</td><td>Alabama</td><td>29</td></tr>
<tr><td>44</td><td>Oregon</td><td>18</td><td>37</td><td>North Carolina</td><td>27</td></tr>
<tr><td>11</td><td>Pennsylvania</td><td>74</td><td>38</td><td>Nebraska</td><td>26</td></tr>
<tr><td>5</td><td>Rhode Island</td><td>99</td><td>39</td><td>Washington</td><td>25</td></tr>
<tr><td>41</td><td>South Carolina</td><td>23</td><td>40</td><td>Arkansas</td><td>24</td></tr>
<tr><td>42</td><td>South Dakota</td><td>22</td><td>41</td><td>South Carolina</td><td>23</td></tr>
<tr><td>27</td><td>Tennessee</td><td>37</td><td>42</td><td>South Dakota</td><td>22</td></tr>
<tr><td>17</td><td>Texas</td><td>48</td><td>43</td><td>Mississippi</td><td>19</td></tr>
<tr><td>46</td><td>Utah</td><td>13</td><td>44</td><td>Oregon</td><td>18</td></tr>
<tr><td>35</td><td>Vermont</td><td>30</td><td>45</td><td>Colorado</td><td>16</td></tr>
<tr><td>15</td><td>Virginia</td><td>54</td><td>46</td><td>Utah</td><td>13</td></tr>
<tr><td>39</td><td>Washington</td><td>25</td><td>47</td><td>Alaska</td><td>11</td></tr>
<tr><td>9</td><td>West Virginia</td><td>81</td><td>48</td><td>Wyoming</td><td>10</td></tr>
<tr><td>23</td><td>Wisconsin</td><td>40</td><td>49</td><td>Montana</td><td>9</td></tr>
<tr><td>48</td><td>Wyoming</td><td>10</td><td>50</td><td>Idaho</td><td>4</td></tr>
<tr><td></td><td></td><td></td><td></td><td>District of Columbia</td><td>148</td></tr>
</table>

Source: Morgan Quitno Press using data from American Medical Association (Chicago, Illinois)
    "Physician Characteristics and Distribution in the U.S." (2001-2002 Edition)
*As of December 31, 1999. National rate does not include physicians in U.S. territories and possessions.

International Medical School Graduates
As a Percent of Nonfederal Physicians in 1999
National Percent = 23.7% of Nonfederal Physicians*

ALPHA ORDER

RANK	STATE	PERCENT
31	Alabama	13.4
45	Alaska	6.1
24	Arizona	16.4
36	Arkansas	11.0
15	California	21.4
47	Colorado	5.8
9	Connecticut	27.0
8	Delaware	27.5
3	Florida	33.9
25	Georgia	16.2
29	Hawaii	15.2
50	Idaho	2.5
5	Illinois	33.8
21	Indiana	17.8
28	Iowa	15.3
22	Kansas	16.6
20	Kentucky	19.0
27	Louisiana	15.4
35	Maine	11.7
7	Maryland	27.7
17	Massachusetts	19.9
6	Michigan	31.2
33	Minnesota	12.3
38	Mississippi	10.5
16	Missouri	20.3
49	Montana	3.9
39	Nebraska	10.4
13	Nevada	21.8
34	New Hampshire	12.1
1	New Jersey	44.7
32	New Mexico	12.7
2	New York	42.1
39	North Carolina	10.4
19	North Dakota	19.4
11	Ohio	26.3
23	Oklahoma	16.5
44	Oregon	6.6
12	Pennsylvania	23.0
10	Rhode Island	26.7
41	South Carolina	10.0
37	South Dakota	10.6
30	Tennessee	13.8
13	Texas	21.8
46	Utah	5.9
43	Vermont	8.2
17	Virginia	19.9
42	Washington	9.3
3	West Virginia	33.9
26	Wisconsin	15.7
48	Wyoming	5.3

RANK ORDER

RANK	STATE	PERCENT
1	New Jersey	44.7
2	New York	42.1
3	Florida	33.9
3	West Virginia	33.9
5	Illinois	33.8
6	Michigan	31.2
7	Maryland	27.7
8	Delaware	27.5
9	Connecticut	27.0
10	Rhode Island	26.7
11	Ohio	26.3
12	Pennsylvania	23.0
13	Nevada	21.8
13	Texas	21.8
15	California	21.4
16	Missouri	20.3
17	Massachusetts	19.9
17	Virginia	19.9
19	North Dakota	19.4
20	Kentucky	19.0
21	Indiana	17.8
22	Kansas	16.6
23	Oklahoma	16.5
24	Arizona	16.4
25	Georgia	16.2
26	Wisconsin	15.7
27	Louisiana	15.4
28	Iowa	15.3
29	Hawaii	15.2
30	Tennessee	13.8
31	Alabama	13.4
32	New Mexico	12.7
33	Minnesota	12.3
34	New Hampshire	12.1
35	Maine	11.7
36	Arkansas	11.0
37	South Dakota	10.6
38	Mississippi	10.5
39	Nebraska	10.4
39	North Carolina	10.4
41	South Carolina	10.0
42	Washington	9.3
43	Vermont	8.2
44	Oregon	6.6
45	Alaska	6.1
46	Utah	5.9
47	Colorado	5.8
48	Wyoming	5.3
49	Montana	3.9
50	Idaho	2.5

	District of Columbia	18.2

Source: Morgan Quitno Press using data from American Medical Association (Chicago, Illinois)
   "Physician Characteristics and Distribution in the U.S." (2001-2002 Edition)
*As of December 31, 1999. National rate does not include physicians in U.S. territories and possessions.

Osteopathic Physicians in 1999

National Total = 42,324 Osteopathic Physicians*

ALPHA ORDER

RANK	STATE	OSTEOPATHS	% of USA
29	Alabama	260	0.6%
47	Alaska	64	0.2%
12	Arizona	1,189	2.8%
38	Arkansas	169	0.4%
8	California	1,982	4.7%
14	Colorado	688	1.6%
33	Connecticut	196	0.5%
36	Delaware	181	0.4%
4	Florida	3,017	7.1%
18	Georgia	535	1.3%
40	Hawaii	105	0.2%
41	Idaho	103	0.2%
10	Illinois	1,713	4.0%
15	Indiana	606	1.4%
13	Iowa	956	2.3%
16	Kansas	557	1.3%
31	Kentucky	210	0.5%
43	Louisiana	98	0.2%
21	Maine	450	1.1%
26	Maryland	317	0.7%
24	Massachusetts	384	0.9%
1	Michigan	4,982	11.8%
30	Minnesota	224	0.5%
33	Mississippi	196	0.5%
9	Missouri	1,793	4.2%
44	Montana	83	0.2%
45	Nebraska	68	0.2%
27	Nevada	273	0.6%
42	New Hampshire	100	0.2%
6	New Jersey	2,532	6.0%
32	New Mexico	208	0.5%
7	New York	2,428	5.7%
28	North Carolina	270	0.6%
49	North Dakota	51	0.1%
3	Ohio	3,336	7.9%
11	Oklahoma	1,220	2.9%
22	Oregon	408	1.0%
2	Pennsylvania	4,939	11.7%
37	Rhode Island	176	0.4%
35	South Carolina	182	0.4%
46	South Dakota	67	0.2%
25	Tennessee	325	0.8%
5	Texas	2,595	6.1%
39	Utah	107	0.3%
48	Vermont	54	0.1%
23	Virginia	391	0.9%
17	Washington	536	1.3%
19	West Virginia	476	1.1%
20	Wisconsin	457	1.1%
50	Wyoming	36	0.1%

RANK ORDER

RANK	STATE	OSTEOPATHS	% of USA
1	Michigan	4,982	11.8%
2	Pennsylvania	4,939	11.7%
3	Ohio	3,336	7.9%
4	Florida	3,017	7.1%
5	Texas	2,595	6.1%
6	New Jersey	2,532	6.0%
7	New York	2,428	5.7%
8	California	1,982	4.7%
9	Missouri	1,793	4.2%
10	Illinois	1,713	4.0%
11	Oklahoma	1,220	2.9%
12	Arizona	1,189	2.8%
13	Iowa	956	2.3%
14	Colorado	688	1.6%
15	Indiana	606	1.4%
16	Kansas	557	1.3%
17	Washington	536	1.3%
18	Georgia	535	1.3%
19	West Virginia	476	1.1%
20	Wisconsin	457	1.1%
21	Maine	450	1.1%
22	Oregon	408	1.0%
23	Virginia	391	0.9%
24	Massachusetts	384	0.9%
25	Tennessee	325	0.8%
26	Maryland	317	0.7%
27	Nevada	273	0.6%
28	North Carolina	270	0.6%
29	Alabama	260	0.6%
30	Minnesota	224	0.5%
31	Kentucky	210	0.5%
32	New Mexico	208	0.5%
33	Connecticut	196	0.5%
33	Mississippi	196	0.5%
35	South Carolina	182	0.4%
36	Delaware	181	0.4%
37	Rhode Island	176	0.4%
38	Arkansas	169	0.4%
39	Utah	107	0.3%
40	Hawaii	105	0.2%
41	Idaho	103	0.2%
42	New Hampshire	100	0.2%
43	Louisiana	98	0.2%
44	Montana	83	0.2%
45	Nebraska	68	0.2%
46	South Dakota	67	0.2%
47	Alaska	64	0.2%
48	Vermont	54	0.1%
49	North Dakota	51	0.1%
50	Wyoming	36	0.1%
	District of Columbia	31	0.1%

Source: American Osteopathic Association
"AOA Yearbook and Directory of Osteopathic Physicians 1999"
*Excludes retired, disabled, foreign and federal osteopaths. Osteopaths practice a system of medicine based on the theory that disturbances in the musculoskeletal system affect other body parts, causing many disorders that can be corrected by various manipulative techniques in conjunction with conventional medical, surgical, pharmacological, and other therapeutic procedures.

Rate of Osteopathic Physicians in 1999

National Rate = 16 Osteopaths per 100,000 Population*

ALPHA ORDER

RANK	STATE	RATE
37	Alabama	6
22	Alaska	10
10	Arizona	25
34	Arkansas	7
37	California	6
15	Colorado	17
37	Connecticut	6
11	Delaware	24
13	Florida	20
34	Georgia	7
24	Hawaii	9
30	Idaho	8
17	Illinois	14
22	Indiana	10
5	Iowa	33
12	Kansas	21
44	Kentucky	5
50	Louisiana	2
3	Maine	36
37	Maryland	6
37	Massachusetts	6
1	Michigan	51
44	Minnesota	5
34	Mississippi	7
5	Missouri	33
24	Montana	9
48	Nebraska	4
16	Nevada	15
30	New Hampshire	8
7	New Jersey	31
20	New Mexico	12
18	New York	13
48	North Carolina	4
30	North Dakota	8
8	Ohio	30
3	Oklahoma	36
20	Oregon	12
2	Pennsylvania	41
14	Rhode Island	18
44	South Carolina	5
24	South Dakota	9
37	Tennessee	6
18	Texas	13
44	Utah	5
24	Vermont	9
37	Virginia	6
24	Washington	9
9	West Virginia	26
24	Wisconsin	9
30	Wyoming	8

RANK ORDER

RANK	STATE	RATE
1	Michigan	51
2	Pennsylvania	41
3	Maine	36
3	Oklahoma	36
5	Iowa	33
5	Missouri	33
7	New Jersey	31
8	Ohio	30
9	West Virginia	26
10	Arizona	25
11	Delaware	24
12	Kansas	21
13	Florida	20
14	Rhode Island	18
15	Colorado	17
16	Nevada	15
17	Illinois	14
18	New York	13
18	Texas	13
20	New Mexico	12
20	Oregon	12
22	Alaska	10
22	Indiana	10
24	Hawaii	9
24	Montana	9
24	South Dakota	9
24	Vermont	9
24	Washington	9
24	Wisconsin	9
30	Idaho	8
30	New Hampshire	8
30	North Dakota	8
30	Wyoming	8
34	Arkansas	7
34	Georgia	7
34	Mississippi	7
37	Alabama	6
37	California	6
37	Connecticut	6
37	Maryland	6
37	Massachusetts	6
37	Tennessee	6
37	Virginia	6
44	Kentucky	5
44	Minnesota	5
44	South Carolina	5
44	Utah	5
48	Nebraska	4
48	North Carolina	4
50	Louisiana	2
	District of Columbia	6

Source: Morgan Quitno Press using data from American Osteopathic Association
   "AOA Yearbook and Directory of Osteopathic Physicians 1999"
*Excludes retired, disabled, foreign and federal osteopaths. Osteopaths practice a system of medicine based on the theory that disturbances in the musculoskeletal system affect other body parts, causing many disorders that can be corrected by various manipulative techniques in conjunction with conventional medical, surgical, pharmacological, and other therapeutic procedures.

Podiatric Physicians in 1999

National Total = 13,318 Podiatric Physicians*

<u>ALPHA ORDER</u>

RANK	STATE	PODIATRISTS	% of USA
27	Alabama	97	0.7%
46	Alaska	24	0.2%
17	Arizona	198	1.5%
38	Arkansas	55	0.4%
2	California	1,522	11.4%
24	Colorado	128	1.0%
12	Connecticut	269	2.0%
43	Delaware	36	0.3%
4	Florida	914	6.9%
14	Georgia	241	1.8%
47	Hawaii	22	0.2%
42	Idaho	39	0.3%
5	Illinois	863	6.5%
14	Indiana	241	1.8%
21	Iowa	152	1.1%
28	Kansas	90	0.7%
30	Kentucky	82	0.6%
26	Louisiana	103	0.8%
36	Maine	59	0.4%
11	Maryland	290	2.2%
10	Massachusetts	439	3.3%
9	Michigan	530	4.0%
22	Minnesota	134	1.0%
43	Mississippi	36	0.3%
20	Missouri	171	1.3%
41	Montana	41	0.3%
35	Nebraska	60	0.5%
38	Nevada	55	0.4%
40	New Hampshire	54	0.4%
6	New Jersey	744	5.6%
36	New Mexico	59	0.4%
1	New York	1,602	12.0%
18	North Carolina	195	1.5%
47	North Dakota	22	0.2%
7	Ohio	688	5.2%
31	Oklahoma	81	0.6%
29	Oregon	85	0.6%
3	Pennsylvania	1,120	8.4%
32	Rhode Island	77	0.6%
33	South Carolina	66	0.5%
45	South Dakota	27	0.2%
22	Tennessee	134	1.0%
8	Texas	569	4.3%
25	Utah	113	0.8%
49	Vermont	16	0.1%
13	Virginia	248	1.9%
19	Washington	192	1.4%
34	West Virginia	65	0.5%
16	Wisconsin	201	1.5%
50	Wyoming	11	0.1%

<u>RANK ORDER</u>

RANK	STATE	PODIATRISTS	% of USA
1	New York	1,602	12.0%
2	California	1,522	11.4%
3	Pennsylvania	1,120	8.4%
4	Florida	914	6.9%
5	Illinois	863	6.5%
6	New Jersey	744	5.6%
7	Ohio	688	5.2%
8	Texas	569	4.3%
9	Michigan	530	4.0%
10	Massachusetts	439	3.3%
11	Maryland	290	2.2%
12	Connecticut	269	2.0%
13	Virginia	248	1.9%
14	Georgia	241	1.8%
14	Indiana	241	1.8%
16	Wisconsin	201	1.5%
17	Arizona	198	1.5%
18	North Carolina	195	1.5%
19	Washington	192	1.4%
20	Missouri	171	1.3%
21	Iowa	152	1.1%
22	Minnesota	134	1.0%
22	Tennessee	134	1.0%
24	Colorado	128	1.0%
25	Utah	113	0.8%
26	Louisiana	103	0.8%
27	Alabama	97	0.7%
28	Kansas	90	0.7%
29	Oregon	85	0.6%
30	Kentucky	82	0.6%
31	Oklahoma	81	0.6%
32	Rhode Island	77	0.6%
33	South Carolina	66	0.5%
34	West Virginia	65	0.5%
35	Nebraska	60	0.5%
36	Maine	59	0.4%
36	New Mexico	59	0.4%
38	Arkansas	55	0.4%
38	Nevada	55	0.4%
40	New Hampshire	54	0.4%
41	Montana	41	0.3%
42	Idaho	39	0.3%
43	Delaware	36	0.3%
43	Mississippi	36	0.3%
45	South Dakota	27	0.2%
46	Alaska	24	0.2%
47	Hawaii	22	0.2%
47	North Dakota	22	0.2%
49	Vermont	16	0.1%
50	Wyoming	11	0.1%
	District of Columbia	58	0.4%

Source: American Podiatric Medical Association, Inc.
    "Podiatric Physicians in Active Practice"

*As of Fall 1999. Includes only Podiatric physicians considered in "active practice." Podiatry deals with the diagnosis, treatment, and prevention of diseases of the human foot. National total does not include four podiatrists in Puerto Rico.

Rate of Podiatric Physicians in 1999

National Rate = 4.9 Podiatrists per 100,000 Population*

ALPHA ORDER

RANK	STATE	RATE
45	Alabama	2.2
21	Alaska	3.9
19	Arizona	4.1
45	Arkansas	2.2
16	California	4.6
31	Colorado	3.2
4	Connecticut	8.2
14	Delaware	4.8
9	Florida	6.0
32	Georgia	3.1
48	Hawaii	1.9
32	Idaho	3.1
6	Illinois	7.1
19	Indiana	4.1
12	Iowa	5.3
28	Kansas	3.4
47	Kentucky	2.1
41	Louisiana	2.4
15	Maine	4.7
10	Maryland	5.6
6	Massachusetts	7.1
11	Michigan	5.4
36	Minnesota	2.8
50	Mississippi	1.3
32	Missouri	3.1
16	Montana	4.6
24	Nebraska	3.6
35	Nevada	3.0
18	New Hampshire	4.5
2	New Jersey	9.1
28	New Mexico	3.4
3	New York	8.8
40	North Carolina	2.5
27	North Dakota	3.5
8	Ohio	6.1
41	Oklahoma	2.4
39	Oregon	2.6
1	Pennsylvania	9.3
5	Rhode Island	7.8
49	South Carolina	1.7
23	South Dakota	3.7
41	Tennessee	2.4
36	Texas	2.8
12	Utah	5.3
38	Vermont	2.7
24	Virginia	3.6
30	Washington	3.3
24	West Virginia	3.6
22	Wisconsin	3.8
44	Wyoming	2.3

RANK ORDER

RANK	STATE	RATE
1	Pennsylvania	9.3
2	New Jersey	9.1
3	New York	8.8
4	Connecticut	8.2
5	Rhode Island	7.8
6	Illinois	7.1
6	Massachusetts	7.1
8	Ohio	6.1
9	Florida	6.0
10	Maryland	5.6
11	Michigan	5.4
12	Iowa	5.3
12	Utah	5.3
14	Delaware	4.8
15	Maine	4.7
16	California	4.6
16	Montana	4.6
18	New Hampshire	4.5
19	Arizona	4.1
19	Indiana	4.1
21	Alaska	3.9
22	Wisconsin	3.8
23	South Dakota	3.7
24	Nebraska	3.6
24	Virginia	3.6
24	West Virginia	3.6
27	North Dakota	3.5
28	Kansas	3.4
28	New Mexico	3.4
30	Washington	3.3
31	Colorado	3.2
32	Georgia	3.1
32	Idaho	3.1
32	Missouri	3.1
35	Nevada	3.0
36	Minnesota	2.8
36	Texas	2.8
38	Vermont	2.7
39	Oregon	2.6
40	North Carolina	2.5
41	Louisiana	2.4
41	Oklahoma	2.4
41	Tennessee	2.4
44	Wyoming	2.3
45	Alabama	2.2
45	Arkansas	2.2
47	Kentucky	2.1
48	Hawaii	1.9
49	South Carolina	1.7
50	Mississippi	1.3
	District of Columbia	11.2

Source: Morgan Quitno Press using data from American Podiatric Medical Association, Inc.
"Podiatric Physicians in Active Practice"
*Includes only Podiatric physicians considered in "active practice." Podiatry deals with the diagnosis, treatment, and prevention of diseases of the human foot. National rate does not include podiatrists in Puerto Rico.

Doctors of Chiropractic in 1999

National Total = 79,674 Chiropractors*

ALPHA ORDER

RANK	STATE	CHIROPRACTOR	% of USA
28	Alabama	764	1.0%
50	Alaska	166	0.2%
10	Arizona	2,476	3.1%
32	Arkansas	541	0.7%
1	California	12,192	15.3%
17	Colorado	1,831	2.3%
26	Connecticut	894	1.1%
47	Delaware	219	0.3%
4	Florida	4,153	5.2%
6	Georgia	3,482	4.4%
34	Hawaii	522	0.7%
38	Idaho	363	0.5%
8	Illinois	2,925	3.7%
25	Indiana	928	1.2%
20	Iowa	1,409	1.8%
31	Kansas	675	0.8%
23	Kentucky	1,085	1.4%
33	Louisiana	533	0.7%
39	Maine	360	0.5%
30	Maryland	679	0.9%
18	Massachusetts	1,813	2.3%
9	Michigan	2,676	3.4%
16	Minnesota	1,863	2.3%
42	Mississippi	334	0.4%
13	Missouri	1,877	2.4%
43	Montana	277	0.3%
41	Nebraska	338	0.4%
37	Nevada	414	0.5%
36	New Hampshire	423	0.5%
7	New Jersey	3,255	4.1%
35	New Mexico	493	0.6%
2	New York	5,757	7.2%
19	North Carolina	1,490	1.9%
46	North Dakota	224	0.3%
13	Ohio	1,877	2.4%
24	Oklahoma	1,062	1.3%
21	Oregon	1,394	1.7%
5	Pennsylvania	3,727	4.7%
48	Rhode Island	201	0.3%
22	South Carolina	1,263	1.6%
40	South Dakota	350	0.4%
27	Tennessee	802	1.0%
3	Texas	4,341	5.4%
29	Utah	700	0.9%
45	Vermont	235	0.3%
11	Virginia	2,185	2.7%
12	Washington	1,993	2.5%
44	West Virginia	267	0.3%
15	Wisconsin	1,875	2.4%
49	Wyoming	176	0.2%

RANK ORDER

RANK	STATE	CHIROPRACTOR	% of USA
1	California	12,192	15.3%
2	New York	5,757	7.2%
3	Texas	4,341	5.4%
4	Florida	4,153	5.2%
5	Pennsylvania	3,727	4.7%
6	Georgia	3,482	4.4%
7	New Jersey	3,255	4.1%
8	Illinois	2,925	3.7%
9	Michigan	2,676	3.4%
10	Arizona	2,476	3.1%
11	Virginia	2,185	2.7%
12	Washington	1,993	2.5%
13	Missouri	1,877	2.4%
13	Ohio	1,877	2.4%
15	Wisconsin	1,875	2.4%
16	Minnesota	1,863	2.3%
17	Colorado	1,831	2.3%
18	Massachusetts	1,813	2.3%
19	North Carolina	1,490	1.9%
20	Iowa	1,409	1.8%
21	Oregon	1,394	1.7%
22	South Carolina	1,263	1.6%
23	Kentucky	1,085	1.4%
24	Oklahoma	1,062	1.3%
25	Indiana	928	1.2%
26	Connecticut	894	1.1%
27	Tennessee	802	1.0%
28	Alabama	764	1.0%
29	Utah	700	0.9%
30	Maryland	679	0.9%
31	Kansas	675	0.8%
32	Arkansas	541	0.7%
33	Louisiana	533	0.7%
34	Hawaii	522	0.7%
35	New Mexico	493	0.6%
36	New Hampshire	423	0.5%
37	Nevada	414	0.5%
38	Idaho	363	0.5%
39	Maine	360	0.5%
40	South Dakota	350	0.4%
41	Nebraska	338	0.4%
42	Mississippi	334	0.4%
43	Montana	277	0.3%
44	West Virginia	267	0.3%
45	Vermont	235	0.3%
46	North Dakota	224	0.3%
47	Delaware	219	0.3%
48	Rhode Island	201	0.3%
49	Wyoming	176	0.2%
50	Alaska	166	0.2%
	District of Columbia	49	0.1%

Source: Federation of Chiropractic Licensing Boards
  "Official Directory" (http://www.fclb.org/directory/index.htm)
As of December 1999. Licensed active doctors. There is some duplication as some doctors are licensed in more than one state.

Rate of Doctors of Chiropractic in 1999

National Rate = 29 Chiropractors per 100,000 Population*

ALPHA ORDER

RANK	STATE	RATE
43	Alabama	17
30	Alaska	27
1	Arizona	52
39	Arkansas	21
11	California	37
4	Colorado	45
30	Connecticut	27
25	Delaware	29
30	Florida	27
4	Georgia	45
6	Hawaii	44
25	Idaho	29
36	Illinois	24
45	Indiana	16
2	Iowa	49
35	Kansas	25
30	Kentucky	27
49	Louisiana	12
25	Maine	29
48	Maryland	13
25	Massachusetts	29
30	Michigan	27
10	Minnesota	39
49	Mississippi	12
17	Missouri	34
23	Montana	31
40	Nebraska	20
37	Nevada	23
14	New Hampshire	35
8	New Jersey	40
29	New Mexico	28
20	New York	32
42	North Carolina	19
14	North Dakota	35
43	Ohio	17
20	Oklahoma	32
7	Oregon	42
23	Pennsylvania	31
40	Rhode Island	20
18	South Carolina	33
3	South Dakota	48
46	Tennessee	15
38	Texas	22
18	Utah	33
8	Vermont	40
20	Virginia	32
14	Washington	35
46	West Virginia	15
13	Wisconsin	36
11	Wyoming	37

RANK ORDER

RANK	STATE	RATE
1	Arizona	52
2	Iowa	49
3	South Dakota	48
4	Colorado	45
4	Georgia	45
6	Hawaii	44
7	Oregon	42
8	New Jersey	40
8	Vermont	40
10	Minnesota	39
11	California	37
11	Wyoming	37
13	Wisconsin	36
14	New Hampshire	35
14	North Dakota	35
14	Washington	35
17	Missouri	34
18	South Carolina	33
18	Utah	33
20	New York	32
20	Oklahoma	32
20	Virginia	32
23	Montana	31
23	Pennsylvania	31
25	Delaware	29
25	Idaho	29
25	Maine	29
25	Massachusetts	29
29	New Mexico	28
30	Alaska	27
30	Connecticut	27
30	Florida	27
30	Kentucky	27
30	Michigan	27
35	Kansas	25
36	Illinois	24
37	Nevada	23
38	Texas	22
39	Arkansas	21
40	Nebraska	20
40	Rhode Island	20
42	North Carolina	19
43	Alabama	17
43	Ohio	17
45	Indiana	16
46	Tennessee	15
46	West Virginia	15
48	Maryland	13
49	Louisiana	12
49	Mississippi	12
	District of Columbia	9

Source: Morgan Quitno Press using data from Federation of Chiropractic Licensing Boards
"Official Directory" (http://www.fclb.org/directory/index.htm)
*As of December 1999. Licensed active doctors. There is some duplication as some doctors are licensed in more than one state.

Physician Assistants in Clinical Practice in 2001

National Total = 39,989 Physician Assistants*

ALPHA ORDER

RANK	STATE	PA'S	% of USA
35	Alabama	277	0.7%
37	Alaska	255	0.6%
17	Arizona	735	1.8%
49	Arkansas	56	0.1%
2	California	3,929	9.8%
12	Colorado	927	2.3%
16	Connecticut	793	2.0%
48	Delaware	95	0.2%
5	Florida	2,147	5.4%
8	Georgia	1,358	3.4%
47	Hawaii	96	0.2%
41	Idaho	214	0.5%
13	Illinois	923	2.3%
34	Indiana	285	0.7%
22	Iowa	504	1.3%
25	Kansas	470	1.2%
21	Kentucky	529	1.3%
36	Louisiana	276	0.7%
28	Maine	384	1.0%
11	Maryland	1,107	2.8%
14	Massachusetts	892	2.2%
7	Michigan	1,657	4.1%
20	Minnesota	594	1.5%
50	Mississippi	38	0.1%
33	Missouri	308	0.8%
43	Montana	181	0.5%
26	Nebraska	463	1.2%
39	Nevada	224	0.6%
40	New Hampshire	223	0.6%
24	New Jersey	490	1.2%
30	New Mexico	341	0.9%
1	New York	4,894	12.2%
6	North Carolina	2,125	5.3%
42	North Dakota	198	0.5%
10	Ohio	1,162	2.9%
19	Oklahoma	610	1.5%
29	Oregon	371	0.9%
4	Pennsylvania	2,245	5.6%
44	Rhode Island	125	0.3%
32	South Carolina	336	0.8%
38	South Dakota	245	0.6%
23	Tennessee	492	1.2%
3	Texas	2,511	6.3%
31	Utah	337	0.8%
45	Vermont	123	0.3%
18	Virginia	654	1.6%
9	Washington	1,171	2.9%
26	West Virginia	463	1.2%
15	Wisconsin	856	2.1%
46	Wyoming	113	0.3%

RANK ORDER

RANK	STATE	PA'S	% of USA
1	New York	4,894	12.2%
2	California	3,929	9.8%
3	Texas	2,511	6.3%
4	Pennsylvania	2,245	5.6%
5	Florida	2,147	5.4%
6	North Carolina	2,125	5.3%
7	Michigan	1,657	4.1%
8	Georgia	1,358	3.4%
9	Washington	1,171	2.9%
10	Ohio	1,162	2.9%
11	Maryland	1,107	2.8%
12	Colorado	927	2.3%
13	Illinois	923	2.3%
14	Massachusetts	892	2.2%
15	Wisconsin	856	2.1%
16	Connecticut	793	2.0%
17	Arizona	735	1.8%
18	Virginia	654	1.6%
19	Oklahoma	610	1.5%
20	Minnesota	594	1.5%
21	Kentucky	529	1.3%
22	Iowa	504	1.3%
23	Tennessee	492	1.2%
24	New Jersey	490	1.2%
25	Kansas	470	1.2%
26	Nebraska	463	1.2%
26	West Virginia	463	1.2%
28	Maine	384	1.0%
29	Oregon	371	0.9%
30	New Mexico	341	0.9%
31	Utah	337	0.8%
32	South Carolina	336	0.8%
33	Missouri	308	0.8%
34	Indiana	285	0.7%
35	Alabama	277	0.7%
36	Louisiana	276	0.7%
37	Alaska	255	0.6%
38	South Dakota	245	0.6%
39	Nevada	224	0.6%
40	New Hampshire	223	0.6%
41	Idaho	214	0.5%
42	North Dakota	198	0.5%
43	Montana	181	0.5%
44	Rhode Island	125	0.3%
45	Vermont	123	0.3%
46	Wyoming	113	0.3%
47	Hawaii	96	0.2%
48	Delaware	95	0.2%
49	Arkansas	56	0.1%
50	Mississippi	38	0.1%
	District of Columbia	187	0.5%

Source: The American Academy of Physician Assistants
"Projected Number of PAs in Clinical Practice as of January 1, 2001"
(http://www.aapa.org/research/clinprac2001.html)
*Projected.

Rate of Physician Assistants in Clinical Practice in 2001

National Rate = 14.2 PA's per 100,000 Population*

ALPHA ORDER

RANK	STATE	RATE
44	Alabama	6.2
1	Alaska	40.7
27	Arizona	14.3
49	Arkansas	2.1
35	California	11.6
11	Colorado	21.6
9	Connecticut	23.3
31	Delaware	12.1
29	Florida	13.4
23	Georgia	16.6
42	Hawaii	7.9
24	Idaho	16.5
43	Illinois	7.4
48	Indiana	4.7
21	Iowa	17.2
20	Kansas	17.5
30	Kentucky	13.1
44	Louisiana	6.2
4	Maine	30.1
12	Maryland	20.9
28	Massachusetts	14.0
22	Michigan	16.7
31	Minnesota	12.1
50	Mississippi	1.3
47	Missouri	5.5
14	Montana	20.1
5	Nebraska	27.1
36	Nevada	11.2
18	New Hampshire	18.0
46	New Jersey	5.8
16	New Mexico	18.7
7	New York	25.8
6	North Carolina	26.4
3	North Dakota	30.8
38	Ohio	10.2
19	Oklahoma	17.7
37	Oregon	10.8
17	Pennsylvania	18.3
34	Rhode Island	11.9
41	South Carolina	8.4
2	South Dakota	32.5
40	Tennessee	8.6
33	Texas	12.0
26	Utah	15.1
13	Vermont	20.2
39	Virginia	9.2
15	Washington	19.9
8	West Virginia	25.6
25	Wisconsin	16.0
10	Wyoming	22.9

RANK ORDER

RANK	STATE	RATE
1	Alaska	40.7
2	South Dakota	32.5
3	North Dakota	30.8
4	Maine	30.1
5	Nebraska	27.1
6	North Carolina	26.4
7	New York	25.8
8	West Virginia	25.6
9	Connecticut	23.3
10	Wyoming	22.9
11	Colorado	21.6
12	Maryland	20.9
13	Vermont	20.2
14	Montana	20.1
15	Washington	19.9
16	New Mexico	18.7
17	Pennsylvania	18.3
18	New Hampshire	18.0
19	Oklahoma	17.7
20	Kansas	17.5
21	Iowa	17.2
22	Michigan	16.7
23	Georgia	16.6
24	Idaho	16.5
25	Wisconsin	16.0
26	Utah	15.1
27	Arizona	14.3
28	Massachusetts	14.0
29	Florida	13.4
30	Kentucky	13.1
31	Delaware	12.1
31	Minnesota	12.1
33	Texas	12.0
34	Rhode Island	11.9
35	California	11.6
36	Nevada	11.2
37	Oregon	10.8
38	Ohio	10.2
39	Virginia	9.2
40	Tennessee	8.6
41	South Carolina	8.4
42	Hawaii	7.9
43	Illinois	7.4
44	Alabama	6.2
44	Louisiana	6.2
46	New Jersey	5.8
47	Missouri	5.5
48	Indiana	4.7
49	Arkansas	2.1
50	Mississippi	1.3

District of Columbia 32.7

Source: Morgan Quitno Press using data from The American Academy of Physician Assistants
"Projected Number of PAs in Clinical Practice as of January 1, 2001"
(http://www.aapa.org/research/clinprac2001.html)
*Projected. Rates calculated using 2000 Census population figures.

Registered Nurses in 2000

National Total = 2,201,813 Registered Nurses*

ALPHA ORDER					RANK ORDER			
RANK	STATE	NURSES	% of USA		RANK	STATE	NURSES	% of USA
22	Alabama	34,073	1.5%		1	California	184,329	8.4%
49	Alaska	4,914	0.2%		2	New York	160,009	7.3%
24	Arizona	32,222	1.5%		3	Texas	126,436	5.7%
33	Arkansas	18,752	0.9%		4	Florida	125,439	5.7%
1	California	184,329	8.4%		5	Pennsylvania	123,997	5.6%
26	Colorado	31,695	1.4%		6	Illinois	101,660	4.6%
25	Connecticut	32,073	1.5%		7	Ohio	100,144	4.5%
45	Delaware	7,337	0.3%		8	Michigan	79,353	3.6%
4	Florida	125,439	5.7%		9	Massachusetts	75,795	3.4%
12	Georgia	55,881	2.5%		10	North Carolina	69,057	3.1%
42	Hawaii	8,518	0.4%		11	New Jersey	67,280	3.1%
44	Idaho	8,230	0.4%		12	Georgia	55,881	2.5%
6	Illinois	101,660	4.6%		13	Missouri	53,730	2.4%
18	Indiana	46,244	2.1%		14	Virginia	50,359	2.3%
27	Iowa	31,020	1.4%		15	Tennessee	49,626	2.3%
30	Kansas	23,779	1.1%		16	Wisconsin	47,895	2.2%
23	Kentucky	33,655	1.5%		17	Minnesota	47,102	2.1%
21	Louisiana	37,275	1.7%		18	Indiana	46,244	2.1%
37	Maine	13,072	0.6%		19	Maryland	45,323	2.1%
19	Maryland	45,323	2.1%		20	Washington	43,482	2.0%
9	Massachusetts	75,795	3.4%		21	Louisiana	37,275	1.7%
8	Michigan	79,353	3.6%		22	Alabama	34,073	1.5%
17	Minnesota	47,102	2.1%		23	Kentucky	33,655	1.5%
32	Mississippi	21,338	1.0%		24	Arizona	32,222	1.5%
13	Missouri	53,730	2.4%		25	Connecticut	32,073	1.5%
46	Montana	7,327	0.3%		26	Colorado	31,695	1.4%
34	Nebraska	16,399	0.7%		27	Iowa	31,020	1.4%
41	Nevada	10,384	0.5%		28	South Carolina	29,226	1.3%
40	New Hampshire	11,321	0.5%		29	Oregon	27,121	1.2%
11	New Jersey	67,280	3.1%		30	Kansas	23,779	1.1%
38	New Mexico	11,932	0.5%		31	Oklahoma	21,905	1.0%
2	New York	160,009	7.3%		32	Mississippi	21,338	1.0%
10	North Carolina	69,057	3.1%		33	Arkansas	18,752	0.9%
47	North Dakota	7,039	0.3%		34	Nebraska	16,399	0.7%
7	Ohio	100,144	4.5%		35	West Virginia	15,523	0.7%
31	Oklahoma	21,905	1.0%		36	Utah	13,229	0.6%
29	Oregon	27,121	1.2%		37	Maine	13,072	0.6%
5	Pennsylvania	123,997	5.6%		38	New Mexico	11,932	0.5%
39	Rhode Island	11,542	0.5%		39	Rhode Island	11,542	0.5%
28	South Carolina	29,226	1.3%		40	New Hampshire	11,321	0.5%
43	South Dakota	8,511	0.4%		41	Nevada	10,384	0.5%
15	Tennessee	49,626	2.3%		42	Hawaii	8,518	0.4%
3	Texas	126,436	5.7%		43	South Dakota	8,511	0.4%
36	Utah	13,229	0.6%		44	Idaho	8,230	0.4%
48	Vermont	5,829	0.3%		45	Delaware	7,337	0.3%
14	Virginia	50,359	2.3%		46	Montana	7,327	0.3%
20	Washington	43,482	2.0%		47	North Dakota	7,039	0.3%
35	West Virginia	15,523	0.7%		48	Vermont	5,829	0.3%
16	Wisconsin	47,895	2.2%		49	Alaska	4,914	0.2%
50	Wyoming	3,849	0.2%		50	Wyoming	3,849	0.2%
						District of Columbia	9,583	0.4%

Source: U.S. Department of Health and Human Services, Health Resources and Services Administration
   "The Registered Nurse Population" (February 2001)
*Preliminary as of March 2000. Does not include 494,727 registered nurses not employed in nursing.

Rate of Registered Nurses in 2000

National Rate = 782 Nurses per 100,000 Population*

RANK	STATE	RATE
33	Alabama	766
31	Alaska	784
46	Arizona	628
41	Arkansas	701
49	California	544
37	Colorado	737
12	Connecticut	942
13	Delaware	936
30	Florida	785
42	Georgia	683
40	Hawaii	703
44	Idaho	636
25	Illinois	819
34	Indiana	761
5	Iowa	1,060
16	Kansas	885
24	Kentucky	833
23	Louisiana	834
6	Maine	1,025
21	Maryland	856
1	Massachusetts	1,194
28	Michigan	798
10	Minnesota	957
35	Mississippi	750
8	Missouri	960
26	Montana	812
9	Nebraska	958
50	Nevada	520
14	New Hampshire	916
27	New Jersey	800
43	New Mexico	656
22	New York	843
19	North Carolina	858
4	North Dakota	1,096
17	Ohio	882
45	Oklahoma	635
29	Oregon	793
7	Pennsylvania	1,010
3	Rhode Island	1,101
38	South Carolina	728
2	South Dakota	1,128
18	Tennessee	872
47	Texas	606
48	Utah	592
10	Vermont	957
39	Virginia	711
36	Washington	738
19	West Virginia	858
15	Wisconsin	893
32	Wyoming	780

RANK	STATE	RATE
1	Massachusetts	1,194
2	South Dakota	1,128
3	Rhode Island	1,101
4	North Dakota	1,096
5	Iowa	1,060
6	Maine	1,025
7	Pennsylvania	1,010
8	Missouri	960
9	Nebraska	958
10	Minnesota	957
10	Vermont	957
12	Connecticut	942
13	Delaware	936
14	New Hampshire	916
15	Wisconsin	893
16	Kansas	885
17	Ohio	882
18	Tennessee	872
19	North Carolina	858
19	West Virginia	858
21	Maryland	856
22	New York	843
23	Louisiana	834
24	Kentucky	833
25	Illinois	819
26	Montana	812
27	New Jersey	800
28	Michigan	798
29	Oregon	793
30	Florida	785
31	Alaska	784
32	Wyoming	780
33	Alabama	766
34	Indiana	761
35	Mississippi	750
36	Washington	738
37	Colorado	737
38	South Carolina	728
39	Virginia	711
40	Hawaii	703
41	Arkansas	701
42	Georgia	683
43	New Mexico	656
44	Idaho	636
45	Oklahoma	635
46	Arizona	628
47	Texas	606
48	Utah	592
49	California	544
50	Nevada	520

	District of Columbia	1,675

Source: U.S. Department of Health and Human Services, Health Resources and Services Administration "The Registered Nurse Population" (February 2001)

Preliminary as of March 2000. Rates do not include registered nurses not employed in nursing.

Dentists in 1998

National Total = 149,350 Dentists*

<table>
<tr><th colspan="4">ALPHA ORDER</th><th colspan="4">RANK ORDER</th></tr>
<tr><th>RANK</th><th>STATE</th><th>DENTISTS</th><th>% of USA</th><th>RANK</th><th>STATE</th><th>DENTISTS</th><th>% of USA</th></tr>
<tr><td>27</td><td>Alabama</td><td>1,785</td><td>1.2%</td><td>1</td><td>California</td><td>20,404</td><td>13.7%</td></tr>
<tr><td>45</td><td>Alaska</td><td>427</td><td>0.3%</td><td>2</td><td>New York</td><td>13,189</td><td>8.8%</td></tr>
<tr><td>25</td><td>Arizona</td><td>2,036</td><td>1.4%</td><td>3</td><td>Texas</td><td>8,656</td><td>5.8%</td></tr>
<tr><td>35</td><td>Arkansas</td><td>1,004</td><td>0.7%</td><td>4</td><td>Illinois</td><td>7,475</td><td>5.0%</td></tr>
<tr><td>1</td><td>California</td><td>20,404</td><td>13.7%</td><td>5</td><td>Pennsylvania</td><td>7,295</td><td>4.9%</td></tr>
<tr><td>21</td><td>Colorado</td><td>2,516</td><td>1.7%</td><td>6</td><td>Florida</td><td>7,084</td><td>4.7%</td></tr>
<tr><td>22</td><td>Connecticut</td><td>2,400</td><td>1.6%</td><td>7</td><td>New Jersey</td><td>5,837</td><td>3.9%</td></tr>
<tr><td>48</td><td>Delaware</td><td>331</td><td>0.2%</td><td>8</td><td>Ohio</td><td>5,712</td><td>3.8%</td></tr>
<tr><td>6</td><td>Florida</td><td>7,084</td><td>4.7%</td><td>9</td><td>Michigan</td><td>5,511</td><td>3.7%</td></tr>
<tr><td>14</td><td>Georgia</td><td>3,126</td><td>2.1%</td><td>10</td><td>Massachusetts</td><td>4,393</td><td>2.9%</td></tr>
<tr><td>36</td><td>Hawaii</td><td>941</td><td>0.6%</td><td>11</td><td>Virginia</td><td>3,649</td><td>2.4%</td></tr>
<tr><td>40</td><td>Idaho</td><td>637</td><td>0.4%</td><td>12</td><td>Maryland</td><td>3,477</td><td>2.3%</td></tr>
<tr><td>4</td><td>Illinois</td><td>7,475</td><td>5.0%</td><td>13</td><td>Washington</td><td>3,434</td><td>2.3%</td></tr>
<tr><td>18</td><td>Indiana</td><td>2,693</td><td>1.8%</td><td>14</td><td>Georgia</td><td>3,126</td><td>2.1%</td></tr>
<tr><td>30</td><td>Iowa</td><td>1,499</td><td>1.0%</td><td>15</td><td>North Carolina</td><td>3,036</td><td>2.0%</td></tr>
<tr><td>31</td><td>Kansas</td><td>1,258</td><td>0.8%</td><td>16</td><td>Wisconsin</td><td>2,890</td><td>1.9%</td></tr>
<tr><td>24</td><td>Kentucky</td><td>2,042</td><td>1.4%</td><td>17</td><td>Minnesota</td><td>2,798</td><td>1.9%</td></tr>
<tr><td>26</td><td>Louisiana</td><td>1,983</td><td>1.3%</td><td>18</td><td>Indiana</td><td>2,693</td><td>1.8%</td></tr>
<tr><td>42</td><td>Maine</td><td>585</td><td>0.4%</td><td>19</td><td>Tennessee</td><td>2,632</td><td>1.8%</td></tr>
<tr><td>12</td><td>Maryland</td><td>3,477</td><td>2.3%</td><td>20</td><td>Missouri</td><td>2,538</td><td>1.7%</td></tr>
<tr><td>10</td><td>Massachusetts</td><td>4,393</td><td>2.9%</td><td>21</td><td>Colorado</td><td>2,516</td><td>1.7%</td></tr>
<tr><td>9</td><td>Michigan</td><td>5,511</td><td>3.7%</td><td>22</td><td>Connecticut</td><td>2,400</td><td>1.6%</td></tr>
<tr><td>17</td><td>Minnesota</td><td>2,798</td><td>1.9%</td><td>23</td><td>Oregon</td><td>2,068</td><td>1.4%</td></tr>
<tr><td>34</td><td>Mississippi</td><td>1,017</td><td>0.7%</td><td>24</td><td>Kentucky</td><td>2,042</td><td>1.4%</td></tr>
<tr><td>20</td><td>Missouri</td><td>2,538</td><td>1.7%</td><td>25</td><td>Arizona</td><td>2,036</td><td>1.4%</td></tr>
<tr><td>44</td><td>Montana</td><td>457</td><td>0.3%</td><td>26</td><td>Louisiana</td><td>1,983</td><td>1.3%</td></tr>
<tr><td>33</td><td>Nebraska</td><td>1,034</td><td>0.7%</td><td>27</td><td>Alabama</td><td>1,785</td><td>1.2%</td></tr>
<tr><td>41</td><td>Nevada</td><td>628</td><td>0.4%</td><td>28</td><td>South Carolina</td><td>1,592</td><td>1.1%</td></tr>
<tr><td>39</td><td>New Hampshire</td><td>647</td><td>0.4%</td><td>29</td><td>Oklahoma</td><td>1,548</td><td>1.0%</td></tr>
<tr><td>7</td><td>New Jersey</td><td>5,837</td><td>3.9%</td><td>30</td><td>Iowa</td><td>1,499</td><td>1.0%</td></tr>
<tr><td>38</td><td>New Mexico</td><td>690</td><td>0.5%</td><td>31</td><td>Kansas</td><td>1,258</td><td>0.8%</td></tr>
<tr><td>2</td><td>New York</td><td>13,189</td><td>8.8%</td><td>32</td><td>Utah</td><td>1,238</td><td>0.8%</td></tr>
<tr><td>15</td><td>North Carolina</td><td>3,036</td><td>2.0%</td><td>33</td><td>Nebraska</td><td>1,034</td><td>0.7%</td></tr>
<tr><td>49</td><td>North Dakota</td><td>309</td><td>0.2%</td><td>34</td><td>Mississippi</td><td>1,017</td><td>0.7%</td></tr>
<tr><td>8</td><td>Ohio</td><td>5,712</td><td>3.8%</td><td>35</td><td>Arkansas</td><td>1,004</td><td>0.7%</td></tr>
<tr><td>29</td><td>Oklahoma</td><td>1,548</td><td>1.0%</td><td>36</td><td>Hawaii</td><td>941</td><td>0.6%</td></tr>
<tr><td>23</td><td>Oregon</td><td>2,068</td><td>1.4%</td><td>37</td><td>West Virginia</td><td>781</td><td>0.5%</td></tr>
<tr><td>5</td><td>Pennsylvania</td><td>7,295</td><td>4.9%</td><td>38</td><td>New Mexico</td><td>690</td><td>0.5%</td></tr>
<tr><td>43</td><td>Rhode Island</td><td>547</td><td>0.4%</td><td>39</td><td>New Hampshire</td><td>647</td><td>0.4%</td></tr>
<tr><td>28</td><td>South Carolina</td><td>1,592</td><td>1.1%</td><td>40</td><td>Idaho</td><td>637</td><td>0.4%</td></tr>
<tr><td>46</td><td>South Dakota</td><td>339</td><td>0.2%</td><td>41</td><td>Nevada</td><td>628</td><td>0.4%</td></tr>
<tr><td>19</td><td>Tennessee</td><td>2,632</td><td>1.8%</td><td>42</td><td>Maine</td><td>585</td><td>0.4%</td></tr>
<tr><td>3</td><td>Texas</td><td>8,656</td><td>5.8%</td><td>43</td><td>Rhode Island</td><td>547</td><td>0.4%</td></tr>
<tr><td>32</td><td>Utah</td><td>1,238</td><td>0.8%</td><td>44</td><td>Montana</td><td>457</td><td>0.3%</td></tr>
<tr><td>47</td><td>Vermont</td><td>336</td><td>0.2%</td><td>45</td><td>Alaska</td><td>427</td><td>0.3%</td></tr>
<tr><td>11</td><td>Virginia</td><td>3,649</td><td>2.4%</td><td>46</td><td>South Dakota</td><td>339</td><td>0.2%</td></tr>
<tr><td>13</td><td>Washington</td><td>3,434</td><td>2.3%</td><td>47</td><td>Vermont</td><td>336</td><td>0.2%</td></tr>
<tr><td>37</td><td>West Virginia</td><td>781</td><td>0.5%</td><td>48</td><td>Delaware</td><td>331</td><td>0.2%</td></tr>
<tr><td>16</td><td>Wisconsin</td><td>2,890</td><td>1.9%</td><td>49</td><td>North Dakota</td><td>309</td><td>0.2%</td></tr>
<tr><td>50</td><td>Wyoming</td><td>240</td><td>0.2%</td><td>50</td><td>Wyoming</td><td>240</td><td>0.2%</td></tr>
<tr><td></td><td></td><td></td><td></td><td></td><td>District of Columbia</td><td>592</td><td>0.4%</td></tr>
</table>

Source: American Dental Association
    "Distribution of Dentists, by Region and State, 1998"
*Professionally active dentists. Total does not include 1,714 dentists in territories nor dentists in the Armed Forces stationed overseas.

Rate of Dentists in 1998

National Rate = 55 Dentists per 100,000 Population*

ALPHA ORDER

RANK	STATE	RATE
43	Alabama	41
6	Alaska	69
39	Arizona	44
46	Arkansas	40
10	California	62
8	Colorado	63
2	Connecticut	73
39	Delaware	44
29	Florida	48
43	Georgia	41
1	Hawaii	79
23	Idaho	52
10	Illinois	62
35	Indiana	46
23	Iowa	52
29	Kansas	48
23	Kentucky	52
38	Louisiana	45
33	Maine	47
7	Maryland	68
5	Massachusetts	71
18	Michigan	56
15	Minnesota	59
49	Mississippi	37
33	Missouri	47
23	Montana	52
10	Nebraska	62
50	Nevada	36
19	New Hampshire	55
4	New Jersey	72
46	New Mexico	40
2	New York	73
46	North Carolina	40
29	North Dakota	48
27	Ohio	51
35	Oklahoma	46
8	Oregon	63
13	Pennsylvania	61
19	Rhode Island	55
43	South Carolina	41
35	South Dakota	46
29	Tennessee	48
39	Texas	44
15	Utah	59
17	Vermont	57
22	Virginia	54
14	Washington	60
42	West Virginia	43
19	Wisconsin	55
28	Wyoming	50

RANK ORDER

RANK	STATE	RATE
1	Hawaii	79
2	Connecticut	73
2	New York	73
4	New Jersey	72
5	Massachusetts	71
6	Alaska	69
7	Maryland	68
8	Colorado	63
8	Oregon	63
10	California	62
10	Illinois	62
10	Nebraska	62
13	Pennsylvania	61
14	Washington	60
15	Minnesota	59
15	Utah	59
17	Vermont	57
18	Michigan	56
19	New Hampshire	55
19	Rhode Island	55
19	Wisconsin	55
22	Virginia	54
23	Idaho	52
23	Iowa	52
23	Kentucky	52
23	Montana	52
27	Ohio	51
28	Wyoming	50
29	Florida	48
29	Kansas	48
29	North Dakota	48
29	Tennessee	48
33	Maine	47
33	Missouri	47
35	Indiana	46
35	Oklahoma	46
35	South Dakota	46
38	Louisiana	45
39	Arizona	44
39	Delaware	44
39	Texas	44
42	West Virginia	43
43	Alabama	41
43	Georgia	41
43	South Carolina	41
46	Arkansas	40
46	New Mexico	40
46	North Carolina	40
49	Mississippi	37
50	Nevada	36

District of Columbia	114

Source: Morgan Quitno Press using data from American Dental Association
    "Distribution of Dentists, by Region and State, 1998"
*Professionally active dentists. Total does not include 1,714 dentists in territories nor dentists in the Armed Forces
stationed overseas.

Percent of Population Lacking Access to Dental Care in 2000

National Percent = 5.8% of Population*

ALPHA ORDER			RANK ORDER		
RANK	STATE	PERCENT	RANK	STATE	PERCENT
11	Alabama	10.1	1	South Carolina	23.3
47	Alaska	0.9	2	Tennessee	20.6
23	Arizona	5.0	3	New Mexico	18.8
28	Arkansas	4.8	4	Idaho	14.6
44	California	1.2	5	Mississippi	13.5
40	Colorado	2.6	6	Utah	12.6
36	Connecticut	3.0	7	Oregon	12.5
10	Delaware	11.4	8	Nevada	12.0
20	Florida	5.6	9	Michigan	11.5
19	Georgia	5.9	10	Delaware	11.4
31	Hawaii	4.1	11	Alabama	10.1
4	Idaho	14.6	11	Maine	10.1
23	Illinois	5.0	13	Rhode Island	8.9
39	Indiana	2.8	14	Washington	8.8
45	Iowa	1.0	15	Texas	8.6
30	Kansas	4.3	16	North Carolina	8.1
21	Kentucky	5.2	17	South Dakota	7.6
23	Louisiana	5.0	18	Pennsylvania	6.3
11	Maine	10.1	19	Georgia	5.9
38	Maryland	2.9	20	Florida	5.6
42	Massachusetts	1.8	21	Kentucky	5.2
9	Michigan	11.5	21	Missouri	5.2
48	Minnesota	0.6	23	Arizona	5.0
5	Mississippi	13.5	23	Illinois	5.0
21	Missouri	5.2	23	Louisiana	5.0
34	Montana	3.6	23	North Dakota	5.0
43	Nebraska	1.3	27	New York	4.9
8	Nevada	12.0	28	Arkansas	4.8
36	New Hampshire	3.0	29	Ohio	4.4
45	New Jersey	1.0	30	Kansas	4.3
3	New Mexico	18.8	31	Hawaii	4.1
27	New York	4.9	32	Oklahoma	4.0
16	North Carolina	8.1	33	Wisconsin	3.8
23	North Dakota	5.0	34	Montana	3.6
29	Ohio	4.4	35	Virginia	3.3
32	Oklahoma	4.0	36	Connecticut	3.0
7	Oregon	12.5	36	New Hampshire	3.0
18	Pennsylvania	6.3	38	Maryland	2.9
13	Rhode Island	8.9	39	Indiana	2.8
1	South Carolina	23.3	40	Colorado	2.6
17	South Dakota	7.6	41	West Virginia	2.1
2	Tennessee	20.6	42	Massachusetts	1.8
15	Texas	8.6	43	Nebraska	1.3
6	Utah	12.6	44	California	1.2
48	Vermont	0.6	45	Iowa	1.0
35	Virginia	3.3	45	New Jersey	1.0
14	Washington	8.8	47	Alaska	0.9
41	West Virginia	2.1	48	Minnesota	0.6
33	Wisconsin	3.8	48	Vermont	0.6
50	Wyoming	0.5	50	Wyoming	0.5
				District of Columbia	1.1

Source: Morgan Quitno Press using data from U.S. Dept. of Health and Human Services, Div. of Shortage Designation
"Selected Statistics on Health Manpower Shortage Areas, As of December 31, 2000"
*Percent of population considered under-served by dental practitioners. An under-served population does not have primary medical care within reasonable economic and geographic bounds.

Employment in Health Care in 1998

National Total = 12,004,643 Employees*

RANK	STATE	EMPLOYEES	% of USA
23	Alabama	182,547	1.5%
50	Alaska	22,858	0.2%
25	Arizona	164,033	1.4%
33	Arkansas	112,209	0.9%
1	California	1,101,663	9.2%
26	Colorado	155,838	1.3%
22	Connecticut	182,923	1.5%
45	Delaware	41,202	0.3%
4	Florida	664,002	5.5%
12	Georgia	287,417	2.4%
46	Hawaii	40,214	0.3%
44	Idaho	44,523	0.4%
7	Illinois	528,234	4.4%
14	Indiana	277,712	2.3%
28	Iowa	150,487	1.3%
30	Kansas	133,895	1.1%
24	Kentucky	170,859	1.4%
21	Louisiana	208,057	1.7%
37	Maine	66,943	0.6%
20	Maryland	222,901	1.9%
9	Massachusetts	391,308	3.3%
8	Michigan	430,756	3.6%
15	Minnesota	258,570	2.2%
32	Mississippi	114,360	1.0%
13	Missouri	280,702	2.3%
47	Montana	38,051	0.3%
35	Nebraska	83,553	0.7%
41	Nevada	52,646	0.4%
40	New Hampshire	56,206	0.5%
10	New Jersey	356,812	3.0%
38	New Mexico	65,186	0.5%
2	New York	974,686	8.1%
11	North Carolina	331,932	2.8%
43	North Dakota	45,894	0.4%
6	Ohio	553,286	4.6%
27	Oklahoma	150,647	1.3%
31	Oregon	128,264	1.1%
5	Pennsylvania	650,500	5.4%
39	Rhode Island	59,324	0.5%
29	South Carolina	142,653	1.2%
42	South Dakota	48,237	0.4%
17	Tennessee	253,226	2.1%
3	Texas	812,285	6.8%
36	Utah	74,125	0.6%
48	Vermont	32,784	0.3%
16	Virginia	254,570	2.1%
19	Washington	228,101	1.9%
34	West Virginia	86,895	0.7%
18	Wisconsin	248,488	2.1%
49	Wyoming	23,694	0.2%

RANK	STATE	EMPLOYEES	% of USA
1	California	1,101,663	9.2%
2	New York	974,686	8.1%
3	Texas	812,285	6.8%
4	Florida	664,002	5.5%
5	Pennsylvania	650,500	5.4%
6	Ohio	553,286	4.6%
7	Illinois	528,234	4.4%
8	Michigan	430,756	3.6%
9	Massachusetts	391,308	3.3%
10	New Jersey	356,812	3.0%
11	North Carolina	331,932	2.8%
12	Georgia	287,417	2.4%
13	Missouri	280,702	2.3%
14	Indiana	277,712	2.3%
15	Minnesota	258,570	2.2%
16	Virginia	254,570	2.1%
17	Tennessee	253,226	2.1%
18	Wisconsin	248,488	2.1%
19	Washington	228,101	1.9%
20	Maryland	222,901	1.9%
21	Louisiana	208,057	1.7%
22	Connecticut	182,923	1.5%
23	Alabama	182,547	1.5%
24	Kentucky	170,859	1.4%
25	Arizona	164,033	1.4%
26	Colorado	155,838	1.3%
27	Oklahoma	150,647	1.3%
28	Iowa	150,487	1.3%
29	South Carolina	142,653	1.2%
30	Kansas	133,895	1.1%
31	Oregon	128,264	1.1%
32	Mississippi	114,360	1.0%
33	Arkansas	112,209	0.9%
34	West Virginia	86,895	0.7%
35	Nebraska	83,553	0.7%
36	Utah	74,125	0.6%
37	Maine	66,943	0.6%
38	New Mexico	65,186	0.5%
39	Rhode Island	59,324	0.5%
40	New Hampshire	56,206	0.5%
41	Nevada	52,646	0.4%
42	South Dakota	48,237	0.4%
43	North Dakota	45,894	0.4%
44	Idaho	44,523	0.4%
45	Delaware	41,202	0.3%
46	Hawaii	40,214	0.3%
47	Montana	38,051	0.3%
48	Vermont	32,784	0.3%
49	Wyoming	23,694	0.2%
50	Alaska	22,858	0.2%
	District of Columbia	48,190	0.4%

Source: U.S. Bureau of the Census
    "County Business Patterns 1998 (NACIS)" (http://tier2.census.gov/cbp_naics/index.html)
*Includes employees at establishments exempt from as well as subject to the federal income tax. Includes
employees at those establishments within the North American Industry Classification System (NACIS) classifications
621 (ambulatory health care services), 622 (hospitals) and 623 (nursing and residential care facilities). See
Facilities Chapter for establishments.

VII. PHYSICAL FITNESS

Users of Exercise Equipment in 1999

National Total = 45,207,000 Users

ALPHA ORDER

RANK	STATE	USERS	% of USA
29	Alabama	539,000	1.2%
NA	Alaska*	NA	NA
24	Arizona	756,000	1.7%
31	Arkansas	424,000	0.9%
1	California	5,502,000	12.2%
17	Colorado	900,000	2.0%
34	Connecticut	336,000	0.7%
47	Delaware	65,000	0.1%
4	Florida	2,355,000	5.2%
11	Georgia	1,255,000	2.8%
NA	Hawaii*	NA	NA
42	Idaho	192,000	0.4%
6	Illinois	2,109,000	4.7%
25	Indiana	736,000	1.6%
27	Iowa	562,000	1.2%
32	Kansas	395,000	0.9%
19	Kentucky	830,000	1.8%
20	Louisiana	785,000	1.7%
41	Maine	200,000	0.4%
12	Maryland	1,231,000	2.7%
14	Massachusetts	939,000	2.1%
9	Michigan	1,441,000	3.2%
18	Minnesota	850,000	1.9%
36	Mississippi	283,000	0.6%
23	Missouri	779,000	1.7%
38	Montana	263,000	0.6%
33	Nebraska	337,000	0.7%
35	Nevada	301,000	0.7%
39	New Hampshire	214,000	0.5%
8	New Jersey	1,527,000	3.4%
40	New Mexico	210,000	0.5%
2	New York	3,229,000	7.1%
10	North Carolina	1,393,000	3.1%
43	North Dakota	185,000	0.4%
5	Ohio	2,177,000	4.8%
30	Oklahoma	482,000	1.1%
22	Oregon	780,000	1.7%
7	Pennsylvania	1,857,000	4.1%
46	Rhode Island	116,000	0.3%
20	South Carolina	785,000	1.7%
44	South Dakota	157,000	0.3%
26	Tennessee	618,000	1.4%
3	Texas	3,056,000	6.8%
28	Utah	548,000	1.2%
45	Vermont	144,000	0.3%
13	Virginia	1,059,000	2.3%
16	Washington	931,000	2.1%
37	West Virginia	264,000	0.6%
15	Wisconsin	935,000	2.1%
48	Wyoming	33,000	0.1%

RANK ORDER

RANK	STATE	USERS	% of USA
1	California	5,502,000	12.2%
2	New York	3,229,000	7.1%
3	Texas	3,056,000	6.8%
4	Florida	2,355,000	5.2%
5	Ohio	2,177,000	4.8%
6	Illinois	2,109,000	4.7%
7	Pennsylvania	1,857,000	4.1%
8	New Jersey	1,527,000	3.4%
9	Michigan	1,441,000	3.2%
10	North Carolina	1,393,000	3.1%
11	Georgia	1,255,000	2.8%
12	Maryland	1,231,000	2.7%
13	Virginia	1,059,000	2.3%
14	Massachusetts	939,000	2.1%
15	Wisconsin	935,000	2.1%
16	Washington	931,000	2.1%
17	Colorado	900,000	2.0%
18	Minnesota	850,000	1.9%
19	Kentucky	830,000	1.8%
20	Louisiana	785,000	1.7%
20	South Carolina	785,000	1.7%
22	Oregon	780,000	1.7%
23	Missouri	779,000	1.7%
24	Arizona	756,000	1.7%
25	Indiana	736,000	1.6%
26	Tennessee	618,000	1.4%
27	Iowa	562,000	1.2%
28	Utah	548,000	1.2%
29	Alabama	539,000	1.2%
30	Oklahoma	482,000	1.1%
31	Arkansas	424,000	0.9%
32	Kansas	395,000	0.9%
33	Nebraska	337,000	0.7%
34	Connecticut	336,000	0.7%
35	Nevada	301,000	0.7%
36	Mississippi	283,000	0.6%
37	West Virginia	264,000	0.6%
38	Montana	263,000	0.6%
39	New Hampshire	214,000	0.5%
40	New Mexico	210,000	0.5%
41	Maine	200,000	0.4%
42	Idaho	192,000	0.4%
43	North Dakota	185,000	0.4%
44	South Dakota	157,000	0.3%
45	Vermont	144,000	0.3%
46	Rhode Island	116,000	0.3%
47	Delaware	65,000	0.1%
48	Wyoming	33,000	0.1%
NA	Alaska*	NA	NA
NA	Hawaii*	NA	NA
	District of Columbia*	NA	NA

Source: The National Sporting Goods Association
"NSGA Sports Participation Survey, January-December 1999 (Copyright 2000, reprinted with permission)
*Not available.

Participants in Golf in 1999

National Total = 27,005,000 Golfers

<table>
<tr><td colspan="4">ALPHA ORDER</td><td colspan="4">RANK ORDER</td></tr>
<tr><td>RANK</td><td>STATE</td><td>GOLFERS</td><td>% of USA</td><td>RANK</td><td>STATE</td><td>GOLFERS</td><td>% of USA</td></tr>
<tr><td>26</td><td>Alabama</td><td>339,000</td><td>1.3%</td><td>1</td><td>California</td><td>3,251,000</td><td>12.0%</td></tr>
<tr><td>NA</td><td>Alaska*</td><td>NA</td><td>NA</td><td>2</td><td>New York</td><td>1,939,000</td><td>7.2%</td></tr>
<tr><td>21</td><td>Arizona</td><td>431,000</td><td>1.6%</td><td>3</td><td>Illinois</td><td>1,518,000</td><td>5.6%</td></tr>
<tr><td>35</td><td>Arkansas</td><td>162,000</td><td>0.6%</td><td>4</td><td>Texas</td><td>1,469,000</td><td>5.4%</td></tr>
<tr><td>1</td><td>California</td><td>3,251,000</td><td>12.0%</td><td>5</td><td>Ohio</td><td>1,440,000</td><td>5.3%</td></tr>
<tr><td>23</td><td>Colorado</td><td>426,000</td><td>1.6%</td><td>6</td><td>Pennsylvania</td><td>1,263,000</td><td>4.7%</td></tr>
<tr><td>30</td><td>Connecticut</td><td>326,000</td><td>1.2%</td><td>7</td><td>Michigan</td><td>1,234,000</td><td>4.6%</td></tr>
<tr><td>47</td><td>Delaware</td><td>10,000</td><td>0.0%</td><td>8</td><td>Florida</td><td>1,217,000</td><td>4.5%</td></tr>
<tr><td>8</td><td>Florida</td><td>1,217,000</td><td>4.5%</td><td>9</td><td>Wisconsin</td><td>781,000</td><td>2.9%</td></tr>
<tr><td>14</td><td>Georgia</td><td>673,000</td><td>2.5%</td><td>10</td><td>North Carolina</td><td>753,000</td><td>2.8%</td></tr>
<tr><td>NA</td><td>Hawaii*</td><td>NA</td><td>NA</td><td>11</td><td>Minnesota</td><td>696,000</td><td>2.6%</td></tr>
<tr><td>33</td><td>Idaho</td><td>197,000</td><td>0.7%</td><td>12</td><td>Missouri</td><td>691,000</td><td>2.6%</td></tr>
<tr><td>3</td><td>Illinois</td><td>1,518,000</td><td>5.6%</td><td>13</td><td>New Jersey</td><td>674,000</td><td>2.5%</td></tr>
<tr><td>16</td><td>Indiana</td><td>606,000</td><td>2.2%</td><td>14</td><td>Georgia</td><td>673,000</td><td>2.5%</td></tr>
<tr><td>19</td><td>Iowa</td><td>532,000</td><td>2.0%</td><td>15</td><td>South Carolina</td><td>620,000</td><td>2.3%</td></tr>
<tr><td>43</td><td>Kansas</td><td>96,000</td><td>0.4%</td><td>16</td><td>Indiana</td><td>606,000</td><td>2.2%</td></tr>
<tr><td>22</td><td>Kentucky</td><td>430,000</td><td>1.6%</td><td>17</td><td>Washington</td><td>599,000</td><td>2.2%</td></tr>
<tr><td>39</td><td>Louisiana</td><td>152,000</td><td>0.6%</td><td>18</td><td>Massachusetts</td><td>597,000</td><td>2.2%</td></tr>
<tr><td>46</td><td>Maine</td><td>47,000</td><td>0.2%</td><td>19</td><td>Iowa</td><td>532,000</td><td>2.0%</td></tr>
<tr><td>25</td><td>Maryland</td><td>377,000</td><td>1.4%</td><td>20</td><td>Virginia</td><td>451,000</td><td>1.7%</td></tr>
<tr><td>18</td><td>Massachusetts</td><td>597,000</td><td>2.2%</td><td>21</td><td>Arizona</td><td>431,000</td><td>1.6%</td></tr>
<tr><td>7</td><td>Michigan</td><td>1,234,000</td><td>4.6%</td><td>22</td><td>Kentucky</td><td>430,000</td><td>1.6%</td></tr>
<tr><td>11</td><td>Minnesota</td><td>696,000</td><td>2.6%</td><td>23</td><td>Colorado</td><td>426,000</td><td>1.6%</td></tr>
<tr><td>38</td><td>Mississippi</td><td>154,000</td><td>0.6%</td><td>24</td><td>Nebraska</td><td>407,000</td><td>1.5%</td></tr>
<tr><td>12</td><td>Missouri</td><td>691,000</td><td>2.6%</td><td>25</td><td>Maryland</td><td>377,000</td><td>1.4%</td></tr>
<tr><td>32</td><td>Montana</td><td>210,000</td><td>0.8%</td><td>26</td><td>Alabama</td><td>339,000</td><td>1.3%</td></tr>
<tr><td>24</td><td>Nebraska</td><td>407,000</td><td>1.5%</td><td>27</td><td>Utah</td><td>335,000</td><td>1.2%</td></tr>
<tr><td>37</td><td>Nevada</td><td>157,000</td><td>0.6%</td><td>28</td><td>Oregon</td><td>332,000</td><td>1.2%</td></tr>
<tr><td>42</td><td>New Hampshire</td><td>100,000</td><td>0.4%</td><td>29</td><td>Tennessee</td><td>327,000</td><td>1.2%</td></tr>
<tr><td>13</td><td>New Jersey</td><td>674,000</td><td>2.5%</td><td>30</td><td>Connecticut</td><td>326,000</td><td>1.2%</td></tr>
<tr><td>40</td><td>New Mexico</td><td>121,000</td><td>0.4%</td><td>31</td><td>Oklahoma</td><td>233,000</td><td>0.9%</td></tr>
<tr><td>2</td><td>New York</td><td>1,939,000</td><td>7.2%</td><td>32</td><td>Montana</td><td>210,000</td><td>0.8%</td></tr>
<tr><td>10</td><td>North Carolina</td><td>753,000</td><td>2.8%</td><td>33</td><td>Idaho</td><td>197,000</td><td>0.7%</td></tr>
<tr><td>44</td><td>North Dakota</td><td>78,000</td><td>0.3%</td><td>34</td><td>West Virginia</td><td>177,000</td><td>0.7%</td></tr>
<tr><td>5</td><td>Ohio</td><td>1,440,000</td><td>5.3%</td><td>35</td><td>Arkansas</td><td>162,000</td><td>0.6%</td></tr>
<tr><td>31</td><td>Oklahoma</td><td>233,000</td><td>0.9%</td><td>36</td><td>Vermont</td><td>159,000</td><td>0.6%</td></tr>
<tr><td>28</td><td>Oregon</td><td>332,000</td><td>1.2%</td><td>37</td><td>Nevada</td><td>157,000</td><td>0.6%</td></tr>
<tr><td>6</td><td>Pennsylvania</td><td>1,263,000</td><td>4.7%</td><td>38</td><td>Mississippi</td><td>154,000</td><td>0.6%</td></tr>
<tr><td>44</td><td>Rhode Island</td><td>78,000</td><td>0.3%</td><td>39</td><td>Louisiana</td><td>152,000</td><td>0.6%</td></tr>
<tr><td>15</td><td>South Carolina</td><td>620,000</td><td>2.3%</td><td>40</td><td>New Mexico</td><td>121,000</td><td>0.4%</td></tr>
<tr><td>41</td><td>South Dakota</td><td>109,000</td><td>0.4%</td><td>41</td><td>South Dakota</td><td>109,000</td><td>0.4%</td></tr>
<tr><td>29</td><td>Tennessee</td><td>327,000</td><td>1.2%</td><td>42</td><td>New Hampshire</td><td>100,000</td><td>0.4%</td></tr>
<tr><td>4</td><td>Texas</td><td>1,469,000</td><td>5.4%</td><td>43</td><td>Kansas</td><td>96,000</td><td>0.4%</td></tr>
<tr><td>27</td><td>Utah</td><td>335,000</td><td>1.2%</td><td>44</td><td>North Dakota</td><td>78,000</td><td>0.3%</td></tr>
<tr><td>36</td><td>Vermont</td><td>159,000</td><td>0.6%</td><td>44</td><td>Rhode Island</td><td>78,000</td><td>0.3%</td></tr>
<tr><td>20</td><td>Virginia</td><td>451,000</td><td>1.7%</td><td>46</td><td>Maine</td><td>47,000</td><td>0.2%</td></tr>
<tr><td>17</td><td>Washington</td><td>599,000</td><td>2.2%</td><td>47</td><td>Delaware</td><td>10,000</td><td>0.0%</td></tr>
<tr><td>34</td><td>West Virginia</td><td>177,000</td><td>0.7%</td><td>48</td><td>Wyoming</td><td>9,000</td><td>0.0%</td></tr>
<tr><td>9</td><td>Wisconsin</td><td>781,000</td><td>2.9%</td><td>NA</td><td>Alaska*</td><td>NA</td><td>NA</td></tr>
<tr><td>48</td><td>Wyoming</td><td>9,000</td><td>0.0%</td><td>NA</td><td>Hawaii*</td><td>NA</td><td>NA</td></tr>
<tr><td></td><td></td><td></td><td></td><td colspan="2">District of Columbia*</td><td>NA</td><td>NA</td></tr>
</table>

Source: The National Sporting Goods Association
"NSGA Sports Participation Survey, January-December 1999 (Copyright 2000, reprinted with permission)
*Not available.

Participants in Running/Jogging in 1999

National Total = 22,366,000 Runners/Joggers

ALPHA ORDER

RANK	STATE	RUNNERS	% of USA
22	Alabama	393,000	1.8%
NA	Alaska*	NA	NA
27	Arizona	332,000	1.5%
31	Arkansas	226,000	1.0%
1	California	3,680,000	16.5%
24	Colorado	368,000	1.6%
35	Connecticut	139,000	0.6%
46	Delaware	22,000	0.1%
4	Florida	909,000	4.1%
9	Georgia	670,000	3.0%
NA	Hawaii*	NA	NA
36	Idaho	125,000	0.6%
5	Illinois	895,000	4.0%
15	Indiana	468,000	2.1%
28	Iowa	311,000	1.4%
34	Kansas	162,000	0.7%
16	Kentucky	463,000	2.1%
19	Louisiana	432,000	1.9%
47	Maine	16,000	0.1%
10	Maryland	623,000	2.8%
21	Massachusetts	409,000	1.8%
11	Michigan	597,000	2.7%
29	Minnesota	305,000	1.4%
33	Mississippi	177,000	0.8%
17	Missouri	458,000	2.0%
39	Montana	101,000	0.5%
32	Nebraska	224,000	1.0%
41	Nevada	90,000	0.4%
38	New Hampshire	117,000	0.5%
12	New Jersey	574,000	2.6%
43	New Mexico	63,000	0.3%
3	New York	1,386,000	6.2%
8	North Carolina	680,000	3.0%
44	North Dakota	38,000	0.2%
7	Ohio	796,000	3.6%
26	Oklahoma	336,000	1.5%
18	Oregon	445,000	2.0%
6	Pennsylvania	847,000	3.8%
40	Rhode Island	98,000	0.4%
13	South Carolina	486,000	2.2%
42	South Dakota	83,000	0.4%
29	Tennessee	305,000	1.4%
2	Texas	1,770,000	7.9%
20	Utah	415,000	1.9%
45	Vermont	32,000	0.1%
14	Virginia	472,000	2.1%
23	Washington	384,000	1.7%
37	West Virginia	120,000	0.5%
25	Wisconsin	364,000	1.6%
NA	Wyoming*	NA	NA

RANK ORDER

RANK	STATE	RUNNERS	% of USA
1	California	3,680,000	16.5%
2	Texas	1,770,000	7.9%
3	New York	1,386,000	6.2%
4	Florida	909,000	4.1%
5	Illinois	895,000	4.0%
6	Pennsylvania	847,000	3.8%
7	Ohio	796,000	3.6%
8	North Carolina	680,000	3.0%
9	Georgia	670,000	3.0%
10	Maryland	623,000	2.8%
11	Michigan	597,000	2.7%
12	New Jersey	574,000	2.6%
13	South Carolina	486,000	2.2%
14	Virginia	472,000	2.1%
15	Indiana	468,000	2.1%
16	Kentucky	463,000	2.1%
17	Missouri	458,000	2.0%
18	Oregon	445,000	2.0%
19	Louisiana	432,000	1.9%
20	Utah	415,000	1.9%
21	Massachusetts	409,000	1.8%
22	Alabama	393,000	1.8%
23	Washington	384,000	1.7%
24	Colorado	368,000	1.6%
25	Wisconsin	364,000	1.6%
26	Oklahoma	336,000	1.5%
27	Arizona	332,000	1.5%
28	Iowa	311,000	1.4%
29	Minnesota	305,000	1.4%
29	Tennessee	305,000	1.4%
31	Arkansas	226,000	1.0%
32	Nebraska	224,000	1.0%
33	Mississippi	177,000	0.8%
34	Kansas	162,000	0.7%
35	Connecticut	139,000	0.6%
36	Idaho	125,000	0.6%
37	West Virginia	120,000	0.5%
38	New Hampshire	117,000	0.5%
39	Montana	101,000	0.5%
40	Rhode Island	98,000	0.4%
41	Nevada	90,000	0.4%
42	South Dakota	83,000	0.4%
43	New Mexico	63,000	0.3%
44	North Dakota	38,000	0.2%
45	Vermont	32,000	0.1%
46	Delaware	22,000	0.1%
47	Maine	16,000	0.1%
NA	Alaska*	NA	NA
NA	Hawaii*	NA	NA
NA	Wyoming*	NA	NA
	District of Columbia*	NA	NA

Source: The National Sporting Goods Association
"NSGA Sports Participation Survey, January-December 1999 (Copyright 2000, reprinted with permission)
Not available.

Participants in Swimming in 1999

National Total = 57,916,000 Swimmers

ALPHA ORDER

RANK	STATE	SWIMMERS	% of USA
22	Alabama	905,000	1.6%
NA	Alaska*	NA	NA
17	Arizona	1,055,000	1.8%
31	Arkansas	554,000	1.0%
1	California	7,473,000	12.9%
27	Colorado	676,000	1.2%
26	Connecticut	772,000	1.3%
48	Delaware	22,000	0.0%
4	Florida	3,365,000	5.8%
16	Georgia	1,127,000	1.9%
NA	Hawaii*	NA	NA
40	Idaho	209,000	0.4%
6	Illinois	2,342,000	4.0%
14	Indiana	1,339,000	2.3%
30	Iowa	642,000	1.1%
37	Kansas	374,000	0.6%
23	Kentucky	867,000	1.5%
20	Louisiana	985,000	1.7%
34	Maine	422,000	0.7%
12	Maryland	1,595,000	2.8%
11	Massachusetts	1,629,000	2.8%
9	Michigan	1,820,000	3.1%
24	Minnesota	853,000	1.5%
34	Mississippi	422,000	0.7%
13	Missouri	1,392,000	2.4%
39	Montana	262,000	0.5%
33	Nebraska	426,000	0.7%
42	Nevada	172,000	0.3%
36	New Hampshire	381,000	0.7%
8	New Jersey	1,893,000	3.3%
45	New Mexico	114,000	0.2%
3	New York	4,276,000	7.4%
10	North Carolina	1,643,000	2.8%
43	North Dakota	171,000	0.3%
7	Ohio	2,171,000	3.7%
32	Oklahoma	549,000	0.9%
29	Oregon	670,000	1.2%
5	Pennsylvania	3,279,000	5.7%
38	Rhode Island	278,000	0.5%
28	South Carolina	671,000	1.2%
46	South Dakota	110,000	0.2%
18	Tennessee	1,050,000	1.8%
2	Texas	4,362,000	7.5%
25	Utah	834,000	1.4%
44	Vermont	139,000	0.2%
15	Virginia	1,286,000	2.2%
19	Washington	1,049,000	1.8%
41	West Virginia	177,000	0.3%
21	Wisconsin	976,000	1.7%
47	Wyoming	47,000	0.1%

RANK ORDER

RANK	STATE	SWIMMERS	% of USA
1	California	7,473,000	12.9%
2	Texas	4,362,000	7.5%
3	New York	4,276,000	7.4%
4	Florida	3,365,000	5.8%
5	Pennsylvania	3,279,000	5.7%
6	Illinois	2,342,000	4.0%
7	Ohio	2,171,000	3.7%
8	New Jersey	1,893,000	3.3%
9	Michigan	1,820,000	3.1%
10	North Carolina	1,643,000	2.8%
11	Massachusetts	1,629,000	2.8%
12	Maryland	1,595,000	2.8%
13	Missouri	1,392,000	2.4%
14	Indiana	1,339,000	2.3%
15	Virginia	1,286,000	2.2%
16	Georgia	1,127,000	1.9%
17	Arizona	1,055,000	1.8%
18	Tennessee	1,050,000	1.8%
19	Washington	1,049,000	1.8%
20	Louisiana	985,000	1.7%
21	Wisconsin	976,000	1.7%
22	Alabama	905,000	1.6%
23	Kentucky	867,000	1.5%
24	Minnesota	853,000	1.5%
25	Utah	834,000	1.4%
26	Connecticut	772,000	1.3%
27	Colorado	676,000	1.2%
28	South Carolina	671,000	1.2%
29	Oregon	670,000	1.2%
30	Iowa	642,000	1.1%
31	Arkansas	554,000	1.0%
32	Oklahoma	549,000	0.9%
33	Nebraska	426,000	0.7%
34	Maine	422,000	0.7%
34	Mississippi	422,000	0.7%
36	New Hampshire	381,000	0.7%
37	Kansas	374,000	0.6%
38	Rhode Island	278,000	0.5%
39	Montana	262,000	0.5%
40	Idaho	209,000	0.4%
41	West Virginia	177,000	0.3%
42	Nevada	172,000	0.3%
43	North Dakota	171,000	0.3%
44	Vermont	139,000	0.2%
45	New Mexico	114,000	0.2%
46	South Dakota	110,000	0.2%
47	Wyoming	47,000	0.1%
48	Delaware	22,000	0.0%
NA	Alaska*	NA	NA
NA	Hawaii*	NA	NA
	District of Columbia*	NA	NA

Source: The National Sporting Goods Association
   "NSGA Sports Participation Survey, January-December 1999 (Copyright 2000, reprinted with permission)
Not available.

Participants in Tennis in 1999

National Total = 10,921,000 Tennis Players

ALPHA ORDER

RANK	STATE	PLAYERS	% of USA
15	Alabama	238,000	2.2%
NA	Alaska*	NA	NA
24	Arizona	141,000	1.3%
38	Arkansas	49,000	0.4%
1	California	1,596,000	14.6%
28	Colorado	130,000	1.2%
27	Connecticut	131,000	1.2%
41	Delaware	23,000	0.2%
6	Florida	443,000	4.1%
5	Georgia	533,000	4.9%
NA	Hawaii*	NA	NA
47	Idaho	7,000	0.1%
4	Illinois	589,000	5.4%
12	Indiana	295,000	2.7%
17	Iowa	205,000	1.9%
35	Kansas	71,000	0.7%
21	Kentucky	163,000	1.5%
16	Louisiana	220,000	2.0%
31	Maine	100,000	0.9%
19	Maryland	185,000	1.7%
14	Massachusetts	247,000	2.3%
13	Michigan	273,000	2.5%
30	Minnesota	107,000	1.0%
34	Mississippi	82,000	0.8%
22	Missouri	156,000	1.4%
36	Montana	68,000	0.6%
29	Nebraska	122,000	1.1%
42	Nevada	21,000	0.2%
39	New Hampshire	42,000	0.4%
8	New Jersey	435,000	4.0%
44	New Mexico	19,000	0.2%
2	New York	978,000	9.0%
11	North Carolina	296,000	2.7%
45	North Dakota	17,000	0.2%
9	Ohio	370,000	3.4%
26	Oklahoma	132,000	1.2%
23	Oregon	153,000	1.4%
7	Pennsylvania	438,000	4.0%
37	Rhode Island	64,000	0.6%
10	South Carolina	332,000	3.0%
46	South Dakota	16,000	0.1%
33	Tennessee	92,000	0.8%
3	Texas	654,000	6.0%
18	Utah	191,000	1.7%
43	Vermont	20,000	0.2%
25	Virginia	137,000	1.3%
32	Washington	94,000	0.9%
40	West Virginia	35,000	0.3%
20	Wisconsin	167,000	1.5%
NA	Wyoming*	NA	NA

RANK ORDER

RANK	STATE	PLAYERS	% of USA
1	California	1,596,000	14.6%
2	New York	978,000	9.0%
3	Texas	654,000	6.0%
4	Illinois	589,000	5.4%
5	Georgia	533,000	4.9%
6	Florida	443,000	4.1%
7	Pennsylvania	438,000	4.0%
8	New Jersey	435,000	4.0%
9	Ohio	370,000	3.4%
10	South Carolina	332,000	3.0%
11	North Carolina	296,000	2.7%
12	Indiana	295,000	2.7%
13	Michigan	273,000	2.5%
14	Massachusetts	247,000	2.3%
15	Alabama	238,000	2.2%
16	Louisiana	220,000	2.0%
17	Iowa	205,000	1.9%
18	Utah	191,000	1.7%
19	Maryland	185,000	1.7%
20	Wisconsin	167,000	1.5%
21	Kentucky	163,000	1.5%
22	Missouri	156,000	1.4%
23	Oregon	153,000	1.4%
24	Arizona	141,000	1.3%
25	Virginia	137,000	1.3%
26	Oklahoma	132,000	1.2%
27	Connecticut	131,000	1.2%
28	Colorado	130,000	1.2%
29	Nebraska	122,000	1.1%
30	Minnesota	107,000	1.0%
31	Maine	100,000	0.9%
32	Washington	94,000	0.9%
33	Tennessee	92,000	0.8%
34	Mississippi	82,000	0.8%
35	Kansas	71,000	0.7%
36	Montana	68,000	0.6%
37	Rhode Island	64,000	0.6%
38	Arkansas	49,000	0.4%
39	New Hampshire	42,000	0.4%
40	West Virginia	35,000	0.3%
41	Delaware	23,000	0.2%
42	Nevada	21,000	0.2%
43	Vermont	20,000	0.2%
44	New Mexico	19,000	0.2%
45	North Dakota	17,000	0.2%
46	South Dakota	16,000	0.1%
47	Idaho	7,000	0.1%
NA	Alaska*	NA	NA
NA	Hawaii*	NA	NA
NA	Wyoming*	NA	NA
	District of Columbia*	NA	NA

Source: The National Sporting Goods Association
    "NSGA Sports Participation Survey, January-December 1999 (Copyright 2000, reprinted with permission)
*Not available.

Alcohol Consumption in 1997

National Total = 465,680,000 Gallons*

ALPHA ORDER

RANK	STATE	GALLONS	% of USA
25	Alabama	6,339,000	1.4%
48	Alaska	1,191,000	0.3%
17	Arizona	9,177,000	2.0%
35	Arkansas	3,570,000	0.8%
1	California	56,492,000	12.1%
23	Colorado	7,995,000	1.7%
27	Connecticut	5,864,000	1.3%
45	Delaware	1,705,000	0.4%
3	Florida	31,229,000	6.7%
10	Georgia	13,056,000	2.8%
40	Hawaii	2,230,000	0.5%
42	Idaho	1,919,000	0.4%
5	Illinois	21,841,000	4.7%
18	Indiana	9,054,000	1.9%
32	Iowa	4,340,000	0.9%
34	Kansas	3,587,000	0.8%
28	Kentucky	5,485,000	1.2%
21	Louisiana	8,476,000	1.8%
39	Maine	2,236,000	0.5%
20	Maryland	8,514,000	1.8%
11	Massachusetts	12,075,000	2.6%
8	Michigan	16,051,000	3.4%
19	Minnesota	8,857,000	1.9%
30	Mississippi	4,530,000	1.0%
16	Missouri	9,426,000	2.0%
44	Montana	1,730,000	0.4%
37	Nebraska	2,815,000	0.6%
29	Nevada	5,245,000	1.1%
33	New Hampshire	3,854,000	0.8%
9	New Jersey	14,193,000	3.0%
36	New Mexico	3,184,000	0.7%
4	New York	28,095,000	6.0%
12	North Carolina	11,712,000	2.5%
47	North Dakota	1,204,000	0.3%
7	Ohio	17,321,000	3.7%
31	Oklahoma	4,435,000	1.0%
26	Oregon	5,969,000	1.3%
6	Pennsylvania	18,323,000	3.9%
42	Rhode Island	1,919,000	0.4%
24	South Carolina	7,109,000	1.5%
46	South Dakota	1,285,000	0.3%
22	Tennessee	8,099,000	1.7%
2	Texas	33,993,000	7.3%
41	Utah	1,981,000	0.4%
49	Vermont	1,123,000	0.2%
14	Virginia	10,465,000	2.2%
15	Washington	9,813,000	2.1%
38	West Virginia	2,419,000	0.5%
13	Wisconsin	11,477,000	2.5%
50	Wyoming	911,000	0.2%

RANK ORDER

RANK	STATE	GALLONS	% of USA
1	California	56,492,000	12.1%
2	Texas	33,993,000	7.3%
3	Florida	31,229,000	6.7%
4	New York	28,095,000	6.0%
5	Illinois	21,841,000	4.7%
6	Pennsylvania	18,323,000	3.9%
7	Ohio	17,321,000	3.7%
8	Michigan	16,051,000	3.4%
9	New Jersey	14,193,000	3.0%
10	Georgia	13,056,000	2.8%
11	Massachusetts	12,075,000	2.6%
12	North Carolina	11,712,000	2.5%
13	Wisconsin	11,477,000	2.5%
14	Virginia	10,465,000	2.2%
15	Washington	9,813,000	2.1%
16	Missouri	9,426,000	2.0%
17	Arizona	9,177,000	2.0%
18	Indiana	9,054,000	1.9%
19	Minnesota	8,857,000	1.9%
20	Maryland	8,514,000	1.8%
21	Louisiana	8,476,000	1.8%
22	Tennessee	8,099,000	1.7%
23	Colorado	7,995,000	1.7%
24	South Carolina	7,109,000	1.5%
25	Alabama	6,339,000	1.4%
26	Oregon	5,969,000	1.3%
27	Connecticut	5,864,000	1.3%
28	Kentucky	5,485,000	1.2%
29	Nevada	5,245,000	1.1%
30	Mississippi	4,530,000	1.0%
31	Oklahoma	4,435,000	1.0%
32	Iowa	4,340,000	0.9%
33	New Hampshire	3,854,000	0.8%
34	Kansas	3,587,000	0.8%
35	Arkansas	3,570,000	0.8%
36	New Mexico	3,184,000	0.7%
37	Nebraska	2,815,000	0.6%
38	West Virginia	2,419,000	0.5%
39	Maine	2,236,000	0.5%
40	Hawaii	2,230,000	0.5%
41	Utah	1,981,000	0.4%
42	Idaho	1,919,000	0.4%
42	Rhode Island	1,919,000	0.4%
44	Montana	1,730,000	0.4%
45	Delaware	1,705,000	0.4%
46	South Dakota	1,285,000	0.3%
47	North Dakota	1,204,000	0.3%
48	Alaska	1,191,000	0.3%
49	Vermont	1,123,000	0.2%
50	Wyoming	911,000	0.2%
	District of Columbia	1,767,000	0.4%

Source: U.S. Department of Health and Human Services, National Institute on Alcohol Abuse and Alcoholism
    "Volume Beverage and Ethanol Consumption for States" (http://silk.nih.gov/silk/niaaa1/database/consum02.txt)
This is apparent consumption of actual alcohol, not entire volume of an alcoholic beverage (e.g. wine is roughly 11% absolute alcohol content). Apparent consumption is based on several sources which together approximate sales but do not actually measure consumption. Accordingly, figures for some states may be skewed by purchases by nonresidents.

Adult Per Capita Alcohol Consumption in 1997

National Per Capita = 2.5 Gallons Consumed per Adult Age 21 & Older*

ALPHA ORDER				RANK ORDER		
RANK	STATE	PER CAPITA		RANK	STATE	PER CAPITA
42	Alabama	2.1		1	New Hampshire	4.6
5	Alaska	3.1		2	Nevada	4.5
7	Arizona	2.9		3	Delaware	3.2
45	Arkansas	2.0		3	Wisconsin	3.2
20	California	2.6		5	Alaska	3.1
6	Colorado	3.0		6	Colorado	3.0
25	Connecticut	2.5		7	Arizona	2.9
3	Delaware	3.2		7	Florida	2.9
7	Florida	2.9		7	Louisiana	2.9
25	Georgia	2.5		10	Montana	2.8
13	Hawaii	2.7		10	New Mexico	2.8
33	Idaho	2.4		10	Wyoming	2.8
20	Illinois	2.6		13	Hawaii	2.7
36	Indiana	2.2		13	Massachusetts	2.7
36	Iowa	2.2		13	Minnesota	2.7
45	Kansas	2.0		13	North Dakota	2.7
45	Kentucky	2.0		13	Rhode Island	2.7
7	Louisiana	2.9		13	South Carolina	2.7
25	Maine	2.5		13	Vermont	2.7
35	Maryland	2.3		20	California	2.6
13	Massachusetts	2.7		20	Illinois	2.6
33	Michigan	2.4		20	Oregon	2.6
13	Minnesota	2.7		20	South Dakota	2.6
25	Mississippi	2.5		20	Texas	2.6
25	Missouri	2.5		25	Connecticut	2.5
10	Montana	2.8		25	Georgia	2.5
25	Nebraska	2.5		25	Maine	2.5
2	Nevada	4.5		25	Mississippi	2.5
1	New Hampshire	4.6		25	Missouri	2.5
25	New Jersey	2.5		25	Nebraska	2.5
10	New Mexico	2.8		25	New Jersey	2.5
36	New York	2.2		25	Washington	2.5
36	North Carolina	2.2		33	Idaho	2.4
13	North Dakota	2.7		33	Michigan	2.4
36	Ohio	2.2		35	Maryland	2.3
48	Oklahoma	1.9		36	Indiana	2.2
20	Oregon	2.6		36	Iowa	2.2
42	Pennsylvania	2.1		36	New York	2.2
13	Rhode Island	2.7		36	North Carolina	2.2
13	South Carolina	2.7		36	Ohio	2.2
20	South Dakota	2.6		36	Virginia	2.2
42	Tennessee	2.1		42	Alabama	2.1
20	Texas	2.6		42	Pennsylvania	2.1
50	Utah	1.6		42	Tennessee	2.1
13	Vermont	2.7		45	Arkansas	2.0
36	Virginia	2.2		45	Kansas	2.0
25	Washington	2.5		45	Kentucky	2.0
49	West Virginia	1.8		48	Oklahoma	1.9
3	Wisconsin	3.2		49	West Virginia	1.8
10	Wyoming	2.8		50	Utah	1.6
					District of Columbia	4.3

Source: Morgan Quitno Press using data from U.S. Department of Health and Human Services, National Institute on Alcohol Abuse and Alcoholism "Volume Beverage and Ethanol Consumption for States"
*This is apparent consumption of actual alcohol, not entire volume of an alcoholic beverage (e.g. wine is roughly 11% absolute alcohol content). Apparent consumption is based on several sources which together approximate sales but do not actually measure consumption. Accordingly, figures for some states may be skewed by purchases by nonresidents.

Percent of Adults Who Abstain from Drinking Alcohol: 1997

National Percent = 50.1% of Adults*

ALPHA ORDER

RANK	STATE	PERCENT
9	Alabama	63.2
33	Alaska	44.8
12	Arizona	58.9
3	Arkansas	69.4
45	California	38.6
46	Colorado	38.0
47	Connecticut	37.9
29	Delaware	45.8
31	Florida	45.2
15	Georgia	55.4
22	Hawaii	48.9
16	Idaho	52.4
30	Illinois	45.3
17	Indiana	51.5
28	Iowa	46.1
13	Kansas	58.7
6	Kentucky	66.3
21	Louisiana	49.4
34	Maine	44.6
14	Maryland	55.6
49	Massachusetts	35.2
38	Michigan	42.6
24	Minnesota	46.5
8	Mississippi	64.9
18	Missouri	50.8
37	Montana	42.8
39	Nebraska	42.0
48	Nevada	37.1
44	New Hampshire	38.7
40	New Jersey	41.7
26	New Mexico	46.4
24	New York	46.5
10	North Carolina	62.4
27	North Dakota	46.3
6	Ohio	66.3
5	Oklahoma	67.2
36	Oregon	43.3
19	Pennsylvania	50.7
41	Rhode Island	40.6
11	South Carolina	60.3
35	South Dakota	44.5
2	Tennessee	71.3
20	Texas	50.6
1	Utah	71.7
42	Vermont	39.8
32	Virginia	45.1
43	Washington	39.6
4	West Virginia	69.0
50	Wisconsin	29.8
23	Wyoming	47.4

RANK ORDER

RANK	STATE	PERCENT
1	Utah	71.7
2	Tennessee	71.3
3	Arkansas	69.4
4	West Virginia	69.0
5	Oklahoma	67.2
6	Kentucky	66.3
6	Ohio	66.3
8	Mississippi	64.9
9	Alabama	63.2
10	North Carolina	62.4
11	South Carolina	60.3
12	Arizona	58.9
13	Kansas	58.7
14	Maryland	55.6
15	Georgia	55.4
16	Idaho	52.4
17	Indiana	51.5
18	Missouri	50.8
19	Pennsylvania	50.7
20	Texas	50.6
21	Louisiana	49.4
22	Hawaii	48.9
23	Wyoming	47.4
24	Minnesota	46.5
24	New York	46.5
26	New Mexico	46.4
27	North Dakota	46.3
28	Iowa	46.1
29	Delaware	45.8
30	Illinois	45.3
31	Florida	45.2
32	Virginia	45.1
33	Alaska	44.8
34	Maine	44.6
35	South Dakota	44.5
36	Oregon	43.3
37	Montana	42.8
38	Michigan	42.6
39	Nebraska	42.0
40	New Jersey	41.7
41	Rhode Island	40.6
42	Vermont	39.8
43	Washington	39.6
44	New Hampshire	38.7
45	California	38.6
46	Colorado	38.0
47	Connecticut	37.9
48	Nevada	37.1
49	Massachusetts	35.2
50	Wisconsin	29.8

District of Columbia 56.3

Source: U.S. Department of Heath and Human Services, National Institute on Alcohol Abuse and Alcoholism
    "Per Capita and Per Drinker Ethanol Consumption for Selected States, 1986-97"
        (http://silk.nih.gov/silk/niaaa1/database/consum04.txt)
*National average is a simple average of all states.

Apparent Beer Consumption in 1997

National Total = 5,879,132,000 Gallons of Beer Consumed*

ALPHA ORDER

RANK	STATE	GALLONS	% of USA
25	Alabama	88,807,000	1.5%
48	Alaska	13,569,000	0.2%
16	Arizona	121,315,000	2.1%
34	Arkansas	49,949,000	0.8%
1	California	627,850,000	10.7%
24	Colorado	93,210,000	1.6%
32	Connecticut	57,055,000	1.0%
45	Delaware	18,439,000	0.3%
3	Florida	369,357,000	6.3%
9	Georgia	161,788,000	2.8%
39	Hawaii	29,513,000	0.5%
42	Idaho	24,322,000	0.4%
5	Illinois	270,769,000	4.6%
17	Indiana	119,194,000	2.0%
28	Iowa	66,865,000	1.1%
33	Kansas	50,997,000	0.9%
26	Kentucky	75,226,000	1.3%
18	Louisiana	116,143,000	2.0%
41	Maine	26,134,000	0.4%
23	Maryland	95,792,000	1.6%
14	Massachusetts	127,402,000	2.2%
8	Michigan	202,667,000	3.4%
21	Minnesota	104,045,000	1.8%
29	Mississippi	66,745,000	1.1%
15	Missouri	127,040,000	2.2%
43	Montana	23,761,000	0.4%
36	Nebraska	40,276,000	0.7%
31	Nevada	57,686,000	1.0%
38	New Hampshire	36,662,000	0.6%
12	New Jersey	144,225,000	2.5%
35	New Mexico	45,963,000	0.8%
4	New York	312,992,000	5.3%
10	North Carolina	158,271,000	2.7%
47	North Dakota	16,280,000	0.3%
7	Ohio	257,204,000	4.4%
30	Oklahoma	65,561,000	1.1%
27	Oregon	70,741,000	1.2%
6	Pennsylvania	265,867,000	4.5%
44	Rhode Island	22,599,000	0.4%
22	South Carolina	96,207,000	1.6%
46	South Dakota	17,776,000	0.3%
19	Tennessee	114,549,000	1.9%
2	Texas	525,261,000	8.9%
40	Utah	26,707,000	0.5%
49	Vermont	13,238,000	0.2%
13	Virginia	138,220,000	2.4%
20	Washington	112,384,000	1.9%
37	West Virginia	38,145,000	0.6%
11	Wisconsin	147,860,000	2.5%
50	Wyoming	11,800,000	0.2%

RANK ORDER

RANK	STATE	GALLONS	% of USA
1	California	627,850,000	10.7%
2	Texas	525,261,000	8.9%
3	Florida	369,357,000	6.3%
4	New York	312,992,000	5.3%
5	Illinois	270,769,000	4.6%
6	Pennsylvania	265,867,000	4.5%
7	Ohio	257,204,000	4.4%
8	Michigan	202,667,000	3.4%
9	Georgia	161,788,000	2.8%
10	North Carolina	158,271,000	2.7%
11	Wisconsin	147,860,000	2.5%
12	New Jersey	144,225,000	2.5%
13	Virginia	138,220,000	2.4%
14	Massachusetts	127,402,000	2.2%
15	Missouri	127,040,000	2.2%
16	Arizona	121,315,000	2.1%
17	Indiana	119,194,000	2.0%
18	Louisiana	116,143,000	2.0%
19	Tennessee	114,549,000	1.9%
20	Washington	112,384,000	1.9%
21	Minnesota	104,045,000	1.8%
22	South Carolina	96,207,000	1.6%
23	Maryland	95,792,000	1.6%
24	Colorado	93,210,000	1.6%
25	Alabama	88,807,000	1.5%
26	Kentucky	75,226,000	1.3%
27	Oregon	70,741,000	1.2%
28	Iowa	66,865,000	1.1%
29	Mississippi	66,745,000	1.1%
30	Oklahoma	65,561,000	1.1%
31	Nevada	57,686,000	1.0%
32	Connecticut	57,055,000	1.0%
33	Kansas	50,997,000	0.9%
34	Arkansas	49,949,000	0.8%
35	New Mexico	45,963,000	0.8%
36	Nebraska	40,276,000	0.7%
37	West Virginia	38,145,000	0.6%
38	New Hampshire	36,662,000	0.6%
39	Hawaii	29,513,000	0.5%
40	Utah	26,707,000	0.5%
41	Maine	26,134,000	0.4%
42	Idaho	24,322,000	0.4%
43	Montana	23,761,000	0.4%
44	Rhode Island	22,599,000	0.4%
45	Delaware	18,439,000	0.3%
46	South Dakota	17,776,000	0.3%
47	North Dakota	16,280,000	0.3%
48	Alaska	13,569,000	0.2%
49	Vermont	13,238,000	0.2%
50	Wyoming	11,800,000	0.2%
	District of Columbia	14,703,000	0.3%

Source: U.S. Department of Health and Human Services, National Institute on Alcohol Abuse and Alcoholism
"Volume Beverage and Ethanol Consumption for States" (http://silk.nih.gov/silk/niaaa1/database/consum02.txt)
This is apparent consumption and is based on several sources which together approximate sales but do not actually measure consumption. Reported state volumes reflect only in-state purchases. Accordingly, figures for some states may be skewed by purchases by nonresidents.

496

Adult Per Capita Beer Consumption in 1997

National Per Capita = 31.5 Gallons Consumed per Adult 21 Years and Older*

ALPHA ORDER

RANK	STATE	PER CAPITA
34	Alabama	29.2
17	Alaska	34.9
8	Arizona	38.9
43	Arkansas	28.5
40	California	28.6
19	Colorado	34.4
49	Connecticut	24.1
16	Delaware	35.0
18	Florida	34.6
27	Georgia	31.3
15	Hawaii	35.2
29	Idaho	30.6
23	Illinois	32.6
36	Indiana	29.1
21	Iowa	33.4
43	Kansas	28.5
45	Kentucky	27.4
6	Louisiana	39.7
34	Maine	29.2
46	Maryland	26.4
40	Massachusetts	28.6
33	Michigan	29.7
24	Minnesota	32.2
10	Mississippi	36.4
20	Missouri	33.7
7	Montana	39.0
14	Nebraska	35.4
1	Nevada	49.1
2	New Hampshire	44.0
47	New Jersey	25.0
5	New Mexico	40.3
48	New York	24.2
31	North Carolina	30.2
9	North Dakota	36.6
22	Ohio	32.7
40	Oklahoma	28.6
28	Oregon	30.9
29	Pennsylvania	30.6
25	Rhode Island	31.7
12	South Carolina	36.1
13	South Dakota	35.6
32	Tennessee	30.0
4	Texas	40.6
50	Utah	21.6
26	Vermont	31.4
38	Virginia	28.7
38	Washington	28.7
37	West Virginia	29.0
3	Wisconsin	40.8
10	Wyoming	36.4

RANK ORDER

RANK	STATE	PER CAPITA
1	Nevada	49.1
2	New Hampshire	44.0
3	Wisconsin	40.8
4	Texas	40.6
5	New Mexico	40.3
6	Louisiana	39.7
7	Montana	39.0
8	Arizona	38.9
9	North Dakota	36.6
10	Mississippi	36.4
10	Wyoming	36.4
12	South Carolina	36.1
13	South Dakota	35.6
14	Nebraska	35.4
15	Hawaii	35.2
16	Delaware	35.0
17	Alaska	34.9
18	Florida	34.6
19	Colorado	34.4
20	Missouri	33.7
21	Iowa	33.4
22	Ohio	32.7
23	Illinois	32.6
24	Minnesota	32.2
25	Rhode Island	31.7
26	Vermont	31.4
27	Georgia	31.3
28	Oregon	30.9
29	Idaho	30.6
29	Pennsylvania	30.6
31	North Carolina	30.2
32	Tennessee	30.0
33	Michigan	29.7
34	Alabama	29.2
34	Maine	29.2
36	Indiana	29.1
37	West Virginia	29.0
38	Virginia	28.7
38	Washington	28.7
40	California	28.6
40	Massachusetts	28.6
40	Oklahoma	28.6
43	Arkansas	28.5
43	Kansas	28.5
45	Kentucky	27.4
46	Maryland	26.4
47	New Jersey	25.0
48	New York	24.2
49	Connecticut	24.1
50	Utah	21.6

| | District of Columbia | 36.2 |

Source: Morgan Quitno Press using data from U.S. Department of Health and Human Services, National Institute on Alcohol Abuse and Alcoholism "Volume Beverage and Ethanol Consumption for States"
*This is apparent consumption and is based on several sources which together approximate sales but do not actually measure consumption. Reported state volumes reflect only in-state purchases. Accordingly, figures for some states may be skewed by purchases by nonresidents.

Wine Consumption in 1997

National Total = 508,042,000 Gallons of Wine Consumed*

RANK	STATE (ALPHA ORDER)	GALLONS	% of USA	RANK	STATE (RANK ORDER)	GALLONS	% of USA
29	Alabama	4,057,000	0.8%	1	California	97,352,000	19.2%
45	Alaska	1,307,000	0.3%	2	New York	42,931,000	8.5%
19	Arizona	9,021,000	1.8%	3	Florida	35,956,000	7.1%
40	Arkansas	1,908,000	0.4%	4	Illinois	25,720,000	5.1%
1	California	97,352,000	19.2%	5	Texas	23,979,000	4.7%
16	Colorado	9,320,000	1.8%	6	New Jersey	21,679,000	4.3%
15	Connecticut	10,144,000	2.0%	7	Massachusetts	19,337,000	3.8%
38	Delaware	2,154,000	0.4%	8	Pennsylvania	14,989,000	3.0%
3	Florida	35,956,000	7.1%	9	Washington	14,883,000	2.9%
13	Georgia	11,692,000	2.3%	10	Michigan	13,538,000	2.7%
32	Hawaii	2,818,000	0.6%	11	Virginia	12,497,000	2.5%
33	Idaho	2,662,000	0.5%	12	Ohio	12,443,000	2.4%
4	Illinois	25,720,000	5.1%	13	Georgia	11,692,000	2.3%
23	Indiana	6,915,000	1.4%	14	North Carolina	10,869,000	2.1%
39	Iowa	2,142,000	0.4%	15	Connecticut	10,144,000	2.0%
37	Kansas	2,254,000	0.4%	16	Colorado	9,320,000	1.8%
30	Kentucky	3,192,000	0.6%	17	Maryland	9,199,000	1.8%
25	Louisiana	6,069,000	1.2%	18	Oregon	9,139,000	1.8%
34	Maine	2,585,000	0.5%	19	Arizona	9,021,000	1.8%
17	Maryland	9,199,000	1.8%	20	Wisconsin	8,223,000	1.6%
7	Massachusetts	19,337,000	3.8%	21	Minnesota	7,832,000	1.5%
10	Michigan	13,538,000	2.7%	22	Missouri	7,445,000	1.5%
21	Minnesota	7,832,000	1.5%	23	Indiana	6,915,000	1.4%
44	Mississippi	1,514,000	0.3%	24	Nevada	6,331,000	1.2%
22	Missouri	7,445,000	1.5%	25	Louisiana	6,069,000	1.2%
43	Montana	1,603,000	0.3%	26	Tennessee	5,540,000	1.1%
41	Nebraska	1,890,000	0.4%	27	South Carolina	4,522,000	0.9%
24	Nevada	6,331,000	1.2%	28	New Hampshire	4,059,000	0.8%
28	New Hampshire	4,059,000	0.8%	29	Alabama	4,057,000	0.8%
6	New Jersey	21,679,000	4.3%	30	Kentucky	3,192,000	0.6%
36	New Mexico	2,461,000	0.5%	31	Rhode Island	2,865,000	0.6%
2	New York	42,931,000	8.5%	32	Hawaii	2,818,000	0.6%
14	North Carolina	10,869,000	2.1%	33	Idaho	2,662,000	0.5%
49	North Dakota	519,000	0.1%	34	Maine	2,585,000	0.5%
12	Ohio	12,443,000	2.4%	35	Oklahoma	2,553,000	0.5%
35	Oklahoma	2,553,000	0.5%	36	New Mexico	2,461,000	0.5%
18	Oregon	9,139,000	1.8%	37	Kansas	2,254,000	0.4%
8	Pennsylvania	14,989,000	3.0%	38	Delaware	2,154,000	0.4%
31	Rhode Island	2,865,000	0.6%	39	Iowa	2,142,000	0.4%
27	South Carolina	4,522,000	0.9%	40	Arkansas	1,908,000	0.4%
48	South Dakota	599,000	0.1%	41	Nebraska	1,890,000	0.4%
26	Tennessee	5,540,000	1.1%	42	Vermont	1,736,000	0.3%
5	Texas	23,979,000	4.7%	43	Montana	1,603,000	0.3%
46	Utah	1,285,000	0.3%	44	Mississippi	1,514,000	0.3%
42	Vermont	1,736,000	0.3%	45	Alaska	1,307,000	0.3%
11	Virginia	12,497,000	2.5%	46	Utah	1,285,000	0.3%
9	Washington	14,883,000	2.9%	47	West Virginia	1,112,000	0.2%
47	West Virginia	1,112,000	0.2%	48	South Dakota	599,000	0.1%
20	Wisconsin	8,223,000	1.6%	49	North Dakota	519,000	0.1%
50	Wyoming	505,000	0.1%	50	Wyoming	505,000	0.1%
					District of Columbia	2,696,000	0.5%

Source: U.S. Department of Health and Human Services, National Institute on Alcohol Abuse and Alcoholism
"Volume Beverage and Ethanol Consumption for States" (http://silk.nih.gov/silk/niaaa1/database/consum02.txt)
This is apparent consumption and is based on several sources which together approximate sales but do not actually measure consumption. Reported state volumes reflect only in-state purchases. Accordingly, figures for some states may be skewed by purchases by nonresidents.

Adult Per Capita Wine Consumption in 1997

National Per Capita = 2.7 Gallons Consumed per Adult Age 21 Years and Older*

ALPHA ORDER

RANK ORDER

RANK	STATE	PER CAPITA		RANK	STATE	PER CAPITA
40	Alabama	1.3		1	Nevada	5.4
12	Alaska	3.4		2	New Hampshire	4.9
19	Arizona	2.9		3	California	4.4
45	Arkansas	1.1		4	Connecticut	4.3
3	California	4.4		4	Massachusetts	4.3
12	Colorado	3.4		6	Delaware	4.1
4	Connecticut	4.3		6	Vermont	4.1
6	Delaware	4.1		8	Oregon	4.0
12	Florida	3.4		8	Rhode Island	4.0
25	Georgia	2.3		10	New Jersey	3.8
12	Hawaii	3.4		10	Washington	3.8
12	Idaho	3.4		12	Alaska	3.4
18	Illinois	3.1		12	Colorado	3.4
33	Indiana	1.7		12	Florida	3.4
45	Iowa	1.1		12	Hawaii	3.4
40	Kansas	1.3		12	Idaho	3.4
42	Kentucky	1.2		17	New York	3.3
28	Louisiana	2.1		18	Illinois	3.1
19	Maine	2.9		19	Arizona	2.9
23	Maryland	2.5		19	Maine	2.9
4	Massachusetts	4.3		21	Montana	2.6
30	Michigan	2.0		21	Virginia	2.6
24	Minnesota	2.4		23	Maryland	2.5
49	Mississippi	0.8		24	Minnesota	2.4
30	Missouri	2.0		25	Georgia	2.3
21	Montana	2.6		25	Wisconsin	2.3
33	Nebraska	1.7		27	New Mexico	2.2
1	Nevada	5.4		28	Louisiana	2.1
2	New Hampshire	4.9		28	North Carolina	2.1
10	New Jersey	3.8		30	Michigan	2.0
27	New Mexico	2.2		30	Missouri	2.0
17	New York	3.3		32	Texas	1.9
28	North Carolina	2.1		33	Indiana	1.7
42	North Dakota	1.2		33	Nebraska	1.7
37	Ohio	1.6		33	Pennsylvania	1.7
45	Oklahoma	1.1		33	South Carolina	1.7
8	Oregon	4.0		37	Ohio	1.6
33	Pennsylvania	1.7		37	Wyoming	1.6
8	Rhode Island	4.0		39	Tennessee	1.5
33	South Carolina	1.7		40	Alabama	1.3
42	South Dakota	1.2		40	Kansas	1.3
39	Tennessee	1.5		42	Kentucky	1.2
32	Texas	1.9		42	North Dakota	1.2
48	Utah	1.0		42	South Dakota	1.2
6	Vermont	4.1		45	Arkansas	1.1
21	Virginia	2.6		45	Iowa	1.1
10	Washington	3.8		45	Oklahoma	1.1
49	West Virginia	0.8		48	Utah	1.0
25	Wisconsin	2.3		49	Mississippi	0.8
37	Wyoming	1.6		49	West Virginia	0.8
					District of Columbia	6.6

Source: Morgan Quitno Press using data from U.S. Department of Health and Human Services, National Institute on Alcohol Abuse and Alcoholism "Volume Beverage and Ethanol Consumption for States"
*This is apparent consumption and is based on several sources which together approximate sales but do not actually measure consumption. Reported state volumes reflect only in-state purchases. Accordingly, figures for some states may be skewed by purchases by nonresidents.

Distilled Spirits Consumption in 1997

National Total = 329,882,000 Gallons of Distilled Spirits Consumed*

ALPHA ORDER					RANK ORDER			
RANK	STATE	GALLONS	% of USA		RANK	STATE	GALLONS	% of USA
27	Alabama	4,427,000	1.3%		1	California	38,152,000	11.6%
46	Alaska	1,002,000	0.3%		2	Florida	24,258,000	7.4%
21	Arizona	6,214,000	1.9%		3	New York	20,614,000	6.2%
33	Arkansas	2,619,000	0.8%		4	Texas	17,672,000	5.4%
1	California	38,152,000	11.6%		5	Illinois	15,423,000	4.7%
20	Colorado	6,321,000	1.9%		6	Michigan	12,614,000	3.8%
25	Connecticut	4,837,000	1.5%		7	New Jersey	11,937,000	3.6%
40	Delaware	1,453,000	0.4%		8	Pennsylvania	10,768,000	3.3%
2	Florida	24,258,000	7.4%		9	Georgia	10,382,000	3.1%
9	Georgia	10,382,000	3.1%		10	Ohio	10,076,000	3.1%
42	Hawaii	1,310,000	0.4%		11	Massachusetts	9,360,000	2.8%
44	Idaho	1,171,000	0.4%		12	Wisconsin	9,155,000	2.8%
5	Illinois	15,423,000	4.7%		13	North Carolina	7,755,000	2.4%
17	Indiana	6,808,000	2.1%		14	Minnesota	7,701,000	2.3%
34	Iowa	2,567,000	0.8%		15	Maryland	7,341,000	2.2%
35	Kansas	2,436,000	0.7%		16	Washington	6,899,000	2.1%
28	Kentucky	4,108,000	1.2%		17	Indiana	6,808,000	2.1%
22	Louisiana	6,002,000	1.8%		18	Missouri	6,688,000	2.0%
38	Maine	1,767,000	0.5%		19	Virginia	6,407,000	1.9%
15	Maryland	7,341,000	2.2%		20	Colorado	6,321,000	1.9%
11	Massachusetts	9,360,000	2.8%		21	Arizona	6,214,000	1.9%
6	Michigan	12,614,000	3.8%		22	Louisiana	6,002,000	1.8%
14	Minnesota	7,701,000	2.3%		23	Tennessee	5,424,000	1.6%
31	Mississippi	3,238,000	1.0%		24	South Carolina	5,344,000	1.6%
18	Missouri	6,688,000	2.0%		25	Connecticut	4,837,000	1.5%
45	Montana	1,104,000	0.3%		26	Nevada	4,459,000	1.4%
37	Nebraska	1,847,000	0.6%		27	Alabama	4,427,000	1.3%
26	Nevada	4,459,000	1.4%		28	Kentucky	4,108,000	1.2%
29	New Hampshire	4,088,000	1.2%		29	New Hampshire	4,088,000	1.2%
7	New Jersey	11,937,000	3.6%		30	Oregon	3,909,000	1.2%
36	New Mexico	1,941,000	0.6%		31	Mississippi	3,238,000	1.0%
3	New York	20,614,000	6.2%		32	Oklahoma	2,812,000	0.9%
13	North Carolina	7,755,000	2.4%		33	Arkansas	2,619,000	0.8%
48	North Dakota	985,000	0.3%		34	Iowa	2,567,000	0.8%
10	Ohio	10,076,000	3.1%		35	Kansas	2,436,000	0.7%
32	Oklahoma	2,812,000	0.9%		36	New Mexico	1,941,000	0.6%
30	Oregon	3,909,000	1.2%		37	Nebraska	1,847,000	0.6%
8	Pennsylvania	10,768,000	3.3%		38	Maine	1,767,000	0.5%
43	Rhode Island	1,296,000	0.4%		39	Utah	1,492,000	0.5%
24	South Carolina	5,344,000	1.6%		40	Delaware	1,453,000	0.4%
47	South Dakota	993,000	0.3%		41	West Virginia	1,360,000	0.4%
23	Tennessee	5,424,000	1.6%		42	Hawaii	1,310,000	0.4%
4	Texas	17,672,000	5.4%		43	Rhode Island	1,296,000	0.4%
39	Utah	1,492,000	0.5%		44	Idaho	1,171,000	0.4%
50	Vermont	737,000	0.2%		45	Montana	1,104,000	0.3%
19	Virginia	6,407,000	1.9%		46	Alaska	1,002,000	0.3%
16	Washington	6,899,000	2.1%		47	South Dakota	993,000	0.3%
41	West Virginia	1,360,000	0.4%		48	North Dakota	985,000	0.3%
12	Wisconsin	9,155,000	2.8%		49	Wyoming	766,000	0.2%
49	Wyoming	766,000	0.2%		50	Vermont	737,000	0.2%
						District of Columbia	1,843,000	0.6%

Source: U.S. Department of Health and Human Services, National Institute on Alcohol Abuse and Alcoholism
"Volume Beverage and Ethanol Consumption for States" (http://silk.nih.gov/silk/niaaa1/database/consum02.txt)
*This is apparent consumption and is based on several sources which together approximate sales but do not actually measure consumption. Reported state volumes reflect only in-state purchases. Accordingly, figures for some states may be skewed by purchases by nonresidents.

Adult Per Capita Apparent Distilled Spirits Consumption in 1997

National Per Capita = 1.8 Gallons Consumed per Adult 21 Years and Older*

ALPHA ORDER

RANK	STATE	PER CAPITA
36	Alabama	1.5
4	Alaska	2.6
14	Arizona	2.0
36	Arkansas	1.5
28	California	1.7
8	Colorado	2.3
14	Connecticut	2.0
3	Delaware	2.8
8	Florida	2.3
14	Georgia	2.0
33	Hawaii	1.6
36	Idaho	1.5
21	Illinois	1.9
28	Indiana	1.7
44	Iowa	1.3
41	Kansas	1.4
36	Kentucky	1.5
11	Louisiana	2.1
14	Maine	2.0
14	Maryland	2.0
11	Massachusetts	2.1
21	Michigan	1.9
6	Minnesota	2.4
23	Mississippi	1.8
23	Missouri	1.8
23	Montana	1.8
33	Nebraska	1.6
2	Nevada	3.8
1	New Hampshire	4.9
11	New Jersey	2.1
28	New Mexico	1.7
33	New York	1.6
36	North Carolina	1.5
10	North Dakota	2.2
44	Ohio	1.3
47	Oklahoma	1.2
28	Oregon	1.7
47	Pennsylvania	1.2
23	Rhode Island	1.8
14	South Carolina	2.0
14	South Dakota	2.0
41	Tennessee	1.4
41	Texas	1.4
47	Utah	1.2
28	Vermont	1.7
44	Virginia	1.3
23	Washington	1.8
50	West Virginia	1.0
5	Wisconsin	2.5
6	Wyoming	2.4

RANK ORDER

RANK	STATE	PER CAPITA
1	New Hampshire	4.9
2	Nevada	3.8
3	Delaware	2.8
4	Alaska	2.6
5	Wisconsin	2.5
6	Minnesota	2.4
6	Wyoming	2.4
8	Colorado	2.3
8	Florida	2.3
10	North Dakota	2.2
11	Louisiana	2.1
11	Massachusetts	2.1
11	New Jersey	2.1
14	Arizona	2.0
14	Connecticut	2.0
14	Georgia	2.0
14	Maine	2.0
14	Maryland	2.0
14	South Carolina	2.0
14	South Dakota	2.0
21	Illinois	1.9
21	Michigan	1.9
23	Mississippi	1.8
23	Missouri	1.8
23	Montana	1.8
23	Rhode Island	1.8
23	Washington	1.8
28	California	1.7
28	Indiana	1.7
28	New Mexico	1.7
28	Oregon	1.7
28	Vermont	1.7
33	Hawaii	1.6
33	Nebraska	1.6
33	New York	1.6
36	Alabama	1.5
36	Arkansas	1.5
36	Idaho	1.5
36	Kentucky	1.5
36	North Carolina	1.5
41	Kansas	1.4
41	Tennessee	1.4
41	Texas	1.4
44	Iowa	1.3
44	Ohio	1.3
44	Virginia	1.3
47	Oklahoma	1.2
47	Pennsylvania	1.2
47	Utah	1.2
50	West Virginia	1.0

District of Columbia 4.5

Source: Morgan Quitno Press using data from U.S. Department of Health and Human Services, National Institute on Alcohol Abuse and Alcoholism "Volume Beverage and Ethanol Consumption for States"
*This is apparent consumption and is based on several sources which together approximate sales but do not actually measure consumption. Reported state volumes reflect only in-state purchases. Accordingly, figures for some states may be skewed by purchases by nonresidents.

Percent of Adults Who Are Binge Drinkers: 1999

National Median = 14.9% of Adults*

ALPHA ORDER

RANK	STATE	PERCENT
43	Alabama	11.7
8	Alaska	18.9
47	Arizona	8.8
44	Arkansas	10.3
24	California	15.5
17	Colorado	17.2
31	Connecticut	14.0
8	Delaware	18.9
34	Florida	12.9
36	Georgia	12.5
31	Hawaii	14.0
29	Idaho	14.7
4	Illinois	19.7
6	Indiana	19.1
10	Iowa	18.3
42	Kansas	11.8
46	Kentucky	9.8
25	Louisiana	15.0
28	Maine	14.8
21	Maryland	15.9
12	Massachusetts	17.4
7	Michigan	19.0
20	Minnesota	16.3
39	Mississippi	12.1
19	Missouri	16.4
11	Montana	17.6
18	Nebraska	16.6
2	Nevada	21.0
3	New Hampshire	20.0
37	New Jersey	12.3
25	New Mexico	15.0
33	New York	13.9
41	North Carolina	12.0
4	North Dakota	19.7
39	Ohio	12.1
49	Oklahoma	8.1
27	Oregon	14.9
21	Pennsylvania	15.9
23	Rhode Island	15.6
37	South Carolina	12.3
12	South Dakota	17.4
50	Tennessee	7.7
15	Texas	17.3
45	Utah	10.2
12	Vermont	17.4
35	Virginia	12.7
30	Washington	14.4
48	West Virginia	8.6
1	Wisconsin	27.0
15	Wyoming	17.3

RANK ORDER

RANK	STATE	PERCENT
1	Wisconsin	27.0
2	Nevada	21.0
3	New Hampshire	20.0
4	Illinois	19.7
4	North Dakota	19.7
6	Indiana	19.1
7	Michigan	19.0
8	Alaska	18.9
8	Delaware	18.9
10	Iowa	18.3
11	Montana	17.6
12	Massachusetts	17.4
12	South Dakota	17.4
12	Vermont	17.4
15	Texas	17.3
15	Wyoming	17.3
17	Colorado	17.2
18	Nebraska	16.6
19	Missouri	16.4
20	Minnesota	16.3
21	Maryland	15.9
21	Pennsylvania	15.9
23	Rhode Island	15.6
24	California	15.5
25	Louisiana	15.0
25	New Mexico	15.0
27	Oregon	14.9
28	Maine	14.8
29	Idaho	14.7
30	Washington	14.4
31	Connecticut	14.0
31	Hawaii	14.0
33	New York	13.9
34	Florida	12.9
35	Virginia	12.7
36	Georgia	12.5
37	New Jersey	12.3
37	South Carolina	12.3
39	Mississippi	12.1
39	Ohio	12.1
41	North Carolina	12.0
42	Kansas	11.8
43	Alabama	11.7
44	Arkansas	10.3
45	Utah	10.2
46	Kentucky	9.8
47	Arizona	8.8
48	West Virginia	8.6
49	Oklahoma	8.1
50	Tennessee	7.7
	District of Columbia	13.0

Source: U.S. Department of Health and Human Services, Centers for Disease Control and Prevention
   "1999 Behavioral Risk Factor Surveillance Summary Prevalence Report" (June 23, 2000)
Persons 18 and older reporting consumption of five or more alcoholic drinks on one or more occasions during the previous month.

Percent of Adults Who Drink and Drive: 1999

National Median = 2.4% of Adults*

ALPHA ORDER

RANK	STATE	PERCENT
35	Alabama	1.9
32	Alaska	2.1
37	Arizona	1.8
43	Arkansas	1.5
29	California	2.3
10	Colorado	3.6
17	Connecticut	2.9
13	Delaware	3.2
34	Florida	2.0
43	Georgia	1.5
29	Hawaii	2.3
37	Idaho	1.8
3	Illinois	4.4
13	Indiana	3.2
7	Iowa	3.9
18	Kansas	2.8
41	Kentucky	1.6
10	Louisiana	3.6
49	Maine	1.1
24	Maryland	2.4
18	Massachusetts	2.8
15	Michigan	3.1
5	Minnesota	4.1
21	Mississippi	2.7
16	Missouri	3.0
12	Montana	3.4
9	Nebraska	3.7
1	Nevada	5.5
8	New Hampshire	3.8
46	New Jersey	1.3
29	New Mexico	2.3
41	New York	1.6
39	North Carolina	1.7
3	North Dakota	4.4
47	Ohio	1.2
23	Oklahoma	2.5
35	Oregon	1.9
24	Pennsylvania	2.4
22	Rhode Island	2.6
32	South Carolina	2.1
5	South Dakota	4.1
43	Tennessee	1.5
18	Texas	2.8
47	Utah	1.2
24	Vermont	2.4
24	Virginia	2.4
39	Washington	1.7
49	West Virginia	1.1
2	Wisconsin	4.9
24	Wyoming	2.4

RANK ORDER

RANK	STATE	PERCENT
1	Nevada	5.5
2	Wisconsin	4.9
3	Illinois	4.4
3	North Dakota	4.4
5	Minnesota	4.1
5	South Dakota	4.1
7	Iowa	3.9
8	New Hampshire	3.8
9	Nebraska	3.7
10	Colorado	3.6
10	Louisiana	3.6
12	Montana	3.4
13	Delaware	3.2
13	Indiana	3.2
15	Michigan	3.1
16	Missouri	3.0
17	Connecticut	2.9
18	Kansas	2.8
18	Massachusetts	2.8
18	Texas	2.8
21	Mississippi	2.7
22	Rhode Island	2.6
23	Oklahoma	2.5
24	Maryland	2.4
24	Pennsylvania	2.4
24	Vermont	2.4
24	Virginia	2.4
24	Wyoming	2.4
29	California	2.3
29	Hawaii	2.3
29	New Mexico	2.3
32	Alaska	2.1
32	South Carolina	2.1
34	Florida	2.0
35	Alabama	1.9
35	Oregon	1.9
37	Arizona	1.8
37	Idaho	1.8
39	North Carolina	1.7
39	Washington	1.7
41	Kentucky	1.6
41	New York	1.6
43	Arkansas	1.5
43	Georgia	1.5
43	Tennessee	1.5
46	New Jersey	1.3
47	Ohio	1.2
47	Utah	1.2
49	Maine	1.1
49	West Virginia	1.1
	District of Columbia	1.4

Source: U.S. Department of Health and Human Services, Centers for Disease Control and Prevention
"1999 Behavioral Risk Factor Surveillance Summary Prevalence Report" (June 23, 2000)
*Persons 18 and over who "drive after having too much to drink, one or more times in the past month."

Percent of Adults Who Smoke: 1999

National Median = 22.7% of Adults*

ALPHA ORDER

RANK	STATE	PERCENT
19	Alabama	23.5
4	Alaska	27.3
45	Arizona	20.1
5	Arkansas	27.2
48	California	18.7
27	Colorado	22.5
26	Connecticut	22.8
9	Delaware	25.5
41	Florida	20.6
16	Georgia	23.8
49	Hawaii	18.5
37	Idaho	21.5
14	Illinois	24.2
8	Indiana	27.0
19	Iowa	23.5
40	Kansas	21.0
2	Kentucky	29.7
19	Louisiana	23.5
22	Maine	23.3
43	Maryland	20.3
47	Massachusetts	19.3
11	Michigan	25.1
46	Minnesota	19.5
25	Mississippi	22.9
6	Missouri	27.1
44	Montana	20.2
23	Nebraska	23.2
1	Nevada	31.5
32	New Hampshire	22.3
41	New Jersey	20.6
27	New Mexico	22.5
35	New York	21.8
11	North Carolina	25.1
34	North Dakota	22.1
3	Ohio	27.6
10	Oklahoma	25.2
38	Oregon	21.4
24	Pennsylvania	23.1
32	Rhode Island	22.3
18	South Carolina	23.6
27	South Dakota	22.5
13	Tennessee	24.8
30	Texas	22.4
50	Utah	14.0
36	Vermont	21.7
38	Virginia	21.4
30	Washington	22.4
6	West Virginia	27.1
17	Wisconsin	23.7
15	Wyoming	23.9

RANK ORDER

RANK	STATE	PERCENT
1	Nevada	31.5
2	Kentucky	29.7
3	Ohio	27.6
4	Alaska	27.3
5	Arkansas	27.2
6	Missouri	27.1
6	West Virginia	27.1
8	Indiana	27.0
9	Delaware	25.5
10	Oklahoma	25.2
11	Michigan	25.1
11	North Carolina	25.1
13	Tennessee	24.8
14	Illinois	24.2
15	Wyoming	23.9
16	Georgia	23.8
17	Wisconsin	23.7
18	South Carolina	23.6
19	Alabama	23.5
19	Iowa	23.5
19	Louisiana	23.5
22	Maine	23.3
23	Nebraska	23.2
24	Pennsylvania	23.1
25	Mississippi	22.9
26	Connecticut	22.8
27	Colorado	22.5
27	New Mexico	22.5
27	South Dakota	22.5
30	Texas	22.4
30	Washington	22.4
32	New Hampshire	22.3
32	Rhode Island	22.3
34	North Dakota	22.1
35	New York	21.8
36	Vermont	21.7
37	Idaho	21.5
38	Oregon	21.4
38	Virginia	21.4
40	Kansas	21.0
41	Florida	20.6
41	New Jersey	20.6
43	Maryland	20.3
44	Montana	20.2
45	Arizona	20.1
46	Minnesota	19.5
47	Massachusetts	19.3
48	California	18.7
49	Hawaii	18.5
50	Utah	14.0
	District of Columbia	20.6

Source: U.S. Department of Health and Human Services, Centers for Disease Control and Prevention
"1999 Behavioral Risk Factor Surveillance Summary Prevalence Report" (June 23, 2000)
*Persons 18 and older who have ever smoked 100 cigarettes and currently smoke.

Percent of Men Who Smoke: 1999

National Median = 24.2% of Men*

ALPHA ORDER

RANK	STATE	PERCENT
21	Alabama	26.2
24	Alaska	25.3
30	Arizona	23.7
6	Arkansas	29.7
42	California	22.0
38	Colorado	22.7
24	Connecticut	25.3
11	Delaware	27.6
40	Florida	22.2
9	Georgia	28.3
47	Hawaii	20.1
39	Idaho	22.5
16	Illinois	27.0
3	Indiana	31.0
18	Iowa	26.6
26	Kansas	24.3
1	Kentucky	33.9
17	Louisiana	26.8
10	Maine	27.7
41	Maryland	22.1
48	Massachusetts	19.5
18	Michigan	26.6
44	Minnesota	21.7
13	Mississippi	27.4
4	Missouri	30.6
49	Montana	18.5
13	Nebraska	27.4
2	Nevada	32.8
45	New Hampshire	21.6
42	New Jersey	22.0
28	New Mexico	24.1
36	New York	22.8
11	North Carolina	27.6
31	North Dakota	23.4
7	Ohio	29.3
18	Oklahoma	26.6
34	Oregon	22.9
27	Pennsylvania	24.2
32	Rhode Island	23.2
8	South Carolina	28.4
33	South Dakota	23.1
23	Tennessee	25.6
13	Texas	27.4
50	Utah	16.7
36	Vermont	22.8
45	Virginia	21.6
29	Washington	24.0
5	West Virginia	30.2
34	Wisconsin	22.9
22	Wyoming	25.9

RANK ORDER

RANK	STATE	PERCENT
1	Kentucky	33.9
2	Nevada	32.8
3	Indiana	31.0
4	Missouri	30.6
5	West Virginia	30.2
6	Arkansas	29.7
7	Ohio	29.3
8	South Carolina	28.4
9	Georgia	28.3
10	Maine	27.7
11	Delaware	27.6
11	North Carolina	27.6
13	Mississippi	27.4
13	Nebraska	27.4
13	Texas	27.4
16	Illinois	27.0
17	Louisiana	26.8
18	Iowa	26.6
18	Michigan	26.6
18	Oklahoma	26.6
21	Alabama	26.2
22	Wyoming	25.9
23	Tennessee	25.6
24	Alaska	25.3
24	Connecticut	25.3
26	Kansas	24.3
27	Pennsylvania	24.2
28	New Mexico	24.1
29	Washington	24.0
30	Arizona	23.7
31	North Dakota	23.4
32	Rhode Island	23.2
33	South Dakota	23.1
34	Oregon	22.9
34	Wisconsin	22.9
36	New York	22.8
36	Vermont	22.8
38	Colorado	22.7
39	Idaho	22.5
40	Florida	22.2
41	Maryland	22.1
42	California	22.0
42	New Jersey	22.0
44	Minnesota	21.7
45	New Hampshire	21.6
45	Virginia	21.6
47	Hawaii	20.1
48	Massachusetts	19.5
49	Montana	18.5
50	Utah	16.7

| | District of Columbia | 21.4 |

Source: U.S. Department of Health and Human Services, Centers for Disease Control and Prevention
"1999 Behavioral Risk Factor Surveillance Summary Prevalence Report" (June 23, 2000)
Men 18 and older who have ever smoked 100 cigarettes and currently smoke.

Percent of Women Who Smoke: 1999

National Median = 20.9% of Women*

ALPHA ORDER				RANK ORDER		
RANK	STATE	PERCENT		RANK	STATE	PERCENT
24	Alabama	21.1		1	Nevada	30.3
2	Alaska	29.5		2	Alaska	29.5
48	Arizona	16.7		3	Ohio	26.1
5	Arkansas	25.0		4	Kentucky	25.9
49	California	15.5		5	Arkansas	25.0
16	Colorado	22.2		6	West Virginia	24.4
30	Connecticut	20.6		6	Wisconsin	24.4
12	Delaware	23.5		8	Tennessee	24.1
40	Florida	19.1		9	Missouri	23.9
35	Georgia	19.6		10	Michigan	23.8
47	Hawaii	16.9		10	Oklahoma	23.8
30	Idaho	20.6		12	Delaware	23.5
21	Illinois	21.7		13	Indiana	23.4
13	Indiana	23.4		14	New Hampshire	23.0
29	Iowa	20.7		15	North Carolina	22.9
44	Kansas	18.0		16	Colorado	22.2
4	Kentucky	25.9		17	Pennsylvania	22.1
30	Louisiana	20.6		18	Wyoming	22.0
38	Maine	19.2		19	Montana	21.9
43	Maryland	18.6		19	South Dakota	21.9
40	Massachusetts	19.1		21	Illinois	21.7
10	Michigan	23.8		22	Rhode Island	21.5
46	Minnesota	17.3		23	Virginia	21.2
42	Mississippi	19.0		24	Alabama	21.1
9	Missouri	23.9		25	New Mexico	20.9
19	Montana	21.9		25	North Dakota	20.9
36	Nebraska	19.4		25	Washington	20.9
1	Nevada	30.3		28	New York	20.8
14	New Hampshire	23.0		29	Iowa	20.7
36	New Jersey	19.4		30	Connecticut	20.6
25	New Mexico	20.9		30	Idaho	20.6
28	New York	20.8		30	Louisiana	20.6
15	North Carolina	22.9		30	Vermont	20.6
25	North Dakota	20.9		34	Oregon	20.1
3	Ohio	26.1		35	Georgia	19.6
10	Oklahoma	23.8		36	Nebraska	19.4
34	Oregon	20.1		36	New Jersey	19.4
17	Pennsylvania	22.1		38	Maine	19.2
22	Rhode Island	21.5		38	South Carolina	19.2
38	South Carolina	19.2		40	Florida	19.1
19	South Dakota	21.9		40	Massachusetts	19.1
8	Tennessee	24.1		42	Mississippi	19.0
45	Texas	17.8		43	Maryland	18.6
50	Utah	11.3		44	Kansas	18.0
30	Vermont	20.6		45	Texas	17.8
23	Virginia	21.2		46	Minnesota	17.3
25	Washington	20.9		47	Hawaii	16.9
6	West Virginia	24.4		48	Arizona	16.7
6	Wisconsin	24.4		49	California	15.5
18	Wyoming	22.0		50	Utah	11.3
					District of Columbia	19.8

Source: U.S. Department of Health and Human Services, Centers for Disease Control and Prevention
"1999 Behavioral Risk Factor Surveillance Summary Prevalence Report" (June 23, 2000)
Women 18 and older who have ever smoked 100 cigarettes and currently smoke.

Percent of Adults Overweight or Obese: 1999

National Median = 56.2% of Adults*

RANK	STATE	PERCENT
4	Alabama	60.9
3	Alaska	61.1
45	Arizona	51.6
8	Arkansas	58.8
34	California	54.8
50	Colorado	47.9
43	Connecticut	52.6
29	Delaware	55.5
20	Florida	56.9
19	Georgia	57.6
48	Hawaii	50.2
33	Idaho	55.2
20	Illinois	56.9
23	Indiana	56.7
11	Iowa	58.4
26	Kansas	56.1
10	Kentucky	58.5
12	Louisiana	58.3
34	Maine	54.8
30	Maryland	55.4
47	Massachusetts	50.3
6	Michigan	59.6
27	Minnesota	55.9
1	Mississippi	62.3
18	Missouri	57.7
42	Montana	52.7
16	Nebraska	57.8
41	Nevada	53.7
49	New Hampshire	50.1
36	New Jersey	54.5
32	New Mexico	55.3
40	New York	54.0
15	North Carolina	57.9
5	North Dakota	60.1
20	Ohio	56.9
16	Oklahoma	57.8
36	Oregon	54.5
25	Pennsylvania	56.2
39	Rhode Island	54.2
12	South Carolina	58.3
7	South Dakota	59.3
24	Tennessee	56.6
12	Texas	58.3
46	Utah	50.9
44	Vermont	52.3
9	Virginia	58.7
38	Washington	54.4
2	West Virginia	62.0
28	Wisconsin	55.7
30	Wyoming	55.4

RANK	STATE	PERCENT
1	Mississippi	62.3
2	West Virginia	62.0
3	Alaska	61.1
4	Alabama	60.9
5	North Dakota	60.1
6	Michigan	59.6
7	South Dakota	59.3
8	Arkansas	58.8
9	Virginia	58.7
10	Kentucky	58.5
11	Iowa	58.4
12	Louisiana	58.3
12	South Carolina	58.3
12	Texas	58.3
15	North Carolina	57.9
16	Nebraska	57.8
16	Oklahoma	57.8
18	Missouri	57.7
19	Georgia	57.6
20	Florida	56.9
20	Illinois	56.9
20	Ohio	56.9
23	Indiana	56.7
24	Tennessee	56.6
25	Pennsylvania	56.2
26	Kansas	56.1
27	Minnesota	55.9
28	Wisconsin	55.7
29	Delaware	55.5
30	Maryland	55.4
30	Wyoming	55.4
32	New Mexico	55.3
33	Idaho	55.2
34	California	54.8
34	Maine	54.8
36	New Jersey	54.5
36	Oregon	54.5
38	Washington	54.4
39	Rhode Island	54.2
40	New York	54.0
41	Nevada	53.7
42	Montana	52.7
43	Connecticut	52.6
44	Vermont	52.3
45	Arizona	51.6
46	Utah	50.9
47	Massachusetts	50.3
48	Hawaii	50.2
49	New Hampshire	50.1
50	Colorado	47.9
	District of Columbia	50.9

Source: U.S. Department of Health and Human Services, Centers for Disease Control and Prevention
   "1999 Prevalence Report for New Body Weight Measures" (2000)
Persons 18 and older. This table reflects a revised definition of overweight and differs from previous years. It is now defined as a Body Mass Index (BMI) of 25.0 to 29.9 and obese is defined as a BMI of 30.0 or more regardless of sex. BMI is a ratio of height to weight. As an example, a person 5' 8" and weighing 185 pounds has a BMI of 28. See http://www.cdc.gov/nccdphp/dnpa/bmi/bmi-adult.htm.

Percent of Adults Who Have Not Had Their Blood Pressure Checked in the Past Two Years: 1999
National Median = 5.4% of Adults*

ALPHA ORDER			RANK ORDER		
RANK	STATE	PERCENT	RANK	STATE	PERCENT
33	Alabama	4.8	1	New Mexico	9.7
19	Alaska	6.2	2	Idaho	9.4
12	Arizona	7.2	3	Texas	8.7
14	Arkansas	6.7	4	Oregon	8.5
6	California	8.0	5	Nevada	8.1
7	Colorado	7.8	6	California	8.0
33	Connecticut	4.8	7	Colorado	7.8
46	Delaware	3.8	8	Indiana	7.7
26	Florida	5.4	8	Wyoming	7.7
40	Georgia	4.4	10	Utah	7.6
48	Hawaii	3.5	11	Wisconsin	7.4
2	Idaho	9.4	12	Arizona	7.2
16	Illinois	6.5	13	Washington	7.1
8	Indiana	7.7	14	Arkansas	6.7
26	Iowa	5.4	14	Montana	6.7
38	Kansas	4.5	16	Illinois	6.5
23	Kentucky	5.6	17	New York	6.4
41	Louisiana	4.2	17	Virginia	6.4
29	Maine	5.2	19	Alaska	6.2
49	Maryland	3.4	19	West Virginia	6.2
42	Massachusetts	4.1	21	South Dakota	5.7
31	Michigan	4.9	21	Vermont	5.7
23	Minnesota	5.6	23	Kentucky	5.6
37	Mississippi	4.7	23	Minnesota	5.6
31	Missouri	4.9	25	New Hampshire	5.5
14	Montana	6.7	26	Florida	5.4
26	Nebraska	5.4	26	Iowa	5.4
5	Nevada	8.1	26	Nebraska	5.4
25	New Hampshire	5.5	29	Maine	5.2
30	New Jersey	5.0	30	New Jersey	5.0
1	New Mexico	9.7	31	Michigan	4.9
17	New York	6.4	31	Missouri	4.9
46	North Carolina	3.8	33	Alabama	4.8
38	North Dakota	4.5	33	Connecticut	4.8
44	Ohio	3.9	33	Oklahoma	4.8
33	Oklahoma	4.8	33	South Carolina	4.8
4	Oregon	8.5	37	Mississippi	4.7
44	Pennsylvania	3.9	38	Kansas	4.5
50	Rhode Island	3.3	38	North Dakota	4.5
33	South Carolina	4.8	40	Georgia	4.4
21	South Dakota	5.7	41	Louisiana	4.2
42	Tennessee	4.1	42	Massachusetts	4.1
3	Texas	8.7	42	Tennessee	4.1
10	Utah	7.6	44	Ohio	3.9
21	Vermont	5.7	44	Pennsylvania	3.9
17	Virginia	6.4	46	Delaware	3.8
13	Washington	7.1	46	North Carolina	3.8
19	West Virginia	6.2	48	Hawaii	3.5
11	Wisconsin	7.4	49	Maryland	3.4
8	Wyoming	7.7	50	Rhode Island	3.3
				District of Columbia	3.9

Source: U.S. Department of Health and Human Services, Centers for Disease Control and Prevention
   "1999 Behavioral Risk Factor Surveillance Summary Prevalence Report" (June 23, 2000)
*Persons 18 and older.

Percent of Adults Who Have Not Been Tested in Past Year for HIV: 1999

National Median = 62.3% Have Not Been Tested in Past Year*

ALPHA ORDER

RANK	STATE	PERCENT
39	Alabama	57.2
12	Alaska	66.0
9	Arizona	67.6
18	Arkansas	64.5
NA	California**	NA
27	Colorado	61.6
20	Connecticut	64.4
28	Delaware	61.4
31	Florida	60.5
37	Georgia	57.6
48	Hawaii	50.1
3	Idaho	71.4
NA	Illinois**	NA
38	Indiana	57.4
15	Iowa	65.7
25	Kansas	62.0
41	Kentucky	56.7
46	Louisiana	53.3
34	Maine	59.7
24	Maryland	63.1
2	Massachusetts	72.1
21	Michigan	64.3
10	Minnesota	67.5
29	Mississippi	60.6
41	Missouri	56.7
8	Montana	68.7
11	Nebraska	66.8
14	Nevada	65.8
33	New Hampshire	59.9
21	New Jersey	64.3
17	New Mexico	65.2
47	New York	52.5
45	North Carolina	53.7
29	North Dakota	60.6
1	Ohio	73.3
32	Oklahoma	60.0
16	Oregon	65.6
23	Pennsylvania	64.1
35	Rhode Island	59.0
41	South Carolina	56.7
36	South Dakota	57.8
40	Tennessee	57.1
26	Texas	61.9
6	Utah	69.9
7	Vermont	68.9
44	Virginia	54.7
5	Washington	70.2
12	West Virginia	66.0
4	Wisconsin	70.5
18	Wyoming	64.5

RANK ORDER

RANK	STATE	PERCENT
1	Ohio	73.3
2	Massachusetts	72.1
3	Idaho	71.4
4	Wisconsin	70.5
5	Washington	70.2
6	Utah	69.9
7	Vermont	68.9
8	Montana	68.7
9	Arizona	67.6
10	Minnesota	67.5
11	Nebraska	66.8
12	Alaska	66.0
12	West Virginia	66.0
14	Nevada	65.8
15	Iowa	65.7
16	Oregon	65.6
17	New Mexico	65.2
18	Arkansas	64.5
18	Wyoming	64.5
20	Connecticut	64.4
21	Michigan	64.3
21	New Jersey	64.3
23	Pennsylvania	64.1
24	Maryland	63.1
25	Kansas	62.0
26	Texas	61.9
27	Colorado	61.6
28	Delaware	61.4
29	Mississippi	60.6
29	North Dakota	60.6
31	Florida	60.5
32	Oklahoma	60.0
33	New Hampshire	59.9
34	Maine	59.7
35	Rhode Island	59.0
36	South Dakota	57.8
37	Georgia	57.6
38	Indiana	57.4
39	Alabama	57.2
40	Tennessee	57.1
41	Kentucky	56.7
41	Missouri	56.7
41	South Carolina	56.7
44	Virginia	54.7
45	North Carolina	53.7
46	Louisiana	53.3
47	New York	52.5
48	Hawaii	50.1
NA	California**	NA
NA	Illinois**	NA
	District of Columbia	49.7

Source: U.S. Department of Health and Human Services, Centers for Disease Control and Prevention
"1999 Behavioral Risk Factor Surveillance Summary Prevalence Report" (June 23, 2000)
*Persons 18 to 64 years old. Does not include HIV testing for blood donations.
**Not available.

Number of Days in Past Month When Physical Health was "Not Good": 1999

National Median = 3.2 Days*

RANK	STATE	DAYS		RANK	STATE	DAYS
	ALPHA ORDER				**RANK ORDER**	
2	Alabama	4.0		1	Kentucky	4.1
45	Alaska	2.8		2	Alabama	4.0
50	Arizona	0.9		2	Arkansas	4.0
2	Arkansas	4.0		2	West Virginia	4.0
18	California	3.3		5	New Mexico	3.7
18	Colorado	3.3		5	North Carolina	3.7
24	Connecticut	3.2		7	Oregon	3.6
18	Delaware	3.3		7	Wisconsin	3.6
14	Florida	3.4		9	Maine	3.5
41	Georgia	2.9		9	Mississippi	3.5
49	Hawaii	2.4		9	Missouri	3.5
24	Idaho	3.2		9	Nevada	3.5
24	Illinois	3.2		9	Washington	3.5
32	Indiana	3.1		14	Florida	3.4
14	Iowa	3.4		14	Iowa	3.4
47	Kansas	2.6		14	Michigan	3.4
1	Kentucky	4.1		14	Tennessee	3.4
18	Louisiana	3.3		18	California	3.3
9	Maine	3.5		18	Colorado	3.3
32	Maryland	3.1		18	Delaware	3.3
24	Massachusetts	3.2		18	Louisiana	3.3
14	Michigan	3.4		18	New York	3.3
47	Minnesota	2.6		18	Texas	3.3
9	Mississippi	3.5		24	Connecticut	3.2
9	Missouri	3.5		24	Idaho	3.2
32	Montana	3.1		24	Illinois	3.2
32	Nebraska	3.1		24	Massachusetts	3.2
9	Nevada	3.5		24	New Jersey	3.2
32	New Hampshire	3.1		24	Pennsylvania	3.2
24	New Jersey	3.2		24	South Carolina	3.2
5	New Mexico	3.7		24	Utah	3.2
18	New York	3.3		32	Indiana	3.1
5	North Carolina	3.7		32	Maryland	3.1
41	North Dakota	2.9		32	Montana	3.1
32	Ohio	3.1		32	Nebraska	3.1
38	Oklahoma	3.0		32	New Hampshire	3.1
7	Oregon	3.6		32	Ohio	3.1
24	Pennsylvania	3.2		38	Oklahoma	3.0
38	Rhode Island	3.0		38	Rhode Island	3.0
24	South Carolina	3.2		38	South Dakota	3.0
38	South Dakota	3.0		41	Georgia	2.9
14	Tennessee	3.4		41	North Dakota	2.9
18	Texas	3.3		41	Vermont	2.9
24	Utah	3.2		41	Wyoming	2.9
41	Vermont	2.9		45	Alaska	2.8
46	Virginia	2.7		46	Virginia	2.7
9	Washington	3.5		47	Kansas	2.6
2	West Virginia	4.0		47	Minnesota	2.6
7	Wisconsin	3.6		49	Hawaii	2.4
41	Wyoming	2.9		50	Arizona	0.9
					District of Columbia	2.7

Source: U.S. Department of Health and Human Services, Centers for Disease Control and Prevention
   "1999 Behavioral Risk Factor Surveillance Summary Prevalence Report" (June 23, 2000)
Persons 18 and older.

Number of Days in the Past Month When Mental Health was "Not Good": 1999

National Median = 2.9 Days*

ALPHA ORDER				RANK ORDER		
RANK	STATE	DAYS		RANK	STATE	DAYS
6	Alabama	3.6		1	Kentucky	4.7
15	Alaska	3.2		2	Nevada	4.1
50	Arizona	0.7		3	Oregon	3.9
15	Arkansas	3.2		4	New Mexico	3.8
10	California	3.3		5	Maryland	3.7
10	Colorado	3.3		6	Alabama	3.6
32	Connecticut	2.8		7	Mississippi	3.5
10	Delaware	3.3		8	Michigan	3.4
27	Florida	2.9		8	Texas	3.4
19	Georgia	3.1		10	California	3.3
49	Hawaii	2.2		10	Colorado	3.3
19	Idaho	3.1		10	Delaware	3.3
32	Illinois	2.8		10	New Hampshire	3.3
19	Indiana	3.1		10	Utah	3.3
32	Iowa	2.8		15	Alaska	3.2
46	Kansas	2.4		15	Arkansas	3.2
1	Kentucky	4.7		15	Louisiana	3.2
15	Louisiana	3.2		15	Wisconsin	3.2
40	Maine	2.7		19	Georgia	3.1
5	Maryland	3.7		19	Idaho	3.1
32	Massachusetts	2.8		19	Indiana	3.1
8	Michigan	3.4		19	Virginia	3.1
32	Minnesota	2.8		19	Washington	3.1
7	Mississippi	3.5		24	North Carolina	3.0
27	Missouri	2.9		24	Tennessee	3.0
40	Montana	2.7		24	West Virginia	3.0
32	Nebraska	2.8		27	Florida	2.9
2	Nevada	4.1		27	Missouri	2.9
10	New Hampshire	3.3		27	New Jersey	2.9
27	New Jersey	2.9		27	New York	2.9
4	New Mexico	3.8		27	Vermont	2.9
27	New York	2.9		32	Connecticut	2.8
24	North Carolina	3.0		32	Illinois	2.8
45	North Dakota	2.5		32	Iowa	2.8
48	Ohio	2.3		32	Massachusetts	2.8
46	Oklahoma	2.4		32	Minnesota	2.8
3	Oregon	3.9		32	Nebraska	2.8
40	Pennsylvania	2.7		32	South Dakota	2.8
40	Rhode Island	2.7		32	Wyoming	2.8
40	South Carolina	2.7		40	Maine	2.7
32	South Dakota	2.8		40	Montana	2.7
24	Tennessee	3.0		40	Pennsylvania	2.7
8	Texas	3.4		40	Rhode Island	2.7
10	Utah	3.3		40	South Carolina	2.7
27	Vermont	2.9		45	North Dakota	2.5
19	Virginia	3.1		46	Kansas	2.4
19	Washington	3.1		46	Oklahoma	2.4
24	West Virginia	3.0		48	Ohio	2.3
15	Wisconsin	3.2		49	Hawaii	2.2
32	Wyoming	2.8		50	Arizona	0.7
					District of Columbia	2.8

Source: U.S. Department of Health and Human Services, Centers for Disease Control and Prevention
   "1999 Behavioral Risk Factor Surveillance Summary Prevalence Report" (June 23, 2000)
Persons 18 and older.

Safety Belt Usage Rate in 1999

National Rate = 67.0% Use Safety Belts*

RANK	STATE	PERCENT		RANK	STATE	PERCENT
ALPHA ORDER				RANK ORDER		
40	Alabama	57.9		1	California	89.3
37	Alaska	60.6		2	New Mexico	88.4
16	Arizona	71.1		3	Maryland	82.7
44	Arkansas	57.2		3	Oregon	82.7
1	California	89.3		5	Washington	81.1
26	Colorado	65.2		6	Hawaii	80.3
14	Connecticut	72.9		7	Nevada	79.8
30	Delaware	64.4		8	North Carolina	78.1
38	Florida	59.0		9	Iowa	78.0
11	Georgia	74.2		10	New York	76.1
6	Hawaii	80.3		11	Georgia	74.2
40	Idaho	57.9		12	Montana	74.0
25	Illinois	65.9		12	Texas	74.0
43	Indiana	57.3		14	Connecticut	72.9
9	Iowa	78.0		15	Minnesota	71.5
33	Kansas	62.6		16	Arizona	71.1
39	Kentucky	58.6		17	Michigan	70.1
24	Louisiana	67.0		18	Virginia	69.9
31	Maine	64.3		19	Vermont	69.8
3	Maryland	82.7		20	Pennsylvania	69.7
46	Massachusetts	52.0		21	Nebraska	67.9
17	Michigan	70.1		22	Utah	67.4
15	Minnesota	71.5		23	Rhode Island	67.3
45	Mississippi	54.5		24	Louisiana	67.0
35	Missouri	60.8		25	Illinois	65.9
12	Montana	74.0		26	Colorado	65.2
21	Nebraska	67.9		26	South Carolina	65.2
7	Nevada	79.8		28	Wisconsin	65.1
40	New Hampshire	57.9		29	Ohio	64.8
32	New Jersey	63.3		30	Delaware	64.4
2	New Mexico	88.4		31	Maine	64.3
10	New York	76.1		32	New Jersey	63.3
8	North Carolina	78.1		33	Kansas	62.6
48	North Dakota	46.7		34	Tennessee	61.0
29	Ohio	64.8		35	Missouri	60.8
36	Oklahoma	60.7		36	Oklahoma	60.7
3	Oregon	82.7		37	Alaska	60.6
20	Pennsylvania	69.7		38	Florida	59.0
23	Rhode Island	67.3		39	Kentucky	58.6
26	South Carolina	65.2		40	Alabama	57.9
50	South Dakota	38.6		40	Idaho	57.9
34	Tennessee	61.0		40	New Hampshire	57.9
12	Texas	74.0		43	Indiana	57.3
22	Utah	67.4		44	Arkansas	57.2
19	Vermont	69.8		45	Mississippi	54.5
18	Virginia	69.9		46	Massachusetts	52.0
5	Washington	81.1		47	West Virginia	51.9
47	West Virginia	51.9		48	North Dakota	46.7
28	Wisconsin	65.1		49	Wyoming	45.7
49	Wyoming	45.7		50	South Dakota	38.6
					District of Columbia	77.9

Source: U.S. Department of Transportation, National Highway Traffic Safety Administration
"Traffic Safety Facts 1999" (http://www.nhtsa.dot.gov/people/ncsa/factshet.html)
*As of December 1999.

VIII. APPENDIX

Population Charts

Population in 2000

National Total = 281,421,906*

RANK	STATE	POPULATION	% of USA
23	Alabama	4,447,100	1.6%
48	Alaska	626,932	0.2%
20	Arizona	5,130,632	1.8%
33	Arkansas	2,673,400	0.9%
1	California	33,871,648	12.0%
24	Colorado	4,301,261	1.5%
29	Connecticut	3,405,565	1.2%
45	Delaware	783,600	0.3%
4	Florida	15,982,378	5.7%
10	Georgia	8,186,453	2.9%
42	Hawaii	1,211,537	0.4%
39	Idaho	1,293,953	0.5%
5	Illinois	12,419,293	4.4%
14	Indiana	6,080,485	2.2%
30	Iowa	2,926,324	1.0%
32	Kansas	2,688,418	1.0%
25	Kentucky	4,041,769	1.4%
22	Louisiana	4,468,976	1.6%
40	Maine	1,274,923	0.5%
19	Maryland	5,296,486	1.9%
13	Massachusetts	6,349,097	2.3%
8	Michigan	9,938,444	3.5%
21	Minnesota	4,919,479	1.7%
31	Mississippi	2,844,658	1.0%
17	Missouri	5,595,211	2.0%
44	Montana	902,195	0.3%
38	Nebraska	1,711,263	0.6%
35	Nevada	1,998,257	0.7%
41	New Hampshire	1,235,786	0.4%
9	New Jersey	8,414,350	3.0%
36	New Mexico	1,819,046	0.6%
3	New York	18,976,457	6.7%
11	North Carolina	8,049,313	2.9%
47	North Dakota	642,200	0.2%
7	Ohio	11,353,140	4.0%
27	Oklahoma	3,450,654	1.2%
28	Oregon	3,421,399	1.2%
6	Pennsylvania	12,281,054	4.4%
43	Rhode Island	1,048,319	0.4%
26	South Carolina	4,012,012	1.4%
46	South Dakota	754,844	0.3%
16	Tennessee	5,689,283	2.0%
2	Texas	20,851,820	7.4%
34	Utah	2,233,169	0.8%
49	Vermont	608,827	0.2%
12	Virginia	7,078,515	2.5%
15	Washington	5,894,121	2.1%
37	West Virginia	1,808,344	0.6%
18	Wisconsin	5,363,675	1.9%
50	Wyoming	493,782	0.2%

RANK	STATE	POPULATION	% of USA
1	California	33,871,648	12.0%
2	Texas	20,851,820	7.4%
3	New York	18,976,457	6.7%
4	Florida	15,982,378	5.7%
5	Illinois	12,419,293	4.4%
6	Pennsylvania	12,281,054	4.4%
7	Ohio	11,353,140	4.0%
8	Michigan	9,938,444	3.5%
9	New Jersey	8,414,350	3.0%
10	Georgia	8,186,453	2.9%
11	North Carolina	8,049,313	2.9%
12	Virginia	7,078,515	2.5%
13	Massachusetts	6,349,097	2.3%
14	Indiana	6,080,485	2.2%
15	Washington	5,894,121	2.1%
16	Tennessee	5,689,283	2.0%
17	Missouri	5,595,211	2.0%
18	Wisconsin	5,363,675	1.9%
19	Maryland	5,296,486	1.9%
20	Arizona	5,130,632	1.8%
21	Minnesota	4,919,479	1.7%
22	Louisiana	4,468,976	1.6%
23	Alabama	4,447,100	1.6%
24	Colorado	4,301,261	1.5%
25	Kentucky	4,041,769	1.4%
26	South Carolina	4,012,012	1.4%
27	Oklahoma	3,450,654	1.2%
28	Oregon	3,421,399	1.2%
29	Connecticut	3,405,565	1.2%
30	Iowa	2,926,324	1.0%
31	Mississippi	2,844,658	1.0%
32	Kansas	2,688,418	1.0%
33	Arkansas	2,673,400	0.9%
34	Utah	2,233,169	0.8%
35	Nevada	1,998,257	0.7%
36	New Mexico	1,819,046	0.6%
37	West Virginia	1,808,344	0.6%
38	Nebraska	1,711,263	0.6%
39	Idaho	1,293,953	0.5%
40	Maine	1,274,923	0.5%
41	New Hampshire	1,235,786	0.4%
42	Hawaii	1,211,537	0.4%
43	Rhode Island	1,048,319	0.4%
44	Montana	902,195	0.3%
45	Delaware	783,600	0.3%
46	South Dakota	754,844	0.3%
47	North Dakota	642,200	0.2%
48	Alaska	626,932	0.2%
49	Vermont	608,827	0.2%
50	Wyoming	493,782	0.2%
	District of Columbia	572,059	0.2%

Source: U.S. Bureau of the Census
    "First Census 2000 Results" (December 28, 2000, http://www.census.gov/main/www/cen2000.html)
*Resident population.

Population in 1999

National Total = 272,690,813*

ALPHA ORDER

RANK	STATE	POPULATION	% of USA
23	Alabama	4,369,862	1.6%
48	Alaska	619,500	0.2%
20	Arizona	4,778,332	1.8%
33	Arkansas	2,551,373	0.9%
1	California	33,145,121	12.2%
24	Colorado	4,056,133	1.5%
29	Connecticut	3,282,031	1.2%
45	Delaware	753,538	0.3%
4	Florida	15,111,244	5.5%
10	Georgia	7,788,240	2.9%
42	Hawaii	1,185,497	0.4%
40	Idaho	1,251,700	0.5%
5	Illinois	12,128,370	4.4%
14	Indiana	5,942,901	2.2%
30	Iowa	2,869,413	1.1%
32	Kansas	2,654,052	1.0%
25	Kentucky	3,960,825	1.5%
22	Louisiana	4,372,035	1.6%
39	Maine	1,253,040	0.5%
19	Maryland	5,171,634	1.9%
13	Massachusetts	6,175,169	2.3%
8	Michigan	9,863,775	3.6%
21	Minnesota	4,775,508	1.8%
31	Mississippi	2,768,619	1.0%
17	Missouri	5,468,338	2.0%
44	Montana	882,779	0.3%
38	Nebraska	1,666,028	0.6%
35	Nevada	1,809,253	0.7%
41	New Hampshire	1,201,134	0.4%
9	New Jersey	8,143,412	3.0%
37	New Mexico	1,739,844	0.6%
3	New York	18,196,601	6.7%
11	North Carolina	7,650,789	2.8%
47	North Dakota	633,666	0.2%
7	Ohio	11,256,654	4.1%
27	Oklahoma	3,358,044	1.2%
28	Oregon	3,316,154	1.2%
6	Pennsylvania	11,994,016	4.4%
43	Rhode Island	990,819	0.4%
26	South Carolina	3,885,736	1.4%
46	South Dakota	733,133	0.3%
16	Tennessee	5,483,535	2.0%
2	Texas	20,044,141	7.4%
34	Utah	2,129,836	0.8%
49	Vermont	593,740	0.2%
12	Virginia	6,872,912	2.5%
15	Washington	5,756,361	2.1%
36	West Virginia	1,806,928	0.7%
18	Wisconsin	5,250,446	1.9%
50	Wyoming	479,602	0.2%

RANK ORDER

RANK	STATE	POPULATION	% of USA
1	California	33,145,121	12.2%
2	Texas	20,044,141	7.4%
3	New York	18,196,601	6.7%
4	Florida	15,111,244	5.5%
5	Illinois	12,128,370	4.4%
6	Pennsylvania	11,994,016	4.4%
7	Ohio	11,256,654	4.1%
8	Michigan	9,863,775	3.6%
9	New Jersey	8,143,412	3.0%
10	Georgia	7,788,240	2.9%
11	North Carolina	7,650,789	2.8%
12	Virginia	6,872,912	2.5%
13	Massachusetts	6,175,169	2.3%
14	Indiana	5,942,901	2.2%
15	Washington	5,756,361	2.1%
16	Tennessee	5,483,535	2.0%
17	Missouri	5,468,338	2.0%
18	Wisconsin	5,250,446	1.9%
19	Maryland	5,171,634	1.9%
20	Arizona	4,778,332	1.8%
21	Minnesota	4,775,508	1.8%
22	Louisiana	4,372,035	1.6%
23	Alabama	4,369,862	1.6%
24	Colorado	4,056,133	1.5%
25	Kentucky	3,960,825	1.5%
26	South Carolina	3,885,736	1.4%
27	Oklahoma	3,358,044	1.2%
28	Oregon	3,316,154	1.2%
29	Connecticut	3,282,031	1.2%
30	Iowa	2,869,413	1.1%
31	Mississippi	2,768,619	1.0%
32	Kansas	2,654,052	1.0%
33	Arkansas	2,551,373	0.9%
34	Utah	2,129,836	0.8%
35	Nevada	1,809,253	0.7%
36	West Virginia	1,806,928	0.7%
37	New Mexico	1,739,844	0.6%
38	Nebraska	1,666,028	0.6%
39	Maine	1,253,040	0.5%
40	Idaho	1,251,700	0.5%
41	New Hampshire	1,201,134	0.4%
42	Hawaii	1,185,497	0.4%
43	Rhode Island	990,819	0.4%
44	Montana	882,779	0.3%
45	Delaware	753,538	0.3%
46	South Dakota	733,133	0.3%
47	North Dakota	633,666	0.2%
48	Alaska	619,500	0.2%
49	Vermont	593,740	0.2%
50	Wyoming	479,602	0.2%
	District of Columbia	519,000	0.2%

Source: U.S. Bureau of the Census
  "State Population Estimates" (December 29, 1999, http://www.census.gov/population/estimates/state/st-99-3.txt)
Includes armed forces residing in each state.

Male Population in 1999

National Total = 133,276,559 Males

ALPHA ORDER

RANK	STATE	MALES	% of USA
23	Alabama	2,097,319	1.6%
47	Alaska	325,077	0.2%
20	Arizona	2,364,468	1.8%
33	Arkansas	1,232,955	0.9%
1	California	16,579,707	12.4%
24	Colorado	2,010,784	1.5%
29	Connecticut	1,592,801	1.2%
45	Delaware	366,275	0.3%
4	Florida	7,330,099	5.5%
10	Georgia	3,791,130	2.8%
41	Hawaii	592,037	0.4%
39	Idaho	624,504	0.5%
5	Illinois	5,916,083	4.4%
14	Indiana	2,891,620	2.2%
30	Iowa	1,397,208	1.0%
32	Kansas	1,305,408	1.0%
25	Kentucky	1,923,606	1.4%
22	Louisiana	2,103,825	1.6%
40	Maine	611,437	0.5%
19	Maryland	2,513,133	1.9%
13	Massachusetts	2,977,965	2.2%
8	Michigan	4,799,912	3.6%
21	Minnesota	2,353,020	1.8%
31	Mississippi	1,326,704	1.0%
16	Missouri	2,649,479	2.0%
44	Montana	438,758	0.3%
38	Nebraska	814,663	0.6%
35	Nevada	921,070	0.7%
42	New Hampshire	590,941	0.4%
9	New Jersey	3,946,443	3.0%
37	New Mexico	856,048	0.6%
3	New York	8,770,974	6.6%
11	North Carolina	3,710,119	2.8%
48	North Dakota	315,167	0.2%
7	Ohio	5,441,233	4.1%
27	Oklahoma	1,639,559	1.2%
28	Oregon	1,637,721	1.2%
6	Pennsylvania	5,765,533	4.3%
43	Rhode Island	476,331	0.4%
26	South Carolina	1,875,030	1.4%
46	South Dakota	360,485	0.3%
17	Tennessee	2,646,694	2.0%
2	Texas	9,887,415	7.4%
34	Utah	1,058,639	0.8%
49	Vermont	292,120	0.2%
12	Virginia	3,358,569	2.5%
15	Washington	2,862,019	2.1%
36	West Virginia	870,356	0.7%
18	Wisconsin	2,580,153	1.9%
50	Wyoming	240,943	0.2%

RANK ORDER

RANK	STATE	MALES	% of USA
1	California	16,579,707	12.4%
2	Texas	9,887,415	7.4%
3	New York	8,770,974	6.6%
4	Florida	7,330,099	5.5%
5	Illinois	5,916,083	4.4%
6	Pennsylvania	5,765,533	4.3%
7	Ohio	5,441,233	4.1%
8	Michigan	4,799,912	3.6%
9	New Jersey	3,946,443	3.0%
10	Georgia	3,791,130	2.8%
11	North Carolina	3,710,119	2.8%
12	Virginia	3,358,569	2.5%
13	Massachusetts	2,977,965	2.2%
14	Indiana	2,891,620	2.2%
15	Washington	2,862,019	2.1%
16	Missouri	2,649,479	2.0%
17	Tennessee	2,646,694	2.0%
18	Wisconsin	2,580,153	1.9%
19	Maryland	2,513,133	1.9%
20	Arizona	2,364,468	1.8%
21	Minnesota	2,353,020	1.8%
22	Louisiana	2,103,825	1.6%
23	Alabama	2,097,319	1.6%
24	Colorado	2,010,784	1.5%
25	Kentucky	1,923,606	1.4%
26	South Carolina	1,875,030	1.4%
27	Oklahoma	1,639,559	1.2%
28	Oregon	1,637,721	1.2%
29	Connecticut	1,592,801	1.2%
30	Iowa	1,397,208	1.0%
31	Mississippi	1,326,704	1.0%
32	Kansas	1,305,408	1.0%
33	Arkansas	1,232,955	0.9%
34	Utah	1,058,639	0.8%
35	Nevada	921,070	0.7%
36	West Virginia	870,356	0.7%
37	New Mexico	856,048	0.6%
38	Nebraska	814,663	0.6%
39	Idaho	624,504	0.5%
40	Maine	611,437	0.5%
41	Hawaii	592,037	0.4%
42	New Hampshire	590,941	0.4%
43	Rhode Island	476,331	0.4%
44	Montana	438,758	0.3%
45	Delaware	366,275	0.3%
46	South Dakota	360,485	0.3%
47	Alaska	325,077	0.2%
48	North Dakota	315,167	0.2%
49	Vermont	292,120	0.2%
50	Wyoming	240,943	0.2%
	District of Columbia	243,020	0.2%

Source: U.S. Bureau of the Census
"Population Estimates for the U.S., Regions, and States by Selected Age Groups and Sex" (ST-99-9, March 9, 2000)
(http://www.census.gov/population/estimates/state/st-99-09.txt)

Female Population in 1999

National Total = 139,414,254 Females

ALPHA ORDER

ALPHA ORDER

RANK	STATE	FEMALES	% of USA
22	Alabama	2,272,543	1.6%
49	Alaska	294,423	0.2%
21	Arizona	2,413,864	1.7%
33	Arkansas	1,318,418	0.9%
1	California	16,565,414	11.9%
24	Colorado	2,045,349	1.5%
28	Connecticut	1,689,230	1.2%
45	Delaware	387,263	0.3%
4	Florida	7,781,145	5.6%
10	Georgia	3,997,110	2.9%
42	Hawaii	593,460	0.4%
40	Idaho	627,196	0.4%
6	Illinois	6,212,287	4.5%
14	Indiana	3,051,281	2.2%
30	Iowa	1,472,205	1.1%
32	Kansas	1,348,644	1.0%
25	Kentucky	2,037,219	1.5%
23	Louisiana	2,268,210	1.6%
39	Maine	641,603	0.5%
19	Maryland	2,658,501	1.9%
13	Massachusetts	3,197,204	2.3%
8	Michigan	5,063,863	3.6%
20	Minnesota	2,422,488	1.7%
31	Mississippi	1,441,915	1.0%
17	Missouri	2,818,859	2.0%
44	Montana	444,021	0.3%
38	Nebraska	851,365	0.6%
36	Nevada	888,183	0.6%
41	New Hampshire	610,193	0.4%
9	New Jersey	4,196,969	3.0%
37	New Mexico	883,796	0.6%
3	New York	9,425,627	6.8%
11	North Carolina	3,940,670	2.8%
47	North Dakota	318,499	0.2%
7	Ohio	5,815,421	4.2%
27	Oklahoma	1,718,485	1.2%
29	Oregon	1,678,433	1.2%
5	Pennsylvania	6,228,483	4.5%
43	Rhode Island	514,488	0.4%
26	South Carolina	2,010,706	1.4%
46	South Dakota	372,648	0.3%
16	Tennessee	2,836,841	2.0%
2	Texas	10,156,726	7.3%
34	Utah	1,071,197	0.8%
48	Vermont	301,620	0.2%
12	Virginia	3,514,343	2.5%
15	Washington	2,894,342	2.1%
35	West Virginia	936,572	0.7%
18	Wisconsin	2,670,293	1.9%
50	Wyoming	238,659	0.2%

RANK ORDER

RANK	STATE	FEMALES	% of USA
1	California	16,565,414	11.9%
2	Texas	10,156,726	7.3%
3	New York	9,425,627	6.8%
4	Florida	7,781,145	5.6%
5	Pennsylvania	6,228,483	4.5%
6	Illinois	6,212,287	4.5%
7	Ohio	5,815,421	4.2%
8	Michigan	5,063,863	3.6%
9	New Jersey	4,196,969	3.0%
10	Georgia	3,997,110	2.9%
11	North Carolina	3,940,670	2.8%
12	Virginia	3,514,343	2.5%
13	Massachusetts	3,197,204	2.3%
14	Indiana	3,051,281	2.2%
15	Washington	2,894,342	2.1%
16	Tennessee	2,836,841	2.0%
17	Missouri	2,818,859	2.0%
18	Wisconsin	2,670,293	1.9%
19	Maryland	2,658,501	1.9%
20	Minnesota	2,422,488	1.7%
21	Arizona	2,413,864	1.7%
22	Alabama	2,272,543	1.6%
23	Louisiana	2,268,210	1.6%
24	Colorado	2,045,349	1.5%
25	Kentucky	2,037,219	1.5%
26	South Carolina	2,010,706	1.4%
27	Oklahoma	1,718,485	1.2%
28	Connecticut	1,689,230	1.2%
29	Oregon	1,678,433	1.2%
30	Iowa	1,472,205	1.1%
31	Mississippi	1,441,915	1.0%
32	Kansas	1,348,644	1.0%
33	Arkansas	1,318,418	0.9%
34	Utah	1,071,197	0.8%
35	West Virginia	936,572	0.7%
36	Nevada	888,183	0.6%
37	New Mexico	883,796	0.6%
38	Nebraska	851,365	0.6%
39	Maine	641,603	0.5%
40	Idaho	627,196	0.4%
41	New Hampshire	610,193	0.4%
42	Hawaii	593,460	0.4%
43	Rhode Island	514,488	0.4%
44	Montana	444,021	0.3%
45	Delaware	387,263	0.3%
46	South Dakota	372,648	0.3%
47	North Dakota	318,499	0.2%
48	Vermont	301,620	0.2%
49	Alaska	294,423	0.2%
50	Wyoming	238,659	0.2%
	District of Columbia	275,980	0.2%

Source: U.S. Bureau of the Census
"Population Estimates for the U.S., Regions, and States by Selected Age Groups and Sex" (ST-99-9, March 9, 2000)
(http://www.census.gov/population/estimates/state/st-99-09.txt)

Population in 1998

National Total = 270,248,003*

ALPHA ORDER

RANK	STATE	POPULATION	% of USA
23	Alabama	4,351,037	1.6%
48	Alaska	615,205	0.2%
21	Arizona	4,667,277	1.7%
33	Arkansas	2,538,202	0.9%
1	California	32,682,794	12.1%
24	Colorado	3,968,967	1.5%
29	Connecticut	3,272,563	1.2%
45	Delaware	744,066	0.3%
4	Florida	14,908,230	5.5%
10	Georgia	7,636,522	2.8%
41	Hawaii	1,190,472	0.4%
40	Idaho	1,230,923	0.5%
5	Illinois	12,069,774	4.5%
14	Indiana	5,907,617	2.2%
30	Iowa	2,861,025	1.1%
32	Kansas	2,638,667	1.0%
25	Kentucky	3,934,310	1.5%
22	Louisiana	4,362,758	1.6%
39	Maine	1,247,554	0.5%
19	Maryland	5,130,072	1.9%
13	Massachusetts	6,144,407	2.3%
8	Michigan	9,820,231	3.6%
20	Minnesota	4,726,411	1.7%
31	Mississippi	2,751,335	1.0%
16	Missouri	5,437,562	2.0%
44	Montana	879,533	0.3%
38	Nebraska	1,660,772	0.6%
36	Nevada	1,743,772	0.6%
42	New Hampshire	1,185,823	0.4%
9	New Jersey	8,095,542	3.0%
37	New Mexico	1,733,535	0.6%
3	New York	18,159,175	6.7%
11	North Carolina	7,545,828	2.8%
47	North Dakota	637,808	0.2%
7	Ohio	11,237,752	4.2%
27	Oklahoma	3,339,478	1.2%
28	Oregon	3,282,055	1.2%
6	Pennsylvania	12,002,329	4.4%
43	Rhode Island	987,704	0.4%
26	South Carolina	3,839,578	1.4%
46	South Dakota	730,789	0.3%
17	Tennessee	5,432,679	2.0%
2	Texas	19,712,389	7.3%
34	Utah	2,100,562	0.8%
49	Vermont	590,579	0.2%
12	Virginia	6,789,225	2.5%
15	Washington	5,687,832	2.1%
35	West Virginia	1,811,688	0.7%
18	Wisconsin	5,222,124	1.9%
50	Wyoming	480,045	0.2%

RANK ORDER

RANK	STATE	POPULATION	% of USA
1	California	32,682,794	12.1%
2	Texas	19,712,389	7.3%
3	New York	18,159,175	6.7%
4	Florida	14,908,230	5.5%
5	Illinois	12,069,774	4.5%
6	Pennsylvania	12,002,329	4.4%
7	Ohio	11,237,752	4.2%
8	Michigan	9,820,231	3.6%
9	New Jersey	8,095,542	3.0%
10	Georgia	7,636,522	2.8%
11	North Carolina	7,545,828	2.8%
12	Virginia	6,789,225	2.5%
13	Massachusetts	6,144,407	2.3%
14	Indiana	5,907,617	2.2%
15	Washington	5,687,832	2.1%
16	Missouri	5,437,562	2.0%
17	Tennessee	5,432,679	2.0%
18	Wisconsin	5,222,124	1.9%
19	Maryland	5,130,072	1.9%
20	Minnesota	4,726,411	1.7%
21	Arizona	4,667,277	1.7%
22	Louisiana	4,362,758	1.6%
23	Alabama	4,351,037	1.6%
24	Colorado	3,968,967	1.5%
25	Kentucky	3,934,310	1.5%
26	South Carolina	3,839,578	1.4%
27	Oklahoma	3,339,478	1.2%
28	Oregon	3,282,055	1.2%
29	Connecticut	3,272,563	1.2%
30	Iowa	2,861,025	1.1%
31	Mississippi	2,751,335	1.0%
32	Kansas	2,638,667	1.0%
33	Arkansas	2,538,202	0.9%
34	Utah	2,100,562	0.8%
35	West Virginia	1,811,688	0.7%
36	Nevada	1,743,772	0.6%
37	New Mexico	1,733,535	0.6%
38	Nebraska	1,660,772	0.6%
39	Maine	1,247,554	0.5%
40	Idaho	1,230,923	0.5%
41	Hawaii	1,190,472	0.4%
42	New Hampshire	1,185,823	0.4%
43	Rhode Island	987,704	0.4%
44	Montana	879,533	0.3%
45	Delaware	744,066	0.3%
46	South Dakota	730,789	0.3%
47	North Dakota	637,808	0.2%
48	Alaska	615,205	0.2%
49	Vermont	590,579	0.2%
50	Wyoming	480,045	0.2%
	District of Columbia	521,426	0.2%

Source: U.S. Bureau of the Census
"State Population Estimates" (December 29, 1999, http://www.census.gov/population/estimates/state/st-99-3.txt)
Includes armed forces residing in each state. This updates earlier 1998 population estimates.

IX. SOURCES

American Academy of Physicians Assistants
950 North Washington Street
Alexandria, VA 22314-1552
703-836-2272
Internet: www.aapa.org

American Cancer Society, Inc.
1599 Clifton Road, NE.
Atlanta, GA 30329-4251
800-227-2345
Internet: http://www.cancer.org

American Dental Association
211 E. Chicago Ave.
Chicago, IL 60611
312-440-2500
Internet: www.ada.org

American Hospital Association
One North Franklin
Chicago, IL 60606-3421
312-422-3000
Internet: www.aha.org

American Medical Association
515 North State Street
Chicago, IL 60610
312-464-5000
Internet: http://www.ama-assn.org

American Osteopathic Association
142 East Ontario Street
Chicago, IL 60611
800-621-1773
Internet: www.am-osteo-assn.org

American Podiatric Medical Association
9312 Old Georgetown Road
Bethesda, MD 20814-1698
301-581-9221
Internet: www.apma.org

Bureau of Labor Statistics
Census of Fatal Occupational Injuries
2 Massachusetts Ave., NE
Washington, DC 20212
202-691-6175
Internet: http://stats.bls.gov/oshhome.htm

Census Bureau
3 Silver Hill and Suitland Roads
Suitland, MD 20746
301-457-2800
Internet: http://www.census.gov

Centers for Disease Control and Prevention
1600 Clifton Road, NE.
Atlanta, GA 30333
404-639-3534 (Public Affairs)
800-458-5231 (AIDS Clearinghouse)
Internet: http://www.cdc.gov

Federation of Chiropractic Licensing Boards
901 54th Ave., Ste. 101
Greeley, CO 80634-4400
970-356-3500
Internet: www.fclb.org

Health Care Financing Administration
U.S. Department of Health and Human Services
7500 Security Boulevard
Baltimore, MD 21244
410-786-3000
Internet: http://www.hcfa.gov

InterStudy
P.O. Box 4366
St. Paul, MN 55104
800-844-3351
Internet: www.hmodata.com

National Center for Health Statistics
U.S. Department of Health and Human Services
6525 Belcrest Road
Hyattsville, MD 20782-2003
301-458-4636
Internet: http://www.cdc.gov/nchswww/

**National Institute on Alcohol Abuse
and Alcoholism**
National Institutes of Health
6000 Executive Boulevard
Bethesda, MD 20892-7003
301-443-9970
Internet: www.niaaa.nih.gov/

National Highway Traffic Safety Admin.
400 Seventh Street, SW
Washington, DC 20590
202-366-9550
Internet: www.nhtsa.dot.gov

National Sporting Goods Association
1601 Feehanville Drive, Ste 300
Mt. Prospect, IL 60056-6035
847-296-6742
Internet: www.nsga.org

Smoking and Health Office
Centers for Disease Control and Prevention
4770 Buford Hwy, NE., Mail Stop K-50
Atlanta, GA 30341-3724
770-488-5701
www.cdc.gov/nccdphp/

X. INDEX

X. INDEX (continued)

X. INDEX (continued)

CHAPTER INDEX

HOW TO USE THIS INDEX

Place left thumb on the outer edge of this page. To locate the desired entry, fold back the remaining page edges and align the index edge mark with the appropriate page edge mark.

Other books by Morgan Quitno Press:

- *State Statistical Trends (monthly journal)*
- *State Rankings 2001 ($52.95)*
- *Crime State Rankings 2001 ($52.95)*
- *City Crime Rankings, 7th Edition ($39.95)*

Call toll free: 1-800-457-0742 or
visit us at www.statestats.com